Handbook *of* Home Health Care Administration

Fourth Edition

Marilyn D. Harris, RN, MSN, CNAA, BC, FAAN

Former Executive Director
Abington Memorial Hospital Home Care
Willow Grove, Pennsylvania

JONES AND BARTLETT PUBLISHERS
Sudbury, Massachusetts
BOSTON   TORONTO   LONDON   SINGAPORE

World Headquarters

Jones and Bartlett Publishers	Jones and Bartlett Publishers Canada	Jones and Bartlett Publishers International
40 Tall Pine Drive	2406 Nikanna Road	Barb House, Barb Mews
Sudbury, MA 01776	Mississauga, ON L5C 2W6	London W6 7PA
978-443-5000	CANADA	UK
info@jbpub.com		
www.jbpub.com		

Production Credits
Acquisitions Editor: Penny M. Glynn
Production Manager: Amy Rose
Senior Production Editor: Linda S. DeBruyn
Associate Production Editor: Karen C. Ferreira
Editorial Assistant: Amy Sibley
Marketing Manager: Edward McKenna
Manufacturing Buyer: Amy Bacus
Cover Design: Bret Kerr
Composition: Modern Graphics
Printing and Binding: Malloy Lithographing

Library of Congress Cataloging-in-Publication Data

Handbook of home health care administration / Marilyn D. Harris, editor.—4th ed.
p. ; cm.
Includes bibliographical references and index.
ISBN 0-7637-3251-6
1. Home care services–Administration.   2. Home care services–United States–Administration.
[DNLM: 1. Home Care Agencies–organization & administration.   2. Home Care Services–organization & administration. WY 115 H236 2004] I. Harris, Marilyn D.
RA645.3.H355 2004
362.1'4—dc22

                                                                                    2003025355

The authors have made every effort to ensure the accuracy of the information herein. However, appropriate information sources should be consulted, especially for new or unfamiliar procedures. It is the responsibility of every practitioner to evaluate the appropriateness of a particular opinion in the context of actual clinical and administrative situations and with due considerations to new developments.

Printed in the United States of America
08 07 06 05 04   10 9 8 7 6 5 4 3 2 1

In 2004, I celebrate my 50th anniversary as a nurse. There was no way for me to know, or even imagine, in 1954 the many challenges and changes that I would experience during my career. During these years, I have had the opportunity to meet and work with professionals in agency, regional, state, national, and international communities. I learned valuable lessons and formed personal and professional relationships that continue today.

It is my honor to serve as the editor of the fourth edition of *Handbook of Home Health Care Administration,* and to dedicate this book to:

- Each individual who has been, and continues to be, a valuable part of my personal history of nursing and home health and hospice care
- The home care and hospice professionals who contributed their expertise and time to share important information in this new edition
- My colleagues, administration, and staff at Abington Memorial Hospital Home Care who worked with me as a team to provide high-quality, compassionate home health and hospice care to thousands of patients each year
- My husband, Charles, for his support of my nursing endeavors

---

Acknowledgments

I express my special thanks and appreciation to the staff at Jones and Bartlett Publishers who were involved with this new edition of the textbook. Their expertise and support were invaluable in bringing this new edition to reality.

Dr. Penny Glynn for the invitation to edit another edition of the textbook

Linda DeBruyn, Senior Production Editor

Karen Ferreira, Associate Production Editor

Amy Sibley, Editorial Assistant

Eileen Ward, Director of Special Markets

Table of Contents

Foreword

Home care and hospice have changed dramatically over the last few years, not only as a result of the 1997 Balanced Budget Act, but also as a result of the implementation of outcome-based quality improvement (OBQI) initiatives. Today's home care and hospice administrators face a number of unique challenges that are intensified in an environment of technological advances.

As our population ages, we will be faced with an unprecedented growth in the number of elderly patients who will become a priority for our health care systems. Much of the burden—or rather, privilege—of providing care for the aging population will fall on home health organizations. Most home health veterans agree that home care will play an increasingly central role because of its lower cost and increases in technology. In addition, anecdotal evidence supports the idea that both young and aged individuals prefer to be cared for in their homes.

The home care industry is entering a new era, one in which society increasingly defines the industry in terms of its quality-focused processes, and measures the industry in terms of the benchmarks it has achieved. The most successful home care and hospice agencies will be those who take a proactive approach to adapting to these changes.

In the midst of all of these changes, Marilyn D. Harris (MSN, RN, CNAA, BC, FAAN) has once again stepped up to the "plate" and hit a home run. With the fourth edition of *Handbook of Home Health Care Administration*, Ms. Harris has demonstrated again her expertise in pulling together the movers and shakers of home care and hospice. The contributing authors don't just share their experiences in home care—they offer sound advice for the future. This "handbook," which has become a classic within the home care industry, includes information regarding legal and legislative issues, case management processes, and state-of-the-art technology. Also featured are chapters regarding the importance of audits and credentialing, clinical and quality management, and ready-to-use reproducible forms and tools with guidelines for their implementation. New chapters include areas such as HIPAA (the Health Insurance Portability and Accountability Act) and compliance issues, cultural competency in home care, and home telehealth. An additional bonus is Chapter 71, which contains tips for success from experienced administrators that are beneficial to both novice and seasoned managers. The book is an excellent review resource for a home health certification exam.

While countless books are devoted to unique or specific areas of home care, Marilyn Harris has drawn on her many years of research and experiences and created an outstanding compendium of home care excellence. She has pulled together a "blue chip" reference source, not only for administrators and clinical educators, but also for accountants, lawyers, and consultants, to name a few. Harris's *Handbook of Home Health Care Administration* is sure to become an essential guide for the coming transitional years.

Ruth Constant, Ed.D., MSN, CHCE, FHHC
President and CEO, Beaumont, Port Arthur, and Wichita Home Health Agencies
Victoria, Texas
Chairman of the Board of Directors
National Association for Home Care
Washington, DC

Introduction

The number and types of challenges that administrators of home health care and hospice programs face on a daily basis continue to escalate. The challenges include implementation of new federal laws and regulations; updates to certification, accreditation, and professional standards; the shortage of professionals and other personnel to fill budgeted positions; positions on hold because of budget shortfalls; decreased payment by federal and private insurers; and more!

Although home care services are available to all age groups, individuals who are aged 65 years and older continue to use the majority of the services. To meet the needs of patients of all ages and their families, current and future administrations, supervisors, staff, consultants, and students in nursing and home health care administration need the most up-to-date information about a wide array of topics to meet the challenges they encounter each day. The chapters in this edition include new and updated information related to the myriad issues that are important to everyone involved with the administration of home health care and hospice services.

The strategic consensus report of the National Consensus Conference on the Educational Preparation of Home Care Administrators (Cary, 1989) contains 12 cluster areas of knowledge and skills recommended for home care administrators (Exhibit 1). Primary areas reflect the essential knowledge and skills that a home health administrator needs to achieve a beginning competency level. Secondary areas reflect knowledge needed to identify priorities and resources. The contributors to this book address all of these areas except public health science.

Scalzi and Wilson (1990, 1991) completed a study to identify the relative amount of time spent, and the relative importance attributed to, specific job activities of nurse executives. The 184 nurse executives who participated in the study identified 11 curriculum areas by time spent and by practice settings, including home care, long-term care, occupational health, and acute care. The nurse executives in home care identified a stronger need for legal, health care policy, financial, and marketing acumen. They indicated that they spent more time on clinical activities (Table 2).

In 2003, Dr. Scalzi gave me permission to use her ranking tool. I asked a convenience sample of several administrators in various areas of the United States to share relevant information as to the time spent on these areas of importance in 2003. Table 3 includes the 2003 results for home care administrators as compared with those from 1990. It is not unexpected to note that resource management moved from number 9 on the 1990 list to number 1 in 2003, and that organizational strategy moved from number 6 to number 2. The management of resources (financial and human) and organizational strategies are essential to surviving and thriving in the 21st century.

Exhibit 1 Cluster Areas of Knowledge and Skill Recommended for Home Care Administration

- Finance/fiscal
- Human resource development
- Legal/ethical
- Management information systems
- Marketing
- Nursing science
- Operations
- Organization/management
- Policy
- Public health science
- Quality management
- Research

In an attempt to refine the clusters, the panel generated primary and secondary areas within each where appropriate.

1. *Primary areas* were defined as reflecting the essential knowledge and skill areas for a home health administrator to achieve a beginning competency level. As illustrated in the previous section, educational institutions are to assume the major responsibility for this content, with service organizations playing a minor role.
2. *Secondary areas* were defined as those for which a home care administrator needs some knowledge to identify priorities and resources as the basis for developing further competencies. As illustrated in the secondary areas, education and service organizations have equal responsibility for reinforcing this content.

Table 1 reflects the primary and secondary areas within the clusters generated by the consensus panel.

Source: Copyright © Ann H. Cary, PhD, RN., (1989)

The chapters in this book address the areas of need that home care administrators identified as being important and as requiring the most time.

The original idea for this book started with an identified need for an in-house manual to be used by the students who come to Abington Memorial Hospital Home Care (AMHHC) for a practicum in home health administration. Many times, administrators, the clinical educator, supervisors, and other staff spend a significant amount of time explaining to students the programs and services of the agency and describing the services that are offered, types of funding, and other important issues. The purpose of this book is to present an overview of the administration of home health and hospice services.

Each chapter could be expanded into a book-length publication, and as a result not all topics are addressed in detail. However, the principles that apply to one discipline can be applied to others. For example, accreditation standards and documentation principles apply to therapy and paraprofessional services as well as to nursing. Current references, including many websites, are listed. Older references were retained when they provided a historical perspective and continue to be relevant. Some authors have included a bibliography in addition to the reference list so that interested readers can pursue a particular topic in more detail.

All of the contributors to this book are involved in some aspect of home health or hospice care. They include staff members, board members, nurse practitioners, consultants, accountants, lawyers, teachers, supervisors, administrators, and representatives from both national and

Table 1 Primary and Secondary Areas of Knowledge and Skill within 12 Individual Clusters

Cluster	Primary Areas	Secondary Areas
1. Finance/fiscal	p1 Read and interpret financial statements p2 Prepare a basic budget p3 Develop a basic budget p4 Develop financial controls	s1 Basic principles of economics (costing) s2 Basic principles of accounting s3 Principles of finance (resource) utilization, capital acquisition, cash flow management s4 Reimbursement systems s5 Ratio analysis s6 Small business administration (examples: payroll, taxes, banking, prudent buyer concept)
2. Human resource development	p1 Personnel practices (recruitment, retention, evaluation, termination, compensation) p2 Job analysis/staffing p3 Efficiency/effectiveness (productivity) p4 Supervision (orientation, evaluation, coaching, mentoring, maintenance, development)	s1 Staff development (orientation, continuing education, on-the-job/in-service training) s2 Personnel/legal aspects s3 Team building s4 Leadership
3. Legal/ethical		s1 Business law (introduction to corporate law, tort, labor relations, regulatory, legal reporting requirements) s2 Issues/ethical decision making, including confidentiality s3 Legal aspects of personnel administration
4. Management information systems	p1 Basic systems analysis/manual and automated information p2 Efficient use of management information systems, including system confidentiality p3 Computer literacy	s1 Appreciate technological state of the art
5. Marketing	p1 Apply appropriate models/theories to target populations	s1 Marketing theory (basic)
6. Nursing science		s1 Nursing theories s2 Family developmental theories s3 Communication and teaching/learning theories s4 Social/psychological theories

continues

Table 1 continued

Cluster	Primary Areas	Secondary Areas
7. Operations	p1 Program/product line design theory p2 Competencies in aggregate-based clinical care p3 Identify researchable problems p4 Problem-solving process p5 Behavioral objectives p6 Standards of practice p7 Community assessment/needs assessment p8 Program planning process—assessment/planning/implementation/evaluation p9 Community interactions/networking	s1 Patient delivery systems s2 Reimbursement/regulatory activities s3 Grantsmanship, applied s4 Case management/continuity of care s5 Policy and procedure development s6 Planning processes—types, models
8. Organization/management	p1 Principles and functions of management (controls, policy and procedure) p2 Organizational behavior (board/stockholder consultation, negotiation, collaboration, leadership, motivation, conflict management, implementing change) p3 Organizational structure	s1 Contract management
9. Policy	p1 Knowledge of health care delivery systems p2 Knowledge of public policy and implications p3 Legal/ethical implications of public policy p4 Case management/continuity of care p5 Political involvement	s1 Community standards s2 Regulations and regulatory bodies (Occupational Safety and Health Administration, Health Care Financing Administration), state licensure, etc. s3 Legislation/reimbursement s4 Entitlement programs s5 Standards of practice s6 Local/state/national advocacy programs and organizations

Table 1 continued

Cluster	Primary Areas	Secondary Areas
10. Public health science	p1 Epidemiology, population, and demography p2 Health behaviors—culture, risk factors/reductions, wellness concepts p3 Community theory	s1 Major health problems
11. Quality management (QM)	p1 Risk-management problems (prevention strategies/identification of risk, legal parameters, laws affecting home care) p2 QM theory—structure, process, outcome, design of QM program p3 Implement, evaluate QM program p4 Standards of practice p5 Infection control p6 Developing standards	s1 Community standards s2 Applicable regulations s3 Credentialing/licensure/certification/accreditation
12. Research	p1 Basic statistics (prerequisite) p2 Research designs p3 Analyze research reports p4 Interpret and apply findings p5 Knowledge of research process (prerequisite) p6 Basic research skills p7 Biostatistics p8 Support research/collaborate with researchers	

Source: Copyright © Ann H. Cary, PhD, RN. (1989)

Table 2 Rank of Curriculum Areas by Time Spent

Area of Need	Home Care	Overall Average
Law and health care policy	3.07	2.95
Finance	2.79	2.56
Marketing	2.67	2.51
QA	2.53	2.55
Organizational behavior	2.52	2.67
Organizational strategy	2.51	2.61
Risk management	2.31	2.39
Clinical nursing	2.26	2.14
Resource management	2.25	2.22
Management information systems	2.23	2.18
Ethics	2.11	2.11

Note: Low = 1; High = 4.

Source: Courtesy of Cynthia C. Scalzi, PhD, RN, University of Pennsylvania, Philadelphia, Pennsylvania, with permission.

state organizations. Contributors represent various auspices and sizes of home health care agencies and geographical areas.

Some of the chapters could be included in more than one part of the book. For example, I included Disease Management Programs in Part VIII: Strategic Planning/Marketing/Survival Issues, but it also includes Clinical Issues (Part III) and Financial Issues (Part VI).

Part I provides an overview of home health administration. It includes a brief history and a description of the types of agencies.

Part II addresses standards for home health agencies. Agency standards, including certification, accreditation, certificate of need, and licensure, are described. Professional standards such as credentialing of staff and administrators are included. The benefits of membership in national and state organizations are described by the staff of these organizations. The administrative staff or board members for four acrediting organizations shared current information for each of their organizations. The proposed revisions to the Medicare Conditions of Participation (COPs) were not available when this book went to press. The existing Medicare

COPs are included in Chapter 3. Readers must reference the proposed revisions to the COPs, to be released later in 2004 (http://www.access.gpo.gov/nara/cfr), for changes to the existing COPs.

Part III explores a limited number of clinical issues that affect service delivery or cost identification. Documentation, patient classification systems, patient outcome systems, nursing diagnoses, maternal and child health programs, high-technology issues, and others are presented from the administrator's viewpoint. There is increased emphasis on determining and documenting the competency of personnel, including staff, contractors, and volunteers. Authors share their strategies and methods for meeting the challenge of competency evaluation of personnel, and for providing culturally and linguistically appropriate services.

Part IV describes the components of a quality assessment/performance improvement program and service evaluation, evidence-based practice, planning for quality care, benchmarking, and outcome-based quality improvement.

Part V lists selected management issues that are important to home care administrators. Such

Table 3 Comparison of Rank of Area by Importance and Time Spent by Home Care Administrators in 2003 and 1990

Area of Need	2003 Home Care Importance		1990 Home Care Administrators
Resource management	3.76	(Increase of 1.51)	2.25
Organizational strategy	3.72	(Increase of 1.21)	2.51
Finance	3.40	(Increase of .61)	2.79
Organizational behavior	3.08	(Increase of .50)	2.52
Risk management	3.06	(Increase of .75)	2.31
MIS	3.00	(Increase of .77)	2.23
Marketing	2.88	(Increase of .21)	2.67
QA	2.80	(Increase of .27)	2.53
Ethics	2.60	(Increase of .49)	2.11
Law and health care policy	2.50	(Decrease of .55)	3.07
Clinical nursing	2.37	(Increase of .11)	2.26

Note: Low = 1; High = 4.

issues as a current policy and procedure manual, staffing, productivity, labor relations, human resource management, discharge planning, case management, staff education, long-term care, and managed care are addressed. The challenges and opportunities related to transitioning nurses to home care are shared by two experts in this process.

Part VI deals with financial issues. The current insurance/litigation climate, budgets, reimbursement, management information systems, and how to read and interpret financial audits are explored in detail.

Part VII addresses legal, ethical, and political issues. Contracts, informed consent, and liability are discussed. Administrators must be aware of the many legislative and regulatory issues that affect home care at both state and national levels. The authors provide information about the political process and how personnel in home health agencies can participate in the process. Ethical concerns surface at the clinical and administrative levels. A myriad of concerns are explored from theoretical and practical viewpoints. Two new chapters address home health compliance issues and the Health Insurance Portability and Accountability Act (HIPAA).

Part VIII includes strategic planning, marketing, and survival issues. Topics include disease management programs, corporate restructuring, use of the Internet, and marketing strategies.

Part IX addresses areas of opportunity for administrative staff to serve as resource personnel and innovators. Student and volunteer programs are two areas of administration that may not be present in all agencies, but these programs present multiple opportunities for collaborative relationships with other agencies or educational institutions. The physician's role in home health and hospice care are addressed. Other topics include research, publishing, and applying for grants.

Home care administrators are assuming responsibility for an ever-widening array of health care services in the community. Day care, community nursing centers, and community/interfaith parish nurse programs are logical extensions of the administrator's range of expertise as more and more services move into the community. Several authors share their expertise and experiences with these emerging responsibilities. Others attempt to put the administration of home health, hospice, and expanded programs into perspective and share their viewpoints on administration in today's economic, political, and health care climate. A new chapter describes an extension of bereavement support. Safe Harbor is a specific program for bereaved children, teens, and their families. Parish nurse programs are increasing in number throughout the country. One author describes how nurses in faith communities work as partners with home care and hospice nurses to meet the needs of their members and friends.

Part X attempts to put the administration of home health and hospice care into perspective. In addition to the editor, several experienced administrators share their strategies and advice on how to be a successful administrator in the 21st century.

Although issues are addressed on a chapter-by-chapter basis, many of the topics overlap one another. For example, ethical issues are mentioned in the chapters on discharge planning and high-technology procedures. Financial issues surface in reference to budgeting, reimbursement, and documentation. Productivity is common to staffing, budgeting, and ethical issues. Disease management programs can be viewed from a clinical, financial, and/or survival perspective.

Today's home health care climate is ever-changing. Information included in this book was current as of January 2004. Readers are encouraged to review the most recent guidelines and regulations, specifically in such areas as reimbursement, certification and accreditation standards, documentation requirements, and Medicare COPs, to keep informed of important changes that may have occurred since this book went to press.

As an administrator, I had many new experiences during the past 3 years in my role as director of home health and hospice care. For example, I had the opportunity to talk with colleagues throughout the United States through the sharing of benchmarking reports. The staff planned for and implemented a computerized clinical documentation system. My responsibilities also expanded to include planning and implementing health care services that are taken into the community. I worked with community organizations and other hospital department directors and staff to plan for, establish, and open a community health center where direct care is provided by nurse practitioners, and educational and health promotion programs are offered in response to requests for health information. I was also a member of a planning committee for implementing a community/interfaith parish nurse resource center. The opportunities to meet the health care needs of the community we serve by providing high-quality health care services to individuals in a compassionate, caring, and cost-effective manner are endless.

It is my hope that each reader will find this publication to be a ready reference for the multifaceted aspects of home health care administration. I welcome your comments and look forward to hearing from many of you.

Marilyn D. Harris

REFERENCES

Cary, A. 1989. *Strategies for a collaborative future: The consensus report for the National Consensus Conference on the Educational Preparation of Home Care Administrators.* Washington, DC: Catholic University of America School of Nursing.

Scalzi, C., and D. Wilson. 1990. Empirically based recommendations for content of graduate nursing administration programs. *Nursing & Health Care* 11(10): 522–525.

Scalzi, C., and D. Wilson. 1991. Future preparation of home health nurse executives. *Home Health Care Services Quarterly* 12(1): 13, 21.

List of Contributors

EDITOR:

Marilyn D. Harris, MSN, RN, CNAA, BC, FAAN
Former Executive Director
Abington Memorial Hospital Home Care
Hatboro, Pennsylvania

CONTRIBUTORS:

Diana Acker, RN
Nurse Manager
Abington Memorial Hospital Home Infusion
Willow Grove, Pennsylvania

Carol Easley Allen, PhD, RN
Chair and Professor
Department of Nursing
Oakwood College
Huntsville, Alabama

Emily Amerman, MSW, BA
Executive Director
Living Independently for Elders (LIFE)
Philadelphia, Pennsylvania

Pamela A. Andresen, PhD, RN
Director
Loyola University Nursing Center
Loyola University Chicago
Chicago, Illinois

Ida M. Androwich, PhD, RN, BC, FAAN
Professor, Health Promotion, Primary Care,
   Health Systems, and Dietetics
Director, Health Systems Management
Marcella Niehoff School of Nursing
Loyola University Chicago
Maywood, Illinois

Theresa Sekan Ayer, MS, RN, CNAA
President, Ayer Associates, Inc.
Board Chair, Community Health Accreditation
   Program
Tucson, Arizona

Donna R. Baldwin, MSN, RN
Executive Director, Home Health Agency
Baptist Trinity Home Care and Hospice
Memphis, Tennessee

Edward R. Balotsky, PhD
Assistant Professor of Management
Saint Joseph's University
Haub School of Business
Department of Management
Philadelphia, Pennsylvania

Judith A. Bellome, MSEd, RN
Director of Marketing
Southview Home Care
Kansas City, Kansas

Lazelle E. Benefield, PhD, RN
Associate Professor
Harris School of Nursing
Texas Christian University
Fort Worth, Texas

Linda A. Billows, MS, RN
Consultant, Home Health
Marblehead, Massachusetts

Brian M. Block, MA, ARM
Director of Risk Management
Brown & Brown
Bethlehem, Pennsylvania

Thomas D. Brown, RPh, MBA
Pharmacy Manager
Abington Memorial Hospital Home
    Infusion
Willow Grove, Pennsylvania

Nancy B. Brundy, MSW
Director of External Affairs, Institute on
    Aging
Past Chair, National Adult Day Services
    Association
Institute on Aging
San Francisco, California

Paulette D. Bryan, MSW, MLSP
Education and Training Consultant
National Adult Day Services Association
Herndon, Virginia

John I. Buck, BBS
President, Advantage Home Care, Inc.
Chair, National Association for Home
    Care Accreditation Program
Washington, DC

Irma Camaligan, RN
Director of Patient Services
Midpoint Health Care Services, Inc.
East Orange, New Jersey

Jennifer W. Campbell, MSW, MA
Adjunct Faculty
Graduate School of Social Work and Social
    Research
Bryn Mawr College
Bryn Mawr, Pennsylvania

Karen L. Carney, BA
President, Carney Communication
Director of Marketing, Hospice of the North
    Shore
Danvers, Massachusetts

Ann H. Cary, PhD, MPH, RN, A-CCC
Director of Graduate Distance Learning
    Programs
School of Public Health and Health
    Sciences
School of Nursing
University of Massachusetts–Amherst
Amherst, Massachusetts

Diane Cass, MS, RNC, CCRC
Clinical Research Coordinator
Cardiovascular Consultants of Maine
Auburn, Maine

Karen Cassidy, EdD, MBA, MSN, RN
Health Care Consultant
Louisville, Kentucky

Thomas E. Cesar, MPM
President and Chief Executive Officer
Accreditation Commission
    for Health Care, Inc.
Raleigh, North Carolina

Carol A. Clarke, MA, RN
President and Owner
Clarke Health Care Consultants
Community Health Accreditation Program
    Site Visitor
Seminole, Florida

Judith A. Conley, MSN, RN
Vice President, Clinical Services
The Connecticut Hospice
Branford, Connecticut

**Ruth Constant, EdD, MSN, RN, CHCE,
    FHHC**
Board Chair, National Association for Home
    Care and Hospice
President and Administrator
Beaumont, Port Arthur, and Wichita Home
    Health Service Agencies
Victoria, Texas

Todd R. Cote, MD
Medical Director, Home Care
The Connecticut Hospice
Branford, Connecticut

Kathryn S. Crisler, MS, RN
Research Associate
Center for Health Services Research
University of Colorado Health Sciences
    Center
Denver, Colorado

Elissa Della Monica, MSN, RN, CNA, BC
Executive Director
Abington Memorial Hospital Home Care
Willow Grove, Pennsylvania

D. Scott Detar, CPA, BS
Partner, Maillie Falconiero & Company, LLP
Oaks, Pennsylvania

Janna L. Dieckmann, PhD, RN
Assistant Professor
University of North Carolina at Chapel Hill
    School of Nursing
Chapel Hill, North Carolina

Cheryl E. Easley, PhD, RN
Dean and Professor
College of Health and Social Welfare
University of Alaska, Anchorage
Anchorage, Alaska

Jessica S. Eichner, MS, SPHR
Vice President, Human Resources
VNA Services and Foundation, Western
    Pennsylvania
Butler, Pennsylvania

Joann K. Erb, PhD, RN
Education and Research Coordinator
Abington Memorial Hospital Home Care
Willow Grove, Pennsylvania

E. Michael Flanagan, JD, BS
Partner, Health Care Practice Group
Weil, Gotshal & Manges, LLP
Washington, D.C.

Rosemary Franco, RN
Assistant Vice President of Nursing
The Connecticut Hospice
Branford, Connecticut

Ann K. Frantz, BSN, RN
Vice President Clinical Services
Noninvasive Medical Technologies
Auburn Hills, Michigan

Andrea Gendelman, BSN, RN
Staff Nurse
Skilled Nursing Inc.
Blue Bell, Pennsylvania

Patricia Gerrity, PhD, RN, FAAN
Associate Dean
College of Nursing and Health Professions
Drexel University
Philadelphia, Pennsylvania

Joie Glenn, MBA, RN, CAE
Executive Director
New Mexico Association for Home and
    Hospice Care
Albuquerque, New Mexico

Margaret Golden, MBA, RN
Executive Director
Midpoint Health Care Services, Inc.
East Orange, New Jersey

David R. Goldfarb, MBA, CPA Certificate
Senior Vice President of Finance and Human
    Resources
The Connecticut Hospice
Branford, Connecticut

Pearl Beth Graub, MSW
Director of Professional Services for Long
  Term Care
Philadelphia Corporation for Aging
Philadelphia, Pennsylvania

Val J. Halamandaris, JD
President
National Association for Home Care and
  Hospice
Washington, DC

Carolyn J. Humphrey, MS, RN, FAAN
Editor in Chief, *Home Healthcare Nurse*
President, C. J. Humphrey Associates
Louisville, Kentucky

Rosemary Johnson-Hurzeler, MPH, RN, HA
President and Chief Executive Officer
The Connecticut Hospice, Inc.
Branford, Connecticut

Elizabeth R. Kane, MA, RNC
Director of Professional Services
Abington Memorial Hospital Home Care
Willow Grove, Pennsylvania

Katherine K. Kinsey, PhD, RN, FAAN
Associate Professor and Independence
  Foundation Chair
Director, LaSalle Neighborhood Nursing
  Center
LaSalle University
Philadelphia, Pennsylvania

Ronny J. Knight, MBA, FHFMA
Senior Vice President, Planning and
  Reimbursement
The Connecticut Hospice
Branford, Connecticut

Linda H. Krulish, PT, MHS
President, Home Therapy Services
Redmond, Washington

Mary Pat Larsen, BSN, RN, CHCE
Administrator
Sun Plus Home Health
San Diego, California

Jane Isaacs Lowe, PhD, MSW
Senior Program Officer
The Robert Wood Johnson Foundation
Princeton, New Jersey

Carolyn S. Markey, RN, AS
President and Chief Executive Officer
Visiting Nurse Association of America
Boston, Massachusetts

Sharon D. Martin, MSN, APRN, BC
Associate Professor of Nursing
Saint Joseph's College
Standish, Maine

Kathleen Carlson Mebus, MSN, RN, CAE
Director, State Legislation
The Hospital and Healthsystem Association of
  Pennsylvania
Harrisburg, Pennsylvania

**Paula Milone-Nuzzo, PhD, RN, FAAN,
  FHHC**
Professor and Director of the School of
  Nursing
Associate Dean for International Partnerships
  for the College of Health and Human
  Development
The Pennsylvania State University
State College, Pennsylvania

Mary Curry Narayan, MSN, RN, CS, CTN
Senior Consultant
Visiting Nurse Service Network
Chantilly, Virginia

Ann Marie O'Connell, MBA
Director of Human Resources
Visiting Nurse Association of Boston
Boston, Massachusetts

Karen Beckman Pace, PhD, RN
Senior Scientist, Home Health Care Quality
  Improvement
Delmarva Foundation
Easton, Maryland

Carol Ann Parente, MSN, RN, CRNP
Adult Nurse Practitioner
Abington Memorial Hospital Home Care
Willow Grove, Pennsylvania

**Donna Ambler Peters, PhD, RN,
   FAAN**
Professor, College of Nursing
St. Petersburg College
St. Petersburg, Florida

Vern A. Peterschmidt, BS Accounting
President
Peterschmidt & Associates
Albuquerque, New Mexico

**Barbara Kovalcin Piskor, MPH, RN,
   CNAA, BC**
President, BKP HealthCare Resources
Pittsburgh, Pennsylvania

Maryanne L. Popovich MPH, BSN, RN
Executive Director, Home Care Accreditation
   Program
Joint Commission on Accreditation of
   Healthcare Organizations
Oakbrook Terrace, Illinois

Deborah A. Randall, JD
Member, Health Law Group
Arent Fox
Washington, D.C.

Joseph W. Ruane, PhD, MA
Professor of Sociology and Health Policy
University of the Sciences in Philadelphia
Philadelphia, Pennsylvania

Nancy DiPasquale Ruane, MA, RN
Community Health Specialist
Philadelphia, Pennsylvania

Virginia Saba, EdD, RN, FAAN, FACMI, LL
Distinguished Scholar, Adjunct
Georgetown University
Washington, D.C.

Patricia A. Sevast, BSN, RN
Clinical and Operations Consultant
American Express Tax and Business Services,
   Inc.
Timonium, Maryland

Peter W. Shaughnessy, PhD
Professor and Director of Center for Health
   Services Research
University of Colorado Health Sciences
   Center
Denver, Colorado

Ann P. Sherwin, JD, MSN, RN
Attorney
Havertown, Pennsylvania

Larri A. Short, JD, MA
Member, Health Law Group
Arent Fox
Washington, D.C.

Myra L. Skluth, PhD, MD
Associate Medical Director, The Connecticut
   Hospice
Chief of the Section of General Internal
   Medicine–Norwalk Hospital
Norwalk, Connecticut

David B. Smith, PhD
Professor, Department of Health
   Administration
Temple University
Philadelphia, Pennsylvania

Suzanne P. Smith, EdD, RN, FAAN
Editor in Chief, *Journal of Nursing
   Administration*
Bradenton, Florida

Carol-Rae Green Sodano, EdD
Dean, School of Adult and Continuing
   Education
Barry University
Miami, Florida

Richela Stoddard-Johnston, BSN, RN, IBCLC
Pediatric Home Care Nurse
Abington Memorial Hospital
    Home Care
Willow Grove, Pennsylvania

Judith Lloyd Storfjell, PhD, RN
President, Lloyd Consultants, LLC
Associate Professor
College of Nursing
University of Illinois at Chicago
Chicago, Illinois

Julie Tennant, MEd, BSN, RN
Community Health Accreditation Program
    Site Visitor
Alexandria, Virginia

Linda Q. Thede, PhD, RN, BC
Consultant, Nursing Informatics Education
Aurora, Ohio

Brian C. Thomas, MSN, RN
Vice President for Industry Relations
BeyondNow Technologies
Overland Park, Kansas

Miriam Cannon Wagner, BSN, RN
Clinical Research Consultant
Harleysville, Pennsylvania

Peggie Reid Webb, MS, RN
Supervisor of Clinical Services
Visiting Nurse and Homemaker Services, Inc.
Mount Holly, New Jersey

Kathleen E. Williams, MSN, RN, BC
Project Manager
Surgical Information Systems, Inc.
Alpharetta, Georgia

Leona Wilneff, BSN, RN
Assistant Vice President of Home Care
The Connecticut Hospice
Branford, Connecticut

Alexis A. Wilson, PhD, MPH, RN
Administrator
Clinical Information Management
MultiCare Health System
Tacoma, Washington

Kristy Wright, MBA, BSN, RN, FAAN
President and Chief Executive Officer
VNA Services and Foundation—Western
    Pennsylvania
Butler, Pennsylvania

Wendy Yallowitz, MSW
Program Associate
The Robert Wood Johnson Foundation
Princeton, New Jersey

Joan Reynolds Yuan, MSN, RNC, CPHQ
Director of Education and Quality Assessment/
    Performance Improvement
Abington Memorial Hospital Home Care
Willow Grove, Pennsylvania

PART I

Home Health Administration

CHAPTER 1

Home Health Administration: An Overview

Janna L. Dieckmann

DEFINITION OF HOME HEALTH CARE

Home health care is the provision of health care services to people of any age at home or in other noninstitutional settings. Contemporary home health care is based on nursing service models developed within the visiting nurse association movement beginning in the late 19th century. Home health care has continued to evolve and change in response to social, economic, political, and scientific innovation through the 20th century and into this new millennium. As health care professionalism has grown and differentiated, many health care occupations have become linked to home health care, including occupational therapy, home economics, social work, nutrition services, and beginning during World War II, physical therapy. Auxiliary workers, today called home health aides and homemakers, have frequently been part of home health care services. Physicians have a complex history in home care. Although medical practitioners have always made home visits and have generally been gatekeepers for reimbursement for home health services for their patients, direct physician participation within the home health multidisciplinary team has varied. During the last 60 years, medicine has usually been more detached from proliferating home care agencies, although some physicians continue to participate fully in home health care. Other services, including transportation, laboratory services, home-delivered meal programs, and more, have usually been secured from outside agencies, although these have occasionally been directly incorporated into home health care agencies.

Two key goals of home health care have remained constant during more than a century of change: direct provision of health care services to those at home and the education of both client and family toward the goals of health and independence from formal care systems. Contemporary home health care reflects most strongly the impact of the government-funded medical programs that began in the 1960s, Medicare and Medicaid. Nevertheless, public health initiatives, private insurance benefit regulation, and newly emerging health problems contribute to a constantly changing picture. Home health care services secured in a particular case ultimately depend on the complex interaction among client, family, and community needs as well as client-professional goals and the payment sources available to fund service organizations such as home health care agencies.

From a historical perspective, in 1982, four prominent national organizations involved in home health care provision—the Council of Home Health Agencies and Community Health Services, National League for Nursing; the National Home Caring Council (formerly the National Home Care Council); the National Association of Home Health Agencies; and the Assembly of Outpatient and Home Care Institutions of the American Hospital Association—provided a formal definition of home health care:

Home health service is that component of comprehensive health care whereby services are provided to individuals and families in their places of residence for the purpose of promoting, maintaining, or restoring health or minimizing the effects of illness and disability. Services appropriate to the needs of the individual patient and family are planned, coordinated, and made available by an agency or institution, organized for the delivery of health care through the use of employed staff, contractual arrangements, or a combination of administrative patterns. (McNamara, 1982, 61)

Later definitions of home health care have suggested a core agreement over time, but differ in specificity. The most specific is the 1996 regulatory definition of a home health agency from the Health Care Financing Administration (HCFA), now the Centers for Medicare and Medicaid Services (CMS):

A home health agency (HHA) is a public agency or private organization, or a subdivision of such an agency or organization, that meets the following requirements:

A. It is primarily engaged in providing skilled nursing services and other therapeutic service, such as physical therapy, speech-language pathology services, or occupational therapy, medical social services, and home health aides services.
1. An HHA must make available part-time or intermittent skilled nursing services and at least one other therapeutic service on a visiting basis in a place of residence used as a patient's home.
2. An HHA must furnish at least one of the qualifying services directly through agency employees, but may furnish the second qualifying service and additional services under arrangement with another HHA or organization.

B. It has policies established by a professional group associated with the agency or organization (including at least one physician and one registered nurse) to govern the services and provides for supervision of such services by a physician or a registered nurse.
C. It maintains clinical records on all patients.
D. It is licensed in accordance with State or local law or is approved by the State or local licensing agency as meeting the licensing standards, where applicable.
E. It meets other conditions found by the Secretary of Health and Human Services to be necessary for health and safety.

For services under hospital insurance, the term "home health agency" does not include any agency or organization that is primarily for the care and treatment of mental disease.

The American Nurses Association, in its 1999 *Scope and Standards of Home Health Nursing Practice*, articulated the perspective of the professional caregiver in its definition of home health care:

Home health nursing refers to the practice of nursing applied to a client with a health condition in the client's place of residence. Clients and their designated caregivers are the focus of home health nursing practice. The goal of care is to initiate, manage, and evaluate the resources needed to promote the client's optimal level of well-being and function. Nursing activities necessary to achieve this goal may warrant preventive, maintenance, and restorative emphases to prevent potential problems from developing.

The definition of home health care provided by the Joint Commission on the Accreditation of Healthcare Organizations (2003) defines briefly the expected type of services and recipients of care:

Home health services are those services provided by health care professionals on a per-visit or per-hour basis to patients who have or are at risk of an injury, an illness, or a disabling condition or who are terminally ill and require short-term and/or long-term interventions by health professionals.

DESCRIPTION OF HOME HEALTH CARE

Home health care begins with the client, the individual identified as requiring home nursing or therapy services. Although this identified individual is the focus of the home health care services, professional goals for client development are implemented in the context of family and community. The family, neighbors, and other members of the client's informal support system generally provide the 24-hour care and support necessary during the client's period of illness or dependency. Formal services from home health agencies or the community's social service network can only supplement what family and friends provide. The more dependent the client, the greater the skill and commitment demanded from the informal caregiving system. If family and friends are unable to provide adequate care, and clients require more intensive services than available from the home health agency, consideration of nursing home, sheltered care, inpatient hospice, or other institutional placement becomes critical.

Because of this interactive reliance on informal supports in home health care, it is most practical to define a family in a flexible manner. Traditional definitions of family that include only close biological relatives are inadequate and can limit the search for caregiving resources. In community practice, the term *family* must include anyone the client so identifies. In addition to the nuclear family, persons included may be a significant other, distant relatives, a boarder who has lived in the home for years, close friends, or neighbors who perceive a mutual obligation with the client. This flexible definition of family increases the pool of available

helpers for the dependent client, but it also requires that nursing and other home health care workers incorporate the needs of this extended family system into plans of care. In providing care, nursing considers both the learning needs of support system members and the psychosocial supports required to maintain their caregiving roles. It is not enough to provide instruction; meeting the needs of the informal support system requires complex coordination and problem solving as well.

The client's community may facilitate or detract from the provision of professional care and fulfillment of home health care service objectives. Communities vary from densely concentrated urban neighborhoods, to sprawling suburban towns, to lonesome rural back roads. Although a client may be isolated from supports in any environment, the concentration of people and services, the availability of transportation, and the proximity and diversity of pharmacy and grocery services constitute quantitative differences in the challenges faced by home health care clients and families.

The community, and the membership of the client and the family within it, have further effects on the client and family system and their presenting needs for home health care. The client's and family's socioeconomic background and class status frequently influence their access to care. The family's cultural and ethnic background may influence its expectations for health and health care services and its ability to meet those needs within the American health care system. Individuals, families, and communities have particular ways of defining health, illness, and dying that home health care professionals must recognize and address. For example, many religious groups have prohibitions of which formal caregivers should be aware. Home care professionals must acquire the ability to practice within diverse cultural parameters.

Health professionals, usually trained to hospital goals and values, find differences at every step toward home care. The most obvious difference cannot be minimized: The home, in all its many variations, has replaced the hospital. Rather than clients adapting to the foreign environment of the hospital, it is home health care providers themselves who must adapt to the family and community. Home care nurses are liaisons, expert consultants who adapt complex treatment plans to homes. This may involve, for example, obtaining equipment, making referrals to other services, or negotiating with physicians to alter medication programs.

INITIATION OF HOME HEALTH CARE SERVICES

Home health clients are visited by home care agencies after referrals are made for the clients' care. Referrals may originate from the client, the family, a community social service agency, a local physician, or almost anyone else. Many home care referrals are initiated by a nurse or discharge planner attached to a hospital. These referrals are made to home health agencies from hospitals when client needs for continuing care are identified during the hospitalization or while the client is under care at an ambulatory clinic or emergency department. Other referrals are received from nursing homes, community clinics and physicians' offices, area agencies on aging, and social work agencies.

A referral to home health care services usually includes client demographic information, family contacts, diagnoses, medications, and proposed treatment measures ordered by the physician. Professional disciplines to be provided to the client are specified. This referral is often not overly complex, generally focusing on the basic, immediate needs of the client. Nevertheless, it is most helpful for the referral to include a brief medical and surgical history for the client, recent laboratory findings, baseline vital sign readings, and history and course of the present illness. Because the client's social context suggests both needs for and limitations of care, knowledge of client and family strengths and weaknesses pertaining to the illness and home management will provide a head start for home health agency professionals. Thus comments and recommendations from members of the multidisciplinary team will contribute

to accurate and relevant home care service decisions.

Clients' functional abilities are a consideration for home care payers: Are clients able to care for themselves? Are they able to ambulate? Are they substantially confined to the home? Contemporary payment sources for home care require that clients receiving services be homebound. Although the definition of homebound status has varied, it has generally been interpreted to mean that the client's health and functional impairment is so great that he or she is unable to seek health services outside the home. Additional variables, such as the presence or absence of a safe environment and a reliable caregiver, may influence whether services can be provided in the home.

Organizations that provide home care may be voluntary agencies including visiting nurse associations, proprietary agencies, official health departments, social service agencies, or hospital-based home care departments. Whatever the organizational structure, most agencies visit postacute home health care clients within 24 hours of the initial referral. This first visit will probably be the most complex of the entire service period. During this admission visit, the nurse conducts an assessment and evaluation of the client and family, assesses the environmental milieu, analyzes the impact of disease(s) on the client, identifies functional impairments of the client, determines the client's knowledge of and adherence to prescribed treatment for the disease, and identifies client/family desires for care and eventual goals. Nurses establish the groundwork for needed services, ensuring the safety of clients until the next home care visit. Physical therapists or speech therapists may also take primary responsibility for a home health care case. Active participation of clients and families in establishing the goals of treatment and plan of care is sought and utilized to the fullest extent.

Clients receive services for variable periods of time, from a single visit to service durations of several weeks, months, or even years. Duration of care will depend on the focus of care, whether brief post-hospital stabilization, home rehabilitation, or long-term home care services. Visit patterns are usually directed by reimbursement regulations, resulting in varying patterns of care controlled from outside the client-provider nexus. Under Medicare, visits continue until the client's plan of care is addressed. This period is usually short, most often a few weeks in length. Clients requiring technical interventions, especially those requiring urinary catheter management, may receive intermittent services over several years. Case management systems within health maintenance organizations or managed care health plans are often the most restrictive, sometimes allowing only two or three visits to complete all instruction and services, even for cases such as new insulin-dependent diabetics. Other reimbursement sources demand specialized requirements, resulting in varying patterns of care. An example is maternal-child programs with state or federal public health initiatives. In these programs, at-risk infants and their families may be visited monthly during the first year of life. In long-term home care programs for the aged, where available, nursing visits may be spaced at long intervals to provide skilled management of chronic conditions. Home-based hospice program visits may be frequent (sometimes daily), particularly for clients in late stages of a terminal disease.

Home care professionals work with clients and families to establish plans of care that address the long-term goals of the case, working toward incremental change during each visit. Medicare's original focus was comprehensive improvement in client health status; in recent years, care focus has been pointedly limited to the single primary diagnosis, generally the primary diagnosis identified during the qualifying hospitalization. In both approaches, the home health care nurse utilizes many resources to facilitate client and family progress. Services of additional multidisciplinary team members, such as the physical therapist, occupational therapist, social worker, speech therapist, and home health aide, may be utilized for the client's benefit. If rehabilitation goals predominate in the

case, physical therapy or speech therapy may be the only discipline providing services. Home health care professionals communicate with the client's physician to coordinate the treatment plan to reflect client status changes (e.g., progress in rehabilitation, difficulty in wound healing, or persistent challenges of the terminal phase of illness).

The home health care team relies heavily on ongoing services provided by the community's formal support network as well as the family's own informal support system. Ongoing support systems are essential to prepare the client for discharge from home health care and to provide needed services when skilled care through the home health agency is terminated. The nurse or other professional will make, or suggest that the client or family make, appropriate referrals to formal care networks. The nurse will also seek to develop and support informal systems based in the family, neighborhood, religious, or social groups.

Although actual home health care service outcomes vary significantly among clients and families, case discharge usually occurs when the client has met the goals of care. Some clients progress easily and completely to meet mutually set goals for care, whereas others may achieve only partial outcomes. The client and family are prepared for discharge during the entire period of home health care provision by being taught the skills required to resume independent management of health care needs. At the time of discharge, the nurse or other home health care provider usually notifies the physician and other involved services that the case is closed. Discharged cases are reopened when clients are referred for new problems or exacerbations of health problems that were previously addressed.

EARLY SOURCES FOR HOME HEALTH CARE

An appreciation of the history of home health care accomplishments is important to understand its current status, including both the strengths and the limitations of the field (Exhibit 1–1). The

Exhibit 1–1 Chronology of Home Health Care in the United States

1813	Ladies' Benevolent Society of Charleston, South Carolina, is founded to provide relief of distress and aid to the sick poor.
1832	The Nurse Society of Philadelphia provides care for sick poor in their homes.
1859	First District Nursing Association established in Liverpool, England, by William Rathbone.
1875	First United States nurse training schools using the Nightingale model.
1877	New York City Mission sends trained nurses into homes of the sick poor.
1886	Visiting Nurse Society of Philadelphia and the Boston Instructive District Nursing Association are established.
1893	Henry Street Nurses Settlement founded on the lower east side of New York City by Lillian Wald and Mary Brewster. This agency is now known as the Visiting Nurse Service of New York.
1898	First municipal home care nurse employed in the United States at Los Angeles to visit the sick poor.
1901	Fifty-eight organizations provide public health nursing, employing 130 nurses.
1907	Alabama legally approves employment of public health nurses by local boards of health.
1909	*Visiting Nurse Quarterly*, first ongoing specialty journal in the field, begins publication.
1909	Metropolitan Life Insurance Company offers home nursing to its industrial policyholders.
1912	National Organization for Public Health Nursing (NOPHN) is founded.
1912	Rural Nursing Service of the American Red Cross is established, later renamed the Town and Country Nursing Service.
1916	A total of 1,922 public health nursing organizations employ 5,150 nurses, a 30-fold increase over 1901 figures.
1921	The Sheppard-Towner Act provides federal matching funds for prenatal and infant care programs supporting home care by nurses.
1922	Public health nursing organizations totaling 4,040 employ 11,550 nurses, double the 1916 total.
1925	Kentucky Committee for Mothers and Babies, later the Frontier Nursing Service, is founded by Mary Breckenridge.
1925	The first NOPHN statement of qualifications for public health nurses is published.
1931	A total of 4,250 public health nursing agencies employ 15,850 nurses, demonstrating only slight growth since 1922.
1935	Government funding of public health nursing emphasizes health departments over nonofficial agencies.
1935	A joint committee of the American Nurses Association and NOPHN to Study Health Insurance and Its Implications for Nursing forms to seek health insurance funding for nursing care.
1935	The Association of State and Territorial Directors of Nursing forms.
1944	The first basic nursing program is accredited as including sufficient public health nursing content.
1947	The first "coordinated" home medical care program is established at Montefiore Hospital, Bronx, New York.
1950	A total of 25,100 public health nurses are employed.
1950	The Red Cross Rural Nursing Service is discontinued.
1953	NOPHN merges with other organizations to form the National League for Nursing (NLN).
1953	Publication of *Public Health Nursing* ends.
1953	Life insurance companies cease supporting home nursing service.
1955	A total of 27,100 public health nurses are employed.
1956	A feasibility study is conducted for Blue Cross reimbursement for home nursing care in New York City.

Continues

Exhibit 1–1 Chronology of Home Health Care in the United States (continued)

1960	The Kerr-Mills legislation provides Medical Aid for the Aged, including a home care benefit in selected states.
1966	Home health services under Medicare and Medicaid begin providing support for official and nonofficial agencies in caring for the sick.
1982	The National Association for Home Care forms from the combination of the National Association of Home Health Agencies and the NLN Council of Home Health Agencies/Community Health Services.
1983	The Health Care Financing Administration implements medical prospective payment, restricting hospital admissions and length of stay and ultimately increasing the acuity of home care clients.
1983	Medicare hospice care benefit is implemented.
1988	*Duggan et al. v. Bowen et al.,* 691 F. Supp. 1487 (D.C. 1988) is decided (the Staggers lawsuit).
1993	The Word Organization for Care in the Home and Hospice is organized.
1997	Balanced Budget Act of 1997, which included a change in Medicare reimbursement to incorporate the Interim Payment System.
2000	The Medicare Prospective Payment System (PPS) becomes effective.
2003	The Medicare Prescription Drug, Improvement and Moderinization Act of 2003. (PL-108-173)

Compiled by Janna Dieckmann

history of home health care is also an ongoing case study in organizational styles and reimbursement patterns resulting from past patterns of social and economic change. For example, in the early 1900s, home health care was provided by public health and visiting nurses as part of the public health campaign that improved the health of all Americans. Home health care has frequently changed direction, often suddenly and sharply, as the direct result of changing reimbursement practices, which mirror the contemporary experience. Analysis and review of the history of home health care have implications for health care services in the early decades of the 21st century. An opportunity to avoid the pitfalls of the past emerges when similar patterns in the present are identified. The following brief sketch is but a beginning.

Until the 20th century, care of the sick was usually informal, provided by household members, almost always women. Historians today are aware of early experiments in home health nursing that developed during the early 19th century in the United States. Reflecting then contemporary ideas, these programs focused on moral elevation as well as illness intervention. The Ladies' Benevolent Society of Charleston, South Carolina, provided charitable works to the poor and ill beginning in 1813. In Philadelphia, lay nurses who attended a short training program were sent to care for the newborns and postpartum mothers of all social strata. Significant in time and place, programs such as these do not seem to have spread, and their influence on the development of visiting nurse associations and organized home health care in the late 19th century is unclear.

Florence Nightingale's innovations in training English nurses to replace untrained lay nurses influenced the late 19th century pattern of nursing education and service provision in the United States. William Rathbone established the first District Nursing Association in 1859 in Liverpool, England. It was not until 1877, however, that district nursing utilizing graduates of the new nurse training schools was introduced into the United States. Early visiting nurse programs were founded in Boston, Buffalo, Philadelphia, and New York City.

During the late 19th century, nurses who had graduated from the early training programs usually worked in private duty nursing or held a few positions as hospital administrators and instructors. The new field of public health nursing began to employ a few nurses, often adopting the model of service provision used by the private duty nurse in middle- and upper-class homes. Whereas private duty nurses lived with the clients and their families, the public health nurses visited several families in one day, providing personal care to the sick and health teaching to families. Many of these voluntary agencies hired only one nurse. Agency administration and direct supervision of the nurses were the responsibility of the agency board, usually composed of wealthy or socially prominent women of the community. Their charitable community service was to direct both health care and good works by the nurse.

At the turn of the century, public health nursing was defined as "primarily family health work of an educational and preventive character but including restorative work" (Dock and Stewart, 1925, 213), which utilized a large and comprehensive plan for uplifting the general health level through outreach to the community. Although services were offered to individuals and families, especially the poor and immigrants, the public health nurse sought to ensure the health of the community as a whole.

Visiting nursing proved successful in the United States at meeting the public health challenges of that era. High incidence and mortality rates of communicable diseases such as tuberculosis, diphtheria, and typhoid fever affected the entire population. Increased urbanization and industrialization also increased human diseases. The community's health in the late 19th century benefited from the new scientific explanations of disease, and the public health nurse became the agent for preventive education to the lay public. Nursing interventions, improved urban sanitation, economic improvements, and better nutrition were the bases for significant reductions in the incidence of deadly communicable disease by 1910.

Early visiting nurse agencies also sought to develop innovative services, whose ongoing maintenance and income support they expected to shift to government auspices. In New York City, Lillian Wald and her coworkers at the Henry Street Nurses' Settlement (later the Visiting Nurse Services) initiated several new programs. Like visiting nurses, other nursing specialties emerged from public health nursing practice, such as school nursing and occupational health nursing. In this period, these specialties were closely connected to visiting nursing and home health care. Clients identified within the school or work setting were visited in the home, where health promotion and family education were the focus of the nurses' efforts.

Both nurses and lay supporters of the new visiting nurse agencies sought means to expand the visiting nurse movement through exchange of information and development of a professional identity. Publication of the *Visiting Nurse Quarterly* in 1909 established a professional medium of communication for clinical and organization concerns. Establishment of the National Organization for Public Health Nursing (NOPHN) in 1912, whose membership included both nurses and lay supporters, provided an accessible network for the developing leadership in the field. The organizational focus of the NOPHN was "improving the educational and service standards of the public health nurse, and promoting public understanding of and respect for her work" (Rosen, 1958, 381). The NOPHN was soon a dominant force in public health nursing and endured until 1953, when it merged with other nursing organizations to form the National League for Nursing. The loss of this distinct specialty organization, which had joined public health and visiting nurses, remains an obstacle to unifying the specialty of public health/community health nursing.

Rapid growth of the practice field highlighted the need to provide effective educational preparation for current and future public health nurses. Education for public health nursing was initiated separately from the established nurse training schools beginning around 1906. These certificate programs offered lectures in public health nursing theory and practice in a program that might be familiar to contemporary nurses. Public health and community health nursing did not become a regular part of most baccalaureate nursing education programs until much later.

Mechanisms for payment for home health care services were initially much simpler than today. Often through its social networks, the visiting nurse agency board of trustees raised funds to support the work with the poor and needy. However, clients were encouraged to pay a small fee for nursing services, even as little as a nickel, reflecting social welfare concerns against promoting economic dependency by providing charity. An innovation at the time of its creation in 1909, the special nursing service provided by the Metropolitan Life Insurance Company for its policyholders served as a model for life insurance company sponsorship of nursing care. Nurses in existing agencies, or in agencies developed specifically by the life insurance companies, provided home care services in a significant amount until the early 1950s.

Agencies such as the American Red Cross also provided home care in areas outside the larger cities. Through the Rural Nursing Service, later the Town and Country Nursing Service, the Red Cross developed and passed to local voluntary or public administration almost 3,000 generalized programs of public health nursing services.

Beginning in Los Angeles in 1898, municipalities, and eventually the federal government, took on the task of providing financial support for home health care. Government-funding emphasis gradually began to shift to official health departments. Although the economic impact of the Depression in the 1930s reduced both charitable and public funding for home health care that resulted in cutbacks in personnel and traditional services, New Deal legislation created new employment opportunities for nurses in official health programs. As had the Sheppard-Towner Act of 1921, which targeted improvements in maternal and child health care, Public Health Title VI of the 1935 Social Security Act

focused available financial resources toward the nonofficial voluntary agencies.

Mobilization for World War II brought significant changes in nursing education. An increasing emphasis on baccalaureate nursing programs saw the first inclusion of public health nursing in the required coursework. By the mid-1950s, the National League for Nursing required public health nursing courses, but only in baccalaureate-level programs. Clinical practice in all types of public health nursing, including home health care, remains absent from many diploma and associate degree programs and is not a formal category for the nurse licensure examinations.

The influence of the NOPHN in connecting different agencies and in increasing the spread of knowledge and information relating to practice had gradually decreased by the late 1940s. The challenges of securing financial support for the NOPHN and the popular trend toward centralization of professional nursing organizations laid the groundwork for the end of the organization. In 1953, the NOPHN merged with other specialty nursing organizations to constitute the National League for Nursing. At that time, the journal *Public Health Nursing* (first called *Visiting Nurse Quarterly*) ceased publication.

The early 1950s saw other significant changes in visiting nurse sponsorship and organization. Insurance companies, including Metropolitan Life and John Hancock, and the American Red Cross, discontinued their support of home health care and the voluntary agencies that had provided the nursing services. With the decrease in the incidence rate of acute, communicable diseases and distinct and progressive increases in chronic illness prevalence, the sponsoring life insurance companies doubted their financial ability to continue to support home nursing care.

During the 1930s and again in the 1950s, the organization form of home health care service delivery was also reconsidered. Concern over duplication and a desire for excellent, comprehensive service provision fueled a movement toward combination agencies, defined as a merger of official and voluntary nursing services in a geographical area to provide joint public health and home health care nursing service. Although this was a long-sought and innovative format, declining municipal income and services severely threatened some combination agencies during the 1970s. Some previously combined services were separated into their components for reasons of economic survival. A second organizational form emerged in hospital-based home care, particularly influenced by the coordinated home medical care program of Montefiore Hospitals, Bronx, New York, which began in 1947. Visiting nurse agencies spearheaded similar coordinated home care programs, led by the Philadelphia Home Care Program of the Philadelphia Visiting Nurse Society in 1949.

Initiation of Medicare and Medicaid health insurance benefits for the elderly and the poor in July 1966 formed an essential basis for the current home health care structure. Adequate funding for home health care was an infusion to voluntary organizations, resulting in increased breadth and amount of services provided. Where a few hospital-based programs had developed in the late 1940s, many more now operated and were joined by growing numbers of entrepreneurial groups drawn by profit-making opportunities, which recognized that a predictable source of home health care funding was now available. Although in 1960, only 250 official health agencies provided nursing care for the sick on a regular basis, by 1968, 1,328 public health nursing agencies—50 percent of all official agencies—provided this service. Further refinement of Medicare through congressional amendment and administrative control during the 1970s and 1980s progressively refocused the home care benefit on postacute services. This change from 1960s Medicare home care practices constricted medium-term and long-term home health services as well as care of the chronic client.

REASONS FOR THE GROWTH OF HOME HEALTH CARE

Not only has home health care expanded in the last 120 years, but it may continue to grow in response to the expected changes in the contemporary sociopolitical and economic forces influencing the home health care environment. Changing patterns of disease and population aging, emerging economic reimbursement mechanisms, and changing social values draw together to construct the contemporary home health care delivery system.

The change in the distribution of disease since the turn of the century represents the first factor in the growth of home health care. Improved scientific knowledge of disease agents, regular immunizations, availability of antibiotics, provision of basic nutrition to most people, pasteurization of milk, and other factors have decreased the risk of developing and dying of 19th-century disease threats such as communicable diseases, tuberculosis, severe diarrheal illnesses, cholera, and many others. In place of the acute illnesses, chronic illnesses are now the primary causes of death in the United States. These illnesses, such as hypertension, cardiac disease, pulmonary disease, and diabetes, have a long period of development leading to irreversible changes in the body and frequently permanent impairment of the individual's functional abilities. Although early intervention may limit the effect of chronic disease exacerbations, affected individuals generally experience long periods of debility necessitating rehabilitation, during which they may fail to regain their previous abilities. The health care delivery system is faced with making policy decisions about people for whom illness and disease is irreversible, degenerative, and functionally impairing. Chronic illness reduces individual and family resources and decreases the ability to pay privately for needed services. It will be a challenge to society to develop systems that are efficient in meeting client needs and effective in controlling overall costs. Home care has shown promise in being the alternative of choice to meet this large and growing need.

A second and related set of changes affecting the growth of home health care is the changes in the distribution of the population of the United States. This nation is growing older as a whole. Although in 1900 only 4.1 percent of Americans, or 3.1 million individuals, were 65 years or older, by 2000, there were 35.0 million older adults—almost a ten-fold increase. Representing a 12 percent increase in real numbers from 1990 to 2000, the population proportion of adults aged 65 and older declined slightly from 12.6 percent to 12.4 percent in 2000 (U.S. Bureau of the Census, 2001). This change in the population older than 65 years is related to the changes in the distribution of disease toward increased prevalence of chronic illnesses. With decreased mortality due to acute illnesses in the younger population, more individuals are living into their later years, the period in which chronic illness is most likely to appear. Additionally, better treatment of complications of older age and chronic illness mean that, even with serious diseases, people tend to live longer than previously.

Complicating this population trend toward longer life have been changes in the social behavior of families. Changing distribution of employment, economic recession, and improved transportation have dispersed families across the country more than ever before. Fewer relatives live in proximity to elderly individuals, reducing available assistance during illness. Changing patterns of female employment, which have increased the percentage of women in the workforce, have simultaneously reduced the number of female family members available for fulltime care of the chronically ill. As a result of all these functional changes in the family, care of the impaired elderly has required an increased social and governmental responsibility.

A third factor in the growth of home health care, and an indirect effect of the increase in chronic illness prevalence, has been the expansion of rehabilitative services for those at home

with chronic illnesses. Rehabilitation is a longterm process requiring adaptation of the impaired individual to the home environment. This adaptation may require the assistance of a variety of professional services. Home health care has expanded its utilization of the therapies—physical therapy, occupational therapy, and speech therapy—in home rehabilitation efforts. Social work also has a place in the care of the home-bound individual. When individuals require a diversity of services, overall utilization of home health care increases.

Changing reimbursement patterns have had such a profound effect on the outline of services provided under home health care that reimbursement is said to set the direction for home health care. Although analysis of home health care development substantiates this position, this fourth reason for the rise in home health care has had an especially strong impact since the passage of Medicare and Medicaid home care coverage with the 1965 Social Security Amendments. The Medicare focus on shortterm, intermittent interventions has limited funding to develop new concepts for long-term home care management. Furthermore, Medicare reimbursement has made home health care a profitable venture for proprietary agencies and hospitals. This has multiplied the number of agencies in a given area both with and without certificates of need. Competition has thus far led to home health care growth, but it has also opened the question of quality assurance and the adequacy of specific training of staff in home health care skills in the new agencies.

The search for health care cost containment has sometimes encouraged the growth of home health care, a fifth reason for its expansion. Changes in Medicare reimbursement for hospitalization toward prospective payment in the early 1980s, popularly known as the diagnosis-related group system, have given fiscal encouragement to limit the length of acute hospitalizations. A result has been the discharge to nursing home or private home of individuals who, in earlier years, may have remained in the acute care institution. The phrase *sicker and quicker* has been used to describe the situation of those released to home care under this policy. Increased acuity of home care clients implies more frequent skilled visits, more time-consuming visits as a result of increased complexity, and clients at greater risk for decompensation and rehospitalization. A shift of care from acute institutions to home care provides only a beginning for still further changes in home health care.

The optimistic belief that cost containment motives will increase home health care utilization is tempered by at least two different problems. On the one hand, the desire for overall cost containment in health services, instead of increasing reimbursement to encourage hospital discharge, is paradoxically curtailing home health care services. The Medicare Prospective Payment System, Medicare intermediaries, and managed care programs have attempted to limit strictly the client categories reimbursed under regulations of skilled care, intermittent service, homebound status, and other client variables. Managed care also emphasizes linkages between achievement of specific client care outcomes and reimbursement. On the other hand, some experts have questioned whether the real total cost of care for the client has been identified to compare with costs of acute hospital care. Lost income to the family caregiver, cost of physical maintenance of the home, and other informal costs have not usually been part of the comparison equation. Is home health care cheaper than institutional alternatives? An answer to this question will depend on the manner in which patient, family, and community variables are weighed and considered.

Earlier acute care discharge combined with increased home care availability of sophisticated biomedical equipment leads to the sixth factor increasing home health care. Complex services once rarely seen in the home, such as renal hemodialysis, ventilators, and infusion therapy, are more frequently an option for clients who prefer to be at home rather than endure long hospital stays. Simplified technology, effective teaching of clients' caregivers, and efficient supplier networks providing diverse equipment have assured complex care a place in the home environment.

A seventh area affecting the growth in home health care is the question of quality of life. The elderly and the chronically ill often prefer to remain in their independent living situations than be institutionalized in, for instance, a nursing home. Many families negatively value institutionalization and separation of the family members. Some cultural and ethnic groups are especially reluctant to treat the chronically ill and elderly in this manner. A desire for self-care as part of significant long-term changes in popular philosophy has also supported increases in home health care. Despite these significant trends in societal values, needed social and economic supports for clients and family caregivers involved in long-term home care are rarely provided.

CONCLUSION

Home health care has become an essential aspect of health care. The challenge will be to draw from home health care's past, to anticipate its future potential, and to provide effective services to contemporary clients and families.

REFERENCES

Centers for Medicare and Medicaid Services, 1996. *Section 200*. Home Health Agency Manual. Washington, DC: U.S. Department of Health and Human Services.

Dock, L. L., and A. M. Stewart. 1925. *A short history of nursing: From the earliest times to the present day.* 2d ed. New York: G.P. Putnam's Sons.

Rosen, G. 1958. *A history of public health.* New York: MD Publications.

U.S. Bureau of the Census. 2001. *The 65 years and over population: 2000, Census 2002 brief.* Available at www.census.gov.

SUGGESTED READING

American Nurses Association. 1986. *Standards of home health nursing practice.* Kansas City, MO: ANA.

American Nurses Association. 1999. *Scope and standards of home health nursing practice.* Washington, DC: ANA.

Brickner, P.W. 1978. *Home health care for the aged: How to help older people stay in their own homes and out of institutions.* New York: Appleton-Century-Crofts.

Buhler-Wilkerson, K. 1983. False dawn: The rise and decline of public health nursing in America, 1900–1930. In *Nursing history: New perspectives, new possibilities,* edited by E.G. Lagemann, 89–106. New York: Teachers College Press.

Buhler-Wilkerson, K. 1985. Public health nursing: In sickness or in health? *American Journal of Public Health* 75: 1155–1161.

Buhler-Wilkerson, K. 1991. Home care the American way: An historical analysis. *Home Health Care Services Quarterly* 12: 5–17.

Buhler-Wilkerson, K. 2001. *No place like home: A history of nursing and home care in the United States.* Baltimore, MD: Johns Hopkins.

Clemen-Stone, S., et al. 2001. *Comprehensive family and community health nursing: Family, aggregate, and community practice.* 6th ed. St. Louis, MO: Mosby.

Division of Nursing, Bureau of Health Professions, Health Resources and Services Administration, Public Health Service. 1985. *Consensus conference on the essentials of public health nursing practice and education.* Washington, DC: U.S. Department of Health and Human Services.

Fitzpatrick, M.L. 1975. *The National Organization for Public Health Nursing, 1912–1952: Development of a practice field.* New York: National League for Nursing.

Fry, S.T. 1983. Dilemma in community health ethics. *Nursing Outlook* 31: 176–179.

Gardner, M.S. 1932. *Public health nursing.* New York: Macmillan.

Heinrich, J. 1983. Historical perspectives on public health nursing. *Nursing Outlook* 31: 317–320.

McNamara, E. 1982. Home care: Hospitals discover comprehensive home care. *Hospitals.* 56(21): 60–66.

Melosh, B. 1982. *"The physician's hand": Work culture and conflict in American nursing.* Philadelphia: Temple University Press.

Monteiro, L.A. 1985. Florence Nightingale on public health nursing. *American Journal of Public Health* 75: 181–186.

Mundinger, M.O. 1983. *Home care controversy: Too little, too late, too costly.* Rockville, MD: Aspen.

Roberts, D.E., and J. Heinrich. 1985. Public health nursing comes of age. *American Journal of Public Health* 75: 1162–1172.

Stanhope, M., and J. Lancaster. 2000. *Community health nursing: Promoting health of aggregates, families, and individuals.* 5th ed. St. Louis, MO: Mosby.

Stewart, J.E. 1979. *Home health care.* St. Louis, MO: Mosby.

Wald, L.D. 1915. *The house on Henry Street.* New York: Holt.

White, M.S. 1982. Construct for public health nursing. *Nursing Outlook* 30: 527–530.

Williams, C.A. 1977. Community health nursing—What is it? *Nursing Outlook* 25: 250–254.

CHAPTER 2

The Home Health Agency

Kathleen E. Williams

HISTORICAL OVERVIEW

The informal, sympathetic care of the sick in their homes by relatives and friends has a long history indeed. The delivery of systematic nursing care in the home, based on the best available knowledge of the natural history of disease, is a much more recent undertaking and is a result of Florence Nightingale's program of secular scientific education for nurses (Smith, 1983). Admiring the skills of the Nightingale nurses, William Rathbone supported philanthropic projects aimed at the sick poor in Liverpool. The Nightingale nurses ran and staffed some of the projects (Woodham-Smith, 1970).

This notion of delivering skilled nursing services to the sick poor was also developing in the United States. Philanthropists in this country provided funds for the start-up of voluntary organizations, forerunners of our visiting nurse associations (VNAs), with trained nurses hired to deliver home nursing services similar to those of their English counterparts. Home care in the United States included "an idiosyncratic mix of government, voluntary and entrepreneurial initiatives, vulnerable to shifts in community support and perceptions of need" (Buhler-Wilkerson, 2001). As local health departments developed and expanded in the early years of the 20th century, health officers in charge of these so-called official agencies also added nurses to their staffs. One of the nursing responsibilities was the delivery of services in the home. By the

middle part of this century, a number of these voluntary and official agencies had combined their resources to various degrees to streamline their operations and thus decrease overhead, costs, and service duplication. Such organizations became known, not surprisingly, as combination agencies.

In 1947, another innovative service model was instituted. E. M. Bluestone, a physician at Montefiore Hospital in Bronx, New York, introduced the notion of hospital-based home care. Patients discharged from that hospital were entitled to a wide range of nursing, social, and other related services, all delivered in their own homes (Cherkasky, 1949). Such an arrangement—a health care institution operating a department of home care—is not limited to hospitals any longer. Rehabilitation centers and skilled nursing facilities also offer home health services. These departments of home care are referred to as institution-based agencies. In contrast, those agencies that are not part of an institution are referred to as freestanding agencies.

By the mid-1960s, there were approximately 1,200 of the aforementioned agencies delivering home health services (Mundinger, 1983), most of which were paid for by donations through organizations such as local community chests or by the recipients of the care. The passage of Medicare, and to a lesser extent Medicaid, in the mid-1960s spurred the growth of the home health industry because these federal insurance programs ensure a stable source of income for the agencies that are eligible to participate in them. The growth of the private agency, another type of agency for the delivery of home health services, was further stimulated in 1982 when Congress and the Health Care Financing Administration (HCFA) opened up home health care to the for-profit sector for Medicare reimbursement. Table 2–1 shows the effect of the Medicare program on the growth in numbers of Medicare-certified home health agencies from 1967 to 1997 before passage of the Balanced Budget Act.

Since 1982, the growth in numbers of both hospital-based and proprietary agencies has been pronounced. The growth spurt between 1984 and 1995 was due to the passage of the prospective payment system by Congress and to the clarification of Medicare coverage by HCFA. Increasing numbers of acute care hospitals were diversifying to broaden their revenue base, and home health care was one of the areas targeted for this diversification (Ginzberg et al., 1984). Currently about 7,019 noncertified agencies exist (National Association for Home Care [NAHC], 2001). These noncertified agencies, such as homemaker–home health aide agencies, do not provide the kinds of services necessary to be certified by Medicare.

This chapter provides an overview of various types of home health agencies (voluntary, official, and private) that are similar in administrative structure and sources of funding. The major differences among the aforementioned types of agencies are positioning for tax purposes and financial control or ownership.

RECENT DEVELOPMENTS

The most pronounced effect of the passage of the Balanced Budget Act (BBA) of 1997, which changed the way Medicare reimbursed for home health services, was the decrease in the existence of approximately 3,000 home health agencies, with the number of people receiving home care shrinking by 600,000 in 1 year (Buhler-Wilkerson, 2001). It is estimated that there was a 33 percent reduction in the relative value of home health services received per user of home health services post-BBA (McCall et al., 2003).

Another significant development for home health agencies was the implementation in October 2000 of PPS, a prospective payment system that capitates a 60-day episode of home health modifying the agency payment for clinical and service use needs. PPS is to home health reimbursement as the diagnosis-related group (DRG) payment system is to hospital care reimbursement (Sienkiewicz and Narayan, 2002). This reimbursement is based on the assessment of the patient's 60-day episode of care utilizing Outcome and Assessment Information Set (OASIS) criteria, with patients categorized into one of the home health resource groups (HHRG).

Home health agencies have also begun to embrace technology in the form of operational information technology implementations and upgrades as well as in the field of telehome care. The frequency and number of patient contacts via these telehealth technologies are increasing and are beginning to account for an increasing share of service encounters (Salvatore, 2002). With the increase in technology utilization has come additional governmental regulation in the form of the Health Insurance Portability and Accountability Act of 1996 (HIPAA). HIPAA regulations necessitate that home health agencies manage the privacy and security of their patients' health information (Cichon, 2002).

SCOPE OF HOME CARE

Home care is one of many service components in the arena of long-term care, although it is not limited to long-term care. Other service components of long-term care include, for example, nursing homes and programs for substance abusers, the mentally retarded, the occupationally disabled, and the handicapped. In other words, many different age and population groups require continuing care. Within this long-term care context, however, the phrase *home*

Table 2–1 Medicare-Certified Home Care Agencies, Selected Years, 1967–2000

Year	VNA	Combination	Public	Proprietary	Private Nonprofit	Other	Hospital	Rehab	Skilled Nursing Facility	Total
1967	549	93	939	0	0	39	133	0	0	1,753
1975	525	46	1,228	47	0	109	273	9	5	2,242
1980	515	63	1260	186	484	40	359	8	9	2,924
1985	514	59	1205	1,943	832	4	1,277	20	129	5,983
1990	474	47	985	1,884	710	0	1,486	8	101	5,695
1991	476	41	941	1,970	701	0	1,537	9	105	5,780
1992	530	52	1083	1,962	637	28	1,623	3	86	6,004
1993	594	46	1196	2,146	558	41	1,809	1	106	6,497
1994	586	45	1146	2,892	597	48	2,081	3	123	7,521
1995	575	40	1182	3,951	667	65	2,470	4	166	9,120
1996	576	34	1177	4,658	695	58	2,634	4	191	10,027
1997	553	33	1149	5,024	715	65	2,698	3	204	10,444
1998	460	35	968	3,414	610	69	2,356	2	166	8,080
1999	452	35	918	3,192	621	65	2,300	1	163	7,747
2000	436	31	909	2,863	560	56	2,151	1	150	7,152

Source: HCFA, Center for Information Systems, Health Standards and Quality Bureau, February 2001, Washington, DC.

health care is used in two ways. On the one hand, it is used to refer to the range of in-home services provided to chronically ill people over a long period of time. On the other hand, it is also used to refer to the Medicare-reimbursed home-based services that are primarily for the acutely ill elderly and are skilled, short term, and intermittent (Moyer, 1986). Regardless of how home health is defined, however, nursing care is the foundation of the entire system.

FINANCIAL CATEGORIES

The term *not for profit* is a designation that exempts organizations from taxation on profits or excess income under Section 501 of the Internal Revenue Code of 1954. This excess is put back into the organization, and no part of the net earnings can be used for the private benefit of owners, partners, or shareholders. Thus a voluntary organization such as a VNA or a commnity-owned hospital would usually be not for profit. If a not-for-profit organization wants to engage in activities intended to make a profit or surplus that is shared or distributed, it would have to form holding companies or separate corporate entities to deal with those profit-making actions. Many VNAs and hospitals are doing this in today's competitive market. The term *for profit* or *profit making* is also a designation for tax purposes. Agencies with this designation are called *proprietary agencies*, and they are not eligible for tax exemption under Section 501 of the Internal Revenue Code.

Such designations for tax purposes, however, are not true differentiations of financial status. For example, all business organizations (voluntary and private) must make profits or at least have income equal to expenses in order to continue to exist. Terms such as *government agency, nongovernmental, private, church affiliated*, and the like all refer to control or ownership, not to positioning for tax purposes. A health department is an example of an official government agency created to perform specified public functions, such as drinking water purification, and

services, such as public health nursing. It is maintained from revenues such as taxes and fees collected from the people who are benefitting from its services or functions. Within this context, then, a community-owned agency would usually be not for profit, but a privately owned organization such as a home health agency could be either for profit or not for profit.

RANGE OF HOME HEALTH AGENCIES

The Medicare conditions of participation for home health agencies define a home health agency as a public agency or private organization primarily engaged in providing skilled nursing services and other therapeutic services ("Conditions of Participation," 1968; HCFA, 1996). Common to certified home health agencies, because it is required for participation in the Medicare program, is the professional advisory committee. This group of professional persons establishes policies and governs the services provided by the home health agency. Appropriate professional discipline representation is required in addition to a minimum of one physician and one registered nurse. In recent years, consumer representation has been strongly encouraged by the Medicare auditing agencies. This committee must review the agency's policies on an annual basis and fulfill an advisory function on a timely, regular, and planned basis.

Government-Public Agencies

Government (official) home health agencies are "created and given their power through statutes enacted by legislators" (Stewart, 1979, p. 25). Home health services are frequently provided by the nursing division of state or local health departments. The organizational structure within the nursing divisions varies among agencies, with some agencies opting to have their public health nurses include their home health clients within their overall public health caseload. Other government agencies choose to form home health teams within their nursing departments. These teams' primary function is to provide home health services. Local health departments may have a combination of public health nurses and home health team nurses providing home health services. In addition to home health services, government agencies usually provide services such as disease prevention, health promotion, communicable disease investigation, environmental health, maternal–child health, and family planning.

Fiscal responsibility for the government home health agency rests with the city, county, or state government units or a combination of such organizations. The overall county/city/state budget restrictions can directly influence the provision of health services in a particular area. Home health caseloads of government agencies frequently include a disproportionate number of indigent patients because the agency cannot refuse services based on the client's ability to pay.

Voluntary Agencies

Home health agencies that do not depend on state and local tax revenues but are financed primarily with nontax funds, such as donations, endowments, United Way contributions, and third-party insurance providers (Medicare, Medicaid, and Blue Cross), are referred to as *voluntary agencies*; an example is a VNA. Voluntary agencies are governed by a board of directors of interested individuals, frequently respected members of the surrounding community or service area.

These agencies are considered community-based agencies because they provide services within a fairly well-defined geographical location or community. In recent years, however, traditional VNA boundaries have become less distinct as a result of increased competition for clients. In the past, voluntary agencies could depend on virtually all the home health clients within their own catchment areas, but the growth of proprietary and institution-based home health agencies has now eroded their traditional referral base. The relationship between neighboring VNAs has turned in many instances from cooperation to competition.

Private Agencies

Private home health agencies can be for-profit or not-for-profit organizations. Some proprietary (for-profit) agencies participate in the Medicare home health program as part of national chains and are administered through a corporate headquarters. Recently, there has been a merger of several proprietary chain providers that may forecast a consolidation of the proprietary home health industry into larger, national firms. These larger companies are able to generate sufficient revenues to cover overhead costs (Anderson, 1986).

Although revenues are generated by some proprietary agencies through third-party payers such as Medicare and Blue Cross, other proprietaries rely on private pay clients. These private pay agencies offer services such as private duty nursing to both acutely and chronically ill patients; this is a difference from most Medicare-certified providers, which provide most of their services to clients who have had a recent acute change in their medical condition. These private services are often on an extended-hours basis (2 to 24 hours) rather than on a per-visit basis (O'Malley, 1986). Many agencies also provide hospital-staffing services.

Facility/Institution-Based Agencies

Home health agencies operating as departments in sponsoring health care organizations are certified under Medicare and hold a separate provider number, but they are governed by the sponsoring organization's board of trustees or directors. In the past, home health services provided by institution-based providers consisted of intensive-level services intended for those clients requiring multiple-discipline services and supplies. The client case mix of today's institution-based agencies reflects the change to a more balanced caseload, with clients requiring differing degrees of services. The principal source of referrals for these agencies is the in-patient population of the facility, with discharge planning/social services being the case finder of potential home health clients.

The philosophy of the institution-based agency usually coincides with that of the sponsoring organization. Good continuity of care is frequently cited by these agencies as their primary advantage over other types of home health agencies (Stewart, 1979). This continuity can be sold to the medical staff of the institution by promotion of the fact that the home care of the physicians' clients is being coordinated by persons familiar with the physicians and the institution. Until recently, a fiscal advantage of institution-based home health providers was the allowance by Medicare of the inclusion of a percentage of administrative and general overhead in the calculation of the visit costs. The Medicare home health reimbursement system also recognized the higher costs of office space in hospitals and permitted an add-on amount in the calculation of the visit costs. This add-on was eliminated as a result of tax reform legislation of 1993 (NAHC, 1993). Another advantage enjoyed by the institution-based home health agency is the ability to draw from the resources of the other departments of the facility for service provision as well as for formal and informal consultation services.

Hospice

An agency in which services are provided by a medically supervised interdisciplinary team of professionals and volunteers for terminally ill clients is defined as a hospice by the National Hospice Organization (NHO) (1984). There are variations among home care hospice programs in their structure and staffing, but all profess to foster the provision of palliative and supportive services to the patient and family before and after the patient's demise (Morris and Christie, 1995). This service is unique to hospice agencies because other home health agencies cease services upon the death of the client. The hospice concept was imported from Britain into the United States at New Haven, Connecticut, in the mid-1970s and has grown to more than 2,500 programs (Table 2-2). In the 1990s, new hospices experienced an annual growth of 8 percent. The number of hospice patients has grown at an annual rate of 13 percent, with an estimated 579,801 patients served in 2000 (NHO, 2002).

Hospice services are reimbursed by many health insurance plans, such as Blue Cross/Blue Shield, as well as by the home hospice service Medicare benefit provided in the Tax Equity and Fiscal Responsibility Act of 1982 (Cunningham, 1985). Many hospice agencies have chosen to obtain Medicare certification because of the improved reimbursement schedule outlined by recent regulations. Approximately 75 percent of hospices are Medicare certified or have certification pending. The hospice benefit is also covered by Medicaid in 36 states and the District of Columbia, and has been authorized under the Civilian and Medical Program of the Uniformed Services (NHO, 1995). Structurally, hospices can be institution based, independent agencies, or owned by or affiliated with a certified home health agency.

Homemaker–Home Health Aide Agencies

Agencies providing homemaker–home health aide services are frequently private agencies in which clients pay for the home care services or in which the care is financed by private insurance policies (Stewart, 1979). These agencies can provide home health aides who are Medicare certified; that is, they have completed a Medicare-approved home health aide course of study (75 hours in length) and/or have passed competency evaluation procedures. With these certified aides, homemaker–health aide agencies are able to contract with Medicare-certified home health agencies, which in turn are reimbursed by Medicare for the home health aide services. The Medicare-certified agency pays

Table 2–2   Medicare-Certified Hospices, 1984–2001

Year	HHA	Hospital	Skilled Nursing Facility	FSTG	Total
1984	n/a	n/a	n/a	n/a	31
1985	n/a	n/a	n/a	n/a	158
1986	113	54	10	68	245
1987	155	101	11	122	389
1988	213	138	11	191	553
1989	286	182	13	220	701
1990	313	221	12	260	806
1991	325	282	10	394	1011
1992	334	291	10	404	1039
1993	438	341	10	499	1288
1994	583	401	12	608	1604
1995	699	460	19	679	1857
1996	815	526	22	791	2154
1997	823	561	22	868	2274
1998	763	553	21	878	2215
1999	762	562	22	928	2274
2000	739	554	20	960	2273
2001	690	552	20	1003	2265

Source: Center for Medicare and Medicaid Services (CMS) Health Standards and Quality Bureau, April 2002.
Also found in the 2002 *Hospice Facts and Statistics,* November 2002. Hospice Association of America, Washington, DC.

the homemaker–home health aide agency directly on an hourly basis. Such contracts are lucrative because they are guaranteed income for the homemaker–home health aide agency.

The distinction between homemakers and home health aides can at times be difficult to ascertain because both functions are often provided by a single employee. Homemakers function primarily as house cleaners, whereas the principal duties of home health aides are in the area of personal care, such as bathing. Other, more complex services, such as range-of-motion exercises, can be performed by the home health aide after proper instruction by a registered nurse. Homemaker–home health aide agencies are required to ensure that their personnel complete 12 hours of inservice programs per year to meet Medicare standards. In addition, on-site performance evaluations are conducted by professionals, such as registered nurses.

Other Home Health Care Providers

In addition to the types of home health agencies discussed in this chapter (Table 2-3), there are home health services provided by durable medical equipment companies, high-technology service companies (ventilators, total parenteral nutrition, etc.), home telephone reassurance programs, companion services, and telehome care companies, to name a few. Many of these organizations refer to themselves, even in their titles, as home care. With the increase in consumer awareness of and demand for home care services, and as a result of the aging of the American population, all types of health care services provided in the home may blend with each

Table 2–3   Types of Agencies

Type	Description
Visitng Nurse Associations (VNA)	Freestanding, voluntary, nonprofit organizations governed by a board of directors and usually financed by tax-deductible contributions as well as earnings
Combination	Combined government and voluntary agencies; sometimes included with counts for VNAs
Public	Government agencies operated by a state, county, city, or other unit of local government having a major responsibility for preventing disease and for community health education
Proprietary	Freestanding, for-profit home care agencies
Private Nonprofit	Freestanding, privately developed, governed, and owned nonprofit home care agencies
Other	Freestanding agencies that do not fit into the other categories mentioned
Hospital	Agencies that are operating units or departments of a hospital
Rehab	Agencies that are based in rehabilitation facilities
Skilled Nursing Facility (SNF)	Agencies based in skilled nursing facilities
Hospice	Agency providing palliative care with supportive medical, social, emotional, and spiritual services to the terminally ill as well as support for the patient's family

Source: Compiled by the author from *Basic Statistics about Home Care 2001* (November 2001), National Association for Home Care (NAHC), Washington, DC, and *Hospice Facts and Statistics* (November 2002), Hospice Association of America.

other, thus creating even more confusion among consumers and professionals alike about types of home health agencies.

CONCLUSION

The categorization of types of home health agencies has changed in the past decades, and the future may bring new organizational structures that are now beginning to evolve. These new alliances, formed mostly out of economic necessity and the growth of managed care, may continue to blur the distinctions among types of home health agencies, thus creating even more complexities with which a home health administrator must cope.

REFERENCES

Anderson, H. J. 1986. Two recent home healthcare mergers may signal consolidation. *Modern Healthcare* 16: 118–119.

Buhler-Wilkerson, K. 2001. *No place like home: A history of nursing and home care in the United States.* Baltimore, MD: Johns Hopkins University Press.

Cherkasky, M. 1949. The Montefiore Hospital home care program. *American Journal of Public Health* 39: 163–166.

Cichon, T. 2002. How to conduct a privacy gap analysis. *Home Healthcare Nurse* 20: 711–717.

Conditions of participation. Home health agencies. 1968. *Federal Register* 33: 12090–12098.

Cunningham, R. M. Jr. 1985. The evolution of hospice. Part 1. *Hospitals* 59: 124–126.

Ginzberg, E., et al. 1984. *Home health care.* Totowa, NJ: Rowman & Allanheld.

Health Care Financing Administration (HCFA). 1996. *Medicare Home Health Agency Manual.* HCFA Pub. 11, Transmittal 277 (rev). Washington, DC: U.S. Department of Health and Human Services.

McCall, N., A. Petersons, S. Moore, and J. Korb. 2003. Utilization of home health services before and after the Balanced Budget Act of 1997: What were the initial effects? *Health Services Research* 38: 85–106.

Morris, R., and K. Christie. 1995. Initiating hospice care. *Home Healthcare Nurse* 13: 21–26.

Moyer, N. 1986. Public policy, politics, and home health care. *Home Healthcare Nurse* 4: 7–12.

Mundinger, M. O. 1983. *Home care controversy.* Gaithersburg, MD: Aspen.

National Association for Home Care (NAHC). 1993. *NAHC Report.* Report no. 528. Washington, DC: NAHC.

National Association for Home Care (NAHC). 2001. *Basic statistics about home care.* Washington, DC: NAHC.

National Hospice Organization (NHO). 1984. *The basics of hospice* (pamphlet). Arlington, VA: NHO.

National Hospice Organization (NHO). 1995. *Hospice fact sheet* (pamphlet). Arlington, VA: NHO.

National Hospice Organization (NHO). 2002. *Hospice facts and statistics.* Washington, DC: NHO.

O'Malley, S. T. 1986. Reimbursement issues. In *Home-health care nursing: Administrative and clinical-perspectives,* edited by S. Stuart-Siddal, 23–82. Gaithersburg, MD: Aspen.

Salvatore, T. 2002. A telehealthcare primer for managers. *Home Healthcare Nurse* 20: 127–130.

Sienkiewicz, J., and Narayan, M. 2002. Have you mastered PPS? *Home Healthcare Nurse* 20: 308–317.

Smith, J. A. 1983. *The idea of health.* New York: Teachers College Press.

Stewart, J. E. 1979. *Home health care.* St. Louis, MO: Mosby.

Woodham-Smith, C. 1970. *Florence Nightingale: 1820–1910.* London: Fontana.

PART II

Standards for Home Health Agencies

CHAPTER 3

Medicare Conditions of Participation

Peggie Reid Webb

This chapter presents a discussion of the major regulatory requirement that affects the operation of the Medicare-certified home health agency (HHA): the Medicare conditions of participation (Department of Health and Human Services, 1989, 1991, 1992, 1993a, 1993b, 1997a, 1997b, and more recent updates found at http://www.access.gpo.gov/nara/cfr). The conditions of participation are given in a document by the same name that sets forth the requirements that must be met by an organization to achieve and maintain designation as a Medicare-certified provider of home health services. As home health care agencies struggle to design service delivery systems that can successfully accommodate the demands imposed by an everchanging health care environment, a basic understanding of the conditions of participation remains essential. The following discussion is intended to enhance the reader's understanding of the conditions and how they may be operationalized by the HHA to demonstrate the compliance necessary to remain a Medicare-certified home health agency.

Each of the conditions in Subpart B, Administration, and Subpart C, Furnishing of Services, is later presented as written in Part 484, Conditions of Participation: Home Health Agencies (authority: §§1102, 1861, 1871, and 1891 of the Social Security Act [42 USC 1302, 1395x, 1395hh, and 1395bbb]). With one exception, this is followed by a discussion of the conditions and related policies, procedures, and practices

that reflect the intent of the conditions. A full discussion of §484.38, Condition of Participation: Qualifying to Furnish Outpatient Physical Therapy or Speech Pathology Services, is beyond the scope of this chapter. For detailed information, the reader is referred to the sources (conditions) cited therein.

Although the content of each condition has been extrapolated, the reader should have Part 484, Conditions of Participation: Home Health Agencies, available in its entirety because Subpart A, General Provisions, which defines the basis and scope of the home health agency program, definitions relative to the operation of the home health agency, and personnel qualifications, is not reported in detail here. Furthermore, the appendix, which includes the addenda for states incorporating requirements higher than those imposed by the conditions, is not included in this chapter.

SUBPART B: ADMINISTRATION

§484.10—Condition of Participation: Patient Rights

The patient has a right to be informed of his or her rights. The HHA must promote and protect the exercise of these rights.

(a) Standard: Notice of rights.
  (1) The HHA must provide the patient with a written notice of the patient's rights in

advance of furnishing care to the patient or during the initial evaluation visit before the initiation of treatment.

(2) The HHA must maintain documentation showing that it has complied with the requirements of this section.

(b) Standard: Exercise of rights and respect for property and person.

(1) The patient has the right to exercise his or her rights as a patient of the HHA.

(2) The patient's family or guardian may exercise the patient's rights when the patient has been judged incompetent.

(3) The patient has the right to have his or her property treated with respect.

(4) The patient has the right to voice grievances regarding treatment or care that is (or fails to be) furnished or regarding the lack of respect for property by anyone who is furnishing services on behalf of the HHA and must not be subjected to discrimination or reprisal for doing so.

(5) The HHA must investigate complaints made by a patient or the patient's family or guardian regarding treatment or care that is (or fails to be) furnished or regarding the lack of respect for the patient's property by anyone furnishing services on behalf of the HHA and must document both the existence of the complaint and the resolution of the complaint.

(c) Standard: Right to be informed and to participate in planning care and treatment.

(1) The patient has the right to be informed, in advance, about the care to be furnished and the frequency of visits proposed to be furnished.

  (i) The HHA must advise the patient in advance of the disciplines that will furnish care and the frequency of visits proposed to be furnished.

  (ii) The HHA must advise the patient in advance of any changes in the plan of care before the change is made.

(2) The patient has the right to participate in the planning of the care.

  (i) The HHA must advise the patient in advance of the right to participate in planning the care or treatment and in planning changes in the care or treatment.

  (ii) The HHA complies with the requirements of Subpart I of Part 489 of this chapter relating to maintaining written policies and procedures regarding advance directives. The HHA must inform and distribute written information to the patient, in advance, concerning its policies on advance directives, including a description of applicable State law. The HHA may furnish advance directives information to a patient at the time of the first home visit, as long as the information is furnished before care is provided.

(d) Standard: Confidentiality of medical records.

The patient has the right to confidentiality of the clinical records maintained by the HHA. The HHA must advise the patient of the agency's policies and procedures regarding disclosure of clinical records.

(e) Standard: Patient liability for payment.

(1) The patient has a right to be advised, before care is initiated, of the extent to which payment for the HHA services may be expected from Medicare or other sources and the extent to which payment may be required from the patient. Before the care is initiated, the HHA must inform the patient, orally and in writing, of:

  (i) The extent to which payment may be expected from Medicare, Medicaid, or any other Federally funded or aided programs known to the HHA;

  (ii) The charges for services that will not be covered by Medicare; and

  (iii) The charges that the individual may have to pay.

(2) The patient has the right to be advised orally and in writing of any changes in

the information provided in accordance with paragraph (e)(1) of this section when they occur. The HHA must advise the patient of these changes orally and in writing as soon as possible, but no later than 30 calendar days from the date that the HHA becomes aware of the change.

(f) Standard: Home health hotline.
The patient has the right to be advised of the availability of the toll-free HHA hotline in the State. When the agency accepts the patient for treatment or care, the HHA must advise the patient in writing of the telephone number of the home health hotline established by the State, the hours of its operation, and that the purpose of the hotline is to receive complaints or questions about the local HHAs. The patient also has the right to use this hotline to lodge complaints concerning the implementation of the advance directives requirements.

Clearly, these standards require the HHA to have available for each patient accepted for care written material that delineates the patient's rights while he or she is a recipient of the HHA's care and services. These rights are applicable for all patients accepted for care by the HHA, not just those accepted for care under the Medicare benefit. Written patient rights materials must be provided to the patient before any care is provided to the patient.

These rights are specified in a document, usually titled "Bill of Rights" or "Patient Bill of Rights." The document must be written with clarity in language so that the patient can reasonably be expected to understand it, thus enabling the patient to identify his or her rights while receiving HHA care and services and the recourse available in the event that a patient believes these rights are not being honored. There should be guidelines for a review of the document when the patient has limited facility with English and/or limited vision. If the HHA has a significant population, generally 25 percent or more of the HHA's total patient population, for whom English is a secondary language, it is recommended that the HHA have patient rights materials developed in that population's primary language.

At minimum, the document must address the areas cited in standards (a) through (f). In addition to stating the patient's rights, this document may also be used to inform the patient of his or her responsibilities while receiving care. These responsibilities include, but may not be limited to, notifying the HHA when he or she will not be home for a scheduled visit, providing essential medical/psychosocial information to assist in the development of the plan of care, and providing such other information as necessary to enable the HHA to obtain payment for the service(s) rendered. The bill of rights or some other document, signed and dated by the patient, should be incorporated into the clinical record as evidence that a review of patient rights was completed. Other materials may also be reviewed and, where appropriate, signed by the patient before the initiation of care as part of the presentation of patient rights and/or to demonstrate compliance with applicable state requirements, Additionally, Medicare/Medicaid patients should receive the Outcome and Assessment Information Set (OASIS) Statement of Patient Privacy Rights. Non-Medicare/non-Medicaid patients should receive the Notice About Privacy for Patients Who Do Not Have Medicare or Medicaid Coverage. These documents developed under the direction of the Health Care Financing Administration inform the patient of his or her rights relative to the collection and reporting of OASIS information. These rights include the right to be informed that OASIS data will be collected and how the data will be used; the right to expect that the information collected remains confidential and protected; the right to be informed that disclosure of OASIS information is limited to those purposes allowed by the Federal Privacy Act of 1974; the right to refuse to answer a specific question; and the right to review the assessment document and to request changes in the data reported. The HHAs should establish in writing the process for responding to a patient's request to review, change, or duplicate OASIS information.

Standard (b)(2) states that the patient's family or guardian may exercise the patient's rights when the patient has been judged incompetent. Competence is a legal concept determined by the court. There are often instances, however, in which there are questions regarding the individual's competence in the absence of a legal judgment. In these instances, the question of competence should focus on the patient's decision-making capacity. Suggested criteria for assessing the patient's capacity to make a decision regarding care include the following: the ability to understand relevant facts and values; the ability to weigh a decision within a framework of values and goals; the ability to reason and deliberate about the information received; and the ability to give reasons for the decision considering known facts, the alternatives, and the consequence of the decision to the patient. Whereas competence is a legal absolute, decision-making capacity is relative, dependent on the type of decision that needs to be made vis-à-vis the patient's shifting abilities. To ensure uniformity in determinations about the patient's decision-making capacity, guidelines should be developed for the staff. If the patient's condition necessitates the review of patient rights and planning for care with an individual acting on the patient's behalf, this should be thoroughly documented in the admission note.

Although the bill of rights may be considered a "stand-alone" document, the HHA must demonstrate congruence between its operational practices and the assurances made in the document. The orientation for staff, including contracted providers, should include a thorough review of patients' rights and staff members' responsibilities relative to these rights. The review of policies, procedures, rules of conduct, standards of care, other related materials, and clinical records should provide evidence of the HHA's awareness of and commitment to patient rights. For example, written policy statements and/or procedures should specify how the HHA accepts, registers, and investigates patient grievances and the person(s) responsible for investigating patient grievances. This responsibility should also be identified in the appropriate position description. Reports of grievances and subsequent follow-up actions should be maintained apart from the clinical records. The report should document the specific redress offered the complainant. A periodic review of these reports, as part of the HHA's performance improvement program, should be conducted to determine whether further study is warranted and to ascertain whether practices in specific operational areas—human resources, administrative, financial, or patient services—contribute to a pattern of recurring grievances.

Another example is the existence of policies, procedures, protocol statements, and attendant mechanisms to ensure that the right to be informed and to participate in planning care and treatment is demonstrated as specified in standard (c). Clinical record documentation should consistently reveal recording practices that demonstrate patient–provider interaction in planning for care and evidence that visiting personnel are cognizant of the patient's rights while they are providing care. At minimum, the clinical record should document that the patient was given the opportunity to participate in planning care through mutual determination of the goals or outcomes for care and in the attendant discussion of the disciplines involved in furnishing the care, the treatments/interventions to be provided, the frequency of visits, and the anticipated duration of services. Subsequently, the clinical notes should establish that any modifications to the plan of care, such as a change in a treatment, medication, or visit pattern, and/or the termination or addition of therapeutic service, was discussed with the patient.

Standard (c)(2)(i) requires the agency to ensure that its policies regarding advance directives are made known to the patient before furnishing care and services. Detailed written materials concerning the agency's policies regarding advance directives as well as materials describing applicable state laws must be given to and reviewed with the patient. Evidence that this review has been completed should be documented in the record, whether on a designated form completed as part of the initial evaluation visit or by having the patient or his or her representative sign copies of the advance directive materials for incorporation into the clinical record. Questioning during the interview process should determine whether the patient has an advance directive. The existence of an advance directive, or lack thereof, should be documented in the clinical record. The agency should make known, in writing, community resources that are available to assist the patient who wishes to make an advance directive. The patient must be informed of his or her right to contact the state agency hotline with complaints regarding implementation of the advance directive requirement.

Standard (d) requires the HHA to ensure the confidentiality of the patient's clinical record. If the HHA allows portions of the record to remain in the patient's home, HHA staff must instruct the patient and/or primary caregiver(s) regarding their responsibility to maintain the confidentiality of the clinical record and its contents. There should be documentation in the clinical record to substantiate that, when applicable, such instruction has been furnished by HHA staff. The HHA must be able to demonstrate that medical records are maintained and protected in a manner that meets the requirements of the Health Insurance Portability and Accountability Act (HIPAA).

Standard (e) requires the HHA to notify the patient of those services that will be reimbursed by Medicare or other sources and those services that are not covered. Specifically, the patient must be informed orally and in writing of the information stated in standard (e)(1)(i), (ii), and (iii). Documentation in the clinical record must establish that this requirement has been satisfied. Additionally, in the event that there is a change in the payment information initially discussed with the patient, the HHA must have in place a process to ensure that the patient is notified of the change orally and in writing no later than 30 calendar days from the date the HHA becomes aware of the change.

To demonstrate compliance with standard (f), the HHA must provide written information to the patient about the state hotline number, its purpose, and hours of operation. The HHA must be able to document that this information was given to and reviewed with the patient as part of the admission process.

§484.11—Condition of Participation: Release of Patient Identifiable OASIS Information

The HHA and agent acting on behalf of the HHA in accordance with a written contract must ensure the confidentiality of all patient information contained in the clinical record including OASIS data, and may not release patient information to the public.

The HHA should have polices and procedures in place to assure the confidentiality of all patient information including OASIS data. The use of OASIS data must be limited to its intended purposes—to promote the delivery of appropriate patient care. Written agreements must be maintained if the HHA uses a vendor to transmit OASIS data. This agreement must address the confidentiality of OASIS data. Ultimately, it is the HHA's responsibility if the vendor does not protect the confidentiality of the transmitted data.

§484.12—Condition of Participation: Compliance with Federal, State, and Local Laws; Disclosure and Ownership Information; and Accepted Professional Standards and Principles

(a) Standard: Compliance with Federal, State, and local laws and regulations.

The HHA and its staff must operate and furnish services in compliance with all applicable Federal, State, and local laws and regulations. If State or applicable local law provides for the licensure of HHAs, an agency not subject to licensure is approved by the licensing authority as meeting the standards established for licensure.

(b) Standard: Disclosure of ownership and management information.

The HHA must comply with the requirements of Part 420, Subpart C of this chapter. The HHA also must disclose the following information to the State survey agency at the time of the HHA's initial request for certification, for each subsequent survey, and at the time of any change in ownership or management:

(1) The name and address of all persons with an ownership or control interest in the HHA as defined in §§420.201, 420.202, and 420.206 of this chapter.

(2) The name and address of each person who is an officer, a director, an agent, or a managing employee of the HHA as defined in §§420.201, 402.202, and 420.206 of this chapter.

(3) The name and address of the corporation, association, or other company that is responsible for the management of the HHA and the name and address of the chief executive officer and the chairman of the board of directors of that corporation, association, or other company responsible for the management of the HHA.

(c) Standard: Compliance with accepted professional standards and principles.

The HHA and its staff must comply with accepted professional standards and principles that apply to professionals furnishing services in an HHA.

Standard (a) requires that the HHA comply with all applicable federal, state, and local laws and regulations. It is not sufficient to attempt to meet this standard with a single policy that states "The agency will comply with all applicable federal, state, and local laws and regulations." State practice acts, professional standards of practice, codes, and ethics should be available within the agency, as should any applicable local or state communicable disease reporting requirements, Occupational Safety and Health Administration regulations, employment statutes, and other applicable laws, codes, statutes, and regulations. These materials should serve as additional guidelines for the written materials that direct the HHA's operational practices and performance expectations. Evidence of current licensure must be available for each individual as required by state practice acts. Because the number and type of laws and regulations that may affect the operation of an HHA are continually expanding and changing, it is imperative that the HHA develop and maintain an active information network to keep abreast of the changes promulgated by legislative and regulatory bodies.

Meeting standard (b), factor (1) requires the agency to identify those individuals and entities that must be routinely disclosed to the state agency at the time of the initial certification survey, for each survey, and at the time of any change in the ownership or management of the HHA. The need to communicate the required information to the state agency on a timely basis should not be ignored. Policy statements relative to the management of the agency should specify that disclosure will occur as part of the survey process and whenever there is any change in the ownership or management of the agency, and that updated information will be furnished to the secretary of Health and Human Services, via the state agency, at intervals between recertification or within 35 days of a written request to do so.

Submitting the appropriate information to the state agency on a timely basis requires full understanding of the terminology included in standard (b). A discussion of these terms follows.

As defined in §§420.201, 420.203, and 402.206, ownership interest means the possession of equity in the capital, the stock, or the profits of the HHA. A person with ownership or control interest is defined as one who:

- has an ownership interest totaling 5 percent or more in the HHA
- has an indirect ownership interest (i.e., any ownership interest in an entity that has an

ownership interest in the HHA, including an ownership interest in any entity that has an indirect ownership interest in the HHA, equal to 5 percent or more in the HHA)

- has a combination of direct and indirect ownership interest equal to 5 percent or more in the HHA
- owns an interest of 5 percent or more in any mortgage, deed or trust, note, or other obligation secured by the HHA if that interest equals at least 5 percent of the value of the property or assets of the HHA
- is an officer or director of an HHA that is organized as a corporation
- is a partner in an HHA that is organized as a partnership

To determine whether the ownership interest exceeds the 5 percent reporting requirement and thus must be disclosed, the amount of indirect ownership is computed by multiplying the percentages of ownership in an entity and the HHA. For example, if A owns 10 percent of the stock in a corporation that owns 80 percent of the HHA, A's ownership in the HHA is 8 percent and must be reported. Conversely, if B owns 80 percent of the stock of a corporation that owns 5 percent of the stock of the HHA, B's interest equates to a 40 percent indirect ownership and need not be reported. When there is a need to determine applicability of disclosure for an individual who has ownership or control interest in any mortgage, deed or trust, note, or other obligation, the percentage of the obligation owned is multiplied by the percentage of the HHA's assets used to secure the obligation. For example, if X owns 20 percent of a note secured by 60 percent of the HHA's assets, X's interest in the provider's assets equates to 12 percent and must be disclosed. Conversely, if Y owns 30 percent of a note secured by 10 percent of the HHA's assets, Y's interest equals 3 percent and need not be reported.

The second factor in this standard requires the HHA to disclose the names and addresses of selected persons and/or organizations having a management responsibility for the HHA. This includes the officers and directors of the governing body of the HHA, any agent, or any managing employee. An *agent* is defined as any person who has been delegated the authority to obligate or act on behalf of the HHA. A *managing employee* is one who exercises operational or managerial control over, or directly or indirectly conducts, the day-to-day operation of the agency. Defined in this manner, a managing employee includes, but may not be limited to, a general manager, business manager, administrator, director, supervising physician, or registered nurse.

The third factor states that the agency must also disclose the names and addresses of any entity that is responsible for the management of the agency as well as the name and address of the chief executive officer and the directors of the entity.

There is one other requirement relative to information that must be disclosed by the HHA. §420.203, Disclosure of Hiring of Intermediary's Former Employees, requires the HHA to notify the secretary promptly if it, or its home office (in the case of a chain organization), employs or obtains the services of an individual who, at any time during the year preceding such employment, was employed in a managerial, accounting, auditing, or similar capacity by an agency or organization that currently serves, or at any time during the preceding year served, as a Medicare fiscal intermediary or carrier for the HHA. *Similar capacity* means the performance of essentially the same work functions as those of a manager, accountant, or auditor even though the individual is not so designated by title.

Standard (c) requires the HHA to act to ensure that mechanisms exist to monitor professional staff to verify that their performance meets applicable state practice acts as well as any internally or externally derived professional standards that are used by the HHA for the staff. These mechanisms should be identifiable in the agency's operational procedures and processes. The actions of the HHA relative to demonstrating compliance with this standard should be applicable to those personnel who provide service directly or via contractual arrangement as well as for personnel who, although employed by a facility, provide service to the facility-based HHA's patients.

§484.14—Condition of Participation: Organization, Services, and Administration

Organization, services furnished, administrative control, and lines of authority for the delegation of responsibility down to the patient care level are clearly set forth in writing and are readily identifiable. Administrative and supervisory functions are not delegated to another agency or organization, and all services not furnished directly, including services provided through subunits, are monitored and controlled by the parent agency. If an agency has subunits, appropriate administrative records are maintained for each subunit.

(a) Standard: Services furnished.
Part-time or intermittent skilled nursing and at least one other therapeutic service (physical, speech, or occupational therapy; medical social services; or home health aide services) are made available on a visiting basis in a place of residence used as a patient's home. An HHA must provide at least one of the qualifying services directly through agency employees but may provide the second qualifying service and additional services under arrangements with another agency or organization.

(b) Standard: Governing body.
A governing body (or designated persons so functioning) assumes full legal authority and responsibility for the operation of the agency. The governing body appoints a qualified administrator, arranges for professional advice as required under §484.16, adopts and periodically reviews bylaws or an acceptable equivalent, and oversees the management and fiscal affairs of the agency.

(c) Standard: Administrator.
The administrator, who may also be the supervising physician or registered nurse required under section (d) of this section, organizes and directs the agency's ongoing functions; maintains ongoing liaison among the governing body, the group of professional personnel, and the staff; employs qualified personnel and ensures adequate staff education and evaluations; ensures the accuracy of public information materials and activities; and implements an effective budgeting and accounting system. A qualified person is authorized in writing to act in the absence of the administrator.

(d) Standard: Supervising physician or registered nurse.
The skilled nursing and other therapeutic services furnished are under the supervision and direction of a physician or registered nurse (who preferably has at least 1 year of nursing experience and is a public health nurse). This person, or a similarly qualified alternative, is available at all times during operating hours and participates in all activities relevant to the professional services furnished, including the development of qualifications and the assignment of personnel.

(e) Standard: Personnel policies.
Personnel practices and patient care are supported by appropriate written personnel records. Personnel records include qualifications and licensure that are kept current.

(f) Standard: Personnel under hourly or per visit contracts.
If personnel under hourly or per visit contracts are used by the HHA, there is a written contract between those personnel and the agency that specifies the following:

(1) Patients are accepted for care only by the primary HHA.
(2) The services to be furnished.
(3) The necessity to conform to all applicable agency policies, including personnel qualifications.
(4) The responsibility for participating in developing plans of care.
(5) The manner in which the services will be controlled, coordinated, and evaluated by the primary HHA.

(6) The procedure for submitting clinical and progress notes, scheduling visits, periodic patient evaluation.

(7) The procedures for payment for services furnished under the contract.

(g) Standard: Coordination of patient services.

All personnel furnishing services maintain liaison to ensure that their efforts are coordinated effectively and support the objectives outlined in the plan of care. The clinical record or minutes of care conferences establish that effective interchange, reporting, and coordination of patient care do occur. A written summary report for each patient is sent to the attending physician at least every 60 days.

(h) Standard: Services under arrangements.

Services furnished under arrangements are subject to a written contract conforming with the requirements specified in paragraph (f) of this section and with the requirements of section 1861 (w) of the Act [42 USC 1495x(w)].

(i) Standard: Institutional planning.

The HHA, under the direction of the governing body, prepares an overall plan and budget that includes an annual operating budget and a capital expenditure plan.

(1) Annual operating budget.

There is an annual operating budget that includes all anticipated income and expenses related to items that would, under generally accepted accounting principles, be considered income and expense items. However, it is not required that there be prepared, in connection with any budget, an item by item identification of the components of each type of anticipated income or expense.

(2) Capital expenditure plan.

(i) There is a capital plan for at least a 3-year period, including the operating budget year. The plan includes and identifies in detail the anticipated sources of funding for, and the objectives of, each anticipated expenditure of more than $600,000

for items that would, under generally accepted accounting principles, be considered capital items. In determining if a single capital expenditure exceeds $600,000, the cost of studies, surveys, designs, plans, working drawings, specifications, and other activities essential to the acquisition, improvement, modernization, expansion, or replacement of land plant, building, and equipment are included. Expenditures directly or indirectly related to capital expenditures, such as grading, paving, broker commissions, taxes assessed during the construction period, and cost involved in demolishing or razing structures on land, are also included. Transactions that are separated in time but are components of an overall plan or patient care objective are viewed in their entirety without regard to their timing. Other costs related to capital expenditures include title fees; permit and license fees; broker commissions; architect, legal, accounting, and appraisal fees; interest finance; or carrying charges on bonds, notes, and other costs incurred for borrowing funds.

(ii) If the anticipated source of financing is, in any part, the anticipated payment from Title V (Maternal and Child Health and Crippled Children's Services), or Title XVIII (Medicare), or Title XIX (Medicaid) of the Social Security Act, the plan specifies the following:

(A) Whether the proposed capital expenditure is required to conform, or is likely to be required to conform, to current standards, criteria, or plans developed in accordance with the Public Health Service Act or the Mental Retardation Facilities and Community Mental Health Centers Construction Act of 1963.

(B) Whether a capital expenditure proposal has been submitted to the designated planning agency for approval in accordance with section 1122 of the Act (42 U.C 1320a-1) and implementing regulations.

(C) Whether the designated planning agency approved or disapproved the proposed capital expenditure if it was presented to that agency.

(3) Preparation and plan of budget.

The overall plan and budget is prepared under the direction of the governing body of the HHA by a committee consisting of representatives of the governing body, the administrative staff, and the medical staff (if any) of the HHA.

(4) Annual review of the plan and budget.

The overall plan and budget is reviewed and updated at least annually by the committee referred to in paragraph (ii)(3) of this section under the direction of the governing body of the HHA.

(j) Standard: Laboratory services.

(1) If the HHA engages in laboratory testing outside of the context of assisting an individual in self-administrating a test with an appliance that has been cleared for that purpose by the FDA, such testing must be in compliance with all applicable requirements of Part 493 of this chapter.

(2) If the HHA chooses to refer specimens for laboratory testing to another laboratory, the referral laboratory must be certified in the appropriate specialties and subspecialties of services in accordance with the applicable requirements of Part 493 of this chapter.

The opening paragraph for this condition provides broad guidelines for the organization and administration of the HHA. Demonstration of compliance with the condition requires the HHA to have written materials that delineate the organization's structure and mechanisms for controlling and monitoring all aspects of the HHA's operation, whether it is freestanding, facility based, or a part of a state or local (city or county) health department. The agency may re-

tain management services to strengthen its administrative proficiency, but decision-making responsibilities must remain within the HHA. It should be clear from the review of written materials to whom responsibility for administration and supervision is delegated and that responsibility for accepting patients for care and carrying out the treatment and/or interventions specified in the plans of care is reserved exclusively for the HHA. These responsibilities extend to and must be evident in branch offices operated by the agency, but they may be exercised differently in subunits. It should be noted that in the event that an HHA proposes to open a branch location, the state agency must be notified. The notification must include how the proposed branch meets the definition of a branch office as found in 42 CRF 484.2 as well as a description of how the HHA intends to operate the branch. The HHA will receive written notification of whether the proposed location can be a branch or should be a subunit or independent HHA.

A *subunit* is defined as a semiautonomous unit under the same governing body as the parent agency that serves patients in a geographical area different from that of the parent agency. By virtue of the distance between the subunit and the parent agency, the former is judged incapable of sharing administration, supervision, and services on a daily basis with the parent agency, and therefore must independently meet the conditions. A detailed discussion of characteristics that distinguish a branch office from a subunit is beyond the scope of this chapter. For further information, the reader is referred to Sections 2182 and 2184 of the *State Operations Manual* (Department of Health and Human Services, 1993) and the state agency responsible for certification and survey activities.

Key to understanding the HHA's structure is the organizational chart. A current table of organization should be available that, at minimum, depicts the governing body, group of professional personnel, finance/budget committee, and all current positions, including positions filled by contracted personnel, as well as the relationships that exist among and between staff members, the governing body, and established committees. When applicable, the table of organization should depict the relationship between the HHA's main or home office and any branch office(s) and/or subunit(s) as well as the relationship with a parent agency or other controlling entity. More than one organizational table may be required to portray accurately the HHA and its relationships. The table(s) of organization should include a legend to define the types of relationships represented (supervisory, advisory, reporting, etc.). The document(s) should indicate the date of approval by the governing body. The table of organization should be reviewed against position descriptions to ensure that personnel, reporting, and/or supervisory relationships are consistent with those identified in the position descriptions.

Collectively, the written policy statements, procedures, guidelines, protocols, and other approved documents relative to the specific areas identified in the ten standards in this condition should clearly delineate the operational practices of the agency and the mechanisms for maintaining management accountability down to the patient care level. A discussion of the ten standards and the factors and elements in these standards follows.

To meet the intent of standard (a), the HHA must ensure that at least one of the qualifying services is provided by employees on an hourly or per-visit basis. The term *qualifying service*, as used in this context, should not be confused with the same term used in a reimbursement sense. For Medicare reimbursement purposes, the patient must be admitted to the HHA to receive skilled nursing, physical therapy, and/or speech therapy. Consequently, these three services are known as primary or qualifying services. From a standard compliance standpoint, however, these three disciplines, as well as occupational therapy, medical social services, and home health aide services, are defined as qualifying services.

Health care facility-based agencies may utilize facility personnel to provide a qualifying service as direct employees, but the HHA must be able to demonstrate that this employee is available as needed during the agency's operating hours rather than at the discretion of the facility. Time records should be maintained for all personnel utilized in this manner.

Standard (b) addresses the function of the governing body. The bylaws exist as the document that codifies the governing body as the forum for setting the rules for the performance of the work of the HHA. At minimum, the bylaws, or an equivalent document, should specify the governing body's responsibility to appoint a qualified administrator, to maintain an advisory group of professional personnel, to adopt and subsequently review and revise the bylaws or an equivalent document to ensure that it is accurate, and to oversee the management and fiscal affairs of the agency. Minutes of governing body and committee meetings should provide evidence that the governing body receives sufficient information verbally and via written reports on a timely basis to enhance that body's ability to make decisions that contribute to organizational rationality.

Standard (c) requires the HHA to employ an individual who, subject to the approval of the governing body, develops, organizes, and manages the operation of the HHA by following established policies, procedures, and standards and rules of conduct. The administrator must meet the qualifications cited in the definition of administrator given in Subpart A: General Provisions, §484.2: Definitions, as well as any additional requirements set forth in the position description. Policies, procedures, and the position description should clearly convey the administrator's responsibility and commensurate authority, as delegated by the governing body, for organizational performance. A review of governing body, committee, and/or staff meeting minutes, reports, personnel records, public information materials, and similar sources should provide clear evidence that the administrator is fulfilling his or her mandated responsibilities. That the administrator ensures adequate staff education should be evident from a review of the continuing learning activities of those personnel utilized in the patient care and services program.

The person designated in writing to act in the administrator's absence should be qualified to do so. The individual should hold the requisite qualifications stated in the position description and be oriented to the administrator's role responsibilities. In the absence of the requisite qualifications, the governing body may waive this requirement to allow for the appointment of an individual to act on a temporary basis for the administrator. The decision to do so should be documented in governing body meeting minutes or some other document, such as a letter to the incumbent notifying him or her of the temporary appointment. It is necessary, however, that the incumbent meet the basic requirements set forth in the definition of administrator: to wit, be a licensed physician or registered nurse or have training and experience in health service administration and at least 1 year of supervisory or administrative experience in home health care or related programs.

Standard (d) specifies that the HHA must also employ a supervising physician or registered nurse to whom responsibility and authority are delegated for implementing the patient service program and for ensuring high-quality patient care in accordance with the HHA's purpose, objectives, philosophy, and policies. This responsibility is properly demonstrated through the execution of systematic processes for planning, coordinating, implementing, controlling, and evaluating those components that make up the patient service program. Specific activities for which the incumbent may be responsible or in which he or she may participate include, but may not be limited to, recruitment, selection, orientation, and evaluation of personnel; planning for new programs and/or modifications to existing programs; coaching staff for improved performance; developing and maintaining mea-

surable standards of quality; and participating in strategic planning and decision making. Because a registered nurse usually fills this position, the term *supervising nurse* is used for the remainder of this chapter.

The supervising nurse must be readily available either on site or via a telecommunication system. The manner in which availability is demonstrated is a management decision. Nevertheless, it must be apparent that the supervising nurse is available to the HHA on a full-time basis. The position description, personnel record, or other source must identify the person authorized to act as the qualified alternate for the supervising nurse.

To meet the intent of standard (e), the HHA should have written policies that set forth the existing rules, regulations, benefits, and performance expectations for all personnel. Position descriptions should be established for each category of personnel that set forth the qualifications and duties required for the position. Personnel records must be maintained with materials that verify that each employee, including contracted personnel, possesses the requisite qualifications and that applicable personnel policies, such as health examination, orientation, and performance evaluations, are being followed. A copy of the professional license may be made if this is allowed by state law and agency policy. It is permissible to retain current professional licenses for all personnel in one separate file or a display case. It is recognized that some states prohibit copying of the professional license. In those states, the HHA must identify through the state licensing entity the accepted method(s) for documenting that personnel hold a current license. When a facility-based agency provides service using facility personnel, the credentials for these individuals should also be available.

Many agencies rail against the Medicare requirement to retain a current copy of the driver's license and automobile liability insurance for visiting personnel, citing the need to keep abreast of varying expiration dates as particularly troublesome. It is toward the elimination of one source of irritation and complaint that the reader is reminded that the conditions do not require the agency to maintain current drivers' licenses and automobile liability insurance; rather, in the absence of a state requirement, it is a requirement established by the organization. When such a requirement is established by the HHA, it must be met. It is possible to establish a policy that delineates the expectation that designated personnel will present evidence of a current driver's license and liability insurance at the time of hire, will keep these documents current and available for presentation at the request of the supervising nurse or other designated person, and will notify the HHA of any change in the status of the license without the attendant requirement that the HHA maintain evidence that these documents are indeed current.

Hourly or per-visit contracts should be written with specificity to delineate clearly the manner in which the agency will meet the requirements in standard (f). For example, it is not sufficient simply to state that the agency will control, coordinate, and evaluate the services provided. The contract should identify the processes in place to control, coordinate, and evaluate the services. This includes the identification by title of personnel who are involved in these activities as well as any other relevant activities, such as the quarterly review of records, annual program evaluation, or other quality improvement initiatives. If payment for services is contingent upon the timely receipt of all required clinical record documentation or other materials, this should be stated in the contract. The contract must include a clause that allows the comptroller general of the United States, the Department of Health and Human Services, and their duly authorized representatives access to the contractor's contract, books, documents, and records until the expiration of 4 years after the services are furnished under the contract when the cost or value of services is $10,000 or more over a 12-month period. The contract should also specify the terms and

conditions for renewing and terminating the contract.

It is not necessary for a facility-based agency to have a contract with the facility for the use of facility personnel when these personnel provide care to the agency's patients during their usual hospital working shift. If the personnel provide care outside their usual shift, however, a contract would be necessary. The facility-based agency should develop a written agreement with the facility department or unit that specifies the arrangement that exists for the utilization and supervision of personnel and the provision of patient care. The HHA should maintain a current list of personnel who are available from a facility department.

Coordination of service is the focus of standard (g). At the risk of oversimplification, coordination is patient-focused, outcome-oriented planning and communication. Are the care providers, the caregivers, and the patient, to the extent possible, working in tandem to achieve a stated outcome? Are care providers' visits planned so as not to tire the patient? Are the occupational therapist's efforts to increase independence in activities of daily living (ADLs) supported by the activities of the home health aide to assist rather than perform selected ADLs for the patient? As an aside, effective communication is not one-way communication. Too often, it is assumed that all written communication must emanate from a registered nurse, either the nurse functioning as the primary nurse or the nurse's supervisor. All care providers should be oriented to their responsibility to document pertinent information that fosters the coordination of services. Patient conference minutes, case management notes, and other interdisciplinary communication tools are not the exclusive purview of the registered nurse. Coordination of services is an organizational imperative if positive outcomes are to be achieved in the most cost-effective and cost-efficient manner.

Policy statements and/or procedures should specify the responsibilities of identified direct service and/or supervisory personnel to ensure that coordination of services is a linchpin of patient care. That coordination of services is an active and ongoing process should be verifiable through a review of the clinical records and case conference reports (a copy or summary of case conferences should be retained in the clinical record). Such a review would demonstrate timely initiation of ordered and needed services or communication to the physician regarding the inability to provide the service(s) to afford the physician the option of obtaining the needed services from another source; personnel awareness of the goals for care established for each therapeutic discipline, as evident in the provision of treatments and interventions in a complementary manner; scheduling of visits to foster maximum participation of the patient in the plan of care; timely communication among personnel regarding the patient's response to treatment; any impediment(s) to full implementation of the plan of care and collaborative efforts to remove or minimize the impediment(s); and planning for the termination of service(s).

The record would also contain a succinct summary report to the attending physician at least every 60 days. Subpart A: General Provision, §484.2: Definitions defines the summary report as "the compilation of the pertinent factors from a patient's clinical notes and progress notes that is submitted to the patient's physician." This pertinent information should be reported in a succinct, concise manner. Key words here are *pertinent*, *succinct*, and *concise*. Does the physician really need to know that the home health aide provided "personal care, hair and nail care, and food shopping" or that "RN supervises HHA every 2 weeks"? Why does the physician need to know "Blood obtained for PPT on 2/16/04 and transported to lab per order"? Does the physician take comfort in knowing "PT and OT continue to visit 2 X wk"? Such statements are provider rather than patient focused and are of little value in assessing the patient's response, or lack thereof, to the interventions furnished.

The purpose of the summary report is to furnish the physician with information on which to base decisions about the efficacy of the plan of care and to make necessary modifications to the plan. If the summary is to serve this purpose, not only must it contain precise, objective information, but also it must be sent to the physician at the time the plan of care is developed for recertification. Some agencies send the 60-day summary report on a calendar basis or other 60-day time period established by the organization. Too often, this means that the physician receives the summary report several days or a week or more after the plan has been recertified. This practice effectively defeats the purpose of the summary report. It should be noted that the patient's condition may require a summary report to the physician at other than 60-day intervals, but these instances are infrequent. In such a situation, a progress note to the physician is generally more appropriate. Finally, a well-written summary report serves to support the organization's claim for reimbursement for the services rendered to date.

The summary report should answer questions such as: "What does the physician need to know about the patient's condition and response to assess the effectiveness of the plan of care? In what measurable ways has the patient's condition changed as a result of the interventions provided? If the patient did not respond to a particular intervention, what changes were made in the plan of care, and what were the consequences? Does the patient's response over the past 60 days justify the request to continue service for another 60-day period?" These or similar questions are designed to elicit information that fosters a descriptive portrayal of the patient's response to all the therapeutic interventions provided, to justify the HHA's claim for reimbursement, and, where appropriate, to support the need for continued care.

Standard (h) indicates that the content requirements for contracts arranged with groups or organizations for therapeutic services are the same as those specified in standard (f). Thus, such contracts must address the areas cited in standard (f).

The focus of standard (i) is the agency's budget and capital expenditure plan. The HHA must have an annual budget that includes all anticipated income and expenses, consistent with generally accepted accounting principles, and a capital expenditure plan for at least a 3-year period when expenditures of more than $600,000 are anticipated for acquisition, expansion, or replacement of land, plant, building, and/or equipment. If a capital expenditure plan is necessary, it should conform to the requirements set forth in factor (2) of this standard.

Minutes of meetings or other written materials must document that the overall plan and budget is/was developed under the direction of the governing body by a committee that includes representatives of the governing body and the administrative staff. If the agency staff include physicians, a physician must also be represented on the committee. This standard does not require a physician member of the group of professional personnel to be represented on the committee. The dated minutes should document that the committee responsible for preparation of the budget meets at least annually, under the direction of the governing body, to update the annual plan and budget. Governing body minutes should document discussion, review, and approval of the annual plan and budget. For the facility-based HHA, it may be necessary to delineate the sequence of events that occur as a matter of course for the development of the annual budget for the facility to demonstrate how agency administrative representation is ensured when the budget committee exists as a standing committee of the facility's governing body.

Standard (j) requires the HHA to have evidence that it furnishes laboratory services in compliance with Part 493, Laboratory Services. For most agencies, obtaining a Clinical Laboratory Improvement Amendment (CLIA) waiver is sufficient to allow for the performance of certain tests that are waived. These tests are defined as simple laboratory examinations and procedures that are cleared by the FDA for home use,

employ methodologies that are so simple and accurate as to render the likelihood of erroneous results negligible, or pose no reasonable risk of harm to the patient if the test is performed incorrectly. Examples of tests that may be performed under the CLIA waiver are as follows:

- dipstick or tablet reagent urinalysis (nonautomated) for the following:
  1. bilirubin
  2. glucose
  3. hemoglobin
  4. ketone
  5. leukocytes
  6. nitrite
  7. pH
  8. protein
  9. specific gravity
  10. urobilinogen
- fecal occult blood
- ovulation tests (visual color comparison tests for human luteinizing hormone)
- urine pregnancy tests (visual color comparison tests)
- erythrocyte sedimentation rate (nonautomated)
- hemoglobin-copper sulfate (nonautomated)
- blood glucose by glucose monitoring devices cleared by the FDA specifically for home use
- spun microhematocrit
- hemoglobin by single analyte instruments with self-contained or component features to perform specimen/reagent interaction, providing direct measurement and readout (e.g., HemaCue).

A discussion of the conditions and requirements that must be met by the HHA that furnishes a wider range of laboratory services is beyond the scope of this chapter. The reader is referred to Part 493, Laboratory Services. If the HHA furnishes laboratory services under arrangement, the HHA must ensure that the contracting laboratory meets the requirements of Part 493, Laboratory Services. The HHA should ensure that the referral laboratory is appropriately certified.

§484.16—Condition of Participation: Group of Professional Personnel

A group of professional personnel, which includes at least a physician and one registered nurse (preferably a public health nurse), and with appropriate representation from other professional disciplines, establishes and annually reviews the agency's policies governing the scope of services offered, admission and discharge policies, medical supervision and plans of care, emergency care, clinical records, personnel qualifications, and program evaluation. At least one member of the group is neither an owner nor an employee of the agency.

(a) Standard: Advisory and evaluation function.

The group of professional personnel meets frequently to advise the agency on professional issues, to participate in the evaluation of the agency's program, and to assist the agency in maintaining liaison with other health care providers in the community and in the agency's community information program. The meetings are documented by dated minutes.

To meet this condition, there must be a committee composed of professionals who meet the stated representation requirements and actively function in an advisory and evaluation capacity. Additional representatives may be elected or appointed at the agency's discretion. The purview of the group of professional personnel includes the establishment and annual review of all policies governing the agency's patient care and service program, including program evaluation as well as evaluation of the qualifications of personnel utilized in the program. It is not necessary for the group to establish personnel qualifications or some types of policies when this responsibility is reserved for a higher authority. This frequently occurs in public health agencies operated by state, county, or city health departments. In this instance, the group should

review these materials and make such recommendations as the group believes are appropriate. It should be noted that the governing body, having assumed full legal authority and responsibility for the operation of the agency, must approve or reject newly developed and/or revised policies and personnel qualifications. Facility-based agencies may have to involve additional personnel in the chain of command to the governing body or other established committees authorized to act for the governing body on these specific matters. The group is also responsible for ensuring that the annual program evaluation is completed, reviewed, approved, and subsequently submitted to the governing body.

It is the agency's responsibility to ensure that the group comprises individuals who are willing and available to participate on the committee. Agency bylaws or an equivalent document should provide for the election or appointment of members and for the replacement of members who are unable to participate actively on the committee. To ensure full representation at each meeting, it may be appropriate to have more than one representative for each required discipline. Should a member, particularly the physician member, not be present as planned, there should be documentation to establish that the member was afforded the opportunity for input regarding agenda topics and that his or her comments, concerns, or questions were subsequently communicated to the group.

Meeting minutes must document that the group has fulfilled its mandated responsibilities. Additionally, the minutes should document that, as necessary, the members, acting in an advisory capacity, provide guidance and technical assistance in their particular area of competence for the purpose of strengthening the agency's program. Furthermore, the minutes of the group's meetings should substantiate that the actions of the group are designed to ensure that the community served, broadly defined to include consumers, referral sources, physicians, and community organizations, is knowledgeable about and supportive of the work and objectives of the agency as evidenced by a willingness to use the agency's services.

Because of its mandated responsibilities, it is recommended that the group of professional personnel meet on a quarterly or semiannual basis. It is questionable if an annual meeting is sufficient to keep the members informed of activities of the HHA, obtain professional advice on external and internal issues impacting the agency, and assure that this body functions effectively.

§484.18—Condition of Participation: Acceptance of Patients, Plan of Care, Medical Supervision

Patients are accepted for treatment on the basis of a reasonable expectation that the patient's medical, nursing, and social needs can be met adequately by the agency in the patient's place of residence. Care follows a written plan of care established and periodically reviewed by a doctor of medicine, osteopathy, or podiatric medicine.

(a) Standard: Plan of care.
The plan of care developed in consultation with the agency staff covers all pertinent diagnoses, including mental status, types of services and equipment required, frequency of visits, prognosis, rehabilitation potential, functional limitations, activities permitted, nutritional requirements, medications and treatments, any safety measures to protect against injury, instructions for timely discharge or referral, and other appropriate items. If a physician refers a patient under a plan of care that cannot be completed until after an evaluation visit, the physician is consulted to approve additions or modification to the original plan. Orders for therapy services include the specific procedures and modalities to be used and the amount, frequency, and duration. The therapist and other agency personnel participate in developing the plan of care.

(b) Standard: Periodic review of plan of care.
The total plan of care is reviewed by the attending physician and HHA personnel as often as the severity of the patient's condition requires, but at least once every 60 days or more frequently when there is a beneficiary elected transfer; a significant change in condition resulting in a change in the case mix assignment; or a discharge and return to the same HHA during the 60 day episode.

Agency professional staff promptly alert the physician to any changes that suggest a need to alter the plan of care.

(c) Standard: Conformance with physician's orders.
Drugs and treatments are administered by agency staff only as ordered by the physician. Verbal orders are put in writing and signed and dated with the date of receipt by the registered nurse or qualified therapist (as defined in 484.4 of this chapter) responsible for furnishing or supervising the ordered services. Verbal orders are accepted by personnel authorized to do so by applicable state and federal laws and regulations as well as by the HHA's internal policies.

At the risk of oversimplification, this condition requires the HHA to demonstrate how it will ensure that patients are accepted for care only after an analysis of externally and internally derived information supports an expectation that the patient will benefit from the agency's services and that care and services will be provided under the general supervision of the patient's physician in a manner consistent with the agency's established policies and procedures. The HHA must have written policies and procedures stating the process for accepting and evaluating referrals, designate those practitioners who may act as the patient's physician, specify the criteria that are considered in determining whether the patient may be accepted for care, and determine the manner in which the physician's orders may be communicated to the agency to ensure the prompt initiation of care. If the HHA accepts orders from a podiatrist or dentist, the orders must be within the respective practitioner's scope of practice as defined within the applicable state practice act. Written policy and/or procedures should address the electronic transfer of physician's orders, mechanisms for the timely certification and recertification of the plan of care with authenticated and dated physician orders, and the procedures for receipt and countersignature of the physician's verbal order.

The agency's mechanism for conduct of the initial evaluation visit should ensure that the patient assessment is completed on a timely basis by staff holding the requisite skills to perform this activity. The initial evaluation visit must include those activities necessary to document compliance with 484.55 Condition of Participation: Comprehensive Assessment of Patients. The patient assessment has become critically important because of the increasingly complex needs of a diverse home care population. The subsequent analysis of assessment data with interdisciplinary collaboration as warranted must be sufficient to determine the most appropriate course of care for the patient to achieve desired outcomes. Collectively, the HHA's processes should convey a sound understanding of the agency's obligations once the patient is accepted for care as well as recognition of the physician's responsibility for medical supervision.

The Health Care Financing Administration's (HCFA's) Form 485 (Home Health Certification and Plan of Treatment) is widely used as the plan of care, with HCFA Form 487 (Addendum to Plan of Treatment or Medical Update) being used to provide additional information as necessary. As a point of clarification, it should be noted that the terms *plan of care* and *plan of treatment* are synonymous. However, the plan of care should not be confused with the nursing care plan. The nursing care plan is a nursing document. The Conditions of Participation do not require the use of a nursing care plan. The decision to use this document rests with the HHA.

Agency policy should require the plan of care to contain the information specified in standard (a) with modification of the plan as necessary after completion of the initial evaluation visit by professional personnel. Policy statements should also require professional staff to collaborate with the attending physician to evaluate the patient's response to the plan of care and to modify the plan as needed throughout the course of care. The treatments and interventions ordered should be specified for each discipline with a visit frequency that is appropriate to meet the goals established for each therapeutic service. The goals or outcomes identified on the plan of care should be concise and reasonable considering the time-limited nature of the Medicare benefit. The clinical record should establish that, to the greatest degree possible, the goals were developed jointly with the patient or individual designated to act on the patient's behalf. The visit frequency may be ordered using a visit range. The review of clinical records, however, should verify that visit ranges are used to allow the staff to adjust visits readily to meet the patient's needs rather than to accommodate the ebb and flow of staff levels and patient census.

In sum, the plan of care should reflect an aggressive treatment program for the attainment of the highest possible level of independent functioning for the patient. It should exist as a dynamic rather than a static document, ever changing in reaction to the patient's documented responses. A review of the plan(s) of care in the clinical records must document that these requirements are met.

Standard (b) requires the review of the total plan of treatment as often as the severity of the patient's condition requires, but at least every 60 days or when certain events occur as specified in this standard. A perfunctory review is a disservice to the patient and frequently results in a plan of care that is a less-than-accurate prescription for care. Written procedures should require the professionals who have provided care to participate in this review to ensure that the plan is an accurate prescription for care vis-à-vis the patient's status. The agency should have written procedures to ensure the thoroughness and timeliness of this review. It is recommended that this review occur in conjunction with the continuing 60-day review of records required by §484.52 and discussed later in this chapter. The agency should also have established procedures to determine the accuracy of the plan of care when the patient is hospitalized during any certification period.

To demonstrate compliance with standard (c), HHA policy and procedure should require, and the clinical records should document, that care and services are provided only as ordered by the physician. Written policies should specify the necessity for a physician's order whenever there is a change in the plan of care, with the order being authenticated by the physician on a timely basis as identified in agency policy. This includes changes in the frequency of visits. After all, the attainment of the goals established for care is predicated on the provision of specified interventions at specified intervals; any change in this frequency in effect changes the plan of care and as such must be approved by the physician. To minimize the need to contact the physician each time there is a change in the visit pattern, consideration should be given to the use of visit ranges and a specified number of as-needed visits for identified potential problems that would necessitate additional visits.

As stated earlier in this section, all plans of care must be signed and dated by the physician. Policy statements should identify those professionals who may accept the physician's verbal order and require the physician's countersignature to be obtained as soon as possible. The phrase *as soon as possible* should be defined in writing by the HHA as within a reasonable time frame considering any applicable state law or regulation and/or accrediting body requirement.

Compliance with standard (c) requires that agency staff check the patient's medication regimen and promptly report any problems to the physician. There must be written policies relative to the administration and monitoring of drugs and biologicals. The clinical record must contain a current drug profile that identifies physician-ordered medications as well as any over-the-counter (OTC) medication the patient is taking. At minimum, the profile should include the medication name, dose, route of administration, frequency, date ordered, and date discontinued. The profile should include the signature of the registered nurse(s) who initiates or

updates the profile. Unless required by agency policy, it is not necessary for the physician to approve the patient's use of OTC medication. The physician would be notified if the use of an OTC medication is contraindicated or problematic, however.

Mechanisms should exist to ensure that monitoring of the patient's medication regimen occurs with a degree of regularity sufficient to recognize drug allergies or sensitivity, ineffective drug therapy, and/or adverse reactions and to implement promptly and appropriately actions for any untoward response. It is not unusual for the medication regimen to be altered by the physician during the course of care, but it is not necessary for agency staff to obtain written confirmation of the veracity of changes in the regimen that occur as a consequence of communication between the patient and the physician and/or the physician and the pharmacist. Certainly, the staff member would consult the physician if there are questions concerning a new or changed medication. The changes or additions should be noted on the medication profile in the clinical record and included in the plan of care when it is developed for recertification.

§484.20—Condition of Participation: Reporting OASIS information

HHAs must electronically report all OASIS data collected in accordance with 484.55.

(a) Standard: Encoding OASIS data.

The HHA must encode and be capable of transmitting OASIS data for each agency patient within 7 days of completing an OASIS data set.

(b) Standard: Accuracy of encoded OASIS data.

The encoded OASIS data must accurately reflect the patient's status at the time of the assessment.

(c) Standard of transmittal of OASIS data.

The HHA must:

(1) Electronically transmit accurate completed, encoded, and locked OASIS data for each

patient to the State agency or HCFA OASIS contractor at least monthly.

(2) For all assessments completed in the previous month, transmit OASIS data in a format that meets the requirements of paragraph (d) of this section.

(3) Successfully transmit test data to the State agency or HCFA OASIS contractor beginning 3/26/99 and no later than 4/26/99.

(4) Transmit data using electronic communications software that provides a direct telephone connection from the HHA to the State agency of HCFA OASIS contractor.

(d) Standard: Data format.
The HHA must encode and transmit data using the software available from HCFA or software that conforms to HCFA standard electronic layout, edit specification, and data dictionary, and that includes the required OASIS data set.

The standards in this Condition define the HHA's responsibilities relative to the collection and transmission of the data collected during the comprehensive patient assessment. This OASIS data is collected at specified time periods: the start of care, resumption of care, follow-up, transfer to an inpatient facility with or without discharge, discharge to the community, and death at home. The data must be encoded and locked within 7 days of completing the OASIS data set. The data must be transmitted to the State agency or HCFA OASIS at least monthly in a format that meets CMS electronic data and edit specifications. The agency should institute policies and procedures to assure the accuracy of the data collected and transmitted. The procedures should include a mechanism for correcting errors.

SUBPART C: FURNISHING OF SERVICES

§484.30—Condition of Participation: Skilled Nursing Services

The HHA furnishes skilled nursing services by or under the supervision of a registered nurse in accordance with the plan of care.

(a) Standard: Duties of the registered nurse.
The registered nurse makes the initial evaluation visit, regularly reevaluates the patient's nursing needs, initiates the plan of care and necessary revision, furnishes those services requiring substantial and specialized nursing skill, initiates appropriate preventive and rehabilitation nursing procedures, prepares clinical and progress notes, coordinates services, informs the physician and other personnel of changes in the patient's condition and needs, counsels the patient and family in meeting nursing and related needs, participates in inservice programs, and supervises and teaches other nursing personnel.

(b) Standard: Duties of the licensed practical nurse.
The licensed practical nurse furnishes services in accordance with agency policies; prepares clinical and progress notes; assists the physician and registered nurse in performing specialized procedures; prepares equipment and materials for treatments, observing aseptic technique as required; and assists the patient in learning appropriate self-care techniques.

This condition requires the HHA to have written policies that clearly designate the scope of skilled nursing services offered, including those services characterized as specialty nursing services; the manner in which these services are provided, supervised, and evaluated; and the mechanisms for ensuring that skilled nursing service is furnished in accordance with the plan of care and agency policies. Position descriptions, policy statements, and procedures should delineate the duties and performance expectations for the registered nurse and for the licensed practical nurse when this category of personnel is used for service. These duties should be consistent with state practice acts and should reflect current standards generally for professional nursing and specifically for nursing practice specialties. Agency policy should specify under what circumstances, if any, the initial evaluation visit may be made by a therapist instead of the registered nurse.

The clinical record must document the provision of skilled nursing care consistent with the plan of care and agency policy and procedures. The clinical record should demonstrate that the nurse understands the legal implications of clinical recording and documents accordingly (documentation is discussed further under §484.48, Condition of Participation: Clinical Records). Because the registered nurse is delegated the responsibility for coordination of services, the clinical record should document communication with the nursing staff and other providers to ensure that there is continuity of care among the nursing staff and the other disciplines involved with the patient. This is not to suggest that the responsibility to document interdisciplinary communication rests solely with nursing. Evidence to the contrary notwithstanding, the nurse is not endowed with an inalienable right to function as secretary for other members of the health team. Rather, it is the nurse's responsibility, often working in cooperation with the supervising nurse, to ensure that communication for coordination and evaluation of patient care does occur throughout the period when services are provided.

It should be clear from the review of clinical records that the difference between the registered nurse and the licensed practical nurse is recognized. The decision to assign the licensed practical nurse should be based on the patient's needs, not the HHA's need for a nurse to make a visit. The HHA that routinely assigns the licensed practical nurse to make visits without sound criteria for assignment does so at its own peril.

§484.32—Condition of Participation: Therapy Services

Any therapy service offered by the HHA directly or under arrangement is given by a qualified therapist or by a qualified therapist assistant

under the supervision of a qualified therapist and in accordance with the plan of care. The qualified therapist assists the physician in evaluating level of function, helps develop the plan of care (revising as necessary), prepares clinical and progress notes, advises and consults with the family and other agency personnel, and participates in in-service programs.

(a) Standard: Supervision of physical therapist assistant and occupational therapy assistant.

Services furnished by a qualified physical therapist assistant or qualified occupational therapy assistant may be furnished under the supervision of a qualified physical or occupational therapist. A physical therapist assistant or occupational therapy assistant performs services planned, delegated, and supervised by the therapist; assists in preparing clinical notes and progress reports; and participates in educating the patient and family and in in-service programs.

(b) Standard: Supervision of speech therapy services.

Speech therapy services are furnished only by or under supervision of a qualified speech pathologist or audiologist.

This condition requires the HHA to establish written materials that govern the scope of each therapy service offered. The policies and related procedures should ensure that services are provided by or under the supervision of a qualified therapist. Policy statements should also specify the manner in which therapy services will be supervised, coordinated, and evaluated. The process for achieving these objectives should be congruous with the processes identified in any contractual arrangements for these services. Position descriptions should establish the requisite qualifications and duties for the therapist and assistant. These duties should include the functions identified in this condition and should be consistent with applicable state practice acts and professional standards. The manner in which therapy assistants are supervised should be defined in writing and be consistent with applicable state regulations and/or practice acts. For the speech therapist who is completing the clinical fellowship year, the HHA must define in writing how this individual will be supervised by a qualified speech/language pathologist. The position description and other related materials should ensure that the qualified therapist possesses the skills, knowledge, and ability to develop and implement in collaboration with the physician, as appropriate, a therapy program directed toward the attainment of measurable, functionally defined patient outcomes. A review of the clinical records must document that therapy services are provided consistent with the plan of care and with applicable policies and procedures.

The requirement that contracted therapists, and assistants if utilized, participate in in-service programs is frequently disregarded. At minimum, the HHA must be able to demonstrate that these personnel have attended in-service programs on Occupational Safety and Health Administration requirements and other applicable regulatory requirements. It is incumbent upon the HHA to be able to provide evidence that this requirement is considered in planning for and evaluating the provision of therapy service. The agency should maintain a record of the therapy staff's participation in continuing education activities, including in-service programs. Contracted providers should be held accountable for maintaining evidence of participation in in-service education.

§484.34—Condition of Participation: Medical Social Service

If the agency furnishes medical social services, those services are given by a qualified social worker or by a qualified social work assistant under the supervision of a qualified social worker and in accordance with the plan of care. The social worker assists the physician and other team members in understanding the significant social and emotional factors related to the health problems, participates in the development of the plan of care, prepares clinical and progress notes, works with the family, uses appropriate community resources, participates in discharge planning and in-service programs, and acts as a consultant to other agency personnel.

This condition requires the HHA to have written materials that clearly establish the scope of medical social services offered and the manner in which services will be provided, coordinated, supervised, and evaluated. Written policies and/or procedures, position descriptions, and contracts, if applicable, should specify the mechanisms that exist to ensure that the provision of medical social service meets the requirements in this condition as well as applicable state practice acts and professional standards. When social work assistants are utilized, policies, procedures, job descriptions, and contracts, if applicable, should specify the plan for providing supervision by a qualified social worker.

A review of clinical records should establish that the social service interventions are provided as ordered in the plan of care and that staff conform to agency policies when providing services. When indicated, the clinical record should document the social worker's efforts to assist other team members to understand the impact of social and emotional problems on the patient's ability to participate effectively in the plan of care. Where appropriate, the clinical records and/or case conference should also establish the social worker's involvement in discharge planning. The statement made earlier regarding the therapist's participation in continuing education activities, including in-service programs, is applicable to the social work staff as well.

§484.36—Condition of Participation: Home Health Aide Services

Home health aides are selected on the basis of such factors as a sympathetic attitude toward the care of the sick; ability to read, write, and carry out directions; and maturity and ability to deal effectively with the demands of the job. Aides are closely supervised to ensure their competence in providing care. For home health services furnished (either directly or through arrangements with other organizations) after August 14, 1990, the HHA must use individuals who meet the personnel qualifications specified in §484.4 for home health aide.

(a) Standard: Home health aide training.

(1) Content and duration of training.

The aide training program must address each of the following subject areas through classroom and supervised practical training totaling at least 75 hours, with at least 16 hours devoted to supervised practical training. The individual being trained must complete at least 16 hours of classroom training before beginning the supervised practical training.

(i) Communication skills.

(ii) Observation, reporting, and documentation of patient status and the care or service furnished.

(iii) Reading and recording temperature, pulse, and respiration.

(iv) Basic infection control procedures.

(v) Basic elements of body functioning and changes in body functioning that must be reported to an aide's supervisor.

(vi) Maintenance of a clean, safe, and healthy environment.

(vii) Recognizing emergencies and knowledge of emergency procedures.

(viii) The physical, emotional, and developmental needs of and ways to work with the populations served by the HHA, including the need for respect for the patient, his or her privacy, and his or her property.

(ix) Appropriate and safe techniques in personal hygiene and grooming that include:

(A) Bed bath;

(B) Sponge, tub, or shower bath;

(C) Shampoo (sink, tub, or bed);

(D) Nail and skin care;

(E) Oral hygiene; and

(F) Toileting and elimination.

(x) Safe transfer techniques and ambulation.

(xi) Normal range of motion and positioning.

(xii) Adequate nutrition and fluid intake.

(xiii) Any other task the HHA may choose to have the home health aide perform.

"Supervised practical training means training in a laboratory or other setting in which the trainee demonstrates knowledge while performing tasks on an individual under the direct supervision of a registered nurse or licensed practical nurse."

(2) Conduct of training.

(i) Organizations.

A home health aide training program may be offered by any organization except an HHA that, within the previous 2 years, has been found

(A) Out of compliance with requirements of paragraph (a) or paragraph (b) of this section;

(B) To permit an individual who does not meet the definition of home health aide as specified in §484.4 to furnish home health aide services (with the exception of licens-ed health professionals and volunteers);

(C) Has been subjected to an extended (or partial extended) survey as a result of having been found to have furnished substandard care (or for other reasons at the discretion of HCFA or the state);

(D) Has been assessed a civil penalty of not less than $5,000 as an intermediate sanction;

(E) Has been found to have compliance deficiencies that endanger the health and safety of the HHA's patients and has had a temporary management appointed to oversee the management of the HHA;

(F) Has had all or part of its Medicare payments suspended; or

(G) Under any Federal or State law within the 2-year period beginning October 1, 1988:

(1) Has had its participation in the Medicare program terminated;

(2) Has been assessed a penalty of not less than $5,000 for deficiencies in Federal or State standards for HHAs;

(3) Was subject to suspension of Medicare payments to which it otherwise would have been entitled;

(4) Had operated under temporary management that was appointed to oversee the operation of the HHA and to ensure the health and safety of the HHA's patients; or

(5) Was closed or had its residents transferred by the State.

(ii) Qualifications for instructors.

The training of home health aides and the supervision of home health aides during the supervised practical portion of the training must be performed by or under the general supervision of a registered nurse who possesses a minimum of 2 years of nursing experience, at least 1 year of which must be in the provision of home health care. Other individuals may be used to provide instruction under the supervision of a qualified registered nurse.

(3) Documentation of training.

The HHA must maintain sufficient documentation to demonstrate that the requirements of this standard are met.

(b) **Standard: Competency evaluation and in-service training.**

(1) Applicability.

An individual may furnish home health aide services on behalf of an HHA only after the individual has successfully completed a competency evaluation program as described in this paragraph. The HHA is responsible for ensuring that the individuals who furnish home health aide service on its behalf meet the competency evaluation requirements of this section.

(2) Content and frequency of evaluations and of in-service training.

(i) The competency evaluation must address each of the subjects listed in paragraphs (A)(1)(ii) through (xiii) of this section.

(ii) The HHA must complete a performance review of each home health aide no less frequently than every 12 months.

(iii) The home health aide must receive at least 12 hours of in-service training during each 12 month period. The in-service training may be furnished while the aide is furnishing care to patients.

(3) Conduct of evaluation and training.

(i) Organizations.

A home health aide competency evaluation program may be offered by an organization except as specified in paragraph (a)(2)(I) of this section. The in-service training may be offered by any organization.

(ii) Evaluators and instructors.

The competency evaluation must be performed by a registered nurse. The in-service training generally must be supervised by a registered nurse who possesses a minimum of 2 years of nursing experience, at least 1 year of which must be in the provision of home health care.

(iii) Subject areas.

The subject areas listed at paragraphs (a)(1)(iii), (ix), (x), and (xi) of this section must be evaluated after observation of the aide's performance of the tasks with a patient. The other subject areas in paragraph (a)(1) of this section may be evaluated through written examination or after observation of a home health aide with a patient.

(4) Competency determinations.

(i) A home health aide is not considered competent in any task for which he or she is evaluated as unsatisfactory. The aide must not perform that task without direct supervision by a licensed nurse until after he or she receives training in the task for which he or she was evaluated as unsatisfactory and passes a subsequent evaluation with satisfactory rating.

(ii) A home health aide is not considered to have successfully passed a competency evaluation if the aide has an unsatisfactory rating in more than one of the required areas.

(5) Documentation of competency evaluation.

The HHA must maintain documentation which demonstrates that the requirements of this standard are met.

(6) Effective date.

The HHA must implement a competency evaluation program that meets the requirements of this paragraph before February 14, 1990. The HHA must provide the preparation necessary for the individual to successfully complete the competency evaluation. After August 14, 1990, the HHA may use only those aides that [sic] have been found to be competent in accordance with §484.36(b).

(c) **Standard: Assignment and duties of the home health aide.**

(1) Assignment. The home health aide is assigned to a specific patient by the registered nurse. Written patient care instructions for the home health aide must be prepared by the registered nurse or other appropriate professional who is responsible for the supervision of the home health aide under paragraph (d) of this section.

(2) Duties. The home health aide provides services that are ordered by the physician in the plan of care and that the aide is permitted to perform under State law. The du-

ties of a home health aide include the provision of hands-on personal care, performance of simple procedures as an extension of therapy or nursing services, assistance in ambulation or exercises, and assistance in administering medications that are ordinarily self-administered. Any home health aide services offered by an HHA must be provided by a qualified home health aide.

(d) **Standard: Supervision.**

(1) If the patient receives skilled nursing care, the registered nurse must perform the supervisory visit required by paragraph (d)(2) of this section. If the patient is not receiving skilled nursing care, but is receiving another skilled service (that is, physical therapy, occupational therapy, or speech/language pathology services); supervision may be provided by the appropriate therapist.

(2) The registered nurse (or another professional described in paragraph (d)(1) of this section) must make an on-site visit to the patient's home no less frequently than every 2 weeks.

(3) If home health aide services are provided to a patient who is not receiving skilled nursing care, physical or occupational therapy, or speech/language pathology services, the registered nurse must make a supervisory visit to the patient's home no less frequently than every 60 days. In these cases, to ensure that the aide is properly caring for the patient, each supervisory visit must occur while the home health aide is providing patient care.

(4) If home health aide services are provided to an individual who is not employed directly by the HHA (or hospice), the services of the home health aide must be provided under arrangements, as defined in section 1861 (w)(1) of the Act. If the HHA (or hospice) chooses to provide home health aide services under arrangements with another organization, the HHA's (or hospice's) responsibilities include, but are not limited to:

(i) Ensuring the overall quality of the care

provided by the aide.

(ii) Supervision of the aide's services as described in paragraphs (d)(1) and (d)(2) of this section; and

(iii) Ensuring that home health aides providing services under arrangements have met the training requirements of paragraph (a) and/or (b) of this section.

(e) Standard: Personal care attendant: evaluation requirement.

(1) Applicability. This paragraph applies to individuals who are employed by HHAs exclusively to furnish personal care attendant services under a Medicaid personal care benefit.

(2) Rule. An individual may furnish personal care services, as defined 410.170 of this chapter on behalf of an HHA after the individual has been found competent by the State to furnish those services for which a competency evaluation is required by paragraph (b) of this section and which the individual is required to perform. The individual need not be determined competent in those services listed in paragraph (a) of this section that the individual is not required to furnish.

This condition sets forth the requirements that must be met when the HHA provides home health aide services. Specifically, the standards and factors in the condition specify those entities that may conduct a training and competency evaluation program, content areas for training and where that training may occur, the qualifications for instructors, the manner in which competency must be demonstrated and evaluated, and the requirements for the assignment and supervision of the home health aide.

For clarity, and to avoid repetition of the detailed information reported in the condition, the discussion of training and competency requirements is divided into the following subject areas: training, competency, and performance review requirements; instructors and evaluators; and in-service training. This section concludes with a discussion of the assignment, duties, and supervision of the qualified home health aide.

Training, Competency, and Performance Review Requirements

The agency must ensure that those individuals who provide home health aide services, either directly or via contractual arrangements, have successfully completed a state-established or other training program that meets the requirements set forth in standard (a) and a competency evaluation or state licensure program that meets the requirements set forth in standard (b) or a competency evaluation program that meets the requirements set forth in standard (b). The training program may be provided by any organization except a certified HHA that within the previous 2 years has been found out of compliance with standard (a), Home Health Aide Training, or standard (b), Competency Evaluation and In-Service Training.

If the HHA requires its home health aides to complete a training program, materials must be maintained that clearly establish that each home health aide completed a training program of appropriate length and content that was conducted by qualified instructors as defined in standard (a)(2)(ii) and discussed later in this section. These materials should make a clear distinction between what was taught in the classroom setting and what was taught during the supervised practical training. If the home health aide position description and/or the home health aide service policy statements require the aide to perform other tasks in addition to the basic skills specified in standard (a)(2)(iii), the manner in which these tasks will be taught and evaluated should also be documented.

To reiterate, it is imperative that the documentation of training be reported in detail because the determination that a training program did not meet the required specifications will result in a deficiency cited for standard (a), Home Health Aide Training. A deficiency for this standard prohibits the agency from conducting a training program for a 2-year period. If the deficiency is cited while a training program is in progress, the HHA may complete that program but may not begin another program for 24 months after receipt of written notice of the condition-level deficiency.

Most of the admonitions stated for the training program are applicable to the competency evaluation as well. A competency evaluation must be completed successfully before the individual may provide service as a home health aide. The competency evaluation must encompass all the subject areas listed in standard (a)(1)(ii) through (xii). The candidate's competence in four task areas must be evaluated by observation of task performance with a patient or mock patient. The four task areas are, as cited in standard (a), home health aide training: (iii) reading and recording temperature, pulse, and respiration; (ix) appropriate and safe techniques in personal hygiene and grooming that include (A) bed bath, (B) sponge, tub, or shower bath, (C) shampoo (sink, tub, or bed), (D) nail and skin care, (E) oral hygiene, and (F) toileting and elimination; (x) safe transfer techniques and ambulation; and (xi) normal range of motion and positioning. The remaining subject areas may be evaluated through written examination, through oral examination, or after observation of the home health aide applicant with a patient. These areas are, as listed in standard (a), home health aide training: (i) communication skills; (ii) observation, reporting, and documentation of patient status and the care or service furnished; (iv) basic infection control procedures; (v) basic elements of body functioning and changes in body functioning that must be reported to an aide's supervisor; (vi) maintenance of a clean, safe, and healthy environment; (vii) recognizing emergencies and knowledge of emergency procedures; and (viii) the personal, physical, emotional, and developmental needs of and ways to work with the populations served by the HHA, including the need for respect for the patient, his or her privacy, and his or her property. As an aside, it should

be noted that the competency evaluation for an individual who will be utilized to furnish personal care attendant services under the Medicaid personal care benefit may be limited to the evaluation of competency in those areas in standard (a)(1)(ii) through (xii) that the individual may be required to furnish.

Written materials should specify the method(s) used to test the home health aide applicant's competency in all the subject areas listed in standard (a)(ii) through (xiii). The tool(s) used to document competency should allow a reviewer to ascertain the specific tasks, ability, or knowledge area tested as well as the rating (satisfactory or unsatisfactory) attained by the person being evaluated. If competence is reported with a score, the score should be readily identifiable as either a satisfactory or an unsatisfactory rating. Furthermore, the materials should document that competency testing for standard (a)(iii), (ix), (x), and (xi) was performed with a patient or mock patient rather than a mannequin. An individual cannot be considered competent in any task for which he or she is evaluated as unsatisfactory. The HHA should establish in writing the mechanisms used to ensure that the individual who receives an unsatisfactory rating in any task does not perform that task except under the direct supervision of a licensed nurse until such time as he or she is evaluated again and receives a satisfactory rating. The method by which the aide subsequently attains the satisfactory rating should also be detailed in writing.

There is one other requirement germane to the training and competency of home health aides. The definition of *home health aide* in Subpart A of the conditions of participation, §484.4, Personnel Qualifications, states:

> An individual is not considered to have completed a training and competency evaluation program, or a competency evaluation program, if since the individual's most recent completion of this program(s) there

has been a continuous period of 24-consecutive months during none of which the individual furnished services described in §409.40 of this chapter for compensation.

As defined in §409.40, home health services means the following items and services:

- part-time or intermittent nursing care provided by or under the supervision of a registered professional nurse
- physical therapy, occupational therapy, or speech therapy
- medical social services provided under the direction of a physician
- part-time or intermittent services of a home health aide
- medical supplies (other than drugs and biologicals) and the use of medical appliances
- in the case of an HHA that is affiliated or under common control with a hospital, medical services provided by an intern or a resident under a teaching program as provided in §409.15

§409.42 sets forth conditions and requirements that must be met for the services identified in §409.40 and listed here to be covered by Medicare Part A. §409.15 specifies the criteria for interns and residents providing medical services as specified in (f) as just noted.

The HHA must conduct a performance review of the home health aide no less frequently than every 12 months. The performance review interval and the individual(s) responsible for this review should be identified in the personnel policies or in other written material. In the absence of any state, statutory, or contractual requirements or the HHA's own policies, it is not necessary for the home health aide to complete a competency evaluation as all or part of the performance review.

Instructors and Evaluators

The training of the home health aides, including the supervised practical portion of the training, must be performed by or under the general supervision of a registered nurse who has a minimum of 2 years of nursing experience, at least 1 year of which must be in the provision of home health care. Under the general supervision of the qualified registered nurse, other individuals may function as instructors in the training program. These individuals include, but are not limited to, physical therapists, speech/language pathologists, medical social workers, psychologists, and registered dietitians. This general supervision is demonstrated through documented evidence of the qualified registered nurse's responsibility for the content and conduct of the training program.

The competency evaluation must be performed by a registered nurse. In-service training must be provided under the general supervision of a registered nurse who has a minimum of 2 years of nursing experience, at least 1 year of which must be in the provision of home health care. The agency should maintain materials to document that the nurse(s) who function as instructors and evaluators hold the requisite qualifications. The qualifications of other professionals who participate in the training program should also be available.

In-Service Training

As stated in standard (b)(2)(ii), the home health aide must receive at least 12 hours of in-service training per calendar year. To ensure that this requirement is met, it is recommended that in-service programs be scheduled at regular intervals throughout the year or during periods when the agency historically has a lower than usual census. In-service programs should be designed to enhance the skills and knowledge required for successful performance or to introduce or review new or revised policies, procedures, and/or position descriptions. Of course, these new or revised materials will have been reviewed by the group of professional personnel.

In-service training may be furnished while the aide is providing care to patients. If the HHA allows the in-service requirement to be met while the aide is furnishing patient care, there should be guidelines for staff to determine what may be taught in the patient-care setting, who may provide the instruction, and how the learned task or skill is to be documented (for the purposes of meeting the in-service training requirement). As with other health care personnel, a record should be maintained of the aide's participation in in-service programs.

Assignment and Duties of the Home Health Aide

The HHA must ensure that the assignment of the home health aide to furnish care is based on the patient's need for personal care assistance identified, usually by the registered nurse, as part of the initial or a subsequent patient assessment. The home health aide furnishes care following the written instruction of the registered nurse or, where appropriate, the therapist. The instructions must specify not only what is to be done, but also how frequently it should be done. Because the home health aide is assigned to a patient to attain a specified outcome, in the majority of instances it is not appropriate for the designated tasks to be completed on an as-needed basis. It is assumed that the assigned tasks must be performed with some regularity if the desired outcome(s) is to be achieved. Throughout the course of care, the written instructions must be updated as frequently as necessary to ensure that the home health aide's duties are reflective of the patient's current needs.

There are numerous formats available to document the provision of home health aide service. Care should be taken, however, to ensure that the home health aide written instruction form is consistent with the format used by the home health aide to document the care furnished. Too often these formats contain different task definitions; therefore, it is difficult to ascertain that the aide has in fact completed all assigned tasks. An inability to establish clearly that the home health aide did indeed complete all the assigned tasks may present an area of risk for the HHA.

When the home health aide is expected to perform simple exercises as an extension of the therapy program, it is not sufficient to write on the assignment form "Exercises as per the therapist's instructions." The therapist must prepare written instructions for the exercises that the aide is to perform. A copy of the instructions should be available in the clinical record. It should be clear that the assigned exercises are not those that require the knowledge and skill of a therapist or therapy assistant. The HHA should have in place mechanisms to ensure that the home health aide who is assigned can competently perform the assigned duties as written by the registered nurse or therapist as appropriate.

A review of the assignment format and clinical record documentation should provide evidence that the patient's needs and the capabilities of the caregivers in the patient's support system as well as the capabilities of the aide were considered in the assignment of the aide and the duties to be performed. The goals or outcomes for the service should be evident. As noted earlier in this chapter, goals should be established for the services that are concise, realistic, and developed jointly with the patient or individual designated to act on the patient's behalf. The review of assignment formats should also document adherence to agency policies relative to the assignment and duties of the home health aide.

Supervision of the Home Health Aide

When home health aide service is furnished in conjunction with skilled nursing or physical therapy, occupational therapy, or speech therapy, the registered nurse must make a supervisory visit to the patient's residence at least every 2 weeks. When only physical therapy, occupational therapy, or speech therapy is being provided while the patient receives home health aide services, the supervisory visit may be made by a skilled therapist (not a therapy assistant) every 2 weeks at the patient's residence. (In this instance, although skilled nursing care is not being provided, the HHA has the option to require a registered nurse to make the home health aide supervisory visit every 2 weeks. Such a visit would be considered an administrative cost and could not be billed as a skilled nursing visit.) When only home health aide service is provided, a registered nurse must make a supervisory visit to the patient's residence at least every 60 days.

When home health aide service is provided in addition to skilled nursing, physical therapy, occupational therapy, or speech therapy, the supervisory visit may be made while the aide is present to observe and assist, as appropriate, or when the aide is absent to assess relationships and to determine whether the goals for care are met. Standard (d), Supervision does not specify a frequency interval for the presence of the home health aide when the supervisory visit is made; nevertheless, the HHA may want to specify such an interval in its policy to ensure that the registered nurse or therapist periodically supervises the aide while care is being provided. When home health aide service is the only service being provided, however, the registered nurse must make the supervisory visit when the aide is furnishing patient care.

Agency policy/procedure statements must set forth the agency's requirements regarding supervision of the home health aide. These requirements should be consistent with the requirements identified in Standard (d), Supervision. At minimum, the policy statements should specify the professional(s) who may complete the supervisory visit, the frequency for supervision and any circumstance that affects the frequency of supervision (e.g., patient receiving home health aide service only), the focus or purpose of the supervisory visit, and the necessity to document the supervisory visit in the clinical record. It is not acceptable to conduct this supervision via telephone or in any setting other than the patient's residence.

The clinical record must clearly establish that the agency policy for supervision is being followed. The clinical records must contain written reports of supervisory findings. The supervisory visit notation should specify whether the aide was absent or present and should provide an objective assessment of relationships vis-à-vis the goals established for the service or the aide's

performance of the assigned duties. Where applicable, the supervisory note or other format should document actions taken in response to information learned or observations made during the observation visit.

The HHA should institute mechanisms to ensure the routine comparative review of the format completed by the home health aide and the home health aide assignment format to ensure that the home health aide is completing each of the assigned duties. Often, the comparative review reveals that the home health aide performed duties that were not assigned, discontinued assigned duties, and/or did not perform all the assigned duties.

§484.38—Condition of Participation: Qualifying to Furnish Outpatient Physical Therapy or Speech Pathology Services

An HHA that wishes to furnish outpatient physical therapy or speech pathology services must meet all the pertinent conditions of this part and also must meet additional health and safety requirements set forth in §§405.1717 through 405.1719, 405.1721, 404.1723, and 405.1725 of this chapter to implement Section 1861(p) of the Act.

§484.48—Condition of Participation: Clinical Records

A clinical record containing pertinent past and current findings in accordance with accepted professional standards is maintained for every patient receiving home health services. In addition to the plan of care, the record contains appropriate identifying information; name of the physician; drug, dietary, treatment, and activity orders; signed and dated clinical and progress notes; copies of summary reports sent to the attending physician; and a discharge summary. The HHA must inform the attending physician of the availability of a discharge summary. The discharge summary must be sent to the attending physician upon request and must include the patient's medical and health status at discharge.

(a) Standard: Retention of records.
Clinical records are retained for 5 years after the month the cost report to which the records apply is filed with the intermediary unless state law stipulates a longer period of time. Policies provide for retention even if the HHA discontinues operations. If a patient is transferred to another health facility, a copy of the record or abstract is sent with the patient.

(b) Standard: Protection of records.
Clinical record information is safeguarded against loss or unauthorized use. Written procedures govern use and removal of records and the conditions for release of information. The patient's written consent is required for release of information not authorized by law.

The clinical record maintained for each patient accepted for care must, at minimum, contain the information specified in the first paragraph. The record should also include any other documents as required by the HHA, such as the Patient Bill of Rights and consent forms. A review of the clinical records should establish that all required documents are in the record and that these documents are uniformly used and properly completed. The clinical record should be organized in a manner that provides for a chronology of events pertaining to interactions between the patient and members of the health team and that facilitates the incorporation, review, and retrieval of clinical record information. Collectively, the clinical recording documents must clearly establish the provision of physician-directed, coordinated, patient outcome–oriented care and concomitantly must substantiate the agency's claim for reimbursement and minimize the risk of exposure to liability through the documented provision of care in the amount, frequency, and duration ordered and in a manner that meets professional practice standards.

Although the description of the required content is self-explanatory, the need for and distinctions among the clinical note, progress note, and summary report should be clear to all service providers. These three clinical recording methods are defined in Subpart A, General Provisions. A clinical note is defined as "a notation of a contact with a patient that is written and dated by a member of the health team, and that describes signs and symptoms, treatments and drugs administered and the patient's reaction and any changes in physical or emotional condition." A progress note is defined as "a written notation, dated and signed by a member of the health team, that summarizes facts about care furnished and the patient's response during a given period of time." As noted earlier, a summary report is defined as "the compilation of the pertinent factors of a patient's clinical notes and progress notes that is submitted to the patient's physician."

Whatever the clinical recording system, every patient visit report should meet the definition of a clinical note. When clinical information is reported with a flow-sheet format, the format should allow for the reporting of not only objective findings, but also the patient's response to the intervention(s) furnished. As a general rule, a progress note is written at 30- or 60-day intervals; it should be prepared as frequently as warranted by the patient's condition or as specified in agency policy, however. The summary report is prepared and sent to the attending physician at least every 60 days during which the patient receives care. This report contains pertinent information ascertained from the clinical and progress notes. To ensure that the records are up to date, consideration should be given to the routine concurrent review of a random sample of the clinical records (this activity could be completed as part of the continuing review of clinical records required in condition 484.52, Evaluation of the Agency's Program).

Standard (a) requires the agency to have written policies for the retention of clinical records. The policies should be consistent with applicable state laws, including those pertaining to the retention of records of minors and the records of patients involved in litigation. The policy should recognize the need to retain the records in the event that the agency discontinues operations. Finally, the policies should ensure that, when a patient is transferred to another facility for continuing care, a copy of the record or an abstract is sent with the patient.

To meet the intent of standard (b), the agency must establish policies and attendant mechanisms ensuring that safeguards are in place to preserve and protect the clinical record yet meeting the need to have the records readily available for personnel who are caring for the patient. The policies should support the patient's right to confidentiality of medical records. Those individuals who may have access to the record should be identified, as should any restrictions on their access. When patient information is maintained via an automated system, mechanisms must be in place to limit access to this information. Policy statements should specify under what circumstances the clinical record, or parts thereof, may be removed from the protected environment maintained by the agency. When visiting staff are allowed to remove the clinical record or parts of the record from the agency, the agency should establish its expectation for the continued protection of the record. That the patient's consent is required for the release of information not authorized by law should be evident in written policies with supporting evidence in the clinical record. The content of any format used to obtain consent and procedures for obtaining this consent should include consideration of legal and ethical issues.

§484.52—Condition of Participation: Evaluation of the Agency's Program

The HHA has written policies requiring an overall evaluation of the agency's total program at least once a year by the group of professional personnel (or a committee of this group), HHA staff, and consumers or by professional people outside the agency working in conjunction with

consumers. The evaluation consists of an overall policy and administrative review and a clinical record review. The evaluation assesses the extent to which the agency's program is appropriate, adequate, effective, and efficient. Results of the evaluation are reported to and acted upon by those responsible for the operation of the agency and are maintained separately as administrative records.

(a) Standard: Policy and administrative review.

As part of the evaluation process, the policies and administrative practices of the agency are reviewed to determine the extent to which they promote patient care that is appropriate, adequate, effective, and efficient. Mechanisms are established in writing for the collection of pertinent data to assist in evaluation.

(b) Standard: Clinical record review.

At least quarterly, appropriate health professionals, representing at least the scope of the program, review a sample of both active and closed clinical records to determine whether established policies are followed in furnishing services directly or under arrangement. There is a continuing review of clinical records for each 60-day period that a patient receives home health services to determine adequacy of the plan of care and appropriateness of continuation of care.

This condition requires the HHA to conduct an overall evaluation of the agency's total program at least once a year. Those who may participate in the evaluation are identified in the condition. The objectives for the evaluation are to determine the extent to which the agency's program is appropriate (i.e., demonstrates the agency's mission and purposes), adequate (i.e., fosters attainment of the agency's goals and objectives), effective (i.e., significantly and positively affects those served by the agency), and efficient (i.e., demonstrates the most judicious use of financial, human, and information resources). Policy statements should ensure that the scope of the evaluation is sufficiently broad to achieve the evaluation objectives and to ensure that the written evaluation report, including findings and recommendations, is promptly reviewed by the advisory group of professional personnel or a committee acting for the group and is subsequently promptly submitted to the governing body and administrator for review and action. The agency should have a written plan for the evaluation that allows for the collection and review or analysis of information pertaining to the organization, activities, costs, and outcomes of the agency's programs.

Standard (a) requires a policy and administrative review. This review should be coupled with an analysis of personnel and patient service activity data to determine the degree to which the policies and administrative practices of the agency support the provision of high-quality patient care as defined with the agency's measures of quality. The mechanisms for collecting and compiling data (patient service, personnel, financial, etc.) to assist in the evaluation must be delineated in writing.

As part of the evaluation process, standard (b) mandates a review of a sample of open and closed clinical records on a quarterly basis. The review should be conducted by professionals representing the therapeutic services offered by the HHA during the quarter under review; other professionals may participate in the review at the agency's behest, however. The focus of the review is to ensure that services are provided in a manner that demonstrates compliance with professional practice acts, the plan of care, and the agency's written policies and procedures. The format used by the review should be designed to focus on these areas. It is not necessary that professionals conducting the review meet as a group, but the agency must be able to demonstrate that the time of the review of selected records does not exceed any three-month period.

The findings from the review of clinical records should be summarized and reported in writing. The summary report should indicate the methodology for selecting the records, the number of records reviewed, and recommendations. The number of records should be sufficient to constitute a representative sample, but the condition no longer requires that a designated number of records be reviewed each quarter. Action plans for the short- and long-term correction of identified problems should be developed and implemented with appropriate follow-up to assess the effectiveness of the plan.

In addition to the quarterly review of records, standard (b) requires the review of the clinical record every 60 days that the patient receives home health services to determine the adequacy of the plan of care and the appropriateness of the continuation of care. Personnel responsible for completing this review should be identified in the position description or in procedures specifying how the review is to be accomplished. These procedures should ensure that the review is completed on a timely basis and that action is promptly taken whenever evidence of inadequacy or inappropriateness is found. This review should occur as part of the process to develop the plan of care for recertification and to aid in the preparation of the summary report.

The annual program evaluation and the quarterly review of clinical records should be part of the agency's comprehensive quality assurance program. These and other activities should provide objective data that can be used to define and measure quantitatively the quality of the care and services provided by the agency.

§484.55—Condition of Participation: Comprehensive Assessment of Patients

Each patient must receive, and an HHA must provide, a patient-specific comprehensive assessment that accurately reflects the patient's current health status and includes information that may be used to demonstrate the patient's progress toward achievement of desired outcomes. The comprehensive assessment must identify the patient's continuing need for home care and meet the patient's medical, nursing, rehabilitative, social, and discharge planning needs. For Medicare beneficiaries, the HHA must verify the patient's eligibility for the

Medicare home health benefit including home-bound status, both at the time of the initial assessment visit and at the time of the comprehensive assessment also incorporate the use of the current version of the Outcome and Assessment Information Set (OASIS) items, using the language and groupings of the OASIS items, as specified by the Secretary.

(a) Standard: Initial assessment visit.

(1) A registered nurse must conduct an initial assessment visit to determine the immediate care and support needs of the patient; and, for Medicare patients to determine eligibility for the Medicare home health benefit, including homebound status. The initial assessment visit must be held either within 48 hours of referral, or within 48 hours of the patient's return home, or on the physician-ordered start of care.

(2) When rehabilitation therapy service (speech/language pathology, physical therapy, or occupational therapy) is ordered by the physician, and if the need for that service establishes program eligibility, the initial assessment visit may be made by the appropriate rehabilitation skilled professional.

(b) Standard: Completion of the comprehensive assessment.

(1) The comprehensive assessment must be completed in a timely manner, consistent with the patient's immediate needs but no later than 5 calendar days after the start of care.

(2) Except as provided in paragraph (b)(3) of this section, a registered nurse must complete the comprehensive assessment and for Medicare patients, determine eligibility for the Medicare benefit including homebound status.

(3) When physical therapy, speech/language pathology, or occupational therapy is the only service ordered by the physician, a physical therapist, speech-language pathologist or occupational therapist may complete the comprehensive assessment, and for the Medicare home health benefit, including homebound status. The occupational therapist may complete the comprehensive assessment if the need for occupational therapy establishes program eligibility.

(c) Standard: Drug regimen review.

The comprehensive assessment must include a review of all medications the patient is currently using in order to identify any potential adverse effects and drug reactions, including ineffective drug therapy, significant side effects, significant drug interactions, duplicate drug therapy, and non-compliance with drug therapy.

(d) Standard: Update of the comprehensive assessment.

The comprehensive assessment must be updated and revised (including the administration of the OASIS) as frequently as the patient's condition warrants due to a major decline or improvement in the patient(s) health status, but no less frequently than:

(1) The last 5 days of every 60 days beginning with the start of care date unless there is
   (i) Beneficiary elected transfer
   (ii) Significant change in condition resulting in a new case mix assignment; or
   (iii) Discharge and return to the same HHA during the 60-day episode

(2) Within 48 hours of the patient return to the home from a hospital admission of 24 hours or more for any reason other than diagnostic tests.

(3) At discharge.

(e) Standard: Incorporation of OASIS data items.

The OASIS data items determined by the Secretary must be incorporated into the HHA's own assessment and must include record items, demographic and patient history, living arrangements, supportive assistance, sensory status, integumentary status, neuro/emotional/behavioral status, activities of daily living, medications, equipment management, emergent care, and date items collected at inpatient facility admission or discharge only.

Collectively, these standards address the content of the comprehensive assessment, who may conduct the initial assessment, and the time period for collecting OASIS data. A comprehensive assessment, which includes the OASIS data items, must be completed for all patients who receive services from a Medicare-certified HHA except for patients who are:

- Under age 18;
- Receiving maternity services;
- Receiving housekeeping or chore services only; or
- Receiving only personal care services until further notice.

A comprehensive assessment including the OASIS data items must be completed for Medicare, Medicaid, managed care, and private pay patients. Medicaid patients receiving services under a waiver program or demonstration, to the extent they do not fall into one of the exception categories listed above, must also receive a comprehensive assessment that includes the OASIS data items. The OASIS data items are not intended to be the only items in a comprehensive assessment. A comprehensive assessment may include additional items that are necessary to determine the most appropriate care for the patients as well as professional practice standards.

The initial assessment visit is also intended to verify that the patient meets the HHA's admission polices as well as, when applicable, Medicare coverage criteria. To qualify for coverage the patient must be confined to home (homebound); service must be provided under a plan of care established and approved by a physician; the patient must be under the care of a physician; and, the patient must need skilled nursing on an intermittent basis or physical therapy or speech therapy services or has a continued need for occupational therapy.

This condition mandates that the registered nurse conduct the initial assessment visit; however, the conduct of the initial assessment visit is not exclusively reserved for the registered nurse. A physical therapist or speech/language pathologist may conduct the initial evaluation when physical therapy or speech/language pathology, respectively, is the only service ordered. The HHA's policies should specify under which circumstances, if any, a physical therapist or speech/language pathologist is expected to compete the initial assessment visit. If the therapist is permitted to complete the initial comprehensive assessment visit for therapy patients, the HHA must have procedures in place to assure an accurate review of the patient's medication regimen. The initial evaluation visit conducted by the registered nurse to complete the comprehensive assessment may also be the initial evaluation visit specified in Section 484.30(a).

The HHA should have policies and procedures relative to the comprehensive assessment of patients. The materials should assure that the assessments are completed by qualified personnel at the mandated intervals and that patients accepted for services meet the HHA's admission policies.

CONCLUSION

The Medicare-certified HHA must demonstrate compliance with conditions of participation on an ongoing basis regardless of organizational structure or design. To that end, the administrator must consistently act to ensure that the agency's policies, procedures, standards of practice, protocols, and other materials that delineate operational practices and expectations adequately and appropriately reflect the applicable requirements as set forth in the conditions of participation.

REFERENCES

Department of Health and Human Services, Health Care Financing Administration. 1999, August. 42 CFR Part 484. Medicare program: Home health agencies: Conditions of participation and reduction in recordkeeping requirements; interim final role. *Federal Register* 54: 33354–33373.

Department of Health and Human Services, Health Care Financing Administration. 1991a, July. 42 CFR Part 484. Medicare program: Home health agencies: Conditions of participation. *Federal Register* 56: 32967–32975.

Department of Health and Human Services, Health Care Financing Administration. 1991b, September. 42 CFR Parts 409, 418, 484. Medicare program: Medicare coverage of home health services, Medicare conditions of participation, and home health aide supervision. *Federal Register* 56: 49154–49172.

Department of Health and Human Services, Health Care Financing Administration. 1992, February. 42 CFR Part 493. Medicare program: Laboratory services. *Federal Register*, 57.

Department of Health and Human Services, Health Care Financing Administration. 1993a, January. 42 CFR Part 493. Medicare program: Laboratory services. *Federal Register*, 58.

Department of Health and Human Services. 1993b, October. *State operations manual*. Provider Certification Transmittal no. 260, B-25. Washington, DC: Health Care Financing Administration.

Department of Health and Human Services, Health Care Financing Administration. 1997a. Medicare and Medicaid program; Revision of the conditions of participation for home health agencies and use of the Outcome and Assessment Information Set (OASIS) as part of the revised conditions of participation for home health agencies. *Federal Register*, 62(46): 11004–11035.

Department of Health and Human Services, Health Care Financing Administration. 1997b. Medicare and Medicaid program; Use of the OASIS as part of the conditions of participation for home health agencies. *Federal Register*, 62(46): 11035–11064.

Department of Health and Human Services. *http://www.access.gpo.gov./nara/cfr*

CHAPTER 4

The Joint Commission's Home Care Accreditation Program

Maryanne L. Popovich

The Joint Commission on Accreditation of Healthcare Organizations (JCAHO) is a private, not-for-profit organization dedicated to improving the quality and safety of health care provided to the public. This goal is realized through fulfillment of its roles as standard setter, evaluator, accreditor, and consultant. The joint commission is widely recognized for its dynamic leadership role in developing standards. The survey and accreditation processes have been progressively updated to address the important changes and issues in the delivery of health services. The joint commission believes that its standards should:

- focus on those functions and aspects of care, treatment, and services that are essential to safe and quality patient care
- provide a framework of guidance for accredited organizations and those seeking accreditation
- represent a consensus on the state of the art in expected organization performance
- state, to the extent possible, objectives or principles rather than specific mechanisms for meeting requirements
- be reasonable, applicable, and surveyable

The original home care standards were developed over a 2-year period under the guidance of a national home care advisory committee. Several field reviews were conducted to obtain provider and consumer input into the draft standards, with 16 home care organizations participating in pilot testing before the standards were finalized. The first standards became effective June 1, 1988. Since then, there have been several revisions of the standards that have resulted in new standards manuals. These standards apply to both freestanding and hospital-based home care organizations, and they address the provision of various types of home care services. An organization is eligible to apply for a survey if it provides at least one of the following services in the patient's residence:

- Home health services are those services provided by health care professionals on a per-visit or per-hour basis to patients who have or are at risk of an injury, an illness, or a disabling condition or who are terminally ill and require short- and/or long-term intervention by health professionals.
- Personal care and support services are those services provided on a per-visit or per-hour basis to meet the identified needs of patients who have or are at risk of an injury, an illness, or a disabling condition and who require assistance in personal care, activities of daily living, and maintenance and management of household routines.
- Pharmaceutical services are those services provided directly by an organization, or through written agreement or contract with another organization. These services pro-

cure, prepare, preserve, compound, dispense, and/or distribute pharmaceutical products and monitor the patient's clinical status.

- Equipment management includes the selection, delivery, set-up, and maintenance of equipment to meet patients' needs, including the education of patients in the equipment's use.

- Clinical respiratory services are those services provided by respiratory care practitioners to patients who have or are at risk of an injury, an illness, or a disabling condition or who are terminally ill and require short- and/or long-term care intervention by health care professionals; such services are associated with the provision of equipment management services and may include, but need not be limited to, physical assessment, monitoring of vital signs, oximetry testing, and/or the administration of therapeutic treatments.

- Hospice includes an organized program that consists of services provided and coordinated by an interdisciplinary team at a frequency appropriate to meet the needs of patients who are diagnosed with a terminal illness, and have a limited life span. The hospice specializes in providing palliative management of pain and other physical symptoms and meeting the psychosocial and spiritual needs of the patient and the patient's family or other primary care person(s). The program also includes a continuum of interdisciplinary team services across all settings where hospice care is provided, the availability of 24-hour access to care, utilization of volunteers, and bereavement care to the survivors, as needed, for an appropriate period of time.

THE HOME CARE STANDARDS

The survey and accreditation decision processes are based on an organization's demonstration of compliance with the standards in the *2004–2005 Comprehensive Accreditation Manual for Home*

Care (CAMHC) (Joint Commission, 2003). This standards manual is divided into two sections: Section 1 consists of five chapters that focus on an organization's important patient-focused functions, and Section 2 includes six additional chapters that focus on important organizational functions that support how patient care is delivered. Although all the standards are considered important in the delivery of care or service, the following summary highlights those key concepts and standards in each chapter.

Ethics, Rights, and Responsibilities

Standards in this chapter address the right of patients to make informed decisions regarding their care, including the right to formulate advance directives. The standards also require the organization to inform patients of their rights and to establish a mechanism for resolving patient complaints. In addition, the standards include requirements for an organizational mechanism to address ethical issues arising in the care of patients and for organizations to adopt ethical business practices.

Provision of Care, Treatment, and Services

These standards set the expectations for an organization's processes related to patient assessment. The organization should collect relevant assessment data for every patient, analyze the data to determine the patient's needs, and make decisions regarding patient care and services. Assessment should occur at admission and then at appropriate points throughout the course of care or service.

The standards in the chapter continue with requirements for processes that guide the care and services received by patients. The standards require an organization to plan the services that each patient receives. The care planning process should identify the patient's problems and needs, care and/or treatment goals or expected outcomes, and the actions and interventions to achieve these goals.

The standards require that care not only be planned, but also implemented to meet the patient's problems and needs. In addition, the patient's response to care or service needs to be monitored throughout the course of care. The standards also require that care and services be provided in accordance with standards of practice.

Additional standards relate to the educational needs of an organization's patients and their families. The standards require organizations to develop a systematic approach to patient education. An education program should help patients understand and cope with their health status and care options. Organizations should encourage patients and their families to be involved in care decisions and to learn care skills. The standards also identify specific topics that should be included in a patient education program.

The standards also address the responsibility that an organization must accept in providing care and services in a continuous and coordinated manner and that is appropriate for the patient's needs over the entire course of time that the patient is served by the organization. The standards require an organization to define its scope of services and only accept patients whose needs can be met by the organization. The standards establish expectations for continuity of care from admission through discharge. The standards also expect that the care be coordinated with all care providers, both within the organization and external care providers.

Medication Management

This chapter outlines in detail the various processes, systems, and practices to assure effective and safe medication management. It incorporates all functions from selection and procurement of drugs to administration and effective patient monitoring for efficiency of the therapy.

Improving Organization Performance

Standards in this chapter evaluate the organization's ability to monitor and improve the quality of its services through a planned and organization-wide approach. These standards require improvements to be planned and prioritized. The standards also address how processes are designed or redesigned; how and what data are collected, measured, and assessed; and how and when improvements are made. Whenever possible, the organization should consider staff and customer input as well as incorporate benchmarking and comparative data sources in its improvement activities. The standards also address the creation of a methodology for effective identification and analysis and resolution of sentinel or adverse events.

Leadership

These standards address the authority and responsibilities of the organization's leadership, which includes the governing body, management, and supervisors. Leaders should provide the framework for planning, directing, coordinating, providing, and improving patient care and services. The standards examine the role of leadership in setting the mission and priorities, strategic planning, budget approval, annual evaluation of the organization's performance, as well as requiring effective resource and staff allocation. The standards require that the organization comply with applicable laws and regulations. Other standards address personnel and organizational management, development, implementation and review of policies and procedures, and development of written agreements. There are also several standards that relate directly to the role of the leaders in performance improvement.

Environmental Safety and Equipment Management

These standards address the organization's responsibility to provide care and service in a safe and effective manner. The organization should plan for and implement safety practices for both patients and staff. The organizations are required, as applicable to the care, treatment, and services provided, to manage environments, including the patient's home, the home care organization's office, warehouses, pharmacies, and vehicles. The standards require an organization's program to consider fire safety, emergency preparedness, personal safety, basic home safety, and safe handling of medical gases and hazardous materials and wastes. In addition, the standards require an appropriate equipment management program, including routine and preventive maintenance, to ensure that the equipment used by patients and staff is safe and in working order, and that equipment is appropriately set up in the home.

Management of Human Resources

The focus of these standards is the organization's need to provide adequate and appropriate staff to perform both organizational and patient care functions. The standards require the organization to define levels of experience, education, training, licensure, and qualifications for each category of staff. The organization should develop job descriptions for all staff. In addition, organizations are required to develop an education program for all staff that includes orientation and ongoing training, as well as an assessment of staff competence both at hire and on an ongoing basis. Depending on staff categories, the training needs and expectations may differ. Organizational staff may include permanent, full-time staff, part-time and on-call staff, contracted staff, and volunteers.

Management of Information

These standards examine the processes that an organization has established to manage information. Information management should be planned and prioritized. The standards require that information be timely, accurate, and accessible. When appropriate, the organization must ensure that data are secure and confidential. In addition, these standards set the expectations for what should be included in the patient care record. The standards also identify data that are to be collected and aggregated into meaningful information and trended over time to support information

sharing and communication to the appropriate individuals.

Surveillance, Prevention, and Control of Infection

These standards require an infection control program that includes the following specific processes: surveillance, identification, prevention, control of infections, and reporting. The program must include organizational policies and procedures addressing areas such as personal hygiene, precautions, aseptic procedures, communicable infections, reporting of patient and staff infections, and appropriate cleaning, disinfection, and/or sterilization of equipment and supplies. Policies and procedures should be based on infection trends and patterns, new scientific knowledge, and regulatory changes. The standards require that these policies and procedures be implemented across the organization. Data related to the infection control program should be collected, analyzed, and acted upon when appropriate.

THE SURVEY PROCESS

Health care professionals who have both management and clinical experience in home care conduct home care surveys. The background of the assigned surveyor and the duration of the survey are predicted by the type and volume of services provided. Agencies that provide intermittent or private duty nursing, home health aide, and/or homemaker services will have a survey conducted by a home health nurse surveyor. Organizations providing home infusion therapy, including both nursing and pharmaceutical services, are surveyed by a home health nurse and a pharmacist surveyor. Organizations only providing pharmaceutical products are surveyed by a pharmacist surveyor. Home medical equipment (HME) companies are surveyed by individuals with direct experience in owning and/or managing an HME business. If an HME supplier also provides clinical respiratory services, the organization will be surveyed by a respiratory care practitioner. A nurse surveyor will survey hospice services. The duration of the survey is related to the types of services provided by the organization, the volume of patients/clients, and the organizational structure with respect to branch offices and contracted services.

The accreditation process is initiated when an organization submits an application for survey. Initial applications should be submitted at least 4 to 6 months before the requested month of the survey. Approximately 4 to 6 weeks before the survey, the organization is notified of the dates of the survey and the name(s) of the surveyor(s). The surveyors contact the organization 1 to 2 weeks before the survey to establish a tentative agenda for the survey. All surveys begin with an opening conference, in which surveyors summarize the purpose of the survey and the methods used to conduct the survey. At this time, they will review the proposed schedule of survey activities. This is also an opportunity for key staff members to be introduced to the surveyors.

At the end of each survey day, a short briefing is held with key managers. This meeting is designed for the surveyors and management staff to review the findings of that day, to answer any questions, and to review the schedule for the following day. An exit conference is planned for the last hour of the final day of the survey. This is the surveyors' closing statement and a time for the surveyors to identify all their findings. It is also an opportunity to discuss any findings, including recommendations, before the surveyors leave the site. In addition to the exit conference, the organization has the option to request a summation conference for all staff, in which the surveyors highlight the major findings of the survey.

Survey activities include the following:

- management and governing body member interviews
- staff interviews (including hospice volunteers and contracted staff) from a variety of professional disciplines or job cate-

gories; the staff to be interviewed are selected by the surveyor(s)
- home visits to current patients; typically, a surveyor will visit two to three patients for each day of the survey (patients to be visited are selected by the surveyor and should reflect a variety of services provided)
- documentation review, including administrative, personnel, and clinical policies and procedures; orientation, in-service, and continuing education; competence assessment materials; governing body bylaws, charter, and/or articles of incorporation; governing body minutes; contracts and/or written agreements; performance improvement materials; personnel records; sample patient admission packets; patient education materials; promotional materials; equipment maintenance records; and pharmacy dispensing records
- random home care record review, including both current and discharged patients who represent a variety of diagnostic categories, services provided, branch offices (if applicable), and professional disciplines involved in the care
- review of equipment and warehouse and delivery vehicles (when applicable)
- review of the pharmacy (when applicable)

For initial or focused surveys, the surveyors will evaluate the organization's ability to meet the standards for a period of at least 4 months. During the triennial resurvey process, the surveyors may evaluate evidence of compliance with the standards over the previous triennial period; it is expected, however, that the organization will demonstrate compliance with the standards for a period of 12 months before resurvey. The CAMHC includes important policies regarding accreditation that home care organizations are expected to meet, the standards and their elements of performance, guidelines that surveyors use to score compliance with the standards, examples of how an organization may choose to be in compliance with the standards, examples of how standards may be met, and the rules relative to the aggregation of information resulting from the analysis of standards compliance.

UNSCHEDULED, UNANNOUNCED, AND RANDOM UNANNOUNCED SURVEYS

Either an unscheduled or an unannounced survey may take place when the joint commission becomes aware of circumstances within an accredited organization that suggest a potentially serious standards compliance problem. The survey can either evaluate all the organization's services or be restricted to only those areas in which a serious standards compliance problem may exist.

On July 1, 1993, the joint commission began to conduct unannounced surveys at any time from the ninth to the thirteenth month of accreditation to a random 5 percent sample of accredited organizations in each of the joint commission's seven accreditation programs. Random unannounced surveys are conducted by one surveyor for 1 day. The surveyor will direct his or her attention to the five performance areas that the previous year's national aggregate data identified as being most problematic for similar types of organizations. Results of random unannounced surveys can affect an organization's accreditation status.

THE ACCREDITATION DECISION PROCESS

The accreditation decision for an organization is based on its demonstrated compliance with the standards in the CAMHC, and is awarded for a period of 3 years. Compliance with each standard is measured using a 0 through 2 scoring system. A score of 0 represents insufficient compliance with a standard, and a score of 2 indicates satisfactory compliance. If the organization receives requirements for improvements, the joint commission requires formal follow-up from the organization within a specified time frame. The organization will have 90 days to submit evidence of standards compliance.

Upon completion of a survey, the surveyor returns his or her findings to the joint commission's headquarters, where JCAHO staff review the documentation and scoring to ensure consistency in the interpretation of the standards, and to recommend an accreditation decision. The joint commission awards the following categories of accreditation:

- Accredited
- Provisional Accreditation
- Conditional Accreditation
- Preliminary Denial of Accreditation
- Denial of Accreditation
- Preliminary Accreditation

The designation of *Accredited* is awarded to organizations that demonstrate compliance with all standards at the time of the on-site survey, or successfully submit "Evidence of Standards Compliance" (ESC) to demonstrate that it has resolved any standards considered not compliant at the time of the on-site survey.

Provisional Accreditation is awarded to an organization where the ESC fails to fully address all standards that were scored not compliant, the ESC is not submitted within the required timeframe, or the Measure of Success submission does not demonstrate substantial compliance.

Conditional Accreditation is awarded when an organization's survey reveals that the number of standards that are scored "not compliant" meets the Conditional Accreditation threshold that has been determined for that specific program. The organization must undergo an on-site follow-up survey.

Preliminary Denial of Accreditation is awarded when an organization's survey reveals that the number of standards that are scored "not compliant" meets the Preliminary Denial of Accreditation threshold that has been determined for that specific program.

Denial of Accreditation is awarded after an organization exhausts all appeal opportunities.

Preliminary Accreditation is available only under the Early Survey Option.

EARLY SURVEY POLICY

Some organizations may choose to be surveyed under the Joint Commission Early Survey Policy. If an organization elects this survey option, it must be eligible and agree to receive two surveys. There are currently two early survey tracks from which to choose.

For Option 1, the organization is eligible for survey up to 2 months before operations begin. On the first survey, evaluation is limited to standards as they relate to the physical structure and organizational components of the home care organization's operations. Six months later, the organization receives a full survey, in which it is evaluated against all the standards, including implementation of its processes, policies, and procedures.

For Option 2, the organization must be in operation and have serviced at least 10 patients by the time of the initial survey. The first survey is a full survey, but some standards are scored lower because the required 4-month track record may not have been met. The organization will receive a decision of accreditation with requirement for improvements based on this limited track record issue, or actual noncompliance with standards. About 6 months later, the organization receives another full survey, including those track-record requirements that were not evaluated during the initial survey. The organization will probably maintain their original accreditation status unless serious compliance problems exist.

DEEMED STATUS OPTION FOR MEDICARE CERTIFICATION

For a home health agency or hospice to receive Medicare or Medicaid reimbursement, it must first be surveyed and certified by a state agency as complying with the conditions of participation set forth in the federal regulations developed by the Centers for Medicare and Medicaid Services (CMS), previously known as HCFA. If a national accrediting body, such as the joint commission, provides CMS with reasonable assurance that a home health agency or hospice that it accredits meets the federal conditions of participation, CMS may deem that the home health agency or hospice meets certification requirements. This recognition is known as *deemed status*.

The joint commission first submitted application to achieve such recognition for its home care accreditation program to HCFA (now CMS) in 1988. This application included a comprehensive comparison of the conditions of participation with the joint commission's home care standards as well as a detailed analysis of the accreditation decision-making process. As part of its review, HCFA also evaluated surveyor selection, training, and supervision; survey process methods; and the joint commission's general administrative policies and procedures. A final rule regarding deemed status for joint commission–accredited home health agencies was published in the *Federal Register* on June 30, 1993, and made effective September 28, 1993 ("Medicare and Medicaid Programs," 1993).

To ensure comparability between the federal certification and the joint commission evaluation processes, the joint commission agreed to several changes in its process for those home health agencies wishing to use accreditation for Medicare certification. Some changes are reflected in the standards of the CAMHC. In addition, the joint commission agreed to use the CMS functional assessment instrument and certain sampling procedures for those home health agencies that wish to elect the deemed status option. Lastly, as required by law, any survey that was to be used for home health agency certification must be unannounced.

For those agencies interested in having the joint commission's evaluation serve in lieu of the state survey, the organization must elect the deemed status option, allowing the joint commission to conduct an unannounced survey. During an initial or regular triennial survey in which the organization takes the deemed status option, all applicable joint commission standards as well as the Medicare conditions of participation are surveyed. If a joint commission surveyor surveys the organization during the interim years of the triennial accreditation cycle, only those standards that are comparable with the Medicare conditions of participation are evaluated. Deemed status is available for Medicare certification of hospices as well. Similar to home health, the survey is unannounced and the organizations are surveyed against the hospice conditions of participation.

The alterations to the standards and survey process do not change the fundamental intent of the joint commission accreditation approach, but rather are designed to provide congruency with the related regulatory requirements and procedures. Joint commission accreditation is, and will remain, voluntary. Seeking deemed status is an option available to interested home health agencies, not a requirement. Agencies desiring Medicare approval may choose to be surveyed by an accrediting body, such as the joint commission, or by state surveyors. The joint commission award letters, decision reports, and decision grids make the distinction that an agency has elected the deemed status option and has undergone an annual unannounced survey for the purposes of satisfying Medicare certification requirements.

BENEFITS OF ACCREDITATION

Accreditation is a visible demonstration of an organization's commitment to providing high quality care to the patients it serves. Some of the benefits of accreditation include the following:

- improved patient care by incorporation of standards that reflect maximum achievable expectations into daily practices
- provision of an objective, on-site evaluation based on nationally recognized standards
- individualized consultation and education by highly trained surveyors with experience in the home care field
- enhancement of community confidence, including discharge planners, consumers, case managers, and physicians who recognize joint commission accreditation
- reimbursement or recognition from third-party payers that require accreditation
- enhanced team morale and pride in achieving accreditation
- improved risk management for the organization
- fulfillment of licensure requirements in some states

CONCLUSION

Accreditation represents an objective, rigorous evaluation by health care professionals using nationally recognized standards for the provision of home care services. Achieving accreditation signifies the commitment of the organization and its staff to continuous improvement in quality, performance, and patient safety.

REFERENCES

Joint Commission on Accreditation of Healthcare Organizations. 1990. *Committed to quality: An introduction to the Joint Commission on Accreditation of Healthcare Organizations.* 4th ed. Oakbrook Terrace, IL: Joint Commission.

Joint Commission on Accreditation of Healthcare Organizations. 2003. *2004–2005 comprehensive accreditation manual for home care.* Oakbrook Terrace, IL: Joint Commission.

Medicare and Medicaid programs: Recognition of the Joint Commission on Accreditation of Healthcare Organizations standards for home care organizations. 1993. *Federal Register* 58: 35007–35017.

CHAPTER 5

CHAP Accreditation: Standards of Excellence for Home Care and Community Health Organizations

Theresa Sekan Ayer

The Community Health Accreditation Program, Inc, (CHAP) is the oldest organization accrediting community and home care agencies. It began providing this service in 1965 as part of the National League for Nursing (NLN), but in 1987 it was separately incorporated, with the NLN becoming the "principal member" of CHAP. In 2001 the NLN sold its principal membership in CHAP to a New York businessman. In 2002, through a settlement with this businessman, CHAP was able to become fully independent, governed solely by its voluntary board of directors. CHAP's primary goal continues to be setting the highest possible standards for health care professionals working in home and community health services. Since its inception in the late 19th century, the NLN has been a strong advocate of measures that promote consumer health. The NLN's creation of a consumer-driven accreditation program more than 30 years ago demonstrated great foresight, anticipating the expansion of home and community care that would occur in the last half of the 20th century.

CHAP is structured to demonstrate its commitment to quality and its belief that true quality can be achieved only by focusing on the needs of the consumer. CHAP is the only accrediting body in the nation that relies on standards of excellence to assess all areas of an organization: clinical excellence, client satisfaction, risk management, fiscal viability, and overall strength of management. Most important, CHAP is the only accrediting body in the nation that has offered public access to accreditation findings since its inception.

On May 29, 1992, the Department of Health and Human Services (DHHS) formally recognized CHAP's ability to ensure the quality of home health care services provided to Medicare and Medicaid clients by granting it deemed status for home health care (DHHS, 1992). Thus CHAP became the first private accrediting body to be given this distinctive authority. The term *deemed status* signifies that home health care agencies meeting CHAP's accreditation standards will be determined to have met the federal government's conditions of participation in the Medicare and Medicaid programs. CHAP was the first accrediting body, public or private, to implement the home health survey and certification provisions of the Omnibus Budget Reconciliation Act of 1987 (P.L. 100-203). In 1999 CHAP became the first accrediting body to achieve deeming authority for hospice organizations (DHHS, 1999). The following year (2000) home health deeming authority was renewed (DHHS, 2000). In most areas, CHAP standards exceed the federal regulations.

The goal of this chapter is to give the reader an understanding of the benefits of accreditation, the key concepts related to CHAP accreditation, and an overview of the CHAP process. Integral to

CHAP's accreditation process is its consultative nature. Holding firmly to its standards, CHAP takes the approach of improving the organization being reviewed. Also integral to this process is the strong focus on consumers as recipients of care. A basic CHAP tenet is the belief that both the provider and the recipient of care need to be directly involved in the development and evaluation of services. All CHAP standards and processes are organized to promote high-quality management and services that will result in positive/expected client outcomes in its accredited organizations.

PURPOSE OF ACCREDITATION

The process of accreditation promotes the coordination and integration of quality health care delivery by all disciplines. It fosters the best possible use of available health personnel and a climate for ongoing self-study and improvement. Accreditation distinguishes the excellent organization from its competition because independent experts and peers from across the country have judged it as meeting or exceeding quality standards. This process identifies for the consumer those agencies that have measurable quality indicators for structure, process, and outcomes.

BENEFITS OF ACCREDITATION

An organization must understand the value of accreditation to justify the commitment of the critical resources required to complete the steps of any accreditation process. Accreditation becomes an organizing concept to foster staff and organizational efficiency and effectiveness in care delivery. It is therefore important for all participants to understand the benefits of accreditation.

Benefits to Clients

Involving selected clients or former clients in the process of accreditation helps them appreciate the complexity of an organization's functioning. The accreditation process clarifies to clients how services and programs are coordinated and how they relate to the organization's resources. Involving consumers in accreditation is a major, yet inexpensive, management initiative. Clients are fully aware of the products and services of the organization and have established an interpersonal relationship with the staff and management team. The interpersonal relationship that the organization strives to foster may well help identify new or improved services or products.

Benefits to Staff

There are also benefits of accreditation that relate specifically to the organization's staff providing services. All types of organizations, from the most traditional to the most innovative, need to focus on securing a solid market for their services. All staff represent the first line of marketing and selling of an organization's services and products. Positive interactions with staff can form the basis for the development of strong advocates for the organization and home care. One serious negative interaction can destroy an organization's reputation.

The accreditation process can help an organization define and develop a market in concert with professional practice standards. The accreditation process links the philosophy and expectations of the organization with the strength and potential of individual professionals. Accreditation also provides a mechanism for staff within a discipline and across disciplines to work collaboratively. The accreditation standards clarify roles and provide a mechanism by which all staff can share in the process of setting priorities within and among services and programs. Staff develop an organization-wide perspective on issues and can be less parochial in their vision. They see how the organization might evolve to better serve their clients and community while also improving its financial health.

Benefits to the Organization

As previously mentioned, it is essential that accreditation become a major benefit for the organization itself, separate from the benefits to clients and the staff who work for the organization. Accreditation must serve the organization. It must be a wise, acceptable investment from the point of view of both the individual providers of care and the management team, from the governing body to the first-line managers. The process of accreditation can focus the organization's future development, if it commits to using the process proactively for continuous growth. It is an ongoing investment in improvement of services and in the integrity of the organization. Results range from enabling the organization to develop a visionary strategic plan and marketing strategy to developing continuing education programs specifically to meet evolving care technologies. Accreditation may also serve to foster business relationships among various corporations within a community. Organizations are continuously examining the potential for joint ventures and diversification of services within a community. Meeting national standards and developing a blueprint for quality services through the accreditation process ensure the organization's credibility in its promise of high-quality services.

Summary

CHAP's accreditation process is one that will demand continuous commitment to services and programs by all levels of staff within the organization. Benefits of accreditation developed by the organization demand an ongoing commitment of time and energy to improve organization functioning. The benefits of accreditation for the future effectiveness and fiscal solvency of the organization cannot be overestimated. When it becomes a "way of life," accreditation means continual quality improvement. Involvement of staff in the accreditation process results in improved services, decreased staff turnover, increased referrals, and increased staff productivity. The accreditation process can actually become a revenue-generating source for the organization.

THE CHAP PHILOSOPHY

The CHAP philosophy states that "The accreditation process should clearly separate excellent organizations and programs from those meeting only minimal standards. This Philosophy promotes the availability of quality home and community-based health care through organizations' voluntary commitment to accreditation" (CHAP, 2003). This basic principle of a voluntary commitment to excellence by home and community health organizations emphasizes the need for organizational commitment to quality operations and systems to successfully achieve CHAP accreditation. It is CHAP's firm belief that any health care accreditation process should distinctly identify superior organizations that are driven by consumer concerns, be easily understood and administered, evaluate the total system, and be a participative and instructive process for the organizations seeking accreditation.

THE CHAP MISSION AND PURPOSE

CHAP's current mission states that the organization will be an innovative, effective leader providing quality accreditation services to community-based organizations (CHAP, 2003). CHAP strives to provide leadership for enhancing the health and well-being of diverse communities. This is achieved through the development of standards of excellence that ensure the management of ethical, humane, and competent care in home, community, and public health settings. CHAP's purpose is to (CHAP, 2003):

- objectively validate the excellence of community health care practice through consistent measurement of the delivery of quality services
- motivate providers to achieve continuous improvement by adhering to standards of excellence
- assist the public in the selection of community health services and providers with demonstrated excellence

- lead by example through organizational excellence and quality performance

THE OBJECTIVES OF CHAP

CHAP's accreditation program was developed in response to fears and concerns by consumers about the quality of home care services. This vital consumer focus has been apparent in every aspect of CHAP's organization and function since its inception in the mid-1960s. CHAP's board of directors, which establishes broad policy, includes consumer representatives. The content of the standards and the site-visit process focus on excellence and quality through an unrelenting commitment to the consumer. The site-visit findings are made available directly to the public. The primary objectives of CHAP's innovative programs and research activities are to:

- develop and maintain state-of-the-art, consumer-oriented, national standards of excellence focusing on outcomes for the full range of services and products provided by home care and community health organizations
- identify home and community health organizations exhibiting excellence as measured by CHAP's standards
- stimulate continual improvement in the quality of home and community health care
- distinguish excellent community-based health care providers
- facilitate consumer access to accredited organizations
- assist accredited organizations in achieving and maintaining excellence
- stimulate innovation and creativity in home care and community health service delivery
- foster the long-term viability of accredited home care and community health service delivery
- ensure that purchasers and consumers have information readily available to make informed decisions regarding home care and community health services

- promote the development and dissemination of new knowledge in the field of home and community health care through ongoing research
- stimulate continuing growth and development of the home care and community health industry

THE GOVERNANCE OF CHAP

CHAP is a nonprofit corporation governed by an independent board of directors. This board is composed of volunteers who represent the organization and are responsible for setting policy for the staff to implement and goals to achieve. The board is self-perpetuating, with members nominated to the board by other directors or staff for specific terms of office.

Consumers have played an important role on CHAP's board of directors. This is a unique feature of CHAP among accrediting bodies in that it has been a vital component since CHAP's first board was convened. The first chair was Carolyne K. Davis, former head of the Health Care Financing Administration. Since then the board has included experts in the field of quality improvement, representatives of business and insurance, large and small home and community health providers, national industry consultants, and individual consumers.

The CHAP Board of Review, the actual accreditation decision-making body, is also composed of volunteers, serving for specific terms. Members include health care experts and all types of community health service professionals from accredited organizations. This ensures that those reviewing the site-visit findings understand CHAP standards and goals, and so are able to determine the quality of care and services in the organizations seeking or renewing CHAP accreditation.

PUBLIC DISCLOSURE UNDER CHAP

CHAP firmly believes that consumers have the right to direct, immediate access to site-visit findings for agencies from which they are contemplating purchasing services. One of the first actions taken by CHAP's board of directors was to adopt a policy of full public disclosure of accreditation reports directly to the public. CHAP was the first accrediting body to make this information available to the public. It is the only accrediting body that makes this information available for all the organizations it accredits, regardless of the service standards under which they are accredited. This is a marked departure from the procedures of any other accrediting body.

Upon request, whether via CHAP's toll-free number or in writing, CHAP provides consumers with basic information about the organization and its services and a summary of key findings of the organization's most recent site visit.

EXPERT SITE VISITORS

CHAP's site visitors have a diverse range of pertinent experience and education. To ensure that CHAP's high standards are met and maintained and to help participating organizations be viable for the long term, CHAP site visitors are experts in the areas of home and community health management as well as service delivery. The site visitors view themselves as consultants with the management team of the organization being visited. Their aim is to provide enlightened management practices in every aspect of organization operations, from marketing strategy, financial performance, and human resource capabilities to strategic plans for new product lines to ensure future growth.

CHAP'S CONSUMER FOCUS FOR QUALITY IMPROVEMENT

CHAP standards require that a client satisfaction survey be completed for each program. In addition, evidence that the results of these surveys are incorporated into the program must be demonstrated to the site visitors. Not only do CHAP site visitors make home visits and talk with the clients, but they also telephone previously served clients who are willing to speak candidly about the services they have received.

KEY CONCEPTS IN CHAP ACCREDITATION: STANDARDS OF EXCELLENCE

CHAP is committed to setting and maintaining the highest standards in the industry—the CHAP Standards of Excellence,—not merely minimum safety standards. CHAP's total commitment to consumer values is reflected throughout its standards, which identify the key attributes of organizations providing excellent care. CHAP accredits only those agencies capable of meeting these standards, which emphasize clinical competency, client outcomes and satisfaction, organizational management, and financial viability. CHAP Standards of Excellence for home and community health providers are blueprints for achieving excellence in every element of the home care business and were designed to reflect the ever-changing complexion of the industry. Four guiding principles form the framework for all CHAP standards. These principles address the structure and function of the home care organization, the quality of its services and products, the adequacy of all types of resources, and its ability to sustain itself over the long-term. (See Exhibit 5-1.)

These four principles form the basis for the core standards and all service-specific standards, and are applicable to all home care and community health organizations and programs (for the convenience of Medicare-certified home health and hospice agencies, the standards are cross-referenced to the Medicare conditions of participation). The core standards, which cover general management, administration, and financial viability of the organization, are the same for all entities. These standards cover the following areas:

- educational qualifications and credentialing of all levels of management
- the organization's policies and procedures for public disclosure and client rights
- human resources management

Exhibit 5-1 CHAP Standards of Excellence "Guiding Principles"

I. The organization's structure and function consistently support its consumer-oriented philosophy, mission, and purpose.

II. The organization consistently provides high-quality services and products.

III. The organization has adequate human, financial, and physical resources to accomplish its stated mission and purpose.

IV. The organization is positioned for long-term viability.

(CHAP, 2002)

- ongoing quality improvement mechanisms, including client satisfaction surveys and outcomes monitoring, and the incorporation of the results into each program or service
- staffing patterns (appropriateness of workload for service delivery)
- contracts and agreements
- adequacy of financial controls and resources including cash flow
- adequacy of financial information systems
- strategic planning and evaluation
- risk assessment and management
- marketing strategies and initiatives
- data collection and effective incorporation of data
- management information systems
- corporate climate and support of innovation

The service-specific standards, again based on the four guiding principles, have been developed for each of the following services:

- community nursing centers
- home care aide services (for organizations providing only aide services)
- home health (professional and paraprofessional services)
- hospice services
- home infusion nursing

- home medical equipment
- pharmacy services (including infusion therapy)
- private duty services
- public health services
- supplemental staffing

All service-specific standards address the following areas in the context of each service:

- overall program/service management
- qualifications, education, and supervision of professional staff
- qualifications, training, and supervision of paraprofessional staff
- quality improvement/utilization review activities
- level of client satisfaction through surveys and site visitor–client interviews
- quality of clinical services and records
- client home visits
- staff interviews
- inter- and intraorganizational coordination of services
- client outcomes and benchmarking
- service/program planning and evaluation
- service/program fiscal viability
- infection control and safety
- service/program fostering of a climate of and direction for innovation

CHAP has established and refined a set of clear, consistent standards to suit the service mix of any particular applicant organization by combining the core standards with the service-specific standards. Each organization may then concern itself only with the set(s) of standards pertinent to its particular service mix. Home care and community health organizations that meet these standards demonstrate their commitment to the delivery of high-quality services and products while enjoying the unique benefits of CHAP accreditation.

EXAMPLE OF CHAP STANDARDS: OUTCOME MEASURES

Several years ago, CHAP incorporated outcome measures into its standards. How an agency makes a difference is a significant part of what the site visitors look for. To illustrate, CHAP's Core Standard CII states the overall principle that an organization must consistently provide high-quality services and products. Under the umbrella of this principle, Core Standard CII.6 requires an organization to have a comprehensive performance improvement process. Ten criteria support this standard; for instance, CII.6c requires client-focused quality assessment and improvement activities. There are 13 elements under this criterion, including outcomes specific to the primary diagnosis. CII.6d requires that quality of services be defined and measured in terms of client outcomes (CHAP, 2002, pp. 24–25). These include, at a minimum, the group of clients who are the recipients of service, the expected behavior or result of service, the time frame for expected results, and the realistic percentage of clients who are likely to demonstrate expected outcomes within the specified time frame. As spelled out in the criteria, the site visitors look to see documentary evidence that the outcome objectives include the specified items, that each program has at least two client outcome objectives, and that the client outcomes are monitored, measured, and analyzed.

BENCHMARKING/OUTCOMES MANAGEMENT

CHAP's commitment to accreditation with a strong consumer focus led to its development of outcomes management software for home care. It began with a $1.2 million grant from the W. K. Kellogg Foundation, with which it conducted groundbreaking research that resulted in a system of benchmarks for home care across three broad areas: (1) consumer, (2) clinical, and (3) organizational. In 1995, risk and financial management parameters were added. These five "pulse points," as they were named, became a software program. Benchmark ratings are a powerful tool for assessing the strengths and weaknesses of an organization and for seeing where an organization stands in relation to the industry as a whole. These ratings can be used to drive internal quality improvement and to secure both industry and consumer recognition. Benchmark ratings highlight problem areas, so that quality improvement efforts can be directed where they are most needed. By providing a focused vision of what home care should provide, a benchmarking program gets everyone aiming at the same mark.

Benchmarking or outcomes management can assist in the accreditation process by helping an organization document its quality improvement efforts. Not only does outcomes management provide a quantifiable profile of services for reports to internal or external governing/oversight bodies, but it can also provide an invaluable comparative analysis of organizational outcomes among similar organizations. Outcomes management can also provide organizations with the tools to monitor compliance with CHAP Standards of Excellence. Outcomes management is now a requirement for CHAP-accredited home health organizations, although no specific software is mandated. Finally, outcomes' management can assist in increasing consumer satisfaction, improve reimbursement, and increase contract procurement from managed care organizations. In the late 1990s, as other businesses developed outcomes monitoring and benchmarking software, CHAP decided to sell its software and focus more of its resources on the accreditation process as a whole.

THE ADVANTAGES OF CHAP ACCREDITATION

Among the advantages of CHAP accreditation are the following:

- customized clinical and management consultation to help an organization strengthen all facets of its operations
- increased efficiency and productivity
- systematic and comprehensive evaluation of an organization's performance from top to bottom
- a quality audit that ensures accountability to consumers and payers (insurance companies and businesses)

- a complete self-study review before an on-site accreditation visit
- the ability to market to consumers using the CHAP gold seal, which has been endorsed by major consumer groups
- access to payers requiring accreditation
- customized financial profiles
- participation in regional meetings of top managers of CHAP-accredited organizations
- assistance with local media
- involvement in developing and setting CHAP standards and policies
- potential involvement in state-of-the-art national home care research and the ability to benefit from the findings of this research
- discounts on meetings, publications, and videos

OVERVIEW OF THE ACCREDITATION PROCESS

Accreditation by CHAP is accomplished through a simple four-step process: application and contract, self-study, site visit, and determination of accreditation status by the Board of Review. (See Exhibit 5-2.)

Application and Contract

The completed application form, which includes a profile of the organization, is sent to CHAP with an application fee. The organizational profile allows the CHAP staff to determine the applicable fees for each organization. Once the fees have been determined, CHAP will send a contract to the applicant organization outlining the specific elements of the accreditation fee.

Exhibit 5-2 CHAP's Four-Step Process

- Application and contract
- Self-study
- Site visit (survey)
- Determination of accreditation status

The contract covers the 3-year term of the accreditation cycle. The core standards, appropriate service-specific standards, and a self-study guide are sent to the organization separately but at the same time that the contract is sent.

Self-Study

The self-study guides an organization through a unique process of self-evaluation. The self-study is completed to prepare for the site visit, and it must be submitted to CHAP within 4 to 6 months of receipt of the contract. The self-study is a step-by-step guide to the self-assessment of administration, clinical services, planning processes, and financial operations and is beneficial to any organization. The self-study allows the organization to compare itself with the CHAP standards and become acquainted with the purpose of the accreditation site visit without having to purchase additional manuals. It addresses the clinical and business aspects of the organization by looking at the quality of services and products, the availability of resources, the fiscal viability of the organization, and its attention to consumers. Information from the self-study assists CHAP in planning for and conducting the site visit. When completed with input from all levels and types of staff, it reflects the collective vision of management, staff, and consumers.

Site Visit

CHAP evaluates the quality of home and community health organizations through announced and unannounced site visits. Activities include administrative and clinical document reviews, home visits, and telephone surveys to assess client satisfaction. CHAP requires agencies to perform regular client satisfaction surveys and to use the results to improve services.

Unannounced site visits to organizations using CHAP's deeming authority from Medicare are made by a team of trained site visitors specifically chosen for their specialized expertise. Visits average 4 or 5 days in length; the actual time for each organization is determined according to its size and complexity. The visits are designed to be a consultative learning experience. On arrival, site visitors establish a schedule with the organization's management staff that includes a review of appropriate documents such as policies, board and management meeting minutes, and clinical records to ensure the quality of the organization's clinical services and products, the financial health of the organization, and its strategic plan. Considerable attention is given to interviews with staff, advisory committee members, and governing body members. Clients receive significant direct attention through interviews, home visits, and telephone surveys to ensure that the organization is committed to CHAP's consumer-oriented, outcome-based standards.

Findings of the site visitors are discussed at an exit conference. Consultation is always available from the site visitors regarding specific recommendations or areas in which the organization would like help. The consultation is always provided after the exit conference so that it does not interfere with the evaluation process.

Determination of Accreditation Status

The board of review (BOR) evaluates the self-study and the site-visit report and determines the accreditation status of the applicant organization, including any required actions, recommendations, or commendations. Once accredited, an organization receives additional site visits depending on the findings of the initial site visit. The BOR determines the timing for the next site visit. The site-visit interval may be as long as 36 months for organizations with outstanding services and systems.

TYPES OF ORGANIZATIONS ELIGIBLE FOR CHAP ACCREDITATION

CHAP accreditation is available for all types of organizations, including nonprofit, proprietary, voluntary, government, facility based, and freestanding; that is, organizations providing health care services or products for the home or community sites are eligible for CHAP accreditation.

CHAP also welcomes young providers of community or home-based services. An organization only 6 months old may apply for CHAP accreditation and use the self-study as a tool for developing internal systems and processes.

CONCLUSION

The decision by an organization to seek accreditation is a serious one. It demands commitment from management and staff at all levels because it is the path to continuous quality improvement. Initiatives and activities focused on internal improvements lead to results that affect the client positively, which is the ultimate goal of accreditation. Consumers and payers alike recognize that, when an organization has met rigorous national standards, it is more likely to have the consistent positive outcomes that consumers seek. The accreditation process provides a challenge to organizations to accept responsibility for their growth and development. Working through the accreditation process shows the standards to be more than abstract principles. The process, from application by the organization to the decision of the board of review, is one of continuous growth.

REFERENCES

Community Health Accreditation Program, Inc. 2003, March. CHAP philosophy, mission and purpose. *CHAP Policy and Procedure Manual*, Administration Policy A.1.

Community Health Accreditation Program, Inc. 2002.

CHAP core standards: Millennium edition 2002. New York: CHAP.

Department of Health and Human Services, Health Care Financing Administration. 2000, February. [HCFA—2059–FN] RIN 0938–AJ69, Medicare and Medicaid programs: Reapproval of the deeming authority of the Community Health Accreditation Program, Inc. (CHAP) for home health agencies (HHAs). *Federal Register* 65(35): 8725–8727.

Department of Health and Human Services, Health Care Financing Administration. 1999, April. [HCFA–2029–FN], RIN 0938–AJ42, Medicare program: Recognition of the Community Health Accreditation Program, Inc.

(CHAP) for hospices agency, *Federal Register* 64(75): 19376–19379.

Department of Health and Human Services, Health Care Financing Administration. 1992, May. Medicare program: Recognition of the Community Health Accreditation Program standards for home care organizations. *Federal Register* 57: 22773–22780.

SUGGESTED READING

Ayer, T. S. (2002). CHAP accreditation: The "other" home care accrediting body. *Home Health Care Management and Practice*, 14(4): 284–288.

Ayer, T. S. (2002). Frequently asked questions about CHAP accreditation. *Home Healthcare Nurse,* 20: 4.

Community Health Accreditation Program, Inc. 2002. *CHAP home health standards of excellence.* New York: CHAP.

Further information is also available at *www.chapinc.org.*

CHAPTER 6

Accreditation for Home Care Aide and Private Duty Services

John I. Buck

HISTORY

The National Council for Homemaker Services was incorporated in 1962 to promote high-quality homemaker services and to set standards for the field. The first set of standards was developed in 1965. In 1967, the National HomeCaring Council was cited in the *Federal Register* as the national standard-setting body for paraprofessionals. The training of homemaker/home health aides was a primary concern and led to the publishing of a training manual in 1967. That evolved into the *Model Curriculum and Teaching Guide for the Instruction of Homemaker–Home Health Aides*, first published in 1978 (Department of Health and Human Services, 1978). The accreditation program itself was developed in 1971. Initially, the process consisted of the review of self-study and other written documentation, but a comprehensive site-visit survey was added in 1976. Over the years, this accreditation program became recognized in many states across the country, where it was designated as a requirement for participation in various Title III, Title XX, or Medicaid programs. In 1986, the National HomeCaring Council left New York and joined the Foundation for Hospice and Homecare in Washington D.C. In 1994, the council adopted the format of the home care aide

standards and self-study (Foundation for Hospice and Homecare, 1994) to private duty nursing services. That accreditation option became available in 1995, and the first private duty nursing service was accredited through the National HomeCaring Council in 1996.

In 1997 the Foundation for Hospice and Homecare merged with the National Association for Home Care (NAHC), and in May 1998, NAHC established the Home Care University as a new affiliate. The credentialing division of the Home Care University now administers the accreditation for home care aide services and private duty services using the standards established by the National HomeCaring Council. In 1999, the Home Care Aide Association of America published the *Code of Ethics for Home Care Aides* (Exhibit 6-1).

STRUCTURE

The accreditation program consists of two components. The standards committee is responsible for setting and reviewing standards to reflect current practice norms. The established standards are subject to approval by the foundation board. The standards committee meets periodically to keep up with the evolving field of home care.

Original chapter written by Ken Wessel, who was the chair of the accreditation commission.

HOME CARE AIDE
ASSOCIATION OF AMERICA

Code of Ethics
for
Home Care Aides

—Basic Principles—

I.

The safety and well-being of the client is the main concern in all decisions and actions.

II.

The highest level of honesty and integrity shall be maintained in all dealings with clients and the employer.

III.

Qualty services shall be provided in a conscientious, competent, client-centered manner.

IV.

The person and property of the client shall be respected with confidentiality, security, kindness, and recognition of the client's individuality.

V.

All activities shall be carried out according to employer policies and any laws that apply with any actual or possible violation reported to the employer immediately.

Guidelines for Client's Rights

Clients have the right to:
- be served by dependable and responsible caregivers;
- receive services as contracted;
- be treated with respect, consideration, and kindness;
- have honest handling of personal property and money;
- have privacy and modesty respected;
- have confidentiality of financial, medical, emotional, family or other personal problems, or information about the client/family;
- have acceptance of cultural and religious practices;
- refuse any treatment or services;
- dismiss any health team member for unsafe care practices, uncooperative attitude and/or careless work habits; and
- not be abused physically, verbally, emotionally, or sexually by caregivers.

Guidelines for Home Care Aide's Rights

As a Home Care Aide, I have the right to:
- be treated with respect and kindness;
- provide services in a safe work environment;
- be trained for tasks performed; and
- not be abused physically, verbally, emotionally or sexually by the client/family.

©1999 National Association for Home Care

Exhibit 6–1 Code of Ethics for Home Care Aides
Source: Home Care Aide Association of America. Washington, DC.

The second component is the accreditation commission. This group consists of home care professionals, representatives of consumer groups, and volunteers. The commission meets several times a year to review and make recommendations on accreditation applications. The foundation board can grant accreditation status based on these recommendations.

STANDARDS

Standards for home care aide and private duty nursing services are listed in Exhibit 6–2.

PROCESS

The accreditation process is the same for both home care aide and private duty services. That

---

Principle Standards:

I. There is a legally constituted authority responsible for governance and performance.
II. There is compliance with legislation, which relates to prohibition of all forms of discriminatory practices.
III. There is responsible fiscal management.
IV. There is responsible human resource management, which complies with all applicable laws and regulations and includes recruitment, selection, retention, and termination of all staff and volunteers; there are written personnel policies, job descriptions, and wage scales established for each job category.
VI. There is written eligibility criteria for service. There are written policies and procedures for admission, discharge, and referral for other resources. A written confidential client record is maintained.
VIII. There is an annual evaluation of all aspects of the service and a process for quality improvement.
IX. There is ongoing interpretation of the service through community outreach and education.
X. There is a written statement of clients' rights and clear evidence that it is fully implemented.
XI. There is a written policy and procedure of responsible safety management in the care

environment: To ensure the well-being of the patient; to ensure the well-being of the caregiver(s); and to be prepared in cases of emergencies in the home.
XII. There are policies and procedures to prevent, detect, and report violations of laws, regulations, and unlawful conduct and establish ethical business practices by all employees of the organization.

Home Care Aide Services Standards:

V. Every Home Care Aide is to receive training for each task to be performed for the client.
VII. There is supervision and management of the home care aide service, which ensures safe, effective and appropriate care to each individual or family served.

Private Duty Standards:

V. There is a professional case management service for all individuals and families served.
VII. There is professional registered nurse supervision of nursing personnel in the field to ensure safe, effective, and appropriate care to each individual or family served.

Source: Courtesy of the Home Care University, Washington, D.C.

Exhibit 6–2 Standards for Home Care Aide and Private Duty Services process consists of application, self-study, a site visit, and accreditation commission review. Every organization must meet the principle standards, which form the basis of the organization's delivery and operations compliance. For those providers who are interested in only home care aide accreditation, they must also complete Standard V, indicating the level(s) of home care aide provided, and Standard VII of the home care aide standards. The process allows for the organization to apply for and receive accredited status for any single level of home care aide. However, all levels of home care aide services are evaluated if more than one level is provided. Likewise, for organizations interested in only private duty accreditation, Standards V and VII of those standards must be completed in addition to the principle standards. Providers wanting home care aide and private duty services accredited must complete both sets of standards in addition to the principle standards.

To be eligible to apply, the organization must have been in operation with the service to be accredited for at least 1 year. The organization must directly employ the direct care staff. All similar services in an organization are surveyed regardless of funding source. Call the Home Care University at (202) 547-3576 or fax at (202) 547-4322 to fill out an application.

The Accreditation Commission selects two peer reviewers to analyze the self-study, perform a 2-day site-visit survey of the agency, and submit a report to the accreditation commission. These reviewers have been trained by the council and are always principals in home care agencies that have been accredited.

The first part of the self-study involves the applicant mailing questionnaires to a small sample of agency consumers. These questionnaires cover areas of customer satisfaction and clinical competence. They are returned directly to the Accreditation Commission when completed and are reviewed by the two surveyors and the commission.

The major part of the self-study consists of the applicant completing the 30-page self-study document. The document expands on the 12 standards and requires checking responses and narrative answers as well as listing supporting documentation being submitted by the agency. The council suggests forming a broad-based committee among agency staff and board members to complete the self-study.

The completed self-study is forwarded to the Home Care University, and copies are sent to each peer reviewer for evaluation. They begin the completion of a reviewer's instrument that is used to score the self-study and the site-visit survey. The lead reviewer will contact the agency when necessary to discuss any omissions or areas that need clarification. A site visit is scheduled, and the agency is asked to make a variety of board and staff members available for interviews.

During the 2-day site visit, the reviewers confirm documentation, evaluate selected personnel and case records, and interview staff and selected board members. The surveyors use this time to compare their analyses of the self-studies and resolve any contradictions that may have occurred. At the end of the site visit, the peer reviewers will conduct an exit interview with the agency director and give an overview of the findings. They will also submit a written report to the commission that lists areas of concern as well as suggested recommendations and commendations. The commission staff will forward these written concerns to the agency and give the agency an opportunity to respond in writing before the meeting of the accreditation commission.

The accreditation commission will meet several times throughout the year to review agencies that have gone through this process. Whenever possible, one of the surveyors will present the agency to the commission in person. Compliance with each standard is reviewed and voted on in turn. Each standard can be rated as noncompliance, partial conformity, substantial conformity, or full conformity. The commission is assisted by numerical ratings in the reviewer's instrument. When all standards are rated, the results are evaluated in the aggregate, and an accreditation decision is made. Possible outcomes are to deny accreditation, postpone accreditation, grant provisional accreditation, or accredit. If information is missing and can be obtained by the next commission meeting, postponement would be appropriate. Provisional accreditation could be granted if remedial action was required and could be anticipated within a specific time frame. These decisions are communicated to the agency along with final recommendations and commendations made by the commission. An appeals process is in place for agencies that believe the standards were not properly applied.

The accreditation process operates on a 3-year cycle. Full self-studies and site visits are required at that interval. Interim reports are to be submitted midterm to ascertain whether there have been any substantive changes in the agency.

RECENT DEVELOPMENTS

In 1995, the home care aide self-study was computerized and the self-study now can be completed and submitted on a floppy disk. Currently, this is only available for IBM-compatible computers using Microsoft Word for Windows. Future plans are to make this available on the Internet.

In 1999 the Home Care University began to modernize the National HomeCaring Council standards. A new Standard XII, Compliance and Business Ethics, was added to help assure the consumer that accredited agencies were complying with laws, regulations, and program require-

ments and operating in an ethical manner. In 2002 the remainder of the standards were reviewed and new industry developments, such as the inclusion of Americans with Disabilities Act (ADA), Family Medical Leave Act (FMLA), and sexual harassment in Standard II, and a more process improvement orientation to Standard VIII, were introduced.

CONCLUSION

The Home Care University believes

> organizations that meet its standards deliver safe, effective, cost efficient service essential to the protection of the consumer and the community and that their standards provides a much needed guide to the consumer in assessing the quality of the provider organization.

Voluntary accreditation by the Home Care University helps a home care provider demonstrate its administrative and clinical competence to the consumer and community it serves, as well as contractor and other payer sources. As the oldest set of home care standards in the United States, time and again they have proven that care delivered using these standards does produce sufficient consumer protection and a high quality of care to make the organization stand out as one of the best. Clients appreciate the standards value and reward the organization with the respect and recognition that they are a caring organization worthy of the consumer's trust.

REFERENCES

Department of Health and Human Services (DHHS). 1978. *Model curriculum and teaching guide for the instruction of homemaker–home health aides.* Publication No. HSA 80-5508. Rockville, MD: DHHS.

Home Care Aide Association of America. Washington, DC.

Home Care University. 1994. *Self-study manual.* Washington, DC: National HomeCaring Council.

CHAPTER 7

ACHC: Accreditation for Home Care and Alternate Site Healthcare Services

Thomas Cesar

HISTORY

The Accreditation Commission for Health Care, Inc. (ACHC) is an independent, private, 501(c)(3) organization. ACHC was established in 1986 through the efforts of the Association for Home and Hospice Care of North Carolina, and the North Carolina State Government Divisions on Aging, Social Services, Public Health, and Facility Services.

This was done in response to the need for relevant, patient-focused, clearly written accreditation standards for in-home aide services. The purpose of those initial accreditation standards was to enhance and support the quality of health care services received by the patient. The values that supported the development of the initial standards continue to guide the organization today.

ACHC has gained respect and recognition as the accrediting organization uniquely committed to supporting those directly responsible for health care delivery. It has adopted a participatory approach to standards development that actively solicits the input of those providers and organizations most knowledgeable about current approaches to care. The result has been the development and promulgation of standards that are quality driven, practical in application, and effective in assuring optimum care delivery to the patient. In addition, the entire accrediting process is designed to positively impact the way care is delivered through an approach that is collaborative, educational, and genuinely patient focused.

In 1993, ACHC began to expand into other accreditation arenas with the addition of accreditation standards for in-home nursing services. In 1996, ACHC expanded its vision geographically and began offering accreditation services nationally. In the last 16 years, the demand for ACHC to expand into other health care accrediting arenas has led to the development of standards for home health, home medical equipment, specialty pharmacy, mail order medical supply, hospice, rehabilitation technology supplier services, home infusion, respiratory nebulizer medications, and women's services.

MISSION, PURPOSE, VALUES, CORE COMPETENCY, AND QUALITY POLICY

ACHC is dedicated to supporting in the quality of home care and alternate site health care services. The following points underscore the company's ideology to fulfill its commitment to consumers and providers:

- Mission: To support health care organizations and providers in optimizing wellness through standards that promote the effective and efficient delivery of quality services and products.

- Purpose: To help our customers succeed.
- Values: Integrity, Relevance, Innovation, Enhancing Outcomes, Excellence in all Things, Flexibility Without Compromising Quality, and Concern for the Entire Health care Continuum.
- CORE Competency: Home care and alternate site services accreditation standards. A collaborative, relevant approach to the entire accreditation process.
- Quality Policy–ISO 9001-2000: The Accreditation Commission for Health Care is committed to developing and improving health care accreditation programs and services, enhancing employee skills and efficiencies, continually improving of our quality management systems and processes, sustained fiscal growth and improved market presence.

BOARD OF COMMISSIONERS

ACHC is managed by its board of commissioners, which can include up to 29 members. The board employs a president/chief executive officer (CEO) and staff to manage the daily operations. ACHC has 50 contract surveyors that conduct the on-site reviews. The current board makeup includes members from a number of health care services including home care aide services, private duty nursing, home health, pharmacy, home medical equipment, respiratory therapy, hospice, rehabilitation, women's services, pharmacy, and consumer representatives. In addition, ACHC commissioners include the public at large, general business, and manufacturers of health care products.

There are seven standing committees of the board of commissioners. These include the Executive, the Accreditation Review, the Ethics, the Finance, the Standards and Procedures, the Nominations, and the Advisory committees. The chairperson of the board appoints the members of the committees. The board meets quarterly and has decision-making authority for approval of accreditation of customers and all matters of policy and strategy.

ACCREDITATION PROGRAMS

ACHC offers programs tailored specifically to the home care and alternate site health care industry.

- Aide Program: Aide service (i.e., home care aide organization) encompasses all levels including personal care services, chores, companion sitters, and homemakers.
- Home Infusion Program: The infusion therapy continuum of care includes intravenous (IV) drug mixture preparation, IV administration, therapy monitoring, patient counseling, and education. It is the administration of medications using intravenous, subcutaneous, and epidural routes. The IV therapies include IV antibiotics, prescribed primarily for diagnoses such as steomyelitis, sepsis, cellulites total patenteral nutrition, pneumonia, sexually transmitted diseases, and others.
- The ACHC home infusion scope of services section includes infusion nursing, pharmacy services, clinical respiratory care, home medical equipment, rehab technology supplier, and post-mastectomy fitter services.
- Home Medical Equipment Program: Home medical equipment/durable medical equipment includes home health care products, medical supplies, and/or respiratory therapy services provided to a patient in a home. ACHC accredits home medical equipment services, clinical respiratory care, rehab technology services, and post-mastectomy fitter services.
- Hospice Program: Hospice is the care of terminally ill patients in a health care setting that emphasizes quality of life through patient and family involvement in the

home or inpatient environment. End of life care involves a team approach for medical care, pain management, and emotional and spiritual support. ACHC accredits standard hospice services, inpatient services, and pharmacy services.

- Women's Health Care Program: Women's health encompasses the physical and psycho-social needs for women's personal care products and services such as post-mastectomy, including prosthesis fitting, compression therapy, and hair loss, as well as pregnancy, child birth, and incontinence. ACHC accredits fitter services.
- Home Health Program: Home health care replicates the hospital situation in the home for noncritical patients and gives the primary care givers and/or family an opportunity to participate in the care planning process. The integrated continuum of care covers the patient from physician, to hospital, to the home. Home health includes Medicare-certified and noncertified services provided to a patient in a home setting. The primary focus is to help patients recover from acute or chronic illnesses and improve independence in daily activities. ACHC accredits nursing services, physical therapy services, occupational therapy services, speech therapy services, medical social services, clinical respiratory care, and home care aide.
- ACHC accredits Private Duty Agencies with standards in the Home Health program. Private Duty is supportive care provided by homemaker aides and/or registered nurses. A client can purchase private duty care with or without a physician's order. It can include nonmedical services for people who simply need help with daily tasks of living due to aging, chronic conditions, or a disability.
- Specialty Pharmacy Services: A specialty pharmacy company is one that dispenses medications, usually self-injectable, or biotechnology drugs to a patient's home, physician's office, or clinics specializing in certain chronic disease states. Exam-

ples of specialty pharmacy drugs include human growth hormone, Avonex, Rebetron, Remicade, and Viracept Epivir.
- Mail Order Medical Supply: This involves the storage and delivery of home medical equipment and/or medical supplies designed to meet the needs of a client requiring the product for their medical management in the home care setting. A physician generally prescribes these services. The items sold are usually disposable or semi-durable in nature.
- Rehabilitation Technology Supplier Services: Rehabilitation technology supplier services are defined as the application of enabling technology systems designed to meet the needs of a specific person experiencing any permanent or long-term loss or abnormality of physical or anatomical structure or function. These services, prescribed by a physician, primarily address wheeled mobility, seating and alternative positioning, ambulation support and equipment, environmental control, augmented communication, and other equipment and services that assist the person in performing their activities of daily living.
- Respiratory Nebulizer Medications: A Respiratory Nebulizer Medications program applies to a pharmacy that dispenses aerosolized single patient dose respiratory medications. The medications may be prepackaged or compounded by the pharmacy. They are usually delivered directly to the client's home. These medications usually benefit a targeted patient population with a chronic disease such as emphysema, chronic bronchitis, or asthma.

STANDARDS DEVELOPMENT

ACHC has adopted a participatory approach to standards development. Task force groups are made up of providers and state and national association representatives. Standards are focused on patient safety, quality health care, and relevance to the particular health care market being served.

The interpretation given after each criterion provides an explanation of the standard to assist the applicant in determining acceptable evidence. The format and writing style of the standards are in clear, comprehensive language.

The standards are divided into a common core for all manuals and a scope of services section unique to each manual. Core standards are arranged into seven sections: (1) organization and administration; (2) program/service operations; (3) fiscal management; (4) personnel management; (5) client service/care management; (6) quality outcomes/improvement; and (7) risk management for infection and safety control. The scope of services section in each manual covers skilled clinical services unique to that particular program category.

SELF-ASSESSMENT/PRELIMINARY EVIDENCE

The applicant organization uses each standard to conduct a self-assessment to determine its level of compliance and makes necessary changes to assure compliance with standards for policy requirements, internal processes, and the quality of services performed.

The preparation time will vary with each organization depending upon its resources and its ability to stay focused on a systematic plan of evaluating compliance with ACHC standards and making the necessary changes in policy and practice.

It is suggested that the applicant provider utilize a team approach. For internal use only, ACHC standards may be reproduced and distributed among the team members. The staff should read thoroughly the sections that contain Accreditation Policies and Procedures, the Interpretive Guide to Standards, Instructions for Organizing Evidence, and the Preliminary Evidence Report.

An action plan is developed that the staff can follow to conduct a self-assessment and for correcting areas that need to be implemented or improved. Staff participation in this stage is required. Policies should address the actual processes of business operations and how delivery of services is carried out.

It is also suggested that the team meet on a regular scheduled basis to determine progress and to exchange ideas. This stage will take time, but is designed to help the company identify strengths and weakness so that appropriate corrective actions can be made. These meetings can also be used to plan periodic audits on different topics to realistically assess progress. Specific areas may exist that may need more attention prior to the survey visit.

Completion of survey preparation means that the company can demonstrate that its organization fulfills its mission, practices what its policies detail, and is in substantial compliance with ACHC standards. At this point it is time for the applicant to submit the Preliminary Evidence Report and schedule the on-site visit.

The Preliminary Evidence Report is submitted with the application. The policies submitted will be forwarded to the assigned surveyor(s) to conduct a desk review. The policies will be reviewed approximately 2 to 3 weeks prior to the survey visit. Initial scoring is accomplished with this review.

The applicant organization may submit additional supporting evidence prior to the survey visit or label and make available at the time of the visit without losing credit for evidence presented.

SURVEY SITE VISIT

Surveys are usually scheduled and announced. However, ACHC conducts triennial surveys that are unannounced. All surveys provide significant consultative and educational services.

During the site visit, the surveyor(s) will conduct a review of the following: personnel files, client records, budgetary information, policies and procedures, the quality improvement plan, and operational and service delivery outcomes. Interviews will be done with staff and clients.

Typical Agenda for the Site Visit

On the First Day

Conduct an opening conference.

Interview the leader and/or executives of the organization and representative of the board and/or advisory committee.

Interview the quality improvement coordinator.

Interview the program or clinical supervisor.

Review contracts and interview the business manager/accounting clerk.

Select and review personnel records.

Select and review client records.

Select clients to be interviewed.

Develop the agenda for visits and interviews.

(For some small organizations, the survey may be only one day.)

On the Second Day

Visit and interview clients (some interviews may be done by telephone).

Interview staff members.

Interview case managers (when applicable).

Interview service supervisors.

Interview an intake worker who describes the company's services to the public.

Review documented outcomes of quality improvement activities.

Review minutes of staff meetings, board meetings, and planning sessions.

Exit Conference.

Additional Days May Be Added as Necessary

Depending on the number of programs, the services offered, and the size of the organization, a surveyor or team of surveyors might conduct visits to a number of branch locations or such similar activities for several days.

Expert Advice

ACHC surveyors have a diverse range of business and clinical expertise. The average length of time in their chosen fields is 15 years. Their aim is to provide guidance into the best business and clinical practices and to instill the continuous quality improvement ethic into management of ACHC applicants.

SCORING AND THE REVIEW COMMITTEE

Once data are collected, the sum of actual points divided by the total possible points related to each standard results in a compliance percentage threshold that is averaged for each section. Standards related to supervision of services and contracts must be in compliance for accreditation. The organization must score a minimum threshold of 85 percent for each section and for each service provided to earn accreditation.

Completed data collection and scoring tools are forwarded to the ACHC Accreditation Services, along with documented surveyor comments. The ACHC staff completes a Scoring Summary including the data collection and scoring tools, and comments made by the surveyor, which is forwarded to the Accreditation Review Committee for determination.

The Accreditation Review Committee represents the third level of peer review prior to the committee's decision. The committee activities include a review of the overall survey-documented evidence, the scoring summary, and an evaluation of the surveyor recommendations.

Review committee decisions are reported to the board of commissioners at least quarterly. The review committee will approve, defer, or deny accreditation.

The office sites and services for which accreditation has been granted are described in a letter of accreditation approval included with the certificate of accreditation. Additional copies of the certificate are provided for all branch locations included in the survey process.

Accreditation is awarded for a period of 3 years from the first of the month following the date a decision is rendered (anniversary date). Accreditation is contingent upon receipt of total fees and continuing compliance with the standards and the Accreditation Policies and Procedures.

ACHC reserves the right to make announced or unannounced on-site visits at any time during a 3-year accreditation cycle to determine continuing compliance with standards. If an interim visit results in the need for a full survey, the organization will be responsible for appropriate fees.

Organizations must accurately describe only the program(s) and services accredited by ACHC when advertising its accreditation status to the general public. False or misleading advertising shall be grounds for withdrawal of accreditation.

CONCLUSION

There are several advantages of ACHC accreditation. The process itself helps an organization assess company policies and practices with a view to improving programs and services. Accreditation strengthens staff accountability and directs supervisors to focus on goal management. Approval affords a competitive advantage when bidding or negotiating services contracts, increases morale and pride of employees, and alerts the public that national standards have been met. Most importantly, it assures the community that quality patient care is the company's priority. ACHC's cooperative problem-solving approach is a major benefit of the program, and successful completion of the accreditation process is the goal.

REFERENCES

Accreditation Commission for Health Care, Inc. 2002. *Setting standards in accreditation*, Raleigh, NC: ACHC.

Accreditation Commission for Health Care, Inc. 2004–2005. *Home health accreditation manual*, 4th edition, Raleigh, NC: ACHC.

CHAPTER 8

Certificate of Need and Licensure

E. Michael Flanagan

At first glance, a health care entrepreneur's interest in home health as a business is understandable. The product to be furnished is readily identifiable, and labor rather than material intensive. This means that the anticipated capital outlay for start-up costs should be minimal.

It is only when the entrepreneur confronts the complex and often confusing array of federal and state laws and regulations governing home health agencies (HHAs) that the hidden costs of establishing a home care program are realized.

This chapter discusses two aspects of this regulatory scheme: certificate of need (CON) and licensure. The impact of CON and licensure requirements on HHAs varies dramatically depending on the state in which the HHA operates.[1] It is important from the standpoint of marketing feasibility, however, to understand the specific requirements of the jurisdiction in which one plans to establish a home health program.

Finally, because many states have merged their state licensure function with their responsibilities concerning certification of new Medicare providers, some discussion of Medicare certification will be inevitable in this chapter, even though that topic is covered in more detail elsewhere in this book.

HHA CON REQUIREMENTS

Background

When Congress passed the National Health Planning and Resources Development Act of 1974,[2] it sought to rationalize the distribution of health services throughout the United States and to give individual states a legal mechanism to make prospective determinations of need for new health care services. These laudable objectives proved more problematic in practice than originally envisioned, and the 29 years since the enactment of the law have seen the once energetically federal initiative become a creature of state law. Federal funding for health planning is nonexistent today, and many states have repealed their CON laws and substituted more stringent licensure requirements for health care facilities.

The establishment of an HHA historically has required a limited capital expenditure. Moreover, the existence of CON requirements for HHAs in certain states has failed to demonstrate a positive correlation between restricted market entry and lower costs per unit of service.[3] Consequently, a number of states have reconsidered the need to include HHAs in their CON laws, and at least four states (Texas, Tennessee, California, and Florida) have eliminated HHAs from CON review in recent years.[4] The Medicare program's recent transition to the Prospective Payment Sysem (PPS) will probably convince more states in the future to eliminate HHAs from CON review because of the perceived constraints on the growth of HHAs due to fixed payments based on episodes of care.

Impact on Feasibility Study

When someone decides to explore the possibility of entering the home health care market as a provider of services, essentially two options are available. The first is acquisition of part or all of an existing home health care business. The second is the creation of a new HHA that will compete for a share of the existing market. The presence of a CON law for HHAs in the state of intended operation is often the single most important determinant in deciding whether to go forward with the project in that state and under which option.

Some form of feasibility study is desirable for any prospective entrant into the home health care business. The first consideration identified in a creditable feasibility study will be barriers to entry into the market. For example, some states (including Georgia, Alabama, Kentucky, and Mississippi) have at one time or another imposed moratoriums on the issuance of new HHA CONs. This would mean that the only opportunity for entry in these states would be the acquisition of an existing Medicare-certified HHA or establishment of a private-pay HHA (i.e., an agency that provides no services to Medicare or Medicaid beneficiaries), if that is not a reviewable event under state law.[5]

A potential barrier to entry has arisen within the past few years because of federal government cutbacks in funding for state Medicare survey agencies and the general sense in federal and state government that there are an excessive number of HHAs in existence already. It is obvious that acquisition of an existing HHA under these circumstances would be preferable to fighting bureaucratic indifference to obtain a new provider certification.

For all of the reasons just noted, if the state of operation in the new entrant's business plan is not predetermined, the existence of CON requirements could lead to the selection of a different state. Such a move is not without risk.

Selecting a Non-CON State

The selection of a non-CON state will have the immediate beneficial effect of eliminating the need for significant start-up costs for consulting, legal, and accounting expenses related to obtaining CON approval. On the other hand, absence of CON means that other competitors (including local hospitals) can invade the market at any time and steal away referral sources and valued employees.

Survival in such a competitive environment is difficult. Hospitals more than likely will have their own facility-based HHAs to capture their own home health referrals. At the same time, these hospitals will put pressure on their staff physicians to refer patients to the hospital-based agency. In addition, national chain home health providers are generally more active in these markets because their size allows them to endure the financial strains of longer start-up periods.

Thus the decision to pursue a non-CON state is not a panacea. In fact, certain state HHAs (Florida and Georgia, for example) have fought to preserve their state CON programs for HHAs motivated in large measure by their belief that CON is the only way to preserve the freestanding community-based HHA. In Florida, the HHAs lost that battle a few years ago as the law was permitted to sunset.

Acquiring an HHA in a CON State

Recognizing the difficulties of surviving in a non-CON state, it may be advisable to explore acquisition opportunities in a CON state.[6] In most CON states, the acquisition of an HHA's stock or a transfer of assets is considered a change of ownership. As such, unless the change of ownership is accompanied by a change in the scope of services or service area, it will be determined to be a nonreviewable event.[7]

It is often the case, however, that the state health planning agency will require notice of the change of ownership at some time in advance of the event.[8] Thus the recommended manner of proceeding is to identify the intended acquisition, negotiate the purchase offer, and then send a formal letter of intent to acquire the HHA to the state health planning agency. The letter should also request written confirmation that the acquisition is a nonreviewable event under the state CON law. Once the confirmation letter is received, the need to focus on CON issues is at an end unless a later modification of service or service area necessitates review.

If the acquisition entails simply a transfer of part or all of the existing agency's stock, the transaction might not even fall under the CON law's change of ownership rules. Thus, as in all potential CON matters, a careful review of the law and regulations could avoid unnecessary headaches.[9]

Obtaining a CON

This discussion is not for the faint of heart. Under the best of circumstances, obtaining a CON in a conscientiously regulated state can be a brutal affair involving intense political influence wielding and courtroom battles with established HHAs in the affected service area.

Based on experience, it can be anticipated that obtaining a CON will add $100,000 to $200,000 to agency start-up costs. This figure can rise significantly if an adversely affected HHA files suit to enjoin issuance of the CON. In one of the more famous CON wars, Johnson & Johnson waged a major campaign to obtain HHA CONs in Florida several years ago. The widely publicized assault on the state CON program ultimately brought the Florida Association of Home Health Agencies into the fray on the side of the state health planning agency. After having the regulatory basis upon which need determinations had been made in Florida since 1975 declared invalid,[10] Johnson & Johnson abandoned the effort, having spent approximately $3 million in a losing cause.

If you are still undaunted by the bleak prospects of obtaining a CON, then the first step to take would be to examine the CON law and regulations to determine whether there is any way validly to claim entitlement to an exemption from the review requirement.

Exemptions may be available for a number of reasons based on your particular circumstances. We have already discussed the exemption based on change of ownership. Some states have so-called "grandfather" provisions in the CON law that exempt from review existing HHAs that have been providing home health services continuously in the state since a time before the effective data of the CON law. The "grandfather" provision that was a part of the Florida licensure law[11] until repealed in 1990 furnishes an excellent illustration of this type of exemption:

> Any home health agency operating and providing services in the state and having a provider number issued by the U.S. Department of Health, Education and Welfare on or before April 30, 1976 shall not be denied a license on the basis of not having received a Certificate of Need.[12]

Historically, Florida administered its CON program on a district-by-district basis, each district comprising one or more counties. Because of this, HHAs that were Medicare certified and operational in the state before April 30, 1976, successfully used the "grandfather" provision to expand their service areas. By simply demonstrating to the state health planning agency that it had seen one or more patients in the expansion district before the effective date, the HHA was able to obtain a determination that it would be exempt from review and able to serve that entire district as fully as any other preexisting HHA already serving the district.

Another exemption category applies to health maintenance organizations (HMOs) that seek to furnish home health services directly. Many states generally exempt HMOs from the coverage of their CON laws[13] when they are furnishing otherwise covered health care services to their members only. It is unclear, however, whether the exemption would apply to all services that the HMO furnishes directly.

Obviously, exemptions are exceptions to the rule that new HHAs must submit to CON review. If no exemption is available and acquisition is not feasible, it is important to have some understanding of the typical CON-review process so that a strategy can be developed to ensure the best chance of a favorable outcome.

A Typical CON-Review Process

All state CON laws differ in certain respects concerning the formalities of the review process, but here an attempt is made to outline a typical review sequence based on Maryland law.

The first step in the filing of a CON application is the submission of a letter of intent to the health planning agency.[14] If you are unfamiliar with the process generally, a telephone call to the agency would be advisable. Experience indicates that health planning staff persons can be extremely helpful in guiding applicants through the maze of red tape that invariably accompanies CON actions.

The letter of intent is designed to alert the agency of an impending CON application. It usually includes the following information: a description of the proposed project, the nature and scope of new health services to be offered, the location of the project, and the estimated total project cost.[15] The letter of intent normally sets in motion a time period within which to file the CON application. Under Maryland law, the CON application must be submitted at least 60 days after the submission of the letter of intent,

but the application must be received before the expiration of 180 days from the date of submission of the letter of intent.[16] If the application is received too early, it can be held over until the next review period after the expiration of the 60 days. If no application has been received by the expiration of the 180 days, the letter of intent is null and void, and the applicant must start over.[17] Time requirements vary from state to state, so it is essential to know your particular state's rules.

It is also important to realize that a CON application takes a good deal of time and effort to complete and that the burden of proving entitlement to a CON rests squarely on the applicant. If you are serious about obtaining a CON, it is advisable at this point to hire a consultant who specializes in completing and justifying CON applications. It is also a good idea at this time to start lining up whatever political assistance is available to you to begin the necessary lobbying effort to convince the state health planning agency of the need for a new HHA.

Once the application is submitted, the planning agency reviews it for completeness and assigns a docket number.[18] The agency will then notify the applicant in writing of the docketing and will also publish notice of the docketing in a newspaper of general circulation in the area of the proposed project.[19]

Some state planning programs (such as Maryland's) have routine review cycles into which similar applications are batched for the purpose of comparative review. In other words, if three new HHA CON applications are submitted in the same month, they will be assigned together to the same batching cycle, and their individual merits will be assessed in comparison with one another. Thus if only one new HHA is justified in the area, the best applicant of the three will be selected.

Parties that will be affected by the project (referred to in CON laws as *interested persons* or *interested parties*)[20] are entitled to request an evidentiary hearing to be conducted by the planning agency.[21] As a general rule, the hearing must be requested within a certain time period after the notice of docketing is published. The evidentiary hearing is conducted in a fashion similar to a courtroom trial, with counsel representing the parties, oral testimony including examination and cross-examination of witnesses, and a written report by the presiding officer with findings of fact and conclusions of law.[22] The final action of the evidentiary hearing is the issuance by the presiding officer of a proposed order, which will become final after the parties to the hearing have had an opportunity to file written objections and to give oral testimony before final action on the application.[23] The final order in most instances is a grant or denial of the application.

Regardless of whether the application is submitted to an evidentiary hearing or to comparative or individual review, its merits will be judged against certain parameters of need established by the state health planning program. These considerations will generally include the identification of a need for such a service in the state health plan,[24] the need of the population served or to be served (a supplemental analysis to the general need determinations included in the state health plan), the availability of less costly or more effective alternatives for addressing the unmet needs identified by the applicant, the immediate and long-term financial viability of the project, and the adequacy of staffing, community, and professional support for the project.[25]

The decision of the planning agency concerning the application must be issued within a certain time period of docketing.[26] The planning agency can decide to grant the application, to deny it, or to grant it subject to specific conditions.[27] The decision must be in writing, setting forth the reasons for the action.

Assuming that the project has been approved either completely or with acceptable conditions, you might be lulled into thinking that your new HHA is home free. This, however, may be only the beginning of the ordeal. The final decision has created a new class of participants in the CON process called aggrieved parties. An *aggrieved party* is essentially an interested party who has been adversely affected by the final decision.[28] An aggrieved party (which obviously includes the applicant if the decision was a denial) has the right to file exceptions and present arguments to the majority of commissioners making the decision in order to seek reconsideration of the final decision.[29]

Finally, an aggrieved party has the right to take a direct judicial appeal within a specified time frame of the date of the final decision.[30] The judicial appeal is normally made to the trial court level of the state court system, but the review of the case is normally limited to the record that has been developed in the administrative process. Furthermore, any decision at the trial court level may be appealed to the highest appellate level of the state courts and ultimately (carrying the process to its most sublimely ridiculous extent) to the U.S. Supreme Court if a sufficiently national issue can be demonstrated.

SUMMARY

It should be clear from the tenor of the foregoing presentation that it is the opinion of this author that the CON process is an ineffective tool to ensure the appropriate distribution of health care resources. It is tedious, expensive, and ultimately incapable of preventing the granting of unnecessary projects to those with the will and financial and political backing to outlast the process. It is, however, a mandatory precondition to the establishment of a new HHA in 18 states and the District of Columbia. Thus if there is no alternative to submission to the CON process, the foregoing information should prove useful.

HHA LICENSURE

Background

Because in states that have HHA licensure laws the license requirement is not used as a barrier to entry into the marketplace, there is no need to go into elaborate detail about the nuances of the licensure process. The political, practical, and economic realities of licensure are unambiguous: If the HHA meets certain conditions established by the state, it will be issued a license; if not, the HHA will not be permitted to operate until the conditions are met.

In some states, such as California and New York, the licensure laws are so stringent and are enforced so rigorously that, from the standpoint of economic feasibility, they may constitute a barrier to the establishment of a new HHA. The California and New York experiences, however, are clearly the exception.

Of the 39 state licensure laws (including those of the District of Columbia) for HHAs, virtually all have requirements that track closely with the Medicare program's conditions of participation.[31] In fact, most states have unified their state licensure and Medicare certification functions into one office, which coordinates survey activities for both.

Before the Omnibus Budget Reconciliation Act of 1980, if an HHA was established in a state that had no HHA licensure law, the HHA was prohibited from participating in the Medicare program unless it had obtained status as a charitable organization under section 501(c)(3) of the Internal Revenue Code. This restriction was apparently based on the assumption that for-profit HHAs are inherently suspect without a state regulatory body in existence to police their operations. The 1980 legislation abolished such distinctions as a matter of federal law, but at least one state (New York) retained the restriction as a matter of state law until a few years ago.

State HHA licensure laws have generally been administered without much controversy, but it is important to understand your state's law (if any) so that potential problem areas can be anticipated.

Typical Licensure Law

Most states that have HHA licensure laws make it a criminal offense for anyone to operate an HHA without a license. In many instances, however, the licensure requirement applies only to those HHAs that intend to participate in the Medicare or Medicaid program. An HHA that is treating only private insurance or private pay patients might not be required to be licensed. The licensure law sets out minimum operational standards for HHAs operating in the state that must be met at all times. An applicant for initial licensure must furnish certain information to the licensing office on forms provided by the office, including the names and addresses of each officer and director of the HHA and of certain owners.[32]

Upon receipt of the application, the licensing office will schedule a survey to ensure that the HHA meets all requirements. The timing of the licensure survey in relation to the operational start-up of the HHA varies from state to state. It is important to make contact with the licensure office in advance of the survey to ascertain the level of activity the survey team is expecting to see by the date of the survey. Most states will not permit the HHA to see a patient before the license is issued. Others will expect to review a patient chart or two and thus will require some minimal visit activity before the licensure survey.

Essentially, the survey team will be seeking to determine that the key personnel of the HHA have the requisite skill level, that the required scope of services will be provided either directly or through contractual arrangements, that the HHA complies with all applicable state and federal laws, that the HHA has appropriate liability insurance to cover all employees and contractual indemnity to cover services provided under arrangement, and that the HHA has the requisite recordkeeping capability.[33]

If the HHA passes the survey, the state will issue a license for a 1-year period. Most states require that the annual application for relicensure be submitted well in advance of the expiration date (generally 60 days) so that any reinspection can be done and a new license issued before the expiration date. In at least one state (Florida), an administrative fine of $100 per day is levied against any HHA submitting its relicensure application less than 60 days before the expiration date.

If the HHA fails to meet licensure requirements, it will be denied a license. This decision is subject to appeal under the state's Administrative Procedures Act.

Finally, under certain circumstances the state can issue a provisional license (of normally 90 days in duration) to an HHA that is not in substantial compliance if the HHA has submitted an acceptable plan of correction to resolve the areas of noncompliance.[34]

Once the license is issued, it must be displayed in a place viewable by the general public.[35] If the HHA decides to relinquish the license voluntarily, or if it is denied, revoked, or suspended under administrative action, the HHA must provide requisite notice to the patients, their authorized representatives, attending physicians, and third-party payers.[36]

The licensing agency has the right to investigate complaints and to ensure that the HHA is maintaining compliance with all licensure requirements including the governing authority of the HHA,[37] proper personnel,[38] staff supervision and training,[39] and the maintenance and safeguarding of clinical records.[40]

Some Legal and Practical Considerations About Licensure

Although licensure issues do not often arise as legal problems, some points about licensure in the context of CON and Medicare certification should be kept in mind.

As has already been mentioned, in CON states for HHAs, a CON or a formal exemption determination is a precondition to the issuance of a license. It is also true in many states, however, that the continuing viability of the CON is dependent on uninterrupted licensure. Thus if for some reason the HHA license is suspended or revoked, or if the agency ceases to operate for any period of time, the state, or more likely, a competing HHA, could assert that the CON has lapsed. It is important, therefore, that any licen-

sure defects be rectified as soon as possible to avoid threatening the CON.

Licensure problems also seem to arise almost magically when an HHA is forced to fire one of its key employees. An unannounced inspection always seems to follow shortly on the heels of a terminated administrator. Accordingly, if it becomes necessary to fire a key employee, it is often wise to alert the licensure office that the action is pending and that you have taken appropriate steps to hire a qualified replacement. A preventive phone call could save you the aggravation of being visited by licensing inspectors carrying an order to show cause as to why the HHA should not be closed down for being improperly staffed.

Another problem with the license as it affects CON is the fact that health planning authorities look to the license to ascertain the HHA's service area. In states in which the service area is not clearly articulated in the CON, the counties or subdivisions listed on the HHA's license are looked upon as the best evidence of the HHA's service area. Thus whenever a licensure form needs to be completed that asks for any identification of service area (for example, single county or multicounty), to the extent that your answer is not clearly inconsistent with your CON approval, always select the most expansive definition.

Finally, it should be kept in mind that licensure is a precondition to Medicare certification, and although the two offices generally work closely together they do not always coordinate their efforts carefully enough. If a new HHA obtains Medicare certification before licensure is effective, or if licensure is lost for any period of time, the HHA will be forced to forfeit all payment for Medicare services furnished during the period without licensure.

CONCLUSION

If you are interested in becoming involved in the ownership and operation of an HHA, and you are still convinced after reading this chapter, press on. As the chapter indicates, there are often ways to circumvent the costly and time-consuming burdens of confronting the CON process head on. Licensure, on the other hand, must be faced, but it is not nearly so cumbersome or threatening a process. The important principle to keep in mind in dealing with CON and licensure issues is that anticipation and prevention of problems can save enormous headaches and expenses that come as a result of reacting to crises. Before you go flailing head-long into the regula-

tory process that encompasses home health care, establish a business plan, do a marketing feasibility study, retain competent advisors who are knowledgeable in the area, and develop a good working relationship with the government agencies that will determine your entitlement to CON and licensure. The game plan is to accomplish your objectives with the least possible expenditure of your resources. In the present home health care marketplace, there is no substitute for cost consciousness.

NOTES

1. At the present time, 39 states and the District of Columbia have CON and/or licensure requirements for HHAs. It should be noted, however, that not all states that have one requirement have the other. Thus 39 states and the District of Columbia have HHA licensure laws, and 18 states and the District of Columbia have HHA CON laws, but 3 of the HHA CON states (Vermont, Alabama, and West Virginia) have no HHA licensure laws. Furthermore, state legislatures are continually reviewing the need for such laws, particularly CON. Notably, the Florida legislature in 1992 reenacted the state licensure and CON laws by a narrow margin, but included a sunset provision in the new law that caused it to expire on July 1, 1997.

2. P.L. 93-641, 88 Stat. 2225 (January 4, 1975).

3. See generally Anderson, K.B., de Kass, D.S. (1986). *Certificate of need regulation of entry into home health care.* Washington, DC: Bureau of Economics.

4. Tennessee had repealed its CON requirements for HHAs but reinstated them after a rapid expansion of new HHAs in the state threatened to destabilize the entire industry. California has dropped its CON program in its entirety.

5. Most of the 21 CON states require review only if the HHA intends to seek reimbursement from the Medicare or Medicaid programs. Some jurisdictions, including Tennessee, West Virginia, and the District of Columbia, require CON review for all in-home services without regard to payment source.

6. Acquisitions of existing HHAs in non-CON states do occur when the purchaser is seeking to acquire an established patient base and/or goodwill.

7. See, for example, Md. Ann. Code section 19-115 (i)(2)(iii); The Code of Maryland Regulations (COMAR) section 10.24.01.03A(I).

8. Ibid.

9. We are aware of one instance in which a new entrant fought a long, costly, and ultimately successful battle to obtain a new HHA CON only to realize later that it would have been entitled automatically to a CON under the CON law's grandfather provision.

10. Florida had been using the so-called "rule of 300" to make need determinations for new HHAs. The rule of 300 would prevent a new HHA from obtaining a CON unless it could demonstrate that all the existing agencies in the relevant market area had an average daily census of 300 patients. The rule was ultimately struck down by the Florida state courts as having been adopted without proper reliance on any empirical data justifying such a criterion.

11. Because in states having CON laws governing HHAs CON approval is a precondition to licensure, it is not uncommon that certain provisions in the licensure law will have a bearing on CON requirements. This is a point to bear in mind when determining whether to pursue CON.

12. Fla. Stat. Ann. section 400.,504 (1980). (Repealed by laws c. 90-319, § 10, effective July 3, 1990.)

13. See, for example, Md. Stat. Ann. section 19-124(b)(ii).

14. See COMAR section 10.24.01.07C.

15. COMAR section 10.24.01.07C(2).

16. COMAR section 10.24.01.07C(3) and (5).

17. Ibid.

18. COMAR section 10.24.01.08C.

19. COMAR section 10.24.01.08D.

20. Under Maryland law, an interested party includes, among others, the applicant, local health planning agency, and any person who can demonstrate any adverse impact brought about by the approval of the project. COMAR section 10.24.01.01B(16).
21. COMAR section 10.24.01.10D.
22. COMAR section 10.24.01.11.
23. COMAR section 10.24.01.09.
25. The state health plan is a document that sets present and projected need for the distribution of certain health care services and equipment throughout the state. Need is normally projected for a 5-year period.
25. COMAR section 10.24.01.08G(3).
26. See COMAR section 10.24.01.09D. In Maryland, the time period is 150 days if an evidentiary hearing is held and 90 days if not.
27. Ibid.
28. COMAR section 10.24.01.01B(2).
29. COMAR section 10.24.01.09D(6)(b).
30. COMAR section 10.24.01.09E.
31. For a comparative illustration of the various state HHA licensure laws and key elements of Medicare conditions of participation, see The "black box" of home care quality, a report presented by the chair of the Select Committee on Aging, House of Representatives, 99th Cong., 2d sess. Prepared by the American Bar Association (August 1986).
32. See COMAR section 10.07.10.04B.
33. See COMAR section 10.07.10.04. Most licensure laws require HHAs to provide skilled nursing services and at least one of the following: physical therapy, occupational therapy, speech therapy, medical social services, or home health aide.
34. COMAR section 10.07.10.05.
35. COMAR section 10.07.10.07.
36. COMAR section 10.07.01.06.
37. See COMAR section 10.07.01.08.
38. See COMAR section 10.07.01.09.
39. See COMAR section 10.07.01.10.
40. See COMAR section 10.07.01.11.

CHAPTER 9

Credentialing: Organizational and Personnel Options for Home Care

Ann H. Cary, PhD MPH RN A-CCC

CREDENTIALING AND CREDIBILITY

Credentialing is a process of assurance and monitoring that takes many forms in home care. This chapter provides an overview of credentialing options from both organizational and personnel perspectives, and reference sites for examining specific characteristics of each to ensure timely information. Credentialing processes and criteria change frequently as the industry is in a state of flux; therefore, you are encouraged to obtain "real-time" information from Web sites and communicate directly with the vendor.

> Credentialing is a term applied to processes used to designate that an individual, program, institution or product has met established standards set by an agent (governmental or nongovernmental) recognized as qualified to carry out this task. The standards may be minimum and mandatory or above the minimum and voluntary. Licensure, registration, accreditation, approval, certification, recognition or endorsement may be used to describe different credentialing processes, but this terminology is not applied consistently across different settings and countries. Credentials are marks or "stamps" of quality and achievement communicating to employers, payers, and consumers what to expect from a "credentialed" (person), specialist, course, or program of study, institution of higher education, hospital or health service, healthcare product, technology, or device. (Styles and Affara, 1998, p. 44)

Credentialing serves four purposes (Cary, 2003)

1. public protection
2. quality
3. consumer choice
4. competitive advantage

As such, any entity providing credentialing services and a credential should stand the test of meeting these four criteria. In the era of consumer choice, patient safety, and quality improvement, credentialing mechanisms are being scrutinized for relevance, effectiveness, and efficiency as stewards of these purposes.

What oversight exists for the credentialing vendors in the industry? Both governmental and voluntary oversight is currently available. The federal-level Center for Medicare and Medicaid Services (CMS) uses "deeming" as an oversight mechanism for credentialing organizations providing accreditation to providers of home care services. The deeming authority is provided by the Balanced Budget Act of 1997 (BBA) and subsequent Balanced Budget Refinement Act (BBRA) (1999) to CMS, who is authorized to establish and monitor national accreditation entities such as the Community Health Accreditation Program, Inc. (CHAP) and The Joint Commission on Accreditation of Healthcare Organizations (JCAHO). It can then accredit the compliance of home care agencies with Medicare requirements or conditions of participation (COP). The six areas deemed are: (1) quality assurance, (2) antidiscrimination, (3) access to services, (4) confidentiality and accuracy of enrollee records, (5) information on advance directives, and (6) provider participation rules (CHAP, 2003) Each state chooses a mechanism for regulating the existence of a home care agency operating in the state. From a voluntary perspective, the National Commission for Certifying Agencies (NCCA) accredits the certifying bodies for a number of professions and specialties. The American Board of Nursing Specialties (ABNS) and American Board of Medical Specialties (ABMS) accredit certification organizations for nursing and medicine, respectively. The American National Standards Institute (ANSI) is the U.S. International Organization for Standardization (ISO) member that accredits standards developers in particular subject areas (www.ansi.org, 2003). Health care organizations are beginning to realize the value of seeking ISO certification by meeting the ISO standards for processes that drive their performance improvement concerns. Although a newcomer to the health industry, the international recognition of this credential for organizations brings value-added characteristics recognized in a globally competitive environment. These are some of the "credentialers of credentialers" striving to provide oversight and a "checks-and-balance" approach to ensure the integrity of the credentialing industry.

All credentialing bodies need to be viewed by the public as credible. A natural component of credibility is meaningful public member representation on credentialing governing boards. Avoiding credentialing abuses such as restrictive markets and pricing are keys to credibility. Transparency in governance and operations processes allows for judgments of credibility.

The Consumer Advocacy Center (CAC) proposes five areas for investigation in choosing a credentialing body for the (home care) organization or the provider (Swankin, 1999):

1. Is the credentialing organization credible?
2. Is the credentialing organization accountable?
3. Is the credential meaningful?
4. Does the public understand the meaning of the credential?
5. Is periodic compliance or continuing competence required?

Clearly you are being asked to perform due diligence during your selection of a credentialing body for the organization or personnel in the organization, and to be able to defend your choice should the need arise.

ACCREDITATION AND RECOGNITION OF THE ORGANIZATION AND SERVICES

Agency administrators are constantly challenged to place well-qualified individuals in agency positions. Several sources of guidelines from federal, state, and local jurisdictions exist as well as others from organizations that promote agency accreditation. The trends in licensure and certification requirements for the agencies can be determined only by monitoring adaptations in state licensure laws for home health and/or hospice agencies. This chapter reviews options for both the minimum standards and distinctive credentials proposed for the agency and personnel.

Separate chapters in this book provide details of structures, processes, and outcomes for four of the five voluntary accreditations available for home care organizations and services. All use a standards-driven approach that means that standards and criteria define the scope of measurement and evidence to judge compliance with the accreditation requirements. The goal of these standards is to improve outcomes rather than to tell organizations how to achieve the outcomes. Standards are revised periodically as new evidence supports the need for change. Typically there is a fixed period for transitioning to revised standards, so it behooves an applicant to know the timeline for applicable standards. Although all are voluntary, those with deemed status (JCAHO, CHAP) have regulatory and reimbursement consequences and are considered proxy for mandatory regulatory requirements. Re-accreditation and monitoring reports are required, and the trend is for "unannounced" appraisals after the initial accreditation is earned. Typically a branded symbol achieves universal recognition of the accreditation status—Magnet, Gold Seal, and so forth. All require application and program fees. Eligibility for application typically requires that a period of operational time be met or that a threshold number of cases, patients, and/or visits be satisfied. All accreditation bodies do not provide the scope of credentialing for the same services, so you might consider matching the array of services covered by the accrediting body with the services you provide.

A new player, the Magnet Recognition Program, sponsored by the American Nurses Credentialing Center (ANCC), offers a voluntary credential of excellence in nursing services to all health care organizations including home health care. Magnet recognition is predicated on the achievement of excellence in scoring ranges of the 14 Standards of Nursing Administration, criteria to explicate each, and ample evidence to demonstrate the highest level of service. The recognition program is evidence based, relying on studies of hospitals (McClure and Hinshaw, 2002). However, it offers a powerful exemplar of recognition for the highest standards of care delivery, productive work environments, patient care outcomes, and nurse satisfaction. The home care industry has been slow to earn this credential, and organizations would be wise to seek more information about the Magnet credential with its ability to differentiate excellence in care delivery and nursing work environments (ANCCB, 2003).

Figure 9-1 lists credentialing organizations applicable for home care organizations and services as well as their contact information at the time of publication. You are advised to contact the organizations at the time of interest to obtain the most current information about their programs and requirements.

CERTIFICATION OF HOME CARE PERSONNEL

The current COP guidelines for home health care agencies specify the nature of credentialing requirements for agency personnel to minimally meet the federal standards for Medicare approval. Readers are advised to consult the Web site, www.access.gpo.gov/nara/cfr, in order to obtain the most recent version of CMS requirements for home health personnel. As of this printing, the 1991 guidelines applied but were under revision. To provide a sense of the guidelines as of late 2003, they are included here for home health care personnel.

Home health agencies are directed to utilize only individuals whose practices are congruent with professional standards in the specific health disciplines. CMS has issued the rules and regulations for home health aide training and competency requirements. The regulatory standards for nonadministrative personnel are diverse within titles and between professional and semiprofessional categories. Mechanisms for determining qualifications include licensure, certification, work and educational experience, proficiency examination grades, and competency training. As new therapies are included in reimbursement packages, standards for these specialists will need to be developed. The ANA issued a Scope and Standards of Practice for Home Health Nurses in 1999 and another for nursing administration in 2003. ANCC sponsors the certification exams for each. Agency-specific standards plus state practice acts have constituted major credentialing options for providers.

Federal qualifying standards for nonadministrator personnel, initially published in 1985 and amended in the document 42 CFR Part 484 in 1989 and 1991, include the following designations:

Figure 9–1 Accreditation Organizations for Home Health Care and Home Care Services

ACCREDITATION COMMISSION FOR HEALTH CARE, INC (ACHC)
www.achc.org
5816 Creedmoor Road, Suite 201
Raleigh, NC 27612
919-785-1214; e-fax 734-939-6272
National in scope, hospice and home care as well as other services, not "deemed," independent private, not for profit.

AMERICAN NURSES CREDENTIALING CENTER (ANCC)
MAGNET RECOGNITION PROGRAM
www.nursecredentialing.org
600 Maryland Ave. SW, Suite 100 West
Washington, DC 20024
202-651-7261; fax 202-488-8190
International in scope, hospice, home health care, health care services, not "deemed," independent, not for profit.

COMMUNITY HEALTH ACCREDITATION PROGRAM, INC. (CHAP)
www.chapinc.org
39 Broadway, Suite 710.
New York, NY 10006
800-656-9656; fax 212-480-8832
National in scope, home and community-based health care organizations, "deemed," independent, not for profit.

JOINT COMMISSION ON ACCREDITATION OF HEALTHCARE ORGANIZATIONS (JCAHO)
www.jcaho.org
One Renaissance Blvd.
Oak Brook Terrace, IL 60181
630-792-5000; fax 630-792-5005
International in scope, home and hospice and health care services, "deemed," independent, not for profit.

NATIONAL ASSOCIATION FOR HOME CARE ACCREDITATION FOR HOMEMAKER/HOME CARE AIDE SERVICES ADMINISTERED BY HOME CARE UNIVERSITY, AN AFFILIATE OF THE NATIONAL ASSOCIATION FOR HOME CARE AND HOSPICE (NAHC)
www.nahc.org
228 Seventh St.
Washington, DC 20003
202-547-7424; fax 202-547-3540
National in scope, home and hospice aides and services, private duty nursing, not "deemed," independent, not for profit.

- Skilled nursing is provided by or through the direction of a registered nurse. The registered nurse must have graduated from an approved professional school of nursing and be licensed as a registered nurse in the state of practice.

- Licensed practical nurse standards require that the person be a licensed practical (vocational) nurse in his or her state of practice.
- Physician standards include holding a Doctor of Medicine, Doctor of Osteopa-

thy, or Doctor of Podiatry and legal authorization to practice medicine and surgery in the current state of practice

- Physical therapists need to maintain current licensure as physical therapists in their state of practice. The educational preparation, training opportunities, and qualifying examination criteria for those trained within and outside the United States are clearly described.

- Physical therapy assistant standards include state licensure to practice where applicable, experience, and proficiency examination demonstration. For exceptions see § 484.4.

- Occupational therapist standards include any combination of graduation from an approved and accredited school, eligibility for the National Register Examination of the American Occupational Therapy Association, or the combination of experience and satisfactory grade performance on a proficiency examination. For exceptions see § 484.4.

- Occupational therapy assistants must be certified as assistants by the American Occupational Therapy Association or have 2 years of experience as an occupational therapy assistant and demonstrate a satisfactory proficiency score on examinations conducted, approved, or sponsored by the U.S. Public Health Service. For exceptions see § 484.4.

- Social worker standards include a master's degree from a school of social work accredited by the Council on Social Work Education and 1 year of experience in a health care setting.

- Social work assistants must have a baccalaureate degree in social work or a related field and have had at least 1 year of social work in a health-related setting or a combination of 2 years of experience as a social work assistant and achievement of a satisfactory grade on a government-sponsored examination. For exceptions see § 484.4.

- Speech/language pathologist or audiologist requirements include the necessary education and experience to obtain a certificate of clinical competence granted by the American Speech and Hearing Association or having met the educational requirements and currently accumulating the supervised experience necessary for certification.

- Home health aide personnel qualifications, training, and competency requirements changed in the 1990s. Home health aides must have successfully completed a state-established or other type of program that meets the requirements specified in § 484.36(a) and a competency evaluation or state licensure program that meets the requirements in § 484.36(b) or (e). If an individual has not furnished services for a continuous period of 24 consecutive months after meeting the requirements, he or she will no longer be considered qualified. The training program requires a minimum of 75 hours of classroom and supervised practical training. Sixteen hours of classroom training must have been completed before a minimum of 16 hours of supervised practical training. In addition, the home health aide must receive at least 12 hours of in-service training each calendar year.

- Personal care attendants have also been addressed in the revised conditions of participation [§ 484.36(e)] in 1991. Standards and competency evaluation requirements for personal care attendants providing personal care services on behalf of a home health agency are the same as those for home health aides.

Concurrent monitoring and support for maintenance and improvement of personnel capabilities are discussed in COP items relating to participation in in-service programs, orientation programs, and reviews of the currency of personnel employment requirements. Contract personnel are obligated by the agency to be held to the same qualifications as noncontract personnel (DHHS, 1991).

The CHAP standards for nonadministrative personnel are broad in nature. Employment qualifications and responsibilities are congruent with education and experience, provider needs, professional standards, and regulatory guidelines (CHAP, 2003).

Joint commission standards demand that home care personnel have qualifications and abilities equivalent to patients' and/or clients' needs and the skills necessary for the level of care required (Joint Commission, 2003). Both organizations promote standards for staff development in keeping with professional, licensure, or certification criteria.

CREDENTIALING OPTIONS FOR HOME CARE ADMINISTRATORS

At present, there are multiple options for the home care administrator to achieve nationally recognized validation of professional administrative competency. All have eligibility, fee, performance measures, and renewal requirements. Readers are urged to review the Web sites for each credentialing organization in Figure 9-2.

Nursing Administration Certification

The ANCC sponsors a two-level voluntary certification process for licensed registered nurses in administrative (nurse manager and executive-level) positions (ANCC, 2003a). Although applicants do not need to be ANA members, the first level of certification in nursing administration (CNA, BC) requires that the applicant hold a baccalaureate or higher degree in nursing. In addition, the applicant must have held a nurse manager or nurse executive position for the equivalent of 24 months, full time within the past 5 years, and have had 20 contact hours of continuing education applicable to nursing administration within the last 2 years. It is a requirement that a passing score on the written certification examination also be achieved. Recertification is required after 5 years.

The advanced level of certification in nursing administration, advanced (CNAA, BC), recognizes the executive nurse's administrative tasks and functions. Requirements include a master's degree (if it is a nonnursing master's degree, the baccalaureate must be in nursing) and holding an executive position for 24 months within the last 5 years (congruent with published tasks listed for the advanced level). Additionally, 30 contact hours of continuing education applicable to nursing administration during the previous 2 years is required in the absence of a master's degree in nursing administration. A passing score on a written examination is required. Consultants and educators may apply for certification by meeting specific guidelines in the certification manual. Recertification is obtained every 5 years either by providing evidence of continuing education or by obtaining a passing score on the examination.

A third credentialing option by ANCC (2003) for managers in home health care is through certification as a clinical specialist in home health nursing (APRN, BC). A clinical specialist is described as proficient in planning, implementing, and evaluating programs, resources, services, and research for health care delivery to complex clients. Expertise in the process of case management, consultation, collaboration, and education of clients, staff, and other professions is also expected of this clinical specialist. Eligibility requirements include an active registered nurse license and a master's or higher degree in nursing. Since its inception in 1975, more than 150,000 nurses have received all types of specialty certification through the ANCC.

Admission to the American College of Health Care Executives

The American College of Healthcare Executives (ACHE) is a voluntary professional society composed of members who have demonstrated career paths in health services administration. Affiliates of ACHE receive recognition through advancement in status as a diplomate (CHE®), and ultimately a fellow (FACHE). Each level

Figure 9–2 Credentialing Resources for Administrators in Home and Hospice Care

AMERICAN COLLEGE OF HEALTHCARE EXECUTIVES
www.ache.org
One North Franklin, Suite 1700
Chicago, IL 60606-4425
312-424-2800

AMERICAN NURSES CREDENTIALING CENTER
www.nursecredentialing.org
600 Maryland Ave, SW, Suite 100 West
Washington, DC 20024
202-651-7000

HOME CARE UNIVERSITY-CHCE PROGRAM
www.nahc.org
228 Seventh St. SE
Washington, DC 20003
202-547-7424

---

has certain requirements for acceptance and recertification (ACHE, 2003). Admission as an associate is characterized by an initial commitment to health services administration.

Diplomate status is the college's first credentialed status (board certified in health care management-CHE), which confers recognition of the health management administrator's knowledge and capacity for competence in the field. It acknowledges leadership in the health care community as well as life-long learning. Applicants must be currently employed in a health care management position with significant responsibilities; provide two references from an ACHE Fellow and an additional Fellow or ACHE diplomate; pass a written examination in health care management; and have demonstrated leadership in civic or community activities and health care. Evidence of having met 20 hours of category I or II continuing education is also required. Recertification is every 3 years by meeting recertifying criteria.

An application for advancement to Fellow status (FACHE) can occur after the individual occupies diplomate status for 3 years. Eligibility requirements include a current position in health care management of sufficient duties and responsibilities; leadership and civic affairs participation; continuing education of 30 hours; and three references from current ACHE Fellows of the college. Individuals who advance to the Fellow status have successfully completed a Fellow project as approved by the ACHE credentials committee. Fellow status is reserved for those making distinctive contributions in the field of health care management. Recertification is every 3 years by meeting the extant criteria. Individuals occupying home care management positions are eligible for application to the ACHE credentialing process.

Certified Home/Hospice Care Executive

The Home Care University (HCU), an affiliate of the NAHC, offers a comprehensive certification option for home/hospice care executives (CHCE). This credential is limited to those who successfully complete the application, attestation to the NAHC Code of Ethics (1982), testing, and recertification process. The practice of home care and hospice executives is defined as follows:

Home care and hospice executives set expectations; develop plans; and manage, assess, improve and maintain the organizations' activities. The areas of practice span finance, reimbursement, legal and regulatory issues; organization planning and management; human resources; quality and risk management; public relations and marketing; ethics and information management. (NAHC, 2002, p. 2)

Eligibility requirements vary (NAHC, 2002):

- *Individuals with a master's degree*—3 years of home care and/or hospice experience
  1. *Executive level*—12 consecutive months full time within the last 3 years, or
  2. *Management level*—24 consecutive months full time within the last 4 years
- *Individuals with a bachelor's degree*—4 years of home care and/or hospice experience
  1. *Executive level*—18 consecutive months full time within the last 3 years, or
  2. *Management level*—30 consecutive months full time within the last 4 years
- *Individuals with an associate degree or professional licensure in a health-related field*—5 years of home care and/or hospice experience
  1. *Executive level*—24 consecutive months full time within the last 3 years, or
  2. *Management level*—36 consecutive months full time within the last 4 years.

For executives, managers, and surveyors in related organizations the experience requirements are different, and the reader is encouraged to contact NAHC for complete information for this category of applicants.

After individuals achieve initial certification, recertification of the CHCE credential is required every 4 years by retesting or meeting continuing education and professional activity requirements.

The CHCE examination is composed of 165 questions, of which 150 are scorable and 15 are pretest questions. All questions are multiple-choice, four-option responses. The pretest questions are not counted toward the candidate's score. Scaled scores on an examination range from 300 to 600, with the passing score being 500 (NAHC, 2002).

It is expected that the number of home care and hospice executives seeking these various forms of credentialing will grow rapidly. Funding sources and regulators are recognizing the value of continuous performance improvement in industry leadership as important to assuring protection of the public.

CONCLUSION

Home care services are provided in diverse and remote sites from the institutional setting; there are unique challenges in financial management, quality control, risk management, supervision and delegation methods, policy implementation, and organizational development. Reimbursement mechanisms place special demands on home care systems and their operations. The skills of providers are distinct and much more complex than simply moving personnel from a hospital to a home care delivery mode, where independence and resourcefulness are critical to success. The evolution of integrated health care systems redefines the role and challenges of home and hospice executives daily.

The rationale for the creation of a certification process for administrators of home health and hospice goes beyond the assumption that the challenges to these executives reflect a diverse knowledge level. First, states are beginning to mandate certain credentials for administrators in home health agencies for their agencies to be licensed. Second, most other recognized delivery models (hospitals, nursing homes, and public health agencies) have some type of credentialing process in place to recognize the unique qualifications and knowledge of professionals in these respective systems. Certification is a profession's endorsement of these individuals. Home health and hospice administrators as an aggregate require a specific professional endorsement and unique opportunity. Third, home health administrators represent diversity of educational background and professional and nonprofessional experiences. Parameters must be in place to offer boards, consumers, corporate headquarters, certifying agencies, and organizational personnel a measure of comparable worth in the credentials of administrators. Fourth, there is a new professional breed of health care manager known as the gatekeeper of health care: the physician administrator. Although the executive medicine/physician manager model is not currently in vogue for freestanding home health agencies, experiences of managed care organizations and hospital-based agencies show that the competition for administrator positions in health care is intensifying with a newly prepared breed of physician manager.

As hospitals and multisystem entities move toward more fully integrated corporations, many income-producing ventures will emerge. By taking advantage of these opportunities, health care organizations will involve members of the medical staff in equity and management participation. One of the characteristics of a profession is its ability to regulate itself and to set its standards of practice. A certification process is a dimension that can build the image of home care administrators as professionals. This has the dis-

tinct advantage to administrators to be recognized as professional peers by others who are distinguished in the health industry.

The unique certification process for administrators of home health and hospice agencies enhances professional distinction. In selecting certification options, many questions clarifying philosophy, sponsorship, eligibility, and impact arise. These questions reflect the issues inherent in designing, implementing, and evaluating a certification process that aims to recognize professional achievement and protect the public. Agency administrators can contribute to the caliber of the process by verbalizing suggestions and concerns, volunteering to serve on organizational committees implementing the process, validating with other professionals the successes and pitfalls of their own certification process, participating in feasibility studies as well as job analysis studies that can form the foundation for revisions, and challenging collegial creativity to generate ideas for measuring professional distinction. Although this idea may not be a popular one with all administrators, it offers the opportunity for self-regulation and a demonstration of skill and achievement not currently attributed in a standard way to home care administration. This avenue of change can create unparalleled opportunities for professional enhancement.

REFERENCES

American Nurses Association. 2003. *Scope and standards for nurse administrators,* 2nd ed., Washington, DC: ANA.

American Nurses Association. 1999. *A statement on the scope of home health nursing practic,* Washington, DC: ANA.

American Nurses Credentialing Center. 2003a. *2003 certification catalog,* Washington, DC: ANCC.

American Nurses Credentialing Center. 2003b. *Magnet Recognition Program™ manual, 2003–2004,* Washington, DC: ANCC.

Community Health Accreditation Program. 2003. *Standards of excellence for home care organizations,* New York: CHAP.

Cary, A. H. 2003. Public health nursing credentialing and the pseudoshortage. *Public Health Nursing* (20)2: 1–2.

Department of Health and Human Services (DHHS), Health Care Financing Administration. 1989. 42 CFR Part 484. Medicare program: Home health agencies: Conditions of participation and reduction in record keeping requirements; interim final rule. *Federal Register* 54: 33354–44473.

Department of Health and Human Services (DHHS). 1991. Conditions of participation: Home health aide services (§ 484.36–42 CFR Part 484). *Federal Register* 56: 32967–32975.

Joint Commission on Accrediation of Healthcare Organizations. 2003. *2004–2005 Comprehensive Accreditation Manual for Home Care.* Oakbrook Terrace, IL: Joint Commission.

McClure, M., and Hinshaw, A. S. 2002. *Magnet hospitals revisited*, Washington, DC: American Nurses Publishing, Inc.

National Association for Home Care. 1982. *Code of ethics*, Washington, DC: NAHC.

National Association for Home Care. 2002. *Professional certification for home care and hospice executives: Candidates information handbook*, Washington, DC: NAHC.

Styles, M. M. and Affara, F. A. 1998. *ICN on regulation: Towards 21st century models*, Geneva, Switzerland: International Council of Nurses.

Swankin, D. 1999. What drives nurse credentialing? In A. H. Cary and C. Wharton (eds.), *Quality assurance through credentialing*, Washington DC: American Nurses Credentialing Center, Institute for Research, Education and Consultation: 27–35.

RESOURCES

http://www.achc.org, May 16, 2003.
http://www.ache.org, May 16, 2003.
http://www.ansi.org/standards_activities/overview, May 16, 2003.
http://www.chapinc.org/chap-info.htm, May 15, 2003.

http://www.jcaho.org, May 16, 2003.
http://www.nahc.org, May 16, 2003.
http://www.nursecredentialing.org, May, 16, 2003.

CHAPTER 10

The Relationship of the Home Health Agency to the State Trade Association

Joie Glenn

An individual can satisfy basic needs for food and shelter, but he or she must have contact with other human beings to be complete. People joining together for a common purpose is the basis of institutions, trade, and professional associations. Group participation fulfills human needs; it stimulates economic activity and provides a way for people to work together for mutual benefit.

Modern associations have their roots in trade associations that existed thousands of years ago. Throughout the ages, people have banded together for mutual protection and advancement. In ancient Chinese, Japanese, and Indian civilizations, evidence exists of class trade groups that operated for the betterment of members. Trade groups in the Roman empire served regulatory protective functions and applied the concept of apprentice training. Seagoing Phoenician merchants protected their vessels from pirates by sailing together, and the Aramaeans formed large caravans to protect themselves from bandits while they transported goods over land.

Craft guilds and merchant guilds grew rapidly to serve an important function in society in general during the transition from ancient to medieval times. In England, the guilds-craft were formed to safeguard the rights of craftspeople and artisans and to set quality standards for their work. Guilds-merchants, associations of traders and merchants, protected members and in-

creased profits. Early guilds served important functions by encouraging new industries, improving processes, and promoting individual skill and training.

During early U.S. history, mercantilism was the dominant economic force. Carryovers from guilds existed particularly among craftspeople, and a degree of cooperation was found with colonial political authorities.

A parallel exists between the period of transition from medieval guilds to modern associations and the progress of civilization because education and prosperity became more widespread. Governments improved, inventions were ingenious, and communication and transportation became available to the masses rather than only to a privileged few.

Several associations existed in the United States before 1800, some of which are functioning still today. Most associations of home health agencies, however, are comparatively young. As the home health industry has grown, individual agencies have experienced a need to join together to accomplish through the group what they could not alone.

ASSOCIATION STRUCTURE

The democratic process is epitomized in the organizational structure of most home health agency associations. Associations represent,

Original chapter written by Mary Kay Pera.

protect, promote, and are a reflection of their members. The members are the foundation of any association. Ultimate decision making regarding rights and duties occurs at the membership level. The function of the association is to carry out the policies and programs that reflect the views of the majority of the membership. Members choose their leaders, who in turn set the policies of the association.

The leadership of the association is most often called the *board of directors* or *board of trustees*. The board is essentially the association's most important committee. These members are expected to be knowledgeable about the needs of the association and to use this knowledge to transact the business and supervise the affairs of the association so that its purpose may be achieved.

Officers are elected from the members of the board of directors either by the members of the board or by the membership, according to the policies of the association. The elected officers usually form the *executive committee*, which acts as a liaison and functions for the board between meetings.

Committees, which are usually appointed by the chief elected officer, represent the membership by providing input into the decision-making process and ensuring that the diverse interests of the membership are made known. The number, size, and type of standing committees vary according to the objectives of the association, and ad hoc committees are used to address time-sensitive issues related to an ever-changing regulatory and legislative environment. The number, size, and type of committees vary according to the objectives of the association.

Staff members implement the policies and programs of the association. The chief staff person is hired by and reports to the board of directors through the executive committee.

The organizational structure of an association must allow for continued flexibility and responsiveness to member needs. Priorities change according to member needs. A strong, vital organization anticipates and accepts change.

WHAT ASSOCIATIONS DO

The reasons for the existence of home health agency associations are as numerous as the agencies themselves. Typically, however, there are some broad activities that an agency might expect from its association, depending on the availability of resources to support that agency.

Home health associations are in the education business and recognize they are competing with numerous educational opportunities for the provider community. Through seminars, workshops, teleconferences, virtual educational offerings, and other such programs, associations focus on delivering the most reliable and credible education when and where it is needed. Many provide continuing education credits, awards, or certificates for completion of educational programs.

The majority also are involved with government relations programs. Action at the state and federal levels in both the legislative and the regulatory branches can affect the operation of the agency and the care that agency provides to patients. For example, a decision on Medicare by Congress, which is the Medicare agency's biggest payer, could alter significantly the provision of care by that agency.

The association opens the lines of communication, education, and persuasion between the association membership and the legislators and regulators. It becomes a two-way street. The association keeps members up to date on government action and the legislators and regulators informed about home health industry issues and concerns. At times, news from Capitol Hill is fast breaking. The association monitors events as they develop and disseminates information at once, placing the member agency at an advantage over the nonmember agency. Some associations have also formed political action committees through which the membership can support political candidates and incumbents who share their views.

One of the most valuable resources in association membership is the opportunity to meet colleagues in an informal setting and to exchange experiences. It is comforting to know "you are not alone" and helpful to learn what has worked and not worked for others. Many new ideas for resolutions to problems are spin-offs from ideas of others.

Communication is a key function of home health agency associations. The Internet and information technology tools have profoundly enhanced dissemination of time-sensitive information and education to the membership. Government and industry partners rely more and more on associations to provide up-to-date information. Through publications such as the newsletter, membership directory, annual report, position papers, or other bulletins, associations disseminate information to the membership and/or the general public in a print format or on their Web sites. Publicity and public relations activities are also a part of the association's communication program, which members can often use as promotional material in their local areas.

Another program that is part of many home health associations is setting professional standards for home health agencies. The membership has a stake in each agency providing quality home health care. Through standardization of professional home health care, a direct short- and long-term benefit occurs to the members as well as the consumers they serve.

Some associations are also involved in collecting data about the home health industry, researching trends, and reporting outcomes. The ultimate test of an association's effectiveness, however, is not how many or what types of programs it offers but whether the association is meeting the needs and purposes of the membership.

GETTING THE MOST OUT OF MEMBERSHIP

The home health agency that is actively involved in its trade association is the agency that is likely to benefit most from membership. Involvement can take place at many different levels. Each agency must determine its reasons for

belonging to the association and choose the appropriate level of involvement to meet those identified needs.

Participation at the board level requires the greatest amount of involvement in and commitment to the association. The board of directors is involved in policymaking, program planning, initiating change, and getting things done. A successful director is knowledgeable about home health, sensitive to the diverse needs of the membership, flexible, courageous, and, after deliberation, decisive on the issues. By virtue of election to the board, the member is recognized as a leader in the association, is on the cutting edge of the industry, and has the opportunity to affect the direction that the association and industry take.

Committees afford another major opportunity for involvement in the association. Committees are the backbone of the association and the means by which it functions. Service on a committee, which is generally for a year at a time, provides the members with a framework to bring issues before the association for consideration and action. The member with expertise in a given area is often welcomed on a committee that has a responsibility in that area. For example, the member with a strong background and interest in finance would be valuable to the association on the finance committee; a member with legislative or regulatory expertise could contribute to the association on a legislative committee.

An agency may choose not to participate on the board or a committee but remain involved in the association, deriving maximum benefits from membership. An involved association member has a number of important responsibilities. The member should:

- stay informed on the issues by reading all the information disseminated by the association
- learn to know the association's leadership and communicate individual issues and concerns to those people
- share experience with what has and has

not worked and solicit experiences from others

- respond to requests for data on agency operations (every member's input is vital when the association is assessing industry-wide trends)
- ask questions (all questions are worth asking, no matter how insignificant they may seem)
- initiate requests for information (make the association accountable for responding to individual agency needs)
- attend educational programs (provide suggestions for additional, meaningful programs)
- respond to requests from the leadership for calls and letters to legislators (elected officials pay more attention when they hear from large numbers of constituents on a given issue)

The association can also be an invaluable resource in times of difficulty. An agency administrator may think that his or her agency is alone in facing a particular dilemma, only to learn, upon calling the association, that many others are experiencing a similar difficulty. Even if the solution is not immediately found, it is comforting to know that you are not alone.

In approaching the association for assistance, there are certain steps that should be taken. First, identify the problem. Second, be specific about what you are requesting of the association. Third, supply supporting information, such as copies of correspondence, pertinent records, or details of what transpired while you were attempting to resolve the situation on your own. It is helpful to follow up any discussion of the sequence of events with a letter.

CONCLUSION

Membership in an association can yield substantial benefits to a home health agency. The collective wisdom of individual agencies is absolutely essential to compete in the complex health care environment. Individual agencies working alone can make progress, but it is the association with others of similar interest, the sharing of ideas and resources, and the discussion, modification, and filtration that can result in the greatest accomplishments. This, of course, is the essence of belonging to an association.

RESOURCE

American Society of Association Executives (ASAE)
1575 I St., NW
Washington, DC 20005-1103
202-626-2723
www.asaenet.org

CHAPTER **11**

The National Association for Home Care and Hospice

Val J. Halamandaris

The National Association for Home Care and Hospice (NAHC), the nation's largest and most broadly based organization representing home care and hospice professionals, is an aggressive advocate in Washington, D.C. Committed to principles and activities designed to foster an environment where home care and hospice can thrive, the association works to support the dedicated efforts of home care and hospice providers who are helping Americans live dignified, independent lives regardless of age or physical ability. Its membership represents the full spectrum of the home care and hospice industry. Members benefit from comprehensive direct services designed to meet their specific needs.

NAHC is a trade association representing the interests of nearly 7,000 home care agencies, hospices, and home care aide organizations. Its members are primarily corporations or other organizational entities as well as state home care associations, medical equipment suppliers and other vendors, and schools. What these entities have in common is the provision of health care and supportive services on an outreach basis to the ill and infirm in their homes. NAHC also offers individual memberships. Increasingly, professionals such as social workers, nurses, and physical therapists who are employed by home care and hospice agencies are joining one of the forums established by NAHC to serve the specific needs of these fields.

HOW NAHC WORKS

As the nation's voice for home care, NAHC presents a united front promoting trend-setting ideas, programs, and legislation on behalf of all those involved in home care, from the nurse, therapist, and home care aide to the patient and his or her family. The components of home care include skilled nursing, home care aide services, social work, therapy, physician services, adult day care, respite care, Meals-on-Wheels, transportation services, hospice, and many others. Because there are so many components of home care, NAHC retains a professional team of lobbyists, lawyers, policy specialists, and researchers, all of whom combine their efforts as watchdogs of this old-turned-new-again area of health care.

NAHC remains in close contact with the White House, Congress, the Centers for Medicare and Medicaid Services (CMS), the Veterans Administration, and other government agencies; the courts; the state capitals; private enterprise, such as insurance companies, corporate executives, and benefits managers; as well as many others. NAHC also nurtures a close, friendly relationship with the media, both local and national.

CODE OF ETHICS

NAHC has a tough code of ethics to which association members subscribe. NAHC's code of ethics has been copied or adapted by many state organizations. The code of ethics is shown in Exhibit 11-1.

NAHC'S MISSION

NAHC's mission, like that of its members, can be summarized in the statement "We're bring-

Exhibit 11–1 NAHC's Code of Ethics

Preamble

The National Association for Home Care and Hospice (NAHC) was founded with the intention of encouraging the development and the delivery of the highest quality of medical, social and supportive services to the aged, infirm and disabled.

In the process of bringing these essential services to the needy, the Association and its members seek to establish and retain the highest possible level of public confidence.

This Code of Ethics, adopted by the NAHC Board of Directors in September 1982, serves as a statement to the general public that the Association and its individual members stand for integrity and the highest ethical standards.

This Code of Ethics serves to inform members and the general public as to what are acceptable guidelines for ethical conduct for home care agencies and their employees.

It is inherent in the promulgation of this Code of Ethics that the Association and its members covenant to protect and preserve the basic rights of their patients and to deal with them in an honest and ethical manner.

Finally, the Code of Ethics serves as notice to government officials that the Association expects its members to abide by all applicable laws and regulations. It is a precondition of membership in the Association that they do so and failure to comply will result in expulsion from membership in the Association in addition to other penalties prescribed by law.

The Code of Ethics is intended to serve as a guideline to agencies in the following areas:
A. Patient Rights and Responsibilities
B. Relationships to Other Provider Agencies
C. Responsibility to the National Association for Home Care and Hospice
D. Fiscal Responsibilities
E. Marketing and Public Relations
F. Personnel
G. Legislative
H. Hearing Process

Source: Courtesy of the National Association for Home Care and Hospice, Washington, DC.

ing health care back home where it belongs." NAHC is dedicated to the proposition that Americans should receive the health care and social services they need in their own homes insofar as this is possible. NAHC advances the proposition that senior citizens and other vulnerable groups should be assisted to live in independence through the intervention of home care services so that institutionalization is a last resort. NAHC seeks to reverse the current institutional bias that has led to hundreds of thousands, possibly millions, of fragile children and chronically ill seniors being placed in nursing homes or retained in hospitals when they could receive equal or better care at home. NAHC believes that home care and hospice keep families together and is devoted to doing anything in its power to preserve the sanctity of the American family.

NAHC'S VALUES

NAHC's values, from which are derived its mission and specific objectives, include the development of a more caring society; the commitment to preserving the family unit; the preservation of the rights of the underprivileged, ill, and disabled; the protection of the environment; the promotion of wellness, health, and the universal right of access to the highest quality of health care for all; and the promotion of honesty, integrity, and quality.

NAHC'S GOALS

NAHC has 15 goals that include serving as a unified voice for home care and hospice and providing direct services to its members. The specific goals and steps to achieve them are detailed here.

1. *Serve as the unified voice for the home care and hospice community* by making NAHC the information hub for hospice and home care services; disseminating NAHC's values and its broader mission to the general public, Congress, the media, community leaders, and trend setters; and broadening the scope of NAHC membership and representation to include nontraditional service providers, physicians, and organizations that provide specialized care.

2. *Provide direct needed services to the members* by conducting a "service audit" to identify the most and least valuable and effective services offered and to create new member benefits as indicated by member need; including as new benefits local marketing, advocacy, fundraising, and public relations as well as a professional placement service and a travel service; and expanding NAHC staff and resources to accommodate this growth.

3. *Heighten the political visibility of home care and hospice interests* by forming a grassroots political network and encouraging NAHC members to become involved, identifying key legislators at federal, state, and local levels and educating and honoring them; recruiting celebrities as spokespersons; and involving the NAHC board of directors in these efforts.

4. *Influence the legislative, judicial, and regulatory processes with respect to issues of importance to hospice and home care* by exposing legislators to home care issues by taking them on home visits, visiting home care agency offices, and educating key legislative staff persons; providing financial support to key legislators; educating and supporting key regulatory contacts; including regulatory programs as part of the Policy Conference and setting up demonstration projects on regulatory issues; educating and supporting and honoring key judicial officials; and creating a forum of home care attorneys, using the Center for Health Care Law (CHCL) as the clearinghouse for home care and hospice case law.

5. *Sponsor research and gather and disseminate home care and hospice data* by establishing a National Center for Home Care and Hospice Research to act as a clearinghouse, to set national research and funding priorities, to create a home care and hospice library, and to gather all existing relevant data; generating private funds for home care and hospice research; and supporting grant requests from state associations for home care and hospice, universities, and provider organizations.

6. *Promote home care and hospice as central components of the health care delivery system* by commissioning public opinion surveys on patient satisfaction with home care, disseminating the results of these surveys, influencing educational curricula to make the home the primary setting for patient education, contacting and publicizing celebrities who have personal experience with home care and hospice, recruiting movie and television writers and producers to generate wider exposure for home care, and working with special interest groups to incorporate home care information in their consumer education materials.

7. *Foster, develop, and promote high standards of patient care in home care and hospice services* by working with consumer groups to rewrite the Medicare conditions of participation; developing a model licensure law; working with universities and others to develop new standards to keep pace with medical technology and to develop an outcome-driven quality assurance program; disseminating and enforcing the NAHC code of ethics and developing an industry "seal of approval"; and encouraging home care agencies to seek accreditation and supporting "deemed status" for the Joint Commission on Accreditation of Healthcare Organizations and the Community Health Accreditation Program.

8. *Provide expert advice and assistance to members with respect to management, legal, and operational issues* by clearly

defining the limits of NAHC's membership benefits and establishing a fee-for-service consulting service, providing members with a list of outside experts, developing workbook and audio-video packages of information, providing more management seminars, and continuing the certification program for home care executives.

9. *Disseminate information to the media and general public to promote the acceptance of home care and hospice services and to support caregivers who are family, neighbors, and friends* (sometimes called the informal system of care) by launching a national media campaign, building on National Home Care Month and National Hospice Month; developing a syndicated newspaper column and publishing books identifying home care's values and celebrating its heroes; developing programming for television and radio, including human interest pieces about home care clients and caregivers, topics for talk shows, and subjects for sitcoms; publicizing opinion polls to show the public's preference for home care and to promote the values of home care, family solidarity, community service, and the development of a more caring society; and promoting home care as a valuable work setting to high schools and colleges.

10. *Expand private insurance and other third-party sources for financing hospice and home care services* by working to ensure that home care is a mandated benefit in state laws and national programs and is covered among employers who self-insure; developing a model home care and hospice insurance policy, a model long-term care insurance policy, and consumer information about how to select a good home care and hospice insurance policy; educating and recruiting state insurance commissioners; commending insurance companies whose policies cover home care services; and establishing a national case management company.

11. *Promote collaboration among national,*

state, and local organizations relating to home care and hospice services and issues by working with the other coalitions to enact long-term care legislation based on home care, supporting state affiliates and developing a grassroots lobbying network at both state and national levels, and working with civic organizations to promote the broader values of home care.

12. *Initiate, sponsor, and promote educational programs* by presenting seminars and conferences on management issues, new technologies, legal issues, case management, hospice, private duty, and other non-Medicare issues and providing programming to assist state associations (e.g., workshops on how to lobby).

13. *Represent the interests of caregivers (nurses, home care aides, physicians, and therapists) who work in the home care field and encourage individuals to choose a career in home care and hospice services* by preparing publications and videotapes to distribute to schools on home care and hospice as career choices; developing a program for home care organizations to "adopt" a school; taking children on home care visits; providing volunteer opportunities; helping create scholarship programs for those who work in home care; seeking funds to support federal and state job training programs in home care; encouraging home care organizations to provide improved employee benefits to all staff such as health insurance and child care programs; and seeking an amendment to Medicaid allowing welfare recipients to retain health benefits if they work in home care.

14. *Protect the legal rights of hospice and home care beneficiaries, providers, and their employees* by increasing the staff resources in CHCL to create a forum of attorneys and establishing CHCL as the clearinghouse and coordinator of home care case law, preparing publications and audio-video presentations for both consumers and providers to help them understand their legal rights and obligations,

working with state associations to create model legislation, and promoting CHCL with consumer groups and the media.

15. *Promote the independence of home care clients and seek their assistance to help shatter the myth that dependency is the necessary state for the aged and disabled in America* by supporting the growth of adult day and respite care services; supporting the development of in-home educational activities for chronically ill children, the disabled, and the sick elderly; identifying role models of active and successful elderly and disabled; and supporting intergenerational programs such as Foster Grandparents.

GOVERNANCE

Under its articles of incorporation, NAHC has four volunteer elected officers and one paid appointive. The bylaws create the appointive office of association president. NAHC's president is a member of the NAHC board of directors. The appointive office does not vote. All officers are elected and serve for a term of 2 years. The bylaws limit officers to no more than two consecutive elected terms.

The NAHC Board of Directors is made up of 25 members. Each of the 10 geographic regions of the United States elects one board member. The regions are as follows:

Region I, Connecticut, Maine, Massachusetts, New Hampshire, Rhode Island, and Vermont

Region II, New York, New Jersey, Puerto Rico, and the U.S. Virgin Islands

Region III, Delaware, the District of Columbia, Maryland, Pennsylvania, Virginia, and West Virginia

Region IV, Alabama, Florida, Georgia, Kentucky, Mississippi, North Carolina, South Carolina, and Tennessee

Region V, Illinois, Indiana, Michigan, Minnesota, Ohio, and Wisconsin

Region VI, Arkansas, Louisiana, New Mexico, Oklahoma, and Texas

Region VII, Iowa, Kansas, Missouri, and Nebraska

Region VIII, Colorado, Montana, North Dakota, South Dakota, Utah, and Wyoming

Region IX, Arizona, California, Hawaii, Nevada, American Samoa, and Guam

Region X, Alaska, Idaho, Oregon, and Washington

In addition, NAHC has 10 sections. Each elects its own representative to the board, as detailed here:

1. The official section consists of official agencies (city, county, or state health departments).
2. The voluntary section consists of visiting nurse associations and community-based voluntary agencies.
3. The proprietary section is made up of those agencies organized on a for-profit basis.
4. The institution-sponsored section comprises those agencies sponsored by and/or affiliated with a hospital, nursing home, or other institution.
5. The private, not-for-profit section is made up of those agencies whose incorporation status is nonprofit and privately held.
6. The home care aide section is for providers of home care aide services.
7. The hospice section is for providers of hospice services.
8. The state association section comprises the presidents and executives of the affiliated state associations for home care and hospice. When working as a body, the state association members form the Forum of State Associations, which recognizes NAHC as the official national organization representing home care and hospice.

9. The corporate section is composed of multientity providers.
10. The pediatric section was established by the board of directors in 1991 to represent members in this fast-growing part of the home care industry.

The NAHC board of directors also includes five officers: chair, vice chair, secretary, treasurer, and president. Sectional or regional directors are responsible for presiding at their respective meetings and for bringing their constituents' concerns to the board's attention.

The board of directors is the chief policymaking body of the association and, through the programmatic budget, determines the organization's activities and their schedules and funding. The board develops and approves NAHC's legislative, regulatory, and hospice agenda each year, known as its Blueprint for Action.

COMMITTEES

NAHC has an executive committee consisting of four officers and three board members. It has the authority to exercise powers of the board between board meetings. The finance committee is composed of seven members The NAHC treasurer is chair of this committee, which is charged with developing the NAHC budget and monitoring NAHC's financial affairs. The membership committee comprises seven people who advise the board and staff on membership recruitment and retention. The bylaws committee consists of seven members and makes recommendations to the board on possible amendments to the bylaws. The government affairs committee is made up of seven members and helps develop legislative policy. Regulatory policy is developed by a subcommittee of the government affairs committee. The information resources and quality assurance committee, comprising seven members, is responsible for data collection and education. The annual meeting committee plans NAHC's largest event, generally held in October of each year. Finally, the nominating committee is made up of 10 members, representing each of NAHC's 10 sections,

who are elected by the full NAHC membership each year. Its job is to select two candidates to run in opposition for each NAHC board position. The committee is balanced by auspice. It also chooses award winners.

In addition to these committees, NAHC has in the past created certain ad hoc committees, such as the Congressional action committee and the long-term care committee. These committees have been highly successful. They have helped NAHC gather facts and establish and revise its policies. All committees issue reports and make recommendations to the entire NAHC board, which reserves to itself the power of making policy decisions.

COMMUNICATIONS AND INFORMATION DISSEMINATION

NAHC communicates with home care providers in a variety of ways.

Newsletters and Newspapers

The weekly *NAHC Report* gives NAHC members an in-depth understanding of specific legislative and regulatory issues and provides a medium for the communication of late-breaking news items related to NAHC positions.

Homecare News is NAHC's monthly newspaper to keep members informed about activities within NAHC as well as national, regional, and local news affecting the home care industry. It also serves as an information exchange among state associations.

Magazines

Caring addresses the interests and problems of infirm adults, fragile children, disabled persons, and those completing life, with the principal focus on home and hospice care as a solution to many of these problems.

Electronic Communications and Information Services

NAHC maintains a full-featured World Wide Web site (http://www.nahc.org) to facilitate the gathering, analysis, and dissemination of information about home care on both a national and an international level to the home care industry and those interested in home care.

Education and Certification

NAHC provides education and fosters the dissemination of information through its meetings. Each year the educational programs include the annual meeting, financial managers, and a policy conference.

Annual Meeting

The annual meeting provides for the dissemination and exchange of information relating to home care and hospice, encourages interaction among participants at educational and social events, and provides assistance with problem solving in clinical, professional, and management concerns for home care and hospice providers.

Policy Conference

Educational programs are presented on pressing legislative and regulatory topics. Legal workshops are held in conjunction with the policy conference to provide attendees with information about the latest legal issues.

Financial Managers

A special conference on the unique financial concerns affecting home care and hospice agencies is presented yearly. This popular conference serves to promote and assist in the development and improvement of training for financial managers in home care and hospice agencies. It also serves to highlight financial areas that need a legislative or legal change.

Home Care Executives Certification

NAHC provides a certification program for qualified home care and hospice executives to recognize knowledgeable leaders in the industry. It is known as CHCE for Certified Home Care Executive.

DEPARTMENTS

CHCL

The CHCL preserves and protects the legal rights of fragile children, infirm adults, disabled persons, and those who are dying; preserves and protects the legal rights of NAHC, its members, and patients of home care and hospice programs in the community; educates NAHC members as to their legal rights and responsibilities; and increases access to the appropriate legal avenues as a means of ensuring enforcement of the rights of patients and the responsibilities of others. The CHCL provides initial generalized legal advice to members and fee-oriented services to members and nonmembers needing extensive individual legal representation. In addition, the CHCL provides counseling with regard to issues under the purview of NAHC's Regulatory Affairs Department in relation to federal regulations.

The CHCL actively explores and initiates legal action in concert with state associations to ensure fair and reasonable administration and reimbursement of Medicaid programs in each state. Educational activities include development of publications and presentations.

Government Affairs Department

This department initiates and works toward the enactment of legislation to meet the needs of all Americans, including home care as an acute and long-term care benefit. It advocates for the interests of NAHC members with respect to proposed federal legislation that affects or could affect the home care and hospice fields. The department also disseminates timely updates on legislative issues affecting the professions to NAHC members. It assists NAHC members in becoming involved in government relations and political action and organizes and coordinates their efforts, and it assists state associations, regions, and sections in crisis situations involving government affairs issues. It assists other organizations that have similar interests in forming coalitions targeted to achieve legislative results that are of mutual interest. Finally, this department heightens the political visibility of NAHC and its affiliate services and increases home care and hospice coverage by private insurance companies. Each year, the Government Affairs Department develops a Blueprint for Action that contains NAHC's positions on legislative issues and disseminates it to NAHC members, the media, the executive branch, and Congress.

Regulatory Affairs Department

The Regulatory Affairs Department preserves and protects the rights of fragile children, infirm adults, disabled persons, and the dying before regulatory agencies as well as the rights of NAHC, its members, and patients of home care and hospice organizations before these agencies. It educates NAHC members as to their rights and responsibilities before regulatory agencies and represents NAHC members and patients in their dealings with fiscal intermediaries, other third-party payers, and regulatory bodies. This department reduces the paperwork burden and helps bring about greater efficiency in the health care system. It obtains CMS's technical assistance to promote home care and hospice as a mandatory basic benefit, along with long-term care, in health care materials to empower home care agencies with information for grassroots efforts to promote home care services. Each year, in conjunction with the regulatory affairs committee, the department develops a Regulatory Affairs Blueprint for Action and implements the Blueprint for Action plan recommendations.

Research Department

The Research Department develops and disseminates home care and hospice data and analyzes, coordinates, monitors, and promotes research related to hospice and home care services. Specific research objectives include continuing to work toward the development of a home care patient classification system and alternative payment system options; conducting research that will assist home care agencies and hospice organizations; carrying out home care and hospice literature searches; developing NAHC as a

clearinghouse for all research; researching and publishing comparative data relating to the operation of hospices and home care organizations to establish some comparative standards; monitoring, analyzing, and reporting on various national quality assurance projects; and fostering the utilization of standard definitions for home care terminology.

AFFILIATE ORGANIZATIONS

In an effort to recognize the direction of the home care industry, NAHC has established affiliate organizations to provide a vehicle for communication and problem solving for unique types of providers.

Hospice Association of America

This program represents the interests of individuals and families in need of hospice services, promotes the concept of hospice with the media and public, and represents the interests of hospice providers.

Home Care Aide Association of America

This program establishes paraprofessional services as an integral part of home and hospice care within the organization, the industry, and relevant government agencies. It promotes national acceptance of a common title, standardized training, and a career ladder for home care and hospice paraprofessionals. Finally, it provides assistance to agencies in technical and programmatic areas in the development and administration of paraprofessional services.

Hospital Home Care Association of America (HHCAA)

This program assists all providers with effective agency operational issues because hospital systems are in the process of reorganization. It also assists agencies with personnel management issues, information management, billing, and regulatory compliance and in maintaining quality through programs that promote a customer satisfaction-driven philosophy, efficient and effective program management, and cost-containment that helps agencies recognize costs for each service. Finally, it assists members with their efforts to influence legislation and national policy in the best interests of the entire home care field.

Pediatric Home Care Association of America

This program represents the unique delivery and financial issues surrounding home care and hospice for pediatric patients. A core group of dedicated pediatric agencies lead the way in new service and product development and serve to educate other providers on meeting the needs for this population.

Home Health Nurses Association (HHNA)

The mission of HHNA is to promote continuing excellence in the care of home care and hospice patients through the education of staff, students, and the public. HHNA consists of individual nurse members.

Proprietary Home Care Association of America

This program provides a forum within NAHC focusing on issues and concerns of special interest to proprietary home care providers. It enhances agency operations, promotes quality care and customer satisfaction, develops cost-effective strategies to compete in the health care marketplace, and represents the interests of proprietary providers before policymakers, the media, and the public.

World Homecare and Hospice Organization

This program, establishing a worldwide trade association for providers and professionals who deliver health and social services to clients in the home setting, shares information among service providers and their representative groups from nations around the world. It influences public policy in particular countries to improve public support and enhance home care services. This program also educates, trains, and assures quality among service providers to improve the quality of home care services across the globe, and it increases public awareness of and support for home care services around the world. Every 5 years NAHC designates its annual meeting to be an international meeting exploring the world of home care and hospice in other nations.

Home Medical Equipment Association of America (HMEAA)

The mission of the HMEAA is to advance the interests of home medical equipment providers of services, equipment, and supplies. HMEAA identifies issues of concern to its membership and it serves as a forum to present member views while advancing industry changes for HME providers and beneficiaries.

RESOURCE

National Association for Home Care and Hospice
228 Seventh Street, SE
Washington DC 20003
202-547-7424
NAHC has a catalog of publications.

CHAPTER 12

The Visiting Nurse Associations of America

Carolyn S. Markey

The need for home health care has grown dramatically in recent years, due to an aging population and efforts to reduce the cost of inpatient hospital care. The Visiting Nurse Associations of America (VNAA), founded in 1983, is the official national membership organization of not-for-profit, freestanding, community-based home health agencies. Visiting Nurse agencies (VNAs) created the profession of home healthcare over 120 years ago. Representing nearly half of all the not-for-profit home health care organizations in the nation, VNAs, in over four hundred locations, perform a unique and vital role.

VISITING NURSE CONCEPT

The "visiting nurse" concept, developed by Lillian Wald and William Rathbone, is based on the principle that, in many cases, the sick, disabled and elderly benefit most from care given at home by compassionate professionals. In 1880, the first Visiting Nurse agency in the United States was established in Albany, New York. From this modest beginning, a network of VNAs has grown, with more than 400 currently operating across the country assisting 4 million people per year in small-town settings as well as major metropolitan areas. In recent years, home care has become widely recognized as a desir-

able and cost-effective alternative to institutional care, but long before "home care" became a part of the national vocabulary, the VNAs were already making a difference.

VNAA: A VISION FOR ITS MEMBERS

The vision of the VNAA includes:

- To distinguish VNAs as the leader in the most significant sector of the health care industry: home health
- To affect change in regulations and legislation that supports VNAs and their mission
- To achieve prominence as a comprehensive national network, ensuring service excellence through national standards
- To anticipate and respond to changes in the marketplace with innovative use of full-service technology
- To remain driven by our core value: serving patients by putting their needs first

VNAA MISSION

The purpose of the VNAA is to "support, promote and advance VNAs in their mission to serve their communities." VNAA carries out this goal by serving their members through work in the following areas:

- Member services
- Government relations
- Public imaging
- Business development

WHO IT SERVES

The VNA's staff care for people of all ages—from infants to the elderly—and offer comprehensive services that begin with child/maternal health programs at birth and end with hospice care at death. The lifelong care given by visiting nurses makes them indispensable to their communities and patients. This is particularly true of the special programs VNAs make available for underserved populations, including the elderly, the chronically and terminally ill, and children and adults living with HIV/AIDS.

In addition to care for individual patients in their homes, VNAs provide an array of public services and work as health educators in many different settings. Local VNAs run adult daycare centers and hospice facilities. They administer Meals-on-Wheels programs and sponsor a variety of wellness clinics, from blood pressure screenings to immunizations.

The VNA staff facilitate support groups for patients with cancer and Alzheimer's and Parkinson's diseases, as well as their caregivers. On a daily basis, visiting nurses are out in the community, meeting with people in schools, churches and synagogues, neighborhood centers, and the workplace. Through the wide variety of programs they offer, VNAs play a major role in bringing health issues to the attention of the public by encouraging health promotion and disease prevention. Many of these public services are provided at no charge. The VNAs are widely relied on by doctors and government agencies to handle basic needs such as publicizing and delivering immunizations. In many cases, the VNA is the only local agency with the resources, expertise, and knowledge of the community to provide this help.

In their commitment to holistic health care, many VNAs also offer homemaker and chore services that help patients remain in their homes and live independent lives. These services may include cooking, housekeeping, shopping, transportation, personal care, and other nonmedical services.

FINANCING OF VNA SERVICES

Tax-deductible contributions as well as reimbursement from insurance, Medicare, Medicaid, and private payments finance VNA services. VNAs are governed by voluntary boards of directors who are leaders in their communities, a structure that ensures agencies address the specific health care needs of their local populations. VNAs are committed to providing some charitable care to their communities that may take the form of wellness clinics, disease prevention programs, and some indigent care as well.

At a time when the rising cost of health care is a major concern, the VNAs have continued to deliver cost-effective care and to serve all sectors of society, including the indigent. Medicare accounts for approximately 70 percent of the reimbursement VNAs receive for their services. The 1997 Balanced Budget Act mandated changes in Medicare reimbursement that increased the financial pressures on the VNAs, reducing overall revenues by 25 percent.

A growing demand for home health care services has further strained the ability of VNAs to meet their mission of service to all. We have seen a number of VNAs close their doors due to insufficient funds in recent years. We cannot afford to lose a system that is essential to the delivery of home health care for millions of Americans. VNAA is committed to working on behalf of VNAs to support their cause.

In recent years, the VNAA has emerged as a respected voice on Capitol Hill. VNAA and VNA leaders were instrumental in bringing about Medicare reimbursement reform that rewards VNAs for their cost-effective service. In 2003, VNAA fought for and won the elimination of a patient co-pay for Medicare-covered services. The Medicare reimbursement implemented in 2000 will likely reverse the trend of revenue loss experienced by VNAs as a result of the 1997 Balanced Budget Act. Despite this achievement, many VNAs continue to operate with deficits that will take years to erase.

WORKING WITH THE COMMUNITY FOR QUALITY CARE

With their long history of providing care, VNAs are recognized as an important resource in their communities. This role has taken on greater significance in the past two decades as health care has become increasingly decentralized and continuity of care has become the exception rather than the norm. Where does an elderly woman concerned about her risk of heart disease turn? Or the caregiver for a chronically ill relative? Or the young mother who needs assistance and education after the birth of a high-risk baby? In many communities, these people turn to the VNA, not just for nursing care, but for health information and referrals for other services.

Beyond the medical and support services VNAs provide for individuals and their families, they play a significant part in bringing together public and private organizations to meet the needs of their communities. They work with local groups and other nonprofits in sponsoring educational programs. They collaborate with government agencies and corporations to deliver health care through clinics and other programs aimed at reaching a wide segment of the population. The VNA is often the one organization capable of providing information and coordinating services for individuals who need assistance in managing a short or long-term illness.

Other home health agencies currently operating in the field—public health agencies, hospital-based organizations, and private for-profit and nonprofit agencies—typically have not established a presence in the community comparable to that of the VNAs. These organizations do not have the same history of working with other agencies and serving as an educational resource, nor have they demonstrated the same record of delivering cost-effective care. The VNAs are unique in their ability to collaborate with other agencies and in their commitment to meeting all the needs of their patients.

USING TECHNOLOGY TO ENHANCE EFFECTIVENESS

Technology continues to have a major impact on health care, from revolutions in medical procedures to the availability of medical information via the Internet. Many of the new technologies have the potential to enable VNAs to deliver quality care in a more efficient manner. These include the use of telemedicine and laptops in the field, to cite just one example. In addition, the Internet is an important resource capable of creating an even stronger network of VNAs across the country. Through the sharing of information and administrative services on the Internet, local VNAs will save time and money, allowing them to focus on service for patients in their areas.

The VNAA currently operates a Web site (www.vnaa.org) with information for both members and customers seeking information about the local VNA services. This Web site includes listings of all member VNAs, links to medical information, and updates on government regulations for member agencies. The VNAA seeks to expand its Web presence substantially to provide a wider array of services for member agencies, including online required training for professionals and paraprofessionals, best practice sharing, online third-party billing, data collection, and group purchasing. Each of these initiatives will save VNAs money by reducing administrative costs. Meeting professional requirements through online instruction, for example, will free staff from arranging for and presenting education courses, a time-consuming and expensive task. The expanded Web site will also enable the VNAs to share expertise and solutions to problems commonly encountered. The result will be greater financial stability for VNAs and an enhanced quality of care for patients.

The improved Web site will have benefits for the general public as well. Through the site, the organization offers referrals to local agencies, information on the scope of home care available, and details of coverage by insurance agencies and Medicare. It also provides information and support for caregivers who may be overwhelmed by the responsibility of caring for a chronically ill patient or aging relative. Experience has demonstrated that there is a growing need for such information and support as the number of caregivers continues to increase.

PROVIDING SUPPORT FOR MEMBER AGENCIES

The VNAA draws its strength from individual members at the grassroots level and serves as a vehicle for promoting the interests of member agencies to the media, the marketplace, and legislators in Washington, D.C., and state capitals. By using its strength as a national alliance of home health agencies, the organization aims to be the leader in a growing sector of the health care industry, to ensure excellence through national standards, to respond to changes in the marketplace with innovative use of technology, and to remain committed to its mission of serving patients by putting their needs first.

Some of the benefits for VNAA member agencies include:

- Interactive VNA-only listserve
- Industry news and calls to action via e-mail
- Purchasing and third-party payer contracts
- Business partnerships with major corporations
- Wellness and disease prevention programs
- Web-based education and resources

CONCLUSION

As the home health care profession, created by visiting nurses, enters its second century, the challenges are significant. To meet these challenges, the VNAA plans to enhance legislative efforts on behalf of member VNAs, to continue to develop strategic alliances in the marketplace, to implement an expanded Web site, and to provide services that will allow members to achieve their mission of quality home health care for patients, families, and the communities they serve.

PART III

Clinical Issues

CHAPTER 13

Self-Care Systems in Home Health Care Nursing

Joan Reynolds Yuan

If there was ever a time when nurses must be able to articulate what nursing is, it is now. In this time of cost containment, nursing shortage, and reengineering, nurses must be clear on when nursing is required. In this health care revolution, we cannot be locked into the Medicare illness model of home care. In a system that seeks cost-effective, positive outcomes, maintaining or improving health is a priority and falls under the purview of nursing. According to Orem (2001), "a requirement for nursing in an adult is the health-associated absence of the ability to maintain continuously that amount and quality of self-care that is therapeutic in sustaining life and health, in recovering from disease or injury, or in coping with their effects" (p. 82). Because practice in a profession is based on theory, this chapter addresses systems of care based on Orem's nursing theory, its clinical applicability to home health care nursing, and its implications for nursing administration in a home health agency.

In the current cost-conscious environment, there are many changes occurring in health care and home health nursing. According to the American Nurses Association's (ANA) *Scope and Standards of Home Health Nursing Practice* (1999), regardless of the growing demand for home health nursing services, practice will continue to be grounded in evidence-based clinical knowledge and skills within the framework of family, home, and community concepts (p. 2). Community health nurses have long practiced the concept of self-care. Since Lillian Wald conceptualized community health nursing at the turn of the century, self-care has been incorporated into the practice of this specialty. Home health care nursing is recognized as a unique and significant type of community-based nursing practice. The nurse generalist in home health care primarily provides care to individuals, families, and caregivers (ANA, 1999). Consumer involvement is important in the development of the plan of care in community health nursing because the goals and desired outcomes ultimately will be the responsibility of individuals (ANA, 1985).

Home health care nursing, a type of community-based nursing, focuses on the right and responsibility of the patient and family to be included in the planning of care. The Medicare condition of participation concerning patient rights (§ 484.10) mandates "The patient has the right to participate in the planning of the care. [The home health agency] must advise the patient in advance of the right to participate in planning the care or treatment and in planning changes in the care or treatment" (U.S. Government Printing Office, 2002a).

Orem's theory of self-care has significance for home health care. According to Orem (2001), self-care is the practice of activities that are initiated and performed for oneself to maintain life, health, and well-being (p. 43). Self-care requisites are descriptive of the kinds of purposive self-care that are required. Universal self-care requisites are common to all human beings, adjusted for such factors as age, developmental state, and environment; examples are the maintenance of sufficient intake of air, water, and food (Orem, 2001, p. 48).

Developmental self-care requisites are associated with developmental processes and conditions or events that affect development. These include the provision of care to prevent the occurrence of deleterious effects of certain conditions on human development (Orem, 2001, p. 48). Health deviation self-care requisites exist for persons who are ill or injured, have specific forms of pathology, and are under medical treatment (Orem, 2001, p. 48). Self-care agency is the complex acquired ability to meet one's continuing requirements for care that regulates life processes, and maintains or promotes integrity of human structure and functioning and human development (Orem, 2001, p. 522). Dependent care agency is the "ability of mature or maturing persons to know and meet some or all of the self-care requisites of adolescent or adult persons who have health-derived or health-associated limitations of self-care agency, which places them in socially dependent relationships for care" (Orem, 2001, p. 284). Nurses must have the ability to view their patients as self-care and dependent care agents and to diagnose patients' abilities to engage in continuous and effective care.

Orem (2001) describes nursing, a helping art, as "the complex ability to accomplish or to contribute to the accomplishment of a person's usual and therapeutic self-care by compensating for or aiding in overcoming the physical or psychic conditions or disabilities that cause the person (1) to be unable to act, (2) to refrain from acting, or (3) to act ineffectively in self-care" (p. 189). The components of the nursing focus become the guides for nursing action. The self-care that the patient can or cannot manage and the reasons why are evaluated by the nurse when he or she selects among appropriate methods of helping. These methods include acting for or doing for another, guiding another, supporting another, providing an environment that pro-

motes personal development, and teaching another (Orem, 2001, p. 56).

Considering the concept that the nurse and/or patient can act to meet the patient's self-care requisites, three nursing systems have been identified: wholly compensatory, partly compensatory, and supportive-educative (Orem, 2001). In designing the system of care, the home care nurse analyzes the self-care needs identified in the comprehensive assessment. The need for a wholly compensatory nursing system is identified when the patient is unable to engage in those self-care actions requiring self-directed and controlled ambulation and manipulative movement or is under the prescription to refrain from such activity. Three subtypes have been identified: persons who are unable to engage in any form of deliberate action, persons who are aware and may be able to make decisions about self-care but who cannot or should not perform actions requiring ambulation and manipulative movements, and persons who are unable to make rational judgments and decisions about self-care but who are ambulatory and may be able to perform some measures of self-care with continuous guidance and supervision (Orem, 2001, p. 352). Frequently, the helping method utilized by the nurse in this system is acting and doing for another. The nurse must be able to design and manage effective care systems to meet the universal, developmental, and health deviation self-care requirements of these patients. This includes providing guidelines and supervising others who can contribute to the wholly compensatory care system (Orem, 2001).

In the partly compensatory system, both nurse and patient perform care measures or other actions involving manipulative tasks or ambulation. The distribution of responsibility varies with the patient's limitations in ambulation or manipulative activities, the knowledge and skill required, and the patient's psychological state. In this system, all five helping methods may be utilized (Orem, 2001).

The third system, supportive-educative, is used when the patient is able to perform or can and should learn to perform therapeutic self-care measures but cannot do so without assistance. Helping methods include support, guidance, provision of a developmental environment, and teaching (Orem, 2001).

Historically, the home health care nurse has cared for patients with many functional limitations in a way that would be considered wholly compensatory. Systems of care have been designed to include care provided by family, friends, and neighbors as well as by professional and ancillary staff. The number of patients in this population is growing at a time when society is unprepared to care for them. With the current reimbursement structure, a frequently seen phenomenon is that patients are discharged home from the hospital quicker and sicker. This occurs at a time when many of the traditional supports are unavailable as a result of the increased numbers of women in the workforce outside the home, the migration of family members to other parts of the country, and the limited physical and financial resources of many of the young-old who are attempting to care for the old-old. Some of the patients in the wholly compensatory level have chronic problems, and third-party payers will not reimburse for services provided. This is an area that must be addressed by the nursing administration. Is there an agency servicing the community that can provide home health aide, homemaker, and companion services that are affordable to the people in the community?

Many of the people currently being discharged home from the hospital have needs that must be addressed by highly skilled professionals. With advances in technology, patients are now at home with equipment such as ventilators. In many instances, family members will assume responsibility for the provision of care that was designed by the nurse in the wholly compensatory system. The home health care nurse is responsible for the coordination of services. Not only is this good nursing practice, but it is also mandated in § 484.30 of the Medicare conditions of participation for Medicare reimbursement (U.S. Government Printing Office, 2002b). Services provided by the agency, such

as physical therapy, occupational therapy, speech therapy, social services, and home health aide, must be coordinated. Additionally, services that may not be provided by the agency, such as respiratory therapy, and the provision of specialized equipment must also be coordinated. It is imperative that regardless of the mix of disciplines and services provided, the patient's status where possible improves. In this time of public reporting of outcomes, agencies need to be positioned with positive outcomes.

The nursing administrator considers the special needs of the population in the community served by the agency. For example, some communities adjacent to a children's hospital may require private duty nurses for children home on ventilators. Although the structure of a non-profit organization may not support this activity, a reorganization into various corporations could. Some patients in the wholly compensatory system are terminally ill and could benefit from hospice care. During the course of a terminal illness, a patient may shift from one system to another. This is affected by the reimbursement system. Although a patient is terminally ill and could benefit from nursing in a supportive-educative system, it is possible that these services would not be third-party reimbursable because of strict interpretation of regulations such as homebound status. In these instances, other sources of reimbursement should be investigated.

Many of the patients seen at home by the home health care nurse are in a partly compensatory nursing system. Frequently, this skilled, hands-on care is reimbursed by third-party payers. Patients who are receiving services in the home, such as intravenous therapy, are often able to participate in their care and can become independent in such activities as the administration of intravenous antibiotics. It continues to be the responsibility of the nurse to carry out such activities as monitoring the intravenous site for infection or infiltration and changing the catheter. Patients in this system may require multiple services. For example, a patient recovering from a cerebrovascular accident may be able to perform some self-care activities but, to become rehabilitated, may require extensive services including all the therapies.

Other patients admitted to service in a home health agency are in a supportive-educative system. In this system, the patient's requirements for assistance relate to decision making, behavior control, and acquiring knowledge and skills (Orem, 2001, p. 354). Changes in the patient's knowledge, understanding, or behavior should be documented. In this system, the nurse's role is frequently consultative. Some patients require information about the disease process, medication regimen, and safety factors in the home setting.

Preventive health care is an important area for home health care nurses. Three levels of prevention are recognized: (1) primary, (2) secondary, and (3) tertiary. Primary prevention is required before the onset of disease and is directed to the promotion of integrity of structure and functioning and prevention of disease (Orem, 2001, p. 199). Every person requiring nursing care has requirements at the primary level of prevention. Universal self-care and developmental self-care, when therapeutic, constitute prevention at the primary level (Orem, 2001, p. 201). Home health care nurses select, or assist the patient in selecting, methods for meeting self-care requisites that promote and maintain health and development and prevent specific disease. Secondary prevention is required after the onset of disease and is directed to the prevention of com-plications and prolonged disability. Tertiary prevention is appropriate when there is disability and limited functioning. It is directed toward bringing about effective functioning in accord with existing abilities. Health deviation self-care, when therapeutic, is health care at the secondary or tertiary level of prevention (Orem, 2001, p. 201). According to Orem's theory, self-care measures are utilized to regulate and prevent effects of the disease, complications, and prolonged disability or to adapt functioning to compensate for the adverse effects of permanent dysfunction.

CONCLUSION

As we venture into an era of cost containment and increasing demand and short supply of nurses, let us be clear about the value and domain of nursing. Value comes not only from managing health, but also from preventing disease: It is essential that the nursing administration of a home health agency be knowledgeable of the benefits of self-care and have the personnel necessary to design nursing systems. The self-care deficit theory can be utilized in the provision of care to those in the community who require skilled nursing services. Nursing administration must have a system in place to track the outcome of these nursing interventions provided through the nursing system design. This information will be crucial to survival in this health care environment.

REFERENCES

American Nurses Association. 1985. *A guide for community-based nursing services*. Kansas City, MO: ANA

American Nurses Association. 1999. *Scope and standards of home health nursing practice*. Washington, DC: ANA.

Orem, D. 2001. *Nursing concepts of practice*. 6th ed. St. Louis, MO: Mosby.

U.S. Government Printing Office. 2002a. Code of Federal Regulations (42 CFR 484.10). Available from U.S. Gov-ernment Printing Office via GPO Access at *http://www.access.gpo.gov/nara/cfr/* (accessed April 26, 2003).

U.S. Government Printing Office. 2002b. Code of Federal Regulations (42 CFR 484.30). Available from U.S. Government Printing Office via GPO Access at *http://www.access.gpo.gov/nara/cfr/* (accessed April 26, 2003).

CHAPTER 14

Home Health Care Documentation and Record Keeping

Elissa Della Monica and Elizabeth R. Kane

Documentation is one of the ultimate challenges facing home health care administrators today. Changes in the health care environment have created a need for cost-effective, outcome-based systems of documentation. As hospitals aggressively work to decrease hospital length of stay, patients are being discharged "quicker and sicker." The increase in the acuity level of patients has necessitated clear, concise, accurate documentation with evidence of coordination of the multiple services needed to care for the patient.

This chapter presents home health care documentation and record keeping in their entirety. The regulatory bodies governing home health care, specifically the documentation requirements of the Medicare program, are addressed. Discussion includes the components of a clinical record, reasons for documentation, and current trends in documentation systems. Upon completion of this chapter, the reader will possess a basic knowledge of home health documentation and record keeping.

THE CHANGING HEALTH CARE ENVIRONMENT

As alluded to, the delivery of health care is engulfed in an era of change. The 1980s were filled with numerous legislative and regulatory changes that had a major impact on the home care industry. The 1990s have seen the most dramatic changes with the conversion of Medicare patients to managed care, capitated risk contracts, and the change in Medicare from cost reimbursement to prospective payment. In 1982, the Tax Equity and Fiscal Responsibility Act was passed, which mandated that the Department of Health and Human Services (DHHS) institute the system of prospective reimbursement. The diagnosis-related group system of classification and reimbursement resulted in patients being discharged from hospitals in the acute or early recovery phase of an illness. The need for home care services increased because patients were discharged from hospitals requiring intensive levels of home care services. The industry as a whole realized significant increases in services and increasing Medicare expenditures at an average annual rate of 25 percent (National Association for Home Care, 1991).

In 1985, the (then) Health Care Financing Administration (HCFA) now Centers for Medicare and Medicaid Service (CMS) introduced the standardized plan of treatment forms commonly known as Forms 485, 486, and 487 (DHHS, 1966). The introduction of these forms began a period of restrictive interpretation of the Medicare HHA manual. Throughout the country, agencies experienced an increase in medical and technical denials, all based on lack of supporting documentation. Physician orders, progress notes, flow sheets, and assessment forms were closely scrutinized by the fiscal intermediary for homebound status, accuracy in completion of forms, and reasonable and necessary provision of services before agencies were reimbursed for skilled visits. The stringent interpretation of the existing regulations necessitated a dramatic increase in the need for perfect documentation.

In 1989, HCFA (CMS) was forced to revise the Medicare HHA manual. The revisions were the result of the lawsuit brought by Representative Harley Staggers (D,WV) and NAHC. The revisions resulted in a much less restrictive interpretation of the Medicare regulations, enabling nurses and other disciplines to provide medically needed home care services to homebound individuals. The fiscal intermediaries were no longer permitted to make a coverage decision based solely on the reviewer's general inferences about similar diagnoses; rather, decisions had to be based on objective clinical evidence regarding the patient's individual need for care (Harris, 1990).

With the rewrite of the Medicare HHA manual, home health agencies, through the mechanism of documentation, were now able to justify the need for more diverse, less restrictive home care services. Agencies could now provide case management services for patients requiring multidisciplinary management and evaluation of the care plan, venipuncture, and insulin administration for patients for whom there was no able or willing caregiver to administer the drug.

The importance of documentation cannot be stressed enough. The HHA manual revisions place even greater emphasis on the need for quality documentation. It is imperative that home health administrators recognize the impact of documentation on the continued viability of their organization.

REGULATIONS GOVERNING HOME HEALTH CARE DOCUMENTATION

All Medicare-certified home health agencies are governed by the Medicare conditions of partici-

pation (COPs) (HCFA, 1989). An agency is certified as a Medicare provider based on the agency's compliance with the COPs. There are various COPs that govern home health care documentation. The revision to the COPs as listed in the *Federal Register*, March 10, 1997, requires a home health agency to participate in the collection and use of Outcome and Assessment Information Set (OASIS). During the Medicare certification review site visit, all agencies must show that they are in compliance with the standards.

The COPs contain numerous standards that direct an agency's clinical record policy (HCFA, 1991). These are shown in Appendix 14-A. Agencies seeking Accreditation from the Joint Commission on Accreditation of Healthcare Organizations are required to comply with the Medicare COPs and the standards for home health care services as outlined in the Joint Commission's *Accreditation Manual for Home Care* (2002). Hospital-based HHAs are required to seek joint commission accreditation as part of the hospital's accreditation process. The *Accreditation Manual for Home Care* contains a listing of the standards as well as scoring guidelines that direct an agency in how to comply with the intent of the standards. This manual is highly recommended for those seeking accreditation. In addition, managed care companies are beginning to require accreditation as a stipulation for contracting.

The Community Health Accreditation Program (CHAP) is the oldest organization accrediting community and home care agencies. CHAP accreditation is not mandatory, however. Agencies applying for CHAP accreditation must complete a self-study report verifying compliance with the standards as outlined in the manual. The self-study report is an intensive self-evaluation tool that addresses both business and clinical aspects of the organization (CHAP, 2002). The report is reviewed by an expert panel of administrators. A site visit by a few members of the panel is conducted to verify accuracy of the self-study report. An important component of the site visit consists of an extensive analysis of clinical documentation.

CHAP and Joint Commission standards were both developed to provide a means by which community health organizations could ensure excellence. CMS issued regulations deeming agencies accredited by the Joint Commission (HCFA, 1993) and CHAP (DHHS, 1992) to meet the certification requirements for the Medicare program. Thus, agencies that opt for deemed status are no longer subject to routine inspection by Medicare state survey agencies. The joint commission and CHAP surveyors are required to complete the Federal Functional Assessment Instrument as part of the unannounced periodic site visit.

CLINICAL RECORD POLICY

As previously stated, the prime source of funding for many agencies is Medicare. Hence the COPs are the primary tool with which agencies develop their documentation policies. Clinical record and documentation policies are a must for all HHAs. The clinical-record policy addresses protection and retention of records, contents of the clinical record, requirements for the written plan of treatment, requirements for verbal orders, and record-review policy. The clinical-record policy is specific to the agency and describes the system of documentation that an agency is utilizing. The record policy is one that should be strictly adhered to because it will form the basis on which the documentation system is reviewed. During the Medicare certification process and the Joint Commission and CHAP review processes, an agency will be reviewed to verify compliance with its own policies (e.g., if the policy states that verbal orders will be signed and incorporated into the chart in 2 weeks, then it had better be done).

It behooves an administrator to develop a clinical-record policy that does not place restraints on the agency. The policy should describe what is actually occurring in the management of the clinical-record system. Time limits for return of forms from physicians should be avoided because forms are frequently lost or delayed in the physician's office or mail. Nevertheless, agencies should strive to get all verbal orders and plans of treatment signed and incorporated into the record within 1 to 2 weeks or according to state laws. All other agency forms, progress notes, and assessment forms should be incorporated into the record within 1 week.

An example of a clinical-record policy is found in Appendix 14-B. The policy is specific to the agency because it describes the various forms that constitute the clinical-record system. The policy clearly describes the agency's procedures for the protection and retention of records. The policy indicates that the agency is in compliance with the Medicare COPs.

REASONS FOR DOCUMENTATION

During routine daily activities, a home health nurse spends approximately 35 percent of his or her time on documentation and 65 percent on patient care. For nurses, whose primary focus is the care of the patient, the amount of time spent on documentation seems to be counterproductive. Despite the frustrations felt by many home health nurses, the importance of documentation cannot be overemphasized.

Why do we document? There are many reasons, but the primary reason that comes to the mind of home health administrators is reimbursement. Documentation is the method through which the patient's need for home health services is presented (Jacob, 1985). Ineffective, poor documentation could jeopardize the financial stability of the organization. Medicare and other third-party payers may require that documentation be submitted for review before reimbursing the agency. The documentation must objectively inform the reviewer and/or insurance case manager of the clinical status of the patient, inclusive of a description of the services being provided.

The plan of care is a universal form developed and distributed by CMS. The forms are known as Form 485 (Physician's Plan of Care), Form 486 (Medical Update and Patient Information), and Form 487 (Addendum) (DHHS, 1966). The forms contain all the necessary data elements for a physician's plan of care as outlined in the

COPs. The forms were developed to elicit specific information to enable the reviewer to make Medicare coverage determinations. Currently, the fiscal intermediaries no longer require that the physician's plan of care be submitted for review before paying the claim. The intermediary, however, can at any time request the plan of care as well as any other documents in the record. The reviewer will closely analyze the form for inconsistencies in the clinical picture (e.g., Is the diagnosis consistent with the treatment? Are there realistic and measurable goals? Is the care intermittent? Is the patient homebound? Do the clinical diagnosis, treatment, and services ordered support the statement on homebound status? Does the number of visits reflect overutilization of services?). If the reviewer detects any inconsistencies in the plan of care on comparison with the clinical notes, the determination may be made that the care was not reasonable and necessary, and the claim may be denied.

The Medicare fiscal intermediaries are conducting their review through a process called *focused medical review (FMR)*. FMR is the process of targeting and directing medical review efforts on Medicare claims where there is the greatest risk of inappropriate program payment (DHHS, 1966). There has been a significant increase in the use of FMR as a result of concerns by the intermediary about appropriate utilization of services. Through the process of FMR, the fiscal intermediary collects data from a variety of sources and conducts data analysis to identify practice patterns, aberrations, potential areas of inappropriate utilization, and patterns of noncovered services (NAHC, 1996). Although FMR is a process by which the fiscal intermediaries research and analyze data for aberrations, it is also the means by which reviewers determine whether services were reasonable and necessary. FMR is the current mechanism that Medicare uses for coverage decisions. The primary tool that is used in this review process is the clinical record, which is requested by the issuance of a computerized Form 488.

Aside from the physician's plan of care, Medicare and other third-party payers frequently review progress notes, assessment forms, and verbal orders. Quality documentation should include observations written in both clinical and measurable terms (Jacob, 1985). This enables the reviewer and/or case manager to assess changes in the patient's condition. Descriptive, accurate documentation is essential to ensure reimbursement. As previously stated, the professional caregiver is directly accountable for reimbursement. It is only through the mechanism of documentation that an agency receives payment for services.

The second reason for documenting is to prove that quality care was rendered. In home care, the clinical record is the primary tool for assessing the quality and appropriateness of care. The clinical record is a mechanism of proof that the practitioner provided quality services. An agency evaluates for quality via the quarterly record review. The agency is responsible for developing criteria or standards on which to base the clinical record review. The criteria should be well-defined and stated in measurable terms. The clinical record will be evaluated to verify compliance with the established criteria.

Good documentation reflects good care. If the required data do not appear in the clinical record, the quarterly record review may show deficiencies in the care provided to the patient. Remember: Care that is not documented is presumed not to have been done.

The third reason for documentation is to show evidence of coordination of services and continuity of care. Charting shows how several disciplines arrange for continuity and comprehensive care without duplication of services (Stanhope and Lancaster, 1984). The medical record gives members of the health care team a way to communicate with each other. This is accomplished through the formulation of discipline-specific care plans. Short- and long-range goals should be identified indicating expected outcomes for each discipline. These goals should be realistic, measurable, and achievable and should provide guidance in developing a discipline-specific care plan.

A care plan gives direction to patient care by showing all caregivers the goals that are established for a patient, and it gives clear direction for all caregivers to work toward achieving these goals. The plan of care and progress notes provide for continuity of care by informing other professionals of what has been accomplished in the care of the patient. It also informs the caregiver of the plans for future visits.

The coordination of services is documented in the progress note. As addressed in the Medicare COPs, all HHAs are required to show evidence of coordination of multiple services. This is accomplished by the performance and documentation of conferences. A multidisciplinary team conference must establish that there is effective interdisciplinary coordination of the plan of care. These conferences should include all disciplines involved in the care of the patient with reference to goals and expected outcomes.

There should also be evidence of coordination of services from administrative to supervisory clinical staff. Coordination between administrative and clinical staff is documented during patient care conferences and should include reference to the current status of the patient, changes in the plan of care, the ability to achieve the goals as stated in the plan of care, and plans for discharge. The administrative staff may also get involved in a clinical case conference when there is an issue that cannot be resolved at the clinical level. It is imperative that a progress note be documented with evidence of anticipated plans and expected outcomes.

During the Medicare certification visit and the Joint Commission and/or CHAP survey, the surveyor will request evidence of coordination of services at all levels. It behooves all agencies to monitor documentation of coordination of services closely as they are explicitly outlined in the COPs and the Joint Commission and CHAP standards.

The fourth reason to document is that it is a requirement of all professionals involved in the care of patients. Standards I through VI in *Clin-*

ical Nursing Practice (ANA, 1991) addresses documentation as follows:

Standard I, assessment: The nurse collects client health data.

Standard II, diagnosis: The nurse analyzes the assessment data in determining diagnosis.

Standard III, outcome identification: The nurse identifies expected outcomes individualized to the client.

Standard IV, planning: The nurse develops a plan of care that prescribes interventions to attain expected outcomes.

Standard V, implementation: The nurse implements the interventions identified in the plan of care.

Standard VI, evaluation: The nurse evaluates the client's progress toward attainment of outcomes.

Good documentation also establishes the professional's and the agency's credibility. If a chart is poorly written and lacks appropriate terminology and measurable terms, it gives an unfavorable impression of the skill and knowledge of the professional caring for the patient (Jacob, 1985). Hence hospitals, physicians, and community agencies may be reluctant to refer patients.

The fifth reason for documentation addresses the liability issue. As previously stated, professional caregivers are required to show evidence of the care that was rendered. The Medicare COPs and the Joint Commission and CHAP standards all speak to the necessity of the physician's order before care is initiated and throughout the service period. Professional caregivers are required to report all changes in the patient's medical status to the physician. The caregiver may be held liable if there is no evidence of communication with the physician and no evidence of verbal orders to cover changes in the original plan of care.

Home health care workers are also accountable to the Medicare program in documenting provision of skilled services mandated by the federal regulations. An agency may be held liable for fraud and abuse if it cannot demonstrate through documentation that skilled services were provided to a homebound patient and that services were reasonable and necessary for the care of the client.

At all times, agencies must be prepared for an unannounced visit from the Medicare surveyor to certify an agency for participation in the Medicare program or an unannounced visit from the fiscal intermediary to conduct a coverage compliance review. The primary focus of these reviews is to conduct an intensive review of the client records to verify compliance with the federal regulations. State Medicaid reviewers may also conduct unannounced visits per the state statutory regulations. As of July 1993, the Joint Commission initiated unannounced surveys to ensure compliance with selected standards. It is imperative that home health administrators be aware of the quality and appropriateness of their staff's documentation because they are ultimately responsible for deficiencies that may be found.

THE KEY TO SUCCESSFUL DOCUMENTATION

The key to successful documentation lies in the caregiver's ability to paint a picture of the patient for the reviewer. This will enable the reviewer to understand the reason why services were rendered to the client. The reviewer's first introduction to the patient is the physician's plan of care. The plan of care must contain enough information to enable the reviewer to make a coverage determination. As discussed, agencies are using the standard Medicare certification and plan of care forms developed by CMS. There are three separate pages to the CMS forms. Form 485 is the actual plan of treatment and is the only form that must be sent to the physician for signature. CMS Form 486 is

the medical update and patient information form. This form is a dual-purpose form. It is completed by the agency to provide Medicare with supplemental information that will enable the reviewer to make the coverage determination. It is also used as a summary/progress report that is sent to the physician every 60 days, a transfer abstract, and a discharge summary. Form 487 is an addendum for additional writing space to complete the forms.

There are a few key factors in completing the forms according to Medicare specifications. The diagnosis must be a clear diagnosis that conforms in terminology to that of the ninth revision of the *International Classification of Diseases* (ICD-9) published by the DHHS (Jones et al., 1993). The primary diagnosis listed should be the primary reason for which the patient is receiving home health services, which may be different from the primary diagnosis listed on the referral. Other diagnoses should be listed in order of importance. All diagnoses and surgical procedures should contain an ICD-9 code with date of onset and exacerbation. (A note of caution: Avoid chronic diagnoses such as Alzheimer's disease, for which there is a reasonable probability that skilled intervention will not effect a change in the patient's clinical status.)

The treatment orders should be listed per discipline. The orders must be clear and specific to the diagnosis, indicating frequency and duration. For example, ranges may be used when the stability of the condition is such that variations in frequency of treatment are required.

Orders for medication should include dose, frequency, and method of administration. New or changed drug status should be listed after the medication. This indicates to the reviewer the medications for which the patient will need instruction and review.

Goals, rehabilitation potential, and discharge plan should be specific to the diagnosis. The summary of clinical findings should include the clinical status of the client on admission to service and on recertification and the status of the patient over the last 60 days. The physician's signature must be original; a stamp of the physician's signature is not acceptable.

CMS Form 486 (medical update and patient information) is an optional form to evaluate the effectiveness of care. Current Medicare regulations state that Form 486 need not be completed on a routine basis unless requested by the fiscal intermediary for review. Agencies are still required to complete a summary progress report that is sent to the physician every 60 days. Once an agency chooses to eliminate Form 486, it must make provisions to meet this Medicare COP.

In summary, the physician's plan of treatment is the reviewer's first introduction to the patient. It must show that services are coordinated and directed toward a common goal while summarizing the clinical status of the patient from the perspective of all the disciplines.

DOCUMENTATION OF SKILLED CARE

As previously stated, nurses, therapists, and social workers must document evidence that the patient is in need of skilled care. The initial evaluation is documented on assessment forms specific to each discipline. In addition to the assessment form, an agency may or may not require a clinical note. This initial evaluation documentation is important because it contains a brief description of the event or accident that rendered the patient homebound and in need of skilled services. The initial nursing note should contain pertinent findings of the nurse's physical assessment; identification of the need for instruction, observation, or treatment; review of medications, including a preliminary assessment of the patient's understanding of the purpose and signs and symptoms of reaction to the medication; identification of the need for home health aide services; identification of patient goals that are measurable and realistic; anticipated frequency and duration; and homebound status. Documentation includes that the patient has reviewed the bill of rights and has verbalized understanding of the bill of rights. There

must also be documentation addressing the existence of an advance directive. Additionally, there must be evidence of explanation of Health Insurance Portability and Accountability Act (HIPAA) regulations. Instruction to the patient on how to formulate an advance directive is also recommended.

Per the 2002 Joint Commission standards, the initial visit should include documentation of a nutrition and safety assessment. The nutrition assessment forms the basis on which the nurse determines the patient's risk for nutritional problems. In addition, the safety assessment must address such things as fire safety, electrical safety, bed and mobility safety, bathroom safety, and medication safety. The use of patient teaching tools is required once a safety problem has been detected.

The physical therapy and occupational therapy evaluation notes should contain a gradient evaluation, which identifies the areas of deficiency; identification of short- and long-range goals; identification of patient-specific therapy program; the frequency and duration of visits; and evidence of homebound status. The speech pathologist evaluation should include the type of test used in the examination, the identified speech disorders, identification of patient goals that are realistic and measurable, the patient-specific therapy program, the frequency and duration of visits and a list of teaching tools given to the patient for practice and reinforcement, and evidence of homebound status. The social service evaluation should include the persons from whom pertinent information is elicited, the patient's participation or lack of participation in the discussion, the overall plan of action and actions to be initiated after the evaluation and before the patient is visited again, short- and long-range goals that are realistic and measurable, the frequency and duration of visits, and evidence of homebound status.

After completing the initial assessment/evaluation, which may or may not be done on a standard assessment/evaluation form, the caregiver is expected to document a clinical note. The clinical note is a dated, written notation by a member of the health care team on contact with a patient. The note contains a description of signs and symptoms, treatment and/or drugs given, the patient's reaction to the treatment, effects of medication, and changes in physical or emotional condition.

Documentation of instructions given to the patient must also appear in the clinical note. Instructions should be broken down to a specific drug, diet, treatment, or exercise. The use of patient teaching tools is highly recommended. Instructions should continue until the patient/family demonstrates the ability to perform the treatment independently or until the patient/family verbalizes understanding of, for example, medication side effects. Once the clinician documents the patient's understanding of the instruction, further instructions do not constitute a need for ongoing skilled care. Remember: Be specific in your documentation of instructions, and do not repeat instructions once the client has become independent.

Skilled nursing must thoroughly document observation and evaluation visits. The nurse must show evidence of changes in the patient's clinical status with notification of the physician of changes in condition. Skilled observation and evaluation visits are usually covered as long as there are significant changes in the patient's clinical status. The nurse should attempt to chart negatively (e.g., describe in descriptive terms such things as the size, depth, and width of the wound; the color and odor of the exudate; the color of the sputum; the congestion of the lungs; the girth of the abdomen; responses to medications; and the severity of pain). Skilled observation and evaluation visits are important to the care of the client. To ensure reimbursement for these visits, the nurse must document all changes in the patient's status and all written changes by the physician on the plan of care (Engelbrecht, 1986).

Documentation of direct skilled care (e.g., catheter changes, treatments, or injections) is simpler because nurses are accustomed to documentation of specific tasks. Once again, nurses must be specific and describe the length and complexity of the treatment. The Medicare reviewer or case manager will be monitoring the complexity of the care to determine whether it could be done by a nonskilled caregiver (e.g., the family or home health aide). Treatments that require daily care over an extended period of time may not be covered because they may not meet the intermittent criterion.

Skilled nursing and therapy visits for management and evaluation of the care plan are reasonable and necessary. Case management is based on the concept that skilled personnel are needed to meet the patient's medical needs, promote recovery, and ensure medical safety even if the patient does not require skilled care.

All factors must be considered in documentation of management and evaluation of the care plan. Factors such as medications, diagnosis, safety, functional limitations, psychosocial issues, orders for multiple disciplines, goals, and rehabilitation potential must be identified. Documentation must demonstrate the relationship between symptoms and conditions creating a level of complexity that necessitates the intervention of a nurse or therapist. Specific goals must be identified addressing expected outcomes of case management services.

The skilled therapy clinical note should contain an assessment of the patient's clinical status from the therapist's viewpoint, an evaluation of progress or regression since the last visit, the specific therapy modality that was carried out during the visit, the response of the patient to the exercise/therapy during the visit, a statement indicating that the therapist is working toward accomplishment of goals, and a list of new problems that the therapist has discovered on the visit. The therapist's documentation must reflect the degree of motion lost and degree to be restored. Distances that the patient ambulated must be recorded in feet, and the degree of independence in transfer must be explicitly described. The speech pathologist must document the response of the client to therapy using percentages, degrees, number of repetitions, and the like.

As stated in the Medicare HHA manual, "Medical Social Service must contribute significantly to the treatment of the patient's medical condition" (DHHS, 1966, p. 15.11). The medical social service clinical note must contain a detailed description of the social problems that are affecting the patient and contributing to the instability of the disease process. The social worker is expected to describe how his or her intervention can improve the overall status of the patient. The documentation must contain the actual steps taken by the social worker to resolve the problem, the outcomes of the social worker's intervention, and plans for future intervention. Social service visits are generally provided at a maximum of one to three visits per patient. Clear, concise, explicit documentation is needed for coverage of medical social service visits.

In general, home health aides are not required to document in a narrative note. It is customary procedure for a home health aide to document on a worksheet outlining the home health aide's responsibilities. The nurse is expected to develop the home health aide plan of care that directs the aide's activities. The nurse is required to supervise the home health aide every 2 weeks and update the plan of care as needed. The supervision note should be included in a clinical note and must include instructions to the home health aide on the plan of care, the home health aide's understanding of the plan, and his or her ability to perform the necessary functions. The nurse should also include the plans for the future and anticipated plans for a change in aide schedule or discharge of aide service.

Another key issue for reimbursable documentation is homebound status. The reason that the patient is homebound must be discussed on admission and at least weekly thereafter. All disciplines involved in the care of the client should speak to the homebound status with a description of why the patient is homebound. Generalized weakness is not a reason for homebound status. Functional limitations should be clearly described and stated in measurable terms. One discipline must be careful to support another discipline's statement on homebound status. For example, nurses and home health aides must not make statements that are contradictory to the therapist's statements. For example, nurses and aides may indicate that the patient is ambulating without difficulty when the therapist is providing service for gait dysfunction. The nurse's statement may disqualify therapy services. Documentation of coordination via multidisciplinary case conferences will obviate this problem.

Remember: The key to successful documentation lies in the caregiver's ability to describe explicitly why the patient needs home health services and how home health services will improve the patient's overall clinical status. At the completion of your documentation, ask yourself: "Was the care I provided to this patient reasonable and necessary? Did I perform care that was ordered by the physician? Does the clinical note indicate that the patient was homebound? Did I improve the health status of the patient?" All these questions must be answered to ensure reimbursement.

CURRENT TRENDS IN DOCUMENTATION

Although the basic principles of documentation remain the same, there has been significant development of documentation systems. In this era of cost containment, HHAs are seeking more efficient, cost-effective means of documentation. In addition, Medicare and managed care insurers are requesting outcome data from agencies. An outcome, as defined by Shaughnessy and Crisler (1995), is a change in patient health status between two or more points in time. For the first time, professionals are requested to evaluate whether the services that were provided had a positive impact on the health status of the patient.

Designed specifically for HHAs, the Outcome and Assessment Information Set (OASIS) is a tool for measuring outcomes (Shaughnessy and Crisler, 2004). OASIS is used in addition to the assessment because it is not a clinical assessment tool. The tool is designed to measure physiological, functional, cognitive, emotional, and behavioral health. The tool is completed on admission; at specific follow-up points, such as a significant change in patient's condition; at re-certification; and at discharge. Medicare at requires that the tool be completed on all patients because this will justify the need for home health services and thus payment for these services. From the agency's standpoint, outcomes analysis will be integral to a quality improvement program because it will form a basis on which to measure the quality and effectiveness of care.

CRITICAL PATHWAYS

Critical pathways are practice guidelines tailored to a specific patient population, such as patients with congestive heart failure. They are intended to promote the appropriate management of potential or defined health problems by providing a guideline for routine patient care. Unlike care plans, critical pathways provide a time frame for the completion of activities. In addition to providing staff with a clinical practice guideline, critical pathways may be used as a documentation tool. Because critical pathways are usually disease specific, variance reports are necessary to address deviations for patient/family goals, outcomes, and staff interventions (Spath, 1993). The critical pathway generally has a predetermined patient outcome that can easily be measured through variance tracking. The use of critical pathways in disease-specific management programs provides consistency and standardization to the clinical staff in the provision of care. Critical pathways are utilized by insurance case managers to assist them in the decision-making process regarding approval of services. As a documentation tool, critical pathways have their limitations because it is difficult to address all the patients' problems, so that staff must document extensively on variance reports.

COMPUTERIZED DOCUMENTATION

Perhaps the most exciting trend in home health documentation lies in the computerization of the clinical record. Through the use of laptop com-puters, the clinical staff have the capability of documenting at the patient's home. Unlike paper charts, the computerized record allows the clinician to access the patient's record, so that all professional disciplines have current patient information. Generally, computerized documentation decreases the tedious redundancy of traditional charting because the clinician need enter patient information only once. This single data entry is sufficient to transfer the data to a variety of forms, such as the care plan and the physician's plan of treatment. Documentation of the clinical note is expedited because the nurse or therapist addresses the interventions previously identified on the care plan. Specific physician orders may also be carried forward from the physician's plan of care. At the completion of a day's documentation, the clinician takes the laptop home and connects it to his or her home phone line. At a preprogrammed time, the laptop transfers the patient data to the main server located in the central office. Later, the updated information is transferred back to the laptop. Then, the clinician has information about new referrals that he or she is expected to admit to service and current information about patients whom they are scheduled to visit.

In addition to improving the efficiency of staff, computerized documentation has numerous advantages. It forces standardization of documentation, thus improving the work of poor documenters. It enables the agency to customize its practice guidelines that direct clinicians to select from a preapproved menu, thus improving patient care. It significantly improves multidisciplinary coordination of care and communication through the use of computerized communication. Continuity of patient care is enhanced because all clinicians have access to current patient information. Linkage with insurance case managers is possible for them to ask for information about patient status. This could significantly decrease the amount of time spent on phone calls to insurance case managers, thus facilitating the precertification and authorization process. In addition, physicians may query for patient information, which facilitates the physician ordering process and decreases the number of phone calls to physicians.

MEDICAL RECORD DEPARTMENT

Abington Memorial Hospital Home Care (AMHHC) professional staff use laptop computers for documentation. A centralized filing system is used for storage of medical records. Active charts are kept in a Centrex circular file and shelf to allow for easy access. Discharged charts from the previous year are stored in a separate filing cabinet. All other discharged records are stored off the premises. Per agency policy, all charts must be kept for 7 years plus the age of majority. Charts are filed in numerical order utilizing a color-coded numbering system. This allows for quick identification of the clinical record. The department is staffed by a medical record coordinator and medical record clerks. The clinical staff are not permitted to access charts without completing a requisition slip. Staff may request a portion of the chart or the entire chart. Charts are not permitted to leave the office, but care plans, demographic sheets, and medication lists can be printed, when applicable, and taken to the patient's home. In general, staff are discouraged from handling the clinical records.

The agency realized numerous benefits as a result of the tight controls on the medical record system. In general, charts are rarely misplaced or misfiled, forms are incorporated into the charts on a timely basis, and charts are maintained in proper order. The indirect benefits associated with a well-run medical record department are a decrease in the stress of visiting staff (because less time is spent on clerical activities), assistance to the supervisory staff when they are seeking patient information, a decrease in the time spent on quality record review (because charts are complete and forms filed in order), improved efficiency in day-to-day operations of the clinical staff, and reassurance among the staff in knowing that the charts are ready for an unannounced survey by Medicare or the Joint Commission.

Clearly, the future of home care documentation lies in the computerization of the medical record. As previously discussed, this is accomplished through laptop technology that supports off-site entry of patient information. Administrators must keep abreast of the current technology because it may prove to be beneficial to the future of agency operations.

CONCLUSION

Quality reimbursable documentation requires the commitment of the entire agency. This commitment must encompass all levels of employees from the chief administrative officer to the visiting staff to the clerical support staff. All levels of employees should be aware of their responsibilities in the documentation process. Administrators have as one of their primary responsibilities the education of the staff on the complexities of the documentation process and making them aware of the importance of documentation. In today's health care environment, documentation, completed accurately, promptly, and efficiently, is the key to an agency's survival.

REFERENCES

American Nurses Association. 1991. *Clinical nursing practice*. Washington, DC: ANA.

Community Health Accreditation Program. 2002. *CHAP home health standards of excellence*. New York: CHAP.

Department of Health and Human Services. 1966 (Reprinted 1971). *Medicare home health agency manual*. Washington, DC: Government Printing Office.

Department of Health and Human Services, Health Care Financing Administration. 1992. Medicare program: Recognition of the community health accreditation program standards for home health organizations. *Federal Register* 57: 22773–22780.

Department of Health and Human Services, Health Care Financing Administration. 1997, March 10. Medicare and

Medicaid program: Revision of the conditions of participation in home health agencies and use of the Outcome and Assessment Information Set (OASIS) as part of the revised conditions of participation for home health agencies. *Federal Register* 62 (46): 11004–11064.

Department of Health and Human Services, Health Care Financing Administration. 1997, March 10. Medicare and Medicaid program: Use of the outcome and assessment information set (OASIS) as part of the revised conditions of participation for home health agencies. *Federal Register* 62 (46): 11035–11064.

Engelbrecht, L. 1986, March. Engelbrecht on documentation. *Home Health Journal*, 7:11.

Harris, M. D. 1990. The 1980s in review. *Home Healthcare Nurse* 8: 10–12.

Health Care Financing Administration. 1989. 42 CFR Part 484. Medicare conditions of participation for home health agencies. *Federal Register* 54: 33367–33373.

Health Care Financing Administration. 1991. 42 CFR Part 484. Medicare program: Home health agencies: Conditions of participation. *Federal Register* 56: 32967–32975.

Health Care Financing Administration. 1993, June 30. Medicare and Medicaid programs: Recognition of the Joint Commission on Accreditation of Healthcare Organizations standards for home care organizations. *Federal Register* 58: 35007.

Jacob, S. R. 1985. The impact of documentation in home health care. *Home Healthcare Nurse* 3: 16–20.

Joint Commission on Accreditation of Healthcare Organizations. 2002. *2003 Comprehensive accreditation manual for home care*. Oakbrook Terrace, IL: Joint Commission.

Jones, N., et al., eds. 1993. *International classification of diseases: Clinical modification*. 4th edition vol. 13. Alexandria, VA: St. Anthony's.

Medicare Home Health Agencies. Conditions of Participation. March 10, 1997. *Federal Register* 62 (46): 11009–11035.

Medicare and Medicaid program: Use of the OASIS as part of the conditions of participation for home health agencies. March 10, 1997. *Federal Register* 62 (46): 11035–11046.

National Association for Home Care. 1991. *NAHC report: Dramatic home health and hospice spending increases testify to NAHC success in the courts and Congress*. Washington, DC: NAHC.

National Association for Home Care. 1996. *NAHC report: Providers experiencing the burdens of FMR*. Washington, DC: NAHC.

Shaughnessy, P., and K. Crisler. 1995. *Outcome based quality improvement*. Washington, DC: National Association for Home Care.

Shaughnessy, P., and K. Crisler. 2004. Effectiveness of a clinical feedback approach to improving patient outcomes. In M. Harris, *Handbook of home health care administration*, 4th edition. Sudbury, MA: Jones and Bartlett.

Spath, P. 1993. Critical paths: A tool for clinical process management. *Journal of the American Hospital Information Management Association* 64: 56.

Stanhope, M., and J. Lancaster. 1984. *Community health nursing*. St. Louis, MO: Mosby.

COP Standards Pertaining to HHA Clinical Record Policy

Subpart A: General Provisions

Clinical records shall be maintained on all patients, in order to participate as a home health agency.

A Clinical Note means a dated, written notation of a contact with a patient that is written and dated by a member of the health team and that describes signs and symptoms, treatment drugs administered and the patient's reaction and any changes in physical or emotional conditions.

484.10 COP: Patient Rights

The patient has the right to be informed of his or her rights. The HHA must protect and promote the exercise of these rights.

484.10 Standard: Notice of Rights

(1) The HHA must provide the patient with a written notice of the patient's rights in advance of furnishing care to the patient or during the initial evaluation visit before the initiation of treatment.
(2) The HHA must maintain documentation showing that it has complied with the requirements of this section.

484.10 (c) Standard: Right to Be Informed and to Participate in Planning Care and Treatment

(1) The patient has the right to be informed in advance about the care to be furnished, and of any changes in the care to be furnished.
  (i) The HHA must advise the patient in advance of the disciplines that will furnish care, and the frequency of visits proposed to be furnished.
  (ii) The HHA must advise the patient in advance of any change in the plan of care before the change is made.
(2) The patient has the right to participate in the planning of the care.
  (i) The HHA must advise the patient in advance of the right to participate in planning the care or treatment and in planning changes in the care or treatment.

484.10 (d) Standard: Confidentiality of Medical Records

The patient has the right to confidentiality of the clinical records maintained by the HHA. The HHA must advise the patient of the agency's policies and procedures regarding disclosure of clinical records.

484.14 COP: Organization, Service, Administration

484.14(g) Standard: Coordination of Patient Services

All personnel providing services maintain liaison to ensure that their efforts effectively complement one another and support the objectives outlined in the plan of care. The clinical record or minutes of case conferences establish that effective interchange, reporting, and coordination of patient care [do] occur. A written summary report for each patient is sent to the attending physician at least every 60 days.

This standard establishes the agency's responsibilities in the coordination of services. There should be evidence in a clinical record of coordination [among] disciplines and coordination through the various levels of authority. Documentation of case conferences [is] an absolute must in all clinical records.

484.18 COP: Acceptance of Patients, Plan of Care, Medical Supervision

484.18(a) Standard: Plan of Care

The plan of care developed in consultation with the agency staff covers all pertinent diagnoses including: Mental status, types of service and equipment required, frequency of visits, prognosis, rehabilitation potential, functional limitations, activities permitted, nutritional requirements, medications and treatments, any safety measures to protect against injury, instructions for timely discharge or referral, and other appropriate items. If a physician refers a patient under a plan of care that cannot be completed until after an evaluation visit, the physician is consulted to approve additions or modifications to the original plan.

Orders for therapy services include the specific procedures and modalities to be used and the amount, frequency, and duration. The thera-

pist and other agency personnel participate in developing the plan of care.

484.18(b) Standard: Periodic Review of Plan of Care

The total plan of care is reviewed by the attending physician and agency personnel as often as the severity of the patient's condition requires, but at least once every 60 days or more frequently when there is a beneficiary elected transfer; a significant change in condition resulting in a change in the case-mix assignment; or a discharge and return to the same HHA during the 60-day episode. Agency professional staff promptly alerts the physician of any changes that suggest a need to alter the plan of care.

484.18(c) Standard: Conformance with Physician's Orders

Drugs and treatments are administered by agency staff only as ordered by the physician. Verbal orders are put in writing and signed and dated with the date of receipt by the registered nurse or qualified therapist (as defined in §484.4 of this chapter) responsible for furnishing or supervising the ordered services.

484.48 COP: Clinical Records

A clinical record containing pertinent past and current findings in accordance with accepted professional standards is maintained for every patient receiving home health services. In addition to the plan of care, the record contains appropriate identifying information; name of physician; drug, dietary treatment, and activity orders; signed and dated clinical and progress notes; copies of summary reports sent to the attending physician; and a discharge summary. The HHA must inform the attending physician of the availability of a discharge summary. The discharge summary must be sent to the attending physician upon request and must include the patient's medical and health status at discharge.

484.48(a) Standard: Retention of Records

Clinical records are maintained for five years after the month the cost report for which the records apply is filed with the intermediary, unless State law stipulates a longer period of time. Policies call for retention even if the agency discontinues operation. If the patient is transferred to another health facility, a copy of the record or abstract accompanies the patient.

484.48(b) Standard: Protection of Records

Clinical record information is safeguarded against loss or unauthorized use. Written procedures govern use and removal of records and conditions for release of information not authorized by law.

Refer to Chapter 3 for entire COPs.

Abington Memorial Hospital Home Care Clinical Records

PURPOSE: To ensure the availability of clinical data and information which is necessary for the provision of home care services in a systematic and confidential manner.

RESPONSIBLE PERSONNEL: Executive Director, Director of Professional Services, Director of Education/Quality Improvement, Director of Finance, supervisors, professional and contract staff, clinical information staff, therapy staff, and billing staff.

OBJECTIVES: To maintain a complete paper clinical record for each patient on service that provides a patient history, plan of care, and record of all services provided to the patient.

To provide a system for maintenance, storage, and disposal of all clinical records.

To ensure the confidentiality, security, and integrity of patient information.

To provide standardization of abbreviations, acronyms, symbols, and codes to ensure consistent interpretation of information.

POLICY: A clinical record is maintained for each patient admitted to service. The patient is assigned a unique number using the unit numbering system. The information is filed in an end-tab fastener folder using color-coded numbers. Clinical records of active patients and discharged records of approximately 6 months are kept in the Clinical Information Department. An additional 6 months to 2½ years of discharged records are stored in a secure storage room. All other clinical records are stored off the premises, in a storage facility (Guardian/Pierce Leahy) that meets legal requirements.

Clinical records are retained for a minimum of 7 years in a protected environment to safeguard against loss or unauthorized use. Records of minors are retained until the age of majority (18) plus an additional 7 years. If the organization discontinues operation, the Pennsylvania Department of Health must be informed of the date of dissolution and the location of the clinical records.

Information from the clinical record will not be disclosed without the patient's consent, except as necessary to provide services and to obtain payment for those services, or in response to a valid subpoena or court order. (Refer to policies regarding release of HIV and Psychiatric Information.)

The final responsibility for the patient records rests with the Executive Director and the governing body.

Source: Reprinted with permission of Abington Memorial Hospital Home Care, Willow Grove, Pennsylvania.

PROCEDURE: *Action*

Rationale

A. ACTIVE RECORDS

1. A clinical record is initiated on every patient admitted for service, and a unique patient number is assigned using the unit numbering system.

1. Accurate information is captured for every patient upon admission, and a number is assigned for efficiency in filing all subsequent forms.

2. Active records are filed numerically in the Clinical Information Dept. on a central file maintained by the clinical information staff.

2. A color-coded numeric filing system provides for optimum efficiency in filing and retrieving information. Central control of files maintains optimum standardization.

3. The contents of the clinical record
   - Home Health Certification Plan of Care: (485, 487, Assessment Verbal Order)
   - Completed by the RN/Therapist Supervisor and signed by the physician. Updated every 60 days. Additions, deletions, or changes are confirmed by a verbal order.
   - Contains medications, diagnoses, DME and supplies, safety measures, nutritional requirements, allergies, functional limitations, activities permitted, mental status, prognosis, orders for discipline and treatments, including interventions specific to patient and patient teaching needs, goals/rehabilitation potential/discharge plans, and clinical summary.
   - Referral and Admission Information:
     - Contains general information, physician information, facility information, medical diagnoses, surgical procedures, intravenous information, equipment/supplies intake lab work orders, patient status, and referral to discipline.
   - Referral and Admission Information is a combination of the Referral Demographic Information and Referral Clinical Information without the OASIS questions.

3. The clinical record contains all data on the patient to guide the care by all disciplines while a patient of the home care services.

PROCEDURE: *Action*   *Rationale*

- Referral Demographic Information:
  - Contains general information, physician information, facility information and OASIS questions.
  - Initiated by the Intake Department. Reviewed and completed by the RN/Therapist.
- Referral Clinical:
  - Contains medical diagnoses, surgical procedures, intravenous information, equipment/supplies, intake lab work orders, and OASIS questions.
  - Initiated by the Intake Department. Reviewed and completed by the RN/Therapist.
- Pay Source Information:
  - Contains pay source, general information, and additional billing information.
  - Initiated by the Intake Department. Reviewed by the RN/Therapist.
- Assessment History:
  - Contains patient/family history, support system, emergency plan, emergency phone numbers, and OASIS questions.
  - Completed by RN/Therapist.
- OASIS General:
  - Contains compilation of all OASIS questions completed by RN/Therapist.
  - Completed at Start of Care, Recertification, Resumption of Care, Transfer, and Discharge.
- Medication Listing:
  - Contains pharmacy name and phone number.
  - Lists medication and nonmedication allergies and/or prior adverse reactions.
  - Lists name of prescription and nonprescription medications, route, dosage, frequency, start date, and discharge date.

PROCEDURE: *Action*   *Rationale*

- – Medication listing is revised and updated as needed by the RN/Therapist.
- • Plan of Care (SN, SW, HHA, PT, OT, ST)
  - – Contains problem list, patient goals, assessments, patient teaching needs, interventions specific to patient needs, and initial teaching and interventions.
  - – Completed by each discipline on admission, and revised as needed.
- • Home Health Aide Plan of Care:
  - – Contains general information, emergency contact, physician's name and phone number, frequency of visits, medication and nonmedication allergies, and interventions.
  - – Completed by RN or therapist when indicated. Revised as needed. Communicated to home health aide by Home Health Aide department.
  - – Home health aide takes the most recent plan of care when he/she visits the patient.
- • Progress Note: (SN, SW, PT, OT, ST)
  - – Contains skilled observation/evaluation/health systems review, clinical measurements, clinical findings, interventions/teachings/assessments, goals, homebound status, and plan for next visit.
- • Document Communications:
  - – Conference reports within the department, physicians, patients, family, and from other disciplines involved in patient's care.
- • HHA Supervisory Visit:
  - – Contains supervision, assessment of home health Aide care plan, attitude of the aide, skill/performance of the aide, plan for next visit.
  - – Completed by RN/Therapist at least every 14 days.

PROCEDURE: *Action*   *Rationale*

- Clinical Assessment (RN, PT, OT, ST):
  - Contains current problem/reason for home care, complete physical and psychosocial assessment, patient condition/admission status, and OASIS questions.
  - Completed by the RN/Therapist.
- Functional Assessment:
  - Contains pertinent OASIS questions.
  - Completed by the RN/Therapist.
  - Contains safety measures and homebound status.
- Home Health Aide Activity Record:
  - Contains a checklist of activities performed by the aide.
  - Completed by the aide for each day of service.
- Social Work Assessment:
  - Contains reason for referral, problem as perceived by patient and family, pertinent medical/social history, clinical summary.
  - Completed by the social worker on admission to service.
- Discharge Summary:
  - Contains patient condition, services provided, progress towards goals/outcomes, continuing needs, OASIS questions, when applicable.
  - Completed by each discipline at time of discharge from service.
  - Upon request, a copy of each discipline discharge summary and Care Plan Goals History Form is sent to the physician.
- Transfer/Referral Summary
  - Contains pertinent information and OASIS questions when applicable, for transfer of patient to another level of care or another organization.

PROCEDURE: *Action*   *Rationale*

- Patient Discharge Instructions:
  - Contains listing of medications, dose, dose schedule, purpose of medication, diet, physical activity limitations, and follow-up appointments.
  - Completed by RN at the time of discharge.
  - Therapy Discharge Instructions are included in the clinical note.
- Patient Authorization and Release Form—signed copy.
- Patient Bill of Rights—signed copy.

4. All clinical records are kept in an end-tab fastener folder and the filing sequence for active clinical records is as follows:
(All forms are to be filed in reverse chronological order, newest on top.)

4. Standardization increases efficiency of filing and retrieving of medical information.

B. DISCHARGED RECORDS

1. When a patient is discharged from service, the following forms are added to the chart:
   - Discharge from Agency
   - Discharge Summaries (SN, HHA, SW, PT, OT, ST), and Care Plan Goal History.

1. The record is kept intact in case the data are needed for future admissions or other reasons.

2. Documentation must be completed within 30 days, except OASIS questions, which need to follow OASIS guidelines.

2. The clinical information staff reviews all discharged records for completeness.

3. The discharged records are filed in the closed record file for approximately 6 months. Discharge records from 6 months to 2½ years are stored in a secure storage room. All records are stored in sprinkler protected rooms.

3. All records are stored in sprinkler protected rooms.

4. Discharged records from previous years are stored off-site in a storage facility that meets legal requirements.

4. Records are still available if needed, but are not using valuable office space.

5. Discharge records are retained for a minimum of 7 years. Records of minors are retained until age of majority (18), plus an additional 7 years.

5. Patient records are retained to meet agency policy and state and federal regulations.

PROCEDURE: *Action*   *Rationale*

C. DOCUMENTATION OF RECORD

1. The nurse, social worker, and therapist complete documentation on the laptop in the Health Information System. The user password and user ID constitutes a valid signature on all documents. Non-laptop nurses and therapists complete worksheets, which are entered into the system by a data entry clerk. All progress notes entered into the system by a data entry clerk must be co-signed by the author or reviewed and co-signed by a supervisor.

   A nurse, social worker, therapist, or supervisor's signature is required on the Home Health Certification and Plan of Care.

2. To insure the accuracy and integrity of the data, the following forms may not be altered in the computer after communication has taken place with the main system:
   - Verbal Orders
   - Assessment Verbal Order
   - Home Health Certification and Plan of Care
   - Progress Notes
   - Document Communications
   - Physical Assessments
   - OASIS Survey

   Changes to the above forms will be handled as follows:
   - Verbal Orders, Assessment Verbal Orders, and Home Health Certification and Plan of Care—a new order needs to be generated.
   - Progress Notes/Physicial Assessment—an addendum needs to be completed, and form needs to be reprinted.
   - Document Communications—a new document communications needs to be completed explaining the change.

2. Maintains system integrity. After consultation with supervisory staff, authorized Medical Records Coders can change the order of diagnosis to accurately reflect appropriate Home Care diagnosis.

   If a clinical data discrepancy occurs within the documentation of the initial physical assessment or OASIS data set, the PPS nurse will correct the data, including the addition or deletion of a diagnosis after consultation with the clinician.

   A document communication will reflect the reason for the correction and the consultation with the clinician.

PROCEDURE: *Action*   *Rationale*

- OASIS Survey—a document communication will explain clarification of clinical OASIS data.

Changes to all other computer generated forms can be made directly to the form in the computer.

3. All entries into the medical record must be dated (month, day, year) and authenticated with credentials. If more than one signature is needed on a document, initials may be used.

     A supervisor, another nurse, social worker, or therapist may sign a document after review.

3. Documentation must be identified to meet legal requirements.

The nurse, social worker or therapist who provided the care is ultimately responsible for the content of the documentation.

4. All entries recorded in the medical record must be legible and accurate.

There is to be no obliteration of entries by erasures, whiting-out, or pasting over. The proper method of error correction in the medical record is as follows:

- Draw one single line through the entry, write error or mistaken entry, initial and date, and write correct information near the entry or where the correct information can be found.

4. All data must be legally acceptable as to accuracy and legibility.

5. The following staff are authorized to make entries in the medical record:

Executive Director	Director of Finance
Director of Professional Services	Billing Staff
	Transcriptionist
Director of Quality Improvement	Medical Social Worker
Clinical Supervisors	Dietician
	Students
Home Care Nurses	Pastoral Care (Hospice)
Contracted Home Care Nurses	Volunteer Director (Hospice)
Physicians	Volunteers
Clinical Educator	
Clinical Link Trainer/Analyst	Home Health Aide Supervisor
Clinical Information Staff	

PROCEDURE:

Action		*Rationale*

Therapist (PT, OT, ST)   Home Health Aide
Therapy Clerk   Clerk
                                          Home Health Aides
                                          (HHA Activity
                                          Records only)

The following are authorized to review the medical record:

Surveyors from: Licensing, Certification, Accrediting Bodies, and PAC (Professional Advisory Committee).

6. Only approved symbols and abbreviations are used in the medical record and there must be an explanatory legend available to personnel authorized to make entries and/or to read the entries. Each abbreviation or symbol must have only one meaning.

    6. Only approved symbols and abbreviations are used to prevent misinterpretation.

7. The department maintains a list of unacceptable abbreviations that the staff are instructed not to use as they present safety concerns. The inappropriate use of these and all other abbreviations are monitored on quarterly record review and review of records for performance appraisals.

    7. The Director of Quality Improvement monitors use of unacceptable abbreviations and takes necessary action to improve performance.

8. Diagnoses are classified according to the International Classification Code of Diseases, Clinical Modification (ICD-9).

    8. Acceptable standard of practice.

D. RETENTION OF RECORDS

1. Medical records shall be kept on file for a minimum of 7 years following the patient's date of discharge.

    1. Patient records are retained to meet Pennsylvania State Rules and Regulations.

   If the patient is a minor, medical records are to be retained until the age of majority (18) and then for an additional 7 years.

2. If the organization discontinues operation, the Pennsylvania Department of Health must be informed of the location of the stored records. The storage facility chosen must provide retrieval services for 5 years after closure. No records can be destroyed until after public notice in the form of both legal notice and display advertisement is placed in a news-

PROCEDURE: *Action*   *Rationale*

paper of general circulation. Former patients or their representatives must be
provided the opportunity to claim their
records prior to destruction.

E. CONFIDENTIALITY OF RECORDS

1. The confidentiality of the medical record will be maintained in accordance with the HIPAA policies. Patients and staff will be instructed to maintain confidentiality of any portion of the record that is left in the home. Staff are instructed to bring patient documents back to the office for disposal.

1. It is the responsibility of the department to maintain confidentiality of the medical record. Ensures compliance with Conditions of Participation 484.10 (d) and HIPAA regulations.

F. PROTECTION OF RECORDS

1. Authorized personnel, including students, volunteers, and cleaning service employees, have access to the Clinical Information Dept.

1. Students are accepted upon recommendation of the educational facility. They are required to sign a statement of confidentiality and contracts are in place with a Business Associate Agreement. Selected volunteers are assigned to the department and are educated on the HIPAA Privacy Rules. Background information on personnel is contained in the Personnel Dept. Volunteer information is in the Volunteer Department. AMH Properties Department is responsible for cleaning service contracts.

2. The Clinical Information Dept. is secured with locked doors and is fire protected with sprinklers.

2. To ensure compliance with Medicare regulations.

3. Building complies with township codes with reference to fire regulations.

3. The agency complies with local ordinances.

G. RELEASE OF MEDICAL RECORDS

1. In response to a subpoena, all portions of the record may be copied in accordance with HIPAA policies.

PROCEDURE: *Action*

Rationale

2. In response to a request from a governmental insurer and third party payor, clinical documents may be copied in accordance with HIPAA policies.

2. Government regulations and third party insurers require release of clinical information to ascertain compliance with regulations and contract specifications also necessary for reimbursement.

3. Staff may copy any portion of the record to facilitate coordination of care.

3. The staff maintain responsibility for the confidentiality for all copies.

4. Copies of the record must be discarded at the Home Care Dept.

4. To ensure confidentiality of patient care documents.

COP 484.48
Origin date: 1/76
Revised date: 12/82; 1/86; 11/88; 2/90; 1/91; 8/91; 7/92; 5/94; 7/94; 2/97; 4/97;
                  2/00; 5/00; 12/00; 1/01; 6/01; 10/01; 4/03
Approved by: Administration/Board/PAC
Originator: Administration
Distribution: Administration/Staff

CHAPTER 15

Computerized Clinical Documentation

Donna R. Baldwin

The home care industry has invested heavily in information management technology and will continue to do so. A significant portion of the expenditures will involve computerized clinical documentation systems, which offer the potential to reduce costs, streamline paperwork, and improve organizational performance. Successful transition from manual charting to computerization, however, is not without challenges. The technology selected must both enhance current operations and enable the organization to prepare for the future. There is no "perfect" computer system, but through critical analysis home care organizations can choose the technology that is most congruent with their operations and can adapt the organizational environment to achieve maximum return on the investment.

DOCUMENTATION PROCESS

Documentation has been cited as one of the most frustrating aspects of home care nursing (Lynch, 1994). Home care nurses are generally more satisfied than nurses in other practice settings, but they are almost unanimous in identifying documentation as a major source of dissatisfaction (Baldwin and Price, 1994). Federal regulations, accreditation standards, and reimbursement procedures dictate the clinical data that must be recorded, and as a result documentation may account for up to 50 percent of the home care nurses' time (Westra and Raup, 1995).

Home care documentation is essentially a paper-driven system, which contributes to the nurses' frustration. Manual documentation is the established norm in health care and may be acceptable in an institutional setting where the patient and the clinical record are available at the same location. Home care, in contrast, is a mobile industry, with care being provided at multiple locations. Clinical data, recorded at the site of care delivery, must be transported to the office for filing, and staff must return to the office to access the clinical record. As a result, the paper-driven system can be both cumbersome and time consuming.

Manual documentation, although accepted, is not always effective in home care. The staff may provide high-quality care, but this is not necessarily reflected in the manual charting, which is often done after the fact. Clinicians habitually postpone charting until the end of the day, resulting in the loss of valuable information through inaccurate or incomplete recall. In addition, the multitude of forms required to meet specific data collection requirements contributes to the duplication of entries and results in a lack of consistency. Each form stands independent of the others, making it difficult to monitor the patient's progress and promote coordination of care.

Computerization has been proposed as the solution to frustration with documentation. Initial attempts were limited to billing software, however, which automated data entry to produce the plan of treatment. The growth and sophistication of claims submission packages simplified the billing process but did little to address the inadequacies associated with manual documentation.

DEFINING COMPUTERIZED CLINICAL DOCUMENTATION

Over the last few years, technology has been introduced in home care to computerize the recording of clinical data. A variety of options are currently available, but not all approaches address the entire scope of clinical documentation. To resolve the problems inherent in the manual process, a computerized system must contain three elements essential for timely, efficient, and effective clinical documentation. The most important requirement is that the computerized system be based on point-of-care entry of clinical data. Clinical staff must be able to enter clinical findings while in the patient's home. This is sometimes referred to as *mobile computing* because it involves the use of portable computers that are carried from one patient's home to another.

A dramatic increase in the use of portable computers in home care has occurred, but many organizations have only implemented their systems for nursing. Because of the reluctance to expand usage to all services providing care in the home, dual systems of documentation are in operation, which hampers care coordination. Therefore, to be completely effective, the computerized documentation systems must encompass all disciplines providing care for the patient.

Computerized documentation also requires that a clinical database be available to the field staff. The entry of clinical data can be automated, but the system will not promote consistency in documentation and enhance care coordination unless the field staff have access to the entire computerized record while at the site of care delivery.

IMPACT OF HEALTH CARE TRENDS ON DOCUMENTATION

The decision to computerize may be based on internal needs and deficiencies associated with the manual process, but health care trends relative to clinical documentation must also be considered. These external factors are the driving forces that affect the organization's information management requirements and contribute to both immediate and future needs.

Regulations and Standards

The most significant regulations affecting home care are the Medicare conditions of participation. These standards are fairly broad regarding patient care, but compliance is validated primarily by review of documentation. Although most computer documentation systems simplify compliance with current regulations the Center for Medicare and Medicaid Services (CMS) is beginning to focus on patient care outcomes rather than compliance with care processes. Therefore, when a system is envisioned, both current and proposed regulatory requirements must be analyzed.

Federal regulations are of paramount importance, but state regulations are often more challenging. Commercial computerized documentation software is generic and may not assist the organization in complying with state regulations. In fact, the software may actually hamper compliance. A primary example is the fact that most commercial systems are designed for charting by exception, so that entry of clinical observations is required only when the clinician determines that the findings are not within normal limits. Some states, however, require complete documentation of clinical findings, even if no problems are noted.

Accreditation standards for home care also place considerable emphasis on documentation. If the home care organization is accredited by either the Joint Commission on Accreditation of Healthcare Organizations or the Community Health Accreditation Program, such standards must be addressed when the computerization project is initiated. For example, Joint Commission-accredited organizations must ensure that the clinical documentation system will promote timely access to information, improve data accuracy, and maintain a balance of security of and ease of access to data (Joint Commission, 2003).

Outcome Measurement

Outcome measurement became a reality for home care in 1999 when CMS mandated that Medicare-certified home health agencies perform patient-specific, comprehensive assessments for all adult, nonmaternity patients. A standard core data set, known as the Outcome and Assessment Information Set (OASIS), was required to be incorporated into a comprehensive assessment to measure patient outcomes uniformly and consistently. Two types of outcome reports are currently available based on OASIS data: Outcome Based Quality Monitoring (OBQM), which consists of 13 Adverse Event Outcomes, and Outcome Based Quality Improvement (OBQI), which includes 41 risk-adjusted or descriptive outcomes.

Home health agencies have learned that compliance with the OASIS regulations can be facilitated with the use of computerized clinical documentation systems that alert clinicians when an assessment is due, automatically incorporate the required "skip" patterns, force completion of OASIS items in order to complete a form, and display prompts to avoid data inconsistencies within an assessment. Many of these systems also permit extraction of agency-specific outcome data to monitor improvement efforts on an ongoing basis.

Integrated Care Delivery

Patient care delivery needs to be integrated both internally and externally, and computerization must foster coordination both within the organization and throughout the continuum of care. Internal coordination requires access to information by all services providing patient care and is most effectively facilitated if all clinical documentation within the home care organization is incorporated into the computerized system. Consideration must also be given to the transfer of data between the clinical software and the billing and payroll programs because visit data may now be interfaced from the clinical documentation system for reimbursement and compensation purposes.

Hospital-based home care organizations and those that belong to a health care system require systems that enhance external integration of data with affiliated care providers. Therefore, the computerized clinical documentation system must have the ability to interface with other automated systems to analyze, predict, and effectively manage patients' health status across the continuum of care.

Reimbursement

Most computerized clinical documentation systems interact with billing programs that were designed based on the traditional Medicare cost-based model. With the implementation of the Medicare Home Health Prospective Payment System, software vendors had to integrate financial and clinical information in order to calculate the Home Health Resource Group (HHRG). Although controversial, many computerized clinical documentation systems allow the clinician to view the HHRG value assigned to each Medicare patient in order to monitor resource utilization.

FRAMEWORK FOR COMPUTERIZING DOCUMENTATION

Implementing computerized clinical documentation can be a project of immense proportions affecting virtually every area of operations within the home care organization. Because of the magnitude of the project, the technology selected must be congruent with the organization, and internal processes must be redesigned based on the enhanced information capabilities. The principles of project management offer a sound structure for technological implementation of a computerized clinical documentation system, but home care organizations that have pioneered such projects have identified issues critical to overall success.

Vision

A computerized clinical documentation system is a valuable tool by which the home care organization can improve information transfer processes. To align technology with operations, however, the organization must have a clear vision of information management expectations. A comprehensive needs assessment, based on both internal and external requirements for information, can serve as a foundation for formulation of goals to guide the organization throughout the computer implementation project. Typical needs and the corresponding goals are listed in Table 15–1.

Technology

Computerized documentation has become a reality in home care as a result of the technological advancements that complement the mobile nature of the industry. The most significant impact was the introduction of portable computers to input and access data. Three different types of portable computers are currently available, and selection depends on the organization's needs, goals, work processes, and financial status. Each type of device has both strengths and limitations, as summarized in Table 15–2.

Application software is the computer program that facilitates the entry and transfer of clinical data. The majority of documentation programs permit data entry via a series of pop-up menus from which the desired options may be selected to verify the existence of a clinical finding. Because of the need to individualize documentation, some programs also offer the ability to enter free-form, narrative documentation. Application software once mandated the type of portable computer that could be used, but documentation programs have since been introduced that operate on more than one type of device.

Selection of technology begins with evaluation of the computer systems currently used within the organization. Although it may be more expedient to select the vendor supplying the organization's current billing system, this decision should be postponed until all available technology is researched. A review of the literature offers reports on product capabilities and vendor performance as well as anecdotal accounts of organizations that have computerized the documentation process. The published reports of successful implementation each identify a different computerized system, however.

The selection process is often based on financial considerations, but the least expensive tech-

---

Table 15–1 Expectations of a Computerized Clinical Documentation System

Needs	Goals
Efficiency	Logical, effective, and efficient work flow Timely, consistent, accurate, and accessible documentation
Productivity	Reduction in paperwork Ability to increase visits made per clinician Reduction in rework
Cost effectiveness	Cost savings Cost avoidance Cost benefits
Staff satisfaction	Increased time for patient care delivery Continued staff retention
Management of information	Integrated, value-added system Effective use of resources
Quality improvement	Compliance with standards Ability to monitor and manage clinical outcomes

Table 15–2 Comparison of Portable Computers

Device	Advantages	Disadvantages
Laptop or notebook computer	Data storage capabilities Ease of text entry Full-screen viewing	Weight/size Cost
Hand-held device	Weight/size Ease of transport Cost	Limited viewing screens Limited viewing capacity
Pen-based tablets	Ease of use Weight/size Ease of training	Cost Standardized pick lists Handwriting recognition unreliable

nology may not be the most cost-effective technology. Financial justification requires in-depth analysis of potential cost savings through staff reduction, elimination of work processes, and better utilization of resources. The possibility of cost avoidance relative to additional equipment and cost benefits from increased staff efficiency also affect calculation of the actual financial expenditures.

An effective strategy in the selection of technology is a site visit to another organization that is an experienced user. By previewing the impact of the system on daily operations and the functionality of the technology, the capabilities of the computerized documentation system can be realistically evaluated. If detailed questions are prepared before the visit, the home care organization can obtain the information necessary to make an informed decision. Responses from the clinical, administrative, and information management staff at the site visit can also be instrumental in planning for computerization. Exhibit 15–1 offers a list of questions that may be asked during a site visit.

Commitment

The hardware and software may be key components of the computerized clinical documentation system, but commitment of the people within the organization is crucial to the success of the project. Involvement of the future users on the implementation team encourages commitment, and essential team members include staff from information systems and all clinical services. Operational areas such as utilization management, quality management, medical records, admissions, reimbursement, and employee compensation may also be represented on the team. If the project implementation team is formed as soon as the decision is made to investigate the possibility of computerizing documentation within the organization, team members can be vital in solicitation of input from staff regarding current needs and expectations and the development of realistic goals. Open communication and consensus decision making within the team further strengthen commitment to the project.

Human Factors

There is a tendency to focus on the technologic requirements associated with computerized documentation, but the ultimate outcome of the project is dependent upon the human factor: the clinical staff who will be using the system to input and access patient data. Because implementation of a computerized clinical documentation system is a major change for the organization, preparations must be made to assist the staff in working through the change process. Clinical staff may accept the need for the change because of frustration with manual

Exhibit 15–1 Information to Be Obtained During a Site Visit

1. Does the processing unit have enough power and speed to support the software?
2. What type of printer is used, and how many pages are printed daily?
3. What brand of portable computers is used, and how much time has been devoted to repairs and maintenance?
4. What is the percentage of "failed" communications, and what are the reasons?
5. What types of standardized and customized reports can be generated by the system, and how are they used?
6. Has there been a problem with collision of data?
7. How has security been established, and what privileges are given to clinicians?
8. How are discipline addendums handled?
9. What is the maximum caseload that can be stored on the portable computer?
10. How is care coordinated within the organization, and how are recertifications prepared?
11. Is there an electronic signature process, and how was it established?
12. How many referrals are received daily, and how do staff receive referral information?
13. How is the clinical documentation system linked to billing and payroll?
14. How was training completed for the staff?
15. What has been the impact of implementation on the management information services department?
16. How have day-to-day operations changed within the organization since the system was implemented?
17. Who is responsible for printing, sorting, and filing paper forms?
18. What policies and procedures had to be modified based on the implementation?
19. Has the number of patient visits per clinician changed since implementation?
20. How has the implementation affected revenues within the organization?
21. What percentage of clinicians enter data at the point of care?
22. How has the quality of care improved?
23. What has been the effect of the implementation on staff morale?
24. Describe the major advantages and disadvantages of using the system.
25. How could the organization further enhance operations based on the system?

charting, but still be hesitant to adapt to revised workflow processes. Therefore, proactive approaches must be implemented before actual installation of the computer system.

A critical area that must be addressed with staff is the entry of clinical data. Transcription usually refers to the entry of written data into a computer database. When a clinician jots down notes during a home visit and returns to the office to write them on the visit note form, however, this is also a form of transcription. Transcription may be acceptable with manual charting, but computerized documentation is based on data entry at the site of care delivery. If staff are not comfortable writing a visit note in the home, they will not adapt well to point-of-care data entry into a portable computer, and the full potential of the documentation system will never be realized. To address this issue, paper forms need to be revised to include checklists and prompts, and the expectation must be established that all visit notes will be completed at the site of care delivery. By the institution of point-of-care data entry with the manual system, the staff are better prepared for the eventual computerization of the process.

Acceptance of a computerized system by the clinical staff is also facilitated by familiarity with the data elements contained within the software. Many commercial computerized documentation systems offer a standardized package of textual data elements and coded options that can be selected by clinicians to enter clinical data. Because clinical staff may be unaccustomed to the standardized forced-choice options or may view the use of such options as "canned" documentation, some vendors allow customization of the options by the organization. Development of organization-specific options to be added to the software requires considerable time and effort on the part of the project implementation team, but can be crucial in overall staff acceptance of the computerized documentation system.

The provision of education and training of the staff may significantly influence the outcome of the project. Vendors offer training as part of the installation package, but such training should be limited to the project implementation team members, who can then serve as trainers for the staff. Only by understanding the basic logic of the software and the capabilities of the system can team members develop an effective educational program based on how the computerized documentation system is to be used within the organization.

Two components essential to staff education are the practical aspects regarding use of a portable computer and use of the documentation software to input and access data. Various training methods may be used, depending on the type of portable computer selected and the complexity of the software. Most organizations, however, have found it beneficial to develop clinically based training programs, offer hands-on experience with the computer outside the clinical setting, and prepare step-by-step training manuals.

Workflow

Investments in computerized documentation technology offer the potential for effective processing of information. Nevertheless, the organization will not benefit from the enhanced capabilities unless the work processes associated with manual documentation are redesigned. The most profound effect on workflow within the organization will be computer entry of clinical data. Because the basic premise of computerized documentation is the entry of data at the site of care delivery, the need for data entry by clerical staff can be reduced and possibly eliminated.

The manner in which care is managed and provided by organizational staff may also be af-

fected. Computerized documentation empowers the field staff to manage and coordinate patient care effectively, thus reducing the need for in-office coordinators or specially trained nurses to complete admission assessments and/or recertifications. Because the logical linking of data and the availability of prompts within the computer software promote data consistency and compliance with standards, the need for comprehensive in-office clinical record review is also decreased. As a result, the clinical practice model and the need for in-office support can be assessed and possibly redesigned based on enhanced technological capabilities.

EXAMPLE OF A SUCCESSFUL COMPUTER IMPLEMENTATION

Trinity HealthCare Services, serving the Memphis area in southwest Tennessee, was one of the first home care organizations to fully automate clinical documentation for all skilled services. As a Joint Commission-accredited, not-for-profit organization affiliated with a health care system, Trinity encompasses three areas of operations: a private-pay division, a home health agency, and a hospice. The initial project to computerize documentation focused on the home health agency, which is Medicare certified but offers services to a growing number of managed care patients. Agency staff include approximately 140 nurses, therapists, and social workers, who use portable computers to input and access clinical data. These skilled professionals, combined with 100 certified nursing assistants, make more than 300,000 visits annually to more than 2,000 patients.

In 1993, Trinity initiated the commitment to computerized documentation to alleviate staff frustration with documentation and paperwork. The clinical practice model adopted by Trinity empowered the staff providing home services to manage and coordinate all aspects of patient care. The staff preferred this model to in-office case management, which they believed fostered task-oriented care. The associated responsibilities created a paperwork burden, however, and the staff desired computerization to facilitate documentation. Additional goals for computerization were identified through analysis of both current and future information management requirements.

Trinity selected Clinical-Link, a software product marketed by Delta Health Systems in Altoona, Pennsylvania, because of the architecture of the software, the inclusion of all disciplines in the documentation format, the ability to enter data by means of both forced-choice options and narrative entries, and the capability of interfacing data with the billing and payroll programs. Data are entered at the site of care delivery using subnotebook computers, which are commonly referred to as laptops. The staff prefer the laptops to other portable devices because of the full screen viewing, the ability to enter text data, and the large data storage capability. Complete computerized records for more than 60 patients can be maintained on each laptop because of the size of the hard drive. Data entry is simplified by the arrangement of forms within activities, as depicted in Figure 15-1. Portability of the laptop was not an issue because each device weighs approximately 3 lb, measures 5 by 7 in, and can operate on a fully charged battery for up to 8 hours.

Data are transferred between the laptops and the host computer via modem communications over telephone lines. Each laptop is equipped with an internal modem card, and the host computer receives data via 16 external modems. Data are automatically transmitted each night from the laptop to the host computer, also known as the server, at a preset time. Once the server processes all updated data, retransmission with each laptop is completed on a predetermined schedule. Only data for patients assigned to the laptop user are transmitted, however. Communications between the laptop and server can also be established on demand if the user needs to obtain additional assignments or patient data.

An additional module, consisting of a standardized nursing care plan based on North American Nursing Diagnosis Association (NANDA) diagnoses, was offered by the vendor, but the staff preferred the basic Clinical-Link structure. Clinicians complete discipline-specific assessments and care plans, but forms for documenting demographic information, diagnoses, medical history, and medications are shared. Pertinent data are then transferred to HCFA Form 485, which serves as a comprehensive plan of care.

At the recommendation of the vendor, Trinity purchased an external library of drug information for inclusion in the documentation software. More than 9,000 medications are contained in the library, which supplies information such as the generic and brand names of the drug, appro-

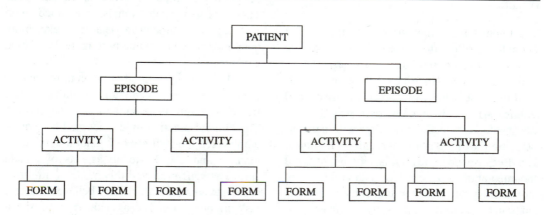

Figure 15–1 Organization of Data within Clinical-Link

priate uses, precautions or warnings, and potential side effects. Nurses can provide drug education while viewing the information on screen and by printing a hard copy of the information for the patient. The use of the drug library has promoted the identification of potential drug interactions and has standardized patient education relative to drug information.

Project Development

Trinity originally planned to limit computer implementation to 17 laptops. As recommended by the literature, additional laptops were to be slowly phased in over the next 3 to 5 years. When flow diagramming the work processes, however, the project implementation team discovered that partial implementation and the resultant parallel documentation systems would actually increase, rather than decrease, costs. Through extensive research, the implementation team prepared a proposal to justify the purchase of 123 additional laptop computers so that point-of-care computerized documentation could be implemented for all skilled services. This included all full-time and part-time nurses, physical therapists, speech therapists, occupational therapists, and social workers. Costs were justified through savings from the elimination of paid office time for the clinical staff, the reduction of data entry and support staff positions, and decreased printing costs; the proposal was approved immediately before the installation in November 1994.

Education for in-office staff was conducted by a vendor representative, but the project implementation team, in conjunction with staff development personnel, designed the training program for the clinical staff. The training program consisted of 20 hours of instruction regarding use of the laptops, organization of data, entry and retrieval of data, and laptop communications, and the clinical staff attended training sessions in groups of eight each week until all laptops were assigned. Training manuals detailing the input of data based on agency operations were also developed and issued to users during the computer classes. Each staff member was expected to transition from paper forms within 6 weeks of completion of the training session. Full implementation of the computerized documentation system was achieved within 5 months of the installation. Exhibit 15–2 offers an overview of the training program.

Some organizations have reported difficulties with implementation of laptops as a result of staff unfamiliarity with computers and lack of typing skills. At Trinity, however, this was not a factor. The staff who had limited computer experience were attentive during the training sessions and found the software to be user-friendly. In contrast, the few staff members who were skilled in computers had greater difficulty because they were hesitant to accept the logic of the software program. To decrease the amount of typing necessary to enter data, the project team developed and added more than 3,000 textual and coded options to the system. Staff were encouraged to use the standardized options but were not restricted from entering additional text.

Security of Information

Because staff would have access to the database of Trinity's patients and their computerized records, security measures had to be implemented to protect the data and prevent unauthorized access. Clinical-Link has internal levels of security based on the privileges assigned to each user, and individual passwords are required to access the system. External levels of security, however, were developed by Trinity to protect the investment in the laptop computers.

When laptops were assigned, the users were required to sign an agreement specifying the care and use of the device. Exhibit 15–3 offers an example of Trinity's laptop agreement.

Clinical Record

Although clinical documentation has been computerized, an electronic clinical record is not

Exhibit 15–2 Computer Implementation: Laptop Training Program

---

Day 1 (8 hours)

Computer basics:
  Computer log-on
  Keyboard and function keys
  Organization of data

E-mail

Discipline assessment:
  Obtaining the assignment
  Selecting the patient
  Assessment activity
  Preparing the orders
  Ready for certification
  Assessment verbal order

Day 2 (8 hours)

Interim orders

Daily visit

Home health aide supervisory visit

Recertification:
  Determining patients requiring recertification
  Recertification activity
  Ready for recertification

Day 3 (4 hours)

Transfer process

Resume care

Discharge:
  Discipline discharge
  Discipline readmit
  Agency discharge

Laptop communications

---

yet a reality. Hard copies of the forms must be printed and filed in a paper record as each form is created and revised. The Clinical-Link system was designed so that the printed form could be reviewed and signed by the staff member who entered the data to validate the entry in the clinical record. Both HCFA and the Joint Commission, however, permit the use of a unique identifier or computer key to authenticate computerized entries for the clinical record if precautions are employed to ensure confidentiality and proper use of the identifier or key. Based on these standards, Trinity developed an agreement for all users to sign, stipulating that they would only use their assigned unique identifier to authenticate entries. The agreement is shown in Exhibit 15–4. As a result of the signed agreements, staff are not required to return to the office daily to sign the computer-generated forms, and this has greatly improved staff efficiency and acceptance of the computerized documentation system. During the implementation, however, written data had to be entered for staff who were not yet assigned laptops. When this occurred, the data entry staff used a special transcription identifier so that the form would be reviewed and signed by the primary author before being filed in the medical record.

The printing of the computer-generated forms was also an issue because of volume. After the nightly communications, by which data are transmitted to the host computer, up to 6,000 forms are printed that require a dedicated duplexing laser printer. Three additional laser printers are available for printing of reports and clinical forms on demand. Originally, forms were printed in batches based on the name of the primary author, and this required additional sorting before filing in the clinical record. Updates to the software have since addressed this problem, so that all forms can now print alphabetically by patient name.

Evaluation

Monitoring of the project was ongoing, but evaluation of the effectiveness of the computer-

Exhibit 15–3 Laptop Agreement

Trinity HealthCare Services
Home Health Agency
Clinical-Link Notebook Computer Agreement

As an employee of Trinity HealthCare Services Home Health Agency, I accept the assignment of *Clinical-Link* Notebook Computer (#_____). I understand that the Notebook is a component of the computer issued by the agency for documentation of clinical information. As a designated *Clinical-Link* Notebook computer user, I make the following agreements:

1. I agree to use the Notebook only for the purpose of documenting clinical information.
2. I agree to follow the instructions that I received regarding the care and use of the Notebook, including:
   a. transporting the Notebook only in the carrying case;
   b. preventing extensive exposure of the Notebook to temperature extremes;
   c. preventing exposure of the Notebook to water or other liquids;
   d. using a proper electrical outlet when connecting the Notebook to AC power; and
   e. never dissembling the Notebook.
3. I understand that, if the Notebook is damaged or lost due to willful neglect or willful abuse, I am financially responsible for repairs and/or replacement up to the full cost of the Notebook.
4. I agree that I will not load nor attempt to load any software programs to the Notebook.
5. I agree that I will perform Nightly Communications each day, unless an exception has been approved by the MIS Department, and I will perform Demand Communications as requested.
6. I agree to bring the Notebook issued to me, as well as additional equipment (e.g., modem, cables) to the MIS Department for maintenance inspection monthly and as requested.
7. In the event that my employment with Trinity HealthCare Services is terminated, I understand that I must return the Notebook to the MIS Department prior to or on my last day of employment.

Employee: _____   **Date:** _____

MIS Manager/Designee: _____   **Date:** _____

Courtesy of Trinity HealthCare Services, Memphis, Tennessee

---

ized documentation system was delayed until 4 months after full implementation. In August 1995, the outcome of the project was analyzed based on the preestablished goals of greater efficiency, increased productivity, cost effectiveness, staff satisfaction, improved management of information, quality improvement, and patient satisfaction.

Efficiency

Efficiency was initially measured in relation to the goal of timely, consistent, accurate, and accessible documentation. Computer entry of data at the point of care ensured that the documentation was timely and eliminated the need for assessment and recertification information to be transcribed in the agency's database by clerical staff. There were problems with modem communications between the laptops and the host computer, but delays were no greater than with submission of written paperwork; furthermore, once the data were transmitted, they were immediately available for review. The consistency of documentation also improved as a result of on-screen prompts, the use of the coded and textual options within the software, and the ability to ac-

Exhibit 15–4 Agreement for the Use of a Unique Identifier

Trinity HealthCare Services
Home Health Agency

Agreement for Use of Unique Identifier for the Authentication
of Entries in the Computer Clinical Record

I acknowledge that, as an employee of Trinity HealthCare Services Home Health Agency, I have been authorized to make entries in the *Clinical-Link* computer system. I further acknowledge that I have been issued a unique identifier to be used when making clinical entries in *Clinical-Link*. I agree that I will keep the unique identifier confidential, and I will only use the unique identifier issued to me to authenticate entries in *Clinical-Link* for which I am the primary author.

To maintain security of the computer system for transcribed entries in *Clinical-Link*, I understand that any entries transcribed for me must be personally reviewed and authenticated by means of my handwritten signature and the date of review.

Employee: _____   Date: _____

Supervisor/Designee: _____   Date: _____

Courtesy of Trinity HealthCare Services, Memphis, Tennessee

---

cess prior assessments and clinical findings. Data were more accurate because software prompts required updating of the plan of care and generation of a physician's order before documentation of an intervention. This resulted in up-to-date plans of care, which significantly reduced the time required for the recertification activity. More important, the documentation was accessible so that current patient information was readily available and staff could view assessments and visit notes entered by other disciplines.

Analysis of workflow patterns was also used to measure efficiency. During the implementation process, workflow was redesigned to eliminate redundancy and streamline operations. Duplication of paperwork was eliminated, work flowed more logically and effectively, and the computer became a valuable tool for review of records and retrieval of management information. For example, the tracking of outstanding assessments and recertifications required a full-time position with the complicated manual

process, but is now a completely automated process with the computerized system.

Because Clinical-Link contains a relational database, all activities must be completed in a timely manner to achieve efficient workflow. The software logic precipitated problems, however, if one discipline did not complete the recertification activity within the required time frame. Some of the staff therefore were not pleased when the computer held them accountable for completing assigned tasks on a timely basis. Management was required to address such situations through the monitoring of computer-generated reports to ensure that efficient workflow was not impeded.

Overall, efficiency of the skilled disciplines improved with Clinical-Link because clinical data were integrated and accessible. Because of Trinity's decision for the nursing assistant services to continue manual charting, however, parallel documentation systems had to be maintained, which affected organizational efficiency.

The skilled services prepare the nursing assistant plan of care using Clinical-Link, but the data have to be transmitted to the host computer and printed in the office and the form transported to the patient's home. Because nursing assistants do not have access to the computer, there are also delays in notifying them regarding newly admitted and discharged patients. It has been realized that greater efficiency could be gained by expanding computerized documentation to include the nursing assistant services, but it has been difficult to justify costs.

Productivity

During August 1995, a visit analysis was completed to determine the impact of computerization on staff productivity. At Trinity, the field staff are paid per visit, and before computer implementation each staff member was compensated for the 5 hours of office time required each week to complete paperwork. After the implementation, reimbursement for office time was eliminated because documentation could be completed in the patient's home. The results of the visit analysis revealed that computerization permitted each staff member to make up to two additional visits per day. The most significant finding, however, was the number of visits completed by the nurses performing the start of care assessments. Before computerization, these nurses typically completed no more than two assessments each day because of the amount of paperwork required. By August 1995, however, up to three assessments could be completed daily.

Productivity was also measured in terms of the time required for documentation because of the concern that the visit times would be significantly lengthened. Overall, the average visit time increased less than 2 minutes. This may have been due to the fact that most of the staff were already accustomed to point-of-care data entry using the manual process. The length of a start of care assessment remained at approximately 90 minutes, but the majority of the documentation is now completed in the home, which allows patient participation in developing the plan of care. In contrast, the manual process required that most of the documentation be done in the office.

Documentation time in relation to the recertification process was significantly decreased. Before computerization, this activity required in-office time to review the clinical record and update the plan of care. Because Clinical-Link facilitates continual updating of the plan of care, the recertification activity now requires less than 15 minutes.

The reduction in rework has also enhanced productivity. Before computerization, extensive review was required to ensure that services were performed as prescribed and that the medication profiles were accurate. The prompts contained in the Clinical-Link system have decreased the problem with documenting orders because a physician's order can be automatically generated each time the plan of care is updated. Medication profiles are a required form for all nursing activities, and as a result accuracy has improved.

Cost Effectiveness

In the proposal for the additional laptops, the project implementation team projected a savings of $7.81 for each nursing visit within 6 months of full implementation. Comparison of financial data for October 1994 and August 1995 revealed that nursing costs had actually decreased by $12.69 per visit. During this 10-month time span, there were unanticipated expenditures, such as the purchase of additional printers and modems and the expansion of the information management department as well as the costs associated with training. The aggregate visit costs, however, were reduced by almost $5.00 per visit. Financial review since August 1995 noted that aggregate visit costs have remained relatively unchanged.

Staff Satisfaction

In October 1994, the nursing staff at Trinity participated in a study to measure their levels of work satisfaction using the Work Characteristics Instrument as the data collection tool.

Responses from the majority of the nurses revealed that, although they perceived their work as moderately to highly exciting, they viewed paperwork and documentation as the most frustrating aspects of their jobs. The survey was repeated in August 1995 to determine the impact of computerization on staff satisfaction. Results revealed that the overall levels of work satisfaction remained relatively unchanged, but the frustration with paperwork was replaced by technological concerns, such as unsuccessful modem communications. The study findings are presented in Table 15–3.

Work satisfaction was also measured in terms of retention. Other organizations that had implemented laptop computers had forewarned Trinity to expect up to a 10 percent turnover in clinical staff. As of August 1995, however, only one part-time therapist had resigned from Trinity because of unwillingness to accept computerized documentation. This resignation was due, in part, to the procedure for completion of the recertification activity, and the procedure has since been revised.

The redesign of work processes could have affected in-office work satisfaction as a result of changes in job functions and workflow. The implementation team prepared for the reduction of positions through attrition, and as job functions changed there was a reallocation of assignments within the organization. This proactive approach was instrumental in maintaining staff satisfaction throughout the organization.

Management of Information

One of the goals at Trinity is effective use of resources regarding the management of information. This was partially accomplished with the improved access to current patient information, but effective use of resources to extract historical data was not achieved. Clinical-Link, like many similar products on the market, does not maintain a complete electronic record. To review and track previous data other than visit notes, interim orders, and communication documents, the paper records must still be retrieved.

To manage information effectively, Trinity sought an integrated system for the retrieval of information. Clinical data interface to the billing system to produce HCFA Form 485 and generate bills; visit data are interfaced to both the billing and payroll systems. Each system maintains a separate database, however, which must be accessed to extract information. Data can be transferred from one system to the other, but the actual interfacing of data between systems has been a challenge. Each system is written in a different programming language, and the data interface is not a completely automated system.

Quality Improvement

To ensure quality, there must be compliance with standards. Computerization has promoted compliance with prompts to remind staff when a recertification activity is due, the ease of generating interim orders, and the ongoing revision of the plan of care. Computerized documentation has also facilitated on-screen review of records, so that the clinical record review process is more effective but less time consuming. Each supervisor completes a random review of visit notes weekly and offers immediate feedback to the staff member, which has resulted in a continual improvement of the quality of documentation.

An important aspect of the quality improvement process is outcome management. At this time, however, only coded data elements can be automatically extracted. As part of the Clinical-Link user group, Trinity has contributed input into the development of an additional module for the monitoring of clinical outcomes. Although the module is not yet available, Trinity has initiated outcome monitoring with the addition of the OASIS data elements to the forced-choice options within the system. Data extraction is not automated, however, and must be completed by means of on-screen review.

Patient Satisfaction

A major concern during computerization was the impact on patient care. Other organizations had reported that laptop computers interfered with the delivery of patient care, but feedback from the Trinity staff suggested the opposite. The staff reported that the use of the laptop promoted patient participation in the care planning

Table 15–3 Work Excitement Survey: Trinity HealthCare Service (Data Are Percentages)

Level of Work Excitement	October 1994	August 1995
Extremely excited	12	12
Very excited	21	19
Moderately excited	18	17
Somewhat excited	17	19
Not too excited	4	3
TOTAL	72	70

process, which in turn increased interaction between the patient and staff. The results of the increased interaction have been evidenced by the responses to patient satisfaction surveys. Since implementation, patient satisfaction ratings have not decreased below 95.0 percent, and as of January 1996 they had reached an all-time high of 96.1 percent.

Decade of Experience

Trinity now has a decade of experience in computerized clinical documentation. Within 2 years of initial implementation, the clinical documentation system was expanded to nursing assistants to improve interdisciplinary communication and promote compliance. This resulted in reduced manual review of the nursing assistant notes and increased compliance at no additional cost. The clinical documentation system was expanded to the other home health agencies within the Baptist Memorial Health Care Corporation (BMHCC) between 1996 and 1998, and adapted for use by hospice in 2002. Approximately 300 clinicians are currently using the documentation system in 7 home health agencies and 8 hospices within BMHCC. The results of the subsequent expansions have been similar to those originally experienced at Trinity.

The original implementation involved the Delta Health Systems Clinical-Link. Siemens has since acquired Delta, and the clinical software has been replaced with Novius Clinical View. The transition was facilitated by the ability to maintain Clinical-Link and Clinical-View simultaneously throughout the transition.

CONCLUSION

Implementation of a computerized documentation system can enable the home care organization to manage clinical data in an accurate and efficient manner that enhances patient care. Organizational expectations must be aligned with technological capabilities, however, to realize the benefits of computerization. Organizations that have pioneered computerization of documentation demonstrate that success of the project also requires a detailed and well-executed plan, active involvement of staff, and the commitment of the entire organization.

REFERENCES

Baldwin, D., and Price, S. 1994. Work excitement: The energizer of home healthcare nursing. *Journal of Nursing Administration* 24: 37–42.

Grimm, C. 1996. Today's hottest technology: Mobile computing. *Remington Report* 4: 6–8.

Joint Commission on Accreditation of Healthcare Organizations. 2003. *2004–2005 Comprehensive accreditation manual for homecare*. Oakbrook Terrace, IL: Joint Commission.

Lynch, S. 1994. Job satisfaction of home health nurses. *Home Healthcare Nurse* 12: 21–28.

National Association for Home Care. 1994. Draft uniform data set for home care and hospice. *Caring* 14: 10–75.

Pierce, C. 1995. The dawn of computer age for home care. *Health Data Management* 2: 61–64.

Shaughnessey, P., et al. 1995. Outcome-based quality improvement in home care. *Caring* 15: 44–49.

Stern, E. 1996. Key management information strategies. *Remington Report* 4: 10–13.

Westra, B., and Raup, G. 1995. Computerized charting: An essential tool for survival. *Caring* 15: 52–57.

CHAPTER 16

Home Telehealth: Improving Care and Decreasing Costs

Ann K. Frantz

INTRODUCTION

In 1912, Willem Einthoven sent a transmission from his new electrocardiogram (ECG) invention over the hospital telephone to his laboratory across the street. This is the first known use of transferring health data over telecommunication lines, also known as *telemedicine*. It wasn't until the early 1990s, however, that the vision of telemedicine debuted in home health care.

Today monitoring and delivery of health data via telecommunication modalities, between the home and health care professional, is referred to as *home telehealth*. Home telehealth encompasses the utilization of many different technologies that collect many types of health data from ECG devices, glucometers, sphygmomanometers, weight scales, and video cameras. A variety of telecommunication modalities are used to transfer health data including plain old telephones (POTs), cable television lines, satellite connections, and the Internet.

As home telehealth technologies have evolved, the purpose and utilization intent have changed. When telehealth technologies were first introduced into home care, research questions regarding utilization included:

- Will clients use the technology?
- Can clients use the technology correctly? (Lenz and Mahmud, 1995)

- Will nurses incorporate telehealth technology into practice? (Remington and Frantz, 2000)

What early researchers found was that telehealth, under certain circumstances, was accepted and used by clients and clinicians. Telehealth study questions evolved to include:

- Does home telehealth affect clinical outcomes? (Britton et al., 1999; Cordisco et al., 1999)
- Does home telehealth affect care costs? (Dimmick et al., 2000; Jerant et al., 2001)

Outcomes studies and demonstration projects continue to indicate that home telehealth can improve clinical outcomes as well as cost effectiveness when used correctly. Telehealth research is beginning to ask more sophisticated questions. For instance, in one recent study, Miranda et al. (2002) found that outcomes associated with telephone encounters between nursing visits for heart failure clients were equal to outcomes reported in studies using more sophisticated telehealth technologies.

Home telehealth is becoming more recognized by clinical professionals. In 1999, the American Nurses Association published *Competencies for Telehealth Technologies in Nursing*. The Home Healthcare Nurses Association (HHNA) has recognized telehealth as a practice intervention and included "Guidelines for Telehealth Integration into Home Care" in the Home Healthcare Nurses Core Curriculum (HHNA, 2001). In addition, the American Telemedicine Association Special Interest Group on Home Telehealth adopted "Home Telehealth Clinical Guidelines" to help guide best practice utilization of telehealth in the home setting (American Telemedicine Association, 2002). Home telehealth appears to be an effective tool; however, professional definition for best practice integration continues to unfold.

HOME TELEHEALTH GOALS AND OUTCOMES

The overall goal of home health care is to help the client and caregiver transition safely and effectively to self-care. Home telehealth is one tool that facilitates achievement of this goal in home care nursing. Three main goals drive home care's need to integrate telehealth into the client's plan of care:

1. Identify early exacerbation/decompensation of the client's condition
2. Reduce unscheduled nurse visits
3. Decrease emergency room visits/acute hospitalizations

Identification of Early Exacerbation/Decompensation

It is common for home care clients to present with multiple comorbidities that confound recovery from an acute event. Managing complex disease entities, various medications, geriatric issues, knowledge deficits, and increased anxiety in an uncontrolled setting is a monolithic task for any nurse. It is difficult for home care nurses to cost effectively make innumerable visits in order to assure that the patient is safe and knowledgeable regarding their care in order to keep from returning to the hospital for the same problem. Home telehealth connects the clinician and client remotely in order to maintain contact and yet minimize extra visits and cost.

Remote vital sign monitoring, also known as *telemonitoring*, allows clinicians to track data points that alert to early client health status changes. Identification of early changes in vital data allows the clinician to intervene before client status decompensates, requiring an emergency room visit or acute hospitalization. When home care nurses visit clients one to two times weekly, trends in vital sign data can be missed. Home telehealth technology is one tool that home care nurses can use to identify early exacerbation.

Identification of early signs and symptoms of exacerbation is the most key goal associated with home telehealth. Whether the signs and symptoms are related to wound infection, congestive heart failure, or asthma, it is important to define what measures indicate early exacerbation.

For example, managing fluid volume in heart-failure patients is key to averting fluid excess in the lungs or congestive heart failure. In order to avoid fluid build-up, the home care nurse must help the patient identify signs and symptoms of early exacerbation. By the time that the patient has gained 2 pounds or more of weight, fluid is compromising cardiac output and the patient may require hospitalization. Helping the patient define their symptoms of early exacerbation is difficult because the signs are vague and ambiguous—fatigue, poor appetite, bloated feeling, or poor concentration. Patients can easily rationalize these symptoms and relate them to causes other than heart failure. Because weight is a sign of late heart-failure exacerbation, placing a telemonitor for heart failure in the home seems inadequate, when the only signs and symptoms of early exacerbation are subjective verbal reports.

Fortunately, an objective measure of thoracic fluid volume, Zo, has become available that indicates changes in fluid as early as 2 weeks before weight gain (Frantz, 2003). Consequently, heart failure home telemonitors that measure thoracic Zo are able to help identify early exacerbation. The physiological parameter being measured must be specific to the disease state, in order to identify changes in status early enough for the home care team to offer a proactive care regimen. (See Figure 16-1.)

Reduce Unscheduled Nurse Visits

Complexity of client conditions combined with a critical nursing shortage mandate that home care management focus on efficiency. Home telehealth technologies offer a method for staying connected with the patient and still maintaining visit frequencies. Telehealth is not intended to replace nurse visits; rather, it is intended to enhance and promote better communication between the nurse and client. Home telehealth thereby allows home care nurses to maintain projected frequency rates without additional unexpected visits that cost time and money.

Decrease Emergency Room Visits and Acute Hospitalizations

The goal of home care is to help the client achieve independent care while remaining at home. Acute care costs associated with the emergency department and acute hospitalizations continue to drive up health care costs. The cost of care at home is significantly less than acute care. Consequently, health care payers, such as the Center for Medicare and Medicaid Services (CMS), track how many home care clients seek emergency room care and require acute hospitalization. These tracking criteria are published for each home care agency as part of the Quality Home Health Initiative at the CMS Web site. Although it has always been an important goal in home care to decrease emergency room access and acute hospitalizations, today health care payers and consumers alike closely scrutinize these goals.

When telehealth is utilized appropriately, client and agency outcomes linked to telehealth initiatives will include:

- *Expeditious client independence.* Telehealth technology that is placed with the appropriate client will promote active participation in care. Automatic data down-

---

Example: Early Signs and Symptoms of Heart Failure Exacerbation

Early S&S Exacerbation	Late S&S Exacerbation	Acute Exacerbation
↓Appetite Fatigue Bloated feeling Fullness in ears ↓ZO	↑Peripheral edema ↑SOB with exertion Weight gain ↑Abdominal girth ↑Pillow use Develops a cough	Pitting edema ↑SOB @ rest Develops S3 Develops crackles SaO2↓ JVD Zo less than 15 ohms

This is when home care nursing intervention must occur to prevent CHF and hospitalization.

Figure 16–1. Home Telehealth Goal: Identification of Early Signs and Symptoms
Source: Courtesy of Ann K. Frantz.

loading often promotes client dependence rather than critical thinking about how, when, and why physiological data changes. Telehealth systems that encourage client participation also promote self-care learning, which greatly facilitates discharge from care with all goals met.

- *Increased client and caregiver satisfaction.* Technology appropriately matched with the client and caregiver's skill set improves care satisfaction. Clients and caregivers enjoy the continuous link to their health care nurse and report reduced levels of anxiety when the technology is available round-the-clock. Mismatched technology can greatly increase anxiety levels and reduce care satisfaction. If clients are unfamiliar with computers, then asking them to learn computer skills during their critical recovery time will only serve to increase stress and reduce satisfaction.
- *Increased nurse job satisfaction.* Home care nurses feel pressure from their clients, caregivers, agency administration, physicians, and themselves to successfully meet care goals. When appropriate home telehealth is introduced as a care tool, not a care substitute, then nurses report increased job satisfaction related to telehealth utilization.
- *Increased physician satisfaction with care delivered.* Simply stated, when clients and caregivers are happy with care, then physicians usually are satisfied. Physicians appreciate referring clients to agencies when there is certainty that the care provided in the home is best practice.
- *Decreased adverse events.* A reduction in adverse events was an unexpected outcome associated with clients using home telehealth. Increased clinician communication and connection with the client appears to minimize adverse events associated with home care.

TYPES, CONNECTIVITY, AND POWER SOURCES OF HOME TELEHEALTH TECHNOLOGIES

Home telehealth technologies range from a simple telephone to sophisticated video imaging systems that are run over a television cable or computer modem. Telehealth systems that utilize video imaging and a two-way connection so that clinician and client may visually communicate in real time with one another, are defined in the American Telemedicine *Home Telehealth Clinical Guidelines* (2002) as "interactive home telehealth." Interactive home telehealth systems have specific issues revolving around client privacy and confidentiality that must be addressed prior to practice integration. Special written consent must be obtained prior to technology setup in the home, because no client should be viewed or heard without their knowledge or consent. In addition, the guidelines for interactive home tele-health include acknowledging additional personnel or visitors that are within viewing or audio range of the encounter. The guidelines also recommend that the interactive home telehealth encounter frequency should be incorporated into the plan of care. Documentation of each client telehealth encounter should be kept in the client's chart.

There are specific guidelines for home telemonitoring also outlined by the American Telemedicine *Home Telehealth Clinical Guidelines* (2002). Policies and procedures need to be written prior to technology integration regarding action that is taken when parameters being monitored deviate from the set ranges. Transmission frequencies must also be incorporated into the client's plan of care. For instance, if the nurse wants the telehealth system to measure weight, blood pressure, and pulse daily, then that action must be included in the plan of care. The client and caregiver must agree to engage in this activity as well.

Guidelines state that measured data elements (blood glucose, blood pressure, or peak flow) for telemonitoring must be clearly defined. In addition, monitored parameters should have access manually and via computer. All data, no matter what type of telehealth system is being used, should have a date and time stamp, and be Health Insurance Portability and Accountability Act (HIPAA) compliant.

If remote sensors are used with home telehealth technology, then the telehealth system is required to indicate:

- When it is out of range for wireless operation
- When there is a low battery status
- That the sensor is working properly

In addition, remote sensors should not irritate the client's skin or interfere with sleep. Remote sensors are not supposed to contain substances that pose a health threat if chewed or licked.

Many different telehealth technology systems and configurations exist. It is important to understand the power and connectivity source so as to assure successful utilization. Most systems require electricity and a telephone outlet. These systems require consideration in remote geographic locations, as there are still areas in North America and around the world that do not have access to electricity or telephonic connections. Many telehealth systems, especially video interactive systems, require a broadband Internet connection. Frequently, clients do not have broadband Internet connectivity in their region, let alone in their home. Cable is another connection modality, but again not every region or home has cable television access. Consequently, prior to telehealth system selection and introduction, connectivity and power issues must be addressed as to what is available in the service area.

Most home telehealth technologies are modular as opposed to fixed systems. A fixed system refers to a technology configured as "one-size-fits-all." The fixed system often comes with a

monitor screen, a sphygmomanometer, and a weight scale attached. The two physiological measurement devices cannot be interchanged based on client need. The modular system, however, typically has a monitor screen and outlets for measurement devices that are selected by the clinician based on client need. If the client is being monitored to identify early changes in asthma status, then a blood pressure cuff and weight scale may not be a good telehealth technology choice. However, a system that uses a peak flow meter and allows the patient to grade breathlessness may be a very successful choice. Telehealth technologies that are modular, often referred to as *plug and play*, offer utilization to a broader scope of clients.

SCOPE OF HOME TELEHEALTH

Historically, home telehealth has targeted the most difficult to manage and most frequently referred diagnoses, such as heart failure and chronic obstructive pulmonary disease. Clients living with these chronic diseases often require intense home care resources and time. As technologies have evolved, the number of projected visits and past care intensity defines clients who benefit from home telehealth. Clients with frequent wound interventions, for instance, can be monitored safely and effectively for caregiver efficacy and progress toward healing via an interactive video telehealth system.

Several home care agencies use telehealth to monitor clients recovering from cardiothoracic surgery. Newly diagnosed and unstable diabetics use telehealth systems to collect and connect blood glucose and nutrition data. Clients living with the care intricacies associated with end stage renal disease are finding benefits via telehealth technologies. Physical therapists are using interactive home telehealth to conduct and evaluate strengthening programs for patients in remote geographic areas. Even hospice care has enlisted home telehealth to connect clinicians with clients, and clients with remote family members.

As telehealth technology becomes more simple and modular, the scope of application in home care becomes increasingly broad. Home telehealth initiatives are currently limited more by cost than any other factor.

EVALUATING HOME TELEHEALTH TECHNOLOGY FOR SUCCESS

Everett Rogers (1995) created a framework from which to predict the successful adoption of new innovations based upon many years of research. Rogers' framework provides five attributes that affect successful innovation adoption. When home care agencies and home care nurses evaluate telehealth technologies, Rogers' five attributes provide a structured approach to assuring success. Five attributes affecting successful innovation technology integration are:

1. Relative advantage
2. Compatibility
3. Complexity
4. Trialability
5. Observability

Relative Advantage

The relative advantage is the degree to which a device or technology is perceived as being better than another. Home care professionals must clearly and succinctly define why one system or telehealth approach is better than another. Relative advantages may provide an economic advantage, social prestige, or professional credibility.

Home telehealth systems can offer economic advantage when the technology is placed with patients who typically require many unscheduled nurse visits that deplete financial reimbursements. In addition, telehealth can offer professional credibility and social prestige when system outcomes demonstrate reduction in emergency room utilization and acute hospitalizations on the home health care quality initiative reports.

Compatibility

Home care clinicians, managers, and administrators must evaluate telehealth technology on many different levels for compatibility. Close scrutiny is required to evaluate whether the technology is compatible with:

- *Professional values and beliefs.* Home telehealth has many assets that lend to enhanced care. However, despite its apparent value, technology removes an integral component of nursing: physical touch. Nurses need to query whether or not they believe that they can deliver care without physical touch. In 1999, Frantz (2001) surveyed 100 home care nurses regarding touch in relation to the use of telehealth. The majority of nurses believed that they could deliver quality care without physical contact "some of the time." The majority of nurses that stated they could not deliver quality care without physical contact were field nurses. This survey has important connotations for home care managers because if the field staff does not believe that telehealth will work, then these values will present significant barriers to successful integration.
- *Client values and beliefs.* Just as professional clinicians must concur with telehealth efficacy, so must the client and caregiver. One telehealth initiative asked stroke caregivers to enter daily client data in order to determine outcomes improvement with care satisfaction. Ninety percent of the caregivers declined to participate because learning how to use the technology required more energy than they believed they had. The study was never completed because the technology requirements and caregiver burden were not compatible.
- *Data value and client need.* One of the greatest barriers to telehealth optimization occurs when clients do not believe that the data they are asked to collect has compat-

ibility with their problems. If clients do not believe that the behavior of measuring weight or blood pressure will keep them healthier, then they will not engage in that activity. Clients measure peak flow to monitor asthma because changes in peak flow indicate a trend toward decompensation. Having the opportunity to intervene early in order to stave off exacerbation has value and is compatible with care goals. However, clients living with heart failure will often stop monitoring blood pressure because changes in blood pressure do not necessarily correlate with heart-failure exacerbation. Tracking weight changes has greater compatibility with care goals and will garner better client adherence. Asking clients to engage in activities that are not compatible with their goals will not drive long-term adherence. DeLusignan et al. (2000) found that heart-failure clients who were given video interactive vital sign monitors quit using the video monitors after 2 months because patients did not perceive video monitoring to be of value in meeting their care goals.

- *End-user capabilities.* The end user of the technology must be able to easily learn how to use the system and successfully give a return demonstration. Assessing the capabilities of the client and professional are both important steps toward assuring successful telehealth implementation.

  Client. Nurses must assess whether the client has sensory capabilities that minimally meet the technology requirements. For instance, technologies need large print on bright screens for older client eyes, as well as large, easy-to-push buttons for older arthritic fingers. In addition, technology alarms must be loud enough for clients with hearing difficulties. The end user's environment must be compatible with the power and connection requirements of the technology.

  Professional. Not all nurses are comfortable using computers. Consequently, telehealth systems that require computer knowledge will require focused education in order for nurses to feel comfortable with the devices. Patients call the nurse when technology problems arise; thus, it is important for the field and on-call staff to have a good working knowledge about the telehealth technology.

- *Budget.* Purchasing or leasing a telehealth system that does not offer a return on investment within the first year of utilization is not compatible with most home care agency budgets. Although the cost of telehealth technologies is decreasing, many systems still are priced over $1,500 per unit, or ask for more than $300 per patient per month in a lease arrangement. If the clients with whom the technology is placed do not incur unscheduled nurse visits, any emergency room visits, or acute hospitalizations during the episode of care, then $300 per month may be cost effective.

  The only method for assuring that telehealth cost does not exceed budget is by defining the target population up front and adhering to the prescription. For example, heart-failure patients often require multiple unscheduled nurse visits that reduce remuneration significantly. At one home care agency, a retrospective review of heart-failure clients indicated that patients requiring unscheduled visits had certain common traits that included New York Heart Failure Class IV, greater than 10 prescription medications, and more than two acute hospitalizations within the last 6 months. When clients presented with these traits at the start of care, an 80 percent chance existed that the costs of care would exceed remuneration. These patients could benefit from an increased connection with the home care nurse; consequently, telehealth investment for these patients made sense (Frantz, 2003).

With the advent of Outcomes Based Quality Improvement (OBQI) reports published from CMS, defining client populations that result in adverse outcomes, such as emergency room visits and acute hospitalizations, is a quick and easy task.

Complexity

The more complex the technology is, the more difficulty clients, caregivers and clinicians will have using it well. Consequently, home telehealth systems must be evaluated for:

- Number of buttons
- Language level associated with the directions for use (should be at a sixth grade reading level or less)
- Familiar items use such as telephone key pads or television remote controls for data entry
- No additional installation required in order to provide connectivity (some systems require an additional telephone line, cable, or computer modem)
- On-call service for technology troubleshooting is one phone call away

Trialability

Home care agencies should request a trial use of the home telehealth system in order to assure that goal attainment is probable. Trials also help evaluate compatibility and complexity issues. Trial periods should be equivalent to the reimbursement period in order to help determine whether a return on investment is possible. Every client needs to be informed that if they choose to have the technology re-

moved, they may call the agency staff at any time.

Observability

Outcomes associated with the telehealth system should be quickly and easily observed. If return on investment or goal attainment is not realized for 12 months after technology implementation, it will be more difficult to justify the telehealth initiative and garner adherence from nurses and clients. Benefits from telehealth technology should be realized within 30 to 60 days of implementation. If benefits are not realized or goals are not met, then the technology is not compatible with the client and goals or the program and care goals are poorly defined.

TAILORING HOME TELEHEALTH

Once program goals have been defined and the telehealth system selected, it is important to remember that each client and caregiver has unique reasons for agreeing to participate in a telehealth initiative. Telehealth success is incumbent on the client's participation. If the client or caregiver is not convinced that the actions required to engage in telehealth are beneficial, then they will become nonadherent.

Designing a tailored approach for each patient helps assure ongoing compliance with the telehealth program. The theory of self-regulation states that individuals will engage in self-regulatory behaviors if they perceive that the behaviors will (1) avoid disruption of usual life activities or (2) promote comfort. In home care, setting care goals are based upon these two theoretical concepts. Heart-failure clients want to stay out of the emergency room (statement 1) and do not want to experience the feeling of drowning in their own fluid (statement 2). Consequently, tailored reasoning for the heart-failure client may be stated as: "You can avoid further hospitalizations or that drowning feeling that you dislike, if you use this telehealth monitor every day."

Tailoring a telehealth plan of care by using the theory of self-regulation as a framework helps to assure adherence. If the nurse, client, and caregiver are unable to define why the telehealth system will specifically benefit them, then the technology may not be a good fit for the home.

CONCLUSION

Home telehealth is an accepted care tool in home care, but technology is only as useful as the individuals using it. Assuring that devices are compatible with clients, caregivers, and clinicians is tantamount to assuring success. In an era of rising costs and a nursing shortage, home telehealth appears to be an enduring practice tool that will help home care improve care and decrease costs.

REFERENCES

American Nurses Association. 1999. *Competencies for telehealth technologies in nursing.* Washington, D.C.: American Nurses Publishing.

American Telemedicine Association. 2002. *Home telehealth clinical guidelines.* Available at *www.americantelemed.org/.icot/hometelehealthguidelines.* (accessed September 2003).

Britton, B. P., Keehner, M. D., Still, A.T., and Walden, C. M., 1999. Innovative approaches to patient care management using telehomecare. *Home Health Care Consultant* 6(12): 11–16.

Cordisco, M. E., Benjaminovitz, A., Hammond, K., and Mancini, K., 1999. Use of telemonitoring to decrease the rate of hospitalization in patients with severe congestive heart failure. *American Journal of Cardiology* 84(7): 860–862.

deLusignan, S., Wells, S., Johnson, P., Meredith, K., and Leatham, E., 2000. Compliance and effectiveness of 1 year's home telemonitoring. *European Journal of Heart Failure* 3(6): 723–730.

Dimmick S. L., Mustaleski, C., and Burgiss, S., 2000. A case study of benefits and potential savings in rural home telemedicine. *Home Healthcare Nurse Journal* 18(2): 124–135.

Frantz, A. 2001. Evaluating technology for success in home care. *Caring* 20(7): 10–12.

Frantz, A. 2003, September 15. *Integrating telehealth into practice: Addressing the issues.* American Telemedicine

Association Home Telehealth Conference. Ft. Lauderdale, Fla.

Home Healthcare Nurses Association. 2001. Core curriculum for Home Healthcare Nurses Association. *Telehealth in Practice*, Chapter 41. Washington, D.C.: National Association of Home Care.

Jerant, A. F., Azari, R., and Nesbitt, T. S. 2001. Reducing the cost of frequent hospital admissions for congestive heart failure: A randomized trial of home telecare intervention. *Medical Care: A Journal of the American Public Health Association* 38(11): 1234–1245.

Lenz, J., and Mahmud, K., 1995. The personal telemedicine system: A new tool for the delivery of health care. *Journal of Telemedicine and Telecare* 1(1): 15–20.

Miranda, M. B., Gorski, L. A., LeFevre, J. G., Levac, K. A., Niederstadt, J. A., and Toy, A. L. 2002. An evidence-based approach to improving care of patients with heart failure across the continuum. *Journal of Nursing Care Quality* 17(1): 1–14.

Remington L., and Frantz, A., 2000. Emerging technologies: The transition from low-tech personal touch to high-tech personal touch. *Remington Report 2000,* March/April: 24–26.

Rogers, E. M., 1995. *Diffusion of innovation.* New York: The Free Press.

CHAPTER 17

Implementing a Competency System in Home Care

Carol Clarke, Irma Camaligan, and Margaret Golden

Changes in health care and advances in medical technology and managed care have significantly impacted the home care industry. Seriously ill patients are being discharged from the hospital after just a few days. Patients who were formerly kept in intensive care units are now receiving home care.

Home care leaders are faced with the overwhelming task of providing care while implementing and maintaining an effective, ongoing staff-competency program. Whether a patient needs high-technology interventions or simple assistance with activities of daily living, he or she needs a competent employee caring for him or her. Employees must be fully qualified for each assignment. Before a home care agency can assign staff to care for a patient, staff competency must be evident. This process begins upon hire and continues through the employee's entire tenure with the agency.

This chapter gives a detailed description of a competency system that works quite well for most agencies. The process begins with an organizational assessment and includes structures, orientation, continuing education, quality improvement, and suggestions on how to maintain and improve staff competency. The concrete examples, competency assessment tools, and accreditation requirements provided will assist you in developing a program for your agency.

ORGANIZATIONAL ASSESSMENT

The best place to start is reviewing your scope of services. Are you an agency devoted to the care of certain groups of patients (e.g., high tech, maternal-child, mental health, or hospice)? Do you primarily care for children, adults, or the elderly? Does your scope of care and services cover a broad range of patient groups? Be sure to include your most prevalent patient types in all your planning efforts.

Consider how many resources your agency is willing and able to devote to this project. At a minimum, it will take 6 months to put the basics in place. One year is more realistic because a competency system requires effective performance improvement and occurrence reporting processes. A team of staff, supervisors, and/or directors will need to devote time to initiate the project. After that, ongoing team effort will be required for planning, assessment, intervention, and follow-up.

Also consider what the agency is willing to pay for. Will employees be expected to attend classes on their own time? Who will teach the orientation and continuing education classes? Who will perform competency assessments? Will all or part of the learning be done through the use of self-study materials? Who will prepare these? Will you need to use a consultant to get your agency started? Will you need to subcontract part of the project? Develop a preliminary budget, and meet with the executive director and/or owner of your agency before proceeding.

Accreditation Requirements

Community Health Accreditation Program (CHAP, 2002a):

CIII.1   The organization has adequate and appropriate human resources to meet caseload and workload demands.

CIII.1b Personnel are employed and assigned responsibilities commensurate with their education and experience.

Joint Commission on Accreditation of Healthcare Organizations (JCAHO, 2001):

HR.4 The organization assesses, maintains, and improves the competence of all staff providing care and services.

The organization designs and implements a competency assessment program which is systematic and allows for a measurable assessment of staff competence. The design of the competence assessment program considers:
- care and services provided by the organization.
- ages and types of populations served.
- defined competencies required for each category of staff based on the care and services provided and populations served.
- defined competencies to be assessed during orientation.
- defined competencies that need to be assessed or reassessed on an ongoing basis, based on techniques or skills needed to provide patient care or services. Information used to design the program may include data from performance evaluations, performance improvement data, assessment of staff

learning needs, infection control data, or aggregate data on competence.
- a defined timeframe for how often competence assessment is performed for each staff member minimally once in the 3-year accreditation cycle and in accordance with law and regulation.
- assessment methods appropriate to determine the skill being assessed.
- identification of the individuals who are qualified to assess competency.
- methods for determining when education, training, and experience are acceptable as evidence of a competence or skill.
- processes for documenting competence.

JOB DESCRIPTIONS

Job descriptions form the basis of any competency system. Have a group of leaders and staff pull out the current job descriptions and look at them critically. Are you using job descriptions tailored for your organization's needs or are you using generic or hospital-based job descriptions? Is the content comprehensive enough to encompass your agency's scope of care and services? Do the competencies reflect current practice? Have you added new skills or services without updating job descriptions? If you do not have job descriptions tailored to your agency's needs, revisions will be required.

Are performance criteria written in general terms, or are they appropriately written in measurable terms, as outlined in Exhibit 17–1? Include a review of the qualifications, physical requirements, and working conditions in your job descriptions. Examples of qualifications, physical requirements, and working conditions for a registered nurse (RN) job description are outlined in Exhibit 17–2. Be sure to include qualifications required by your state and accrediting body.

Are staff familiar with their job description? Do you review performance expectations in orientation? Do staff know who they report to? Do they have a copy of their job description? Do

Exhibit 17–1 Performance Criteria in Job Descriptions

General terminology for certified home health aides (CHHAs)
Assists the patient with activities of daily living

Criteria-based measurable terminology for CHHAs
Competently assists patient in moving from bed to chair or wheelchair
Correctly prepares patient's meals according to plan of care
Dusts and vacuums the rooms the client uses

General terminology for staff RNs
Uses the nursing process

Criteria-based measurable terminology for staff RNs
Competently assesses and documents the patient's biophysical, psychosocial, safety, and educational needs
Designs a comprehensive nursing care plan that is consistent with the medical regimen to meet the patient's needs
Updates the nursing care plan as the patient's needs change, when the patient achieves goals, and/or a minimum of once a month

Source: Courtesy of Clarke Healthcare Consultants, Seminole, Florida.

you require a signature to prove that the employee understands their job description? A sample employee acknowledgement is in Exhibit 17–3.

Consider having the group of staff and leaders who review your job descriptions form a standing committee. Their responsibilities might include ongoing identification of required competencies and a review of all field staff job descriptions at preset intervals. This group may also be responsible to assist in planning ongoing staff development and competency assessment programs.

Qualifications

- Current state license as a registered professional nurse
- At least 1 year of experience as an RN within the past 3 years or documentation of a refresher course within the past year
- Able to meet health standards of employment
- Must maintain current cardio-pulmonary resuscitation certification
- Must successfully complete orientation examinations and competencies

Physical requirements

- Maintains physical capabilities to perform all work-related duties
- Ability to tolerate varied levels of stress

Working conditions

- Frequently handles sharp instruments and contaminated needles
- Cares for physically combative patients
- Potential exposure to hazardous substances (e.g., infections, chemotherapy agents)
- Potential exposure to infectious diseases
- Works in homes and neighborhoods of a variety of socioeconomic groups
- Frequent lifting of patients
- Emotional stress factor inherent in position

Source: Courtesy of Clarke Healthcare Consultants, Seminole, Florida.

Exhibit 17–2 Qualifications, Physical Requirements, and Working Conditions for an RN Job Description

Exhibit 17–3 Employee Job Description Acknowledgement

EMPLOYEE ACKNOWLEDGEMENT

I read and understand the job description above. I know it is my responsibility to follow all aspects of this job description. Further, I know it is my responsibility to ask the supervisor if I have any questions.

Date: **Signature:**

Source: Courtesy of Clarke Healthcare Consultants, Seminole, Florida.

Accreditation Requirements

Community Health Accreditation Program (CHAP, 2002a):

CIII.1c   Job descriptions for each employee category delineate lines of authority and reporting responsibilities, duties to be performed, and educational and experiential qualifications specific to the position.

1)   Employees sign and receive a copy of the specific job description at time of hire or assignment to another position.

2)   Employees identify "chain of command" considerations and state their responsibilities and duties.

3)   Current written job descriptions delineate essential elements of each position.

Joint Commission on Accreditation of Healthcare Organizations (JCAHO, 2001):

HR.2 The organization's leaders define the qualifications for all staff positions.

SUPERVISOR COMPETENCIES

While you are reviewing job descriptions, be sure to review the competencies in the supervisors' job description. You might be surprised to find out that, although your supervisors have excellent clinical experience and are fully competent, their personnel files do not reflect these accomplishments. Once identified, this problem is easily corrected. Have the supervisors submit certificates from educational programs they have attended. Consider asking a "senior" supervisor to act as a preceptor and document the competencies they validate. Successfully completed self-study modules are also acceptable. If newly hired supervisors do not have all the competencies required, simply choose programs and modules that are most appropriate to the scope of care and services that their roles encompass.

Look carefully at the types of performance criteria outlined in the supervisors' job descriptions. The supervisors' leadership competencies are often not well defined. Exhibit 17–4 lists performance criteria that you might want to consider including in your agency's job descriptions.

Evaluate the number and professional qualifications of your agency's supervisors at this time. Do you have enough supervisors to provide adequate supervision? Are your supervisors professionally credentialed to evaluate staff competencies, or do you have staff being evaluated by a supervisor with different professional credentials? For example, the RN supervisor cannot evaluate the therapist's clinical competencies. Do you have professionals of the same discipline available for consultation and review?

Exhibit 17–4 Performance Criteria for Supervisor Job Description

---

- Facilitates professional growth and development of staff by providing orientation and continuing education classes and coaching staff to improve their performance.
- Demonstrates awareness of legal issues by tracking occurrences and taking appropriate steps to reduce risk.
- Effectively supervises and maintains safety standards in accordance with agency policies, to include fire, staff safety, patient safety, and emergency preparedness.
- Submits routine reports, evaluations, patient supervisory visit notes, and staff competency reviews within established time frames.
- Participates in the quality improvement process by identifying opportunities for improvement, completing studies, evaluating results, and taking actions to improve care and services.

Source: Courtesy of Clarke Healthcare Consultants, Seminole, Florida.

Accreditation Requirements

Community Health Accreditation Program (CHAP, 2002b):

HHIII.1e There is adequate supervision of all personnel

1) *Nursing and home health aide services are under the supervision of a registered nurse.*

2) *The supervising RN has at least 2 years of home or community-based health care experience.*

3) *Clinical staff who report to a supervisor of a different discipline have the opportunity for consultation and review with a professional manager in their discipline to ensure adherence to and accountability for professional standards of clinical practice.*

Joint Commission on Accreditation of Healthcare Organizations (JCAHO, 2001):

HR.3.2 The number and qualifications of individuals supervising care and service staff are appropriate to the scope of care and services provided by the organization. For supervisory staff the organization has evidence of:

f. *knowledge and experience appropriate for assigned responsibilities.*

h. *understanding of all care and services that he or she is supervising.*

i. *understanding of all staff responsibilities associated with each level of care he or she is supervising.*

j. *Clinical and supervisory experience in accordance with organizational policy and law and regulation.*

PRE-HIRE PHASE

The prospective employee is required to complete an application and submit credentials to begin the new hire process. Basic requirements include Social Security number, driver's license number, I9, W4, and two references. Submission of the results of a current history and physical, purified protein derivative (PPD), chest radiograph (if PPD is positive), rubella, rubeola, and hepatitis immunity is usually required to meet most agencies' health requirements. Proof of graduation from high school or a graduate equivalency degree is usually required for a home health aide. Some agencies also require a criminal background check. Professional credentials complete the basic requirements for hire. These include an original copy of the RN, LPN, PT, OT, ST license or CHHA/CNA certificate, basic cardiac life support certification, proof of graduation from an accredited school/aide training program, and proof of 1 to 2 years of recent medical-surgical nursing experience (for nurses). Prospective employees are asked to present any other certifications that they have attained, including home health and hospice certification, first aid, Heartsaver, American Nurses Association certifications, intravenous (IV) or peripherally inserted central catheter (PICC) line certifications, chemotherapy certification, and the like. Copies of continuing education units are required.

Keeping track of submitted requirements and credentials is a difficult task. Many agencies have paperwork tracked on various separate forms and computer databases. Exhibit 17–5 is a new hire tracking form for RNs and LPNs that helps simplify this process. There is space for each criterion for identification of the date and person who verified the requirement or credential.

Accreditation Requirements

Community Health Accreditation Program (CHAP, 2002b):

HHIII.1a Qualified personnel are recruited and retained. Documentation is found in personnel and health files.

INTERVIEW PHASE

Once the prospective employee has completed the application process, he or she is scheduled for an interview. The interview phase further evaluates the candidate's degree of cognitive knowledge and clinical experience. After a brief period of socialization and review of the application, the interviewer presents the applicant with a case scenario. He or she then asks the applicant to identify key nursing care issues that require immediate interventions, to prioritize care, and to problem solve a variety of nursing issues. Examples of an RN scenario and a

CHHA scenario follow; naturally, you would design scenarios that represent cases prevalent in your scope of care and services.

Mr. Jones is a 27-year-old patient with a diagnosis of human immunodeficiency virus, cytomegalovirus retinitis, dehydration, and dementia. You are assigned to administer Ganciclovir (DHPG) (300 mg in 100 mL 5 percent dextrose in water over 1 hour) via a Hickman-Broviac catheter. When you arrive at the house, Mr. Jones is upset. He cannot remember if he took his oral medications last evening or this morning. The house is in total disarray. There are dishes in the sink, clutter on the floor, and cups half-filled with juice all over the bedroom. Mr. Jones is unshaven and complaining of tingling of the extremities. Your assessment reveals blood pressure 100/60, heart rate 124 beat/min, respirations 24 per minute, temperature 101.4°F, and breath sounds clear. Mr. Jones has a reddened sacral area and dry skin. He does not remember if he ate breakfast. His roommate, Tom, is at work.

The interviewer asks the RN applicant to do the following:

- List four nursing diagnoses that pertain to this scenario.
- Identify four nursing issues that require immediate intervention.
- Prioritize Mr. Jones's care. What has to be done during this visit?
- Determine what information you must communicate to the physician, the agency, and Tom.
- What will you document in your note, and what other forms will you complete?

Mrs. Smith is an 85-year-old patient. She weighs 92 lbs. At age 75, she broke her hip. Her diagnosis is heart failure. She wears glasses but often forgets to put them on. She is able to walk around by herself. When you arrive at the house one morning, the patient tells you that she fell on the way to the bathroom last night. You notice a new scatter rug in this bathroom. You also see that the patient is wearing new fancy slippers instead of her sneakers.

Exhibit 17–5 New Hire Tracking Form for RNs and LPNs

Page 1 of 2

Credentials, Health Requirements, Interview and Competency Assessment: RN's / LPN's

Employee:	Phone #:	☐Initial Hire ☐Re-hire	
Requirements /Credentials		**Date verified**	**Initials**
Application completed			
RN license ☐Copy obtained ☐Verified on Internet Expir. Date:			
LPN license ☐Copy obtained ☐Verified on Internet Expir. Date:			
Social Security #:			
☐Drivers license copy obtained ☐Other ID:			
☐Car insurance if car is used for work			
☐Physical within the past 12 months Expir. Date:			
☐PPD two step ☐PPD one step Expir. Date:			
☐Chest X-Ray if PPD positive ☐Referred to MD for positive Chest x - ray			
☐Rubella ☐Immune ☐Non Immune			
☐Rubeola ☐Immune ☐Non Immune ☐Birth year			
☐MMR date			
Hepatitis ☐Immune/tite ☐Immune/vaccinated ☐Requested ☐Declined			
☐Criminal background check Date Sent: ☐No disqualifying information			
Malpractice Insurance (1M / 3M)			
Reference #1 ☐Sent/Date: And Received: ☐Written ☐Verbal			
Reference #2 ☐Sent/Date: And Received: ☐Written ☐Verbal			
☐W 4 completed ☐Registration Master completed			
☐I 9 completed			

Interview			
Appearance	cleanliness	☐appropriate	☐inappropriate
	general hygiene	☐appropriate	☐inappropriate
Attitude	eye contact	☐appropriate	☐inappropriate
	body language	☐appropriate	☐inappropriate
Communication	response to questions	☐appropriate	☐inappropriate
	listening ability	☐appropriate	☐inappropriate
	interpersonal skills	☐appropriate	☐inappropriate
	language usage	☐appropriate	☐inappropriate
Situational question	dealing with stress / job demands	☐appropriate	☐inappropriate

Nursing / Home Care **Experience:**

Comments:

Preferred Geographical Areas:

Languages ☐English ☐Spanish ☐Chinese ☐Russian ☐Other:			
Mode of transportation: ☐Auto ☐Public			**Initials**
Availability	☐ Days	From:	To:	
Date:	☐ Evenings	From:	To:	
	☐ Night	From:	To:	
	☐ Weekends	From:	To:	

☐Approved to proceed to orientation

(continues)

Exhibit 17–5 (continued)

Page 2 of 2

Competencies / Certifications		Date Verified	Initials
Home Health			
Hospice			
CPR	Expir. Date:		
Basic IV			
PICC / Midline			
ANA			
Other:			

Exams / Competencies Required **Prior** to Start of Care	Successfully Completed	Initials
Home Care Exam	☐Yes ☐No	
Basic Proficiency & Medication Administration	☐Yes ☐No	
Orientation Learning Module / Class Exam	☐Yes ☐No	
Orientation ☐Acknowledgement signed	☐Yes ☐No	
Orientation ☐Job description signed	☐Yes ☐No	
Orientation ☐HIPAA module completed	☐Yes ☐No	
Orientation ☐Corporate Compliance Commitment signed	☐Yes ☐No	
ID Picture	☐Yes ☐No	

Competencies / Exams Based on Assignments	Successfully Completed	Initials
IV ☐Basic ☐PICC / Midline	☐Yes ☐No	
Pediatrics	☐Yes ☐No	
Maternal Child Health	☐Yes ☐No	
Mental Health	☐Yes ☐No	
Wound Care	☐Yes ☐No	
High Tech: ☐Ventilator ☐EKG	☐Yes ☐No	
Other:	☐Yes ☐No	

Requirements completed for SOC by Personnel / Signature & Date:	
Competencies completed for SOC by SD / DPS / Signature & Date:	

Post Orientation Requirements	Successfully Completed	Initials
Field Review First Day / SOC by RN Supervisor	☐Yes ☐No	
Preceptor Experience (if applicable)	☐Yes ☐No	
Documentation Review by Supervisor / DPS # 1	☐Yes ☐No	
# 2	☐Yes ☐No	
Mandatory Topics Learning Module within the 3 months probationary period	☐Yes ☐No	
Additional Field Reviews (if applicable)	☐Yes ☐No	
Additional personalized requirements:	☐Yes ☐No	
	☐Yes ☐No	
	☐Yes ☐No	

Post Orientation requirements complete SD / DPS / Signature & Date:	

Source: Courtesy of Clarke Healthcare Consultants, Seminole, Florida.

The interviewer asks the CHHA/CNA applicant to do the following:

- Identify what other observations should be made. This should include what you want to look at and what else you want to ask the patient.
- What safety measures should you institute immediately?
- Is there anyone you should talk to about this?
- What will you document in your note?
- Are there any other forms or reports you should complete?

The interviewer rates the applicant's responses based on his or her clinical knowledge, ability to interpret and analyze data, ability to prioritize, and the interventions that he or she anticipates making. Separating the novice from the expert becomes quite easy. This technique also gives the interviewer an indication of how the applicant will think on his or her feet and, more important, whether he or she has common sense. If the prospective employee successfully completes the application phase, he or she is scheduled for the orientation program.

ORIENTATION

The orientation program must be interactive and include an evaluation of cognitive as well as clinical skills. There are several useful methods for presenting the orientation materials. First, hold orientation in a comfortable, well-lit room. Two rooms are preferable: one for lectures and examinations and the other for a skills laboratory. Each participant is given a complete outline of the content to be discussed. The use of a continuous format, with agency forms, job descriptions, and policies included, works the best. A combination of lecture, discussion, demonstration, return demonstration, case studies, and role playing helps these adult learners hear, see, feel, and practice.

Exhibit 17–6 details orientation content required by CHAP and JCAHO. In addition, each agency should carefully evaluate content that applies to their specific agency. Include information relevant to your scope of services. For instance, if you care for a large number of geriatric patients with high risk for falls, prevention strategies should be included in your orientation. If your agency cares for high-tech patients on ventilators, consider including care priorities when orienting staff. Have you included new requirements such as the Health Insurance Portability and Accountability Act (HIPAA) in your orientation? Do you have a contract staff orientation? Be sure to include other state and federal requirements.

Accreditation Requirements

Community Health Accreditation Program (CHAP, 2002a):

CIII.1m *Written policy and procedures detail the orientation process for all new employees. The plan addresses applicable elements pertinent to each job classification.*

HHIII.1d *Home health has a paraprofessional competency program that meets standards established by the Secretary of Health and Human Services.*

1) *Competencies and skills are assessed prior to delivery of services and updated every 12 months.*
2) *Written policies and procedures define the competency evaluation process.*
3) *Competency evaluation is performed by a registered nurse and includes direct observation of all tasks that the paraprofessional is expected to perform.*
4) *Competency checklist is completed and filed in the personnel record.*
5) *There is a 3-month probationary period for all new paraprofessional employees.*
6) *Successful completion of the probationary period is documented, dated, and signed by the employee and the supervisor.*

Exhibit 17–6 Orientation Content

Requirement	Community Health Accreditation Program, CHAP CIII.1m & HHIII.1a	Joint Commission on Accreditation of Healthcare Organizations, JCAHO HR.5.
Philosophy, Mission, Purpose / Goals	X	X
Table of Organization	X	
Lines of authority and responsibility	X	
Hours of work	X	
Job related responsibilities	X	
Baseline skills assessment	X	
Performance standards	X	
Documentation requirements	X	
OSHA compliance / hazardous materials	X	X
Medical Device Act reporting	X	
Infection control standards	X	X
Equal Employment Opportunities Act	X	
Ethical issues identification and resolution process	X	X
Sexual Harassment Act	X	
Salary / hourly wage/independent contractor reimbursement, as applicable	X	
Unemployment compensation	X	
Malpractice coverage, as applicable	X	
Workers Compensation	X	
Collective Bargaining, as applicable	X	
Benefits	X	
Drug testing	X	
Family/State Medical Leave Act	X	
Review of policies and procedures	X	X
Responsibilities and limitations	X	X
Ethics and Confidentiality	X	X
Communication techniques	X	
Supervision Process	X	
Safety	X	X
Client Rights / Confidentiality	X	X
Responding to emergencies	X	X
Role of health team	X	
Types of care and services provided	X	X
Storage of, handling of, and access to supplies, medical gases, and drugs		X
Tests performed by the staff		X
Screening for abuse and neglect		X
Referral guidelines, including guidelines for timeliness and communication		X
Community resources		X
Conflict of interest and professional boundaries		X
Cultural diversity and sensitivity		X
Advance directives		

Source: Courtesy of Clarke Healthcare Consultants, Seminole, Florida.

Joint Commission on Accreditation of Health-care Organizations (JCAHO, 2001):

HR.5 All staff members are oriented to the organization and their responsibilities.

COMPETENCY ASSESSMENT DURING THE ORIENTATION PERIOD

The second phase of the initial orientation involves competency assessments. One commonly used method is written examinations. The purpose of the examinations is to test the applicant's basic cognitive knowledge. The primary examination should be a home care test that covers most of your agency's scope of care and services. For nurses, topics may include assessment, prioritization, care planning, safety, medications, clinical decision making, disease management, nutrition, and use of community resources. For CHHAs/CNAs, observations, basic care modalities, safety, terminology, nutrition, observing, reporting, and patient care are usually included on the test. Nurses whose assignments might involve specialty care may also be asked to take examinations in high technology, pediatrics, intravenous therapy, maternal-child, chemotherapy, and the like to assess their competence. The National League of Nursing (NLN) is a good source for exams.

Prospective employees may also be asked to complete a self-assessment of their knowledge and skills in caring for adult and pediatric patients. Staff are asked to rate their ability as "competent," "some experience," or "no experience." This gives the supervisor a baseline assessment of how the candidate rates his or her own competence. Two things are to be remembered when evaluating the self-assessment. First, the self-assessment represents a comprehensive list that covers most of your agency's scope of care and services. The particular candidate's assignments may never involve the full scope, so review this material in relation to the candidate's experience and possible future assignments. Second, individuals rate their competence based on their own perspective. Some candidates are over-confident and want to impress you. Others are more modest, and their ratings are consistently low. In the end, the only true measures of competence are the ratings done by your own supervisor. Exhibit 17–7 presents sample self-assessments for physical therapists.

The new hire's cognitive and technical skills must be evaluated. Exhibit 17–8 is an example of a CHHA/CNA competency assessment. This basic list is initiated in orientation and completed during the orientation period. It is important to remember that the agency is responsible for supplying competent staff. This includes new hires. Supervisors must be confident that the new employee has the knowledge and skills needed to care for the patient to whom they are assigned.

As discussed previously, competency assessments need to be tailored to your agency's scope of care and services. For example, if your agency cares for high-tech patients, you would include the equipment you use. Be careful to choose the specific knowledge and skills in which the employee must be competent before he or she is assigned to a patient alone. Be realistic, not idealistic, when determining your basic requirements. Exhibit 17–9 is an example of high-tech competency assessments for nurses.

Applicants who do not have any home care experience should be given an opportunity for a preceptor experience. This can be as in-depth and intensive as required. The experienced nurse guides the new applicant through the entire process.

Elements of a preceptor experience for an RN include the following:

- patient status assessment
- initiation of a nursing plan
- updating the care plan
- basic nursing notes
- documentation of changes in patient condition
- client and caregiver education
- discharge planning
- giving/receiving reports

Exhibit 17–7 Sample Self Assessment for Physical Therapy

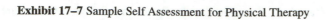

PHYSICAL THERAPY SELF ASSESSMENT

Page 1 of 2

Name: _____ Date: _____

Key: 1. Competent
2. Some experience
3. No experience

COMPETENCE	PEDIATRIC			ADULT			COMMENTS
	1	2	3	1	2	3	
PROCESS RELATED							
Obtain MD orders to meet patient needs							
Medicare regulations							
Documentation							
a) Initial Evaluation							
b) Treatment plan /goals							
c) Visit Note							
d) 60 Day Summary / Progress notes							
e) Discharge Summary							
Occurrence / Incident Report							
Role of PTA, OT, ST, SW, RN, HHA, HCC							
Ordering supplies							
Communication with the case manager							
Supervision of the PTA							
EVALUATION SKILLS							
Manual Muscle test							
Goniometry							
Circumferential measurements							
Muscle tone assessment							
Sensory tests							
Balance assessment							
Postural assessment							
Pain assessment							
Gait analysis							
Joint assessment							
ADL assessment							
Respiratory assessment							
Circulatory status evaluation							
BP, pulse, respirations, temperature							
TREATMENT SKILLS							
Therapeutic exercise							
Joint mobilization							
Muscle re-education							
Balance training							
Gait training							
Transfer training							
ADL training							
Home Exercise Program							

(continues)

Exhibit 17–7 (continued)

SKILL / KNOWLEDGE	ADULT				PEDIATRIC				COMMENTS
TREATMENT SKILLS	1	2	3	4	1	2	3	4	
Home Safety Instruction									
Pain management									
Fall prevention techniques									
Therapeutic interventions:									
a) Joint Replacements: UE LE									
b) Fractures									
c) Back / Neck syndromes / surgery									
d) Prosthetics /Orthotics									
e) CVA									
f) Hemiplegia / paraplegia									
g) Pulmonary therapy									
h) Cardiac rehabilitation									
THERAPEUTIC EQUIPMENT / PROCEDURES									
Crutches / Cane									
Walker									
Wheelchair									
Hoyer Lift									
Continuous Passive ROM / CPM									
Adaptive devices									
Home exercise equipment									
HOME CARE MODALITIES									
Moist heat									
Hydrotherapy									
TENS									
Ultrasound									
Muscle stimulation									
Massage									

Other Areas of Experience	

Comments / Experiences Requested	

Therapist Signature:		Date:
Received for Personnel file by:		Date:
Therapy Reviewer's Signature:		Date:

Source: Courtesy of Clarke Healthcare Consultants, Seminole, Florida.

Exhibit 17–8 Skills Assessment for the Aide

Skills Check	Competent	Needs Improvement	Reviewed	Competent on Re-test	Date	Initials
Take and record pulse						
Take and record temperature						
Take and record respiration						
Bed bath						
Tub and shower safety						
Mouth care						
Hair care						
Nail care						
General skin care						
Shaving						
Shampoo- sink, shower, tub						
Patient positioning						
Range of motion						
Make bed						
Urinal						
Bedpan						
Commode						
Care of an incontinent patient						
Foley catheter care						
Condom catheter care						
Wheelchair						
Cane						
Walker						
Assist with ambulating						
Transfer						
Hoyer lift						
Body mechanics						
Hand washing						
Use of gloves						
Standard precautions						
Disposal of hazardous materials						
Worksheet						
Timecard						
Emergency procedures						
When to call the supervisor						
Identify changes in status						
Occurrences						

Source: Courtesy of Clarke Healthcare Consultants, Seminole, Florida.

Exhibit 17–9 RN PICC Line Competency Assessment

RN PICC LINE INSERTION COMPETENCY

Nurse's Name: _____   Date: _____

PICC line certification certificate from / date:

_____.

Component	Competent	
	Yes	No
Consent		
Patient and caregiver education		
Preparation		
Site Selection		
Insertion		
Dressing		
Documentation		
Sterile technique		
Safety precautions		
Knowledge of complications		
Professional approach with patient and family		

Comments:

_____

_____

_____

_____

_____

_____

I observed _____ RN license number / state _____,

and I certify that she / he is clinically competent in performing the procedure for the insertion of a peripherally inserted central catheter (PICC).

Preceptor Signature: _____ RN license number /state_____

Nurse Signature: _____

Source: Courtesy of Clarke Healthcare Consultants, Seminole, Florida.

- community resources
- laboratory value interpretation
- communication with client, caregiver, physician, and supervisor
- return demonstrations

An LPN preceptor experience would entail the following elements:

- documentation of the client's physical assessment and findings
- implementation of the nursing plan of care
- assisting the RN in evaluating achievement of client goals
- reinforcement of client instructions from the RN or physician
- basic nursing notes
- documentation of changes in patient condition
- giving/receiving reports
- communication with client, caregiver, and RN supervisor
- return demonstrations

If you are planning to use preceptors, be sure to test their competence to precept, too. This usually requires a class outlining responsibilities and competency testing. Role playing is an effective way to ascertain what and how the preceptor will teach. It is important for the preceptors to teach only agency policies. Include the documentation of preceptor competence in the preceptors' personnel files.

At the end of the orientation program, you have a good sense of the new employee's competence. You will also have a basis for making appropriate assignments. The level of the new hire's competence will guide you in planning for additional supervision, if it is necessary.

ONGOING COMPETENCY ASSESSMENT

The fact that the new employee met all your initial requirements for credentials and competencies does not guarantee that he or she will still be competent next month, when he or she is assigned to a new case, or when new equipment or policies are introduced. A good next step, therefore, is to utilize the supervisor visit. This is the ideal time to check the employee's competency. Exhibit 17–10 is a form that can be used to document ongoing nurse competence in the field.

Patient and family satisfaction are assessed at this time. They are asked about the employee's promptness and communication skills, if their rights are respected, and the quality of care they are receiving. It's important to do this when the nurse is not present. For each performance criterion, the supervisor rates the employee as "competent" or "needs improvement." If the employee needs improvement, there is space provided to outline what he or she needs to improve as well as to review his or her behavior, knowledge, or skill, to document competence on retest, and to write comments. You will note there are blanks under performance criteria for additional knowledge and skills required on a particular case. Therefore, if the patient has a tracheostomy, needs suctioning, and has a ventilator you would enter it and validate the employee's competency. These spaces can be used for a variety of topics that meet your agency's or the individual patient's needs.

The supervisor then determines whether the patient's needs are being met by the employee. To complete this process, the supervisor makes an overall comment about his or her assessment of the employee's competence. Check-off boxes are provided to guide the employee in taking actions to improve performance. These include which policy to review, which self-learning package to complete, what class to attend, and with whom the employee should meet. Both the employee and the supervisor sign the form. The employee is given a copy, and one copy is filed in the employee's personnel file.

Exhibit 17–11 is a form that can be used to evaluate ongoing therapist competency in the field. This sample is designed in a different format to meet the needs of this group of employees. It can also be used for therapist contractors.

Exhibit 17–10 RN and LPN Field Competency Review

FIELD REVIEW - RN LPN

Client Observation of Employee

Employee: _____ Client: _____ Date: _____

Prompt: ☐Yes ☐No   Respects Rights: ☐Yes ☐Needs Improvement

Communication: ☐Good ☐Needs Improvement   Quality of Care: ☐Good ☐Needs Improvement

Comments: _____

Competency Review

Performance	Competent	Needs Improvement	Reviewed	Competent on Re-test	Comments
Professional appearance					
Professional demeanor / rapport					
Initiative					
Knowledge: medical condition(s)					
RN: comprehensive assessment					
LPN: physical assessment					
RN: care planning / updating					
LPN: contributes to care plan					
Achievement of goals / outcomes					
Implements care plan					
Organizing / prioritizing					
Medication administration					
Occurrence reporting					
Standard precautions / Infection control					
Hand washing					
Black bag technique					
Equipment maintenance					
Coordinating services					
Collaboration with other disciplines					
Discharge planning					
Patient education – Diagnosis(s)					
Patient education – Health promotion					
Safe transfer / ambulation					
Preventing falls					
Safe home environment					
Body mechanics					
Wound care					
IV care					

Client needs being met by the employee: Yes ☐ No ☐

Comments / Goals: _____

☐ Review policy: _____   ☐ Attend class: _____
☐ Self study module _____   ☐ Meet with: _____
Employee Signature: _____   Supervisor: _____

Source: Courtesy of Clarke Healthcare Consultants, Seminole, Florida.

Exhibit 17–11 Therapist Field Competency Review

FIELD COMPETENCY EVALUATION FOR THERAPISTS

Name:	Date:

Performance Definitions:

E - Exceeds requirements
- Performance far exceeds position requirements and established standards.
- Performance is sustained at this level.

C - Competent
- Performance meets necessary position requirements and established standards.
- Employee achieves position responsibilities in a fully competent manner on a consistent basis.

NI - Needs Improvement
- Performance does not meet the requirements of the position and established standards.
- The employee is responsible to fully implement the improvement plan specifications.

NA - Not Applicable / Not Assessed

Discipline: ☐PT ☐ST ☐OT

Performance Criteria	E	C	NI	NA
Physician Orders Frequency and duration of visits complies with MD orders and are implemented as prescribed				
Assessment, Care Planning, and Treatments Implementation and documentation				
Patient Education Home exercise program, transfer technique, gait instructions, & preventing falls and injuries				
Achievement of goals / outcomes Implementation and documentation				
Vital signs - BP. Pulse, RR				
Vital signs / pain Recognition of pain & abnormal results, appropriate interventions / communication				
Standard precautions / infection control - Hand washing, techniques, equipment, reporting				
Implements safety precautions Home safety assessment, instructions, emergency plans				
Client Satisfaction Prompt, Communication, Respects rights, Quality care				
Professionalism Dress code, ID, hygiene, rapport, attitude, effective communication skills				
Collaboration Communicates appropriate information on a timely basis				

The therapist demonstrated the foregoing skills and was observed to be competent by the therapy supervisor:

_____

_____

_____

_____

_____

Signature of Therapy Supervisor: _____ **Date:** _____

Signature of Contractor : _____ **Date:** _____

Source: Clarke Healthcare Consultants, Seminole, Florida.

Accreditation Requirements

Community Health Accreditation Program (CHAP, 2002a):

CIII.It *Clinical competency evaluations are performed to assess employee basic skills at:*

1) *Time of hire*
2) *Annually*
3) *Special situations as defined by organizational policy*

Joint Commission on Accreditation of Healthcare Organizations (JCAHO, 2001):

HR.4 *The organization assesses, maintains, and improves the competence of all staff providing care and services.*

PERFORMANCE IMPROVEMENT PROGRAM

Ongoing competency assessments of staff are an integral part of the performance improvement program. Statistically valid samplings of these reviews are analyzed. It is even better if you document right in a computer program so that all the results can be compiled. The leadership team can then evaluate competency across all staff groups. The analysis will point out what knowledge and skills most frequently need improvement. It will also reveal the special competencies that are most frequently required. Both CHAP and JCAHO require that the information gained from performance improvement programs be used to improve staff knowledge and skills.

OCCURRENCE AND OUTCOME MONITORING

Occurrence and outcome monitoring statistics should be reviewed by the agency's leaders on a monthly basis. They, too, reveal valuable information about competency. Look for trends that point to possible employee competence issues. These include errors in care or treatment, falls, injuries, infections, admissions to the emergency department or hospital, complaints, wound status deterioration, inadequate client and caregiver education, and the like. Exhibit 17–12 provides an example of a fall prevention competency that could be used for all levels of staff. Implementing this competency is extremely effective in decreasing falls.

CONTINUING EDUCATION

The leader's evaluation of the performance improvement studies, occurrence monitoring, and outcome statistics forms the basis for planning continuing education programs to improve employee competence. Also used is the staff's and supervisor's knowledge of new equipment, new technology, changes in patient mix, mandatory requirements, and employee requests. Each of these criteria points out competence issues that have already appeared or those that are likely to appear. Quarterly planning sessions will help to keep your agency on the cutting edge.

Consider an example of a performance improvement study involving admissions to the emergency department and the hospital. In this scenario, you note an increase in admissions every year during flu season. Further investigation reveals that only 20 percent of the elderly patients you serve had flu shots and that 35 percent of the patients who developed flu were admitted for lengthy hospital stays for pneumonia. Your search also led you to the realization that your staff did little patient education about how to prevent flu. In addition, only 25 percent of the aides assigned to these elderly patients even reported the onset of flu to their supervisors. This scenario plays out in many communities. This type of fact finding gives the agency an excellent opportunity to improve patient care. Classes and/or self-learning programs can be set up to improve employee competence in patient education about preventing flu and responding to the early symptoms of flu. Sharing the improvements realized the next year will help reinforce the employees' positive response to competency training.

Exhibit 17–12 Fall Prevention Competency

Skills Check	Competent	Needs Improvement	Reviewed	Competent on Re-test	Date	Initials
SECTION 1						
Can verbalize at least 2 appropriate strategies in EACH category						
Ambulation						
Transfers						
Environment - Lighting						
Environment - Walkways						
Environment - Stairways						
Environment – Bathroom						
Assistive devices						
Exercise						
Medical Care / Communication with MD						
Medications						
Knowledge - What to do if They Fall						
SECTION 2						
Employee demonstrates correctly:						
Transfer to and from bed						
Transfer to and from chair						
Transfer to and from shower / tub						
Appropriately encourages client to implement and maintain strategies to decrease falls.						

Employee Signature: _____ **Date:** _____

RN Supervisor / SD Initials: _____ **Signature:** _____ **Date:** _____

Source: Courtesy of Clarke Healthcare Consultants, Seminole, Florida.

Several options are open to you when planning continuing education to improve staff competency. Traditionally, classes are offered on a regular basis. To enhance the effectiveness of classes, consider using role playing, demonstrations, case studies, and hands-on practice. Competency testing should be tied to all classes with pre/post-tests, verbal testing, and or return demonstrations. Exhibit 17–13 provides an example of competency testing for wound care. This competency assessment tool might be used when you are not satisfied with outcome monitoring results or when you suddenly increase your case load of wound care patients. Remember, just providing a class, without some form of competency assessment, does not give any assurance that learning took place.

Another widely used educational method is self-learning modules. These work especially well with nurses. A post-test must be part of the module. In all cases, a minimum passing score must be set. Employees who fail the test should be given the opportunity to study and retake the test.

The agency will need to communicate competency requirements clearly to the employees. Each person must be aware of his or her quarterly and annual requirements. Compliance in meeting job category and personal competency requirements must be tracked and shared with employees. Completion of competency requirements should be tied to the employee's annual performance appraisal.

Accreditation Requirements

Community Health Accreditation Program (CHAP, 2002a):

CIII.1a The clinical competency procedures identify learning needs of employees and provide input into staff development/in-service planning.

1) *Competency evaluation tools are tailored to each job category and the services provided.*
2) *Clinical supervisors and/or peer reviewers assess performance of employees during joint visits in the clinical practice setting.*

3) *Competency of supervisors and/or management staff is assessed by the individual's immediate superior and may include peer evaluation as part of the process.*

CIII.1v Staff enhance their job performance through integration of new knowledge and skills.

CIII.1p The organization sponsors a minimum of 12 hours of in-service education for the clinical staff or as stated in organizational policy if the required number of hours exceeds 12 hours.

CIII.1q Continuing Education Units (CEUs) are validated per organizational policy and applicable state

1) *licensure requirements for:Direct care employees*

2) *Contracted care providers*
   a) *Independent contractors*
   b) *Sub contract employees*

HHIII.1g. The organization provides or arranges for documented in-service and continuing education by competent instructors. Part of this education can be furnished while care is being delivered to the patient. The annual minimum requirements are as follows:

1) *Home Health Aides: 12 hours in each 12 month period*
2) *Personal Care Workers: 8 hours*
3) *Chore Workers: 4 hours*

Joint Commission on Accreditation of Healthcare Organizations (JCAHO, 2001):

HR.4.1.1 When competence assessment findings or data from performance improvement activities identify an opportunity for an individual to improve his or her competence, actions are taken to improve the individual's competence.

Exhibit 17–13 RN/LPN Competency Assessment for Wound Care

Skills Check	Competent	Needs Improvement	Reviewed	Competent on Re-test	Date	Initials
ASSESSMENT						
General – location, color, types of drainage, induration, peri-wound area						
Size – width, length, depth, o'clock orientation						
Wound Bed- clean, necrotic, granulation, epithialization						
Undermining / Tunneling						
Pain						
Neurovascular - distal pulse, capillary return, Neuropathy						
INTERVENTION						
Wound Cleaning						
Debridement - types - sharp, irrigation, enzymes, autolytic						
Wound Dressing - choice of & apply						
Implements standard precautions						
Aseptic technique						
Sterile technique						
Pain						
COMPLICATIONS						
Infections - signs and symptoms of superficial and deep incisional infections, organ space, stage 4 pressure sores, Osteomyelitis						
Dehiscence, Evisceration - definition and actions						
PRESSURE SORES						
Risk factors						
Prevention - cushioning; turning / positioning,; strategies to minimize pressure, moisture , friction, and sheer, ROM, activity, nutrition						
Stages – 1, 2, 3, 4, eschar						
DOCUMENTATION						
Visit Note						
Weekly Wound Assessment						

RN / LPN Signature: _____   Date: _____

RN Supervisor / SD Initials: _____   Signature: _____   Date: _____

Source: Courtesy of Clarke Healthcare Consultants, Seminole, Florida.

*HR.6 The organization provides ongoing educa-
tion, including in-services, training, and
other activities.*

POLICIES AND PROCEDURES

Do you have multiple policy and procedure books? Does your staff know what is in them? Where are the policy books kept? If your agency is like most others, the policies are kept in the administrator's or supervisor's office. How can the employees follow policies that they do not know about?

Several solutions can help improve employees' competence related to policies. First, pertinent policies should be part of the orientation. Second, general policies relating to most patient care could be kept in the back of the patient's chart in the home. These include occurrence reporting, medication administration, patient safety, and equipment maintenance, among others. Policies specific to a particular patient are brought to the home by the supervisor and put into the back of the chart; examples include policies relating to ventilators, tracheostomies, suctioning equipment, gastric tubes, and the like.

This system gives the employees a quick reference. Staff caring for the patient should be required to initial all policies in the chart. You can also systematize how you release policies. For example, all policies could be approved by the leadership committee and then released to staff with paychecks. Staff would be responsible for reading and comprehending all releases and would be required to sign a form verifying that they received a specific group of policies, know that they are responsible for reading and comprehending them, and will ask their supervisor if they have any questions. Some policies could be released in a self-learning module so that post-tests could be included.

PERFORMANCE EVALUATIONS

Employee competence is assessed on a more formal basis at the end of the probation period as well as on an annual basis. The review should be signed and dated by the supervisor and the employee. The performance evaluation should include performance criteria listed in the job description, the employee's self assessment, and the employee's development plan and goals. In preparing the performance evaluation, the supervisor uses the competency assessments made during supervisory visits, the employee's compliance in completing ongoing competency requirements, and the employee's competence in reading, comprehending, and signing off on policies.

On the forms shown in Exhibits 17–14 and 17-15, the employee is rated as E (exceeds) if performance far exceeds position requirements and established standards and is sustained at that level. A rating of C (competent) is given if performance meets necessary position requirements and established standards. This employee achieves position requirements in a fully competent manner. The employee receives a rating of NI (needs improvement) when performance does not meet the requirements of the position and established standards. Written comments and a performance improvement plan are required for all performance criteria rated as NI. Employees must improve their competence in these areas to continue employment.

Accreditation Requirements

Community Health Accreditation Program (CHAP, 2002a):

CIII.II An annual written performance evaluation process is completed on all employees by the respective Supervisor and includes active participation by the employee.

Joint Commission on Accreditation of Healthcare Organizations (JCAHO, 2001):

HR.7 The organization evaluates each staff member's ability to meet performance expectations.

Exhibit 17–14 Annual Performance Appriasal–Director of Patient Services

Name:	☐Probationary ☐Annual

Date of hire:	Appraisal Period:	Date of Appraisal:

Performance Definitions:

E – Exceeds requirements	♦ Performance far exceeds position requirements and established standards.
	♦ Performance is sustained at this level.
C – Competent	♦ Performance meets necessary position requirements and established standards.
	♦ Employee achieves position responsibilities in a fully competent manner on a consistent basis.
NI – Needs Improvement	♦ Performance does not meet the requirements of the position and established standards.
	♦ The employee is responsible to fully implement the improvement plan specifications.

Performance Criteria	Self Evaluation			Achievement			Supervisor Comments
	E	C	NI	E	C	NI	
Clinical Expertise Maintains own skills, educates staff to attain and maintain theirs, promotes excellence in practice							
Clinical Performance Ensures that staff implement all aspects of the nursing process & documentation requirements							
Consumer Focus Creates a consumer focus as evidenced by client, patient, family, staff, MCO, & physician satisfaction.							
Budget and appropriate use of Resources Provides input in budget preparation , monitors, adheres to, & justifies expenditures.							
Represents the organization to staff, patients, families, other groups, agencies, and the general public in an appropriate manner							
HR Management Effectively recruits, employs, assigns, supervises, evaluates, and terminates employment of administrative & field personnel along with the RD/ED							
Agency compliance Ensures compliance with all Federal, State, local, OSHA, FDA, CDC, and accrediting regulations.							
Standards, Policies, & Competencies Assists with the development, is familiar with, and consistently implements							
Assignment Management Prioritizes, maintains high productivity, completes assignments, meets responsibilities							
Environment Maintains and promotes a safe work and home environment; ensures an adequate level of supplies							
Quality Service Delivery Communicates effectively with staff, RD, coordinators, supervisors, & ED to ensure quality service delivery.							
Staffing Assesses and evaluates staffing patterns to assure that there are sufficient numbers of qualified staff for care delivered							
Staffing Ensures appropriate staffing and payroll procedures							
Time Management Utilizes time effectively, maintaining a consistent level of productivity, good attendance record							
Professionalism & Communication Appearance, performance communication; creates a positive work environment							
Performance Improvement, Occurrence Reporting, Risk Management, Outcome Achievement, Complaint Resolution, & Infection Control Implements effective strategies to achieve goals							

Employee development plan and goals:

Employee Comments:

Employee Signature: _____ Date: _____

Administrator Signature: _____

Source: Courtesy of Clarke Healthcare Consultants, Seminole, Florida.

Exhibit 17–15 Annual Performance Appraisal–Personnel Assistant

Name:		Probationary ☐ Annual ☐
Date of hire:	Appraisal Period:	Date of Appraisal:

Performance Definitions:

E – Exceeds requirements
- ♦ Performance far exceeds position requirements and established standards.
- ♦ Performance is sustained at this level.

C – Competent
- ♦ Performance meets necessary position requirements and established standards.
- ♦ Employee achieves position responsibilities in a fully competent manner on a consistent basis.

NI – Needs Improvement
- ♦ Performance does not meet the requirements of the position and established standards.
- ♦ The employee is responsible to fully implement the improvement plan specifications.

Performance Criteria	Self Evaluation			Achievement			Supervisor Comments
	E	C	NI	E	C	NI	
Communication / Behavior Demonstrates poised communication with registrants, staff, & clients; effective under stressful situations							
Clerical Functions Maintains accurate, confidential, up-to-date records, reports and files; prepares professional correspondence; performs routine clerical and receptionist functions							
Timely Processing Systems Maintains organized, accurate, timely systems for processing new hires and annual staff requirements for health, credentials, and competency							
Personnel policies Consistently follows and ensures compliance with personnel policies							
Expedites the new hire process by greeting registrants, providing / collecting applications, providing / grading exams, mailing references, and tracking new registrants							
Communication with Supervisor Keeps their supervisor informed of the status of projects/ problems with systems							
Computer Skills Accurately updates personnel holding file and home care master files							
Payroll Assists in preparing and adjusting an accurate weekly payroll, verifies timecards and clinical notes							
Professionalism Consistently demonstrates professionalism through appearance, and performance; remains flexible							
Respect Considers and respects new ideas and divergent points of view, respects the rights, privacy and property of others at all times							
Time Management - Utilizes time effectively, maintains productivity and initiative, prioritizes well, remains organized and focused							
Time and Attendance							
Consistently Attempts to Improve Performance Participates in audits and PI studies , seeks to improve own performance							

Employee development plan and goals:

Employee Comments:

Employee Signature: _____ Date: _____

Administrator Signature: _____

Source: Courtesy of Clarke Healthcare Consultants, Seminole, Florida.

CONCLUSION

Developing a competency system involves establishing standards, hiring appropriate staff, orienting new employees, assessing ongoing competency, tracking data, and implementing systems to improve performance for both individuals and groups. This process is vital to the survival of any organization that wants to provide high-quality care and services.

REFERENCES

Community Health Accreditation Program. 2002a. *Millennium Edition, CORE Standards of Excellence, CORE I.* New York: CHAP.

Community Health Accreditation Program. 2002b. *Millennium Edition, Home Health Standards of Excellence,* New York: CHAP.

Joint Commission on Accreditation of Healthcare Organizations. 2001. *2001–2002 Comprehensive Accreditation Manual for Home Care, Common Home Care Standards, Management of Human Resources,* Oakbrook Terrace, IL: JCAHO.

CHAPTER 18

Meeting the Need for Culturally and Linguistically Appropriate Services

Mary Curry Narayan

With the advent of the millennium, the Department of Health and Human Services (DHHS) and other governmental offices issued a number of documents related to the growing diversity of the United States population and their health care needs. These documents not only describe population trends, but also include a number of health care policies and regulations of which home health administrators must be aware as they plan for the future of their agencies.

This chapter will discuss the main features of these government documents, touch upon some of the literature related to transcultural nursing administration, and suggest strategies that home health care administrators can use in their own agencies to address the trends and regulations related to cultural and linguistic diversity.

GOVERNMENT PROJECTIONS, GUIDELINES, AND MANDATES

Year 2000 Census

Increasingly, people migrate to seek new opportunities and to escape political and geographic turmoil. Advances in transportation make migration less formidable than it was in the past. The U.S. Bureau of the Census (2000, 2001, 2002) confirms that the United States is rapidly becoming more racially, ethnically, culturally, and linguistically diverse. If present trends persist, projections indicate that the diversity of the United States is growing, such that by 2050, the current European-origin, white majority will comprise only about 50 percent of the population (Day, 1996).[1]

Presently, 25 percent of the country's population self-identifies with one of the federally defined minority groups. Over 10 percent of the people living in the United States are foreign-born immigrants, with 50 percent of those originating from Latin American and 25 percent from Asian countries. Almost 20 percent of the American population speaks a language other than English as their first language and for 10 percent that language is Spanish (U.S. Bureau of the Census, 2003).

Unequal Treatment: Confronting Racial and Ethnic Disparities in Health Care

Under the direction of Congress, the Institute of Medicine (IOM) assessed the extent of racial and ethnic disparities in health care, identified potential sources of these disparities, and suggested intervention strategies to remedy the disparities. The IOM issued their report, *Unequal Treatment: Confronting Racial and Ethnic Disparities in Health Care,* in April 2002, concluding that "racial and ethnic minorities tend to receive a lower quality of health care than non-minorities, even when access-related factors,

---

1 All statistical percentages from the 2000 Census are rounded to nearest 5 percent.

such as patients' insurance status and income are controlled" (Smedley et al., 2002, p. 1).

This IOM report sent a shockwave through the health care community. Health professionals were dismayed to find that the outcome of the health care they provide is not congruent with the values they espouse. Yet the evidence is overwhelming. "A large body of published research reveals that racial and ethnic minorities experience a lower quality of health services . . . than White Americans" (Smedley et al., 2002, p. 3). The IOM reported that many sources contribute to these disparities including health systems, health care providers, patients, and utilization managers. Among the findings are:

- Barriers that minorities face to equal access to health care include bias and prejudice, as well as language, geography, cultural dissonance, and financial barriers.
- The conditions in which many clinical encounters take place—characterized by high time pressure, complexity, and pressures for cost-containment—enhance the likelihood that care will be poorly matched to minority patients' needs.
- Evidence suggests that bias, prejudice, and stereotyping on the part of health care providers may contribute to differences in care. "There is considerable evidence that even well meaning whites, who are not overtly biased, and who do not believe that they are prejudiced typically demonstrate unconscious implicit negative racial attitudes and stereotypes" (p. 11).
- Minority patients are more likely to refuse treatment, and this is frequently because of a poor cultural mismatch between the provider and the minority patient, spawning mistrust and misunderstanding of provider instructions.

Home health care administrators, who are committed to just and ethical practices, will find several of the recommendations of the IOM (Smedley et al., 2002, pp. 20–21) helpful to future agency planning:

- Increase health care providers' awareness of disparities.

- Increase the proportion of underrepresented racial and ethnic minorities among health professionals.
- Promote consistency and equity of care through the use of evidence-based guidelines.
- Support the use of interpretation services where community need exists.
- Implement patient education programs to increase patients' knowledge of how to best access care and participate in treatment decisions.
- Integrate cross-cultural education into the training of all health professionals.
- Collect and report data by patient's race, ethnicity, and primary language.
- Include measures of racial and ethnic disparities in performance measurement.

Healthy People 2010

The national health agenda, issued by the DHHS's Office of Disease Prevention and Health Promotion (2000), is a comprehensive set of disease prevention and health promotion objectives for the United States to achieve over the first decade of the new century. Created by scientists both inside and outside of government, *Healthy People 2010* identifies a wide range of public health priorities with specific, measurable objectives. Although there are many focus areas and many specific objectives, there are two overarching goals, one of which is to "eliminate health disparities." (The other overarching goal is to "increase quality and years of healthy life.")

DISCRIMINATION

Policy Guidance on Title VI of the Civil Rights Act

In August 2000, the Office of Civil Rights (OCR) published a policy guidance memorandum, the "Policy Guidance on Title VI of the Civil Rights Act of 1964: Prohibition Against National Origin Discrimination as It Affects Persons with Limited English Proficiency", in the *Federal Register* clarifying the regulatory impact of the 1964 Civil Rights Act on interactions between health care and social service providers and people who have limited or no English speaking skills (OCR, 2000).

Section 601 of Title VI states: "No person in the United States shall, on ground of race, color, or national origin, be excluded from participation in, be denied the benefits of, or be subjected to discrimination under any program or activity receiving Federal financial assistance" (Civil Rights Act of 1964, Public Law 88-352). The guidance memorandum indicates that because language is a core component of national origin, limited English proficient (LEP) clients' right to meaningful communication with health care and social service providers is protected by the Civil Rights Act. It notes that LEP persons "cannot speak, read, write or understand the English language at a level that permits them to interact effectively with health care providers and social service agencies" (OCR, 2000). This excludes them from equal access and services and is in "stark contrast to Title VI's promise of equal access to federally assisted programs and activities" and therefore "constitutes discrimination on the basis of national origin, in violation of Title VI" (OCR, 2000, p. 52762). Therefore, all health care organizations that receive federal funds (Medicare and Medicaid reimbursement for services) must provide appropriately trained interpreter services, at no cost to the patient, when they interact with LEP patients.

The policy guidance memorandum indicates that to ensure LEP clients can communicate effectively with the health care team, health care organizations and providers must:

- Assess the language needs of the population the organization serves.
- Develop a written policy on language access that includes when and how LEP patients' communication needs will be met.
- Never expect a patient's family or friends to interpret for a LEP patient and never allow a minor child to interpret for LEP parents or relatives.
- Assure that all LEP patients are aware of their right to interpreter services—at no

cost to themselves—whenever the health care provider needs to communicate with the patient or the patient needs to communicate with the provider.

- Ensure interpreters are trained in interpretation techniques, medical ethics, and medical terminology and concepts, and can demonstrate competency in both languages.
- Translate written materials, especially vital documents, such as consent forms, required beneficiary notices, and patient rights into all regularly encountered languages.

If a health care provider does not provide language services when LEP persons seek services, the provider could be in violation of Title VI's prohibition of discrimination. The document, however, gives health care providers some flexibility in how stringently they need to comply with these standards. "The failure to take all of the steps outlined . . . will not necessarily mean that [a health care provider] has failed to provide meaningful access to LEP patients" (OCR, 2000, p. 52769). The OCR recognizes that complying with all of these guidelines could be "so financially burdensome as to defeat the legitimate objectives [of a provider's] program" (OCR, 2000, p. 52769). Therefore, the OCR states it will investigate complaints and reports of noncompliance with Title VI by looking at the size of the provider's program, the size of the LEP population the provider serves, the frequency with which different languages are encountered, and the steps that were taken to provide meaningful communication access.

NATIONAL STANDARDS FOR CULTURALLY AND LINGUISTICALLY APPROPRIATE SERVICES

To address the health care needs of culturally and linguistically diverse populations, the Office of Minority Health (OMH) drafted national standards to guide health care organizations in providing care to diverse patient populations. The National Standards for Culturally and

Linguistically Appropriate Services (CLAS Standards) were derived from state and federal regulations, policies, research, and input from health care providers, advocacy groups, and public meetings. The purpose of the 14 standards, published in the December 22, 2000, *Federal Register*, is to "ensure that all people entering the health care system receive equitable and effective treatment in a culturally and linguistically appropriate manner" (OMH, 2000, p. 80872).

Specifically, the purpose of the CLAS Standards is to:

- Improve outcomes, patient satisfaction, and cost-efficient health care services for culturally and linguistically diverse patient populations
- Provide guidance to health care providers on how and when to provide culturally and linguistically appropriate services
- Correct inequities that currently exist in providing services to culturally and linguistically diverse populations
- Improve the health of all Americans, of all racial, ethnic, and cultural groups, no matter what language they speak

Standards 1, 2, and 3 provide guidelines that foster culturally competent care. Cultural competence is the ability of health care providers and organizations to provide effective care to culturally diverse populations. Because the health and illness beliefs, values, and practices of clients may differ from that of the providers, cultural competence implies that health care providers not only respect the clients' cultures, but also adapt care to meet the patients' cultural needs and preferences.

Standards 4 through 7 mirror the OCR's "Policy Guidance on Title VI of the Civil Rights Act of 1964". Whenever LEP patients need to communicate with their health care providers, the providers must secure specially trained medical interpreters and translators.

Standards 8 through 14 recommend specific strategies that organizations should take to assure that care meets patients' cultural and linguistic needs.

The 14 CLAS Standards provide a framework for creating culturally and linguistically appropriate services. Later in this chapter, we will use each of the 14 CLAS Standards as the starting point to suggest strategies home health care administrators can use to develop the cultural and linguistic competence of their own home care agencies.

EFFORTS TOWARD CULTURAL AND LINGUISTIC COMPETENCE

The call to cultural competence is not a new one, though it grew in volume and frequency as we approached and entered into the new millennium. In the 1950s, Madeline Leininger, a nursing theorist, leader, and the founder of the Transcultural Nursing Society, began stressing the importance of cultural care to effective nursing care. She recognized that how health and illness issues are perceived and treated, what care is sought, and what is considered good care are all highly influenced by a person's cultural background and identity.

Leininger (1996) defined "transcultural nursing administration" as the "process of assessing, planning, and making decisions and policies that will facilitate the provision of educational and clinical services that take into account the cultural caring values, beliefs, symbols, references, and lifeways of people of diverse and similar cultures for beneficial or satisfying outcomes." Andrews (1998) clarified health care administrators' need for cultural competence, indicating that "nurses are challenged to develop and practice a new kind of administration that incorporates transcultural concepts," not only to benefit patient care, but as a necessity in managing today's diverse workforce.

Various theorists and authors have offered different models for promoting cultural competence in health care, including Kleinman (1980), Leininger (2002), and Campinha-Bacote (2003). Frusti and associates (2003) describe the Diversity Competency Model and how their large health care organization used the model to promote cultural competence and to build a diverse workforce.

Although there are many effective ways to enhance the cultural and linguistic competence of health care organizations, one of the most helpful tools is undoubtedly the CLAS Standards themselves and the frequently updated, Internet-accessed "Practical Guide for Implementing the Recommended National Standards for Culturally and Linguistically Appropriate Services in Health Care" on the OMH's Web site at www.omhrc.gov/clas/guide3a.asp. This site includes multiple downloadable tools for agency self-assessment and strategic planning.

STRATEGIES FOR ACHIEVING THE CLAS STANDARDS

The 14 CLAS Standards create an outline for delivering culturally and linguistically appropriate services. In the remainder of this chapter, we will consider each standard and suggest strategies that home health care administrators might use to develop the cultural and linguistic competence of their own home care agencies.

1. *Health care organizations should ensure that patients/consumers receive from all staff members effective, understandable, and respectful care that is provided in a manner compatible with their cultural health beliefs and practices and preferred language.*

According to this standard, home health agencies should provide care that is "effective, understandable, and respectful" (OCR, 2000, p. 80874). *Effective care* is defined as care that results in good health outcomes and a high level of patient satisfaction with the agency's services. *Understandable care* means that patients and families understand clinical and administrative information related to their care and that they are aware of their right to choose among care options. The only way this right can be protected is to assure that communication occurs in the language patients and families can comfortably understand.

Respectful care is considerate of the patient's cultural beliefs, values, practices, and linguistic needs. Patients and families should feel comfortable discussing their cultural health beliefs and practices with home health staff. They should not fear ridicule or disregard of their cultural practices. Respectful care also implies that clinicians are familiar with and respectful of the patient's traditional healing beliefs and practices, integrating these approaches into treatment plans whenever possible.

Standard 1 is the umbrella standard for all the other CLAS Standards. Basically, the rest of the standards advise home health agencies on ways agencies can operationalize Standard 1 and can assure effective, understandable, and respectful care.

2. *Health care organizations should implement strategies to recruit, retain, and promote at all levels of the organization a diverse staff and leadership that are representative of the demographic characteristics of the service area.*

Ideally, a home care agency draws its staff from its service area. Staff members, therefore, should be representative of the demographics of the community served. The diversity of the staff should be representative of the diversity of the community at all levels of the agency starting with the governing board and upper-level management. Although a bicultural and bilingual staff does not ensure a culturally and linguistically competent staff, it does facilitate a staff responsive to needs of the ethnic populations served and the languages they speak. According to Cooper-Patrick and associates (1999, p. 583), "Racial concordance of patient and provider is associated with greater patient participation in care processes, higher patient satisfaction, and greater adherence to treatment."

To promote diversity of the home health nursing and therapy workforce, home health care administrators can consider the following strategies:

- Determine the racial, ethnic, and cultural demographics of their staff and the patient population they serve and determine if staff demographics mirror population demographics.

- Target recruitment efforts to professional schools, papers, and journals that are representative of the agency's patient population.
- Work with the nursing and therapy schools in the community to provide appropriate training and mentorship programs. Capitalize on these programs by using them as recruitment tools.
- Create an agency culture that honors the cultural diversity of its staff and is flexible to their cultural and religious holidays, dietary and clothing practices, and patterns of communication.
- Provide upward mobility programs that foster paraprofessional advancement through scholarship programs tied to agency commitment.

3. *Health care organizations should ensure that staff at all levels and across all disciplines receive ongoing education and training in culturally and linguistically appropriate service delivery.*

Cultural competence training consists of education in the attitudes, knowledge, and skills that promote culturally comfortable care. Cultural sensitivity is attitude training. It creates an awareness and respect for the cultural beliefs, values, and practices of others. Cultural competence in health care, on the other hand, means that clinicians and staff adapt the care they provide to the cultural needs and preferences of their patients and families. In order to do this, clinicians need the knowledge and skills to provide culturally appropriate assessments and care planning.

To encourage culturally appropriate care, home health care administrators can:

- Tap into the resources of organizations that are committed to improving cross-cultural health care, such as the Transcultural Nursing Society (http://www.tcns.org/menu/menu6.shtml) or Resources for Cross Cultural Healthcare (http://www.diversityrx.org).

- Include topics that promote cultural knowledge and skills in the agency's staff development plan such as:
  - Patients' civil right, protected by law, to have their cultural and linguistic needs and preferences honored
  - Cultural norms of verbal and nonverbal communication, how these vary across cultures, and how to avoid misunderstandings
  - Impact of American and biomedical cultures on health care providers and how and why providers' practices can be adapted to meet the cultural needs and practices of patients and their families
  - In-depth cultural information about patient populations frequently seen by the agency
  - Strategies for preventing and resolving cultural conflicts between staff members and patients

4. *Health care organizations must offer and provide language assistance services, including bilingual staff and interpreter services, at no cost to each patient/consumer with limited English proficiency (LEP) at all points of contact, in a timely manner during all hours of operation.*

According to this standard, all patients must have "meaningful language access" (OCR, 2000, p. 80875) despite the size of the patient's language group. *Meaningful language access* means that the patient and the clinician can communicate effectively with one another. Medical interpretation, an advanced and complex skill, requires special training and expertise. To assure meaningful communication, the home health agency can:

- Hire bilingual staff who speak the languages most frequently encountered in the agency's service area.

- Arrange for the services of trained medical interpreters through:
  - Agencies that specialize in medical interpretation.
  - Telephone interpretation services (though this should not be the agency's main interpretation resource when a significant percentage of the agency's patient population speaks a language other than English).
  - Bilingual volunteers from the community's cultural and religious communities to serve in the agency's volunteer interpreter pool. (Agency should provide training in medical interpretation techniques to assure competency.)

5. *Health care organizations must provide to patients/consumers in their preferred language both verbal offers and written notices informing them of their right to receive language assistance services.*

The purpose of this standard is to ensure that all patients know they have a right to interpretation services at no cost to themselves. To protect this patient right:

- Intake staff should obtain information about the patient's preferred language and ability to communicate in English.
- Staff should determine, prior to the first visit, if the patient would like to have a medical interpreter present for the admissions visit.
- Agency's *Patient Rights and Responsibilities* document should include a statement that specifically states the patient has a right to interpretation services at no cost to the patient.
- The *Patient Rights and Responsibilities* statement should be translated into all languages spoken by a significant percentage of the population the agency serves.

6. *Health care organizations must assure the competence of language assistance*

provided to limited English proficient patients by interpreters and bilingual staff. Family and friends should not be used to provide interpretation services (except on request by the patient).

This standard addresses two concerns about using untrained interpreters to meet the patient's communication needs. First is that the patient's family and friends make poor interpreters. Patients may be too embarrassed or may not be willing to share certain information with family that conflicts with their sense of modesty or their cultural taboos. Family members may not be comfortable conveying personal or disturbing information the clinician wishes to communicate with the patient. They may filter out information the patient is trying to share with the clinician because they deem it as unimportant. However, because home care patients are frequently so dependent on family and friends to meet their most basic and personal needs, these negative consequences of using family and friends to act as interpreters is not as much of a risk in home care as it is in clinic and acute care settings.

The second concern is that untrained interpreters may not have the skills required to interpret accurately. Medical interpretation is a complex skill. It requires competence in both languages, including the ability to interpret medical terminology. Frequently, word-for-word interpretation does not convey the meaning of a statement from one language to another. According to the OMH (2000, p. 80876), studies show that many bilingual persons do not have the level of language proficiency in one or both languages required for accurate interpretation. The National Council on Interpretation in Health Care recommends that all interpreters receive a minimum of 40 hours of formal training in the techniques, ethics, and cross-cultural issues related to medical interpreting (OMH, 2000, p. 80876).

To assure that interpreters are competent, the home health care agency should:

- Provide training and competency testing for all staff and volunteers who provide interpretation services by contracting with an agency that supplies this kind of training.

- Nonbilingual staff should know when and how to obtain interpretation services for linguistically appropriate home health services.

7. *Health care organizations must make available easily understood patient-related materials and post signage in the languages of the commonly encountered groups represented in the service area.*

Commonly encountered languages are languages spoken by a significant percentage of the provider's target population. The OCR (2000), interpreting the intention of the 1964 Civil Rights Act, defines "languages of commonly encountered groups" as a language that is spoken by 5 percent or greater of an organization's patient population.

To meet the OCR guidelines, the health care agency should:

- Identify the languages most frequently encountered in the agency's service area.
- Translate all required documents—consents, beneficiary notices, patient rights—into any language spoken by 5 percent or more of the patient population.
- If a particular language is spoken by more than 10 percent of the patient population within the agency's service area, in addition to required documents, other resources usually provided to English-speaking patients (e.g., patient education materials), must also be translated into that language.
- Assure that translated materials are linguisitically accurate and culturally appropriate. (Mere literal translation of materials can compromise the purpose and meaning of the educational material.)
- Consider purchasing patient education resources that are already translated into the languages spoken in your service area. For instance, Krames-on-Demand Pat-

ient Education (http://65.201.6.68/krames /Patient.asp?) resources and the *Home Health Care Patient Education Manual* (Narayan, 2003) contain patient education resources already translated into Spanish.

8. *Health care organizations should develop, implement, and promote a written strategic plan that outlines clear goals, policies, operational plans, and management accountability/oversight mechanisms to provide culturally and linguistically appropriate services.*

All health care organizations in the United States are serving ever-increasingly culturally and linguistically diverse populations. Because of this demographic shift, the OMH believes all organizations should tie the CLAS Standards to the mission and strategic plan of the organization. Therefore, home health care administrators should:

- Review the agency's mission statement and strategic plan for congruence with the CLAS Standards.
- Invite community members and staff who represent the diversity of the population the agency serves to participate in the review and planning process.
- Develop a plan with specific, measurable long- and short-term objectives to promote compliance with the CLAS Standards.

9. *Health care organizations should conduct initial and ongoing organizational self-assessments of CLAS-related activites and are encouraged to integrate cultural and linguistic competence-related measures into their internal audits, performance improvement programs, patient satisfaction assessments, and outcomes-based evaluations.*

The OMH encourages agencies to perform CLAS self-audit, using the standards as a guide to determine where the agency is and where the agency needs to go in order to be compliant with the CLAS Standards. Recommendations for self-audit include:

- Use a tool for measuring the degree to which the agency already meets the 14 CLAS Standards, where its strengths and weaknesses are, and what areas need to be addressed in the agency's strategic plan. Tools such as the "Assessment Tool for Measuring Home Health Agency Cultural and Linguistic Competence" (Figure 18-1) or the multiple downloadable assessment forms found on the OMH Web site (http://www.omhrc.gov/clas/guide2a.asp) can help an agency prioritize opportunities for improvement.
- Measure the satisfaction of each of the population groups the agency serves.
- Using the tools that were initially used for self-assessment, perform annual assessments to monitor the degree to which the agency is moving toward its goals for providing culturally and linguistically appropriate services.
- Analyze OASIS OBQI (Outcomes Assessment and Information Set—Outcomes Based Quality Improvement) quality indicators for each patient population the agency is serving to determine if the agency is seeing any racial/ethnic disparities in outcomes.

10. *Health care organizations should ensure that data on the individual patient's/consumer's race, ethnicity, and spoken and written language are collected in health records, integrated into the organization's management information systems, and periodically updated.*

Unless a home care agency knows the cultural and linguistic composition of the population it serves, the organization cannot adequately address the needs of its diverse patient populations, nor can it measure the outcomes of care for each of these populations. To this end, the agency should:

- Collect information about each patient's racial/ethnic group using OASIS M0140.
- Encourage patients to identify racial/ethnic data for themselves rather than having this data identified through staff assumptions.
- Benchmark OASIS's M0140 populations (classification by race/ethnicity) against OASIS quality indicators.
- In addition to M0140's federally defined minority groups, include subclassifications for the particular patient populations special to the agency's service area. For instance, if the agency cares for a significant Somali immigrant population, this population can be subclassified for the agency's purposes from the Black/African-American population.
- Update ethnic/language choices in the information systems documentation to accurately measure shifting demographics and new populations the agency may be serving.
- Collect information about each patient's preferred language and ensure this information is prominent in the patient's record so that all staff providing care for this patient know the patient's language and can take the appropriate steps to meet the patient's linguistic needs.

11. *Health care organizations should maintain a current demographic, cultural, and epidemiological profile of the community as well as a needs assessment to accurately plan for and implement services that respond to the cultural and linguistic characteristics of the service area.*

Health care organizations need to know the cultural and linguistic demographics of the community they serve.

- Assess and then regularly reassess the community profile and needs. (In today's mobile society, the demographic profile of a community can change in a short time.)
- Compare admissions demographics to

Figure 18–1 Assessment Tool for Measuring Home Health Agency Cultural and Linguistic Competence.

Organizational Cultural Competence

Each statement in this checklist considers a structure or process associated with a high degree of cultural and linguistic competence.

Directions: Select A, B, or C for each item listed below. Areas with "Bs" or "Cs" indicate areas that hold opportunities for improvement.

A = Achieved in full   B = Partially achieved   C = No achievement evident

_____ 1.   Leadership within our home health agency support adapting care, whenever appropriate, to meet the cultural health beliefs/practices of the agency's clients.

_____ 2.   Leadership provides financial support and resources, including interpreters and translated materials, to meet the communication needs of our limited English proficient (LEP) clients.

_____ 3.   Our agency's governing board includes members from the diverse cultural/ethnic/linguistic populations within our service area.

_____ 4.   When developing new programs, leadership attempts to develop programs that are accessible and acceptable to the diverse populations within our service area.

_____ 5.   Leadership and clinical staff reflect the cultural and ethnic diversity of the agency's service area.

_____ 6.   Strategies to recruit, retain, and promote employees from the minority groups within our service area are part of the agency's strategic plan.

_____ 7.   Orientation and ongoing education programs include training in cultural awareness and how staff can interact with others—patients and colleagues—in culturally sensitive ways.

_____ 8.   Our staff have been trained in the cultural patterns of the minority groups present in our service area.

_____ 9.   Professional development and training within our agency includes techniques for working with an interpreter most effectively to meet patients' needs.

_____ 10. Competency in delivering care to patients from diverse cultural and ethnic groups is part of employees' performance evaluations.

_____ 11. As part of the referral process, our agency has a mechanism to offer language assistance services to LEP patients/families both verbally and with written notices (so that the first visit is made with an interpreter if preferred by the patient/family).

_____ 12. Our agency keeps an updated list of bilingual staff, bilingual volunteers, and language assistance resources.

_____ 13. Our agency assures that all interpreters used within our agency are trained in medical interpretation (minimum of 40 hours of medical interpretation training is recommended) and demonstrate competence through competency testing.

_____ 14. Bilingual staff, contract staff, or volunteers are available for all the significant languages spoken by patients in our service area, whenever needed to meet a LEP patient's need.

_____ 15. Bilingual staff who assist with meeting the needs of LEP patient populations are compensated for the valuable skill set they bring to the agency and its patients.

_____ 16. Clinical staff plan for interpreters to be present at visits unless the patient prefers a family member/caregiver to provide interpretation.

_____ 17. Clinical staff do not assume bilingual family members/caregivers are appropriate interpreters for LEP patients.

_____ 18. Clinical staff never ask children to interpret a clinical conversation for patients or other family members.

_____ 19. Admission information, including patient rights, consents, and agency information, are available in the languages spoken by a significant percentage of the population within our service area.

_____ 20. Patient education materials are available in the languages our patients speak and have been reviewed to assure they are sensitive to our patients' cultural beliefs, values, and practices.

_____ 21. Our staff have access to books and other resources that describe the cultural patterns of the many cultural/ethnic/religious groups to which our patients may belong.

_____ 22. A cultural assessment is an integral part of our agency's comprehensive assessment tool.

_____ 23. Clinical staff adapt care plans and modify pathways to meet the cultural beliefs/practices of patients from diverse cultural backgrounds.

_____ 24. Our agency has a mechanism for assisting clinicians in resolving cultural conflicts and ethical dilemmas that arise out of the differing ethical frameworks of the clinician and the patient.

_____ 25. Our agency reviews census and social data in order to know the cultural, ethnic, and religious demographics of our service area.

_____ 26. Our agency's patient population reflects the diversity of our service area, indicating that our services are accessible to all the cultural/ethnic/linguistic populations in our geographic area.

_____ 27. Our agency seeks to create services that are sensitive to the needs/preferences of the significant ethnic/cultural/religious populations within our service area.

_____ 28. Our agency has conducted an assessment of our strengths and weaknesses in providing culturally and linguistically appropriate services.

_____ 29. Our agency has a written strategic plan for enhancing agency/staff cultural/linguistic competence.

_____ 30. At least one of our agency's performance improvement projects is related to our agency's attempts to improve on the care we provide to the culturally and/or linguistically diverse populations we serve.

_____ 31. Our agency has policies and/or processes in place that promote culturally and linguistically sensitive care.

_____ 32. Our medical information system database identifies patients who identify with minority populations and who may have special cultural or linguistic care needs.

_____ 33. Our agency's customer satisfaction survey tool identifies the satisfaction rates of the different cultural/ethnic/linguistic populations we serve.

_____ 34. Our OASIS measures identify our outcomes for the different cultural/ethnic/linguistic populations we serve.

Copyright: Mary Curry Narayan, April 2001.

community demographics to assure the agency is meeting the needs of the community and that certain populations are not encountering barriers to care.

- Encourage community members to participate in focus groups that help to identify the needs of the community.

12. Health care organizations should develop participatory, collaborative partnerships with communities and utilize a variety of formal and informal mechanisms to facilitate community and patient/consumer involvement in designing and implementing CLAS related activities.

To assure a home health agency is responsive to the needs of the community, the agency can:

- Make service and marketing decisions in collaboration with representatives of the population it seeks to serve.

- Invite community representatives onto the agency's governing board.
- Invite community representatives to participate in the development of the agency's strategic plan, its CLAS-related quality improvement strategies, and its marketing plan.

13. Health care organizations should ensure that conflict and grievance resolution processes are culturally and linguistically sensitive and capable of identifying, preventing, and resolving cross-cultural conflicts or complaints by patients/consumers.

All staff who respond to grievances need to be aware of the right of all patients and families to culturally and linguistically appropriate services. Agency leadership should:

- Provide education to staff at all levels of the agency in ways to avoid or resolve cultural conflicts.
- Assure that administrators and supervisors who respond to patient complaints and family have mastered the attitudes and techniques associated with culturally sensitive and competent care.
- Pay particular attention to the needs of vulnerable populations who may not be able to, or may be reluctant to, assert their rights because of a language barrier, cultural norms against confrontation, or fear of further discrimination.
- Provide cultural ethics and values education for the Bioethics Committee that may be called upon for guidance when the cultural values of the staff conflict with those of the agency's patients. For instance, staff grounded in Western biomedical ethics may have difficulty when confronted with patients whose ethical principles flow out of an Eastern philosophical framework.
- Ensure the human resources (HR) department of the agency is committed to creating an agency culture that honors the cultural diversity of each staff member. HR department personnel should have training in culturally sensitive conflict management techniques. They should be skilled at addressing issues related to the different cultural beliefs, values, and practices of staff members.

14. *Health care organizations are encouraged to regularly make available to the public information about their progress and successful innovations in implementing the CLAS Standards and to provide public notice in their communities about the availability of this information.*

To promote agency accountability, community involvement, and benchmarking among agencies, the last CLAS Standard recommends the home care agency publish data about its progress in meeting the CLAS Standards and in

serving its patients from diverse cultures who speak diverse languages. In this way, the agency communicates with the community, which can then respond to the efforts of the agency, providing a feedback loop to the agency about the adequacy and appropriateness of its efforts.

SUMMARY

Because of the ever-growing diversity of patient and staff populations, cultural and linguistic competence are critical elements of effective home health agencies and essential attributes of their administrators and staff. A number of government documents outline specific actions that agencies should—or must—take to eliminate racial and ethnic disparities in health care. Among these documents are:

- The U.S. Year 2000 Census
- The Institute of Medicine's (2002) *Unequal Treatment: Confronting Racial and Ethnic Disparities in Health Care*
- The U.S. Department of Health and Human Services' (2000) *Healthy People 2010* Agenda
- The Office of Civil Rights' (2000) *Policy Guidance on Title VI of the Civil Rights Act of 1964: Prohibition Against National Origin Discrimination as It Affects Persons with Limited English Proficiency*
- The Office of Minority Health's (2000) *National Standards for Culturally and Linguistically Appropriate Services*

The *National Standards for Culturally and Linguistically Appropriate Services* (CLAS Standards) furnish a blueprint for developing a culturally and linguistically competent agency. By considering each of the 14 standards a goal to be achieved, agency administrators can measure where their agency stands in relation to each of the standards and where it needs to go. Strategies for reaching each of the standards are implied by considering ways to reach each goal.

Except for the four standards concerning language services—Standards 4 through 7, which require adherence to be in compliance with the

1964 Civil Right Act—the standards are guidelines, not mandates. Nonetheless, they will undoubtedly become increasingly important as regulatory and accrediting bodies adopt them as yardsticks for measuring an agency's ability to provide quality services to diverse populations.

The Office of Minority Health and the Office of Civil Rights both imply that the most important part of showing compliance with these standards is a good faith effort to begin implementing the recommended practices. The CLAS Standards are a map for the journey toward cultural and linguistic competence. They will help agencies consistently provide services that are effective in achieving good outcomes for all patients.

REFERENCES

Andrews, M. 1998. Transcultural perspectives in nursing administration. *Journal of Nursing Administration* 28(11): 30–38.

Campinha-Bacote, J. 2003. *The process of cultural competence in the delivery of healthcare services.* Cincinnati, OH: Transcultural C.A.R.E. Associates.

Cooper-Patrick, L., Gallo, L., Gonzales, J., Vu, H., Powe, N., Nelson, D., Ford, D. 1999. Race, gender, and partnership in the patient-physician relationship. *Journal of the American Medical Association,* 292(6): 583–589.

Day, J. 1996. Population projections of the United States by age, sex, race, and Hispanic origin: 1995 to 2050. *U.S. Bureau of the Census Current Population Reports,* publ. no. P25-1130. Washington, DC: US Government Printing Office.

Frusti, D., I. K. Niesen, and J. Campion. 2003. Creating a culturally competent organization: Use of the diversity competency model. *Journal of Nursing Administration* 33(1): 31–38.

Kleinman, A. 1980. *Patients and healers in the context of culture.* Berkeley: University of California Press.

Krames-On-Demand Patient Education. *http://65.201.6.68/ krames/Patient.asp*? (accessed June 10, 2003).

Leininger, M. 1996. Founder's focus: Transcultural nursing administration: An imperative worldwide. *Journal of Transcultural Nursing* 8(1): 28–33.

Leininger, M. 2002. The theory of culture care and the ethnonursing research method. In Leininger and McFarland, eds., *Transcultural Nursing: Concepts, Theories, Research and Practice,* 3rd ed. pp. 71–98. New York: McGraw-Hill.

Narayan, M. C. 2001. *Assessment tool for measuring home health agency cultural and linguistic competence.* Vienna, VA: Mary Narayan.

Narayan, M. C. 2003. *Home health care patient education manual.* Gaithersburg, MD: Aspen.

Office of Civil Rights, Department of Health and Human Services. 2000. *Federal Register* 65(169): 52762–52774. Policy Guidance on Title VI of the Civil Rights Act of 1964: Prohibition Against National Origin Discrimination as It Affects Persons with Limited English Proficiency.

Office of Disease Prevention and Health Promotion, Department of Health and Human Services. 2002. *Healthy People 2010. http://www.healthypeople.gov/* (accessed June 10, 2003).

Office of Minority Health, Department of Health and Human Services. 2000. *Federal Register* 65(247): 80865–80879. National Standards for Culturally and Linguistically Appropriate Services.

Smedley, B., Stith, A., and Nelson, A. 2002. *Unequal treatment: Confronting racial and ethnic disparities in healthcare.* Institute of Medicine (IOM) Report. Washington, DC: National Academy Press.

U.S. Bureau of the Census. 2000. *Statistical abstract of the United States.* Washington, DC: U.S. Government Printing Office.

U.S. Bureau of the Census. 2001. *Overview of Race and Hispanic Origin. http://www.census.gov/prod/2001 pubs/c2kbr011.pdf* (accessed December 9, 2003).

U.S. Bureau of the Census. 2002. *United States Census 2000 Gateway. http://www.census.gov/main/www/ cen2000.html* (accessed December 9, 2003).

U.S. Department of Health and Human Services. 2000. *Healthy People 2010.* 2nd ed. With Understanding and Improving Health and Objectives for Improving Health. 2 vols. Washington, DC: U.S. Government Printing Office.

CHAPTER 19

Classification: An Underutilized Tool for Prospective Payment

Donna Ambler Peters

The idea of patient classification is not new. It can be traced back to the beginning of contemporary nursing, when Florence Nightingale placed the most acutely ill patients in a ward nearest the nurse's desk and the least ill farthest from the desk (Giovannetti and Thiessen, 1983). More recently, the end product of the grouping of patients has become known as a patient classification system, which has been used in nursing to calculate staffing needs and, more recently, to cost out nursing services. Today, patient classification can be used as an available management tool for prospective payment.

However, classification is not limited to the popular patient classification systems. Classification of nursing diagnoses, for example, has been stimulated by the convening of national conferences on the classification of nursing diagnoses in the early 1970s and the more recent formation of the North American Nursing Diagnosis Association (NANDA) to develop, refine, and promote a taxonomy of nursing diagnoses. Although the NANDA taxonomy is popular, this chapter discusses the Omaha System because it is a nursing diagnosis taxonomy specific for community health. The chapter examines the concept of classification as it applies to patient classification systems and nursing diagnoses. It discusses how a nursing diagnosis taxonomy can be used for clinical management of a home health agency and can be incorporated into a patient classification system for administrative management of an agency. By focusing clinical

and administrative management on defined groups, an agency can be in a better position to deal with prospective payment.

CLASSIFICATION THEORY

Scientific inquiry has two major objectives: to describe a particular phenomenon in the world, and to establish the general principles by which the phenomenon can be explained and predicted. To develop the explanatory and predictive principles, scientifically useful concepts are required. These useful types of concept formations are procedures of quantitative ordering, comparative ordering, and classification (Hempel, 1952).

The classificatory concept depicts a characteristic that any object in the domain under consideration must either have or lack. It is an either/or situation. Ordering concepts, on the other hand, attribute a value to each item in the domain, providing a gradation of the characteristics. Stated another way, the characteristics used in an ordering concept are criteria of precedence and coincidence, whereas the characteristics used in a classification concept are criteria for class membership. The value of the characteristics in an ordering concept may be numerical, giving a quantitative ordering (relative values), or simply ordinal. These concept formations are explained by the theory of classificatory procedures and systems (Hempel, 1965; Sokal, 1974).

In a patient classification system, the class to be divided is patients, and the subclasses are groups of patients with a need for a particular kind of care. In actuality, the concept used is a comparative ordering because the amount of care required falls on a continuum rather than in the dichotomy of requiring care or not requiring care. The characteristics used for placing a patient at the appropriate level on the continuum are usually critical indicators of care that depict greater or lesser needs for care. The greater the needs for care, the higher the level at which the patient is placed. In usage, however, the procedure has been called a classification.

In a nursing diagnosis taxonomy, the class to be divided is nursing diagnosis, and the subclasses are the signs and symptoms that a patient may exhibit. These essential characteristics determine membership in the subclass (i.e., the patient either has the diagnosis or does not have it). The subclasses are not on a continuum, and there is no value (either relative or numerical) assigned to any of the diagnoses. Thus this procedure is defined as a classificatory concept rather than a comparative ordering, which is used by patient classification systems. In addition, because it is the class of nursing diagnoses that is being divided and not patients, as in a patient classification system, a patient having more than one nursing diagnosis may appear in more than one category (i.e., patients are not placed in mutually exclusive categories).

PATIENT CLASSIFICATION SYSTEMS

A patient classification system is a "generic term used to describe a variety of methods for grouping or categorizing patients according to their perceived requirements for nursing care" (Giovannetti and Thiessen, 1983, p. 1). Categorization can be based on natural classifications (patient characteristics) or artificial classifications (critical indicators of care). Classification is done either by rating patient characteristics simultaneously and placing them in a category (prototype design) or by rating the patient on several separate critical indicators of care and combining these ratings to provide an overall rating that determines the category into which the patient is placed (factor evaluation) (Abdellah and Levine, 1978; Bermas and Van Slyck, 1984; Giovannetti, 1979).

There are three basic elements in a patient classification system: (1) a procedure for grouping patients that includes the frequency of classification and the means of reporting these data, (2) a quantification of the nursing care resources associated with each category of care, and (3) a method for calculating staffing for required nursing hours. Such a system can be used to monitor productivity levels, to predict and justify staffing needs in the budgetary process, and to provide a basis for nursing charges (Alward, 1983). It must be emphasized, however, that such a system justifies cost only and cannot justify the care.

Logically, it is reasonable to expect that staffing levels based on a patient classification system will have a positive relationship to the quality of care. In practice, however, three problems are evident: (1) the existence of a patient classification system does not guarantee adequate staff, (2) there is no guarantee that nurses will or can perform in the manner described in the system, and (3) the staffing levels obtained by a patient classification system represent only the quantitative aspect of the complex system of patient care (Brown, 1980; Giovannetti and Thiessen, 1983; Sienkiewicz, 1984).

NURSING DIAGNOSIS TAXONOMY

A nursing diagnosis taxonomy is simply the classification of nursing diagnoses. The nursing diagnoses that make up the taxonomy could be derived either deductively or inductively. To be derived deductively, a distinct group of actual and potential health conditions that are amenable to nursing intervention must exist. Currently, however, there is no consensus on the definitions of these conditions; rather, several models exist, each providing a different orientation to nursing. Nursing diagnoses derived inductively are based on a description of clients' health problems as they are encountered in practice. Developing a taxonomy of these diagnoses is one way of describing the domain of nursing and thus communicating the nature of that service both to other nurses and to those outside the profession, such as patients, other professionals, auditors, and legislators (Roy, 1975). Watson (1994) has gone so far as to state that "if we fail to clarify nursing practice within a nursing paradigm, we are . . . on our way out" (p. 86).

A nursing diagnosis taxonomy for community health nursing was developed by the Visiting Nurse Association of Omaha (Simmons, 1980). This taxonomy is consistent with the general and comprehensive practice of community health nursing, which includes the following tenets: it is not limited to a particular age or diagnostic group; it is continuing, not episodic; it uses a holistic approach for health promotion, health maintenance, health education, coordination, and continuity of care; it recognizes the influence of social and ecological issues; and it utilizes the dynamic forces that influence change (American Nurses Association, 1974; Simmons, 1980). Furthermore, the Omaha System focuses on client needs rather than disciplinary expertise. This focus is important in the interdisciplinary environment of community health and even more significant under prospective payment where the focal point moves from care per visit to care per client episode.

The 44 nursing diagnoses included in the taxonomy were arrived at empirically from the practice of the community health nurses employed by the Visiting Nurse Association of Omaha and seven diverse test sites located throughout the United States. The diagnoses are organized by the four broad domains addressed by community health nurses and other health professionals: environmental, psychosocial, physiological, and health-related behaviors. Each diagnosis is described by a list of signs and symptoms; that is, general statements condensed from assessment data that are patient specific and are used to describe actual problems (diagnoses). For example, one of the problem labels in the health-related behaviors domain is nutrition. There are eight descriptors or signs and symptoms for this problem label, one of which is "weighs 10 percent more than average." The problem may be referenced as health promotion, potential, or deficit/impairment/actual. The patient may be defined as an individual or family (Martin and Scheet, 1992). For example, if a person were more than 10 percent overweight as a result of poor personal eating habits, this would be an actual individual problem. If the person were dependent on the family to buy, prepare, and bring the food to the bedside, however, the problem would be a family problem. If this same person were currently at an appropriate weight but the family was feeding the patient an extreme number of calories for the patient's activity level, this would be a potential family problem.

The Omaha System not only provides nursing diagnoses and specific descriptors for each diagnosis, but also includes a problem rating scale for outcomes and an intervention scheme. The problem rating scale is a five-point Likert type scale that measures the concepts of knowledge, behavior, and status for each identified problem. It provides an evaluation framework for monitoring patient progress on each problem throughout the patient's admission. The intervention scheme is used in conjunction with the problem rating scale. The scheme is an organized framework consisting of three levels of nursing activities designed to address specific client problems using four broad categories of interventions: health teaching, treatments, case management, and surveillance. An alphabetical list of 62 objects of action comprises the second level. The third level is patient-specific information generated by the caregiver (Martin and Scheet, 1992).

CLINICAL MANAGEMENT

Patient classification systems, by definition, are more of an administrative tool than an aid to clinical management. Some improvement in nursing care plans and chart documentation has been seen where classification data are obtained from these documents. The critical indicators of care used in patient classification systems are inadequate criteria for evaluating the quality of care received, however, until a relationship between these indicators and the progress of the patient's condition has been established (Aydelotte, 1973). Furthermore, the tasks, activities, and categories of nursing work found in the systems do not reflect the nature and full character of nursing practice.

Using a classification of nursing diagnoses, however, directly focuses on the care of the client. Nursing diagnosis is the pivotal factor in the nursing process, which is central to community health practice and all nursing actions. Structurally, the nursing process is adapted from the scientific approach to solving problems. It consists of six steps: (1) assessing, (2) diagnosing, (3) identifying outcomes, (4) planning, (5) implementing, and (6) evaluating. Diagnosing is the result of assessment. If there is no nursing diagnosis, then there is no reason to continue to the other components of the process.

Using a nursing diagnosis taxonomy inductively derived from community health practice actually defines that practice. Therefore, because the Omaha System defines community health care, when used correctly it provides for the planning, organizing, and prioritizing of that care. It allows for the sifting and sorting of information in an organized fashion. It actually provides a building block of care; the more difficult and time consuming the case and the more extenuating the circumstances, the more problems will be identified from more domains. By identifying the subsequent problems, the nurse is able to communicate in a logical, concise way to his or her superiors, auditors, payers, and others that this is a difficult case and more time is needed.

It is the classification of the nursing diagnoses that facilitates the organizing and prioritizing of care. The physiological domain, for example, generally provides the structure for those nursing interventions that are closely aligned with the medical regimen. As any nurse working in home health care knows, however, it is those problems that are often the easiest to

handle. The diagnoses under the other three domains are the ones that are often the most difficult and time consuming. For example, the definition of the health-related behaviors domain states that these problems require personal motivation on the part of the client, thereby indicating that resolution of the problem may be more difficult (Simmons, 1980).

Utilizing the Omaha System to show the sequencing of care allows nurses to define and document adequately the complexity of care inherent in these other domains. For example, a patient with tuberculosis may be referred to an agency for monitoring and streptomycin injections. The nurse may begin by using the diagnosis of "respiration: impairment" (physiological domain) to follow the patient's physiological state. Upon assessment, however, it is found that the patient is not taking his medication regularly and is also consuming an excessive amount of alcohol. The diagnosis of "prescribed medication regimen: impairment" (health-related behavior domain) may then be added and a care plan developed to inform the patient of the consequences of not taking the medication and of mixing the medication with alcohol. On subsequent visits the situation may be no better, so that interventions are revised to include family counseling and the involvement of other community agencies. Eventually it is decided that the underlying problem is really alcoholism, and a third diagnosis, "substance use: actual" (also from the health-related behaviors domain), is identified and a relevant plan of care developed. Thus there is a clearly sequenced description of what was done in this case and how it required both changes in interventions and subsequent identification of additional nursing diagnoses from another domain. Additionally, the use of the problem rating scale provides the guide posts to evaluate whether the interventions made a difference in the patient's condition.

Furthermore, when this sequencing of care is done in advance for defined groups of patients, it becomes a standardized approach to care. This standardized approach can be called a *critical path* (defined as a predetermined sequencing and timing of care activities, including nursing, therapies, and medical interventions, through an expected course of care toward an expected outcome) for care that can be examined and compared over time or with other approaches. Critical paths were used by the National Aeronautics and Space Administration space program for activities that were time sensitive toward achievement of the overall goal. They began to be used in health care in the early 1970s. They have become popular today in acute care with the increased importance of meeting outcomes within a designated time frame. With prospective payment, they are being adopted by home care as "care maps" to serve as a baseline for development of a treatment plan (Galloro, 2000).

Critical paths, or care maps, provide staff with guidelines for best practice (i.e., which activities or interventions lead to the best outcomes). Other benefits include standardization of documentation of care, delineation of role responsibility for each discipline involved in care (which also provides for greater interdisciplinary collaboration), improved resource management through comprehensive care planning, and a tool for teaching new staff and students how to care for a specific patient condition.

Most important, critical paths can be a valuable tool for quality improvement. In fact, without tying critical paths to the continuous quality improvement program, an agency may not see an improvement in outcomes or a reduction in costs. The key is the documenting, collecting, analyzing, and reporting of variances from the critical paths, or variance management (Schriefer, 1995). Both positive and negative variances are critical to identifying what works and what needs improvement. Analysis of the variations can be used to revise the critical path, encourage clinical practice to be consistent with the critical path, identify changes to length of stay and resource use, and utilize aggregated data for financial and care analyses (Coffey et al., 1995).

Not all patients can be grouped into critical paths; therefore, for these patients case management is more appropriate. Even for these cases, however, the Omaha System can improve quality within an agency. This scheme makes the nurse ask critical questions, such as: "What data do I need to make a comprehensive assessment? Why am I visiting this case? Do I need to continue visiting? Is this a problem I can do something about, or is it best handled by another discipline or another agency?" It also forces agency administration to examine policy to determine whether there are existing policies or procedures that impede the team concept of care or hamper efficient patient-oriented care. For example, in one agency, usual procedure was to refer cases to the social worker using a referral form. The social worker did not have access to the patient chart. It became apparent, after implementation of the Omaha System, that the social worker needed not only access to the chart, but also more intimate communication with the nurse because both often were working on the same patient problem and a common (supplemental) plan of care.

The building blocks for successful quality improvement programs and for successful competition within prospective payment are data. Improving data collection in community health is important because current data are redundant, lack the key aspects of care, and are expensive to retrieve for any type of analysis. Therefore, information that is needed for guiding practice, setting professional standards, fulfilling payer and surveyor requirements, benchmarking, establishing outcomes, and setting health care policy is missing (Raup and Westra, 1996). These issues have been initially addressed by the Outcome and Assessment Information Set (OASIS) released by Medicare to provide for standard outcome and assessment data across agencies. OASIS is a data collection tool used on all adult Medicare patients that is composed of 89 questions; 79 address a patient assessment of health and functional state and 10 are related to patient demographics. However, OASIS is not a comprehensive assessment and must be integrated exactly as written into an agency's more complete assessment, removing duplicative questions. Without a comprehensive assessment, it is impossible to generate a representative problem list for the patient. Raup and Westra (1996) state that OASIS is easily integrated with the Omaha System and that, combined, they provide a comprehensive assessment care plan and evaluation of patient care. They meet the multiple demands for data and offer the clinical data necessary to provide quality care and shape future policy.

A recent secondary analysis (Kaiser and Hays, 2002) of the clinical data from 205 adult community patient charts determined that adequate and standardized language for naming the patient problems is critical. The findings indicated that providing health care solely on the basis of medical need was insufficient; "that consideration of the client's entire constellation of problems, with their antecedent, concurrent interactions and consequences, provides both direction and support for a family and a forward approach to nursing intervention" (Kaiser and Hays, 2002, p. 28). These researchers found a total of 903 Omaha diagnoses among the 205 patients with a mean number of 4.4 problems per person. These distinct Omaha problem labels provided a representation of more than the singular dimension of an episodic health event and a precision to the language and data elements necessary to describe community care to students, other nurses, policy makers, other health workers, payers, and patients. Also, the standard nomenclature provided in the Omaha System means the same thing to everyone reading the chart, which facilitates both communication and understanding. No longer do supervisors and auditors have to peruse thick charts, trying to identify and evaluate the care rendered. Instead, use of the standard diagnoses, interventions, and outcomes allows anyone to follow the professional caregiver's movement through the problem-solving process. Additional research on the number of Omaha diagnoses per prospective payment group could lead to even more information and assist with the development of more explicit and efficient care maps.

ADMINISTRATIVE MANAGEMENT

Patient classification systems are valuable management tools for staffing, budgeting, monitoring productivity, costing, and program planning. Historically in home health care, however, classification has been more for the purpose of quality management than for resource allocation or costing. This is expected because the Medicare law of 1965 ensured optimal payment to all providers and makes no effort toward cost containment. The law, however, was accompanied by certification regulations that set forth standards for quality aimed at limiting participation in the program to those facilities that provide at least minimum care (Kurowski, 1980; Mundinger, 1983). Thus the motivation for enhancing quality was greater than the motivation for efficient use of resources. Today, with the evolution of prospective payment, the picture is different. With home health care agencies caring for more patients, sicker patients, and more high-technology patients and at the same time facing restrictive managed care agreements and limited prosective payment from Medicare, efficient resource allocation and costing of services are of paramount importance. Some research has been done in home health care to discover possible critical indicators of care for a patient classification system that will predict resource consumption (Ballard and McNamara, 1983; Hardy, 1984; Sienkiewicz, 1984). What is needed, however, is the use of a nursing diagnosis taxonomy as the basis for categorization of patients. Such a taxonomy already exists in the form of the Omaha System, and this taxonomy defines the essence of home health care. Following are some advantages in using such a taxonomy.

Patient classification systems are used for program planning. The Omaha System provides the necessary information as a management tool for program planning. Analysis of specific nursing diagnoses addressed by nurses within a given agency allows the agency to devise and revise its programs systematically according to patient and community needs (Simmons, 1980).

It gives the agency the necessary data to interface with other community agencies and leaders for solving suprasystem problems, such as identifying nutritional needs of patients that are not being met by the local food program. Ideally, categorization of patients would also link quality care to the reimbursement or costing of care, although current patient classification systems are limited in their ability to accomplish this.

The Omaha System as a nursing diagnosis taxonomy for community health both defines reimbursable nursing care under Medicare (facilitation of the medical treatment plan) and provides for a holistic assessment of the patient (Pankratz, 1985). Thus it provides for high-quality nursing care at home while at the same time surviving this world of regulation and cost containment. To prove the viability of this statement, a small, unpublished pilot study was done by this author in 1985 on 41 Medicare patient records in two separate home health agencies to determine whether the goals associated with the identified nursing diagnoses were being achieved under current Medicare law. Charts were selected from the total patient population for 1984 from these two agencies. Criteria for chart selection included Medicare payment, normative discharge (i.e., improved health status), nursing as the primary service used, and inclusion of the nursing diagnosis "integument: impairment." This diagnosis was used as a tracer. The findings indicated that proper use of the Omaha System for planning, documenting, and evaluating care allowed the attainment of 96 percent of the predetermined patient outcomes before the patient was discharged. Unfortunately, the study also showed that often the scheme was not being used at its maximum, resulting once more in inadequate documentation of home health care activities (Table 19–1).

Patient classification requires the use of critical indicators of care or essential characteristics. The Omaha System has been evaluated for its contribution to the essential characteristics that have an effect on nursing workload. In another unpublished study, it was hypothesized that the quantity of nursing care demanded would be a function of the patient's living arrangements and support system, age, sex, ability to perform activities of daily living, prior source of care, presence of surgical intervention, and nursing diagnosis. All the variables except the nursing diagnosis had been measured in previous studies. This study consisted of 68 patient records from two home health agencies. The records were drawn from the total patient population of these agencies for 1984 using a random numbers table. The inclusion of nursing diagnoses with the variable from previous studies helped account for 41.9 percent of the variance in registered nurse visits. Ballard and McNamara (1983), who did not use nursing diagnoses, were only able to explain 31.9 percent of the total variance. In addition, the only variables to enter the regression equation for intensity of nursing visits (number of nursing visits to length of service) were nursing diagnoses. This may indicate that certain problems identified by nurses are especially predictive when one is examining the intensity of service rendered to a patient. Such a finding is important because reimbursement and technological reforms have led to more intense services being provided to home care patients.

Another study (Martin and Scheet, 1985) also indicates that the classification of nursing diagnoses may be an important way of examining the cost of home health care. This study found that the number of nursing diagnoses and race were significant in predicting length of agency service. Hays (1992) found not only that nursing diagnoses were a predictor of direct hours of nursing care, but also that the use of potential and health promotion nursing diagnoses in the Omaha System increased the amount of prediction. Thus there is significant evidence that nursing diagnoses play an important part in the provision of home health care and in allocating resources (money and personnel) for that care. A nursing diagnoses taxonomy per se, however, cannot be used as a patient classification system because it categorizes nursing diagnoses, not patients. In a nursing diagnosis taxonomy, patients cannot be placed into mutually exclusive categories. In addition, a nursing diagnosis tax-

Table 19–1 Nursing Diagnoses Identified and Outcomes Met by Agency A (Visiting Nurse Association) and Agency B (Hospital-Based Agency)

Agency	Problems Identified	Problems Not Identified	Outcomes Met at Discharge*	Outcomes Not Met at Discharge*
A (n = 102)	76 (74.5%)	26 (25.5%)	64 (84.2%)	12 (15.8%)
B (n = 61)	41 (67.2%)	20 (32.8%)	39 (95.1%)	2 (4.9%)
Both (complete charts available)	27 (16.6%)		26 (96.0%)	

* Could not be determined for unidentified problems.

onomy uses the classificatory concepts of class membership, whereas a patient classification system uses the ordering concepts of precedence and coincidence. For example, a patient to be classified in a patient classification system would be evaluated using established critical indicators of care and then would be placed into a level based on the importance or weight of the critical indicators connected with that patient's care. Nursing diagnoses within a taxonomy, however, could be used as the critical indicators of care for placing a patient into a level.

Work has been done on incorporating the Omaha System nursing diagnosis taxonomy into a patient classification system. The Community Health Intensity Rating Scale (CHIRS) was developed by expert groups of community health nurses based on 15 community health parameters inductively derived from the Omaha System. These parameters (Table 19–2) represent content areas of the four domains (environmental, psychosocial, physiological, and health-related behaviors) identified in the Omaha System.

CHIRS also utilizes the nursing process as the organizational structure within each parameter to provide for the definition of the patient's nursing requirements by both essential charac-

teristics and critical indicators of care (i.e., assessment and evaluation steps reflect essential characteristics, and planning and implementation steps reflect critical indicators of care). Essential characteristics for each parameter are noted in Table 19–2. Critical indicators of care for all parameters are nursing diagnoses, other disciplines involved in care, discharge plan, teaching/guidance, monitoring/measurements, referral/coordination, and treatments/care. Incorporating the nursing process necessitated a prototype method of classification to avoid the artificial separation of actions (assessment, planning, implementation, and evaluation), that in reality are not separated. The scale delineates four categories or levels of care (minor, moderate, major, and extreme). Thus it includes 4 patient profiles for each of the 15 parameters, one profile to illustrate the extent of nursing input required for patient care within each level. Each profile includes several elements that define the steps of the nursing process for that level. For example, in the parameter of nutrition, one of the elements in the assessment part of this parameter is weight, as addressed under the nursing diagnosis of nutrition in the Omaha System. This element is defined over the four levels as follows:

Table 19–2 CHIRS Parameters

Parameter	Essential Characteristics
Environmental Domain	
Finances	Financial resources, employment, health insurance, money management
Physical environment/safety	Residence/living conditions, utilities, sanitation, neighborhood, pets, access to commercial services
Psychosocial Domain	
Community networking	Knowledge of resources, availability/use of resources, emergency plan
Family system	Family, family process/roles, caregiving system, social network, interpersonal relationships
Emotional/mental response	Adjustment/coping, emotional state, cultural attitudes, spiritual beliefs, mental status
Individual growth and development	Early development, sense of self, spiritual growth, adaptation to aging
Physiological Domain	
Sensory function	Sensory perception, pain/discomfort
Respiratory and circulatory function	Airway, breathing, cardiovascular status, tissue perfusion, endurance
Neuromusculoskeletal function	Consciousness, orientation, communication, speech, physical mobility
Reproductive/sexual function	Peripartum, sexual organs/menses, sexual practices
Digestion/elimination	Ingestion, assimilation, metabolism, bowel function, bladder habits, renal function
Structural integrity	Skin integrity, immune response
Health-Related Behaviors	
Nutrition	Food selection/preparation, diet, intake, eating, weight
Personal habits	Personal hygiene, exercise regimen, sleep habits, smoking, substance use
Health management	Engagement, technical skill, medications

Level 1, within normal limits for height

Level 2, greater than 10 percent above or below ideal weight

Level 3, greater than 25 percent above or below ideal weight

Level 4, morbid obesity/severe emaciation

In scoring the tool, one rating is made for each parameter by selection of the appropriate patient profile. The overall rating is then calculated using an implicit integration of the ratings assigned to each parameter (Peters, 1988). Initial use of this scale on 560 cases from two different agencies significantly identified four subgroups in regard to the amount of their nursing requirements (Peters, 1988). This was supported in a second study of 237 cases in a third agency (Hays, 1992). In the original study, CHIRS explained 6 percent of the variation in amount of care provided by a nurse (Peters, 1988). In the second study, which was done using a revised factor evaluation form of CHIRS, the amount of variation explained was 10 percent (Hays, 1992).

CHIRS has been tested with several different community health groups, including patients with acquired immunodeficiency syndrome, high-risk prenatal clients and high-risk infants, high-technology and home care clients, and the homeless, and has been adapted for use by school health nurses by Burt et al. (1996). It is also being used internationally with a study currently underway in Turkey. At the University of Nebraska Medical Center College of Nursing and at St. Petersburg College in Florida, CHIRS is used to provide a structure for students in their community health assessments.

In a study of 133 public health nursing clients from a midwestern city/county health department, a composite measure of nursing service was developed, called *nursing effort*, to capture nursing services that were provided both during and outside visits. This measure included the number of nursing visits, number of telephone calls to and on behalf of the client, and number of not home/not found visits. Use of this measure of nursing effort significantly increased the amount of variance explained by CHIRS (Hays, 1995). This indicates that CHIRS recognizes the time spent outside home visits and validates efforts such as phone calls, coordination activities, and other activities of indirect care. This is important because innovative interventions offered under prospective payment, such as electronic interventions and telephone visits, can change the amount of direct contact in the home (Peters and Hays, 1995). Because CHIRS recognizes activities beyond direct care, it may prove to be

a useful tool in measuring and costing services provided.

One means by which prospective payment is postulated to achieve cost savings is by focusing health care services to meet the needs of specific types of consumers or conditions. A secondary analysis of three data sets from these CHIRS studies found that the salient parameters varied depending on the population, indicating that home care is delivered to widely diverse groups and that aggregating data that may appear to go together may obscure important, unique information. No one parameter was significant across all three data sets. Furthermore, of the 12 salient parameters among the three study samples, only half were from the physiological domain, the domain that drives the medical model. (Hays et al., 1996).

This is supported by two other community studies that have found the physiological domain in the Omaha System, the domain most closely aligned to the rendering of medical care, **not** to be the predominant domain in rendering care. In a study of 54 patients at two community-based programs in the rural southwestern United States, it was found that the mean number of Omaha diagnoses was seven, and the most frequently identified were in the psychosocial domain (average 3 per patient). The second domain in which frequent problems were identified was the environmental domain (1.6 per patient) and the physiological domain was third with an average of 1.3 per patient. (Slack and McEwen, 1999). Kaiser and Hays (2002) in their study of 205 patients found that the physiological domain was not even represented among the most common Omaha System problem labels. The researchers indicate that physiological problems were present for many of the patients, such as diabetes, coronary artery disease, and hypertension, but the problems were varied and did not cluster under any of the more specific Omaha labels. The common factor in these studies is clear—the medical diagnosis alone is insufficient to account for care needed by community health patients. The other important information for agencies is that each patient caseload is different, and recognizing the specific types of patients being served by a given agency is key in determining the expertise and abilities needed by staff and what education and credentials are required.

CONCLUSION

Use of a nursing diagnosis taxonomy is valuable in defining, organizing, directing, and communicating home care. It provides the basis for quality and clinical management of care. Its use as a management tool for staffing and costing is limited, however, because it does not place patients into mutually exclusive categories. Nevertheless, research studies indicate that such a taxonomy does provide useful information in allocating resources.

A patient classification system (CHIRS) has been developed that incorporates the Omaha System taxonomy and categorizes patients into four levels of care. This system has the potential to measure costs and determine staffing levels as well as to address the qualitative issues of care. More work needs to be done, but the Omaha System and CHIRS provide agencies with valid and reliable tools for the clinical and administrative management of home care.

The study by Kaiser and Hays (2002) examined the relationship between CHIRS scores and the number of Omaha System problem labels defined for primary patients living in the community. These researchers found a 74.1 percent agreement, meaning that patients with more Omaha System problem labels had higher CHIRS scores, and patients with fewer Omaha System diagnoses had lower CHIRS scores. "This finding indicates that for nearly three-fourths of the clients, the two measures together gave a more complete picture of family need than either measure alone" (p. 26). Therefore, using a patient classification tool such as CHIRS in conjunction with a valid nursing diagnosis taxonomy may be a useful way to quantify, measure, and examine the holistic nature of community health. Once this is accomplished, providing more cost effective and efficient care in this new age of prospective payment becomes more reasonable and attainable.

REFERENCES

Abdellah, F., and Levine, E. 1978. *Better patient care through nursing research.* 2nd ed. New York: Macmillan.

Alward, R. 1983. Patient classification schemes: The ideal vs. reality. *Journal of Nursing Administration* 13: 14–19.

American Nurses Association. 1974. *Standards of community health nursing practice.* Kansas City, MO: ANA.

Aydelotte, M. R. 1973. *Nurse staffing methodology.* DHEW Publication No. (NIH) 73-433. Washington, DC: Government Printing Office.

Ballard, S., and McNamara, R. 1983. Quantifying nursing needs in home health care. *Nursing Research* 32: 236–241.

Bermas, N., and Van Slyck, A. 1984. Patient classification systems and the nursing department. *Hospitals* 58: 99–100.

Brown, B. I. 1980. Realistic workloads for community health nurses. *Nursing Outlook* 28: 233–237.

Burt, C. J., et al. 1996. Preliminary development of the school health intensity rating scale. *Journal of School Health* 66: 286.

Coffey, R. J., et al. 1995. Extending the application of critical path methods. *Quality Management in Health Care* 3: 14–19.

Galloro, V. 2000. Embracing PPS. *Modern Healthcare* 30: 2–4.

Giovannetti, P. 1979. Understanding patient classification systems. *Journal of Nursing Administration* 9: 4–9.

Giovannetti, P., and Thiessen, M. 1983. *Patient classification for nurse staffing: Criteria for selection and implementation.* Edmonton, Alberta: Alberta Association of Registered Nurses.

Hardy, J. A. 1984. A patient classification system for home health patients. *Caring* 3: 26–27.

Hays, B. J. 1992. Nursing care requirements and resource consumption in home health care. *Nursing Research* 41: 138–143.

Hays, B. J. 1995. Nursing intensity as a predictor of resource consumption in public health nursing. *Nursing Research* 44: 106–110.

Hays, B.J., et al. 1996. *The utility of CHIRS parameters in predicting resource consumption among community* health nursing client populations: A secondary analysis. Unpublished manuscript.

Hempel, C. G. 1952. *Fundamentals of concept formation in empirical science.* Chicago: University of Chicago Press.

Hempel, C. G. 1965. *Aspects of scientific explanation and other essays in the philosophy of science.* New York: Free Press.

Kaiser, K. L. and Hays, B. J., 2002. Examining health problems and intensity of need for care in family focused community and public health nursing. *Journal of Community Health Nursing* 19: 17–32.

Kurowski, B. T. 1980. *A cost-effectiveness analysis of home health care: Implications for public policy and future research.* Doctoral dissertation, University of Colorado, Denver.

Martin, K. S., and Scheet, N.J. 1985. The Omaha system: Implications for costing community health nursing. In F. A. Schaffer (ed.), *Costing out nursing: Pricing our product.* New York: National League for Nursing, pp. 197–206.

Martin, K. S., and Scheet, N.J. 1992. *The Omaha system: Application for community health nursing.* Philadelphia: Saunders.

Mundinger, M. O. 1983. *Home care controversy: Too little, too late, too costly.* Gaithersburg, MD: Aspen.

Pankratz, J. D. 1985. *Serving two masters? Professional standards of care and reimbursable care.* Paper presented at the First National Symposium on Home Health Care, Ann Arbor, MI.

Peters, D. A. 1988. Development of a community health intensity rating scale. *Nursing Research* 37: 202–207.

Peters, D. A., and Hays, B.J. 1995. Measuring the essence of nursing: A guide for future practice. *Journal of Professional Nursing* 11: 358–363.

Raup, G., and Westra, B.L. 1996. *Alternate approaches to outcomes data—What provides value?* Paper presented at the Eleventh National Symposium on Home Health Care, Ann Arbor, MI.

Roy, C., Sr. 1975. A diagnostic classification system for nursing. *Nursing Outlook* 23: 90–94.

Schriefer, J. 1995. Managing critical pathway variances. *Quality Management in Health Care* 3: 30–42.

Sienkiewicz, J. I. 1984. Patient classification in community health nursing. *Nursing Outlook* 32: 319–321.

Simmons, D. A. 1980. *A classification scheme for client problems in community health nursing* (DHHS Publication No. HRA 80-16). Washington, DC: Government Printing Office.

Slack, M. C. and McEwen, M. M. 1999. The impact of interdisciplinary case management on client outcomes. *Family Community Health* 22: 30–48.

Sokal, R. 1974. Classification: Purposes, principles, progress, prospects. *Science* 185: 1115–1123.

Watson, J. 1994. Have we arrived or are we on our way out? *Image* 26: 86.

SUGGESTED READING

Iyer, P. W. and Camp, N. H. 1999 *Nursing documentation: A nursing process approach.* Chapter 13. St. Louis, MO: Mosby.

Peters, D. A. 1995. Outcomes: The mainstay of a framework for quality care. *Journal of Nursing Care Quality* 10: 61–69.

Peters, D. A. and McKeon, T. 1998. *Transforming home care: quality, cost, and data management.* Gaithersburg, MD: Aspen.

CHAPTER 20

Analysis and Management of Home Health Nursing Caseloads and Workloads

Judith Lloyd Storfjell, Carol Easley Allen, and Cheryl E. Easley

BACKGROUND

Management of nursing productivity is critical to the financial viability of home health service agencies because nursing wages are usually the largest single budget item, often representing more than half the entire budget. Under fee-for-service payment (payment per visit), the focus of nursing productivity management was on increasing the number of nursing visits per day or month. As reimbursement methodologies shift to episodic payment and capitation, home visit efficiency is still essential, but the amount of nursing intervention required to accomplish a specific outcome may be even more important. In other words, it is increasingly necessary to monitor and control the number of visits per case as well as the number of visits per day. Coupled with this shift in reimbursement is an increasingly diverse client mix that includes not only highly acute cases, but also more long-term cases.

To meet this challenge successfully, home care managers need to establish and monitor nursing productivity standards. These standards, however, must take into account the type and complexity of care required by the client.

PURPOSE OF THE EASLEY-STORFJELL CASELOAD/WORKLOAD ANALYSIS INSTRUMENTS

The Easley-Storfjell Instruments for Caseload/ Workload Analysis (CL/WLA) were designed to give home care nursing managers tools to plan,

monitor, and evaluate nursing activities simply and effectively. They have been used successfully throughout the United States and Canada by a variety of home health and community health agencies since 1977. Their continuing use is due largely to their flexibility and adaptability to various types of settings and clients as well as their ease of use and acceptance by both managers and nursing staff. The following criteria were used in the development of these management tools:

- *Facilitate the supervisory process.* The chief purpose is to assist clinical managers in the assignment of cases, to identify caseload problems and patterns, and to provide a format for supervisory conferences and discussions with staff. By periodic, joint review and the rating of cases, a caseload and workload analysis can be combined easily with other nurse supervisor activities.
- *Be simple to use.* CL/WLA was kept extremely simple so that it would be easily understood by all levels of personnel. Rather than taking extra time from a busy manager's schedule, these instruments should reduce the amount of supervisory time required. Although they are presented here in a manual format, a number of organizations have incorporated them into computer applications.
- *Be flexible.* CL/WLA can be used with a variety of staffing patterns, including

teams and individually managed case-loads. In addition, they can be adapted for use in many types of community health agencies and for various professionals who carry caseloads, including therapists, social workers, and case managers.

- *Include complexity, time, and intervention measures.* These three variables are seen as the key indicators for appropriate staffing and productivity planning.
- *Provide summary reports.* CL/WLA can be summarized by individual, team, office, district, or agency.
- *Be compatible with other tools.* Although the information obtained from CL/WLA is valuable in its own right, it can be augmented by data derived from other analyses, including activity-based costing and management, cost reports, and time studies.
- *Provide management information.* Some management uses of CL/WLA include projecting and evaluating staffing needs and monitoring trends. Findings can be compared with established standards or indicators.

DESCRIPTION OF THE CL/WLA PROCESS

There are two major components of the CL/WLA process: (1) caseload analysis, which involves summarizing the characteristics of individual cases (or clients) carried and/or managed by an individual nurse, and (2) workload analysis, which involves summarizing all activities required of the nurse, including caseload responsibilities. Home health nursing visits vary according to three critical dimensions: (1) the number of visits required to provide care (time), (2) the type of interventions used by the nurse during the visit, and the (3) difficulty or complexity of the care provided.

Therefore, CL/WLA provides a description of a nurse's caseload according to time, type of intervention, and complexity of care factors. Both time and complexity are divided into four levels of intensity according to the frequency of visits and six difficulty of care variables. The third dimension, nursing interventions, is incorporated into the complexity scale.

A nurse performs five major activities (or interventions) during a home visit:

1. assessing the client, environment, and plan of care (using clinical judgment)
2. teaching the client and caregivers
3. providing direct physical care to the client (technical tasks)
4. providing psychosocial support to the client and caregivers
5. coordinating care with other entities and persons (managing the case)

These five interventions are combined with an acuity measure (number of nursing problems) to form a patient classification system. This system has been shown to be both reliable and valid in grouping home care clients according to the complexity (difficulty) of their nursing care needs (Albrecht, 1991). It has also been used successfully independent of the CL/WLA process as a method for measuring complexity of care and to document the major home care nursing interventions (assessment, teaching, physical care, psychosocial support, and coordination/management).

The Easley-Storfjell process for analyzing caseload and workload consists of four steps:

1. Each case is analyzed to predict the number of visits required to accomplish established goals and to determine the complexity of nursing care required.
2. Time and complexity ratings are charted on a visual graph.
3. Time for noncaseload work requirements or duties is calculated.
4. Findings are summarized, and the number of required visits is compared with the number possible according to the workload analysis.

INSTRUCTIONS FOR USE OF CL/WLA INSTRUMENTS

Specific instructions for completing the four steps just outlined follow.

Step 1

The complexity and the number of home visits are seen as the most important variables in assessing the level of nursing care required and the amount of work time needed. Therefore, these two factors are assessed separately.

The amount of time required is assigned a rating from 1 to 4 according to the following scale:

1. 1 visit or fewer per month
2. 2 to 3 visits per month
3. 1 to 2 visits per week
4. 3 to 5 visits per week

This scale can be adjusted by the individual agency according to actual patterns of visit intensity. This scale can also be adapted to include several types of visits (e.g., home or telephone) by assigning units to each type of visit.

The complexity of care (difficulty) is determined by using the patient classification system, which is based on assessing six variables—five nursing interventions and one severity of illness (acuity) indicator:

A. clinical judgment required (assessment needs)
B. teaching needs
C. physical care needs (technical procedures)
D. psychosocial support needs
E. coordination and care management needs
F. number and severity of problems

The complexity variables have also been assigned four categories on a four-point scale from minimal complexity (1) to very great complexity (4). Descriptions of the nursing care requirements for each criterion or level of complexity are shown in Exhibit 20–1. These complexity levels may also be correlated by the agency with its typical levels of nursing practice and ancillary support.

It is often found that the best way to rate cases is through a joint conference between the clinical manager and the staff nurse. This process offers an opportunity for a generalized caseload review and specific planning for each case. During this conference, more accurate information regarding the current status of the client can be

obtained, and care plans and goals can be identified. At the same time, the cases are listed on the caseload analysis roster (Exhibit 20–2) along with the ratings for time and complexity. Space also is provided for recording the length of time a case has been open, the appropriate program area or the client's diagnostic category, and the total number of visits required during the current month.

Step 2

The time and difficulty ratings are then charted on the caseload analysis graph (Exhibit 20–3) to obtain a graphic representation of the entire caseload. This chart, more than any other portion of the CL/WLA, has been beneficial in assisting the individual nurse in "visualizing" his or her caseload by depicting both the complexity and the time requirements of the entire caseload. The average number of monthly visits required by the caseload can also be calculated on this form if it was calculated on the caseload analysis roster.

Step 3

Home health nurses usually have other work responsibilities in addition to their caseload requirements. These assignments and duties also require a commitment of time. The time allocation worksheet (Exhibit 20–4) facilitates the calculation of the time needed for the range of duties that constitute the nurse's total workload. The following specific areas are included on the form:

- personal adjustments (vacation, sick time, holiday, or paid days off)
- supportive activities (supervisor conferences, continuing education, committees, staff meetings)
- special assignments (teaching classes, hospital liaison, preceptoring)
- field activities (clinics, community meetings, committees)

Here again, because of the flexibility designed into the system, organizations can modify this

Exhibit 20–1 CL/WLA Guidelines

TIME DETERMINATION

1. Monthly or less; only 1 visit
2. Biweekly
3. 1–2 times per week
4. 3–5 times per week

COMPLEXITY DETERMINATION

Assign the highest numerical categorical rating (most difficult) in which the case meets two or more of the criteria.
Based on:

A. Clinical judgment/assessment
B. Teaching/education needs
C. Physical care
D. Psychosocial needs
E. Coordination/management
F. Number and severity of problems

1. Minimal
   A. Requires limited judgment, use of common sense, observation of fairly predictable change in patient status
   B. Requires basic health teaching
   C. Requires no or simple maintenance care
   D. Requires ability to relate to patients and families
   E. Requires limited involvement of only one other provider/agency
   F. Few or uncomplicated problems

2. Moderate
   A. Requires use of basic problem-solving techniques, ability to make limited patient assessments
   B. Requires teaching related to common health problems
   C. Requires basic rehabilitation or use of uncomplicated technical skills
   D. Requires use of basic interpersonal relationship skills
   E. Requires limited involvement of two other providers/agencies
   F. Several problems with limited complexity

3. Great
   A. Requires use of well-developed problem-solving skills enhanced by comprehensive knowledge of physical and social sciences, ability to make patient and family assessments
   B. Requires teaching related to illness, complications, and/or comprehensive health supervision
   C. Requires use of complicated technical skills
   D. Requires professional insight and intervention skills in coping with psychosocial needs
   E. Requires extensive involvement of at least one other provider/agency or coordination of several providers/agencies
   F. Several complicated problems

4. Very Great
   A. Requires use of creativity, ability to initiate and coordinate plan for patient or family care, use of additional resources and increased supervisory support, ability to make comprehensive patient and family assessment
   B. Requires teaching related to unusual health problems or teaching/learning difficulties
   C. Requires knowledge of scientific rationale that underlies techniques, ability to modify care in response to patient/family need
   D. Requires ability to intervene in severe psychosocial problems
   E. Requires extensive coordination of multiple providers/agencies
   F. Numerous or complicated problems requiring augmentation of the knowledge base

Source: Courtesy of Storfjell, Allen, and Easley.

Exhibit 20–2 Caseload Analysis Roster

Name _____ Position _____ Date _____

Case Number/Name	Days/Weeks Open	Priority/ Program/ Diagnosis	Complexity Rating	Time Rating	Total Visits Required This Month
1.					
2.					
3.					
4.					
5.					
6.					
7.					
8.					
9.					
10.					
11.					
12.					
13.					
14.					
15.					
16.					
17.					
18.					
19.					
20.					
Totals					
Averages					

Source: Courtesy of Storfjell, Allen, and Easley.

Exhibit 20–3 Caseload Analysis Graph

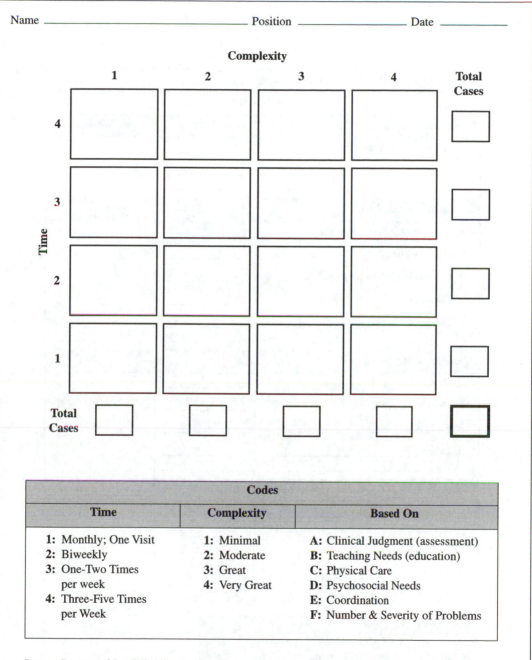

Name ———————————————— Position ——————— Date ————

Complexity

| | 1 | 2 | 3 | 4 | Total Cases |

Time

Time	4				
3					
2					
1					

Total Cases

Codes		
Time	**Complexity**	**Based On**
1: Monthly; One Visit	**1:** Minimal	**A:** Clinical Judgment (assessment)
2: Biweekly	**2:** Moderate	**B:** Teaching Needs (education)
3: One-Two Times per week	**3:** Great	**C:** Physical Care
4: Three-Five Times per Week	**4:** Very Great	**D:** Psychosocial Needs
		E: Coordination
		F: Number & Severity of Problems

Source: Courtesy of Storfjell, Allen, and Easley.

Exhibit 20–4 Time Allocation Worksheet

Name _____ Position _____ Date _____

Time Available (Monthly, Yearly)	_____	

Time Utilization

1. Personal Adjustments:	Hours	Totals
a. Annual Leave/Holiday	_____	
b. Other_____	_____	
_____	_____	_____

2. Supportive Activities:		
a. Supervisor/Nurse Conference	_____	
b. Staff Meetings	_____	
c. Continuing Education/Workshop	_____	
d. Committees	_____	
e. Other_____	_____	
_____	_____	_____

3. Special Assignments:		
a. Classes	_____	
b. Hospital Liaison	_____	
c. Field Advisor	_____	
d. Other_____	_____	
_____	_____	_____

4. Field Activities (Community Service):		
a. Committees/Meetings _____	_____	
_____	_____	
b. Clinics	_____	
c. Other_____	_____	
_____	_____	_____

Total Scheduled Time	
Time Available for Home Visits, Consultation, Documentation, and Follow-Up	

Source: Courtesy of Storfjell, Allen, and Easley.

tool to provide a realistic representation of their specific workload components.

When the time needed for nonclient-related activities is subtracted from the total paid time, the time that remains for client-related activities (caseload duties) can be determined. This includes the time actually spent in the home with clients and time for travel to and from home visits, documentation of care provided, and coordination of care activities.

The information generated from the analysis of individual nurses' workloads can be grouped by team or department. Aggregate workload data are valuable in assessing workload requirements and allocating time for part or all of the nursing staff. By analysis of staff time, it is possible to document staffing needs and to adjust nonclient-related work assignments.

Step 4

Finally, the caseload and workload time requirements are summarized on the top portion of the caseload/workload summary (Exhibit 20–5). The number of home visits that each nurse can make is calculated by dividing the total time available by the average time needed for a home visit. The average time per visit can be determined by doing an actual time study or using organizational productivity standards. If either of these is not available, several studies have shown that an average home visit, including visit support time, often averages about 90 minutes (Storfjell, 1989a). The number of home visits required by the caseload can then be compared with the number of visits possible based on the workload requirements. By subtracting the average number of home visits required by the caseload from the number of visits possible based on available time, a determination can be made easily regarding the reasonableness of caseload requirements.

IMPLICATIONS

Analysis of nursing workloads and caseloads using the CL/WLA approach has implications for home health administrators, managers, and nursing staff as well as the home health industry as a whole.

Administrative Uses

It is important for home health managers to be able to project staffing needs and costs as well as to evaluate utilization of nursing staff. By compilation of data on comprehensive nursing resource demands, staffing needs can be compared with the use of time and the types of services being delivered (Allen et al., 1986).

Through repeated analyses, trends in service delivery can be ascertained. Data provided by workload trends for the entire organization may be used to determine or justify budgetary allocations for nursing staff. In addition, comparisons can be made between service trends and established goals and priorities.

CL/WLA differs from other productivity methodologies because it takes into account the complexity of nursing care required as well as time requirements. The impact of the case complexity as a cost driver can be studied, and case rates can be estimated by type of care adjusted for complexity. This approach to productivity measurement and management meshes well with activity-based costing and management approaches. The CL/WLA tools can be modified to reflect the agency's standard activities and processes. Periodic reviews and updates can be entered into the activity-based costing and management models, and a more precise calculation of costs of products and activities can be tracked.

Clinical Manager Uses

CL/WLA allows clinical managers to base hiring decisions on projections of the nursing care demands of the overall agency's caseload and workload. The complexity profile of a caseload may indicate a need for a particular type of nursing staff, which will obviate underutilization of nursing skills. In this way, nursing costs can be managed effectively based on actual data that

Exhibit 20–5 Caseload/Workload Summary

Name ———————————————— Position ——————— Date ———————

	Total	Average
A. Caseload		
1. Total cases	———————	———————
2. Time factor	———————	———————
3. Complexity factor	———————	———————
4. Total required H.V.'s	———————	———————
5. Average weeks open	———————	———————
6. Program categorical analysis (*priority/program/diagnosis*)		
———————	———————	———————
———————	———————	———————
———————	———————	———————
———————	———————	———————

	Monthly	Yearly
B. Time (monthly, yearly)		
1. Total time available	———————	———————
2. Scheduled time	———————	———————
3. Time available for H.V.'s	———————	———————
4. Time per home visit	———————	———————
5. Number of H.V.'s possible (*divide 3 by 4*)	———————	———————
6. Number of H.V.'s required by caseload	———————	———————
7. Number of H.V.'s to new referrals	———————	———————
8. TOTAL required H.V.'s	———————	———————
9. Excess H.V.'s required (*8 larger than 5*)	———————	———————
10. Additional H.V.'s possible (*5 larger than 6*)	———————	———————
11. Average mileage (*optional*)	———————	———————

Source: Courtesy of Storfjell, Allen, and Easley.

justify the budgetary requirements of nursing staff mix.

Because time utilization is individualized by assessment of all the workload activities for each nurse, many of the pitfalls encountered by assigning average productivity standards to specific individuals are avoided. If an individualized productivity monitoring tool is desired, the number of visits required by the caseload and the number of visits possible according to the workload analysis can be calculated easily on a monthly basis and compared with actual performance.

In addition to general staffing uses, the tools are especially beneficial for supervising individual nurses, especially for evaluating and adjusting individual case assignments. A concentration of high-complexity (social or medical) cases may signal a nurse's need for additional training or support, whereas a caseload complexity rating lower than the nurse's skill level may be the key to restlessness or low morale. Staff development needs can be identified from both individual and aggregate data. For example, if a particular nurse has a high percentage of clients with a certain diagnosis, continuing education in that area might be important.

The average length of time for which cases are open should alert the clinical manager to those nurses who either carry cases too long or close them too quickly. In addition, because initial visits are usually longer than repeat visits (Storfjell, 1989b), nurses with few visits per case may need to have lower productivity standards than nurses with more visits per case. The manager can monitor individual or aggregate productivity data by making a few adjustments to the forms to record and monitor the caseload at regular intervals. This allows the establishment of individual productivity standards based on the specific workload requirements of each nurse.

CL/WLA is also useful when cases are transferred to another nurse or in the orientation of new staff or managers. As home care organizations increase their use of part-time staff and team nursing to improve scheduling flexibility, it is even more important to have a readily available method of allocating cases among a varying group of nursing staff at any given time. The time and complexity ratings provide this capability. The most beneficial use of the CL/WLA process, however, continues to be for providing a framework for clinical managers and direct care providers to communicate and plan client care, including identifying the type of intervention needed, its complexity, and the time required.

Staff Uses

This systematic analysis allows nurses to organize their activities, streamline caseloads, and obtain a realistic picture of workload demands and expectations, all of which lead to greater efficiency, more appropriate time utilization, and increased cost effectiveness. Individual staff members can benefit when a realistic caseload and workload have been defined and goals for service delineated.

Industry Uses

Standards for nursing care based on professional ideals and goals must be established in home care. The model of care that will be recognized in home care nursing will be critically influenced by the patient classification system and the overall dimensions of the workload that are deemed appropriate by those private and public organizations that fund home care services. In addition to facilitating supervision, assisting staff with time management, and providing pertinent data for administrators, the Easley-Storfjell CL/WLA instruments can provide the home care industry with the data necessary to support resource utilization while demonstrating efficiency in management of personnel and finances. The patient classification system standardizes client complexity variables and also provides standard nursing interventions that can be used for quantification of nursing care in research endeavors.

CONCLUSION

Home health care nursing managers are increasingly being required to manage and document the type and quantity of services provided by the agencies that employ them and to reduce costs while increasing or maintaining service quality. The Easley-Storfjell CL/WLA instruments provide a more refined method of analyzing the home health nurse's caseload and workload, thus providing valuable management information for use by administrative, supervisory, and direct service personnel. The reliability and validity of the tools have been demonstrated, but, even more important, experience has shown them to be practical and extremely useful in various types of community health agencies.

REFERENCES

Albrecht, M. N. 1991. Home health care: Reliability and validity testing of a patient classification instrument. *Public Health Nursing* 5: 124–131.

Allen, C. E., et al. 1986. Cost management through caseload-workload analysis. In *Patients and purse strings: patient classification and cost management,* F. Shaffer (ed.). New York: National League for Nursing, 331–446.

Storfjell, J. L. 1989a. Home care productivity: Is the home visit an adequate measure? *Caring* 8: 60–65.

Storfjell, J. L. 1989b. How valuable are nurses' skills? A case for fair pricing in home health care. *Nursing and Health Care* 10: 310–313.

CHAPTER 21

Home Health Care Classification (HHCC) System: An Overview

Virginia K. Saba

ABSTRACT

This paper provides an overview of the Home Health Care Classification (HHCC) System focusing on its two interrelated taxonomies: HHCC of Nursing Diagnoses and HHCC of Nursing Interventions, both of which are classified by 20 Care Components. It highlights the major events that influenced its development, current status, and future uses. The two HHCC taxonomies and their 20 Care Components are used as a standardized framework to code, index, and classify home health clinical nursing practice. Further, they are used to document, electronically track, evaluate outcomes, and analyze home health care over time, across settings, population groups, and geographic locations.

BACKGROUND

Introduction

This section provides the background on the Home Health Care Classification (HHCC) System. It highlights why and how the HHCC System including its two taxonomies were developed. It also describes changes with the introduction of the Medicare Legislation in 1966 in the home health industry, clinical nursing practice, information technology, classification systems, and federal reporting requirements.

HHCC System Development

The Home Health Care Classification (HHCC) System was developed by Saba and colleagues from research conducted at the Georgetown University School of Nursing (Saba, 1991) called the Home Care Project research (1988–1991). It was funded through a cooperative agreement (#17C - 98983/3) by the Health Care Financing Agency (HCFA), now named the Center for Medicare and Medicaid Services (CMS). The purpose of the research was to meet a needed problem in home health which was to develop a means for predicting resource needs and measuring outcomes. The specific goal of the research was to develop a method to assess and classify home health Medicare patients in order to predict their need for nursing and other home care services (resource requirements) as well as to evaluate (measure) their outcomes of care. To accomplish this goal data on actual resource use, which could objectively be measured, were collected and used to predict resource requirements.

The research team consisted of home health nursing experts, a statistician, a systems analyst, and a national advisory committee. They believed that by collecting a large volume of data (national sample) on Medicare patients and resources used for their home health care, a system could be designed to predict care requirements.

They conducted a pilot study, designed a framework, established a methodology, and developed an abstract form consisting of 73 pre-coded variables. They then applied the methodology to a national sample of home health agencies (HHAs) that provided all services and products used to restore, maintain, and promote physical, mental, and emotional health to patients in their homes (Spradley & Dorsey, 1985).

Retrospective research data were collected from 8,967 patient records from a sample of 646 HHAs randomly stratified by staff size, type of ownership, and geographic location. The HHAs represented every state in the nation including Puerto Rico and the District of Columbia. Approximately 5 to 50 recently discharged Medicare patient records for an entire episode of care were abstracted from each of the sample HHAs providing data on the 8,967 patients (Saba, 1991).

The data consisted of all relevant variables considered to be possible predictors of home health care resource requirements. They were collected and analyzed to determine the statistical significance of alternative classification methods. Data were collected consisting of two sets of narrative textual statements focusing on (a) patient problems and/or nursing diagnoses and (b) nursing services, treatments, actions, and/or interventions. Approximately 40,000 narrative statements about patient problems and 72,000 narrative statements representing nursing services provided during their episodes of care were collected from the sample patients.

To code the narrative statements, classification schemes had to be developed, as none of the existing ones were found to be appropriate. Thousands of the statements were keyboarded, using permuted keyword sorts, processed, analyzed, and tested. As a result, two separate vocabularies—nursing diagnoses and nursing interventions—were developed and used to code the narrative statements. The statements, once coded, were analyzed and used to empirically develop the two HHCC System taxonomies classified by the 20 Care Components.

The classified taxonomies (list of terms arranged in a hierarchal format) made it possible to predict home health care services and resource requirements as well as to measure outcomes. One major finding from the research demonstrated that the combined nursing diagnoses and interventions data classified by 20 Care Components were the best predictors of resources used (Saba, 1991; Saba & McCormick, 2001).

Home Health Industry

The Home Care Project addressed several important changes in the home health industry. With the enactment of Medicare and Medicaid Legislation in 1966, the care of the elderly sick at home changed drastically. Home health care was viewed as a cost effective alternative to institutional care and patients were being discharged "sicker and quicker" from in-hospital stays, increasing the demand for acute, complex, home health services. As a result, home health services expanded and the number of HHAs increased from 1,275 in 1966 to over 10,000 in 1997 (National Association of Home Care, 1997). However, there was a lack of uniform data on home health care resources, services, and reimbursement practices. Further, the ambiguities in terminology and policies as well as the lack of standardized definitions among fiscal intermediaries affected the scope of services provided by the HHAs. The Home Care Project was undertaken to address the issue of predicting home health resource requirements and measuring outcomes.

Clinical Nursing Practice Requirements

With the introduction of Medicare Legislation, changes occurred in the documentation of clinical nursing practice requiring the use of nursing classifications for the computer-based patient record (CPR) and/or electronic medical record (EMR) systems. The American Nurses Association (ANA), for years, promoted the need for classification systems to support clinical nursing practice and data to measure the care process. As early as 1980, the ANA introduced the Nursing: Social Policy Statement (1995) which recommended that the nursing process serve as the standards of care for documenting clinical nursing practice (ANA, 1998). In 1990 the ANA passed a resolution adopting the Nursing Minimum Data Set (NMDS) as the core data set that should be used to manage nursing information in CPRs and included in any national database. In 1991, the ANA further approved the North American Nursing Diagnoses Association (NANDA) Taxonomy I Revised (NANDA, 1991) for classifying nursing problems.

In 1989, the ANA formed the Steering Committee on Databases to Support Clinical Nursing Practice renamed in 1998 Committee for Nursing Practice Information Infrastructure (CNPII). The committee was involved in several activities one of which was recognizing classification systems to support nursing practice. In 1991 the Database Steering Committee recognized the first four classification systems under the umbrella of the NMDS and approved them as nursing data standards. The systems were: NANDA Taxonomy I, The Omaha System, Nursing Intervention Classification (NIC), and Home Health Care Classification (HHCC). Since then eight classification systems have been recognized (Coenen, McNeil, Bakken, Bickford, & Warren, 2001). They include: Nursing Outcomes Classification (NOC), Patient Care Data Set (PCDS), Perioperative Nursing Data Set, Nursing Minimum Data Set, Nursing Management Minimum Data Set, International Classification of Nursing Practice (ICNP), Complete Complementary Alternative Medicine Billing and Coding Reference, and the Systematized Nomenclature of Medicine Reference Terminology (SNOMED RT). SNOMED RT is a terminology developed by the College of American Pathologists for all healthcare professionals and recently nursing. The ANA continues to promote the use of nursing information, classifica-

tions, and taxonomies in CPR and EMR systems focusing on clinical nursing practice to prove that "what nurses do makes a difference" (McCormick et al.,1994).

Information Technology

Since the 1950s and 1960s, computer hardware, software, and communication networks changed radically. Computer hardware advanced in size, speed, storage capacity, and processing capability. The multi-user mainframe computer systems of the 1960s advanced to the single desktop (microcomputer) personal computer (PC) of the 1980s, laptop PCs of the 1990s, and hand held PCs of the 21st century. The computer software advanced from programming languages to the windows platform with user-friendly icons, navigation mouse, and generic programs. The computer communication networks advanced from local area networks (LANs), to wide area networks (WANs), to the World Wide Web, and the Internet. The Internet offers unlimited access to resources and offers free electronic mail (e-mail).

Information technology impacted on the health care delivery system, the management of clinical nursing practice, and influenced the need for classification systems for the CPR and EMR systems. Data, data standards, classifications, and taxonomies emerged as essential for the processing of raw data into information and knowledge.

Nursing Classifications

Nursing classifications emerged as critical to the advancement of the profession and were created to name nursing phenomena. They emerged as data sets, taxonomies, or classification systems that could be used to document clinical nursing practice in CPR systems. They were viewed as the foundation for a unified nursing language system (UNLS) and proposed as the basis for the CPR. Nursing data had to be identified to measure patient care. Data had to be processed into nursing information and ultimately into nursing knowledge to advance the science of nursing.

Computer-Based Patient Record Systems

In the early 1990s, the Institute of Medicine (IOM) identified the computer-based patient record (CPR) and CPR system (CPRS). The IOM recommended that standardized classifications and code sets, using a uniform structure be developed for the health care industry (Computer-based Patient Record Institute,1994; Dick & Steen, 1991). The CPRSs were developed to collect, store, process, display, retrieve, and communicate timely data and information in and across health care facilities. To utilize CPRSs, nursing data need to be collected as discrete facts (atomic-level data), stored in a relational database, processed, and transformed into meaningful information. Such systems are needed to ensure the visibility and viability of nursing practice as well as for its advancement.

Home Health CPRS.

The home health CPRS emerged to process federal requirements for participation in their programs. They emerged as information systems critical to the delivery of home health nursing practice, management of care services, and determination of care resources. They were used for the management of the continuum of care from hospital to the home and community. They required classification systems/taxonomies to ensure the comparability of where, why, and when data are collected, processed and aggregated across systems, settings, and geographic populations.

CMS Requirements

The Outcome and Assessment Information Set (OASIS) data set was implemented in 1998 by the newly named CMS as the condition of participation for home health agency Medicare services (Shaughnessy, Crisler, & Schienker, 1997). The OASIS reporting requirement was implemented as a stand-alone instrument that

consisted of 79 core sets of data items for the assessment of patient condition and measurements of patient outcomes. The OASIS was and continues to be aimed at measuring changes in health status from admission until discharge or between two or more points. In the year 2000, the Prospective Payment System (PPS) was added as another requirement of participation. The home health (HHPPS) is a method that extracts from the OASIS a core set of 20 data items that serve as a grouper and payment source for services for an episode of home health care. These two new instruments increased the documentation and reporting requirements for home health services.

CMS reporting rules.

As a result of all the Federal regulations by CMS, the current reporting and reimbursement requirements for Medicare and Medicaid beneficiaries were expanded.. Every Medicare patient admitted to a certified HHA for home health services generally must have the old and new federal forms completed for participation in the program. The forms include (a) HCFA 485: Home Health Certification and Plan of Treatment Form, (b) Outcome and Assessment Information Set (OASIS) Instrument, (c) OASIS Prospective Payment System (HHPPS) Instrument, (d) visit and billing record forms, and (e) a Plan of Care for documenting home visits.

Generally, federal forms are processed in separate CPRSs, whereas, the Plan of Care continues to be documented manually and in a narrative format. The manual method of documenting each visit makes it difficult to predict requirements, measure resources and evaluate outcomes. However, by using the standardized HHCC System taxonomies classified by the 20 Care Components in a CPRS, clinical nursing practice can be documented, coded, tracked and analyzed electronically.

HHCC SYSTEM'S TWO TAXONOMIES

This section describes the HHCC System focusing on its two taxonomies and classification framework. It provides a description of the two taxonomies and care component classes, highlights their definitions, coding structure, current status, educational uses, and research and evaluation studies

Overview

The HHCC System is specifically designed for the documentation of patient care using a CPRS. It consists of two standardized interrelated taxonomies: HHCC of Nursing Diagnoses and the HHCC of Nursing Interventions. These two taxonomies are classified by 20 Care Components that serve as the standardized framework for documenting home health clinical nursing practice. They are used not only to code, index, and classify home health care; but, also, to document, track, and analyze the care over time, across settings, population groups, and geographic locations (Saba, 1994a). (See web site <www.sabacare.com> Tables 1-8).

HHCC of Nursing Diagnoses

The HHCC of Nursing Diagnoses consists of 145 (50 two-digit major categories and 95 three digit subcategories) that depict nursing diagnoses and/or patient problems. The terms in this taxonomy include over 50 unique home health nursing diagnostic terms as well as several of the 104 NANDA terms derived from the Taxonomy I Revised (1991). Further, the NANDA terms were transcribed from verb phrases to noun clauses to conform to the structure of the HHCC terms.

A Nursing Diagnosis is defined as:

> A clinical judgement about an individual, family, or community response to actual and potential health problems/life processes. Nursing Diagnoses provide the basis for the selection of nursing interventions to achieve outcomes which the nurse is accountable (NANDA, p. 5, 1992).

This taxonomy is expanded by using three qualifiers (improve, stabilize, deteriorate).

These qualifiers expand by modifying each diagnostic term to code the expected outcomes and the same qualifiers (improved, stabilized, deteriorated) are used to code actual outcomes.

HHCC of Nursing Interventions

The HHCC of Nursing Interventions consists of 160 (60 two digit major categories and 100 three digit subcategories) that depicts nursing interventions, procedures, treatments, activities, and/or services.

A single nursing action is designed to achieve an outcome for a diagnosis (medical / nursing) for which the nurse is accountable. This taxonomy is expanded by four qualifiers (assess/monitor, care/perform, teach/supervise, manage/refer) that represent a specific type intervention action. These qualifiers enhance and expand by modifying each intervention to code the specific action making a total of 640 terms that comprise the HHCC of Nursing Interventions.

HHCC 20 Care Components

The 20 Care Components classifies the two interrelated HHCC taxonomies and serves as the standardized framework. They are used to computer process and statistically analyze clinical care. The 20 Care Components have been found to be the most clinically relevant assessment classes, best predictors of home health care resource requirements, and the most appropriate framework for classifying home health nursing diagnoses and interventions (Holzemer et al., 1997).

The HHCC 20 Care Components represents a cluster of elements that depict the four health care patterns; health behavioral, functional, physiological, and psychological representing a holistic approach to patient care (Saba, 1994b, 1995; Saba & Sparks, 1998) (see Table 1).

Coding Structure

The two HHCC taxonomies are coded using a five character alphanumeric code based on the

International Classification of Diseases and Health Related Health Problems (ICD-10-CM) and the ICD-10-CM Health Care for Inpatient Procedures called ICD-10-CM-PCS. The 20 Care Components are similar to the chapters used in ICD-10-CM (WHO, 1992). Each vocabulary term consists of a five-character alphanumeric code as follows:

- 1st position: One alphabetic character for the care component
- 2nd & 3rd positions: Two digit code for a core data element (major category representing either a nursing diagnosis or a nursing intervention) followed by a decimal point
- 4th position: One digit code for a subcategory, if used, (representing either a nursing diagnosis or a nursing intervention, if used)
- 5th & last position: One digit code for the qualifier.

An example of a Nursing Diagnosis Coding Structure for an assessed patient problem "Unable to Walk" is classified as "Activity" Component problem, diagnosed as "Physical Mobility Impairment" with the expected outcome/goal 'To Improve Physical Activity Impairment," and coded as A.01.51:

A = Activity (Component)

A.*01.5* = Physical Mobility Impairment (Diagnostic SubCategory)

A.01.51 = To Improve Physical Mobility Impairment

(Expected Outcome/Goal)

An example of a Nursing Intervention Coding Structure for the same assessed patient problem "Unable to Walk" is classified as "Activity" Component activity, the plan of care intervention "Ambulation Therapy," and the intervention qualifier action "Teach" to expand the intervention to "Teach Ambulation Therapy" is coded as A.03.03:

A   = Activity (Component)

A.*03.0* = Ambulation Therapy (Major Diagnostic Category)

A.03.0*3* = Teach Ambulation Therapy (Type Action)

This coding structure facilitates computer processing, provides linkages, and word mappings between the two taxonomies and other health care classifications. It facilitates the design of a clinical pathway, decision support, and evidence-based systems and is essential for the development of decision support and expert systems.

Why Use HHCC Taxonomies

There are several major reasons why the HHCC of Nursing Diagnoses and HHCC of Nursing Interventions taxonomies will continue to be included in home health CPRSs (Saba, 1997). They are used to facilitate the electronic documentation of patient care at the point-of-care, instead of the traditional paper-based method. They are classified by the 20 Care Components that serve as a standardized framework. The Care Components represent four different patterns (Functional, Health Behavior, Physiological, and Psychological) of care and focus on a holistic approach to patient care. They consist of discrete atomic-level data (terms) that use qualifiers to enhance and expand other dimensions of terms (data elements). Data, once collected, are used many times and for many purposes making for more efficient aggregation, summarization, and analysis. The taxonomies use a coding structure of five alphanumeric digits similar to ICD-10 to link and cross- map the terms of the two taxonomies to each other and to other classifications. The codes make it possible to assess, document, and track the care process data during and between visits. They are flexible, adaptable, and expandable. Further, the two classified taxonomies are in the public domain and available to anyone for manual and/or electronic use without any cost but with permission. Web Site <http://www.sabacare.com>.

Table 21–1 HHCC 20 Care Components by Four Clinical Care Patterns

I. Health Behavioral Components			*11.*	Metabolic

I. Health Behavioral Components

1. Medication
2. Safety
3. Health Behavior

II. Functional Components

4. Activity
5. Fluid Volume
6. Nutritional
7. Self-Care
8. Sensory

III. Physiological Components

9. Cardiac
10. Respiratory

11. Metabolic
12. Physical Regulation
13. Skin Integrity
14. Tissue Perfusion
15. Bowel Elimination
16. Urinary Elimination

IV. Psychological Components

17. Cognitive
18. Coping
19. Role Relationship
20. Self Concept

Current Status

The two HHCC taxonomies: HHCC of Nursing Diagnoses and the HHCC of Nursing Interventions were recognized by the ANA in 1991 as appropriate for documenting nursing practice in CPRSs. Since then, they have been registered as a Health Level 7 (HL7) language; integrated into Logical Observations, Identifiers, Names, and Codes (LOINC), the Systematized Nomenclature of Human and Veterinary Medicine Reference Terminology (SNOMED RT), and the Metathesaurus of the Unified Medical Language System (UMLS) of the National Library of Medicine (NLM); indexed in Cumulative Index of Allied and Health Literature (CINAHL); and used as the basis for the International Classification of Nursing Practice (ICNP) developed by the International Council of Nursing (ICN).

The two HHCC taxonomies have been approved by American National Standards Institute Healthcare Informatics Standards Board (ANSI HISB) and listed in its Inventory of Health Care Information (ANSI-HISB,1997) as an approved code set for consideration for the federal legislation entitled Health Insurance Portability and Accountability Act of 1996 (Public Law 104-191). They comply with format standards of (a) Health Level 7 electronic transmission standards, (b) ICD-10 coding structure standard, and (c) The ANA Nursing Information and Data Set Evaluation Center (NIDSEC) standards. Further, they have been translated into Dutch, Chinese, Finnish, German, Korean, Portuguese, Spanish, and they are currently being translated into other languages. The HHCC 20 Care Components have been adapted as the framework for the Patient Care Data Set (PCDS) (Ozbolt, Fruchtnicht, & Hayden, 1994).

Current Uses

The two classified HHCC taxonomies have been accepted by home health nursing. They are being used to document home health care manually and/or electronically for CPRSs. They serve as a language for nursing and other health care providers (physical, occupational and speech therapy, medical social worker, and home health aide). They are used to document integrated care processes, classify and track clinical care, develop evidence based practice models, analyze patient profiles and populations, and predict care needs and resources. They are used for research, educational purposes, and electronic pathways. Several HHAs and/or commercial vendors use the two interrelated HHCC taxonomies with the 20 Care Components to cross- map medical conditions, disease categories, and/or clinical procedure terminologies required by the federal government. Other vendors use selected care components and/or nursing intervention terms to document and determine the cost of specific nursing services.

Educational Uses

During the past ten years the HHCC taxonomies and 20 Care Components have been introduced in several schools of nursing to document clinical nursing practice by students using computer-based software. At the Georgetown University School of Nursing, Sparks, Saba, and faculty tested using the 20 Care Components to structure learning modules and the two HHCC taxonomies to document patient care following the nursing process. The 20 Care Components were used to implement a holistic approach to patient care and to classify the learning modules (Saba & Sparks, 1998). In other universities the HHCC taxonomies are being used to teach basic nursing, community, and home health nursing. In others they are being used to document clinical care using pathways for specific disease conditions by computer at the point-of-care.

Research and Evaluation Studies

Several nursing researchers have conducted studies on the two interrelated HHCC Terminologies categorized by 20 Care Components and/or evaluated their structure and usability. They are described as follows.

Ozbolt, Fruchtnicht, and Hayden (1994) determined that the HHCC System's 20 Care Components were useful as an organizing framework for nursing problems and interventions in the hospital setting. They adapted only the 20 Care Components and expanded them to 22 by splitting Metabolic / Immunological into two and adding Pre / Intra / Post procedure for the Patient Care Data Set (PCDS).

Holzemer and colleagues (1997) conducted a study of 600 patient encounters for 201 patients with AIDs who were hospitalized with pneumonia. They determined that all terms could be categorized using the 20 Care Components and the major categories of Nursing Diagnoses and Nursing Interventions of the HHCC System. They further demonstrated that all Nursing Intervention terms could be coded according to the Type of Nursing Intervention Action qualifiers and concluded that the Action qualifiers had a potential useful attribute for the comparison of patient care among care settings.

Henry and Mead (1997) in a theoretical paper analyzed the HHCC of Nursing Interventions, the Intervention Scheme of the Omaha System, and NIC addressing the activities nurses perform when caring for patients. They conceptualized that one of the three principles of a coding system is the capture of granular information and found that the HHCC was inherently more "granular" (terms more refined), and at atomic level than the Nursing Intervention Classification (NIS).

Henry, Warren, Lange, and Button (1998) compared the evaluation literature related to the six major nursing classifications approved by the ANA, the HHCC, NANDA, NIC, NOC, Omaha System, and ICNP. Their goal was to determine the extent to which they possess the characteristics needed to implement a computer-based system including such criteria as (a) atomic and compositional characters, (b) attributes, (c) hierarchies and inheritance, (d) unique identifiers, (e) definitions. They concluded that none met all criteria but HHCC, Omaha System, and ICNP did meet five of the criteria.

Parlocha and Henry (1998) conducted a research study which tested the usefulness of the

HHCC taxonomies for coding patient problems and nursing interventions of psychiatric patients with major depression disorders in the home health care setting. They found that the HHCC taxonomies could be used to code and classify the majority of problems and interventions and identified several new potential terms for the psychiatric population.

Zielstorff, Tronni, Basque, Griffin, and Welebob (1998) conducted a study cross-mapping patient problems or diagnosis terms from three nomenclatures, the HHCC, Omaha System, and NANDA, term to term, to determine commonalities and differences. They concluded, that at that time, the differences in structure and incompatibilities in the three classifications made cross-mapping impossible. The team found that the Unified Medical Language System (UMLS) lacked concept matches for the majority of terms in the three classifications.

Bakken, Cashen, Mendonca, O'Brien, and Zieniewicz, (2000) studied nursing activities in relations to concept-oriented terminologies and identified three concepts as necessary for each activity; namely, delivery mode, activity focus, and recipient. They conducted research on 1,038 terms found in patient records and found that 73.9 terms could be cross-mapped to ICNP of which 91.3 percent were found in the HHCC and only 63.5 percent in the Omaha System.

Another study conducted by Bakken and colleagues (2000) was to test the adequacy of the semantic structure of Clinical LOINC (Logical Observation Identifiers, Names and Codes) as a terminology model for standardized assessment measures. They dissected 1,096 items from 35 standardized assessment instruments. into the elements of LOINC. The HHCC classified by 20 Care Components was included and considered to be a standardized nursing-sensitive assessment instrument and its three outcome qualifiers as possible measures to evaluate outcomes of health care. They further suggested that care components could be useful for the classification of standardized assessments.

Recent research by Hardiker (2001) from the United Kingdom compared the nursing inter-vention components of the HHCC, NIC and the Omaha System to develop a mechanism for mediating between diverse nursing intervention terminology systems. Of the three terminology systems included in the study, the HHCC of Nursing Interventions had the largest number of terms (640 potential terms through post coordination) and the richest taxonomic structure between nursing interventions (through the classification of minor categories as major categories). The research revealed that although there were some similarities between nursing interventions drawn from different terminology systems, differences for example in content and structure makes direct comparison difficult. The research used a formal terminology system to expose underlying concepts thereby making it possible to map automatically between nursing interventions drawn from the three terminology systems.

The ANA newly named Committee for Nursing Practice Information Infrastructure (CNPII) recently revised the criteria for recognition of nursing language systems (Coenen et al., 2001). The committee expanded the criteria to distinguish between the various existing classifications as data sets, classification systems, and/or nomenclatures. They discussed the need for different health care data standards and the role of the ANA in this effort. The CNPII considered the two HHCC classifications to be taxonomies since they conform to the International Standards Organization (ISO) (1990) definition of a Taxonomy: "Classification according to presumed natural relationships among types and their subtypes (p. 242)." They also determined that they satisfy the ISO definition for a Classification scheme: "An assignment of objects into groups based upon characteristics that have common objects, e.g. origin, composition, structure, function (p.243)".

NEXT STEPS

This section addresses the plans for the next revisions of the two taxonomies. It also describes the innovative uses of the HHCC System Taxonomies in clinical care pathways.

New Release

The two HHCC System taxonomies including the Care Components are currently being revised by the HHCC Terminology Committee. The taxonomies will be expanded to include new terms as reported by vendors, educators, and researchers. It is envisioned that the taxonomies will continue to be enlarged to encompass the scope of services provided by Primary Care Providers (PCPs), clinicians, physicians assistants, and nurse practitioners (NPs), and other advanced practice nurses (APNs). Since the PCPs function in all health care settings, home health, community, and ambulatory care, the new services that they provide are being used to expand the taxonomies. Currently, the non-physician PCPs use only the coded classifications used by physicians for reimbursement and generally omit and exclude patient and/or nursing care since nursing services are not reimbursed by CMS.

Clinical Pathways

The HHCC System taxonomies are being used to develop HHCC Clinical Pathways for the electronic documentation of clinical nursing practice for CPRSs. The HHCC Pathways utilize the 20 Care Components as its framework and the two standardized HHCC System taxonomies to (a) assess and diagnose care needs on admission, (b) document and track care during and between visits/encounters, and (c) evaluate and measure care outcomes on discharge for an episode of illness.

Pathway definition

An electronic pathway is a method such as a summarized worksheet that can be computerized. The electronic pathway format makes it possible to track interventions and actions as well as to facilitate for flexibility and individualized care, while monitoring actions to see if expected outcomes are being met. An electronic pathway can assist in the case management of patient care by providing comprehensive, coordinated, and cost-effective care (Zander, 1988; Spath, 1993).

Clinical pathway uses.

The Clinical HHCC Pathways are used on admission to link the OASIS Instrument, the PPS Instrument, and the HCFA Forms to the patient assessment. The HHCC Pathways are used to identify clinical actions and events for the entire episode and specifically for each visit to determine the patient, family, and resources needed for the care process. The pathway events and actions are planned based on the admission assessment of the patient by component and then tracked during the individual home visits.

The HHCC Pathways are used to measure quality, provide evidence for the evidence-based practice, decision making, bench marking, and standards of cost effective care. Further, they are used to summarize the episode to provide clinical, financial, and research information as well as manage the care provided, determine resources required, and measure the outcome of home health care.

SUMMARY

The HHCC System, consisting of the HHCC of Nursing Diagnoses and the HHCC of Nursing Interventions classified by 20 Care Components, facilitates the documentation of patient care by computer at the point-of-care, and replace the traditional paper-based method. The HHCC System is being used for documenting nursing practice in computer-based systems as well as in nursing education. The HHCC System's two taxonomies make it possible not only to assess and document, but also code, index, classify, link, and map the care process according to the 20 Care Components. These two innovative taxonomies provide coding term structure and the 20 Care Components the classification framework for the CPRSs. They are used to track the clinical nursing care across time, different settings, populations groups, and geographic locations. The collected data can be used many times which allow for improved documentation and analysis.

The two HHCC System taxonomies can be integrated into any home health system and linked electronically to any CPRS designed to collect the data required for federal home health care reporting and reimbursement. The system is being used (a) to improve the efficiency of assessing and documenting home health nursing care, (b) to provide the strategy for evaluating quality and measuring outcomes of care, (c) and

to develop a costing method for reimbursement and payment. They are used to develop electronic clinical pathways, measure practice, and determine care costs. The two HHCC System taxonomies are available on the Internet, offering the world-wide nursing community the means to manage and monitor clinical nursing practice.

Web Site

Download the web site <*http://www.sabacare .com*> to review the two HHCC taxonomies and the 20 Care Components lists, codes, and definitions in Table 1-8.

REFERENCES

American National Standards Institute Healthcare Informatics Standards Board (ANSI-HISB). 1997. *Inventory of health care information standards: Pertaining to the Health Insurance Portability and Accountability Act (HIPAA) of 1996 (P.L. 104–191)*. Washington, DC: ANSI-HISB.(39).

American Nurses Association. 1995. *Nursing: social policy statement*. Kansas City, MO: ANA.

American Nurses Association. 1998. *Standards of clinical nursing practice*. Washington, DC: ANA.

Bakken, S., Cashen, M. S., Mendonca, E. A., O'Brien, A., & Zieniewicz, J. 2000. Representing nursing activities within a concept-oriented terminological system: Evaluation of a type definition. *Journal of the American Medical Informatics Association*, 7(1): 81–90.

Bakken, S., Cimino, J. J., Haskell, R., Kukafka, R., Matsumoto, C., Chan, G. K., & Huff, S. M. 2000. Evaluation of Clinical LOINC (Logical Observation Identifiers, Names, and Codes). *Journal of the American Medical Informatics Association,* 7(6): 529–538.

Coenen, A., McNeil, B., Bakken, S., Bickford, C., & Warren, J. J. 2001. Toward comparable nursing data: American Nursing Association criteria for data sets, classification systems, and nomenclatures. *Computers in Nursing,* 19(6): 240–246.

Computer-Based Patient Record Institute. 1994. *Proposal to accelerate standards development for computer-based patient record systems*. Chicago, IL: CPRI.

Dick, R. S., & Steen, E. B. (eds.). 1991. *The computer-based patient record: An essential technology for health care*. Washington, DC: Institute of Medicine-National Academy Press.

Hardiker N. 2001. Mediating between Nursing Intervention Terminology Systems. In: S. Bakken, (ed). *A medical informatics odyssey: Visions of the future and lessons from the past* (pp., 239–243). Philadelphia: Hanley & Belfus, Inc.

Henry, S. H., & Mead, C. N. 1997. Nursing classifications systems; Necessary but not sufficient for representing "What Nurses Do" for inclusion in computer-based patient record systems. *Journal of the American Medical Informatics Association* (JAMIA), 4(3): 222–232.

Henry, S. H., Warren, J. J., Lange, L., & Button, P. 1998. A review of major nursing vocabularies and the extent to which they have the characteristics required for implementation in computer-based systems. *Journal of the American Medical Informatics Association* (JAMIA), 5(4): 321–328.

Holzemer, W. L., Henry, S. B., Dawson, C., Sousa, K., Bain, C., & Hsieh, S-F. 1997. An evaluation of the utility of the Home Health Care Classification for categorizing patient problems and nursing interventions from the hospital setting. In. U.Gerdin, M. Tallberg, P. Wainwright (Eds.). *NI'99: Nursing Informatics: The impact of nursing knowledge on health care informatics* (pp. 21–26). Stockholm, Sweden: IOS Press.

International Standards Organization. 1990. *International Standard ISO 1087:Terminology, vocabulary*. Deneva, Swiyserland: International Standards Organization.

McCormick, K. A., Lang, N., Zielstorff, R., Milholland, D. K., Saba, V. K., & Jacox, A. 1994. Toward standard classification schemes for nursing languages: Recommendations of the American Nurses Association Steering Committee on Databases to Support Clinical Nursing Practice. *Journal of the American Medical Informatics Association (JAMIA)*, 1(6): 421–427.

National Association for Home Care. 2000. *Basic statistics about home care, 1997*. Washington, DC: NAHC.

North American Nursing Diagnoses Association. 1991. *Taxonomy I: Revised - 1991*. St Louis, MO: NANDA.

North American Nursing Diagnosis Association. 1992. *NANDA nursing diagnoses: Definitions and classification 1992–1993*. St. Louis, MO: NANDA.

Ozbolt, J. Fruchtnicht, J. N., & Hayden, J. R. 1994. Toward data standards for clinical nursing information. *Journal of the American Medical Informatics Association (JAMIA)*, 1(2): 175–185.

Parlocha, P. K., & Henry, S. B. 1998. The usefulness of the Georgetown Home health Care Classification system for coding patient problems and nursing interventions in Psychiatric home care. *Computers in Nursing*, 16(1): 45–52.

Saba, V.K. 1991. *Home Health Care Classification project*. Washington, DC: Georgetown University (NTIS Pub # PB92-177013/AS).

Saba, V. K. 1994a. *Home Health Care Cassification (HHCC) of Nursing Diagnoses and Interventions*. (Revised). Washington, DC: Author.

Saba, V. K. 1994b. Twenty nursing diagnoses home health care components.. In R. M. Carroll-Johnson & M. Paquette (eds.). *Classification of nursing diagnoses: Proceedings of the Tenth Conference* (p. 301). Philadelphia: J. B. Lippincott

Saba, V. K. 1995. A new paradigm for computer-based nursing information systems: Twenty care components. In R.

A. Greenes, H. E. Peterson, & D. J. Proti (eds.). *Medinfo'95 Proceedings* (pp. 1404–1406). Edmonton, Canada: IMIA

Saba, V. K. 1997. Why the Home Health Care Classification is a recognized nomenclature. *Computers in Nursing*, 15(20): S67–S73.

Saba, V. K., & McCormick, A. 2001. *Essentials of computers for nurses: Informatics in the new millennium* 3rd Edition. New York City, NY: McGraw Hill.

Saba, V. K., & Sparks, S. M. 1998. Twenty care components: An educational strategy to teach nursing science. In B. Cesnik, A. T. McCray, & J. R. Scherrer (eds). *Medinfo'98: Proceedings of the Ninth World Congress on Medical Informatics* (pp. 756–759). Amsterdam, Netherlands: IOS Press.

Shaughnessy, P. W., Crisler, K. S. & Schienker, R. R. 1997. *Medicare's OASIS: Standardization Outcome and Assessment Information Set for home health care: OASIS B, March 1997*. Denver, CO: Center for Health Services and Policy Research.

Spath, P. 1993. *Succeeding with Critical Paths*. Forest Grove, OR: Spath & Associates.

Spradley, B. W., & Dorsey, B. 1985. Home health care. In B. W. Spradley (ed.)., *Community health nursing*. Boston, MA: Little, Brown & Co.

World Health Organization. 1992. *ICD-10: International Statistical Classification of Diseases and Related Health Problems: Tenth Revision: Volume 1*. Geneva, Switzerland: WHO.

Zander, K. 1988. Nursing case management: Strategic management of cost and quality outcomes. *Journal of Nursing Administration*, 18, 23–30.

Zielstorff, R. D., Tronni, C., Basque, J., Griffin, L. R., & Welebob, E. M. 1998. Mapping nursing diagnosis nomenclatures for coordinated care. *Image: Journal of Nursing Scholarship*, 30(4): 369–373.

BIBLIOGRAPHY

Bakken, S., Button, P., Konicek, D., Matney, S., Mc-cormick, K., Ozbolt, J., Saba, V. K., Warren, J. J., & Westra, B. 2002. Standardized terminologies, for nursing concepts: Collaborative activities in the United States. *Nursing Informatics 2000 Post-Conference Proceedings.* New Zealand: NZ Press.

Bakken, S., Cashen, M. S., Mendonca, E .A., O'Brien, A., & Zieniewicz, J. 2000. Representing nursing activities within a concept-oriented terminological system: Evaluation of a type definition. *Journal of the American Medical Informatics Association* (JAMIA), 7(1): 81–90.

Button, P., Androwich, I., Hibben, L., Kern, V., Madden, G., Marek, K., Westra, B., Zingo, C. N., & Mead, C. 1998. Challenges and issues related to implementation of nursing vocabularies in computer-based systems. *Journal of the American Medical Informatics Association,* 5(4): 332–334.

Campbell, J. R., & Payne, T. H. 1994. A comparison of four schemes for codification of problem lists. In J. Ozbolt (ed.). *Symposium for Computer Applications in Medical Care* (pp. 201–205). Philadelphia: Hanley & Belfus.

Chute, C. G., Cohn, S. P., Campbell, K. E., Oliver, D. E., & Campbell, J. R. 1996. The content coverage of clinical classifications. *Journal of the American Medical Informatics Association* (JAMIA), 3(3): 224–233.

Cinahl Information Systems. 1998. *CINAHL Subject Heading List.* Glendale, CA: Author.

Coenen, A. M., Marin, H. F., Park, H. A., & Bakken, S. 2001. Collaborative efforts for representing nursing concepts in computer-based systems. *Journal of the American Medical Informatics Association* (JAMIA), 8(3): 202–211.

Giovannetti, P. 1979. Understanding patient classification systems. *Journal of Nursing Administration,* 2, 4–9.

Hardiker, N. R., & Rector, A. L. 1998. Modeling nursing terminology using the GRAIL representation langauge. *Journal of the American Medical Informatics Association* 5(1): 120–130.

Henry, S. B., Holzemer, W. L., Randell, C., Hsieh, S-F, & Miller, T. J. 1997. Comparison of nursing interventions classification and Current Procedural Terminology codes for categorizing nursing activities. *Image: Journal of Nursing Scholarship,* 29, 238–251.

Henry, S. B., Holzemer, W. L., Reilly, C. A., & Campbell, J. R. 1994. Terms used by nurses to describe patient problems: Can SNOMED III represent nursing concepts in the patient record: *Journal of the American Medical Informatics Association* (JAMIA), 1(1): 61–74.

Lamberts, H., & Wood, M. (eds.). 1987. *International classification of primary care (ICPC).* New York: Oxford University Press

Lange, L. 1996. Representation of everyday clinical nursing language in UMLS and SNOMED. In J. J. Cimino (ed.). *1996 AMIA Annual Fall Symposium* (pp. 140–144). Washington DC: Hanley & Belfus.

Marin, H. F., Rodrigues, R. J., Delaney, C., Nielsen, G. H., & Yan, J. (eds.). 2001. *Building standard-based information systems* Washington, DC: Pan American Health Organization.

McCormick, K. A., & Jones, C. B. 1998. Is one taxonomy needed for health care vocabularies and classifications? *Online Journal of Issues in Nursing.* Available *http://www.nursing world.org/ojin/tpc7\-2.html.*

Mortensen, R. A. & Nielsen, G. H. 1996. *International classification of nursing practice (ICNP) (Version 0.2)* Geneva, Switzerland: International Council of Nursing.

Mortensen, R. A., Mantas, J., Manuela, M., Sermeus, W., Nielsen, G. H., & McAvinue. 1994. Telematics for health care in the European Union. In S. J. Grobe, & E. S. P. Pluyter-Wenting (eds.). *Nursing informatics: An international overveiw for nursing in a techological era* (pp. 750–752). Amsterdam: Elsevier

National Library of Medicine. 2002. *Unified Medical Language System: UMLS Knowledge Sources* 13th Edition. Rockville, MD: NLM, NIH, DHHS

Nielsen, G. H. & Mortensen, R. A. 1996. The architecture for an International Classification for Nursing Practice (ICN)), *International Nursing Review,* 43, 175–182.

Nursing Information & Data Set Evaluation Center. 1997. *NIDSEC: Standards and scoring guidelines.* Washington, DC: American Nurses Association

Omnibus Budget Reconciliation Act of 1987 (OBRA, 1987). *Homecare: Omnibus Budget Reconciliation Act of 1987. Public Law 100-203.* Washington, DC.

Parlocha P. K. 1995. *Defining a critical path for psychiatric home care patients with a diagnosis of Major Depressive Disorder* (Doctoral Dissertation). San Francisco, CA: University of California. San Francisco.

Saba, V. K. 1992a. The classification of home health care nursing diagnoses and interventions. *Caring,* 10(3): 50–57.

Saba, V. K. 1992b. Home health care classification. *Caring,* 10(5): 58–60.

Saba, V. K. 2002. Nursing information technology: Classifications and management. In J. Mantas, & A. Hasman (eds.). *Textbook in health informatics* (pp. 21–44). Amsterdam, The Netherlands: IOS Press.

Saba, V. K., & Zuckerman, A. E. 1992. A new home health re classification method. *Caring,* 10(10): 27–34.

Zielstorff, R. D., Cimino, C., Barnett, G. O., Hassan, L., & Blewett, D. R. 1993. The repesentation of nursing terminology in the UMLS meta-thesaurus: A pilot study. In M.E. Frisse (ed.). *Symposium on Computer Applications in Medical Care* (pp. 292–296). New York: McGraw-Hill.

Zielstorff, R. D., Lang, N. M., Saba, V. K., McCormick, K. A., & Milholland, D. K. 1995. Toward a uniform language for nursing in the US: Work of the American Nurses Association Steering Committee on Databases to Support Clinical Nursing Practice. In R. A. Greenes, H. E. Peterson, & Protti, D. J. (eds.). *Medinfo '95 Proceedings* (pp. 1362–1366). Edmonton, Canada: Healthcare Computing & Communications Canada, Inc.

Zielstorff, R. D., Hudgings, C. I., & Grobe, S. J. 1993. *Next-generation nursing information systems: Essential characteristics for professional practice.* Washington, DC: ANA.

CHAPTER 22

Nursing Diagnoses in Home Health Nursing

Carol Ann Parente

THE CONCEPT

The concept of nursing diagnoses may initially strike the home health administrator as more appropriate for clinical use. After all, of what use is an alteration in skin integrity at budget time? The definition and application of nursing diagnoses would definitely seem more valuable to those who provide direct patient services and their immediate supervisors. The nursing diagnosis concept, however, may prove to be valuable indeed to the administrative team, as demonstrated in this chapter. Discussions of nursing diagnoses in recent literature generally focus on their clinical uses and benefits. This chapter, however, discusses the concept, process, and effects of nursing diagnoses from a home health administrative perspective.

Nursing diagnosis represents the continuing steps in the profession's attempts to define its scope and science. Controversy has swirled around the concept since its inception. The debate continues today regarding the appropriateness of identified diagnoses (Jacoby, 1985), the taxonomy selected (Lunney, 1982), and even the idea of diagnoses made by nurses (Shamansky and Yanni, 1983). Some investigators (Sherwood et al., 1988) take issue with specific diagnostic labels, such as *noncompliance* and *knowledge deficit*. Mitchell (1991) proposes that ethical dilemmas surrounding the diagnostic process negate the usefulness of nursing diagnoses and in fact may undermine professional growth.

Proponents focus on the value of a common language, which offers nursing a minimum data set across practice settings and a theoretical and pragmatic foundation for eventual direct reimbursement of nursing activities (Gordon, 1987). More recently, Carpenito (1995b) cites nursing diagnoses as leading to a clearer identification of the body of nursing knowledge, promoting greater accountability and ultimately greater professional autonomy. There has been further growth in attempts to design a uniform nursing language combining nursing diagnosis, nursing interventions and nursing outcomes (Dochterman and Jones, 2003).

In spite of the debate, or perhaps because of it, the concept of nursing diagnoses has continued to gain acceptance and widespread use since the first National Conference on Classification of Nursing Diagnoses, which was convened in St. Louis in the early 1970s. The concept has become well entrenched at all levels of education and in various fields of practice. Indeed, the American Nurses Association (ANA), in its social policy statement of 1980, described nursing as "the diagnosis and treatment of human responses to actual and potential health problems" (ANA, 1980a, p. 9). In 1996, the ANA's social policy statement cited "the application of scientific knowledge to the processes of diagnosis and treatment" as an essential feature of contemporary nursing practice (ANA, 1996, p. 6). The ANA's *Scope and Standards of Home Health Nursing Practice* further elaborates on nursing diagnoses as being derived from the assessment data, validated with the physician, client, family, and other health care practitioners, when possible and appropriate, documented in a manner that facilitates the determination of expected outcomes and plan of care, and include condition-specific, health promotion, and disease prevention aspects (ANA, 1999, p. 9). The ANA clearly sees the nursing diagnostic process as a key nursing function that is vital to providing quality professional nursing care. In addition, many state nurse practice acts now include the nursing diagnosis as part of the defined functions of the professional nurse.

Nursing diagnoses evolved over several paths during the last 30 years. The most commonly accepted format emerged from the North American Nursing Diagnosis Association (NANDA). This group evolved from the National Conference Group on Classification of Nursing Diagnoses. The NANDA diagnosis list may be used by nurses in all clinical fields. Over the years since the first National Conference on the Classification of Nursing Diagnoses in 1973, the list of diagnoses has been revised slowly. Current diagnoses represent the series of conferences and refinements since the first NANDA conference. From the original list of 34, the number of nursing diagnoses has grown to 155 (Dochterman and Jones, 2003). Considering the number of medical diagnoses available, it is clear that the industry is still making the first steps in this area.

Classification of nursing diagnoses in the NANDA system makes use of 11 broad functional patterns: (1) health perception-health management, (2) nutritional-metabolic, (3) elimination, (4) activity-exercise, (5) sleep-rest, (6) cognitive-perceptual, (7) self-perception/ self-concept, (8) role-relationship, (9) sexuality-reproductive, (10) coping/stress/tolerance, and (11) value-belief patterns. Nursing diagnoses in these categories range from the physiological (e.g., altered nutrition in the exchanging cate-

gory) to the spiritual (e.g., spiritual distress) and the psychosocial (e.g., ineffective individual coping). Diagnoses related to activities of daily living are found within the activity-exercise category; sensory input and self-concept diagnoses are located in the self-perception/self-concept category. Knowledge deficit is a diagnosis under the cognitive-perceptual pattern, and the role-relationship pattern includes anticipatory grieving (Gordon, 2002).

Nursing diagnoses differ, however, from our medical colleagues' diagnostic categories by defining actual or potential human responses to health problems (Gordon, 1976) rather than describing specific disease or illness states. Furthermore, the ninth NANDA conference described nursing diagnoses as including individual, family, or community response to actual or potential health problems or life situations (NANDA, 1992). The relationship of nursing diagnoses to medical diagnoses may in one sense be demonstrated in the problem-etiology-symptom format of nursing diagnoses as described by Gordon (1982). Here, the nursing diagnosis is the problem or first part of the diagnostic statement. The etiology, second in the statement format, is shown in relationship to the problem and is often (but not always) the medical illness or treatment. Resulting symptoms form the last part of the diagnosis, and further individualize the nursing diagnosis to reflect a specific patient's problem. An example is as follows: alteration in nutrition, less than body requirements related to chemotherapy resulting in anorexia, and taste changes. The relationship of the nursing diagnosis to the medical diagnosis is one that must be considered carefully by the home health administrator in these days of close scrutiny by third-party payers for reimbursable services.

Another nursing diagnosis group is of particular interest to home health administrators and nursing staffs. The Omaha Visiting Nurse Association (Simmons, 1980), under a 1977 contract with the Division of Nursing, Human Resources Administration, Department of Health and Human Services (DHHS), defined and tested a patient diagnostic and classification scheme. Four domains of nursing endeavor (environmental, psychosocial, physiological, and health behaviors) were defined, and related diagnoses were elaborated. The diagnostic categories resemble the NANDA list in some areas and define other diagnoses with more direct community health impact, such as income and sanitation deficits. The structure of the diagnosis scheme, now known as the Omaha System, is somewhat similar to the NANDA format. The Omaha diagnosis is listed first and is individualized for a particular patient by the use of modifiers, which are specific for each diagnosis. The Omaha System was structured initially to be computerized, further enhancing its usefulness to the home health administrator. This built-in computerization allows the administrator to maximize the information available about an agency's population.

The home health care components (HHCCs; Saba, 1992; see also Chapter 21) represent an adaptation of the NANDA taxonomy I and include classification and coding of both nursing diagnoses and interventions gathered from a national sample of 646 home health agencies. Twenty HHCCs were derived from the data to categorize nursing diagnoses and interventions (Saba, 1992; see also Chapter 21). Diagnoses and interventions are coded under each HHCC as discharge status/goals for diagnoses and actions are coded under interventions. This integration of diagnosis, intervention, and outcome is designed for computerization and retrieval of data that are useful for administrators.

Some authorities (Campbell, 1978; Lunney, 1982) suggest variations on the diagnostic taxonomy in response to patient and nursing needs. Of particular concern are the areas of wellness care and the independent versus interdependent actions of the nurse. Most NANDA diagnoses indicate a problem with the patient's health and/or his or her response to health. The Omaha System does address wellness or health behaviors to some extent. Unfortunately, wellness care is not fully addressed by the diagnostic labels, and equally unfortunately, it is not reimbursable in the current third-party payer environment. Recently, participants at NANDA conferences have developed axes such as unit of analysis (i.e., individual, family, and community), age group, wellness, and illness to be included in taxonomy II of NANDA and to give further dimension to nursing diagnoses. Kelley and colleagues (1995) proposed a trifocal model of nursing diagnoses that includes not only the existence of an identified problem (e.g., a risk or high risk of a particular nursing diagnosis), but also an opportunity for enhancement. This allows the nurse to identify and intervene in an area to promote the patient's health and wellness. The authors suggest that the label "opportunity for enhancement" would facilitate classifications along the illness-wellness axis. These axes may give the community health nurse, researcher, and administrator the opportunity to address the wellness and community issues previously lacking in the NANDA system. Additionally, the NANDA nursing diagnoses have been proposed for inclusion in the next revision of the *International Classification of Diseases* (Carroll-Johnson, 1991). This proposal could have far-reaching implications for home health administrators through enhancing international nurse communications and further validating nursing services, including wellness activities, for reimbursement.

Controversial, too, is the independent response of the nurse in treating certain diagnostic categories (e.g., the NANDA-approved impaired gas exchange). Many of the physiologically based diagnoses are considered to have interdependent responses that are based on both medical and nursing orders (Kim, 1985). Some argue that nurses do not even have the tools to assess such diagnoses (Jacoby, 1985). Gordon's (1995) diagnostic manual clearly suggests medical referral in cases in which a nurse suspects an interdependent diagnosis (e.g., impaired gas exchange). Carpenito (1995b) describes a list of "collaborative" problems as potential complications attached to medical diagnoses (e.g., potential complication: peripheral vascular disease). These problems occur in association with a given pathology and would require both medical and nursing interventions to achieve patient goals. This particular area is less problematic to the home health administrator because the current atmosphere dictates a signed physician's order to cover any nursing activities. When the legislative climate changes to allow direct reimbursement for nursing activities, these interdependent diagnoses may present an administrative challenge.

THE PROCESS

Now that we have described the concept of nursing diagnoses, how do we establish the diagnosis? A larger question also remains: What conceptual framework would give focus and definition to the diagnostic process? To respond to the first question, Gordon (1982) notes that nursing diagnosis is both a label and an action. Diagnosis therefore requires a nursing knowledge base and skill in application of the nursing process. The second question may prove to be more difficult to answer clearly in that no one unified framework has been established for the profession. Consideration must then be given to the nursing agency's and the individual nurse's philosophy and the framework that most closely corresponds to it.

The nursing process involves the methodical examination, definition, and solution of the patient's health problems in relation to nursing. More traditionally, the process is defined as assessment, planning, intervention, and evaluation. The ANA model practice act statement (1980b) inserts the diagnostic step directly after assessment in its discussion of the nursing process. The step-by-step nature of the nursing process and the placement of the nursing diagnosis within it help define and organize the patient's care needs for the staff nurse regardless of the complexity of that patient's problems.

Clearly, the nursing diagnosis is established within the nursing process. The staff nurse, after the initial assessment of the patient, defines problems (the diagnosis) that may be addressed by nursing interventions and may reflect the instructions of the medical regimen, such as knowledge deficit related to a 2g sodium diet.

The diet in the example is prescribed by the physician, and the nurse's evaluation shows that the patient in some way lacks the information to select that diet appropriately. For those nurses who are unfamiliar with the diagnostic categories and their defining characteristics, several pocket-size manuals are available to help clarify and select appropriate diagnoses (Gordon, 2002; Jaffe and Skidmore-Roth, 1993; Kim et al., 1987; NANDA, 1992; Sherwood et al., 1988). By following the definition of the nursing diagnosis, the nurse can proceed to plan and implement interventions based on the problem and the goals set by the patient and nurse. The final step in the process is the evaluation of the effectiveness of the interventions and the overall plan. This step guides the nurse in revision or adaptation of the plan to meet the patient's needs most effectively.

Selection of a particular diagnosis is based on analysis of the patient's nursing assessment data. The focus and definition of the nursing assessment come from a conceptual framework. A variety of frameworks are available for the clinical nurse's examination. Some popular nursing frameworks include Roy's adaptation model, Roger's life process conceptual framework, Neuman's behavioral systems, and Orem's self-care agencies (Orem, 2001; Riehl and Roy, 1980). Many agencies and certainly many individuals use an eclectic approach, some combination of a formalized framework and unspoken concepts that guides their practice. An additional factor in considering a practical conceptual framework for an agency is the demand of third-party payers because, although the patient may have an adaptive or self-care problem, that diagnosis may not represent a reimbursable nursing activity.

Regardless of the framework selected, the nursing assessment must consider all aspects of the patient's care needs. Gordon (2002) suggests a functional approach and considers 11 health patterns that are necessary for a complete assessment in any framework: health perception/health management, nutritional-metabolic pattern, elimination pattern, activity-exercise, cognitive-perceptual pattern, sleep-rest pattern, self-perception/self-concept, role relationship pattern, sexuality-reproductive pattern, coping-stress-tolerance pattern, and value-brief pattern.

Once selected, the nursing diagnosis can be documented in a variety of ways. Particularly useful is the problem-oriented method of charting, which allows the nurse to address each problem separately and systematically. First described by Weed (1971), the problem-oriented method contains four main components: (1) a problem list, (2) a defined database, (3) initial and revised plans, and (4) progress notes. For our purposes, the nursing diagnoses are the problems listed, and the previously discussed nursing assessment is the database. Goals or expected outcomes are listed with the problems and diagnoses, and detailed plans are established on the physician's order forms or plans of treatment.

Progress notes are formulated using the SOAP method (subjective, objective, assessment, and plan). In this format, subjective data represent the patient's point of view, objective data are the evidence collected by the professional, assessment is the professional's analysis of both the subjective and the objective data, and the plan outlines the steps needed to deal with the assessment and the overall problem or diagnosis.

Flow sheets or some other abbreviated form of documentation, such as checklists, may be used with a narrative description of the nursing diagnoses and the subsequent nursing interventions. Depending on the agency's documentation policies and third-party demands, the nurse may document every visit on the flow sheet and record a narrative only when changes occur or as mandated by the agency. This combination may prove to be time saving for the home health nurse while also preserving a graphic flow of the patient's needs. Parameters necessary to measure the patient's progress and the effectiveness of the nursing interventions may be defined individually on the flow sheet for each patient according to his or her diagnoses.

Standardized flow sheets, which reflect parameters necessary to assess and intervene in specific diagnostic categories, can also be established. The standardized flow sheets may be designed to promote a minimum level of nursing care expected by the agency for a certain diagnosis. Items found on the flow sheets may include physical data, such as vital signs, measurements of a wound, or peripheral edema; instruction needs, such as insulin administration and diet instructions; psychosocial data, such as affect; and treatment needs, such as wound dressing changes or catheter changes.

Individualization of the patient's care needs to reflect his or her own nursing diagnosis, etiology, and symptoms may be accomplished if the standardized flow sheets have ample space for the nurse to document the patient's specific requirements.

In this manner, the nurse may overcome the tendency to fit the patient to the diagnosis rather than fit the diagnosis to the patient. Standardized flow sheets may be designed by the agency staff based on their documentation requirements and care plans related to specific nursing diagnoses. Parameters are formatted according to the nursing process and may be adapted from a variety of sources, including clinicians, staff members, nursing texts, and nursing care plan manuals. Many recent projects also identify and classify nursing interventions that can be used as parameters in standardized charting. The National Intervention Classification project, the HHCCs, the International Classification in Nursing Project, and the Omaha System are among many classifications of interventions at various levels of development that may correlate with nursing diagnoses (Snyder et al., 1996). The Agency for Health Care Policy and Research (AHCPR), now the Agency for Healthcare Research and Quality (AHRQ) established by Congress in 1989, has examined both traditional medical and variations of nursing diagnoses, such as urinary incontinence and pressure ulcer treatment (Bergstrom et al., 1994; Fantl et al., 1996).

AHCPR guidelines may also be incorporated into standardized charting formats to reflect current national standards for selected problems. Several nursing investigators have also developed a series of nursing care plans for home care agencies based on nursing diagnoses; these may also serve as reference points for standardized flow sheet parameters (Carpenito, 1995a; Gould and Wargo, 1987; Walsh et al., 1987). The use of standardized flow sheets in conjunction with a nursing diagnosis taxonomy may further contribute to the establishment of outcomes in relation to a quality assurance program.

Computer programs have been designed to provide nurse-friendly formats for individualized clinical information systems for nursing diagnoses and plans of care. Much of this work has been done in acute care settings, but with advancements in portable hardware technologies, including laptop and hand-held computers, the home care arena is showing an expansion in automation of nursing diagnosis-related plans of care (Hannah et al., 1987; see also Chapter 15). These computerized clinical information systems will eventually replace the paper standardized flow sheets currently in use. For data to be retrieved from computerized systems, a standard or structured language must be used. Nursing diagnoses lists approved by NANDA, the Omaha System, or the HHCCs or adapted by a particular agency (see Exhibit 22-1) should help staff avoid confusing or chaotic terminology that prohibits data collection. The inclusion of a nursing diagnosis format in management information systems will additionally link clinical and financial data for home health administrators (Martin et al., 1992). This link will take on increasing importance in the era of health care reform in providing information about costing out of nursing services and utilization of resources.

THE EFFECTS

The effects of nursing diagnoses may be evident in many facets of home health nursing, including administration, clinical practice, and associated research. This is not to say that there are no problems with nursing diagnoses. The taxonomy is often awkward, whether the NANDA system, the Omaha System, or another system is used. In addition, even though there has been almost three decades of work on the taxonomy, the language of nursing diagnoses can and will change as nursing further refines the lists and explores the range of its professional practice. Defining characteristics for the diagnoses may not always be clear to the practicing staff nurse, and there may be some resulting confusion as to the choice of an accurate and appropriate diagnosis (Dalton, 1985). The concurrent assessment and documentation scheme for nursing diagnoses may be cumbersome initially for staff unaccustomed to the concepts of nursing process and diagnosis.

Conversion to a nursing diagnosis system will require considerable staff development efforts. Although more recently educated nurses may find the process easy, older nurses may be unsure and may need guidance from both development and supervisory staff in selection and documentation of a nursing diagnosis. There are also possible legal considerations in nursing diagnoses, such as inaccurate diagnoses or misdiagnoses resulting in improper nursing treatment. In actuality, nursing diagnoses represent the labeling of problems that nurses normally treat; therefore, nurses would be held accountable for their actions whether or not the label or diagnosis is attached (Gordon, 1982).

For the clinical nurse, the advantages of nursing diagnoses include the standardization of the language used to communicate within the profession. The communications link of nursing diagnoses aids home health nurses in validating their practices for themselves, their peers, supervisors, and third-party payers. For the home health nurse, the stresses of independent home care and the many documentation requirements associated with third-party payers can contribute to a burnout problem (Marvan-Hyam, 1986). The nursing diagnosis, which clearly shows the nurse's professional assessment, goals, and interventions, may increase professional self-worth. This may be accomplished by helping the nurse view the nursing process as a proactive problem-solving technique rather than merely reactively carrying out the physician's orders. The use of nursing diagnoses in an agency's documentation system can also help clarify communications among staff members

Exhibit 22–1 Sample Nursing Diagnosis List

Seq	Text	
1	AGEN	
2	#18	Fluid Volume Deficit
3	#24E	Altered Health Maint: Impaired Bone Density
4	#27J	Knowledge Deficit: Chemotherapy
5	#29	Noncompliance
6	#33	Altered Oral Mucous Membranes
7	#38	Self-Bathing—Hygiene Deficit
8	#51	Risk for Activity Intolerance
9	#55	Risk for Fluid Volume Deficit
10	#73	Health-Seeking Behaviors
11	#82	Total Self-Care Deficit
12	#83	Self-Dressing—Grooming Deficit
13	#85	Self-Toileting Deficit
14	RESP	
15	#2	Ineffective Airway Clearance
16	#7	Ineffective Breathing Pattern
17	#21	Impaired Gas Exchange
18	#107	Inability to Sustain Spontaneous Ventilation
19	#108	Dysfunctional Ventilatory Weaning Response
20	CV	
21	#8	Decreased Cardiac Output
22	#19	Risk Fluid Volume Deficit
23	#20	Fluid Volume Excess
24	#24A	Altered Health Maint: Cardiac
25	#24B	Altered Health Maint: HTN
26	#48	Altered Tissue Perfusion
27	GI	
28	#4	Constipation
29	#5	Diarrhea
30	#6	Bowel Incontinence
31	#27E	Knowledge Deficit: GI Bleed
32	#21I	Knowledge Deficit: Ostomy
33	#78	Colonic Constipation
34	#79	Perceived Constipation
35	GU	
36	#24K	Altered Health Maint: Renal Disease
37	#49	Altered Urinary Elimination Pattern
38	#59	Functional Incontinence
39	#60	Reflex Incontinence
40	#61	Stress Incontinence
41	#62	Total Incontinence

continues

Exhibit 22–1 Continued

42	#63	Urge Incontinence
43	#72	Urinary Retention
44	ENDO	
45	#27A	Knowledge Deficit: Diabetes
46	NEURO/PAIN	
47	#1	Activity Intolerance
48	#9	Pain
49	#10	Impaired Verbal Communication
50	#24C	Altered Health Maint: CVA
51	#27D	Knowledge Deficit: Bedbound
52	#28	Impaired Physical Mobility
53	#53	Chronic Pain
54	#57	Hyperthermia
55	#67	Impaired Swallowing (Uncompensated)
56	#68	Risk for Altered Body Temperature
57	#69A	Ineffective Thermoregulation
58	#77	Risk for Aspiration
59	#81	Risk for Disuse Syndrome
60	#86	Dysreflexia
61	#87	Sensory Overload Effects
62	#109	Risk Peripheral Neurovascular Dysfunct.
63	NUTR	
64	#27M	Knowledge Deficit: Enteral Feedings
65	#30	Altered Nutrition: Less than Body Requirements
66	#31	Altered Nutrition: More than Body Requirements
67	#32	Altered Nutrition: Risk for More than Body Requirements
68	#84	Self-Feeding Deficit
69	SAFE	
70	#25	Impaired Home Maintenance Management
71	#26	A Risk for Injury
72	#35	Risk for Infection
73	#74	Risk for Poisoning
74	#75	Risk for Suffocation
75	#113	Altered Protection
76	SKIN	
77	#42	Pressure Ulcer
79	#43	Risk for Impaired Skin Integrity
79	#70	Impaired Tissue Integrity
80	#110	Impaired Skin Integrity
81	PSYCH	
82	#3	Anxiety
83	#11	Ineffective Coping (Individual)
84	#12	Family Coping: Compromised

continues

Exhibit 22–1 Continued

85	#13	Family Coping: Disabling
86	#14	Family Coping: Potential for Growth
87	#15	Diversional Activity Deficit
88	#16	Altered Family Processes
89	#17	Fear (Specify Focus)
90	#22	Anticipatory Grieving
91	#23	Dysfunctional Grieving
92	#36	Powerlessness
93	#37	Rape Trauma Syndrome
94	#39	Self-Esteem Disturbances
95	#40	Sensory Deprivation
96	#41	Sexual Dysfunction
97	#44	Sleep-Pattern Disturbance
98	#45	Social Isolation
99	#46	Spiritual Distress (Distress of Human Spirit)
100	#47	Altered Thought Processes
101	#50	Risk for Violence
102	#52	Impaired Adjustment
103	#56	Hopelessness
104	#64	Unilateral Neglect
105	#65	Altered Sexuality Patterns
106	#66	Impaired Social Interaction
107	#71	Post-Trauma Response
108	#80	Fatigue
109	#88	Decisional Conflict
110	#89	Chronic Low Self-Esteem
111	#90	Situational Low Self-Esteem
112	#91	Body Image Disturbance
113	#92	Personal Identity Disturbance
114	#93	Altered Role Performance
115	#95	Parental Role Conflict
116	#96	Rape Trauma Syndrome: Compound Reaction
117	#97	Rape Trauma Syndrome: Silent Reaction
118	#98	Defensive Coping
119	#99	Ineffective Denial
120	#100	Caregiver Role Strain
121	#101	Risk for Caregiver Role Strain
122	#102	Risk for Self-Mutilation
123	#103	Relocation Stress Syndrome
124	#104	Ineffective Management of Therap. Regimen
125	#111	Depression
126	IV	
127	#27C	Knowledge Deficit: IV Therapy

continues

Exhibit 22–1 Continued

128	#27K	Knowledge Deficit: Central Venous Access Device
129	MATERNAL/CHILD	
130	#24F	Altered Health Maint: Pregnancy
131	#24G	Altered Health Maint: Hyperbilirubinemia
132	#24I	Altered Health Maint: Asthma
133	#24	Altered Prenatal Health Maintenance
134	#26B	Risk for Injury R/T Drug/Alcohol Withdrawal
135	#27F	Knowledge Deficit: Post Partum Care/Breast Feeding
136	#27G	Knowledge Deficit: Post Partum Care/Lactation Suppression
137	#27H	Knowledge Deficit: Infant Care
138	#27I	Knowledge Deficit: Apnea Monitor
139	#34	Altered Parenting (Specify Education)
140	#54	Altered Growth and Development
141	#69	Ineffective Thermoregulation R/T Prematurity
142	#76	Ineffective Breastfeeding
143	#76A	Ineffective Breastfeeding: Breast Engorgement
144	#76B	Ineffective Breastfeeding: Sore Nipples
145	#76C	Ineffective Breastfeeding: Flat Inverted Nipples
146	#94	Risk for Altered Parenting (Specify)
#105		Interrupted Breastfeeding
#106		Ineffective Infant Feeding Pattern

Source: Reprinted with permission of Abington Memorial Hospital Home Care, Willow Grove, Pennsylvania.

when many nurses are needed to see an individual patient; for instance during weekend or vacation coverage. The nursing diagnosis can help clarify priority problems, and when standardized flow sheets or computerized care plans are used the covering nurse can quickly and confidently follow the primary nurse's care plan as outlined by the selected parameters or interventions. Nursing diagnoses can also facilitate communication between the home health and acute and long-term care colleagues to promote continuity of the patient's care. The transition from hospital to home and home to independence or other care mode may be eased if the nursing diagnoses are clear and the goals or expected outcomes are well defined.

Nursing diagnoses and expected outcomes also may be included in the process of develop-

ment of critical pathways. Critical pathways, which are timelines of multidisciplinary activities, plans, and outcomes, describe care for patients in an episode of illness for a specific diagnosis-related group (DRG), such as total hip replacement. Nursing diagnoses for a majority (75 percent) of patients in a DRG could be included in the critical pathway of patients as they move through an illness (Carpenito, 1995a).

In addition, the use of the nursing diagnosis may assist in a peer review process (Warren, 1983). The practice of diagnosing and treating competently can be evaluated by peers reviewing a nursing record that includes a database.

For supervisory staff, the use of a nursing diagnosis taxonomy by clinical nurses can assist them in evaluating nursing competence and accountability. The supervisor may review the nurse's competence via joint home visits, patient care conferences focusing on nursing, diagnosis selection and treatment, or chart review. Areas of staff concern may be identified by both staff and supervisors and converted into staff development programs as appropriate. The usefulness of nursing diagnoses clinically is perhaps most crucial when one considers third-party reimbursement. This issue is clearly valuable to the community health nurse and administrator considering the Medicare regulation stipulating reimbursement for skilled nursing services (DHHS, 1996). Nursing diagnoses can, within the Health Care Financing Administration's constraints regarding time, homebound status, and patient response or progress, assist in documenting areas where nursing contributes significantly to the patient's care and hence is more likely to be considered skilled.

In addition to the benefits of diagnoses for the clinical staff, distinct advantages accrue to the home health administrator from the use of nursing diagnoses within the agency. The administrator may identify many valuable statistics for the provision of cost-effective, quality care based on the staff's use of the nursing diagnoses. As an example, these statistics may show length of service per diagnosis and cost per diagnosis. How long is the mean service period for the patient with an alteration in skin integrity? How much does it cost to care for the average patient with an alteration in mobility? What other services are required for a person with a self-care deficit? What are the most frequently occurring diagnoses for the agency's population base? Analysis of the accumulated data could prove useful in considering the impact of prospective payments in home health care, in planning services and community programs, and in planning staff expansions or reductions.

A sound quality improvement program may also be an outcome of nursing diagnosis use. Reviewers can identify the appropriateness of the diagnoses and the accompanying goals, interventions, and outcomes as documented in the chart. The consistency of a nursing diagnosis taxonomy such as the Omaha System or the NANDA system helps clarify the patient's problems even though the reviewer may see only a "paper patient." The clear identification of the goals and outcomes related to the diagnosis helps the quality assurance process determine the effectiveness of the available nursing services and the nurse's coordination of services required by the patient. A utilization process may also be facilitated by nursing diagnosis statistics gathered on length of service per diagnosis, number and frequency of visits, and number of disciplines involved per diagnosis.

Nursing research could be encouraged within the clinical practice and administrative fields to seek refinements of the diagnostic taxonomies and standardization of interventions and to develop levels of acuity of nursing intensity. These and other research efforts may prove valuable to the home health administrator who seeks to retain an edge in the competitive home health care market.

REFERENCES

American Nurses Association. 1980a. *A social policy statement.* Kansas City, MO: ANA.

American Nurses Association. 1980b. *The nursing practice act: Suggested state legislation.* Kansas City, MO: ANA.

American Nurses Association. 1996. *Nursing's social policy statement.* Washington, DC: ANA.

American Nurses Association. 1999. *Scope and standards of home health nursing practice.* Washington, DC. Author.

Bergstrom N., et al. 1994. December. *Pressure ulcer treatment clinical practice guideline* (Quick Reference Guide for Clinicians No. 15). Rockville, MD: U.S. Department of Health and Human Services, Public Health Service, Agency for Health Care Policy and Research. AHCPR Pub. No. 95-0653.

Campbell, C. 1978. *Nursing diagnosis and interventions in nursing practice.* New York: Wiley.

Carpenito, L. J. 1995a. *Nursing care plans and documentation.* Philadelphia, PA: Lippincott.

Carpenito, L. J. 1995b. *Nursing diagnosis: Application to clinical practice.* Philadelphia, PA: Lippincott.

Carroll-Johnson, R. M., ed. 1991. *Classification of nursing diagnosis: Proceedings of the ninth conference.* Philadelphia, PA: Lippincott.

Dalton, J. 1985. A descriptive study: Defining characteristics of the nursing diagnosis "cardiac output, alterations in: Decreased." *Image* 17: 113–117.

Department of Health and Human Services, Health Care Financing Administration. 1996, April. *Health insurance manual* (HIM II Revisions 277). Washington, DC: Government Printing Office.

Dochterman, J., and D. Jones, eds. 2003. *Unifying nursing languages.* Washington, DC: ANA.

Fantl, J. A., et al. 1996, March. *Managing acute and chronic urinary incontinence* (Quick Reference Guide for Clinicians No. 2, 1996 Update). Rockville, MD: U.S. Department of Health and Human Services, Public Health Service, Agency for Health Care Policy and Research. AHCPR Pub. No. 96-0686.

Gordon, M. 1976. Nursing diagnosis and the diagnostic process. *American Journal of Nursing* 76: 1276–1300.

Gordon, M. 1982. *Nursing diagnosis: Process and application.* New York: McGraw-Hill.

Gordon, M. 1987. Issues in nursing diagnoses. In *Classification of Nursing Diagnoses.* In A. M. McLane (ed.), *Proceedings of the Seventh Conference,* 17–20. St. Louis, MO: Mosby.

Gordon, M. 2002. *Manual of nursing diagnosis.* St. Louis, MO: Mosby-Year Book.

Gould, E. J., and J. Wargo. 1987. *Home health nursing care plans.* Gaithersburg, MD: Aspen.

Hannah, K. J., et al., eds. 1987. *Clinical judgment and decision making: The future with nursing diagnosis.* New York: Wiley.

Jacoby, M. K. 1985. The dilemma of physiological problems: Eliminating the double standards. *American Journal of Nursing* 85: 281–285.

Jaffe, M. S., and L. Skidmore-Roth. 1993. *Home health nursing care plans.* St. Louis, MO: Mosby.

Kelley, J., et al. 1995. A trifocal model of nursing diagnosis: Wellness reinforced. *Nursing Diagnosis* 6: 123–128.

Kim, M. J. 1985. Without collaboration, what's left? *American Journal of Nursing* 85: 281–284.

Kim, M. J., et al. 1987. *Pocket guide to nursing diagnosis.* St. Louis, MO: Mosby-Year Book.

Lunney, M. 1982. Nursing diagnosis: Refining the system *American Journal of Nursing* 82: 456–459.

Martin, K., et al. 1992. The Omaha System, a research-based model for decision making. *Journal of Nursing Administration* 22: 47–52.

Marvan-Hyam, J. 1986. Occupational stress of the home health nurse. *Home Healthcare Nurse* 4: 18–21.

Mitchell, G. 1991. Nursing diagnosis: An ethical analysis. *Image* 23: 101–103.

North American Nursing Diagnosis Association. 1992. *NANDA nursing diagnoses: Definitions and classification.* St. Louis, MO: NANDA.

Orem, D. 2001. *Nursing concepts of practice,* 6th ed. St. Louis, MO: Mosby.

Riehl, J. P., and C. Roy, eds. 1980. *Conceptual models of nursing practice.* New York: Appleton-Century-Crofts.

Saba, V. 1992. The classification of home health care nursing diagnoses and interventions, *Caring* 11: 50–57.

Shamansky, S. L., and C. R. Yanni. 1983. In opposition to nursing diagnosis: A minority opinion. *Image* 15: 47–50.

Sherwood, M. J., et al. 1988. *Determining nursing diagnosis through assessment.* Baltimore, MD: Williams & Wilkins.

Simmons, D. A. 1980. A classification scheme for client problems in community health nursing. Washington, DC: Government Printing Office. DHHS Pub. No. HRA 80-16.

Snyder, M., et al. 1996. Defining nursing interventions. *Image* 28: 137–141.

Walsh, J., et al. 1987. *Manual of home health nursing.* Philadelphia, PA: Lippincott.

Warren, J. J. 1983. Accountability and nursing diagnosis. *Journal of Nursing Administration* 17: 34–37.

Weed, L. L. 1971. *Medical records, medical education and patient care.* Cleveland, OH: Case Western Reserve University Press.

SUGGESTED READING

Ballard, S., and R. McNamara. 1983. Qualifying nursing needs in home health care. *Nursing Research* 32: 236–241.

Carnevali, D., and M. D. Thomas. 1993. *Diagnostic reasoning and treatment decision making in nursing.* Philadelphia, PA: Lippincott.

Carroll-Johnson, R. M., and M. Paquette, eds. 1994. *Classification of nursing diagnosis: Proceedings of the tenth conference.* Philadelphia, PA: Lippincott.

Daubert, E. 1979. Patient classifications systems and outcome criteria. *Nursing Outlook* 27: 450–454.

Giovannetti, T. 1979. Understanding patient classification systems. *Journal of Nursing Administration* 9: 4–9.

Gordon, M. (1995). Manual of Nursing Diagnosis. St. Louis. Mosby-Year Book.

Hardy, J. 1984. A patient classification system for home health patients. *Caring* 3: 26–27.

Harris, M., et al. 1985. A patient classification system in home health care. *Nursing Economics* 3: 276–282.

Kim, M. J., and A. M. McLane, eds. 1984. *Classification of nursing diagnoses, proceedings of the fifth national conference.* St. Louis, MO: Mosby.

Kim, M. J., and D. A. Morita. 1982. *Classification of nursing diagnosis (third and fourth national conferences).* New York: McGraw-Hill.

McLane, A. M., ed. 1987. *Classification of nursing diagnosis.* St. Louis, MO: Mosby.

National League for Nursing (NLN). 1974. *Problem-oriented systems of patient care.* New York: NLN.

Sienkiewicz, J. 1984. Patient classification in community health nursing. *Nursing Outlook* 32: 219–221.

Visiting Nurse Association (VNA) of New Haven. 1980. *Patient classification objective system methodology manual.* New Haven, CT: VNA of New Haven.

CHAPTER 23

Perinatal High-Risk Home Care

Richela Stoddard-Johnston

INTRODUCTION

Home care for women experiencing complications of pregnancy is a rapidly growing specialty. Health care reform in the United States continues to direct the type of home care women with pregnancy complications receive. Ongoing health care reform also provides an opportunity for nurses to expand their scope of practice as they care for the high-risk perinatal patient with complex home care needs. The more recent movement of patient-managed high-technology health care into the home setting has been the result of ongoing health care reimbursements from federal and private insurances, improved technology, and client preference.

High health care costs, along with consumer demand for participation in their care and the availability of new technologies, have prompted the development of home care high-risk programs (Heaman, 1994). National strategies to control health care costs have resulted in the decrease of hospitalization and readmission rates, thereby increasing the use of home care services for many high-risk patients. These special patients are at risk for delivering low birth weight (LBW) infants. LBW infants have high mortality and morbidity rates and increased health care costs (Brooten, 1998). Any strategy that lengthens the gestational period and increases birth weight can result in significant savings of health care costs.

Standards of care that reflect current practices are an important piece necessary to implement a high-risk program. The cost of home care in relation to the cost of a hospital stay per day ranges anywhere from one-fourth to one-fifth the cost. Well-designed programs must evaluate stress factors relating to environment, financial, and psychological needs (Monical, 1998). The home environment produces less stress and enhances the ability to learn thoroughly. Hospitals have the disadvantage of isolating patients from their family support system, and increasing the risk of infection, as well as being extremely expensive. Home care reduces the cost significantly, yielding an equal or better outcome (Coon, 1997). Proper discharge planning must be instituted prior to home care services for the high-risk client, as well as thorough explanation and education by their obstetrician.

MAKING IT WORK

Home-based perinatal high-risk care works because of the increased availability of services placed in the home such as monitoring, highly skilled nurses, social workers, nutritionists, and durable medical equipment (DME) companies. Also the reduction of stress that the patient feels is a big factor, as is the decreased risk of infection. Patient preference dictates that it is preferable to hospital care. Success is dependent on the basic elements of a highly motivated patient, qualified agency providers, and coordination of all services.

There are three basic models of ante-partum home care: (1) hospital-based programs that have developed as a new service within an existing hospital that provides care for the high-risk inpatient, or within an existing hospital-based home care department; (2) small businesses run by nurses who have developed a home-care agency specific to high-risk pregnancies; and (3) government-funded public agencies. The differences between public and private run agencies are important to understand. Public agencies focus on preventive care, health promotion, teen pregnancies, nutritionally at-risk patients, and substance abuse. Private agencies care for women with more acute problems, use more high-tech interventions, and employ high-risk labor and delivery nurses (Heaman, 1998). Advanced practice nurses may function in the role of a discharge planner, an advocate in the development of these special programs, in the home as a coordinator of care, or as a direct caregiver.

MANAGEMENT OF THE MOST COMMON DIAGNOSES

Clients suitable for a high-risk program can be classified into one of the following several groups. Patients with hyperemesis as early as 6 weeks, who have signs and symptoms (s/s) of dehydration and severe weight loss, can be managed with oral or intravenous (IV) antiemetics and IV infusion along with a DME company. All patients need to be seen by a nutritionist for evaluation and a perinatal nurse one to three times per week. Patient teaching is extremely intense and should include other family members. Advancement of oral fluids and diet will be slow over several weeks or even months if on continuous IV hydration. After three trials of peripheral IV insertions, a peripheral inserted central catheter (PICC) line needs to be considered for long-term use to maintain nutrition. Weekly lab work needs to be drawn and evaluated for electrolyte balance.

Gestational diabetics are the second most common types of admissions who need a nutrition evaluation and a perinatal nurse visit for teaching. Initially for the first 1 to 2 weeks a telephone call one to three times a week is needed. The initial visit includes assessing the patient's ability to self-monitor using a glucometer, assessing proper use of supplies, and proper disposal of sharps. Telephone contact includes daily diet review for 1 to 2 weeks (Coon 1997). The nurse on each visit assesses fetal and maternal well-being, evaluates kick counts, measures fundal height, and evaluates blood sugars. Blood sugar parameters should be a fasting < 100 and 2 hours after meals < 120 (Sanborn, 2001).

Pregnancy-induced hypertension (PIH) is the third most frequent type of high-risk patient managed in the home. PIH includes three stages: (1) Pre-eclampsia (renal involvement leading to protienuria), (2) eclampsia (involving the central nervous system leading to seizures), and (3) hemolysis leading to HELLP Syndrome (Hemolysis-Elevated Liver Enzymes-Low Platelets). Frequent visits of one to three times per week, telephone contact, education of self blood pressure monitoring, urine protein evaluation, and maintaining modified to strict bed rest are the standards for proper management. The perinatal nurse teaches the patient to self-monitor fetal activity, reduce stress, and evaluate daily weights, keeping all the data on a weekly flow sheet. Home care management requires blood pressure readings $< 150/100$, headache free, and without epigastric pain.

Preterm labor patients are a less frequent type of high-risk client managed in the home. Clients must be 1 centimeter or less in dilation and have less than 4 to 6 contractions per hour. Cause of preterm labor continues to be difficult to understand. These patients can be maintained at home with a self-uterine monitoring program, bed rest, and medications. Daily assessments either by visit or telephone are done to evaluate contractions, fetal movements, s/s of preterm labor, weight, vital signs, and even cervical exam as ordered by the obstetrician (Heaman, 1998). Use of tocolytic therapy can be used if minimal side effects can be maintained. Due to restricted activity, the client needs to be on a diet high in roughage along with stool softeners. The American College of Obstetricians and Gynecologists (ACOG) considers home uterine monitoring investigational and does not recommend it for routine clinical use.

Multiple gestation clients are managed quite similar to preterm labor clients. The major goal is preventing pregnancy complications through monitoring and patient education of s/s to report (Coon, 1997). Clients are usually maintained on bed rest of various levels with one to two times per week nursing visits, fetal activity monitoring, urine checks, weight recordkeeping, and frequent telephone calls.

Other complications in pregnancy that require management by high-risk home care but that are admitted with less frequency include cervical prolapse, spontaneous rupture of membranes, ante-partum bleeding, cardiac disease (only class I and II accepted in home care according to Coon, 1997), renal disease, pulmonary disease, endocrine disorders, connective tissue disorders, and blood dyscrasias. These are all managed case by case, using the basic guidelines for referrals, assessments, applicable nursing diagnoses (to establish a plan of care), client education, and activity limits.

ADEQUATE SCREENING PROCESS

A physician must evaluate the high-risk patient in order to be referred to a home-based high-risk program. A medical history and a physical need to be completed and forwarded to the agency accepting the patient referral. The patient needs to be educated in the program's process of intervention, family involvement, and follow-up on medical appointments. The patient must be capable and willing to follow the plan of care established for her diagnosis. There needs to be a caregiver and support resources available. The home environment should be evaluated for cleanliness and suitability. Not all patients will be manageable at home or meet criteria (Monical, 1998).

STEPS TO ENTERING A PATIENT INTO A HIGH-RISK HOME CARE SYSTEM

A referral is made by either a physician's office, through hospital-based discharge planning, or an insurance case manager. There should be no acute clinical concerns for the maternal and fetal couple, and there should be an adequate support system in place at home for reduced activity and stress. The availability of a telephone and rapid hospital transportation needs to be in place. Absence of active vaginal bleeding, along with a reassuring biophysical profile of 8 to 10 needs to be confirmed. At this point, insurance authorization and visit protocol along with negotiated costs need to be established. DME companies need to be notified of equipment required and delivery arrangements confirmed.

The first antenatal visit time and date can now be arranged with the patient. As well as advising the client, the nurse will take a history, do a maternal and fetal assessment, evaluate psychosocial adjustments, assess environmental needs, and determine educational requirements (Campbell, 1997).

INITIAL VISIT

When admitting a patient to home care, the nurse completes a thorough physical and psychological assessment to determine how best to care for the client and whether or not she is a candidate for home care. The nurse needs to assess the patient's ability to receive and understand home care instructions. The first visit should include a history of current and past obstetrical information as well as medical, surgical, and family history. The nurse makes an assessment of maternal and fetal well-being along with an assessment of the patient's psychological adjustment to lifestyle changes. Environmental evaluation of accessibility to telephone and transportation needs to be completed. The nurse also assesses the environment for safety and housing standards. Last, the perinatal nurse needs to evaluate the client's knowledge in order to comprehend the teaching required. Information should be given to the client as to the role of the nurse as well as the role of patient. The perinatal nurse's role is to visit one to seven times per week, assess maternal and fetal well-being, review activity reports, educate in the s/s of abnormalities, inform of the disease process, and give care relating to the diagnosis. The client's role is to keep records of fetal activity, medications, temperature, urine dipsticks, intake and output, uterine palpations, maternal pulse, and fluid leakage (Campbell, 1997).

After completing the initial assessment and education, the nurse makes referrals to the appropriate disciplines such as dietician, home health aide, physical therapy, DME vendors, home prenatal education, social work, clergy, lactation specialists, and high-risk parent support group. Finally the perinatal nurse makes a plan of care (POC) based on several applicable nursing diagnoses. The following are the most common: (1) knowledge deficit, (2) altered nutrition, (3) impaired physical mobility, (4) activity intolerance, (5) constipation, (6) infection, and (7) altered role performance (Grohar, 1994).

RISK MANAGEMENT

Many day-to-day, even month-to-month, variations in services are dictated by reimbursements from insurances, rather than addressing patient needs. Home care nurses need to document all patient contacts needed in giving care (home visits, telephone contact, and case conference) to ensure payments reflect the various types of communication home care nurses have with patients. Changes in reimbursement are occurring constantly; therefore, nursing time and contact with patients should be reviewed regularly in order for accurate planning of costs and charges (Brooten et al., 1998).

Before developing a high-risk program, it is important to ensure proper malpractice coverage is in place. In addition, the need for adequately trained staff, current standards of practice, and documentation protocols must be in place. Policies and procedures showing continuing education of the staff need to be current because of increased demand by accrediting agencies for health care professionals to have current competencies. Nurses must also be aware of federal and state regulations relating to home care, as well as being oriented to legal and ethical considerations surrounding the use of equipment, safety issues, coordination of care, admission process, communication, and documentation (Monical, 1998).

PATIENT SATISFACTION EVALUATION

As consumer demand for quality care increases, the evaluation of patient satisfaction with nursing care assumes greater importance in the delivery of nursing care and technical knowledge. Physicians are in a role of introducing women to a high-risk home care program, and they need to provide adequate information for the patient to feel confident and secure in this alternative model of care. The importance of communication in the health care team from discharge planning, insurance- or physician-based referrals, DME companies, and home care cannot be emphasized enough. Patients need to be introduced to the program with the use of teaching booklets, and during care with the use of recordings (Heaman et al., 1994).

CONCLUSION

Home care is a proven, positive method of providing nursing care. It reduces stress on both the patient and family support system while providing care toward the goal of improving maternal and neonatal outcomes (Campbell, 1997). Providing effective ante-partum home care for the high-risk patient requires advanced knowledge and clinical skills in perinatal and home health nursing, as well as an understanding of the structure and protocol of a home health care agency. Nursing care in the home includes case management, maternal and fetal assessment, education of self-monitoring needs, proper use of equipment, and coordination of DME companies and other services, as well as providing psychological support to the client and her family. Advanced practice nurses have an important role to play in developing their competencies, advocating for the development, as well as implementation, and evaluation of their high-risk programs (Heaman, 1998). Advanced practice nurses have clinical expertise that allows for the thorough assessment of patient situations and early interventions to decrease risk, improve outcomes, and potentially decrease the cost of care. The availability of a nurse specialist to answer questions and provide information and support could potentially decrease the numbers of acute hospital admissions and readmissions, again decreasing costs (Armstrong 1996).

As home health care progresses, it is important to remember the benefits available to the high-risk perinatal patient. Perinatal nurses with advanced education, expertise, and skills are the advocates of quality perinatal care in the home. Nursing care of the high-risk client will continue to expand as a result of change in the external health care system, as well as increases in the knowledge of the advantages of home care for clients and families. Individualization of care that addresses the specific needs relating to her condition and home environment can greatly reduce the stress caused by the client's diagnosis. Communication, coordination of services to meet the client's needs, and patient satisfaction measurements are important components for high-risk home care programs to succeed (Grohar, 1994). Nurses have the opportunity to shape the future of health services and enhance programs that not only are cost effective, but also meet consumer needs (Heaman, 1998).

REFERENCES

Armstrong Persily, C. 1996. A model of home care for high-risk childbearing families (women with diabetes in pregnancy). *Nursing Clinics of North America* 31: 327–333.

Brooten, D., et al. 1998. Home care of high risk pregnant women by advanced practice nurses: Nurse time consumed. *Home Healthcare Nurse* 16: 823–830.

Cambell, D. 1997. Home care of the high-risk perinatal. *Home Health Care Management & Practice* 9: 15–22.

Coon, N. 1997. *High-risk perinatal home care manual.* St. Louis, MO: Mosby-Year Book, Inc.

Grohar, J. 1994. Nursing protocols for antepartum home care. *Journal of Obstetric, Gynecologic, and Neonatal Nursing* 23: 687–694.

Heaman, M., et al. 1994. Patient satisfaction with an antepartum home care program. *Journal of Obstetric, Gynecologic, and Neonatal Nursing* 23: 707–713.

Heaman, M. 1998. Antepartum home care for high-risk pregnant women. *AACN Clinical Issues* 9: 362–376.

Monical, W. 1998. Managing high-risk pregnancies at home. *Home Health Care Consultant* 5: 28–31.

Sanborn, N. 2001. *Abington Hospital home care policies and procedures.* Willow Grove, PA: Abington Memorial Hospital Home Care.

CHAPTER 24

High-Technology Home Care Services

Diana Acker and Thomas D. Brown

Health care in the 21st century is a dynamic system that continues to balance patient, insurance, and care providers' needs. Over the past 20 years, we have seen a health care system that was very much inpatient based where hospital providers drove the pricing and reimbursement for services. During this period of time, hospitals were financially secure and built large financial reserves. The cost of health care continued to rise due to the pricing structure and the increasing costs associated with the vast improvements in diagnostic and treatment technologies. The next generation of health care saw an increased presence and influence by insurance providers. As costs continued to increase, patients were forced to rely more on insurance to pay for their health care needs. These insurers were often commercial based and continued to pay the rates established by the provider.

The next step in the evolution was payment based on negotiated, preferred provider rates. This gave birth to the concept of paid provider organizations (PPOs) and health maintenance organizations (HMOs). We saw a shift in reimbursement that forced significant cost-cutting measures to be enacted by care providers in an effort to maintain profits while continuing to provide quality care to patients. Hospitals changed their focus from keeping beds filled as long as possible to a focus on discharge planning and the ultimate goal of decreasing the length of hospital stays. This change in hospital

philosophy has essentially driven the development of the entire home care industry. Home care services have now developed into a significant portion of most hospital business plans. As hospitals continue to work with or develop their home care programs, increased efficiencies are required as the economy of health care continues to change. New ways of decreasing inpatient days are continually being developed. Over the last 10 years, high-technology home care services have been developed and refined to meet the continued demand for a decrease in patient days.

MAJOR CATEGORIES OF HIGH-TECHNOLOGY SERVICES

High-technology home care services can be defined as specialized home care services that employ techniques, supplies, and equipment traditionally reserved for inpatient care facilities. Care is often provided by a multidisciplinary group of health care providers including, but not limited to, specialized nurses, pharmacists, respiratory therapists, discharge planners, social workers, physical therapists, and occupational therapists. High-technology home care services can be broken into several major categories of care including respiratory care, durable medical equipment (DME), infusion services, pharmacy services, and specialized nursing.

RESPIRATORY CARE

Respiratory care services begin with safety evaluation and insurance verification. This ensures that the home environment is appropriate for the intense care that is often required. Equipment used in respiratory care often includes oxygen, ventilators, apnea monitors, nebulizers, and continuous positive airway pressure (CPAP) units. This equipment must be delivered, set up in the patient's home, and maintained according to the manufacturer's recommended standards. The clinical staff is required to customize the equipment to the patient's needs, and dispense and administer supplemental medications. The clinical staff is also responsible for teaching the appropriate caregivers and for monitoring the patient's response to treatment.

DURABLE MEDICAL EQUIPMENT

Durable medical equipment (DME) services often address the daily physical needs of the patient. The DME services attempt to offer the patient a certain degree of independence in their daily living. Specific DME services include evaluating the home situation as they relate to safety issues, evaluating the patient and caregivers' abilities to cope with the patient's needs, and providing insurance verification to assure reimbursement for service. Under the guidance of the physician and physical and/or occupational therapists, equipment is provided, properly fitted for the patient, set up for proper use, caregivers are educated, and the patient's response to the aids are evaluated and monitored. Equipment provided may include walking aids, bathroom aids, wound care supplies, hospital beds, enteral tube feeding supplies, and suction units.

INFUSION SERVICES

Infusion services in home care are the most notable of high-technology services offered. Infusion services are multifaceted and begin by including patient safety evaluation and insurance verification. Clinical services are a collaborative effort between medical, nursing, and pharmacy staff. Clinical services include care planning, provision of specialized infusion equipment, specialized pharmaceutical preparation, patient/caregiver education, and ongoing clinical monitoring of response to therapy. Infusion products provided include:

- antibiotics/antivirals
- intravenous (IV) steroids
- hematologics (i.e., Epogen, Neupogen)
- IV hydration
- chemotherapy
- total parenteral nutrition (TPN)/enteral tube feeding
- blood products (IV immune globulin, clotting factors)
- positive inotropics (milrinone, dobutamine)
- pain management (IV and epidural)
- catheter maintenance

PHARMACY SERVICES

Another important component is pharmacy services. Pharmacists practicing in home infusion play an integral role in planning the care process. They are responsible for obtaining the medication orders from the physician and determining the medication and dose appropriateness. They assist in determining the proper method of administration along with dispensing the often-complex catheter supply orders to accomplish this plan of care. Pharmacists assist in care planning for the patient by monitoring laboratory data to assure the continued safe administration of medication. Pharmacists can also play a key role in determining the optimal drug dose through the use of pharmacokinetic dosing.

SPECIALIZED NURSING CARE

High-technology home care service revolves specifically around nursing care. Nurses in the home infusion specialization bring special skills. They are required to be proficient in all aspects of infusion administration including catheter maintenance procedures and extensive infusion pump programming with troubleshooting experience. Nurses must be able to assess and make recommendations on all aspects of a patient's situation, both physically and psychologically. Nurses must be proficient in assisting the patient's social situation in an effort to maintain a safe and effective environment of care for the patient.

As a whole, high-technology nursing care is generally categorized into disease-specific patient care. Patients with certain conditions are visited by specially trained nurses who view the patient from a holistic approach but are specially trained in a specific disease state. The overall intention of offering these specialized nursing services is to identify patient-specific issues that can be addressed early in an effort to prevent repeated hospital admissions. Nurses provide care to patients with a wide range of disease processes and needs. Examples of infusion services provided by high-technology nurses include antibiotic therapy provided to an orthopedic patient with osteomyelitis, and a pregnant patient with a urinary tract infection. Each patient has specific needs as they relate to their disease process and overall state of health. Other infusion services include hydration provided for young children and care for young and elderly adults for reasons varying from post-chemotherapy vomiting, hyperemesis, or metabolic electrolyte imbalance. Total parenteral nutritional (TPN) can be provided for a patient with an acute post-op abdomen or for the patient with long-term diseases such as Crohn's or mechanical intestinal obstruction. Communication is imperative for the health care team to provide appropriate care and monitoring of the patient in the home care environment.

Two other categories of specialty nursing that a home care nurse may provide include hospice nursing dealing with end-of-life issues and long-term pain management as well as cardiac nursing providing congestive heart-failure patients and their families with the opportunity to treat excessive symptoms at home and avoid hospitalizations through infusion, monitoring,

and teaching. Other types of specialty nursing include wound care, nutrition, and psychological care related to disease processes that require care. The home infusion nurse needs to demonstrate a wide knowledge base of nursing care in a variety of patient needs.

EDUCATION AND DOCUMENTATION RESPONSIBILITIES

Patient and caregiver teaching is a primary focus for high-technology nursing care. Patients and caregivers must understand that they need to take an active part in the care of the patient. The home care staff will provide supplies, drugs, pharmacist dispensing, monitoring, and nursing to provide care services, but the family will have to be involved in the daily care and monitoring. Education handbooks are often issued and prove helpful in providing patients and caregivers a reference when clinical staff is not present. Education needs to be reinforced with each visit. Every patient situation is different, and education needs must be customized. Documentation of education must be completed along with clinical documentation. Patient history and physical exams, usually based on body systems and psychosocial assessment, must be documented with each visit. A current medication list and nutritional assessment must also be included in the patient documentation.

All documentation of patient information including ordered therapy, demographic information, patient history, and ongoing assessments must be kept confidential. The patient's privacy needs to be safeguarded at all times. This can be an arduous task in that the patient information must be available to the nurses as they travel and see their patients, yet it must be kept out of view. All home care staff including customer service representatives and delivery personnel must be cognizant of the need for privacy, specifically in relation to the Health Insurance Portability and Accountability Act (HIPAA) that became effective in April 2003 (see Chapter 51).

BENEFITS OF HIGH-TECHNOLOGY HOME CARE

High-technology home care services are designed to ultimately decrease inpatient hospital days while capturing the patient for future services. With advancement in medical equipment technology, high-technology home care is possible while allowing for the care to be safely and effectively administered. In theory, the patient is kept in the health care network for acute inpatient care, outpatient diagnostic services, and ongoing chronic care. The insurers prefer high-technology home care services because a day of care at home is more cost effective than inpatient days. In essence, home care is utilized to defray the ever-increasing cost of specialized acute care diagnostic equipment and procedures.

Patient satisfaction also tends to increase with the ability to offer high-technology home care services. In previous years, if a patient had certain chronic health care needs, they often spent extended periods of time in a hospital or long-term care facility. Some admissions to an extended care facility were for a lifetime. With the implementation of sophisticated high-technology home care services, chronically ill patients often have the ability to return to their homes with the support of their family and friends. This often allows the chronically ill patient to maintain some sense of normalcy and maintains the "family unit." Chronically ill patients can actually see a decrease in the psychological issues that are prevalent in patients confined to a long-term care facility. High-technology home care can also play a role in avoiding the acquisition and spread of nosocomial infection. With high-technology home infusion, nosocomial infections can be effectively treated while removing the patient from the facility where they may have acquired the infection, thus preventing the transmission to other patients.

CASE STUDY

The true patient impact of high-technology home care services can be demonstrated by presenting a patient case. Joe is a 32-year-old married male with two children. Joe is a carpenter for a local construction company and enjoys motorcycling as a hobby. On July 7, he is involved in a serious motorcycle accident. In the car-versus-motorcycle accident, Joe was severely injured, suffering significant head and back injuries. From the scene, he is flown by emergency medical helicopter to the nearest Level-I trauma center, 32 miles from the scene. Immediately upon arrival, he is taken to the operating room for reconstruction of his cranium with plates and pinning of an L-3 vertebral fracture.

During the several weeks post-operatively, it was determined that Joe was paralyzed from the mid-chest down and would remain a paraplegic. Joe has undergone a second surgery to remove one of the plates in his head due to a potential infection. After the surgery, the area is cultured and the infection is determined to be fungal in nature. In addition to the significant rehabilitation needs, the patient will also require several months of treatment with an intravenous antiviral. Additionally, the patient will require enteral feedings due to his jaw being wired shut from the reconstructive surgery.

In mid-August, case management along with the various medical teams begins to discuss the transfer of the patient to a rehabilitation facility. On August 25, Joe is transferred to a local spinal cord injury rehabilitation center. While he is there, he receives significant physical therapy, occupational therapy, enteral tube feedings, intravenous antiviral therapy, and psychological counseling for depression. On December 5, Joe remains in the rehabilitation center and is making significant progress in his rehabilitation. This is the point in his medical treatment that exemplifies the difference in medical care today versus 15 or more years ago. If Joe's injuries had occurred in the early 1980s, at this point in his treatment, he would be transferred to a long-term care facility in an effort to meet his long-term therapy goals, and he probably would have remained in the facility for the rest of his life. He probably would have had numerous acute care readmissions for various nosocomial infections and probably would have developed significant clinical depression requiring a multifaceted medication regimen.

Since the advent of high-technology home care services, Joe has the opportunity to return to his home. High-technology home care services that Joe will receive include physical therapy, occupational therapy, infusion services for antiviral administration, and DME supplies for the provision of enteral tube feeding, incontinence items, and a wheelchair and hospital bed. There are multiple advantages of the patient returning to his home setting at this time. The advantages include a significant cost savings to the insurer versus keeping the patient in a long-term facility for life. The hospital can benefit because the patient is returning to its system, where he will utilize outpatient services including laboratory and radiology. The patient will also remain in the system for any future acute care hospital admissions.

Probably the most significant advantage in this situation is that the patient will return to his family unit prior to the holiday season. The patient will fare significantly better from a psychological perspective, and this often leads to a better, more medically stable patient. Even though Joe's injuries were devastating when compared to his situation before the accident, through the correct application of acute care, rehabilitation services, and high-technology home care services, Joe will have the best chance to lead a productive, family-supported life.

TYPES OF PROVIDERS OF HIGH-TECHNOLOGY SERVICES

High-technology services continue to expand, with providers entering and exiting the market constantly. The provision of service in some areas is extremely competitive, with many providers seeking a limited number of patients. Providers can be established as hospital-based systems or independent providers. Hospital-based systems have one clear advantage over independent providers in that they have a captured client base. Even though patients ultimately have the right to choose their provider, most patients, if they are comfortable with the care received as an inpatient, will choose to continue service with the hospital-based system. Hospital-based systems can be established as either not-for-profit or for-profit entities of the hospital. Traditionally, the for-profit status often mirrors the main hospital. Decisions of the profit status generally lay with the finance department of the hospital and are often tax based. In hospital-based systems, the long-term plans and goals of the entire hospital must be evaluated. Future service expansion plans must be prioritized as per the long-range plan of the hospital. A complete evaluation of where services are being referred to currently must be conducted.

Independent providers are often established as a for-profit business. The independent provider is a business entity that must compete for business within their particular market sector. Often independent providers must have extensive marketing departments. The marketing departments must provide sales support to insurers, hospitals, and physicians. They must sell their product to entities that do not have access to their own service. They are competing for the business that exists outside of the traditional hospital system. Independent providers can be on the local level with only one or two area branch offices or they may be part of a larger national chain of company-owned or franchise-branch facilities. Extensive evaluation must be conducted prior to entering the high-technology home care market as a provider.

FINANCIAL CONSIDERATIONS

Financial evaluation of current referrals for high-technology home care must be conducted. Is there sufficient patient load to make the entering of the market financially feasible? The structure of the service must also be considered. Is it feasible to purchase an existing service? Partnering/profit-sharing with an independent provider, or start a service from the ground up? Independent providers considering the entry into the market must consider many of the same items as the hospital. Is the local hospital base large enough to provide enough patients? Do the hospitals have existing contracts with a "preferred provider"? Are there enough local physicians to support operations? Are physicians contractually obligated to a specific provider? A survey of local insurance providers is also necessary. What is the structure of the predominant local insurers? Are local insurers accepting and/or establishing contracts with new local providers? Independent providers should also explore and consider a risk sharing agreement with local hospitals.

After the decision has been made to enter the high-technology home care market, a significant amount of due diligence must be completed prior to any organization providing service. Figure 24-1 gives a general overview of what is required to establish a high-technology home care service.

In the establishment of a hospital-based home care service, most of the core items can be accomplished by utilizing existing departments/employees within the hospital. As an independent provider, these functions are initially accomplished by an entrepreneur that is establishing the service. If the founder is not capable of all of these functions, they must partner with individuals who have the knowledge either through direct partnership or on a consultative basis. After an initial feasibility study for the service is completed and the decision has been made to enter the market, the establishment of a finance department is crucial to future success. All accounting procedures for the business must be established to meet audit and tax requirements in an ultimate effort to prevent fraud and abuse.

Collaboration with other departments in the establishment and the relationship between reimbursement and clinical information systems must be completed early into the process. Timely reimbursement for provided services is crucial for the long-term viability of the entire service. The financial sector is also responsible for negotiating and contracting with all insurers. Financial and operating terms of a contract must be established and conveyed to other sectors in the devel-

opment process. The finance department is also key in the development of strict operational and capital planning and budgeting to assure that initial feasibility projections can be met.

HUMAN RESOURCES

The initial feasibility study provides for the quantity and nature of employees required to establish the service. As we move toward the implementation of a service, the human resources department must be established to advertise, interview, and ultimately hire qualified staff required to operate the service. Great care must be taken in selecting employees that will have the ability to carry the business plan of the organization toward a successful result. Hiring certain key employees that have been responsible for establishing similar services will offer invaluable advice and experience. This will also prevent oversights that can often prove to be fatal to a newly established organization. Appropriate budget consideration should be given to hire the specialized talent.

LICENSURE AND ACCREDITATION ISSUES

Health care as a whole is an extremely regulated industry. High-technology home care services are no exception. Accreditation agencies for high-technology home care often include but are not limited to:

> Joint Commission on Accreditation of Healthcare Organizations (JCAHO)
>
> Community Health Accreditation Program (CHAP)
>
> Local boards of pharmacy/nursing
>
> Local departments of health
>
> Drug Enforcement Administration (DEA)
>
> Food and Drug Administration (FDA)

Figure 24–1 General Overview of Requirements to Establish a High-Technology Home Care Service

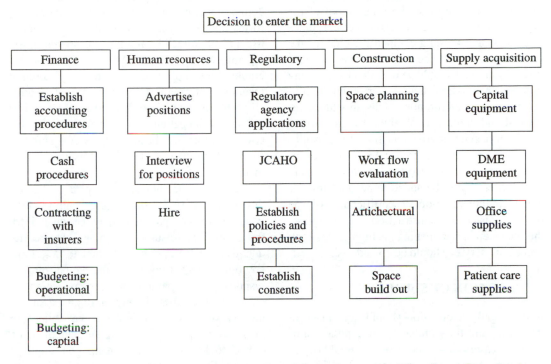

Source: Courtesy of the Abington Memorial Hospital Home Infusion Department, Willow Grove, Pennsylvania.

In establishing a new high-technology home care service, application to and accreditation by appropriate agencies must be established. Insurance reimbursement contracts are often tied to successful accreditation. Also a host of legal issues exist that an organization may face if they fail to obtain the correct licensures required to run a particular high-technology health care service. Often the accreditation process includes a complete review of the organization's policies and procedures in order to assure safe delivery of care to the patient. As part of the accreditation requirements, complete policies and procedures must be established and implemented. These policies and procedures influence the entire operation of the organization. Consents for treatment must also be established for patients to review and agree to prior to offering any high-technology service. This is crucial in protecting the organization from litigation that may arise from any adverse events that occur during the course of care and treatment.

PHYSICAL LOCATION OF SERVICES

The physical space where the organization will conduct business needs to be addressed. Upon evaluation of the initial feasibility study, plans must be made to accommodate the amount of patients expected. Generally a 10 to 15 percent increase in patients is built in for busy periods. Sufficient office and warehouse space must be obtained and the workflow of the operation must be considered. The space planning and work-flow evaluation should culminate with architectural plans that propose the final layout of the organization's workspace. Architectural plans will assist in obtaining competitive bids for the construction work to be done. A 10 percent contingency amount should be included to cover any unforeseen situations that may arise during construction or rehabilitation. Plans should be reviewed and comments obtained by the various regulatory agencies. Adequate time must be allocated to complete the physical construction or rehabilitation of the workspace. An adequate time buffer should be added to account for any delays in construction or certification of the physical space. As construction is in progress, the final step in establishing the high-technology home care service should be considered.

ACQUISITION OF SUPPLIES

Initial supply acquisition should take place at this time, and the purchasing of capital equipment necessary to run the business should begin. Examples include delivery vehicle(s), office furniture, copy machine(s), telephone systems, and an initial supply of patient durable medical equipment. The initial feasibility study for the project should be consulted in an effort to determine the amount of equipment that will need to be purchased or leased and how much will need to be rented. Finally, office supplies and disposable patient care supplies must be purchased and stored.

DAY-TO-DAY OPERATIONS

Operational aspects of high-technology home care services are similar to all other home care services. Figure 24-2 represents an overview of the operational aspects of a high-technology home care service. A physician, case manager, or the patient makes a referral for high-technology care to the agency. Information gathering during the intake process is of utmost importance in providing the appropriate care for the patient and receiving proper reimbursement for services. It is important to obtain accurate demographic information along with therapy information, and it is imperative that an agency use a standardized intake form to prevent missing information. Figure 24-3 serves as an example of a complete intake form. Verification of insurance information is necessary to determine eligibility of the patient to receive the prescribed therapy. If the patient has an insurance plan that covers the therapy, the agency should assure that a contract is negotiated and established with the insurer.

Many insurance plans require prior authorization of services. If timely prior authorization is not obtained, payment may be denied for those services. Insurance policies change frequently; therefore, it is important to determine any out-of-pocket costs that the patient may be responsible for paying. After determining all out-of-pocket costs, if any, a financial agreement should be provided for the patient or guardian to sign. It is important to note the daily out-of-pocket costs and the estimated length of service. Even a relatively small out-of-pocket expense could become significant when compounded over a lengthy course of treatment. This amount may be a large portion of a patient's monthly income. When a patient clearly understands the financial responsibility, a payment plan may be established to assure complete reimbursement.

Orders for clinical care must be verified with the physician. Patient allergies should be investigated and noted and a coordinated plan of care must be established by the entire care team. Clinicians and intake and reimbursement personnel must have input on the plan of care. Many issues can and must be addressed, including: How long will the insurer authorize the therapy? When does the authorization need to be extended or renewed? Based on the therapy, what clinician visit pattern must be established? By what means will the therapy be provided? Are clinician education visits required? How often are they requried? Clinician education of

Figure 24–2 Overview of the Operational Aspects of a High-Technology Home Care Service

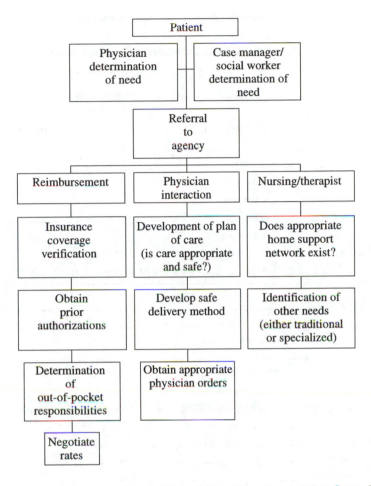

Source: Courtesy of the Abington Memorial Hospital Home Infusion Department, Willow Grove, Pennsylvania.

caregivers is crucial to effective high-technology home care and must include all aspects of care.

The support network for the patient in the home setting must be evaluated by the initial visiting clinician and be part of an ongoing assessment. A patient may believe that they have sufficient help available for care when in fact they do not. It is important to establish a relationship with the person responsible for care at the onset. These discussions can assist the pa-tient, family, and clinician in determining the level of care and interventions needed. Examples of care issues that may arise include a care-giver may work the dayshift and be available to give the once-daily dose of medication at 6:00 P.M. rather than at the hospital schedule of 1:00 P.M. The patient may have been on an every 8-hour dose regimen of medication where the dose is given at 3:00 A.M. in the hospital. The dose time may have to be adjusted to accommodate the patient and caregivers.

Figure 24–3 One Example of a Complete Intake Form

** SEE REVERSE SIDE FOR INSURANCE INFORMATION **

ABINGTON MEMORIAL HOSPITAL HOME INFUSION - PATIENT INTAKE FORM

DATE OF REFERRAL: ___ / ___ / ___   REFERRAL SOURCE: _____

REFERRAL SOURCE CONTACT: _____ PHONE : (_____) _____ - _____

PATIENT INFORMATION:

LAST NAME: _____ FIRST NAME: _____ MIDDLE INT.: _____

ADDRESS: _____

CITY: _____ STATE: _____ ZIP: _____

PHONE: (_____) _____ - _____ HOME WORK OTHER _____

PHONE: (_____) _____ - _____ HOME WORK OTHER _____

D.O.B.: _____ AGE: _____ HEIGHT: _____ WEIGHT: _____ ALLERGIES: NONE KNOWN YES: _____

CAREGIVER: _____ RELATION: _____

CAREGIVER PHONE: (_____) _____ - _____ HOME WORK OTHER _____

HOSPITAL: _____ ROOM #: _____ HOSPITAL ROOM PHONE: (_____) _____ - _____

ALTERNATE DELIVERY ADDRESS: _____

   CITY: _____ STATE: _____ ZIP: _____

   PHONE: (_____) _____ - _____ HOME WORK OTHER _____

EMERGENCY INFORMATION: EMERGENCY CONTACT: _____ RELATION: _____

PHONE: (_____) _____ - _____ HOME WORK OTHER _____

PHYSICIAN INFORMATION:

ORDERING PHYSICIAN: _____ PHONE: (_____) _____ - _____

FOLLOW-UP PHYSICIAN: _____ PHONE: (_____) _____ - _____

CASE INFORMATION: DIAGNOSIS 1: _____ ICD No.: _____

                          DIAGNOSIS 2: _____ ICD No.: _____

THERAPY CATEGORY: ANTIBIOTIC TPN / PPN ENTERAL INOTROPE CATH CARE PAIN INJECTABLE OTHER _____

ACCESS: PERIPHERAL PICC–GROSHONG HICKMAN PORT PICC–OPEN END EPIDURAL PEG-TUBE G-TUBE

   J-TUBE NG-TUBE OTHER _____   DATE OF CATH PLACEMENT/ LAST RE-START: _____

THERAPY DESCRIPTION (MED/CONC/RATE ETC.): _____

START OF CARE AT HOME (DATE AND TIME) _____ DURATION: _____

LAB STUDIES: _____ SCHEDULE: _____

IS THIS THE PATIENT'S FIRST DOSE ? YES NO DON'T KNOW

ADMINISTRATION METHOD: GRAVITY VOLUMETRIC PUMP AMBULATORY PUMP SYRINGE PUMP

            ENTERAL PUMP SYRINGE BOLUS IV PUSH SQ IM OTHER _____

Source: Courtesy of the Abington Memorial Hospital Home Infusion Department, Willow Grove, Pennsylvania.

Figure 24–3 (Continued)

INSURANCE INFORMATION:

INSURANCE 1: _____

CONTACT NAME: _____   CONTACT PHONE: (_____) _____ - _____

GROUP No. : _____   ID No. : _____   DATE OF ELIGIBILITY: _____

BILLING ADDRESS: _____ _____

   CITY: _____   STATE: _____   ZIP: _____

AUTHORIZATIONS:

   THERAPY 1 : _____   PROCEDURE CODE: _____   AUTH. No. _____   AUTH. PERIOD: _____

   THERAPY 2 : _____   PROCEDURE CODE: _____   AUTH. No. _____   AUTH. PERIOD: _____

   THERAPY 3 : _____   PROCEDURE CODE: _____   AUTH. No. _____   AUTH. PERIOD: _____

SPECIAL INSTRUCTIONS: _____

INSURANCE 2: _____

CONTACT NAME: _____   CONTACT PHONE: (_____) _____ - _____

GROUP No.: _____   ID No.: _____   DATE OF ELIGIBILITY: _____

BILLING ADDRESS: _____

   CITY: _____   STATE: _____   ZIP: _____

AUTHORIZATIONS:

   THERAPY 1 : _____   PROCEDURE CODE: _____   AUTH. No. _____   AUTH. PERIOD: _____

   THERAPY 2 : _____   PROCEDURE CODE: _____   AUTH. No. _____   AUTH. PERIOD: _____

   THERAPY 3 : _____   PROCEDURE CODE: _____   AUTH. No. _____   AUTH. PERIOD: _____

SPECIAL INSTRUCTIONS: _____

REFERRAL RECEIVED BY: _____   DATE: _____   TIME: _____

INSURANCE VERIFIED BY: _____   DATE: _____   TIME: _____

REFERRAL ACCEPTED BY: _____   DATE: _____   TIME: _____

COPIES DISTRIBUTED TO:

   PHARMACY MANAGER   NURSE MANAGER   REIMBURSEMENT   PHARMACY   NURSING   DELIVERY

*** ORIGINAL COPY TO PATIENT CHART ! ***

Source: Courtesy of the Abington Memorial Hospital Home Infusion Department, Willow Grove, Pennsylvania.

The high-technology home care clinicians must determine what supplies are needed to provide optimal patient care. Medication, disposable supplies, and durable medical equipment need to be supplied. Durable medical equipment is usually rented by the patient/insurer or it may be purchased by the patient or insurer if it is financially prudent to do so. When equipment is rented, the provider needs to have procedures established to document appropriate cleaning and proper functioning between patient use. Maintaining a system either electronically or manually to track inventory of DME and to inventory medication and disposable supplies is necessary to continue uninterrupted care. After appropriate supplies are gathered and double checked for accuracy, a delivery must be made to the patient. Deliveries may be accomplished by employed delivery staff, hired courier services, or overnight shipping. Regardless of the delivery method employed, policies and procedures must be established to retrieve and properly dispose of biomedical hazardous materials and to retrieve of rental equipment.

The clinical staff must maintain ongoing assessments during the course of therapy. Any assessments must be documented according to current agency policy to assure consistency. Handwritten or electronic notes may be used and must be maintained according to department or accrediting agency policy. Reimbursement staff must keep accurate records of therapy, professional services, and supplies utilized in patient care. Prompt, accurate billing according to contracts will limit errors and maintain consistent cash flow for the agency. It is crucial for the clinician to relay therapy information in a timely manner to assure proper reimbursement for services provided.

SUMMARY

The ultimate goal of high-technology home care is to provide care at home that was once reserved for inpatient facilities. Care is provided in an effort to keep the patient at home where they are more comfortable and surrounded by their family while maintaining their usual routine. Compliance tends to increase and better care outcomes are achieved when therapy meets the schedule and lifestyle of the patient and caregivers. Insurers can decrease costs while quality care is provided. As care continues in the new millennium, we expect to see a continual rise in patients utilizing high-technology home care services.

CHAPTER 25

Discharge of a Ventilator-Assisted Child from the Hospital to Home

Andrea Gendelman

Katie is a bright 5-year-old girl who attends kindergarten. She is a little different from her classmates in that she is wheelchair bound and requires mechanical ventilation. Katie spent her first 9 months of life in a pediatric intensive care unit, where she was successfully weaned to requiring nighttime ventilation and subsequently was discharged to home. This case study illustrates the safe and successful discharge of the ventilator-assisted child from the hospital to home.

The polio epidemics of the 1940s through the 1950s spurred medical advances in mechanical ventilation. With these advances, neonatology and pediatric critical care medicine evolved, becoming adept at treating critically ill infants and children. Some of the infants and children who survive the acute stages of an illness continue to have complex medical problems and disabilities, with an increasing number being dependent on sophisticated technological support, such as mechanical ventilators. Traditionally, children who required this level of support remained in intensive care units, an environment incongruous with normal growth and development. Long-term hospitalization of technology-dependent children is no longer an option as a result of policymaking and reimbursement strategies that limit length of stay and health care expenditures. Home care of the technology-dependent child provides cost-effective care in an environment conducive to meeting the developmental and psychosocial needs of the child and family.

Katie was delivered at full term after an uncomplicated pregnancy, born with an L1-2 myelomeningocele with Arnold-Chiari malformation. She underwent posterior fossa compression and had multiple medical problems including hydrocephalus necessitating placement of a ventriculoperitoneal shunt, upper airway obstruction requiring a tracheostomy at 2 weeks of age, apnea requiring full ventilatory support, and paraplegia. Over the course of a 9-month hospitalization, Katie's condition stabilized, and she demonstrated continued growth and development.

Katie's mother, Ms. M., a single parent and now mother of two, actively participated in Katie's well-infant care shortly after birth. As Katie's condition improved, her mother began learning how to care for her more complex needs. As Katie was successfully stabilized, her mother expressed interest in taking her daughter home. The medical staff recognized that the intensive care unit was not conducive to Katie's further growth and development and felt that she would be an acceptable candidate for home care.

The decision to discharge a ventilator-assisted child to home is intricate. Not every child and/or family is appropriate for home care. The child must be medically stable, as demonstrated by a stable airway, baseline oxygen requirements that do not fluctuate, blood gases that remain within medically acceptable limits, and positive gains on the growth scale. Commensurately, the parents must display the desire and ability to learn to successfully manage the care of the ventilator-assisted child.

Once a family has been identified as appropriate for home care, a discharge plan is formulated. This is accomplished with the input of the following people: the parents, primary physician, primary nurse, social worker and/or discharge coordinator, respiratory therapist, and developmental therapists. This team must consider closely all aspects of the child's care to provide a smooth transition from the hospital to home.

FUNDING FOR HOME CARE

Determining the funding for home care is often the most complex and time-consuming aspect of the discharge process. Katie was covered by her mother's private insurance policy. The policy reimbursed for a maximum of 120 days of patient hospitalization and had a $500,000 major medical benefit. The 120 inpatient days were exhausted, and the remaining 5 months of hospital costs were paid via the major medical portion of the policy. At an average cost of $60,000 per month, $300,000 of the major medical benefit was used for her hospitalization. The remaining $200,000 was targeted for home care.

The social worker contacted the case manager of the insurer to ensure that the remaining major medical funds would be available for home care coverage. Because Katie would have exhausted more than half her major medical funds by her discharge date, the social worker sought a secondary, long-term funding course. An application was submitted to the state Medicaid waiver program for Katie. The waiver program in her state provides reimbursement for the home care of a predetermined number of technology-dependent children. The reimbursement covers durable medical equipment (DME) supplies, and up to 16 hours of nursing care per day depending on the severity of the child's medical needs. The waiver program deems a child eligible for medical assistance regardless of parental income and assets.

The social worker also filed an application for Katie with the Ventilator Assisted Children/Home Program (VAC/HP), a program funded by the Commonwealth of Pennsylvania. The VAC/HP would provide supportive and advocacy services via a case coordinator once Katie was home. The program's administrator would remain available to the discharging institution for assistance with the discharge process.

TEACHING PLAN

The teaching plan for the family can be devised and implemented concurrent with negotiating for home care funding. Ms. M. identified one back-up caregiver to assist in Katie's care in the event that Ms. M. was not available for Katie. Ms. M. and the back-up caregiver completed an extensive teaching plan, that covered:

- anatomy of the respiratory system
- the child's diagnosis as it related to the tracheostomy and mechanical ventilation
- signs and symptoms of infection
- care of the tracheostomy
- pulmonary toilet
- emergency care of the artificial airway
- cardiopulmonary resuscitation
- administration of medications and nutritional supplements via nasogastric tube
- physical and occupational therapy exercises
- operation and maintenance of the ventilator and associated equipment

Before discharge, Ms. M. and the secondary caregiver were required to spend at least 24 consecutive hours in the hospital providing all Katie's care. During the education process, the hospital social worker met with the primary nurse and the respiratory therapist to compile a list of necessary equipment and supplies for home.

SELECTION OF A DME VENDOR

Once the lists of equipment and supplies were complete, the social worker and Ms. M. reviewed the selection of a DME provider. While interviewing possible vendors, the family should consider the following questions:

- Does the vendor guarantee 24-hour service?
- What is the vendor's proximity to the home?
- What is the vendor's response time to service and emergency calls?
- What is the vendor's experience with the population of ventilator-assisted children?
- Will the vendor accept the funding mechanism's reimbursement as payment in full?
- Is the vendor Medicaid certified in the state in which the family resides?

Ms. M. interviewed and identified a DME vendor. The vendor was given an itemized list of the necessary equipment and supplies for Katie. The equipment to be used at home, including the ventilator and its external battery, cascade humidifier, and pulse oximeter, were delivered to the hospital's biomedical department to be evaluated for safety and proper functioning. Before discharge, Katie was placed on the equipment for 1 week to familiarize the mother and caregivers with it and to assess further its safety and performance.

The day before discharge, the vendor delivered and set up all the equipment in Katie's home; disposable supplies sufficient for 1 month were provided. The respiratory therapist reviewed with the mother and home care staff the equipment's maintenance and function. On the day of discharge, the respiratory therapist was present in the home to assess Katie's adaptation to the equipment.

One aspect of the discharge plan that can be easily overlooked is the possible purchase of equipment. Katie's physicians determined that she would require mechanical ventilation for an extended period of time. As a cost-saving measure, the social worker negotiated with the insurer to purchase one complete set of equipment along with the service contract. The rationale behind the purchase of equipment is that the rental of the ventilator alone for 1 year will exceed its purchase price.

HOME NURSING CARE

A major component of home care for a ventilator-assisted child is nursing care. The parents, with insight from the child's physician and social worker, must determine the amount and type of nursing care to be used at home. This will vary because each family is unique in its composition and obligations (parents' careers, other dependents, and the intricacy of the child's care).

Katie's sister was 6 years old, and her mother worked full time. Katie was on the ventilator 12 hours per day and required pulmonary toilet at least every 4 hours. A nursing time study performed in the hospital demonstrated that Katie needed at least 16 hours of direct nursing care per day as well as continuous monitoring. Ms. M. chose to utilize the 16 hours of nursing care per day with one day shift and one night shift. Katie's mother worked a full 8-hour day, Monday through Friday, and had a half-hour commute to work. Ms. M.'s friend and neighbor elected to care for Katie for the hour each day that the nurse and Ms. M. were not available.

Home nursing care for a ventilator-assisted child can be provided by a registered nurse, a licensed practical nurse, and in some cases, a home health aide. Because of the complexity of Katie's care, the medical staff recommended that registered nurses and licensed practical nurses should provide her care at home. Taking into consideration the long-term plan for Katie's home care funding, the discharge team suggested that Ms. M. choose a Medicaid-certified nursing agency. This would ensure consistency of care for Katie when the funding mechanism changed from the major medical benefit to the state Medicaid waiver program.

Selecting a nursing agency can be a difficult task for a family, but with guidance and support from experienced hospital personnel, the family can feel confident in making an informed decision. The social worker assisted Ms. M. in interviewing nursing agencies. Together they outlined a list of considerations that were important to Ms. M.:

- the nursing agency's experience with the pediatric ventilator-assisted population
- the agency's ability to staff the case to the family's satisfaction
- the experience and qualifications of the agency's nurses
- the agency's policies on notification of and coverage for call-outs and vacations
- the agency's philosophy of nursing care
- the family's ability to maintain autonomy in caring for the child at home

After interviewing four nursing agencies, Ms. M. selected one she felt would best meet the family's needs.

For the discharging institution and the family to be assured that the home care nurses are competent in providing the patient care, it is beneficial that as many of the home care nurses as possible be trained by the patient's primary nurse before discharge. It is important that there be an established teaching plan with specific objectives to promote consistency and maximum benefit from the teaching sessions. Katie's nursing case manager and four home care nurses were trained at the hospital.

HOME ASSESSMENT

Before discharge, it is essential to assess that the child's home environment is safe and appropriate. This is best accomplished with a home visit by the social worker and the primary nurse. The visit also provides an opportunity to assist the family in developing concrete plans for the child's care at home. The family may need guidance with decisions such as where physically to locate the child and her necessary equipment. Ms. M. lived in a small, two-bedroom house

with her 6-year-old daughter, and she had initially planned for Katie to share the room with her sister. The nurse/social work team suggested that the rarely used dining room be converted into a room for Katie. This would afford her sister privacy and the ability to sleep through the night undisturbed by Katie's care. A representative from the DME provider visited the home to assess its electrical capabilities and to determine whether additional outlets were necessary.

DEVELOPMENTAL NEEDS

A complete home care plan for the ventilator-assisted child addresses his or her developmental needs. During the child's hospitalization, he or she will most likely be evaluated by the physical, occupational, and speech therapists. If they recommend continued therapies for the child at home, it is advisable to obtain the prescriptions for the therapies and to register the child for those services in the community before discharge.

It was recommended that Katie receive physical, occupational, and speech therapies each once a week for at least the first 6 months she was home. The social worker informed the case worker for the county office of mental health and mental retardation of Katie's history, developmental needs, and therapy recommendations. The case worker agreed to schedule an appointment with the family once Katie was at home for the assessment and evaluation of speech, physical, and occupational therapies.

EMERGENCY RESOURCES

Last, Ms. M. received assistance in compiling a list of emergency resources. The social worker notified the gas, electric, and phone companies as well as the police, fire, and rescue squad that a child on life-support equipment was being discharged into the community. Katie was identified as a priority by each of these service providers in the event of an emergency or interruption of services. Katie's primary nurse suggested that Ms. M. keep a card by every phone, listing emergency telephone numbers and pertinent information about Katie's medical condition. Ms. M. elected to have a phone placed in Katie's room as an added safety measure.

THE HOME NURSING CARE PLAN

The week before discharge, the nursing agency's case manager met with Ms. M. and Katie's primary nurse to develop the home nursing care plan (Table 25–1). The social worker, primary nurse, and agency case manager addressed with Ms. M. the realities of home care for a family with a ventilator-assisted child.

Ms. M. and her family may experience many new stressors during the first few months of Katie's homecoming. Two of the most frequently identified stresses of home care are the disruption in family lifestyle and the lack of privacy due to the constant flow of personnel through the home. Some families manage this by organizing the home in such a manner that the child's care, and therefore the nursing personnel, are confined to certain areas in the home. For example, if nursing personnel care for the child during the night, the child's room is optimally located distant from the family bedrooms. This will foster a maximal degree of privacy for the parents and isolate the rest of the family from the disturbance of the frequent alarms.

Another lifestyle change that families often experience is a sense of social isolation and alienation from friends and family. Parents are unable to partake in social activities because they are often confined to the home to care for their child. Friends and relatives may feel inadequate to assist the parents in caring for their family. It can be difficult for parents to alter nursing shifts or arrange for a skilled caregiver to watch the child when they wish to attend a social event.

Management issues may create added stress on the family. Once the child is home, the role of patient advocate is transferred from the inpatient primary nurse to the parent(s). It is the responsibility of the parents to communicate with the home care nurses, physicians, case managers, therapists, and so forth to ensure the safety and welfare of the child. Parents may feel overwhelmed with providing the day-to-day care and coordinating services. To alleviate some of this stress, some families have learned to delegate responsibilities as part of their management strategy. A primary nurse or night nurse may be given the job of taking inventory and reordering supplies.

Cost containment within the home care setting should be addressed with the family before discharge. In the hospital, disposable items are used once and discarded to reduce the risk of contamination and the incidence of nosocomial infections. During the daily routine, hospital personnel give little thought to the cost of those items. Families with limited home care funds do not have that luxury. Educating the family and other caregivers about supply costs, cleaning, disinfection, and reuse of certain supplies can greatly affect the expenditure of home care dollars.

While discussing fiscal matters, it is important to emphasize the financial implications that the home care setting will have for the family. Uncovered nursing shifts may necessitate that a parent remain at home, therefore missing work and possibly losing wages. Also, the family's utility bills can be expected to increase once the technology-dependent child is home. It is not unusual for the electricity bill to double. Some families have benefited from enrolling in their local electric company's budget payment plan.

The homecoming of a ventilator-assisted child may have a great impact on siblings. Often the child has been hospitalized for a long period of time, and the siblings may not identify the child as a brother or sister. Also, the demanding nature of the child's illness and care may leave a sibling feeling jealous and neglected. These feelings may be exhibited as anger, depression, somatic complaints, behavior disorders, nightmares, and general disequilibrium. Parents, relatives, and health care professionals can assist the sibling(s) in adjusting to the myriad changes that the home care setting brings by including them

Table 25–1 Home Care Plan

Problem	Goals	Assessments	Interventions
Alteration in respiratory status secondary to tracheostomy and need for mechanical ventilation.	Katie will have a patent airway and adequate respiratory function.	Observe Katie for signs of respiratory distress: Restlessness Nasal flaring Retractions Cyanosis Tachypnea	1. Maintain patent #2 Portex tracheostomy tube at all times: • Suction every 2 hours and as needed. • Provide humidification via ventilator. • Change tracheostomy tube weekly (Wednesdays). 2. Maintain ventilator settings as ordered. Maintain humidifier temperature at 30° to 34°C. Empty water traps as needed.
	Katie will eventually be weaned from respiratory support during the day.	Check ventilator settings (rate, inspiratory pressure, oxygen, dial volume, alarms).	3. When going outside on a trip, always take emergency travel bag. This should include: • Tracheostomy tube with strings • Endotracheal tube • Portable suction with suction catheters • Resuscitation bag • K-Y jelly • Saline • Scissors and hemostat
Potential for respiratory infections secondary to tracheostomy.	Katie will be free of respiratory infections and atelectasis.	Assess breath sounds every 4 hours. Observe for signs and symptoms of respiratory infection: change in amount, color, odor, consistency of secretions; decreased aeration; fever; chest congestion; fatigue.	1. Follow good hand washing techniques. Always wash hands before tracheostomy care. 2. Daily tracheostomy care: • Clean tracheostomy site with water (half strength peroxide if crusted). • Change tracheostomy dressing twice daily and as needed. • Change tracheostomy strings every morning and as needed. • Change tracheostomy tube weekly (Wednesdays) with sterile technique and two caregivers. 3. Chest percussion every 4 hours while awake. Instilled 1–2 mL normal saline as needed for thick secretions. 4. Maintain clean technique during suctioning: every 1 to 2 hours while awake, every 4 to 6 hours while asleep. 5. Change disposable ventilator tubing every 3 days (on night shift). 6. Change and disinfect cascade humidifier and nondisposable ventilator parts every 3 days (night shift).
Impaired gas exchange related to respiratory disorder.	Katie will maintain normal gas exchange.	Assess for symmetric chest wall movement and bilateral breath sounds. Monitor heart rate, respiratory rate and oxygen saturation level.	1. Ventilate Katie using a hand-held resuscitation bag if she has signs and symptoms of hypoxia.

Table 25–1 continued

Problem	Goals	Assessments	Interventions
Alteration in growth and development secondary to diagnosis and prolonged hospitalization.	Katie will increase her developmental skills and reach age-appropriate developmental milestones.	Assess developmental skills.	2. Encourage Katie to be independent: Allow her to feed herself, assist in dressing herself. 3. Follow posted daily schedule for activities. 4. Provide play time and encourage development skills. • Gross motor: Encourage full use of upper extremities. Provide passive range of motion exercises to lower extremities, follow prescribed leg and foot splint schedule. • Fine motor: Encourage use of crayons, blocks, etc. • Speech: Encourage Katie to vocalize around tracheostomy. Katie knows some sign language. 5. Speak to Katie about her environment. Introduce new things she has not had the opportunity to experience while in the hospital. Follow through on speech therapist recommendations. 6. Katie will receive physical, occupational, and speech therapy each once per week.
Alteration in nutritional status secondary to poor oral intake and new environment.	Katie will gain weight.	Weigh weekly.	1. Provide high-calorie, high-protein meals with three snacks at 10 A.M., 2 P.M., and bedtime. 2. Allow Katie to eat with the family, sitting at the table in a highchair. Provide favorite foods. 3. Encourage Katie to use a cup. Do not give her a bottle until after meals.
Potential alteration in family functioning secondary to child's prolonged hospitalization and complex needs.	Katie will become an active family member. The M's will be an intact family unit.	Assess family for signs of stress.	1. Allow time for individual attention to Katie and her sister by mother. 2. Encourage Katie and her sister to play together. 3. Provide time for Ms. M. to go out by herself. 4. Provide time for family to socialize as a unit. 5. Allow Katie's sister to participate in Katie's care. 6. Maintain familiar routines for children.

Source: Andrea Gendelman.

whenever appropriate in activities and care, patiently answering their questions, displaying genuine interest in their own activities and achievements, allowing the siblings to spend time together, avoiding displacement of the siblings from their own bedrooms, and maintaining continuity of familiar routines.

CONCLUSION

Experience has shown that, with careful planning, thorough education of the parents and caregivers, and coordination of community resources, a safe and successful discharge for the ventilator-assisted child can be accomplished.

REFERENCES

Parra, M. May 2003. Nursing and respite care. Services for ventilator-assisted children. *Caring* XXII(5): 6–9.

Speer, K. 1999. *Pediatric care planning.* 3rd ed. Springhouse, PA: Springhouse Publishers.

PART IV

Quality Assessment and Improvement

CHAPTER 26

Performance Improvement

Joan Reynolds Yuan

Performance improvement (PI) in home care has evolved from a long series of efforts to monitor and evaluate quality of patient care services. Providers of health care have long been interested in monitoring the quality of patient care services. Around the turn of the century, implicit review was used to investigate morbidity and mortality rates after certain medical procedures or inpatient stays. The next development was audits of the medical record: specific criteria were established and defined, and a standard of expected compliance was determined. Closed records were reviewed for compliance with the predetermined standard, and results were reported to the organization's leaders. This process had no priority setting for problem resolution.

The next evolution, quality assurance through monitoring and evaluation, occurred in a planned and systematic manner. An organization's scope of care was determined by identification of the types of services provided and the types of patients served. Aspects of care were identified and included referral, care planning, treatment procedures, administration of medications, and discharge planning. Clinical indicators were developed and thresholds for evaluation established; if the threshold was not reached, there was no problem. The most common source used to obtain data was the patient record. If the threshold was reached, an opportunity for improvement occurred. Corrective action was taken, and after an appropriate time interval, compliance with the indicator was again evaluated. If the problem was resolved, the cycle was finished; if not, a new plan for resolution was developed.

Although this system was clearly an improvement over chart audits, there were some basic deficits in the process. The establishment of thresholds needed to be realistic and reasonable. For example, a threshold of 85 percent or 90 percent might have been set unless a clinical event would result in serious difficulties or death, such as administration of the wrong drug or extravasation of a vesicant chemotherapeutic agent. The tacit understanding, therefore, was that 10 percent or 15 percent of the time it was all right not to comply with the indicator. In addition, priorities were not established for correction of problems.

Over the last decade, several things have happened that have paved the way for PI in home care. Cost containment strategies—including prospective payment, capitation, and managed care—have shifted health care from institutions to the home. As home care has grown, organizations have faced increased scrutiny and demands for accountability. A need exists to examine outcomes as well as those elements that improve patient care while being cost effective. The degree to which a home care organization carries out its key processes and functions will influence its outcomes (Joint Commission on Accreditation of Healthcare Organizations

This chapter is updated from a chapter written by Nancy Bohnet for the *Handbook of Home Health Care Administration*, 2nd edition (1997).

[JCAHO], 1995). Experts such as W. Edwards Deming (1986), Juran (1989), and Crosby (1984) have promoted quality in American industry for more than a decade. Deming's 14 points for the provision of quality products/services, Juran's quality trilogy (quality planning, quality control, and quality improvement), and Crosby's steps for top-down quality management are all adaptable to health care in general and home care specifically.

The experts all agree that an organization must understand its key functions and processes, measure quality, and build quality into the functions and processes. A home care function is a group of processes with a common goal; a process is a series of goal-directed activities (JCAHO, 1995). For example, patient assessment is a function, whereas obtaining the information about the patient's medication profile is a process. Leadership is a function within an organization, and driving the quality improvement activities is a process.

For an organizational philosophy of quality to be implemented, the leadership must be committed to it. The leadership has the responsibility to improve the system, "to make it possible, on a continuing basis, for everybody to do a better job with greater satisfaction" (Deming, 1986, p. 249). Leaders are responsible for setting the tone for a nonpunitive, respectful environment. Education must be provided to help employees understand improvement techniques and statistical measurement. Those who are to investigate processes and devise ways to improve them must be given the opportunity to do so. Leaders have to be involved at all levels of PI by understanding organizational processes and providing resources for improvement activities in terms of time, people, and information systems.

A different type of leadership is required for PI, one that understands that people must work together both within and across departments and that the people who do the work are in the best position to offer improvement suggestions. Therefore, staff from the entire organization must be involved in improvement activities

(Bohnet, 1995). Not only must the leaders understand the importance of organizational commitment, they must educate the next level down, one level at a time, until every employee has a basic knowledge of PI. Improving quality increases productivity because less time is spent redoing, repairing, and inspecting. When processes are studied, opportunities for streamlining and improvement are often found. An important question to ask is: Do all steps in the process add value to the product or service? Streamlining processes is critical to meeting the needs of the customer for quicker service at lower cost. Additionally, a well-designed process increases work satisfaction (Scholtes et al., 2002).

INITIATION AND IMPLEMENTATION

There are several stages in putting a PI program in place. The first stage, initiation, requires the leaders to study the principles of PI, to educate the managers under them, to identify key functions of the organization, and to develop a quality vision statement. This vision will help everyone understand the commitment to quality and will serve as an organizational guideline during the transition to and actual adoption of PI (Bohnet et al., 1993).

The next stage is implementation, whereby management establishes priorities for examining certain key functions that can be improved. Project teams are chosen, and the work begins. Teams need more specific education about PI (e.g., PI principles, philosophy, and teamwork). Teams must understand the goal for their group's work and should have basic guidelines for productive meetings. Every group should have a leader who understands the process being investigated, as well as a facilitator. The leader prepares and distributes an agenda (an essential item) for each meeting, and the facilitator keeps the meeting on track and on time, also reminding the group of its stated goal and progress toward it. Minutes must be taken for each meeting to record discussions, assignments, and progress. They serve also as a review for the next meeting. Each meeting should be evaluated by the team, and then the next meeting's agenda can be prepared (Scholtes et al., 2002). The first projects undertaken should be relatively simple and quickly implemented. This early win strategy will help gain employee buy-in and familiarize the teams and leaders with the PI process.

In addition to education about PI principles and philosophy, PI tools must be taught to the team as needed. Basic tools used to identify, analyze, and solve problems include brainstorming, multivoting, cause-and-effect diagrams, flow charts, run charts, control charts, histograms, and Pareto charts.

Brainstorming

This technique is used to generate as many ideas as possible in a short period of time. It is important to expand thinking to include all of the dimensions of a problem or solution. Brainstorming is commonly used to identify causes of a problem. The following techniques are useful (Scholtes et al., 2002, pp. 4–14):

1. State the ground rules of the session: No idea is to be criticized or judged, no discussion, don't hold back ideas, hitchhike, or build on the ideas generated.
2. Review the topic to ensure understanding of the issues.
3. Allow several minutes for the group members to gather their thoughts in silence.
4. Call out ideas either as they occur or by turn around the group.
5. Write all ideas on a flip chart for easy visualization.

Multivoting

Multivoting provides a way to determine the most popular items from a list. It is often done after a brainstorming session to identify items needing immediate attention. Following are guidelines to conducting a multivote (Scholtes et al., 2002, pp. 4–15):

1. Number each item on the list.
2. Combine two or more items if the group agrees that they are similar.
3. Renumber items if needed.
4. Have participants choose several items to be addressed and write the numbers on a piece of paper. Select a number of items equal to at least one-third of the total number of items.
5. Tally the votes by a show of hands when each number is called out.
6. Reduce the list by eliminating items with the fewest votes.

Cause-and-Effect Diagrams

This type of diagram helps teams picture a large number of possible causes of a specific outcome (Figure 26–1). Cause-and-effect, fishbone, or Ishikawa diagrams are developed to illustrate causes affecting a process. The problem or condition, the effect, is stated on the right of the diagram. The causes are categorized on the left. In the service sector, it may be useful to categorize using the 4Ps: people, procedures, policies, and plant (such as equipment) (Brassard and Ritter, 1994, p. 25). An example of the use of this tool would be listing the causes of barriers to the implementation of a congestive heart failure (CHF) guideline (Figure 26–2).

Flow Charts

Processes must be understood to be improved. Flow charts depict sequential steps in a process. This enables a team to identify redundancies and misunderstandings and guides the team in creating a more systematic and efficient process. For example, a patient is admitted to home care as illustrated in Figure 26–3. Simple shapes are used for different aspects of the process: ovals for start and end, diamonds for decisions, rectangles for steps, and circles for holding the process (Brassard and Ritter, 1994, p. 57).

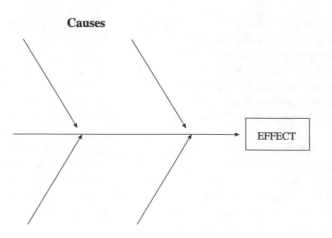

Figure 26–1 Cause-and-Effect Diagram

Run Charts

This type of tool allows a team to look for patterns or trends over time. Patterns of referrals from a particular hospital are depicted in Figure 26–4 as an example. It has a *y* axis (vertical), which indicates a unit of measurement, and an *x* axis (horizontal), which indicates a time or sequence. It is used to monitor a process to see if the average is changing. When monitoring a process, it is expected that an equal number of points will fall above and below the average. A

trend of six or more points steadily increasing or decreasing would not be expected to happen by chance, and would indicate the need to investigate (Brassard and Ritter, 1994, p. 144).

Control Charts

These are run charts with the mean and one to three standard deviations above and below the mean calculated and with upper and lower limits determined. These limits show whether a process is in statistical control. According to

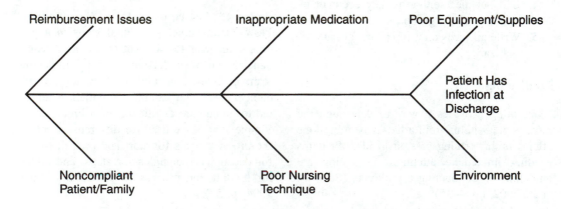

Figure 26–2 Application of a Cause-and-Effect Diagram to a Specific Problem

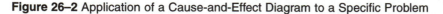

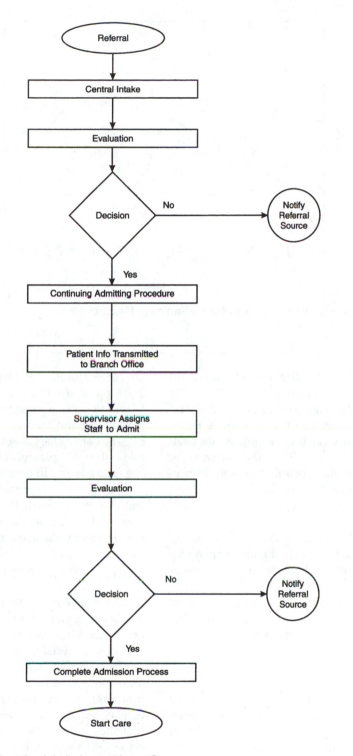

Figure 26–3 Flow Chart for Admission to Home Care

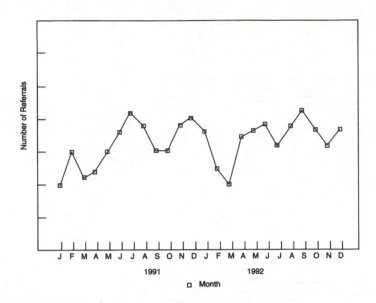

Figure 26–4 Run Chart for Referrals from a Particular Hospital

Deming (1986), "statistical control is a state of random variation, stable in the sense that the limits of variation are predictable" (p. 354). He advises that once statistical control is established, then work can begin to improve the quality (Deming, 1986, p. 354). The run chart for referrals becomes a control chart with the necessary calculations (Figure 26–5).

Histograms

The histogram, a vertical bar graph, displays the frequency with which events occur. It reveals the amount of variation that a process has (Brassard and Ritter, 1994, p. 66). Frequent patient diagnoses in a home care organization are shown as a histogram in Figure 26–6.

Pareto Charts

A Pareto chart is a form of vertical bar graph with the height of the bars arranged in descending order from left to right. The height of the bar reflects the frequency or impact of the problem. The name of this tool is derived from the Pareto Principle: 80 percent of the trouble stems from 20 percent of the problems (Scholtes et al., 2002, pp. 2–20). If the home care organization wishes to develop patient teaching tools for the most common diagnoses, a Pareto chart is useful. The Pareto chart shown in Figure 26–7 indicates that 57 percent of all patients have congestive heart failure and diabetes. This indicates the need to concentrate on those areas first and that more than half the patients in home care will benefit from the work involved in generating patient education materials.

VARIATION AND BENCHMARKING

An important consideration when one is analyzing data is variation. Variation exists in every aspect of the things we do as well as in nature. All variation is caused: A person's weight goes up or down daily, as does his or her performance. Variation is a main factor in the unreliability of a process. "Every process has variation in its outputs because it has variation in its inputs" (Scholtes et al., 2002, pp. 2–21). Common cause variation is the ever-present fluctuation in processes. Special cause correlates with something happening out of the ordinary: snow

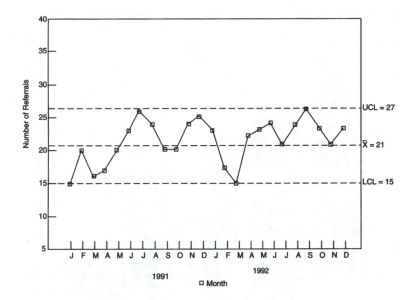

Figure 26–5 Control Chart for Referrals from a Particular Hospital

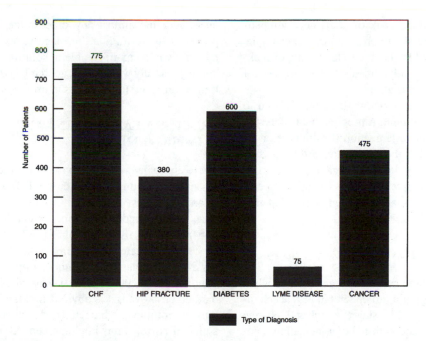

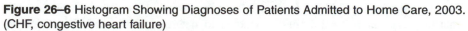

Figure 26–6 Histogram Showing Diagnoses of Patients Admitted to Home Care, 2003. (CHF, congestive heart failure)

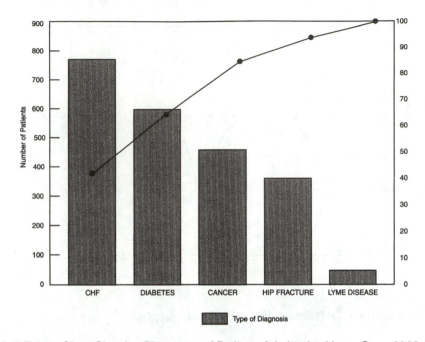

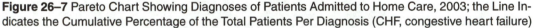

Figure 26–7 Pareto Chart Showing Diagnoses of Patients Admitted to Home Care, 2003; the Line Indicates the Cumulative Percentage of the Total Patients Per Diagnosis (CHF, congestive heart failure)

storms, tornadoes, lack of staff, new competition, or closure of a referral source, for example. Variation may also be due to tampering or making unnecessary adjustments to compensate for common cause variation.

Benchmarking is one method that is used to achieve improvement. A process that is done the best by another organization (health care or industry) is used as the model standard for performance. Learning how an organization carries out its process so well makes it possible to emulate that performance by matching what that organization does.

ACCELERATION

After two to three processes are examined when people are beginning to understand PI, acceleration occurs. At this stage, a cultural change slowly takes place within the organization. People begin to believe that they have good ideas for improvement, that they can make a real differ-ence, and that almost any process can be improved. It is exciting at this stage to see people taking ownership of problem solutions. Most employees truly want to do a good job and are delighted that their input results in improvement.

PROCESS MEASUREMENT AND IMPROVEMENT

There are many systems devised for process assessment and improvement: the PDCA cycle (plan, do, check, and act), FOCUS (find, organize, clarify, understand, and select [or solution]), and the five-stage plan (understand the process, eliminate errors, remove slack, reduce variation, and plan for continuous improvement; Scholtes et al., 2002, pp. 5–9). Regardless of the method employed, it is obvious that the process must be completely dissected and studied before a plan of correction is implemented. After a sufficient time period elapses, the process must be studied to determine whether it has been improved, has stayed at an improved level without slipping, or has other improvement opportunities. According to JCAHO (2002) data are analyzed to judge if design specifications for processes were met; performance expectations for processes were stable; opportunities for improvement existed; action was taken to improve the process; and changes to the process resulted in improvement (p. PI-10).

Measurement is important in PI. The guesses and estimates that often determine management decisions become obsolete. Measurement and the use of statistical tools are used to improve decision making when analyzing processes. "Decisions based on fact have always outperformed decisions based on hunch or empirical judgment" (Juran, 1989, p. 278).

Home care is rich in processes that may be examined and improved. Referrals, admissions, documentation, and billing are aspects of patient care that may be problematic. Reducing redundancies and errors helps increase productivity and drive down costs. Other areas that can be improved include management/billing of supplies, inventory control, billing, and delivery. Obtaining signed orders and laboratory results is important and may not be done in a timely manner. The delay may result in tardy billing or patient record discharge. Staff issues may also be improved, such as weekend and holiday rotation and on-call nursing coverage. Potential problem areas of patient care include care planning, treatment procedures, medication administration, infection control, and care coordination (Bohnet et al., 1993).

CONCLUSION

PI must be driven by top management personnel who must understand an organization's key processes. It involves workers across departments and necessitates the use of tools and statistics. It will work in health care as well as it has in industry. As home care organizations attempt to serve patients better and compete more effectively, many will design or redesign their services to be more efficient, to be attentive to customer expectations, and to improve patient outcomes (JCAHO, 1994). Total quality will be the way to differentiate among health care organizations. Prices will be equal, so that the quality and value of service will distinguish organizations. As consumers evaluate the effectiveness of your services through the outcomes displayed on the Home Health Compare Web site (http://www.medicare.gov/HHCompare/Home.asp) know that the way to improve outcomes is found in process improvement inherent in the outcome-based quality improvement (OBQI) methodology.

REFERENCES

Bohnet, N., et al. 1993. Continuous quality improvement: Improving quality in your home care organization. *Journal of Nursing Administration* 23: 42–48.

Bohnet, N. 1995. Continuous quality improvement in home care. In *Core Curriculum for Home Health Care Nursing*, K. Morgan and S. McClain (eds.). Gaithersburg, MD: Aspen.

Brassard, M., and D. Ritter. 1994. *The memory jogger II*. Salem, NH: GOAL/QPC.

Crosby, P. 1984. *Quality without tears: The art of hassle-free management.* New York: McGraw-Hill.

Deming, W. E. 1986. *Out of the crisis*. Cambridge, MA: Massachusetts Institute of Technology Center for Advanced Engineering Study.

Joint Commission on Accreditation of Healthcare Organizations. 1994. *Forms, charts and other tools for perfor-mance improvement*. Oakbrook Terrace, IL: Joint Commission.

Joint Commission on Accreditation of Healthcare Organizations. 1995. *Framework for improving performance: A guide for home care and hospice organizations*. Oakbrook Terrace, IL: Joint Commission.

Joint Commission on Accreditation of Healthcare Organizations. 2002. *2003 comprehensive accreditation manual for home care*. Oakbrook Terrace, IL: Author.

Juran, J. 1989. *Juran on leadership for quality: An executive handbook*. New York: The Free Press.

Scholtes, P., et al. 2002. *The team handbook,* 2nd ed. Madison, WI: Oriel Incorporated.

CHAPTER 27

Evidence-Based Practice: Basic Strategies for Success

Lazelle E. Benefield

Editor's Note:
The emphasis on best practices based on evidence and research is an increasing focus in all areas of healthcare. This movement has reached home care and is a concept clinicians must understand and apply to their practice. To assist our readers in learning the basics of this concept, this article launches a series of articles to be published in HHN during 2003. Dr. Lazelle Benefield, a researcher, faculty member, and HHN editorial board member, has agreed to coordinate this article series.

—Carolyn J. Humphrey

The integration of the comprehensive assessment using OASIS and examining care outcomes using OBQI has left clinicians' heads spinning. The care provided between assessment and outcomes-interventions has not been closely examined. That is soon to change. This article provides clinicians with an overview of how using best evidence can assist in making up-to-date clinical interventions. Evidence reports and sources to reference best evidence to improve clinical decision making are outlined.

Evidence-based practice is defined as *using the best evidence available to guide clinical decision making.* The expected outcome of this type of practice is improved quality of care and outcomes. Clinicians use evidence reports to "provide a scientific basis for a topic" and then "tie this basis with the clinical realities of practice" (personal communication, CINAHL Information Systems, *Online Journal of Clinical Innovations,* July 26, 2002).

Evidence reports include knowledge synthesis, review, and documentation of how evidence-based practices are used in the clinical area, and can include discussion of the clinical relevance and utility of such practices.

Systematic or integrative reviews, sometimes termed *evidence summaries* (Stevens, 2002), are reports that synthesize research knowledge and typically include a review and analysis of the relevant research to support decision making and best practice. These evidence summaries represent the science of evidence-based practice.

Systematic reviews differ from literature reviews in that systematic reviews use *all* relevant literature from multiple sources, published and unpublished, and there is a more rigorous and systematic appraisal and evaluation (Pettigrew, 2001; Stevens, 2002; West et al., 2002).

Clinical practice guidelines or protocols are another form of evidence reports that are developed when scientific knowledge from these systematic reviews are translated into specific approaches to patient care. Clinicians use established and innovative research and change strategies to incorporate clinical guidelines and protocols into daily practice. Therefore, the goal of using evidence reports is to move toward innovations in nursing practice that make "a difference to clients, to clinical practice, or to other problems with disciplinary importance" (per-

Reprinted from *Home Healthcare Nurse* 2002; 20(12): 803–807.

sonal communication, CINAHL Information Systems, *Online Journal of Clinical Innovations,* July 26, 2002).

WHAT IS INCLUDED IN AN EVIDENCE REPORT?

Evidence reports may include a structured summary statement, a lengthy analysis of the published and unpublished data, the level of evidence quality, recommendations for clinical practice, and the report's sponsor or source.

Research Summary Statement: Succinctly describes what the evidence reports (i.e., the core recommendations).

Analysis of the Scientific Data

This section describes:

- review of the various articles and unpublished reports,
- details of the analysis,
- the target populations that were studied,
- the type of clinical interventions investigated, and
- the strength of the individual and/or collective study results.

Level of Evidence Quality

- The *level of evidence,* sometimes called the level of recommendation for use, (Stetler, 2001) ranks the strength and quality of the study findings.
- *Evidence reports* summarize scientific investigations that vary in depth and research rigor, and the level of evidence is graded to help the clinician judge the relative strength and value of the recommendations.
- In an *integrative* or *systematic review,* where the focus is a summary of the research evidence, the research study analysis is comprehensive and systematically developed. *Clinical practice guidelines, protocols,* or *standards* are translated

from research and will **not** include this type and level of analysis.

Recommendations for Practice: In this section look for practice-focused guidelines or recommendations to inform your clinical interventions.

The Report's Source: This includes governmental or private entities or professional associations as well as the date the evidence report was developed and is ready to be used by clinicians.

EVALUATING THE REPORT

Critique an evidence report considering these questions that are unique to your organization:

- Is this the best available evidence? Look for reports in respected and peer-reviewed sources. Reports should be updated every 3 to 5 years.
- Are the recommendations of value to the population with whom I work? For example, is the evidence review directed toward congestive heart failure management in elders? In women?
- How will the recommendations fit with preferences and values of the clients with whom I work? For example, will the evidence on chronic disease management of diabetes work with the Hispanic seniors in my caseload?

HOW TO LOCATE EVIDENCE REPORTS

Use clinical journals, governmental and private entities, and professional nursing and other health-related specialty organizations in print and/or electronic format to find evidence reports (see Internet Resources for Evidence-Based Practice). Journals focused on evidence synthesis include *Evidence-Based Nursing,* the *Online Journal of Clinical Innovations (OJCI),* and *The Online Journal of Knowledge Synthesis for Nursing (OJKSN).* Clinically focused specialty journals such as *Home Healthcare Nurse* report the usefulness of clinical guidelines and discuss the "how to" of translating the evidence to inform practice.

Public and private entities also disseminate evidence reports. The U.S. Agency for Healthcare Research and Quality (AHRQ) supports the National Guideline Clearinghouse, a repository of clinical practice guidelines. The Cochrane Collaboration, an international not-for-profit research organization, also develops and maintains systematic reviews of the effects of healthcare interventions.

Nursing specialty organizations such as the Oncology Nursing Society support and disseminate evidence-based clinical guidelines. Online sources for clinical practice guidelines are also maintained by nursing and health-related colleges. Of note is the "Evidence-Based Nursing and Health Care Resources" clearinghouse site maintained by the State University of New York at Buffalo.

HOW SHOULD EVIDENCE REPORTS AFFECT MY PRACTICE?

Clinicians want to do the right thing. Incorporating best care practices into daily practice improves care effectiveness and efficiency while providing a practice framework that enhances the likelihood of positive outcomes. Using best practices provides tangible benefits to the patient and caregiver. Using practices shown to be effective and taking into account the patient and caregiver values and goals provides increased quality and promotes positive patient and caregiver outcomes.

Using Evidence Reports: Where to Begin

Identify the area(s) where you know an improvement or an update in clinical interventions is needed. Use the following questions to select priority areas:

- What type of clients do I treat most often?
- On what type of diseases and conditions does my agency focus?
- Which are high-volume or high-risk population groups in the agency?

- What causes high stress to patients/caregivers?
- What processes and procedures cause problems? Ask the patient and caregiver to identify where they see a need for improvement; engage the caregiver in this process.
- What is especially labor intensive to staff and/or caregivers?

Finding and Reviewing the Reports

1. Review the evidence-based practice literature for evidence reports on the topic you've identified. Selecting only one topic or issue helps narrow the focus and lets you maintain energy for the project. If needed, use the online resources listed in this article to update your search skills. Many of the online tutorials are very user-friendly, and this effort will increase your speed and comfort in finding relevant information.
2. Use one or more of the online sources listed in this article to retrieve the evidence report.
3. Select an established clinical practice guideline. This may be listed as a clinical pathway, case management protocol, clinical standard, or evidence-based recommendation.
4. Look for a structured report with clinical relevance and clinical utility. The report's clinical utility and directed implications sections must be clear and concise. The report should delineate key implications for practice.

   A reference librarian in a local nursing or medical school can assist, often without charge, in the search and selection of the report. Contact professors in local colleges of nursing, social work, or physical therapy to guide you in assessing the report's strength and validity.
5. Always determine the relevance of the recommendations to your clinical setting and specific patient environment. Remember, integrating best evidence into clinical decision making involves a consistent, goal-directed, and organized ap-

proach to change; agency managers, individual clinicians, and the patient and caregiver are all involved in the process.

SUMMARY

The nurse's role is to "bridge the divide" (Ingersoll, 2000) between research and best evidence and improve clinical interventions. We strive for healthcare to be safe, effective, patient-centered, timely, efficient, and equitable (Institute of Medicine, 2001). Giving the correct care, in the proper amount and at the proper time, increases the likelihood that we can improve patient outcomes.

To make this happen, we must base clinical changes on valid evidence, focus on what works, and concentrate on improving the delivery of clinical care. Selecting and using evidence reports, especially clinical practice guidelines, is a tested and valid first-step method to making improvements in clinical interventions.

INTERNET RESOURCES FOR EVIDENCE-BASED PRACTICE

Journals

Access may involve a per-article retrieval fee or an individual agency subscription to the online journal. Details are noted at each Web site.

Evidence-Based Nursing (http://ebn.bmjjournals.com/)

The general purpose of Evidence-Based Nursing is "to select from the health related literature those articles reporting studies and reviews that warrant im-mediate attention by nurses attempting to keep pace with important advances in their profession. These articles are summarized in 'value added' abstracts and commented on by clinical experts."

The Online Journal of Clinical Innovations (OJCI) (www.cinahl.com)

The *OJCI* contains systematic reviews of the literature concerning problems of clinical interest. The reviews go beyond "traditional boundaries of research literature" to "encompass knowl-edge gleaned from quality improvement litera-ture . . . and clinical reports." *Priority is placed on key implications for practice.*

The Online Journal of Knowledge Synthesis for Nursing(OJKSN) (www.stti.iupui.edu/ VirginiaHendersonLibrary/OJKSNAbout .aspx)

"OJKSN presents current scientific evidence to inform clinical decisions and ongoing discussions on issues, methods, clinical practice, and teaching strategies for EBP. The journal's purpose is to provide prominent and authoritative evidence supporting clinical decisions and consumer choices in nursing care and to provide a forum for advancing evidence-based practice in nursing."

Clearinghouse and Information Resources

Evidence-Based Nursing and Healthcare Resources (http://ublib.buffalo.edu/ libraries/units/hsl/internet/ebn.html)

This clearinghouse, maintained by the State University of New York at Buffalo, includes links to articles on how to review evidence and evidence reports, classifications of clinical practice guidelines, and professional organizations involved in evidence-based research and dissemination. *Highly recommended.*

Evidence-Based Healthcare Resources

University of Rochester Medical Center, Edward G. Miner Library (www.urmc .rochester.edu/Miner/Links/ebmlinks.html)

A set of links to organizations, tutorials, and search tools for evidence-based practice.

National Guideline Clearinghouse (www.guideline.gov)

". . . a public resource for evidence-based clinical practice guidelines." E-mail alerts are available announcing the latest guidelines. *Highly recommended.*

Canadian Task Force on Preventive Health Care Evidence-Based Clinical Prevention (www.ctfphc.org)

". . . a practical guide to health care providers, planners, and consumers for determining the inclusion or exclusion, content, and frequency of a wide variety of preventive health interventions, using the evidence-based recommendations of the Canadian Task Force on Preventive Health Care (CTFPHC)." E-mail alerts are available announcing the latest guidelines.

Guide to Clinical Preventive Service (www.ahrq.gov/clinic/prevnew.htm)

". . . provides the latest available recommendations on preventive interventions: screening tests, counseling, immunizations, and chemoprophylactic regimens for more than 80 conditions. Reviews and recommendations will be released as they are completed. Recommendations are made by the U.S. Preventive Services Task Force."

The Cochrane Collaboration (www.cochrane.org)

". . . preparing, maintaining, and promoting the accessibility of systematic reviews of the effects of health care interventions." The Cochrane Library distributes the Cochrane Database of Systematic Reviews.

CDC Recommends:

The Prevention Guidelines System (www.phppo.cdc.gov/CDCRecommends/ AdvSearchV.asp)

". . . contains up-to-date and archived guidelines and recommendations approved by the U.S. Centers for Disease Control for the prevention and control of disease, injuries, and disabilities."

Oncology Nursing Society (www.ons.org)

Special project "Evidence-Based Practice Resource Center" includes "a guide to using evidence" as well as comprehensive listing of Web-based resources.

Hospice and Palliative Nurses Association (www.hpna.org/about2.asp)

"The purpose is to exchange information, experiences, and ideas; to promote understanding of the specialties of hospice and palliative nursing; and to study and promote hospice and palliative nursing research."

University of Sheffield, UK School of Health and Related Research (www.shef.ac.uk/?scharr/ir/netting)

"Netting the Evidence is intended to facilitate evidence-based healthcare by providing support and access to helpful organisations and useful learning resources, such as an evidence-based virtual library, software, and journals."

Note: All URLs were current as of September 2002.

REFERENCES

Ingersoll, G. 2000. Evidence-based nursing: What it is and what it isn't. *Nursing Outlook*, 48(4): 152.

Institute of Medicine. 2001. Crossing the quality chasm: A new health system for the 21st century. Committee on Quality of Health Care in America, Institute of Medicine. Washington, DC: National Academy Press.

Pettigrew, W. 2001. Systematic reviews from astronomy to zoology: Myths and misconceptions. *British Medical Journal*, 322: 98–101.

Stetler, C. 2001. Updating the Stetler model of research utilization to facilitate evidence-based practice. *Nursing Outlook* 49(6): 272–278.

Stevens, K. 2002. Star model of evidence-based practice. Cycle of knowledge transformation. Academic Center for Evidence-Based Nursing. Retrieved July 20, 2002 from http://www.acestar.uthscsa.edu.

West, S., King, V., Carey, T., Lohr, K., McKoy, N., Sutton, S., et al. 2002. Systems to rate the strength of scientific evidence. Evidence Report/Technology Assessment No. 47 (Prepared by the Research Triangle Institute-University of North Carolina Evidenced-Based Practice Center under Contract # 290-97-0011). Pub No. 02-C016. Rockville, MD: Agency for Healthcare Research and Quality.

CHAPTER 28

Quality Planning for Quality Patient Care

Marilyn D. Harris and Joan Reynolds Yuan

Home care in the 21st century presents many challenges for administrators, caregivers, and patients. It is an era characterized by an aging population, high cost of health care, high-technology care, consumers who are disgruntled with the health care system, organizations grappling with a changing environment, an increased number of case management programs, and resultant fiscal constraints. How do the administrators of a home care organization ensure that quality health care services are being provided, and why should they care? Nursing is a key service in most skilled home care organizations. Nursing, being an art as well as a science, is known for its caring function. Caring has been described as nursing's central moral ideal (Pater and Gallop, 1994). This professional care and caring must be evident in the design and implementation of the quality program and the quality assessment/performance improvement (QA/PI) plan.

A quality program may be shaped by the Juran (1989) trilogy of processes: quality planning, quality control or quality assurance in nursing peer review activities, and quality improvement. *Quality planning* refers to the activity of developing products or processes required to meet customers' needs. *Quality control* (quality assurance) is a process that evaluates quality performance, compares actual performance with quality goals, and acts on the differences. *Quality improvement* is a process of raising quality performance to unprecedented levels.

Deming (1982) writes in response to the question "How do you go about improving quality and productivity?" that "Best efforts are essential. Unfortunately, best efforts, people charging this way and that way without guidance of principles, can do a lot of damage. Think of the chaos that would come if everyone did his best not knowing what to do" (p. 19). Deming advises that a constancy of purpose needs to be created toward the improvement of products and services. It is the responsibility of the leaders to identify areas that need improvement.

Although quality improvement is a process that utilizes scientific tools, quality planning or choosing quality improvement projects involves not only science, but also caring. Some quality programs are designed with a heavy emphasis on inspection of areas that may have no relevance to the customer. The development of a quality plan is not for the paper chase. In an attempt to ensure the quality and appropriateness of care, the quality program must have clinical relevance and be meaningful to the customer. Often in nursing, it has been said that things would change if the congressperson's mother were the recipient of care. This idea can be applied to the design of a quality plan. Quality takes on a different dimension when it makes a difference in the care provided. We should ask this question when the quality plan is designed: "Would I want my mother to receive care from this organization, and how can I make sure that

316 HANDBOOK OF HOME HEALTH CARE ADMINISTRATION

she would receive what she needs?" The quality plan that is designed with care and a constancy of purpose must be meaningful and workable. In 2004, the administration must be committed to the quality plan that includes the measurement of patient outcomes.

Consumers can share their thoughts on caregivers, attitudes, and perceptions of competency through formal questionnaires or unsolicited letters, but organizations cannot depend on consumers to identify technical problems. Administration has an important role in the structure of the quality program. Crosby (1984) states that senior management is 100 percent responsible for problems with quality and their continuance.

PROFESSIONAL STANDARDS

The American Nurses Association's *Scope and Standards for Nurse Administrators,* Standard 1, Quality of Care and Administrative Practice (ANA, 1996) states that "the nurse administrator systematically evaluates the quality and effectiveness of nursing practice and nursing services administration (p. 17). The ANA (1999) *Scope and Standards of Home Health Nursing Practice*, Standard 1, Quality of Care states that "the home health nurse systematically evaluates the quality and effectiveness of nursing practice" (p. 13). The measurement criteria for the nurse administrator include (p. 17):

- Identifies key quality indicators for monitoring and evaluation
- Analyzes data and information to identify opportunities for improving services, using appropriate internal and external data
- Develops, implements, and evaluates systems and processes that complement the overall system for performance improvement
- Participates in interdisciplinary evaluation teams

The ANA Code of Ethics for Nurses (2001), Provision 7 states that the nurse participates in the advancement of the profession through contributions to practice, education, administration, and knowledge development (p. 22). Home care administrators have the overall responsibility to establish practice standards in their own agencies and to participate actively in the profession's ongoing efforts to foster optimal standards of practice at the local, regional, state, and national levels.

The collection and analysis of nursing data are essential components of managing and providing high-quality home health care in the 21st century. There is a role for each member of the staff of the agency in this process in data collection, development of protocols, or involvement in the implementation of newly published guidelines and protocols. It must be remembered that data collection represents more than just statistics. There is the human side of data collection, the actual benefits to patients and their families as a result of these findings. This aspect of the QA/PI process is brought to life through the words of Doris Schwartz, author of *Give Us to Go Blithely* (1995). Schwartz was honored in 1994 with the Lillian D. Wald Spirit of Nursing Award. In a letter reflecting on her many experiences, Schwartz (1994) recalls that one of her former students talked with her at this awards ceremony and reminded her that she taught epidemiology. The former student related that she hated the idea of math because she did not see its relevance to patient care. What this student remembered Schwartz stating was "We can all rejoice in the statistics that show that infant deaths in our district were reduced last year by six-tenths of a percent, but as caregivers, we need to remember that no mother ever lost six-tenths of a baby." These words put statistics into perspective and present the reality associated with what would otherwise be only numbers.

Too often, quality planning, quality assurance, and quality improvement take second place to putting out the fires. It seems prudent to utilize scarce resources to plan, monitor, and design mechanisms to improve the organization's performance. Administration must be committed to establishing a system to track, evaluate, and improve care. Quality as conformance to requirements is therefore specific and lends credence to the need to meet professional standards (e.g., the ANA's standards for home health [1999]) and to conform to and implement these standards as well as Agency for Health Care Policy and Research (AHCPR), now the Agency for Healthcare Research and Quality (AHRQ). guidelines (DHHS, 1992a, 1992b, 1992c).

ACCREDITATION AND CERTIFICATION CONSIDERATIONS

Quality improvement continues to receive attention at the national level. The Joint Commission on Accreditation of Healthcare Organizations' *2003 Comprehensive Accreditation Manual for Home Care* (2002) includes a chapter titled "Improving Organization Performance." It states "the goal of the Improving Organization Performance function is to design processes well and systematically monitor, analyze, and improve patient outcomes. Essential processes include designing processes; analyzing and monitoring current performance; improving and sustaining improved performance" (PI-1). This approach does not leave anything to chance or subscribe to the attitude "I'll do it when I have time!" Administrative commitment, professional and support staff, time, and dollars are required to have a successful program.

Several years ago the Health Care Financing Administration, now the Center for Medicare and Medicaid Services (CMS), released a draft of proposed revisions to the home health Medicare conditions of participation (COPs) that proposed the elimination of two existing COPs, 484.16 Group of Professional Personnel and 484.52 Evaluation of Agency's Programs, and replacing them with a single, new quality assessment and performance improvement COP. The release of the proposed revisions is scheduled for 2004 after this textbook went to press. Readers must obtain current information through the government Web site (http://www.access.gpo.gov/nara/cfr) and through state and national health care organizations.

PI must be an integral part of home health care each day; this can be accomplished through various methods. During a presentation at the annual meeting of the National Association for Home Care, one of the speakers noted that it is not unusual for 10 years to elapse from the introduction of national standards to their implementation. In light of the national guidelines that have been published, would you want your Congressperson's (or your) mother to receive home health care through an agency that implemented the guidelines in 1 to 2 years or that waited 10 years or more?

IMPLEMENTING GUIDELINES: ONE AGENCY'S EXPERIENCE

The AHCPR (now AHRQ) was established in 1989 by Congress to improve the quality and effectiveness of health care and access to care. At the Abington Memorial Hospital Home Care (AMHHC), each staff nurse received a copy of the AHCPR guidelines for urinary incontinence in adults (DHHS, 1992a, 1992b, 1992c) immediately after they were published in 1992, plus several other guidelines. In 1994, a PI indicator was included in the PI plan, and a PI team was formed to examine the issues of urinary incontinence and Foley catheter use among patients admitted for home care, because urinary incontinence is prevalent in American adults. Also, Foley catheters used for incontinence management are a significant source of urinary tract infections, sepsis, and mortality.

The first phase of the AMHHC's PI effort was the attainment of 100 percent compliance with all instructions related to the care of a Foley catheter for all patients with an indwelling catheter. After this goal had been attained for a 6-month period, the next phase was put in place to assess each patient to determine whether he or she meets the AHCPR guidelines for use of a Foley catheter. This phase included ongoing educational programs for all nursing staff, development of an improved history and physical assessment form (which includes space to record the results of dipstick urinalysis), development of a refined standardized flow sheet for documentation and patient teaching tools, and mailing of an informational letter to all staff and nonstaff referring physicians to advise them of the AMHHC's process to implement the national guidelines for urinary incontinence. This notice to the physicians of the AMHHC's plans was vitally important because their assistance and cooperation are needed in providing patient and family education when a Foley catheter is requested by the patient or family in an attempt to control incontinence but is not the treatment of choice for numerous reasons. Data collection at the AMHHC during 1994 for this population showed that the AMHHC sample closely mirrored the national data. Based on these AMHHC data, the administrative staff are able to measure goal attainment for those AMHHC patients who meet the AHCPR guidelines during each year.

BENCHMARKING

It was important to document improvements and positive outcomes for the AMHHC patients. It was and continues to be beneficial to benchmark against other home health agencies. Benchmarking is a continuous process of comparison, projection, and implementation. It involves comparing your organization with others, discovering and projecting best trends in practices, and meeting and exceeding the expectations of those watching you (Wilson, 2004). Departments can compare performance and practices against those of departments or organizations that have similar characteristics and are identified as best performers. Davis (1994) states that benchmarking opens windows to new ideas and ways of doing business. It highlights the gap between what is and what is possible.

Since 1994, staff at the AMHHC have been involved in an annual benchmarking process as one of the hospital's departments. The administrative staff of each department was asked to identify costs, productivity, and statistics by cost centers for their department. These data were shared with the outside benchmarking organization, which input data into its national database. After the accuracy of these reports was verified, a report was generated that lists other home health care and hospice departments/organizations nationwide that were similar in characteristics and were identified as best performers. The administrative staff reviewed these reports, identified gaps and opportunities for improvement, and developed written questions that were shared with those home care and hospice agencies across the country that agreed to share their information. This process provided for follow-up telephone calls among agency administrative staff to explore answers to specific questions that helped clarify or explain variations in costs, staffing, visit time, and productivity. Once these relationships were established, there was sharing of clinical as well as administrative information.

CONCLUSION

There must be a constancy of purpose to ensure that home health care patients receive quality care. Nursing leaders are obligated to design a quality plan that will measure outcomes and ensure that certification, accreditation, and national, state, professional, and agency standards and guidelines are met. There must also be a commitment to improved quality of care when standards are not met in their agency or when there are opportunities to raise the standards after comparison with the performance of other home care agencies through the benchmarking process.

The development of a quality plan and the related QA/PI activities is vital to quality patient care. This quality focus must also be the very essence of the home health agency's business plan to meet the needs of the myriad customers, who include physicians and third-party payers as well as patients and families. Quality planning for quality patient care will enable administrators to face and meet the multiple challenges in the competitive environment that exists in the 21st century.

REFERENCES

American Nurses Association. 1985 to 2001. *Code of ethics for nurses with interpretative statements.* Kansas City, MO: ANA.

American Nurses Association. 1991. *Standards for organized nursing service.* Washington, DC: ANA.

American Nurses Association 1999. *Scope and standards for nurse adminsitrators.* Washington, DC: ANA, p. 17.

American Nurses Association. 1999. *Standards for home health nursing practice.* Kansas City, MO: ANA.

Crosby, P. 1984. *Quality without tears. The art of hassle-free management.* New York: Plume.

Davis, R. 1994. *Total quality management for home care.* Gaithersburg, MD: Aspen.

Deming, W. 1982. *Out of the crisis.* Cambridge, MA: MIT Press.

Department of Health and Human Services, Public Health Service, Agency for Health Care Policy and Research. 1992a. *Urinary incontinence in adults. Clinical practice guidelines* (AHCPR Pub. No. 92-0038). Rockville, MD: DHHS.

Department of Health and Human Services, Public Health Service, Agency for Health Care Policy and Research. 1992b. *Urinary incontinence in adults. A patient's guide* (AHCPR Pub. No. 92-0040). Rockville, MD: DHHS.

Department of Health and Human Services, Public Health Service, Agency for Health Care Policy and Research. 1992c. *Urinary incontinence in adults. Quick reference guide for clinicians* (AHCPR Pub. No. 92-0041). Rockville, MD: DHHS.

Joint Commission on Accreditation of Healthcare Organizations. 2002. *2003 comprehensive accreditation manual for home care.* Oakbrook Terrace, IL: Joint Commission.

Juran, J. 1989. *Juran on leadership for quality. An executive handbook.* New York: Free Press.

Pater, E., and R. Gallop. 1994. The ethic of care: A comparison of nursing and medical students. *Image* 26: 47–51.

Schwartz, D. 1994, March 16. Personal letter.

Schwartz, D. 1995. *My fifty years in nursing: Give us to go blithely.* New York: Springer.

Wilson, A. 2004. Home health care benchmarking. In M. Harris. *Handbook of Home Health Care Administration,* 4th ed., Sudbury, MA: Jones and Bartlett Publishers.

CHAPTER 29

Program Evaluation

Nancy DiPasquale Ruane and Joseph W. Ruane

Program evaluation measures effectiveness, a major concern of home health agencies. It is used to measure the status quo and to project future changes and anticipated agency responses. External and internal constraints and supports influence program evaluations. Information gathering and analysis provide a basis for rational decision making.

DEFINITIONS AND CHARACTERISTICS

Program

A program is a structured set of activities organized to accomplish a goal. It pursues a comprehensive goal with multifaceted objectives utilizing various levels of human potential and resources. A program activates a prearranged plan of operation, which acts as an outline of the work to be done by the organization. The viability and progress of a program rely on the effectiveness of its evaluation.

Evaluation

Evaluation is the process of assessing qualities or characteristics of an individual, an intervention, a program, or an agency as the basis for making a judgment. The emphasis in evaluation is collecting data designed to delineate the relevant, identifying features of factors under study. It involves a systematic process of determining the extent to which the objectives are achieved.

Evaluation starts with quantitative measurement and goes beyond it to include qualitative description and judgment.

The effectiveness of evaluation can be promoted by attention to the following points:

- Evaluation is a process of analysis.
- Evaluation is a means to an end and not an end in itself.
- Evaluation is a method of gathering and processing evidence that may indicate a need for improvement.
- Evaluation clarifies goals and expected outcomes.
- Evaluation is a process of determining the extent to which goals and objectives are met.
- Evaluation is a system of quality control that determines the effectiveness of the program.
- Evaluation must be focused on utilization to identify what changes must be made to ensure the effectiveness of the program (NLN, 1974).
- Evaluation must be credible.
- Evaluation will stimulate ideological, ethical, and political discussion.

An evaluation has a sponsor. This is the person or organization that requests the evaluation and is responsible for its completion. In a home health agency, the sponsor may be the governing body, fulfilling the mandate of certification and accreditation bodies as well as its desire to provide quality services. There is always an audience for an evaluation. Evaluation needs will not go away. Evaluation has become part of the tools of government. Contracts for program assessment will continue to need well-trained researchers (Miller, 2002). More often, federal and state governments and foundations request evaluations for accountability or for new program funding.

Of course, the findings and recommendations are reported to the sponsor, but there are other recipients of the information. The audience varies and may include the program managers and staff, the recipients of the program services, prospective consumers, special interest groups, professional peer groups, and the community served by the agency (Herman et al., 1987).

Evaluation may be formative or summative. Formative evaluation assesses how well the program is going. It is used throughout the duration of the program for the primary purpose of improving the program operation. Formative evaluation helps determine whether the program is moving toward its goals and objectives. It differs from summative evaluation in timing and audience, which are usually the program management and staff. The emphasis is improvement as the program continues. Summative evaluation focuses on assessing the achievement of the goals and objectives of the program. It is done annually, at other specified intervals, or at the conclusion of the program period. Summative evaluation determines whether the goals and objectives of the program have been attained, and it gives feedback for future planning. It looks at the total impact of the program (Breckon, 1982).

Program Evaluation

Program evaluation is a set of methods, skills, and individualized interpretations used to determine the necessity, compliance, and relevance of an agency's goals and activities. It provides a basis for rational decision making for the future. Program evaluation without sensitive adaptation results in sterile critiques and recommendations without vision.

Program evaluation involves conducting systematic research within an agency to acquire information that can be fed back to enhance the agency's functioning. It is applied research involving problem solving and strategic action (Rothman, 1980). Evaluation research differs from basic research; the latter produces or verifies theories and knowledge and is not aimed at prescribing a solution to a problem. Program evaluation entails such inquiries as needs assessment, agency mission, statement and beliefs, descriptive information about quality of services delivered and client outcomes, and cost analysis. Comparative use of evaluation research can lead to meaningful theory and build upon it.

ISSUES

Relationship to Planning

Program evaluation is part of the cycle of program development. The cycle begins with the planning phase, moves through the implementation phase, and is followed by the review or evaluation phase. This last phase of program development is linked directly into the planning phase, at which point the cycle is reviewed. Figure 29–1 illustrates this cycle. Planning for program evaluation must be incorporated during program planning so that data needed for evaluating program outcomes will be available when the time comes for the actual evaluation (Clark, 1992).

Program evaluation is reactive evaluation for proactive planning. It is like a "mirror image of planning in that it is the process of looking back upon action, making judgment about it in order to provide the necessary information for planning for the future" (Blum, 1979, p. 542). Program evaluation acts as a comet in the heavens. A comet, with energy from its source, has momentum and gains speed as it is propelled through space to fulfill its purpose in the universe. Program evaluation gathers and analyzes data from the program's activities and propels the findings into the future to plan for

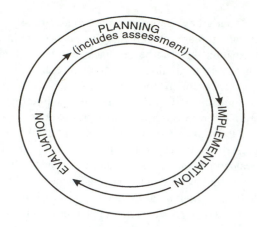

Figure 29–1 Cycle of program development. The cycle starts with the planning phase and moves to the implementation phase, then to the evaluation phase, and then back to the planning phase, at which point the cycle starts again.

Source: Copyright © Nancy D. Ruane

progressive development. This concept is depicted in Figure 29–2, which also illustrates the context and purpose of program evaluation.

The components of quality in health care defined by Donabedian (2003) speak to stakeholder expectations, including patients, in the United States and elsewhere. These components are *efficacy*, the ability to bring about improvements; *effectiveness,* the degree the improvements are attained; *efficiency*, the ability to lower the costs without diminishing improvements; *optimality*, the balancing of improvements against their costs; *acceptability*, conformity to social and ethical principles and norms; and *equity*, the just and fair distribution of health care among all members of the population.

Accountability

Program evaluations are conducted to describe and assess the effects of program activity. This information is essential because the agency, through its governing body, is accountable to the community that it serves. Accountability in-

cludes the quality and extent of the services provided and the funds used to finance the services. In proprietary agencies, the stockholders constitute another group that expects accountability. An effective program evaluation can establish accountability to all its stakeholders.

Relationship to Quality Assurance

Home health care is familiar with accountability. It is the common denominator for quality assurance and program evaluation. Both processes are evaluative in nature and are essential to the existence, growth, and development of an agency. Program evaluation focuses on examining the achievement of the outcome of a set of objectives, activities, and services. This examination leads to recommendations, which feed directly into the planning process. Quality assurance is a proactive set of policies and activities utilized to evaluate the scope and effectiveness of patient care delivery. The recommendations from this evaluation usually result in stronger enforcement of a procedure or a change of procedure to improve quality of care.

INFLUENCES ON PROGRAM EVALUATION

External Influences

Although program evaluation is designed to assess the appropriateness, adequacy, effectiveness, and efficiency of an agency, it is affected by forces over which it has little or no control. These forces may be characteristics of the climate of the industry, the population served by the agency, rules and regulations imposed by legislation, and third-party payers (see Figure 29–2).

Industry

The climate of the industry is influenced by numerous factors. Home health agencies have proliferated overwhelmingly since the late 1970s, especially in those states that do not require a certificate of need. This has placed agencies in adversarial positions with each other. This

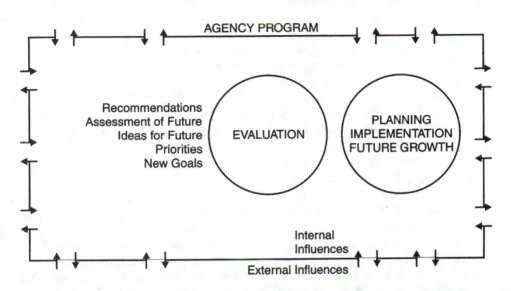

The agency program is an open system that has internal and external influences. The internal influences are contained within the boundary of the agency and affect the program evaluation process. The agency program output crosses over the boundary into the community, usually local but sometimes national. The external influences lie beyond the agency boundary and affect the agency program and its evaluation by crossing over the boundary.

Internal Influences	*External Influences*
Agency philosophy and goals	Patient population
Management	Demographics
Staff	Health status and needs
Policies	Economic status
Procedures	Demand for service
Management information system	Market competition
	Legislation
	Industry trends
	Third-party payers
	Home health associations
	Managed care programs

Figure 29–2 Context and purpose of program evaluation

Source: Copyright © Nancy D. Ruane

climate provides support for performing program evaluation, however, and is a strong influence in urging agencies to go through this process. In addition to the increasing number of agencies, managed care systems, the economic forecast, and future trends of the industry must be researched and understood because their effect is unavoidable.

This force in the industry has prompted some agencies to go beyond the minimum criteria imposed by Medicare. Many agencies utilize the accreditation services of the Community Health Accreditation Program (CHAP) or the Joint Commission on Accreditation of Healthcare Organizations (JCAHO). For hospital-based home health agencies, accreditation by the Joint Commission is not optional because the home health agency is part of the hospital organization. Medicare criteria for program evaluation require the assessment of organizational structure and process. CHAP and the JCAHO, through recent revisions, have expanded the evaluative emphasis to include standards that concern quality health care outcome statements. This shift requires agencies seeking accreditation by these bodies to reflect these standards in their programs.

In addition to these accrediting organizations, there are other industry associations that develop codes of ethics and standards for their membership. Membership in these organizations is voluntary, and the codes and standards are developed by the markets. Nevertheless, the codes and standards do influence the programs of the member agencies by establishing guidelines for quality programs. Indirectly, these guidelines influence the nonmember agencies because they establish informal criteria that are accepted by the industry.

Population Served

The population served by the agency influences the services offered. The demographics, health status, health needs, and socioeconomic levels of the people served by the agency all affect the type and amount of services that will be utilized by the community. Careful monitoring of population shifts, health statistics, and the economy of the region is absolutely necessary and, therefore, is an item to be considered in program evaluation. The reliable use of social indicators permits comparison with other communities and societies.

Rules and Regulations

The mandates imposed by rules and regulations of legislation and third-party payers are the strongest influences on program evaluation. Many states require licensure before an agency can provide any home health services (Warhola, 1980). In some states, only certified home health programs are required to be licensed and the licensing agency is usually the state government. The licensing criteria require the agency to have program evaluation policies and procedures. The state health department evaluates these programs at specified intervals. Usually the agency must complete a self-study report and experience an on-site visit. The criteria used for this internal report mandate that at least organizational structure and process evaluation be completed. This process is in itself a program evaluation.

The third-party payers view program evaluation as a vital indicator of the agency's functioning. Program evaluation is required by Medicare, Medicaid, and Blue Cross, and most commercial insurers use the Medicare certification criteria as a standard for measuring the acceptability of an agency for reimbursement eligibility. Therefore, for an agency to be eligible for reimbursement and to survive as a provider, program evaluation must be included in its policies.

Internal Influences

Influences that the agency develops or can usually control still have an impact on program evaluation. This group of influences includes the agency's philosophy and goals, the quality of its staff, the expertise of its management, and the system of managing all patient information within the agency (see Figure 29–2).

Philosophy and Goals

In the development of an agency, the philosophy and goals, or *mission statement*, are created initially to give substance to the project. From this statement, the agency's founders draw the ideas and direction for the programs. The objectives and policies for the implementation of the programs emanate from the ideas. Directed by the objectives and policies, the program managers guide the staff's activity to provide services. The program objectives, along with the mission statement, give direction to the evaluation because they are included in the criteria used to measure program effectiveness.

Staff

The quality of the members of the staff affects program evaluation because the staff are actors in the performance of the program activity. Inadequately prepared, undereducated staff can lead to ineffectiveness of programs and may become a threat to the program's quality. Control of the quality of the staff begins with the job advertisement, continues through the selection process, and is maintained through employer evaluation and staff development.

Management

The expertise of management influences program planning and implementation as well as program evaluation. The quality of management is essential not only to maintain the program's effectiveness, but also to ensure that the programs are properly planned. Ineffective managers lead to ineffective leadership and ineffective functioning of staff. The program goals will not be achieved, as the evaluation will reveal.

Management Information System

The patient information system is vital to program evaluation. It represents a significant portion of the information that is gathered for analysis in the evaluation process. Therefore, the lack of accuracy and other characteristics of the system influence program evaluation. Tracking of the information can be done by computer

or by hand. In either case, the information must become part of the system and monitored at certain checkpoints for accuracy so that quality and comprehensiveness of care can be demonstrated. For example, effective evaluation must take into account the withdrawals and additions to the patient population; only an accurate system can measure such variations.

DEVELOPMENT OF A PROGRAM EVALUATION SYSTEM

Since the beginning of the home health care movement, evaluation has been an integral part of the fundamental principles and practices of the industry. Evaluation areas are numerous and can be endless. There are relevant issues that must be considered and heeded in approaching evaluation. Investigative areas are selected according to their influences on patients, home health agency management staff, and the community served by the agency. The focus of the evaluation is also dictated by those regulatory and accreditation bodies that set standards for the industry.

Relevant Issues

By law, the Medicare regulations require certified home health agencies to evaluate their programs. The section on evaluation states that the agency must have written policies requiring an overall evaluation of the agency's total program at least once a year. The evaluation must be completed by the professional advisory group of the agency or a committee of that group along with the home health agency staff and consumers. The professional advisory group includes at least one registered nurse (preferably a public health nurse) and one physician as well as appropriate representation from the other professional disciplines that administer the scope of services. Overall policy, administrative, and clinical record reviews are included.

The aim of the evaluation is to assess the extent to which the agency's patient service delivery is appropriate, adequate, effective, and efficient. Each policy and administrative practice and its effect on patient care is reviewed. A report of the evaluation is presented to the governing body for action. The report is maintained as a part of the administrative record.

The agency must have established written mechanisms for the collection of data to assist the evaluation. The data may include numbers of patients receiving each service offered, sources of referral, number of patient visits, criteria for admissions, reasons for discharge, total staff days for each service offered, and number of patients not accepted (with reasons). If other data are available, they may be included because they will broaden and strengthen the statistical picture presented. This section also addresses the clinical record review, which is accomplished through quality assurance and utilization review. The Medicare conditions of participation serve as the basic structure upon which an evaluation program for home health agencies can be built (Stuart-Siddal, 1986).

The JCAHO is a private, nonprofit organization whose purpose is to encourage the attainment of uniformly high standards of institutional health care. Its manual notes that one of its roles is that of evaluator. All hospital-based agencies are required to have Joint Commission accreditation. Other home health agencies may choose to request it. The JCAHO standards require that the program's policies and procedures be reviewed annually and revised as necessary. The time of the last review and/or revision must be indicated. The evaluators are the individuals who are representative of the home care services provided. At least one physician and one registered nurse are among the evaluators. The specific inclusion of a physician as a reviewer is unique to this evaluation.

Through CHAP, the home health agencies participate in a voluntary accreditation process that aims to evaluate and improve the agency's services. To qualify for accreditation, the agency must complete a self-study report and experience an on-site visit (CHAP 2003; NLN, 1993). The CHAP criteria recommend an annual program evaluation, and usually an annual

evaluation is state mandated. CHAP does require an evaluation every 3 years, so an annual self-evaluation assists evaluations in CHAP's 3-year cycle (CHAP, 2003). The evaluation includes the assessment of program services and practice policies, the quality of care delivered by each discipline, the population served, the services and visits provided, and the client/patient outcomes.

The agency must have an overall program evaluation plan that includes strategic planning and marketing, organization and administrative review, programs and service, and staffing policies and practices. This plan should indicate the frequency of each evaluation and the person or group responsible as well as the purpose of the evaluation. CHAP places responsibility for implementing the evaluation on the governing body for the professional advisory group. This annual review prevents the typical demise of reports (i.e., their being ignored and forgotten, left to collect dust on some bookshelf) (Babbie, 2004).

Another mechanism that has a part in controlling the quality of care is licensure. Some states have assumed the responsibility for mandatory regulation. The regulations vary from state to state. The criteria are similar to the criteria for Medicare certification, with minor variations in each state. Generally, states establish agencies composed of a majority of professionals to set the guidelines for licensure. This process gives the states a means to revoke a license and therefore to prevent an agency from continuing in the provider role if compliance with criteria is not demonstrated (Spiegel, 1983).

Considering the nature of the home health care setting, the program evaluation is a mechanism utilized to ensure the delivery of quality care. It is difficult and costly to do comprehensive on-site evaluation of the care as it is being delivered. Other methods of evaluation involving staff and patients are employed to ensure the high quality of certain aspects of the agency's program. The staff participate in evaluating home visits, conducting surveys of other agencies in the area, opinion polling of patients and referral services, and making descriptive reviews and comparative evaluations. Usually the patients are involved in evaluation by answering opinion or attitude polls and by commenting on care received at specific times by specific health professionals.

Areas to Be Evaluated

Program evaluation has four areas of concern: (1) organization, (2) activities, (3) outcomes, and (4) costs. These areas are also known as structure, process, outcome, and fiscal evaluation. Structure deals with the administrative organization, the facilities and equipment, scope of services, the qualifications and profiles of the professional personnel, the characteristics of the patient population, and the policies and procedures governing patient care. Process involves the activities that are planned to occur in the program. Outcome refers to the program or patient objectives in relation to their attainment. The fiscal area focuses on costs and cost accountability (Dever, 1980).

Structure may be considered an input measure of the quality of services based on the number, type, and quality of the resources used in the production of the services. Structure is an indirect measure because it does not consider the activities or actual result. Because of this, structure may be considered an inferior area to evaluation (U.S. House of Representatives, 1976). Structure and its relationship to process and outcomes have sufficient support, however. Donabedian (1978) supported the evaluation of structure on the assumption that, when an agency has good structure, good care will follow. CHAP, in its accreditation program, pays particular attention to the achievement and maintenance of an efficient, effective management structure in the delivery of quality care. Therefore, the evaluation of structure continues to be a relevant area of focus.

Process is an indicator of the quality of care used to assess the activities of the multidisciplinary team and the programs in the management of patients. Process measurement documents the activities that make up a program and the flow of these activities. The specific activities are directed by the agency mission and the policies and procedures that evolve from it. Generally, such measures study the degree of conformity with standards and expectations that are established by the peer groups and leaders of the professions (U.S. House of Representatives, 1976).

Outcome measures the quality of care in which the standard of judgment is the attainment of a specified result. The outcome of patient care is measured by the parameters set by the health professionals providing the care. These professionals are guided by the standards of their professions and are directed by the agency mission, policies, and procedures (U.S. House of Representatives, 1976).

Fiscal evaluation looks at planned and actual expenditures. The planned or budgeted expenditures are compared with the actual expenditures. Another aspect to be examined is whether the actual activities occurred as a result of the expenditure of the resources. Actual costs and possible alternative costs are considered. This evaluation may also involve the study of bookkeeping, billing, banking policies, procedures, and systems.

The sources of information for program evaluation are the patient and family or significant other, the patient's clinical record, the analysis of patient statistics, the administrative and organizational documents, community statistics, and financial records and reports. The patients and their families or significant others can influence the program by choosing to accept or deny services. They also play a significant part in the accomplishment of outcomes by cooperating with health professionals. Assessing the patient's reactions, feelings, and judgments about the program is important to the evaluation of both process and outcome. The opinions of the patient and family can be evaluated by surveys or questionnaires, which are mailed or used in telephone contact. Concrete cost estimates cannot be provided because several factors affect cost, namely cost per respondent associated with the type of method, sample size, length of the questionnaire, time frame in which the data are needed, personnel wages, and other situational conditions (Dillman, 1978; Dillman et al., 1974).

The use of the clinical record as a source of information for program evaluation has been reported in the literature since the 1960s (Helbig et al., 1972). The clinical record reveals information about process and outcome. Along with the analysis of patient statistics, which reveals, at minimum, reasons for admission and discharge, amount and types of services, number of visits, and patients' diagnoses, the evaluator can report a significant amount of information to the governing body.

The documents related to the administration and organization of the agency give the evaluator information from the agency's philosophy and objectives about the most specific patient care policy. Their information forms the framework upon which the program is built and can reveal much about the program's quality. The statistics that describe the community served by the agency are important to the evaluator in developing recommendations. Without knowledge of community needs, it is difficult to recommend changes and plans for the future. Financial records and reports assist the evaluator in realizing the cost effectiveness of the program. Cost accountability is as much a reality as professional accountability. Sufficient information about fiscal evaluation is included in every program evaluation, so that the governing body can make the correct decisions about future programs.

EVALUATION MODELS

To ensure a well-organized evaluation study, an evaluation model is used. Models reinforce conclusions drawn by the evaluator. Without a model, the information presented after an evaluation may be misinterpreted. Typically, the program evaluations performed by home health agencies are summative evaluations, examining goals and objectives of the programs as noted earlier. This type of evaluation is associated

with the use of a model (Fitz-Gibbon and Morris, 1987). The summative evaluation, described earlier in this chapter, is the focus of the following discussion and illustration.

Systems Model

The systems model of evaluation focuses on the process as a working model or social unit capable of achieving a goal. This model is concerned with attaining objectives, coordinating the functioning of units, maintaining resources, and adapting to the environment. The systems model examines other aspects in addition to the goal. Recognizing that organizations have multiple goals, this model considers a single goal attainment in relation to its effect on other goals in the system.

The variables that are described and evaluated are the input, the throughput, and the output. *Input* refers to characteristics and conditions of the people and the resources. *Throughput* refers to human and nonhuman resources and processes. *Output* refers to the product of the system (Baker and Northman, 1979; LaParta, 1975; Schulbert et al., 1969; Stanhope and Lancaster, 1988). Scott (2003) notes that outputs are what organizations produce, goods and services, over which the organization typically has much control. Human service organizations need also to evaluate outcomes or results that represent the product of organizational performance and environmental response. Difficulties that evaluation research must resolve are how to account for variations of input resulting in variations of outcomes, as well as how the characteristics of the output environments affect outcomes (Scott, 2003). The systems model is comprehensive because it considers more elements and describes their interaction with each other.

Structure-Process-Outcome Model

The structure-process-outcome model of Donabedian (1978) was designed primarily for medical care. Because it is applicable to the broader areas of health care, today it is a popular method. The definitions of structure, process, and outcome were presented earlier in this chapter. The rationale of structure evaluation is based on the concept that good care is dependent upon good administration, organization, facilities, and providers. Donabedian (1978) believed that, through review of the patient record and direct observation of care, an evaluative judgment can be made. The activities performed by the provider of care can be labeled good and competent when viewed in the context of a certain patient. Although outcome usually refers to the attainment of a goal for patient recovery, it is also used to convey changes in health status, health-related knowledge, attitude, and behavior. The tracer method, based on the premise that health status and care can be evaluated by viewing specific health problems called *tracers*, is a structure-process-outcome model that uses the results in comparative research (Stanhope and Lancaster, 1996).

Goal Attainment Model

The goal attainment model refers to a method for assessing the effectiveness of a program by measurement of the predetermined goals. The components of the goal attainment model are developing objectives, deciding how to measure the objectives, collecting information, assessing the effects, and analyzing and interpreting data. Shields (1974) developed an example of the goal attainment model. For each goal, the evaluator examines the categories of wherewithal, structure, operations, and outcomes.

Wherewithal refers to resources, materials, equipment, and physical facilities. Structure includes the organizational framework or the administrative structure, lines of authority, committee linkages, and patterns of communication. Operations pertain to processes and procedures for carrying out program goals. Outcome refers to the level of attainment of a goal (Shields, 1974). Effectiveness is directly concerned with goal attainment (Miller, 2002). The criteria applied to outcomes are effectiveness (the attainment of purpose), efficiency or cost

effectiveness, and control (whether unexpected events were associated with the program). The evaluation process is applied to each goal in the program (Stanhope and Lancaster, 1988).

Planned Versus Actual Performance Model

The planned versus actual performance model compares preprogram-targeted objectives with the actual program performance. Realistic goals are established for the evaluation criteria. The establishment of realistic goals is an important issue. The model assumes that the goals that are established are the best available indicators of the actual accomplishments. It can be used widely and regularly once a plan for program evaluation is developed (Dever, 1980).

Summary

The systems model, structure-process-outcome-model, goal attainment model, and planned versus actual performance model described here are the most practical ones for a home health agency to use. Each of these designs may be applied with limited resources and minimal personnel. As a home health agency management tool, program evaluation must demonstrate its worth. The expected results of program evaluation are benefit increase and cost reduction (fiscal evaluation), increase in efficiency and productivity (structure evaluation), improvement in effectiveness (process evaluation), and documented change in health behavior and status of patients (outcome evaluation). Criteria for these evaluations are as varied as the theoretical models used and the constituents requiring the study. This must be kept in mind in selecting an evaluation tool.

PROGRAM EVALUATION TOOLS

An evaluation tool or instrument is used to identify the information to collect and provides the evaluation criteria. There are numerous tools in the literature for conducting a program evaluation (Bulaw, 1986; Herman et al., 1978, 1987;

Kosecaff and Fink, 1982). A review of these tools for the purpose of selection is time and cost effective. A program evaluation tool is a worksheet that indicates those areas to be evaluated, the time of evaluation, the rationale for the evaluation, and the evaluator.

In designing or selecting a tool, the following guidelines provide direction for evaluation (Dever, 1980; Kosecaff and Fink, 1982):

- How well did the program achieve its goals or outcomes?
- Were the program's activities implemented as planned?
- How effective were the activities in achieving the goals?
- Does the program have any unintended adverse or beneficial effects?
- Are the quantity and scope of service provided sufficient to meet the needs of the program participants?
- How quickly does the program respond to requests for service?
- Are patients discharged from the program prematurely?
- Do the patients, families, or significant others who use the program consider it satisfactory?
- What did the program cost?
- How did social, political, and regulatory factors influence the program's development and impact?
- How well was the program managed?
- What is to be changed in the program in the immediate future and in the long-term plan?

In addition to these guidelines, the following criteria assist in ensuring that the assessment by the tool will be valid, accurate, and complete:

- The tool provides useful information about the program that justifies the collection, analysis, and presentation of the data.
- The tool addresses the aspects of concern of the governing body and regulatory agencies.

- The sources of data requested by the tool are sufficiently reliable. There are no biases, exaggerations, omissions, or errors that will cause the tool to become inaccurate or misleading.
- The tool has reliability. Reliability refers to the degree to which the measurements or observations are consistent.
- The tool enables the data to be collected and analyzed in time for the deadline.
- The tool does not restrain the evaluator from obtaining required information.
- The cost requirements for utilization of the tool can be met by the agency.
- The information that the tool produces can be interpreted clearly as desirable or undesirable (Dever, 1980).
- The tool has validity. Each criterion in the tool is based on expert judgment, past experience, and data from research.

COLLECTION OF INFORMATION

After one considers the development or selection of a tool for program evaluation, thought is given to collecting information or data. This involves numerous and important techniques. In the selection of the correct technique for a program, the following factors should be considered. First, the technique should be acceptable to the governing body and management staff; be technically sound to collect data that are reliable, valid, and targeted to evaluation criteria; provide the best data that the budget can afford; and allow sufficient time for collection and analysis of the data before the deadline (Kosecaff and Fink, 1982).

The major methods and strategies that are utilized to collect information are as follows:

- review of the organization of the agency
- critical review of administrative philosophy, goals, objectives, and documents
- clinical record review for quality and utilization of services (the quality assurance and utilization review committee reports

may be used, or the evaluator may review a sampling of clinical records)

- patient care policies and procedures review and evaluation using the current literature of the multidisciplinary health professions as a resource
- review of the goals and objectives of each program for attainment and relevance
- critical review of personnel policies, job descriptions, professional qualifications, and activities
- reports of the Medicare survey, state licensing consultants, or accreditation agencies
- recommendations from the agency committees
- results of patient opinion surveys and patient letters of appreciation and complaint
- results of referral source opinion surveys
- compilation of any patient statistics that can be acquired from the agency information system
- analysis of the proposed and actual budget and the cost report

PROGRAM EVALUATION REPORT

The report is the official record of the program evaluation. The audience of the report should be considered so that the style of writing will be understood. The evaluation findings should be communicated in a comprehensible way without compromising any qualitative and quantitative details. A clear and logical evaluation report increases the credibility of the information presented. The report should include the following:

- an introduction, which briefly describes the program(s) being evaluated, the participants conducting the evaluation, and the approach to the evaluation
- the evaluation model and evaluation tool description, including any limitation (attach a copy of the tool if possible; if not, give some sample items and present infor-

mation about the reliability and validity of the tool)

- a summary of all activities performed in the collection of data and what sources were used
- the results of any analysis that was done to arrive at answers to the evaluation criteria (use graphs and other visual presentations where applicable)
- the evaluation findings, the answers to the evaluation questions, and the evaluator's interpretation of the findings (it is important to point out the strengths and weaknesses of a program and to report the limitations of the findings)
- the recommendations and modifications for the program (prioritize the recommendations so that they may be incorporated readily into the plan)
- a report on the sequence of events in conducting the evaluation and recommendations for future evaluation (this may be appended to the report for the governing body and the management team)

A summary or brief overview of the evaluation report explains the purpose of the evaluation and lists its major recommendations and conclusions. It contains enough detail to be usable and believable but is easy to read. The summary may be placed at the beginning of the evaluation as an introduction. Because the summary may be more widely circulated and read than the complete report, it should be prepared carefully.

The evaluation report may begin with a section devoted to background information concerning the program. A description of the development of the program and its purpose sets the evaluation in context. The amount of detail presented is dependent upon the audience's degree of familiarity with the program (Fitz-Gibbon and Morris, 1987; Kosecaff and Fink, 1982).

It is important to emphasize here that the recommendations of the evaluation report must be communicated effectively to the persons responsible for plan development. The evaluation of a program is one of the ways in which the planners get a sense of how their ideas are being implemented. The relevance of what was planned in the past has a significant influence on what is planned for the future.

Communication of evaluation findings, so that the planner or planning committee has a better comprehension of program effectiveness, is a vital step in the evaluation process (Blum, 1979).

The evaluator(s) can go one step further and present questions about the future to the planners as part of the section on recommendations. These questions can address such subjects as population shifts; prospective payment programs; changes in federal, state, or local regulations regarding health care delivery; consumer movements; and occurrence of a disaster.

SYSTEMATIC APPROACH TO PROGRAM EVALUATION

A program comes into being because an individual, a committee, or other group of concerned persons has an idea for a service that is needed by the community, The idea's creator visualizes a set of goals that, when taken collectively, become the program. The next phase in the development of the program, after the idea is conceptualized, is the stating of goals. Planning and evaluation are continually interfacing. The evaluative process, which begins operation at the outset of the program, is similar to the planning process in the development of the program.

The first step in the evaluative process is to look at the goals of the program. The goals must be clear, specific, and measurable. They should be people oriented. They must address program outcomes. The next step in the evaluative process is to clarify goals. Any goals that are not measurable, people oriented, or stated in outcome terminology should be rewritten. It may be necessary to change the stated measurement in the goal to be more realistic or relevant. The process then moves on to goal activation, or the implementa-

tion of the goals. At this time, the activities of the program are being performed, and the patients are receiving the services. The measurement of the goal effect follows. At this stage, the goal effect is measured through patient statistics and utilization review data. The final step in the evaluative process is the evaluation of the program. This is the judgment concerning the attainment of the program goals.

The planning for program evaluation is also part of the program plan. It is similar to the evaluative process but is more direct, specific, and task oriented. The steps in planning for program evaluation are as follows (Stanhope and Lancaster, 1988):

1. Identify people as evaluators. Usually program personnel, professional advisory board members, and consumers are included.
2. Conduct preliminary meetings to discuss the evaluation's purpose. A decision is reached to do the evaluation in a specific time period. A time line is drawn to indicate who will evaluate each section of the program in the time indicated.
3. Review the literature (this is done by the evaluators who are external to the program).
4. Determine the methods of conducting the evaluation. What evidence is needed to measure the program outcomes?
5. Conduct the evaluation.
6. Determine what committee or individual will write the program evaluation report after receiving recommendations from the evaluators.
7. Determine who will compose the planning group, who will carry out the recommendations for change, and how the change will be accomplished.
8. Present the evaluation report to the governing body, planning group, and community groups. The recommendations are emphasized so that they are not ignored but are received and implemented if possible.

OPERATIONAL CONSIDERATIONS IN PROGRAM EVALUATION

Even though the principles of evaluation are known, a critical aspect of evaluation should be considered. The present climate of the home health industry embodies cost containment. Everyone is seeking to prove cost effectiveness in the delivery of home care services. The federal government has awarded grants to studies to develop cost-effective care techniques, such as prospective payment systems. It may be erroneous to concentrate solely on dollars, however. Although containment is important, we must remember that care of human beings is at least equally important.

Benefits of the Program Evaluation

The central benefits of a program evaluation are the judgments concerning the attainment of the goals of the program. Through evaluation, the program managers and governing body can determine whether the program's purpose is being fulfilled. The feedback, which gives information about goal attainment, also verifies that the program is effective. This knowledge assists the decision makers in planning for future allocation of funds. Competent monitoring or evaluation of the program enables the decision makers to determine whether the achieved goals can be met in a more cost-effective manner.

Fiscal accountability may be another benefit derived from program evaluation. Funds given to operate a program must be spent for the purposes for which they are given, and resources required to undertake economic evaluations are scarce (Drummond et al., 1997). The accountability for the funds requires more than simple auditing of accounting records. The funding agency may take an alternative approach to monitoring; namely, if certain milestones (structure, process, and outcome) are achieved within the stated budget, it is assumed that the money given to the agency has been used appropriately (Alkin and Solman, 1983).

Evaluation can make contributions to the store of knowledge about the program, certain professional activities, and consumer needs. This information can be used to market the program through direct marketing and public relations efforts. It can provide a basis of comparison from which to judge the relative quality of good practice. Accumulated information from many evaluations can serve as a basis for conclusions about what sorts of programs work best.

Program evaluation is an intelligent response to controversy. An accumulation of strong data can resolve a situation beset by diverse opinions. Evaluation also persuades people to pay attention to data concerning what home health agencies are doing. It is the best response to the individuals who continuously push new ideas without substance. Innovations must be tried, but if health professionals never find out which ones are worthwhile, home health agencies will deliver care with a fad-oriented mentality. Each time an evaluation is conducted, additional people acquire evaluation skills. As more people in home health agencies become familiar with evaluation methods, they will be able to collect information and distinguish valuable, effective innovations from ineffective fads (Herman et al., 1987).

Cautions on Evaluation

Much work over the past 30 years has taught us to be cautious in interpreting results of evaluation research or program evaluations. The many stakeholders—program administrators, professionals, evaluators, legislators, directors, consumer advocates, and others—all may view results differently. Evaluators have gradually come to understand the need to use multiple methods in evaluation. The quality of knowledge increases with critical public scrutiny of it (Shadish et al., 1991). The focused evaluation of single agencies, such as those providing home health care, moves us closer to meaningful evaluations and program improvement.

Special Implementation Considerations

The organization of the home health agency may present specific circumstances that directly influence program evaluation. Most home health agencies have only one site. In these agencies, some decentralization is necessary. In such situations, the decentralization is not merely physical. The home health personnel who work in the site offices and neighborhoods are in the best position to know the problems, needs, and resources of the area served by the site office. Therefore, the personnel from that home health agency site, under the direction of the site administrator, should have the responsibility and the authority for determining and carrying out the details of the daily operations and activities. They function, of course, within the overall agency philosophy, goals, and policies. Capable leaders are placed in the administrative positions for the decentralized units. They administer their local programs to the maximum extent feasible.

Program evaluation in the one-site agency is conducted without difficulty because everything to be evaluated is centralized. In the multisite agency, the planning is more tedious. The governing body of a multisite agency has two operations. The first is to evaluate the total agency as one site. With this plan, the evaluator(s) must coordinate the data so that each site is represented in the evaluation of each goal in the program. This approach is difficult to coordinate and requires meticulous attention to ensure accuracy. If the governing body chooses to evaluate each site individually, the evaluator's task is less complicated. Also, this approach will enable the agency to do comparison evaluation studies. These studies will yield valuable information about the differences and similarities in the program as it is delivered to different communities. Program evaluation in a multisite agency is a challenge to the most seasoned evaluator. The information that this evaluation yields can be so rewarding, however, that it negates the frustrations of the experience.

Program Evaluation Tool Formats

There are numerous approaches to presenting a program evaluation tool. Appendix 29–A gives a few approaches. Each format attempts to assess the extent to which the home health care agency's program is appropriate, adequate, effective, and efficient. These formats may be modified as necessary to meet the objectives of the evaluator or evaluation team.

REFERENCES

Alkin, M., and L. Solman. 1983. *The costs of evaluation.* Beverly Hills, CA: Sage.

Babbie, E. 2004. *The practice of social research,* 10th ed. Belmont, CA: Wadsworth.

Baker, F., and J. E. Northman. 1979. Evaluation of a school mental health clinic. In *Program Evaluation in the Health Field,* vol. 2. H. C. Schulbert and F. Baker, eds. New York: Human Sciences Press.

Blum, H. 1979. *Planning for health.* New York: Human Sciences Press.

Breckon, D. J. 1982. *Hospital health education.* Gaithersburg, MD: Aspen.

Bulaw, J. M. 1986. *Administrative policies and procedures for home health care.* Gaithersburg, MD: Aspen.

Clark, M. J. 1992. *Nursing in the community.* East Norwalk, CT: Appleton & Lange.

Community Health Accreditation Program (CHAP). 2003. *Philosophy, mission, purpose, CHAP policy and procedure manual.* Administration Manual 2003. New York: CHAP.

Dever, G. E. A. 1980. *Community health analysis.* Gaithersburg, MD: Aspen.

Dillman, D. A. 1978. *Mail and telephone surveys.* New York: Wiley.

Dillman, D. A., et al. 1974. Increasing mail questionnaire response: A four state comparison. *American Sociological Review* 39: 744–756.

Donabedian, A. 1978. The quality of medical care. In *Health Care Regulation, Economics, Ethics, and Practice,* P. H. Abelson, ed. Washington, DC: American Association for the Advancement of Science.

Donabedian, A. 2003. *An introduction to quality assurance*

in health care, Rashid Bashur, ed. New York: Oxford University Press.

Drummond, M. F., B. O'Brien, G. L. Stoddart, and G. W. Torrance. 1999. *Methods for the economic evaluation of health care programmes*, 2nd ed., New York: Oxford University Press.

Fitz-Gibbon, C., and L. Morris. 1987. *How to design a program evaluation*. Newbury Park, CA: Sage.

Helbig, D., et al. 1972. The care component core. *American Journal of Public Health* 62: 540–546.

Herman, J., et al. 1978. *How to measure program implementation*. Beverly Hills, CA: Sage.

Herman, J., et al. 1987. *Evaluator's handbook*. Newbury Park, CA: Sage.

Joint Commission on Accreditation of Healthcare Organizations. 2004–2005 *Comprehensive accreditation manual for home care, standards manuals for home care -2003*. Oakbrook Terrace, IL: JCAHO.

Kosecaff, J., and A. Fink. 1982. *Evaluation basics*. Beverly Hills, CA: Sage.

LaParta, J. W. 1975. *Health care delivery system: Evaluation criteria*. Springfield, IL: Thomas.

Miller, D. C. 2002. *Handbook of research design and social measurement*, 6th ed. Beverly Hills, CA: Sage.

National League for Nursing. 1974. *Faculty-curriculum evaluation, part II* (Pub. No. 15-1530). New York: NLN.

Rothman, J. 1980. *Using research in organizations*. Beverly Hills, CA: Sage.

Schulbert, H. C., et al. 1969. *Program evaluation in the health field*. New York: Behavioral Publications.

Scott, W. R. 2003. *Organizations: Rational, natural, and open systems*, 5th ed., Upper Saddle River, NJ: Prentice Hall.

Shadish, W. R., et al. 1991. *Foundations of program evaluation: Theories of practice*. Beverly Hills, CA: Sage.

Shields, M. 1974, July. *An evaluation model for science programs*. Nursing Outlook 22: 448.

Spiegel, A. D. 1983. *Home health care*. Owings Mills, MD: National Health Publishing.

Stanhope, M., and J. Lancaster. 1988. *Community health nursing*, 3rd ed. St. Louis, MO: Mosby.

Stanhope, M., and J. Lancaster. 1996. *Community health nursing*, 4th ed. St. Louis, MO: Mosby.

Stanhope, M., and J. Lancaster. 2000. *Community and public health nursing*, 5th ed. St. Louis, MO: Mosby.

Stanhope, M., and J. Lancaster. 2004. *Community and public health nursing*, 6th ed. St. Louis, MO: Mosby.

Stuart-Siddal, S. 1986. *Home health care nursing*. Gaithersburg, MD: Aspen.

U.S. House of Representatives, Committee on Interstate and Foreign Commerce, Subcommittee on Health and the Environment. 1976. *A discursive dictionary of health care*. Washington, DC: U.S. Government Printing Office.

Warhola, C. F. R. 1980. *Planning for home health services* (DHHS Pub. No. [HRA] 80-14017). Washington, DC: U.S. Government Printing Office.

APPENDIX 29–A

Formats for Presenting Program Evaluation Tools

FORMAT 1

Evaluation Area with Outcomes	Outcome Met YES NO	Corrective Action Needed	Suggested Frequency and Month
A. Administration 1. The governing body maintains relevant articles of incorporation			Once a year July
B. Organization 1. The chief executive officer (CEO) keeps the operating chief (OC) up to date			Once a year July
C. Patient Care Policies 1. All patients who fit the admission criteria received care from the agency			Twice a year March September
D. Nursing Services (etc.)			Annually

Continue this format until all areas that are to be evaluated are completed.
Source: Copyright © Nancy D. Ruane.

FORMAT 2

Activity with Outcomes	Evaluation Frequency	Responsible Group/Person	Outcome Met YES NO
A. Organizational Structure	Annually	Governing Body or Ad Hoc Committee	
1. Articles of Incorporation	Annually		
2. Bylaws: The governing body reviews the bylaws annually	Annually		
3. Agency Philosophy: The governing body and staff review the philosophy annually	Annually		
B. Financial Management	Monthly	Finance Committee	

Continue this format until all areas that are to be evaluated are completed.

FORMAT 3

Activity with Outcomes	Minimum Frequency	Responsible Body/Person	Comments
A. Organizational Structure 1. The CEO manages the day-to-day operation of the agency	Yearly and prn	Board of Directors	
B. Administrative Policies	Monthly and prn	Board of Directors	
C. Financial Management 1. The controller prepares for the preparation of monthly financial statements	Monthly	Finance Committee	
D. Community Assessment	Annually	Program Coordinator	
E. Program Services	Quarterly	Professional Advisory Committee, Program Coordinator	

Continue this format until all areas that are to be evaluated are completed.

FORMAT 4

Evaluation Area: List Outcomes under Category	Frequency	Responsible Committee/Person	Outcome Met YES NO
Organization and Administration			
A. Organization Chart The CEO keeps the OC consistent with the agency operation	Annually	Board, CEO	
B. Philosophy and Goals	Annually	Board	
C. Administrative Policies	Annually and prn	Board, CEO	
D. Administrative Procedures	Annually and prn	Board, CEO	
E. Community Needs	Annually	Board, CEO, Consultant	
F. Financial Management	Monthly	Board and Finance Committee	
Program and Services			
A. Program Services	Annually	Board, CEO, Professional Advisory Board	
B. Practice Policies		Procedures Committee	
C. Quality Assurance/ Utilization Review (QA/UR)		QA Committee, UR Committee	

Continue this format until all areas that are to be evaluated are completed.

FORMAT 5

Evaluation Area with Outcomes under Each Category	Frequency	Responsible Body/Person	Outcome Met YES NO	Comments
Structure				
A. Organization The CEO keeps the OC consistent with agency operation	Annually Annually	Board Professional Advisory Board		

B. Administrative
   1. Policies: All patients who meet criteria receive care from the agency
   2. Procedures
	Annually			

C. Community Needs	Annually			
D. Facilities 1. Equipment	Annually			
E. Staff	Annually			
Process				

A. Program Services
   Skilled Nursing
   HHA
   PT
   OT
   MSS
	Twice a year	CEO
		Director of Professional/ Patient Services Staff		

B. Utilization of Services	Four times a year	CEO, Professional Advisory Board		

Continue this format until all areas that are to be evaluated are completed.

CHAPTER 30

Effectiveness of a Clinical Feedback Approach to Improving Patient Outcomes

Peter W. Shaughnessy and Kathryn S. Crisler

Home health care represents one component of the health care continuum. Because Medicare is the dominant payer for home health services, its payment and regulatory practices have impacted considerably the types and number of home health agencies as well as utilization and expenditures. The Omnibus Budget Reconciliation Act of 1980 (P.L. 96–499) encouraged home health utilization and enabled more agencies to particpate in Medicare, resulting in an increase from 2,924 agencies in 1980 to 5,695 agencies in 1990. As a result of a 1987 legal challenge, clarification of Medicare coverage spurred growth to 10,577 agencies by 1997. Through the Balanced Budget Act of 1997 (P.L. 105–33), Congress imposed limits and decreases in payment that became effective under the Interim Payment System (IPS) for Medicare-certified providers until a per-case prospective payment system (PPS) could be implemented, which occurred in October 2000. By 1999, IPS resulted in more than a 50 percent reduction in total home health visits to 112 million, a decline of over 40 percent in visits per patient to 42, and greater than a 50 percent decrease in Medicare expenditures on home health care to $7.9 billion. Agency closures and withdrawals from Medicare reduced the number of agencies by almost one-third to 7,146 by the end of 2000 (Centers for Medicare and Medicaid Services [CMS], 2002).

As these swings in supply, use, and cost were occurring, concerns regarding the lack of evidence on patient-level health effects of such care were heightening. Payers (including Medicare and Medicaid) lacked objective information to assess the effects of these changes on Medicare beneficiaries. As payment lessened and eventually was based on per-case reimbursement, perverse incentives to underserve patients were created. Accreditation and certification programs, such as the Joint Commission on Accreditation of Healthcare Organizations (JCAHO) and the Community Health Accreditation Program (CHAP), as well as state and federal government certification agencies became progressively more outcome oriented. The importance of objectively assessing the impacts of care increased correspondingly for physicians, hospital discharge planners, and case managers. Equally important, home care agencies were increasingly concerned with measuring their own performance relative to other providers or standards. This combination of factors has fueled a powerful movement toward outcome measurement in home care.

This chapter focuses on the research and demonstration work conducted by the Center for Health Services Research at the University of Colorado Health Sciences Center. The research that led to the outcome-based quality improvement approach described here was developed for home health care over nearly a decade with several million dollars in funding from CMS and the Robert Wood Johnson Foundation. The resulting outcome measure system and its application for performance improvement constitute a methodology termed outcome-based quality improvement (OBQI) in home care. The measure system was developed predominantly for adult patients receiving skilled care, although the resulting measures pertain to other types of adult patients. Measures for younger populations as well as specific subgroups of patients will likely be developed in the future.

The focus of the OBQI approach is patient outcomes that occur over a home health care episode. The purpose of the original research was to develop valid and reliable measures of patient outcomes that could be precisely quantified and compared across home health agencies and patients. Subsequent sections of this chapter describe the outcome measures and the results of the demonstrations incorporating the measures into an OBQI system.

The evolution of the outcome measure system and the performance improvement approach based on the measure system has involved a number of separate but integrated activities (Center for Health Services Research, 2002; Shaughnessy, 1991; Shaughnessy et al., 1994a, 1995, 1996, 1997a, 1997b, 2002). These included comprehensive reviews of outcome measures and related papers, documents, and articles published in the research literature and the provider and clinical literature as well as reviews of outcome measures in use or under development by individual agencies or groups of agencies (i.e., in their formative stages). A number of clinical panels were convened to review the outcome measures and approaches at regular intervals.

A variety of data sources were examined for potential information about outcome measurement. Outcome measures were specified first, and data items needed to measure outcome were developed thereafter. Extant sources of information for such data items were examined, including clinical records, claims or billing data, and other administrative data. After an extensive examination of such data sources, we concluded that it would be necessary to develop a new data set to measure properly the outcomes that had

been specified. Several hundred home care agencies throughout the United States participated in the developmental efforts over a period of several years, including various types of research investigations, data item refinement (including validity and reliability testing), and both demonstration and evaluation projects (Center for Health Services Research, 2002; Hittle et al., 2003; Powell et al., 1994; Shaughnessy et al., 1994a, 1995, 2002).

The system described here is currently being implemented nationally by the Medicare program in the context of the public reporting of home health outcomes, the support for agency quality improvement efforts by the Quality Improvement Organizations (QIOs), and the home health agency survey and certification program. The overall system presented in this chapter is therefore intended for application by individual home health agencies and by purchasers of home care who wish to assess what is happening to patient/clients as a result of their financial investment.

TYPES OF OUTCOMES

The fundamental definition of a patient-level outcome is a change in health status between two or more time points. In the current OBQI system, this is the basic or anchoring definition of an outcome. It is termed an *end-result outcome* because it reflects change in patient health status over the course of time, which is the focal point of health care provision. The two time points that are typically used to gauge outcomes in home care are start of care (SOC) and discharge. (Resumption of care following an inpatient stay also can begin a new episode, and transfer to an inpatient facility is a proxy for discharge.) Health status, as noted, is broadly defined, encompassing physiological, functional, cognitive, mental, and social health. Illustrations of end-result outcomes include improvement in ability to ambulate between admission and discharge, decline in dyspnea between admission and 120 days after admission, stabilization or no change in pain interfering with activities between 60 and 180 days, and improvement in ability to manage oral medications between admission and discharge. The third illustration demonstrates that it is not necessary to consider SOC and discharge as the only two follow-up points that define outcomes.

A second type of outcome that has been considered for future use in OBQI is termed an *instrumental outcome* (or *intermediate-result outcome*). An instrumental outcome is a change in patient's (or informal caregiver's) behavior, emotions, or knowledge that can influence a patient's end-result outcomes. Illustrations of instrumental outcomes include change in compliance with the treatment regimen, knowledge of self-care, signs, and symptoms to report to the physician, informal caregiver strain, patient or family satisfaction with care, and motivation to improve. These are termed instrumental outcomes because, although they are outcomes in their own right, their (non)attainment can influence the (non)attainment of end-result outcomes. Instrumental outcomes are critical in home care but are more difficult to measure than end-result outcomes and therefore are not in widespread use in OBQI at the present time.

The third type of outcome is termed a *utilization outcome*. Such outcomes can refer to utilization of nonhome care services that reflect a (typically substantial and untoward) change in health status over time. Illustrations of utilization outcomes include hospital admission and emergent care. These are also termed *proxy outcomes* because they are often (but not always) surrogates for untoward or negative health status changes in patients. Such outcomes have the redeeming feature that they are more straightforward to measure, although statistical risk adjustment is often of paramount importance in comparing such outcomes across different groups of patients.

An outcome measure is a quantification of an outcome. Under the assumption that the outcome under consideration is an end-result outcome, an outcome measure is a quantified change in patient health status between two or more time points. The change referred to in this case is intrinsic to the patient (e.g., the provision of a cane or walker is not intrinsic to the patient and is therefore not an outcome). The change can represent improvement, stabilization, or worsening. Objective measures are superior to subjective measures in that, when one is quantifying outcomes, specific, reliable, and objective health status scales should be used for end-result and instrumental outcomes, and precise information about health care use should be used to measure utilization outcomes.

A wide variety of outcomes and outcome measures were specified in the developmental research that underpins OBQI. Over time, these were culled, modified, or refined from different vantage points, including clinical relevance, reliability, specificity, practicality, utility for quality improvement purposes, and minimization of statistical redundancy. Because the initial objectives focused on specifying measures, all data items followed from the outcome measures. That is, OBQI data items were not first specified and then used to determine which measures would be possible. The primary focus was outcome measures that could be integrated to form a system that would be valid and practical for OBQI, with all other considerations (including data items) being secondary to this purpose.

DATA ITEM SET

The set of data items used in the OBQI system is termed the Outcome and Assessment Information Set (OASIS). It was tailored to home care after investigation of the appropriateness of using data items from other fields (such as the Functional Independence Measure data set in the rehabilitation field and the Minimum Data Set in the nursing home field; Fries et al., 1994; Granger et al., 1993, 1995; Hawes et al., 1995; Morris et al., 1990; State University of New York at Buffalo, 1993, 1995). Extensive modifications of these data sets would have been necessary to adapt them properly to home care; in addition, several of the items did not necessarily provide the information needed to measure the outcomes needed for home care. Nevertheless, the OASIS data set is continuing to undergo re-finement, as is the scope of the OBQI home care measure system. The first release of the OASIS occurred in August 1995 as a special supplement to the National Association for Home Care's *NAHC Report* (NAHC, 1995). This was termed OASIS-A and has been followed by subsequent releases, the most recent of which was termed OASIS-B1 (12/2002).

OASIS is not intended to be a comprehensive assessment instrument; rather, it is a set of data items that are essential for measuring or risk-adjusting outcomes in the home care field. With national implementation of data collection for adult nonmaternity patients in Medicare-certified agencies, CMS required that OASIS items be embedded within the comprehensive assessment instrument of each home care agency, replacing those items in current assessment instruments that address similar concepts. Adding the OASIS items to an existing assessment instrument would have created substantial redundancy because almost all OASIS items correspond to analogous, but typically less precise, items already used for comprehensive assessment (in addition to this redundancy, adding similar items would serve only to increase an already substantial documentation burden in home care).

To measure outcomes, because these have been defined as changes in health status, it is necessary to collect OASIS data items at 60-day intervals until and including time of discharge. Further specifics are available in other research documents and the *OASIS Implementation Manual* available from CMS (Centers for Medicare and Medicaid Services, 1998).

TWO-STAGE CONTINUOUS QUALITY IMPROVEMENT APPROACH

The general framework for OBQI is the two-stage continuous quality improvement (CQI) approach depicted in Figure 30–1. This schematic shows the overall OBQI applications framework. The sequence of events on the left side of the figure constitutes the outcome analysis component, and those on the right side constitute outcome enhancement. In the conduct of the two-stage CQI process, data must be collected at the previously mentioned intervals for all adult patients receiving skilled care.

The outcome analysis component begins with collecting, computerizing, and transmitting OASIS data to a central source. The production of outcome reports is the culmination of this analysis. Using these reports, agency staff can determine which outcomes are inferior and which are exemplary. The outcomes on which the agency staff elect to focus for purposes of subsequent review are called *target outcomes* and constitute the focal point of the outcome enhancement process. In outcome enhancement, each agency is given considerable latitude to conduct its own CQI activities. All activities in this process involve investigating care provided for purposes of reinforcing those care behaviors that produce exemplary outcomes or remedying problems in care that produce inferior outcomes. This usually entails record review for the triggered outcomes to determine specific activities in care provision (e.g., assessment, care planning, intervention, or care coordination/referral) that should be reinforced or remedied. The outcome enhancement activities culminate with a written plan of action specifically targeted at changing or reinforcing care behaviors that produce certain outcomes. The plan of action entails specifying what will be done, how it will be done, who will undertake the activities necessary to change care behaviors, when it will be done, and how the process of implementing change will be monitored. The effectiveness of the enhancement activities, including the final plan of action, can then be assessed by virtue of continued data collection and review of outcome reports for the next time period. This permits agency staff to determine whether outcomes targeted for improvement have in fact improved and whether those targeted for reinforcement have remained the same or improved. The heart of the CQI process, therefore, is producing (evidence-based) outcome reports on a regular basis that can be used to monitor outcomes of care and assess whether changes introduced to remedy problems have improved

Outcome analysis component

Outcome enhancement component

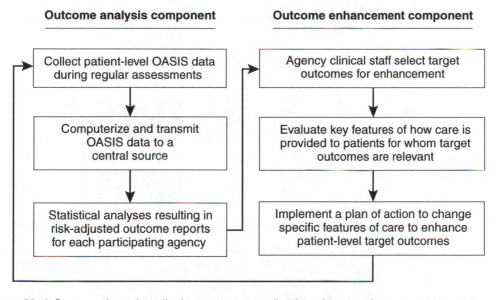

Figure 30–1 Outcome-based quality improvement applications framework

outcomes and whether reinforcement activities implemented to maintain exemplary or superior outcomes have done so.

SAMPLE OUTCOME REPORT

Figure 30–2 contains an excerpt from a hypothetical outcome report for an individual home care agency. It displays results for two improvement measures. Improvement measures that correspond to end-result outcomes, such as improvement in dressing upper body or improvement in management of oral medications (as indicated in Figure 30–2), are constructed from health status scales at two points in time. In this case, the outcome measures correspond to change in upper body dressing or ability to manage oral medications between SOC and discharge. The results indicate that 64.5 percent of patients improved in upper body dressing during the current reporting period (most recent year) for the agency compared with 51.3 percent of patients for the agency's prior period (preceding year) and 57.7 percent of patients from a na-

tional reference group. Two hundred and three patients contributed to the outcome results in the current reporting period, 136 contributed from the prior period, and 11,326 contributed from the national comparison group. The current and prior period outcome results showed a statistically significant difference between the two means (i.e., 64.5 percent versus 51.3 percent; $p = .02$). The comparison with the national reference is significant at $p = .06$. A similar statistical interpretation pertains for improvement in management of oral medications. The outcome reports routinely contain asterisked, double asterisked, or nonasterisked items depending on whether the statistical significance occurs at the .10 level, the .05 level, or not at all (i.e., $p > .10$), respectively. (The p-values correspond to the significance level of a dichotomous indicator of agency versus reference group in a multivariate logistic regression model using several risk factors as well as this dichotomy. Each outcome measure requires its own risk model. The test used for significance of the coefficient of this dichotomy [actually the odds ratio] is a type of chi-square test.)

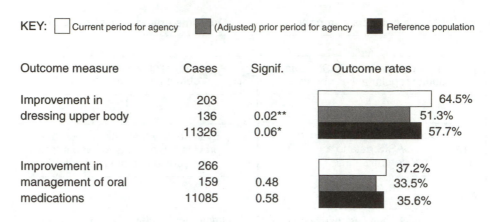

Figure 30–2 Excerpt (using 2 of 41 outcomes) from an agency-level risk adjusted outcome report

RESULTS OF OBQI DEMONSTRATION PROGRAMS

After the developmental research period, including an OBQI pilot conducted in three agencies in Colorado, two large-scale demonstrations were implemented. CMS sponsored a national OBQI demonstration between 1995 and 2000, with funding from both CMS (then HCFA) and the Robert Wood Johnson Foundation. This national demonstration involved 54 home health agencies from 27 states. Demonstration sites included small, medium, and large agencies, both rural and urban, and agencies representing a variety of ownership types. The national OBQI trial was designed to establish a template to (1) collect uniform (OASIS) data on all adult, nonmaternity home health patients to measure and report patient outcomes, (2) utilize outcome measures for quality improvement purposes, and (3) provide a foundation for a systemwide approach to enhancing patient outcomes in home health care. If successful, it would serve as the evidence-based prototype for a national OBQI program for all Medicare-certified home health agencies.

In late 1995, the New York State Department of Health implemented a statewide OBQI demonstration patterned after CMS's national OBQI demonstration that began with 19 and would eventually involve 33 certified agencies

and 24 noncertified agencies. As with the national demonstrations, this 6-year program was administered by the University of Colorado Center for Health Services Research. After training by the research center staff, the agencies participating in the two demonstrations integrated into their day-to-day operation all facets of OASIS and outcome data collection, monitoring, processing, transmission, and OBQI.

Evaluation of the demonstrations was concerned primarily with the impacts of OBQI on patient outcomes and secondarily with the feasibility of implementing the OBQI approach. If outcomes were impacted as a result of the first or succeeding years' outcome reports and outcome enhancement activities, this would suggest that the OBQI framework was feasible to implement in a manner that produced the desired results. The outcome reports provide a straightforward way to evaluate the impacts of each individual agency's OBQI program by comparing target outcome rates for the current period with the risk-adjusted rates for the prior period. Hospitalization was a strongly recommended target outcome during the first round of OBQI for all agencies. For the second target outcome in the first round (and for all target outcomes in subsequent rounds of OBQI), agencies were free to choose from approximately 80 different outcomes contained in either their standard 41-outcome report or, where applicable, two special outcome reports for orthopedic and cardiac patients, respectively.

Hospitalization Outcome Findings

The time periods for each cycle of outcome reporting were approximately 12 months. OBQI impacts on outcomes were assessed by comparing the outcome changes between pairs of consecutive years for all demonstration agency patients. The results comparing risk-adjusted hospitalization rates for Year 1 and Year 2 versus Year 3 for the national and New York state demonstrations are presented in Figure 30–3, along with the Year 3 versus Year 4 comparison for New York state. The risk-adjusted net decrease (not shown in Figure 30–3) of 7.2 percentage points (from 32.5 percent to 25.3 percent) in hospitalization rates from Year 1 to Year 3 for the national demonstration resulted in an overall relative rate of decline of 22 percent over the 3-year period.

Analogous annual decreases in risk-adjusted hospitalization rates occurred for the New York state OBQI demonstration patients as shown in the lower portion of Figure 30–3. The overall relative rate of decline from Year 1 to Year 3 was 20 percent, and the Year 1 to Year 4 change in New York (from 30.1 percent to 22.2 percent, not shown in Figure 30–3) produced a net decrease of 7.9 percentage points and a 4-year overall relative rate of decline of 26 percent.

Other Target Outcome Findings

The results for target outcomes other than acute hospitalization are presented in Figure 30–4. The mean percentage change in outcome rates across all national demonstration agencies in risk-adjusted target outcomes (other than hospitalization) from Year 1 to Year 2 was 7.7 percent, while the percentage change for comparison outcomes was 1.4 percent over this period. The percentage change in target outcomes (other than hospitalization) from Year 2 to Year 3 was 5.8 percent, compared with a 1.1 percent rate of change in comparison outcomes over the same period. Thus, paralleling the findings for the patient-

level hospitalization analyses, the agency-level analyses of target outcome improvement rates over these two successive periods of adjacent years resulted in significant outcome enhancements ($p < .05$) for both time periods. The New York state results presented in Figure 30–4 demonstrate similar significant changes ($p < .05$) in target outcomes other than hospitalization when compared to other outcomes over the successive periods of adjacent years.

In general, (1) the magnitude of the effects of OBQI, (2) the large numbers and variety of patients and providers involved that ensured breadth of experience and statistical power, (3) the parallel findings for the two separate demonstration trials, (4) the continual successes of outcome enhancement for the vast majority of agencies throughout the demonstration, and (5) the information conveyed by clinical staff about the value of OBQI combine to strongly suggest a pervasively favorable impact of OBQI on patient outcomes. The magnitude of the improvements in hospitalization rates and other outcomes was substantial, particularly because home health clinicians had never undertaken this type of quality improvement. Further, as noted in the introduction, the latter stages of these demonstrations were conducted during a time of unprecedented and radical decline in payment (under IPS) accompanied by large reductions in visits per patient and serious threats to agency survival.

Demonstration agency staff generally exhibited a strong sense of ownership of OBQI (and OASIS), reflected by the manner in which they adapted OBQI to their agency's day-to-day operations. Several factors accounted for the successes of the OBQI demonstration programs. First, information obtained, analyzed, and used in feedback reports is precise, understandable, and of practical value for clinicians. Second, when implemented correctly, requisite data items and CQI activities can be integrated into and replace current items and activities rather than add substantially to the day-to-day operational routine of clinical staff. Third, the OBQI applications framework encourages clinical and quality improvement staff to be rigorous and

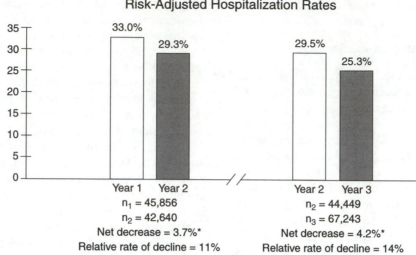

National OBQI Demonstration Findings
Risk-Adjusted Hospitalization Rates

A.

New York State OBQI Demonstration Findings
Risk-Adjusted Hospitalization Rates

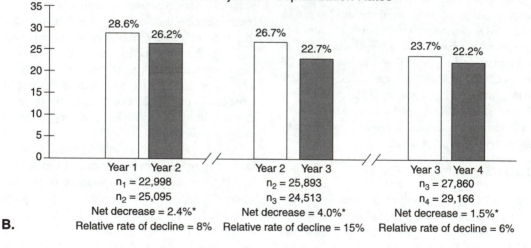

B.

* All net decreases are statistically significant ($p < .001$).

Figure 30–3 (A) Outcome-Based Quality Improvement (OBQI) effects on risk-adjusted hospitalization rates: National OBQI demonstration findings. (B) OBQI effects on risk-adjusted hospitalization rate: New York State OBQI demonstration findings.

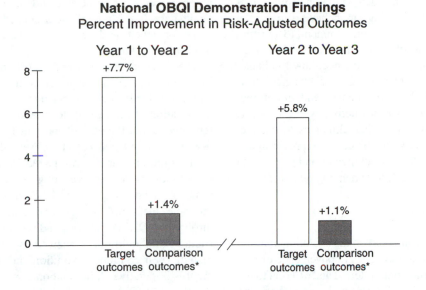

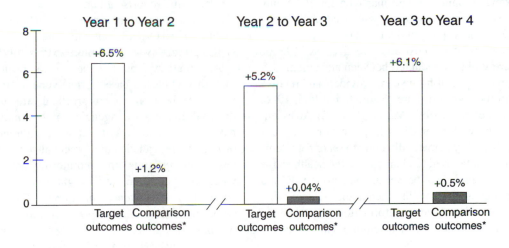

* All mean differences (for pairs of years) were significant (*p* < .05).

Figure 30–4 (A) Combined Outcome-Based Quality Improvement (OBQI)effects on risk-adjusted target outcomes other than hospitalization: National OBQI demonstration findings. (B) Combined OBQI effects on risk-adjusted target outcomes other than hospitalization: New York state OBQI demonstration findings.

innovative in areas such as (1) choosing target outcomes; (2) isolating care behaviors to change in their agency or care environment; (3) writing a focused plan of action that documents which target care behaviors to change, how to change them, who is responsible for changes, how changes will be implemented and monitored, and when these various activities are to occur; and (4) motivating other clinicians to change. Such factors serve as the basis for providing informative feedback to clinicians and give rise to a flexible approach to enhancing outcomes.

CONCLUSION

We are at a unique point in the evolution of home care in the United States. A convergence of factors is occurring, both internal and external to the industry, which will guide and even reshape the provision of home care over the next decade. Home care has moved in the direction of per episode prospective payment, increased penetration by managed care organizations, and outcomes monitoring and management. Following the earlier precedent set by selected analysts and researchers, progressively more comprehensive analyses of the cost and effectiveness of home care will be conducted between and among different types of home care providers and relative to other types of care (Hedrick and Inui, 1986; Kramer et al., 1997, Murtaugh, 1992). An essential ingredient for all such applications is a carefully and systematically derived set of data items that can be used to characterize the health status and care needs of home care patients at SOC and at regular time points thereafter, including discharge. Patient-level information about volume of services (visits) by discipline will also be essential for such analyses.

As home care continues to evolve, it should and will be analyzed more carefully in terms of its costs and benefits. As discussed at the outset of this chapter, a framework is needed that enables us to integrate cost and effectiveness issues in home care so that decision and refinements in the provision of home care can be made at the levels of individual patients/clients, home care agencies, and our home care delivery system, in-

cluding integrating home care with other types of health care. In this regard, we first need a framework for concurrently evaluating the effectiveness of home care.

The outcome analyses and reports presented in the previous section can constitute the foundation for this framework. Such reports provide information at the agency level and at the system level about the effectiveness of home care. Whether the OBQI effects observed in the demonstrations can be replicated or approximated more widely or over longer time periods remains to be seen. The OASIS data set, the outcome measures derived and risk adjusted through the OASIS data set, and the total OBQI framework should not be viewed as work completed. Their continued evolution and improvement is imperative. A foundation now exists for a national OBQI program for home health care, but refinements will be needed intermittently in areas such as revised OASIS data items for OBQI and payment purposes. New outcome measures can be developed and incorporated into outcome reports and adverse event reports. Gaps and areas to improve will naturally be identified as OASIS, outcome measures, and OBQI principles are used more extensively.

Above all, we should adhere to the principle that this evidence-based effectiveness framework must be useful and of practical value to individual home care agencies, not simply to payers or regulators. Without serving the needs of home care agencies in a practical sense, system level reporting and monitoring activities will sink under their own weight. On the other hand, if an effectiveness monitoring (i.e., outcome monitoring) framework is of direct value for purposes of clinical management, quality improvement, case mix monitoring, cost monitoring, and meeting regulatory and other fiscal requirements, the information and reporting system is likely to be diligently and accurately maintained by home health agency staff.

Acknowledgments

The work described in this chapter was funded by the Centers for Medicare and Medicaid Services (Contract #500-94-0054), the Robert Wood Johnson Foundation (Grant #19218), and the New York State Department of Health (Contract #C-015111). The findings of the demonstrations were published in Shaughnessy et al., 2002, Improving patient outcomes of home health care: Findings from two demonstration trials of outcome-based quality improvement. *Journal of the American Geriatrics Society* 50: 1354–1364.

REFERENCES

Center for Health Services Research. 2002. *OASIS and outcome-based quality improvement in home health care: Research and demonstration findings, policy implications, and considerations for future change,* vols. 1–4. Denver, CO: Center for Health Services Research.

Centers for Medicare and Medicaid Services. 1998. *Outcome and assessment information set: Implementing OASIS at a home health agency to improve patient outcomes.* Baltimore, MD: Author.

Centers for Medicare and Medicaid Services. 2002. Data Compendium. Available from http://www.cms.hhs.gov/researchers/pubs/datacompendium (accessed May 16, 2003).

Fries, B. E., et al. 1994. Refining a case-mix measure for nursing homes: Resource utilization groups (RUG-III). *Medical Care* 32: 668–685.

Granger, C. V., et al. 1993. Performance profiles of the Functional Independence Measure. *American Journal of Physical Medicine and Rehabilitation* 72: 84–89.

Granger, C. V., et al. 1995. The Uniform Data System for Medical Rehabilitation: Report of first admissions for 1993. *American Journal of Physical Medicine and Rehabilitation* 74: 62–66.

Hawes, C., et al. 1995. Reliability estimates for the Minimum Data Set for nursing home resident assessment and care screening (MDS). *Gerontologist* 35: 172–178.

Hedrick, S. C., and T. S. Inui. 1986. The effectiveness and cost of home care: An information synthesis. *Health Services Research* 20: 851–880.

Hittle, D. F., et al. 2003. A study of reliability and burden of home health assessment using OASIS. *Home Health Care Services Quarterly* 22(4): 43–63.

Kramer, A. M., et al. 1997. Outcomes and costs after hip fracture and stroke: A comparison of rehabilitation settings. *Journal of the American Medical Association* 277: 396–404.

Morris, J. N., et al. 1990. Designing the national resident assessment instrument for nursing homes. *Gerontologist* 30: 293–307.

Murtaugh, C. 1992. Quality of life, functional status, patient satisfaction. In *Patient Outcome Research: Examining the Effectiveness of Nursing Practice: Proceedings of a Conference* (Pub. No. NIH–93–3411). Washington, DC: U.S. Department of Health and Human Services, Public Health Service, National Institutes of Health.

National Association for Home Care. 1995. Medicare's OASIS: Standardized outcome and assessment information set for home health care. *NAHC Report* (special supplement no. 625, August 11, 1995). Washington, DC: NAHC.

Powell, M. C., et al. 1994. *Technical appendices to the report on measuring outcomes of home health care,* vol. 2. Denver, CO: Center for Health Services Research.

Shaughnessy, P. W. 1991. *Shaping policy for long-term care: Learning from the effectiveness of hospital swing beds.* Ann Arbor, MI: Health Administration Press.

Shaughnessy, P. W., et al. 1994a. Measuring and assuring the quality of home care. *Health Care Financing Review* 16: 35–68.

Shaughnessy, P. W., et al. 1994b. *Measuring outcomes of home health care,* vol. 1. Denver, CO: Center for Health Services Research.

Shaughnessy, P. W., et al. 1995. Outcome-based quality improvement in home care. *Caring* 14: 44–49.

Shaughnessy, P. W., et al. 1996. Home health care: Moving forward with continuous quality improvement. *Journal of Aging and Social Policy* 7: 149–167.

Shaughnessy, P. W., et al. 1997a. Outcomes across the care continuum. Home health care. *Medical Care* 35: 1225–1226.

Shaughnessy, P. W., et al. 1997b. Outcomes across the care continuum. Home health care. *Medical Care* 35 (11 Supplement): NS115–NS123.

Shaughnessy, P. W., et al. 2002. Improving patient outcomes of home health care: Findings from two demonstration trials of outcome-based quality improvement. *Journal of the American Geriatrics Society* 50: 1354–1364.

State University of New York (SUNY) at Buffalo. 1993. *Guide to the Uniform Data Set for Medical Rehabilitation (adult FIM^{SM}).* Buffalo, NY: SUNY-Buffalo.

State University of New York (SUNY) at Buffalo. 1995. *Getting started with the Uniform Data System for Medical Rehabilitation (adult FIM^{SM}).* Buffalo, NY: SUNY-Buffalo.

CHAPTER 31

Implementing Outcome-Based Quality Improvement in the Home Health Agency

Linda H. Krulish

The Outcome and Assessment Information Set (OASIS) and Outcome-Based Quality Improvement (OBQI) offer the home care industry the first real opportunity to measure and globally compare outcomes of care. Although mandatory OASIS data collection by Medicare-certified agencies has been required since July 1999, and OASIS-based reports allowing Outcome-Based Quality Improvement have been nationally available since February 2002, not all agencies have demonstrated an interest in pursuing OBQI. Although the level of commitment to OBQI may be a reflection of an agency's philosophy or stability, specific issues that may influence OBQI involvement include regulatory status, use of OBQI reports in the survey process, public reporting of OBQI outcomes, and OASIS data accuracy.

NO REGULATORY REQUIREMENT FOR OBQI

The Medicare Conditions of Participation (CoPs) do not currently require that agencies access, review, or use the OASIS derived reports for OBQI activities. A notice of proposed rule making was published in March 1997 that would require agencies to incorporate information from OBQI reports into their quality assessment and performance improvement activities. Although this regulation has not yet been published in its final form, a final rule is expected in 2004 that will include some level of mandatory OBQI involvement by agencies.

USE OF OBQI REPORTS IN COMPLIANCE SURVEYS

Although agencies are not currently required to access or use OBQI reports, state surveyors are. Effective May 1, 2003, the home health survey process has changed to require review and incorporation of information from OASIS-based reports. State surveyors have been provided with specific protocols to support a standardized approach to report review and survey follow-up actions, including identification of survey focus areas, chart reviews and in home visits. (See Figure 31–1) Therefore, involvement in OBQI may be undertaken as a means of survey preparation, allowing an agency to identify the potentially problematic areas, patient types, and actual care episodes that surveyors will discover using the new enhanced survey process. Identifying a problem and implementing a plan of action to correct it before the surveyor arrives is the best course of action.

PUBLIC REPORTING OF OBQI OUTCOMES

May 1, 2003, marked the kick-off date for public reporting of OASIS data. As part of the Home Health Quality Initiative (HHQI), the

CMS HHA Training Worksheet
OBQM & OBQI Reports
Pre-Survey Process and Sample Selection

Adverse Event Outcome Report
(for most recent quarter, or longer if necessary to reach 60 patients)

	Any Patients Listed?	Difference ≥ Two Times Ref. Value?	Area for Focus (check box)	Record Review* (check box)	Home Visit*
Tier 1 AE Outcomes					
• Emergent Care for Injury Caused by Fall or Accident at Home	Y☐ N☐	N/A	☐	☐	yes
• Emergent Care for Wound Infections, Deteriorating Wound Status	Y☐ N☐	N/A	☐	☐	yes
Tier 2 AE Outcomes					
• Emergent Care for Improper Medication Administration, Medication Side Effects	Y☐ N☐	Y☐ N☐	☐	☐	Y☐ N☐
• Emergent Care for Hypo/Hyperglycemia	Y☐ N☐	Y☐ N☐	☐	☐	Y☐ N☐
• Substantial Decline in ≥ Three Activities of Daily Living	Y☐ N☐	Y☐ N☐	☐	☐	no
• Discharged to the Community Needing Wound Care or Medication Assistance	Y☐ N☐	Y☐ N☐	☐	☐	no
• Discharged to the Community Needing Toileting Assistance	Y☐ N☐	Y☐ N☐	☐	☐	no
• Discharged to the Community with Behavioral Problems	Y☐ N☐	Y☐ N☐	☐	☐	no

OBQI Outcome Report (for most recent 12-month period)

	≥ 30 Eligible Cases? (check if yes)	Difference from Ref. Value?		Statistically Sig.? (check if yes)	Outcomes for Focus** (check two)**
• Improvement in Upper Body Dressing	☐	≥ 10% lower	Y☐ N☐	☐	☐
• Improvement in Bathing	☐	≥ 10% lower	Y☐ N☐	☐	☐
• Improvement in Transferring	☐	≥ 15% lower	Y☐ N☐	☐	☐
• Improvement in Ambulation/Locomotion	☐	≥ 7% lower	Y☐ N☐	☐	☐
• Improvement in Management of Oral Medication	☐	≥ 10% lower	Y☐ N☐	☐	☐
• Improvement in Dyspnea	☐	≥ 15% lower	Y☐ N☐	☐	☐
• Improvement in Urinary Incontinence	☐	≥ 20% lower	Y☐ N☐	☐	☐
• Acute Care Hospitalization	☐	≥ 10% higher	Y☐ N☐	☐	☐
• Improvement in Pain Interfering w/Activity	☐	≥ 15% lower	Y☐ N☐	☐	☐
• Improvement in Status of Surgical Wounds	☐	≥ 10% lower	Y☐ N☐	☐	☐
• Other					☐

OBQI Case Mix Report (for most recent 12-month period)
Acute conditions or diagnoses statistically sig. & ≥ 15% points higher than ref.***

* Select one to two records and one to two HV w/RR for areas for focus.
** Select one to two HV w/RR for patients eligible for focus outcome.
*** Select one to two HV w/RR and (opt.) one to two RR w/o HV.

CMS HHA Training
Practice Exercise - Worksheet for OBQM and OBQI Reports
February 2003

Figure 31–1 Survey Protocol Worksheet

continues

Department of Health and Human Services (DHHS) began making agency-specific outcome data available to the public in an effort to assist Medicare and Medicaid beneficiaries and their families in making informed healthcare decisions. DHHS also expects that public reporting will motivate home health agencies to aggressively work to improve their patient outcomes.

This "phase one" kick-off included publication of 11 of the 41 OASIS-based OBQI outcome measures for agencies in eight states. (See Figure 31–2.) Comparative outcome rates are

Submission Statistics by Agency (for most recent 6-month period)

Submission Questions		If yes to either probe, investigate:	
Is HHA submitting data less often than monthly?	Y □ N □	• HHA policies/procedures for receiving, tracking, data entering and transmitting OASIS data and correcting clinical records. Do HHA processes follow policies/ procedures?	Y □ N □
Does HHA have >20% rejected records?	Y □ N □	• If another organization (e.g., vendor) submits data for the HHA:	
		- Is there a written contract covering the arrangement?	Y □ N □
		- Does the other organization provide feedback reports to the HHA?	Y □ N □
		• For 4-6 records selected for clinical record review, ask the HHA for a printout of a final validation report showing that at least one assessment (e.g., SOC, F/U, Discharge) was received by the state. (Because the HHA may not yet have submitted data for more recent assessments, it will be necessary to select patient assessments that were completed one to two months prior to the survey.)	
		- Can the HHA provide the requested final validation reports?	Y □ N □
		- Was at least one assessment per record (e.g., SOC, F/U, Discharge) received by the State?	Y □ N □
		• If there is a high percentage of rejected records:	
		- Is there a legitimate reason (e.g., a large batch of records was sent twice, and all records in the second batch were rejected)?	Y □ N □
		- Can the HHA verify that its software conforms to CMS standards?	Y □ N □

Error Summary Report by HHA (for most recent 6-month period)

Do the following errors appear on the report?		Threshold met or exceeded?		If yes, determine if the HHA's processes:
102 (Inconsistent Lock date) (warning)	Y □ N □	≥20%	Y □ N □	Ensure the 7-day lock requirement is met (Assessment forms are completed, reviewed, corrected as needed, and data entered and locked within a 7-day period).
262 (Inconsistent M0090 date; RFA 4 must be done on an every 60-day cycle) (warning)	Y □ N □	≥20%	Y □ N □	Ensure that recertification assessments are completed between day 56 and day 60 of the certification period (HHA has system for notifying clinician that recertification is due and tracks incoming recertification assessments to ensure timely completion).
1003 (Inconsistent effective date sequence) (warning)	Y □ N □	≥10%	Y □ N □	Track submission of complete patient episodes (SOC/ROC and corresponding Transfer or Discharge assessment for each patient).
1002 (Inconsistent record sequence) (warning)	Y □ N □	≥10%	Y □ N □	Track that assessments are submitted in the order they were conducted (e.g., SOC data are entered and submitted prior to recertification data).

Figure 31–1 *continued*

accessible on a Home Health Compare Web site, accessible from the Medicare Web site, www.Medicare.gov, or by phoning 1-800-MEDICARE. Additionally, rates of 3 of the 11 outcome measures were published in major newspapers in the eight phase-one states, listing an agency's performance rates, and comparing them to the average rates of agencies in the state, and in the group of phase one states (see Figure 31–3). Release of outcome rates from

Medicare-certified agencies in all states followed in the fall of 2003.

ACCURACY OF OASIS DATA

Issues related to the accuracy of the OASIS data may be influencing an agency's willingness to commit to OBQI. Agencies are increasingly using OASIS data as the basis for quality and reimbursement functions, including Outcome-Based Quality Monitoring (OBQM), OBQI, and utilization and profitability analysis and modeling. Increasing data use is accompanied by increasing awareness of how slight variations in OASIS scores potentially result in significant

quality reporting or reimbursement consequences. For example, an OASIS score of "2" versus "3" on a single OASIS item may be the difference between the outcome episode being reported as patient *improvement* or *stabilization* on an agency's OBQI report. Such a single level variation may also result in an episode being categorized as an adverse event on an agency's OBQM report. Under the enhanced survey protocols, such a single adverse event may trigger mandatory survey action, including identification of a survey focus area with associated chart audits and home visits. Additionally, a single level variation in score may significantly influence reimbursement, often increasing or

<u>Outcome Measures:</u>

Percentage of patients who get better at getting dressed

Percentage of patients who get better at bathing

Percentage of patients who are confused less often

Percentage of patients who get better at taking their medicines correctly (by mouth)

Percentage of patients who get better at walking or moving around

Percentage of patients who get better getting to and from the toilet

Percentage of patients who get better at getting in and out of bed

Percentage of patients who have less pain when moving around

Percentage of patients who stay the same or don't get worse at bathing

Percentage of patients who need urgent, unplanned medical care

Percentage of patients who had to be admitted to the hospital

<u>Phase 1 States:</u>

Florida

Massachusetts

Missouri

Oregon

New Mexico

South Carolina

West Virginia

Wisconsin

Source: 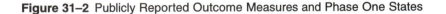 http://www.medicare.gov/HHCompare

Figure 31–2 Publicly Reported Outcome Measures and Phase One States

Figure 31–3 Sample Phase One Ad: *Miami Herald*

decreasing the agency's reimbursement under the Medicare prospective payment system by hundreds of dollars.

Recognition of the potential ramifications related to OASIS scoring is resulting in agencies evaluating their own internal OASIS scoring practices, as well as seeking clarification for current scoring guidelines that lack the clarity or comprehensiveness to allow consistent, reliable, and valid scoring among clinicians nationwide. Lack of confidence in the OASIS data on which the outcome reports are based may be perceived by some organizations as a questionable foundation on which to devote the significant agency resources required by OBQI implementation.

OASIS ANALYSIS AND REFINEMENT

Industry concerns related to ongoing analysis and refinement of the OASIS data set and scoring guidelines have been heard by the Department of Health and Human Services. Industry providers and supporting associations have been offered means to voice concerns and offer recommendations, such as through involvement in ongoing open door forums and provider representation on the OASIS Technical Expert Panel. Providers are encouraged to actively offer concerns and recommendations to facilitate OASIS refinement efforts that are significant and meaningful.

Although it is expected that the OASIS data set and associated uses for quality and reimbursement will continually evolve, there is much that agencies can do immediately to address and improve OASIS data concerns and maximize the value and effectiveness of the OBQI system to the benefit of their patients. Along with standardized data collection, which is the first step of the OBQI cycle (see Figure 31–4), OBQI success requires competent implementation at each step of the cycle:

- OASIS transmission
- outcome report analysis
- target outcome selection
- process-of-care investigation
- plan of action development and implementation

The remainder of this chapter will present practical issues and strategies to consider in efforts to implement or enhance OBQI efforts at each step of the OBQI process.

OBQI STEP ONE: STANDARDIZED OASIS DATA COLLECTION

The OASIS assessments provide the foundational data on which the OBQI system operates. Currently, this OASIS data is being collected during patient assessment visits by thousands of home health nurses and therapists across the country. The realization of OBQI as a key vehicle to continually improve home health patient outcomes requires OASIS data accuracy. The quality of the OASIS data is dependent upon collection by clinicians who possess adequate technical knowledge of OASIS-specific scoring instructions, as well as clinical skills necessary to adequately assess the patient and interpret assessment findings. Data quality will require ongoing competency evaluation and training for involved nurses and therapists, for clinical and technical knowledge and skills related to the OASIS assessment.

Competency Assessment

Related to OASIS data collection, competency assessment can take many forms. The first step is to identify specific knowledge and skills that are required for competent OASIS collection. The next step is to evaluate a clinician's knowledge and/or abilities relative to the OASIS-specific task list. Figure 31–5 presents a sample competency assessment tool listing OASIS tasks for evaluation. The method of evaluation can take the form of self-assessment, written or verbal testing, simulated demonstration, or observed performance during an actual home visit. Figure 31–6 presents a competency assessment tool in the form of a simple written test that can be used to evaluate a clinician's ability to apply scoring guidelines to patient scenarios in order to determine an OASIS response for five different OASIS items. The various methods of competency assessment present a hierarchy of

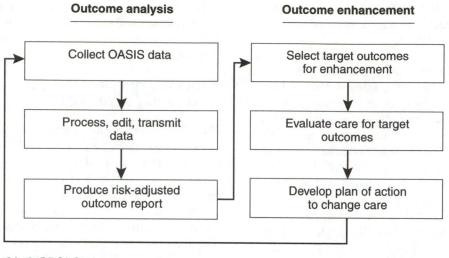

Figure 31–4 OBQI Cycle

approaches, where those offering the truest picture of a clinician's ability to apply OASIS knowledge and skill (the observed performance during an actual home visit) also require the greatest expenditure of agency resources (unreimbursed expense of a supervising staff member during the visit, as well as resources to compare and reconcile clinician and supervisor OASIS scores after the assessment visit). Compare this approach with a self-assessment method, where relatively few agency resources are consumed, but which also result in conclusions that may reflect clinician bias or unawareness of their own lack of skill. A thoughtful combination of various competency assessment approaches will likely provide the most reasonable and effective conclusions on which to formulate appropriate OASIS training.

The agency's competency assessment program should include any clinician who would ever conduct a comprehensive assessment and collect OASIS, at any time point. Based on agency practice, this might include weekend or part-time RNs, contract therapists, or other groups who pose unique challenges for involvement in routine agency testing or inservicing. Applicable staff new to the agency should also

undergo competency assessment and be provided training based on identified needs. Substantial experience in relevant clinical fields, even in the setting of another Medicare-certified home health agency, should not be automatically equated to experience or proficiency with OASIS, because agency practice and expectations related to OASIS training and application vary greatly between organizations.

Resources for OASIS Accuracy Training

In providing training, "accurate" data collection must be defined as *consistent with OASIS scoring guidelines*. In other words, the concept of standardization in data collection must not be disregarded in an effort to select a score that may appear "more correct" for a specific patient situation. The ability of a clinician to reference and consistently apply established scoring guidelines is as critical as the proven validity and reliability of the OASIS items themselves. Neither poor collection practices with a flawless tool nor perfect collection practices with a faulty tool will yield high quality data. As expected OASIS refinement produces outcomes with improved reliability and validity, the skills

Competency Assessment Tool for Comprehensive Assessment Activities Page 1 of 4			
Competency : Patient Selection			
The therapist or nurse:	YES	NO	COMMENTS:
Understands the patient populations requiring the comprehensive assessment			
Understands the patient population exceptions for OASIS data collection			
Competency : Data Collection Time Points			
The therapist or nurse:	YES	NO	COMMENTS:
Lists the various time points at which a comprehensive patient assessment is required			
Describes criteria or events which would define a "major decline or improvement in the patient's health status"			
Identifies the appropriate OASIS items/version required for collection at each specific assessment time points			
Describes the timeliness requirements for completion of the comprehensive assessment at the various time points			
Competency : Data Collection Personnel			
The therapist or nurse:	YES	NO	COMMENTS:
Describes the criteria for determining which agency clinicians may conduct the comprehensive assessment and/or OASIS data collection at various time points			
Competency : Data Collection Rules			
The therapist or nurse:	YES	NO	COMMENTS:
Describes the rules related to collecting data based on the patient's "usual status"			
Describes the rules related to collection of "prior" data (i.e. events occurring within the past 14 days, or ADL status 14 days prior to SOC)			
Describes assessment methods which may be used to collect comprehensive assessment and OASIS data			
Describes the rules related to skip patterns			
Describes the rules related to the use of "not applicable" or "unknown" responses			

Figure 31–5 Sample Competency Assessment Tool

continues

Competency Assessment Tool for Comprehensive Assessment Activities

Page 2 of 4

Competency : OASIS Data Elements

The therapist or nurse:	YES	NO	COMMENTS:
Is familiar with the terminology used in the OASIS data items, as defined in the OASIS implementation manual (i.e. "skin lesion", "incontinence")			
Understands the intent of the OASIS items, as described in the OASIS implementation manual			
Describes assessment strategies which can be utilized to gather OASIS data			

Competency : Determining Eligibility for the Medicare Home Health Benefit

The therapist or nurse:	YES	NO	COMMENTS:
Describes services covered by the Medicare Home Health Benefit, as outlined in the HIM-11			
Describes the eligibility criteria for the Medicare Home Health Benefit			
Can appropriately identify a patient's homebound status			

Competency : Drug Regimen Review

The therapist or nurse:	Is Proficient with regular experience	Is Competent with occasional experience	Has had Some exposure; will need further training	Has had No exposure	Comments:
Identifies the activities required by the drug regimen review					
Identifies the time points at which the drug regimen review is required					
Identifies all medications a patient is currently taking					
Is able to assess for ineffective drug therapy					
Is able to assess for significant side effects					
Is able to assess for significant drug interactions					

Home Therapy Services   Copyright 2000
www.oasisanswers.com

Figure 31–5 *continued*

Competency Assessment Tool for Comprehensive Assessment Activities

Page 3 of 4

Competency : **Drug Regimen Review (cont.)**

The therapist or nurse:	Is Proficient with regular experience	Is Competent with occasional experience	Has had Some exposure; will need further training	Has had No exposure	Comments:
Is able to assess for duplicate drug therapy					
Is able to assess for noncompliance with drug therapy					

Competency : **Assessment of OASIS Domains**

The therapist or nurse:	Is Proficient with regular experience	Is Competent with occasional experience	Has had Some exposure; will need further training	Has had No exposure	Comments:
Assesses Living Arrangements and Supportive Assistance (M0300-M0380) including home safety and identification of caregiver assistance					
Assesses Sensory Status (M0390-M0430) including vision, communication and pain					
Assesses Integumentary Status (M0440-M0488) including identification of skin lesions, and differential identification and assessment of pressure ulcers, stasis ulcers and surgical wounds					
Assessment of Respiratory Status (M0490-M0500) including presence of dyspnea and respiratory treatments utilized at home					
Assessment of Elimination Status (M0510-M0550) including UTI history, catheter/ostomy status, and bowel/bladder incontinence					

Home Therapy Services   Copyright 2000
www.oasisanswers.com

Figure 31–5 *continued*

continues

Competency Assessment Tool for Comprehensive Assessment Activities
Page 4 of 4

Competency : Assessment of OASIS Domains (cont.)

The therapist or nurse:	Is Proficient with regular experience	Is Competent with occasional experience	Has had Some exposure; will need further training	Has had No exposure	Comments:
Assessment of Neuro/Emotional/Behavioral Status (M0560-M0630) including cognitive functioning, and presence of anxiety, depression and high risk problem behaviors					
Assessment of ADL/IADL Function (M0640-M0770) including current and prior functioning for grooming, dressing, bathing, toileting, transferring, ambulation/locomotion, feeding/eating, meal planning/preparation, transportation, laundry, housekeeping, shopping, and telephone use					
Assessment of Medication Management (M0780-M0800) including patient and/or caregiver management of oral, inhalant/mist, and injectable medications					
Assessment of Equipment Management (M0810-M0820) including patient and/or caregiver management of oxygen, IV/infusion, enteral/parenteral equipment and supplies					

Clinician: _____ Date: _____

Assessment method(s):

☐ Self-Assessment (SA)   ☐ Verbal reporting (VR)
☐ Written reporting (WR)   ☐ Skills lab simulation (SLS)
☐ Chart review (CR)   ☐ Direct observation/Clinical Performance (DO)

Assessment by (if applicable): _____

Home Therapy Services   Copyright 2000
www.oasisanswers.com

Figure 31–5 *continued*

Name: _____   **Date:** _____

Instructions: Score each of the following OASIS items (current status only) based on the patient information provided.

1. (M0520) Urinary Incontinence or Urinary Catheter Presence:

☐   0   No incontinence or catheter (includes anuria or ostomy for urinary drainage)

☐   1   Patient is incontinent

☐   2   Patient requires a urinary catheter (i.e., external, indwelling, intermittent, suprapubic)

A healthy patient recovering from a tibial plateau fracture resulting from a motor vehicle accident reports that because she must walk slowly to maintain touch down weight bearing, she has had a few minor urinary "accidents" on her way to the bathroom.

2. (M0680) Toileting: Ability to get to and from the toilet or bedside commode:

Current

☐   0   Able to get to and from the toilet independently with or without a device

☐   1   When reminded, assisted, or supervised by another person, able to get to and from the toilet.

☐   2   **Unable** to get to and from the toilet but is able to use a bedside commode (with or without assistence).

☐   3   **Unable** to get to and from the toilet or bedside commode but is able to use a bed-pan/urinal independently.

☐   4   Is totally dependent in toileting.

    UK   Unknown

A patient's only bathroom is upstairs, and the patient has demonstrated safe independent ambulation with a cane to and from the toilet, including up and down the stairs. Yesterday the physician restricted stair climbing for 1 week, during that time the patient is using a bedside commode.

3. (M0690) Transferring: Ability to move from bed to chair, on and off toilet or commode, into and out of tub or shower, and ability to turn and position self in bed if patient is bedfast.

Current

☐   0   Able to independently transfer.

☐   1   Transfers with minimal human assistance or with use of an assistive device.

☐   2   **Unable** to transfer self but able to bear weight and pivot during the transfer process.

☐   3   Unable to transfer self and **unable** to bear weight or pivot when transferred by another person.

☐   4   Bedfast, unable to transfer but able to turn and position self in bed.

☐   5   Bedfast, unable to transfer and **unable** to turn and position self.

    UK   Unknown

Patient is independent in bed-to-chair transfers and toilet transfers without assistive devices. Requires moderate assistance for tub transfer.

Figure 31–6 Competency Assessment Tool in the Form of a Simple Written Test

continues

4. (M0700) Ambulation/Locomotion: Ability to **safely** walk, once in a standing position, or use a wheelchair, once in a seated position, on a variety of surfaces.

Current

☐   0   Able to independently walk on even and uneven surfaces and climb stairs with or without railings (needs no human assistance or assistive device).

☐   1   Requires use of a device (e.g., cane, walker) to walk alone **or** requires human supervision or assistance to negotiate stairs or steps or uneven surfaces.

☐   2   Able to walk only with the supervision or assistance of another person at all times.

☐   3   Chairfast, **unable** to ambulate but is able to wheel self independently.

☐   4   Chairfast, unable to ambulate and is **unable** to wheel self.

☐   5   Bedfast, unable to ambulate or be up in a chair.

     UK   Unknown

Patient lives alone and is currently ambulating throughout two levels of the house with no assistive device. The patient is observed to frequently rely on the furniture and walls for support during gait.

5. (M0780) Management of Oral Medications: **Patient's ability** to prepare and take all prescribed medications reliably and safely, including administration of the correct dosage at the appropriate times/intervals. **Excludes injectable and IV medications. (Note: This refers to ability, not compliance or willingness.)**

Current

☐   0   Able to independently take the correct oral medication(s) and proper dosage(s) at the correct times.

☐   1   Able to take medication(s) at the correct times if:

                  a: individual dosages are prepared in advance by another person; **or**

                  b: given daily reminders; **or**

                  c: someone develops a drug diary or chart.

☐   2   **Unable** to take medication unless administered by someone else.

☐   NA   No oral medications prescribed.

     UK   Unknown

The patient's medication profile contains 7 oral medications, 6 of which the patient has been safely and independently self-administering for several months. The 7th oral medication is a new tapered dose of Prednisone, for which daily reminders by the patient's caregiver are required to achieve accurate dosing.

Figure 31–6 *continued*

---

related to standardized data collection will need to be refined among the field clinicians who score the OASIS items based on reported and observed patient information.

For training purposes, the source for data collection guidelines should be those formally provided or endorsed by the Centers for Medicare and Medicaid Services (CMS). Currently these include the *OASIS Implementation Manual*, and batches of OASIS-related questions and answers; both available on the OASIS Web site (www.cms.hhs.gov/oasis). Chapter 8 of the *OASIS Implementation Manual* provides a list of general conventions (rules) to observe in

Answers to Competency Assessment: OASIS Accuracy

1. (M0520) Urinary Incontinence or Urinary Catheter Presence:

■   1   Patient is incontinent

Rationale: M0520 identifies the presence of the symptom of urinary incontinence, not the etiology. Urinary incontinence may result from multiple causes, including physiologic dysfunction, cognitive deficits, environmental barriers, or mobility impairments. The cause of the incontinence is not addressed in the item. (See *OASIS Implementation Manual,* pg. 8.78).

2. (M0680) Toileting:

Current

■   2   **Unable** to get to and from the toilet but is able to use a bedside commode (with or without assistance).

Rationale: M0680 identifies the patient's ability to safely ambulate to and from the toilet or bedside commode. Although the patient may have the physical and cognitive function required to get to and from the toilet, the combination of the patient's environment (upstairs bathroom) and the current activity restrictions (no stair climbing) present identified barriers, making the patient currently *unable* to get to the toilet. (See *OASIS Implementation Manual,* pg. 8.96).

3. (M0690) Transferring:

Current

■   0   Able to independently transfer.

Rationale: M0690 identifies the patient's ability to safely transfer in a variety of situations. The patient information reveals that the patient's functional status is not consistent for all of the transfer tasks assessed. The *OASIS Implementation Manual* provides the following instruction: "If ability varies between the transfer activities listed, record the level of ability applicable to the majority of those activities." The patient is independent without assistive device in the majority of the applicable tasks; therefore, the standardized response would report the patient as independent in transfers without assisstive devices. (See *OASIS Implementation Manual,* pg. 8.97).

4. (M0700) Ambulation/Locomotion:

Current

■   1   Requires use of a device (e.g., cane, walker) to walk alone **or** requires human supervision or assistance to negotiate stairs or steps or uneven surfaces.

■   2   Able to walk only with the supervision or assistance of another person at all times.

Rationale: M0700 identifies the patient's ability to safely walk on level and uneven surfaces. While the patient demonstrates the task of walking without the use of an assistive device or supervision, the technique used (relying on support from furniture/walls) demonstrates a dependence on external support (an assistive device) during gait. The patient would be scored a 1 or 2, depending upon the level of safety that is achievable with the use of an assistive device (i.e., if use of the assistive device allowed safe independent ambulation on level surfaces, response 1 would apply; if the patient required continuous supervision/assistance even when using the assistive device, response 2 would apply.) (See *OASIS Implementation Manual,* pg. 8.98).

Figure 31–6 *continued*

continues

Answers to Competency Assessment: OASIS Accuracy *(Continued)*

5. (M0780) Management of Oral Medications:

Current

■   0   Able to independently take the correct oral medication(s) and proper dosage(s) at
                         the correct times.

Rationale: M0780 identifies the patient's ability to prepare and take all prescribed oral medications reliably and safely. The patient information reveals that the patient's ability is not consistent across all medications the patient is currently taking. The *OASIS Implementation Manual* provides the following instruction: "If [the] patient's ability to manage medications varies from medication to medication, consider [the] total number of medications and total daily doses in determining what is true most of the time." Assuming the six "independent" medications represent a majority of the medications and total daily doses, the standardized response would report the patient as independent in management of oral medications. (See *Oasis Implementation Manual*, pg. 8.106.)

Figure 31–6 *continued*

---

collecting and recording OASIS data. Chapter 8 also provides an item-by-item review, outlining definitions, response-specific instructions, and assessment strategies for each of the OASIS items. It should be recognized that unless clinicians are familiar with the information provided in Chapter 8, they will likely not be reporting OASIS scores accurately (i.e., consistent with CMS guidelines). For instance, M0175 asks: "From which of the following Inpatient Facilities was the patient discharged during the past 14 days?" (See Figure 31–7.) Chapter 8 provides specific defining criteria for M0175 response #3 "Skilled Nursing Facility" as a Medicare-certified nursing facility where the patient received a skilled level of care under the Medicare Part A benefit during the 14 days prior to the home health admission. Because the OASIS item itself does not contain this unique definition, without the benefit of the Chapter 8 detail, the clinician is likely to apply a more general definition of *skilled nursing facility*. This would likely result scoring as response #3 patient stays that were not Medicare Part A funded, resulting in "inaccurate" OASIS scoring.

Other resources for data accuracy include questions and answers on the OASIS Web site that address scoring issues and provide further details that are not found in the *Implementation Manual*. For issues not addressed in these written sources, providers may contact their state OASIS Education Coordinator (OEC) to obtain a "formal" response to their issue. Contact information for the OECs by state is available on the OASIS Web site (www.cms.hhs.gov/oasis). Additionally, CMS has sponsored the development of a Web-based training program for OASIS that is intended for agency use and accessible at www.oasistraining.org. In order to allow accurate data collection, OASIS training must include effective dissemination and familiarity with the most current details and instructions available from CMS.

OBQI STEP TWO: OASIS TRANSMISSION

After OASIS data is collected, it is transmitted to the State Assessment Collection Database. The Home Assessment Validation and Entry (HAVEN) is a basic data entry system provided by CMS to agencies free of charge. The HAVEN allows agencies to encode and submit files to the state in a defined format. Some agencies choose to use proprietary software products that offer features beyond those of HAVEN,

OASIS ITEM:

(M0175) From which of the following **Inpatient Facilities** was the patient discharged <u>during the past 14 days</u>? **(Mark all that apply.)**

- ☐ 1 - Hospital
- ☐ 2 - Rehabilitation facility
- ☐ 3 - Skilled nursing facility
- ☐ 4 - Other nursing home
- ☐ 5 - Other (specify) _____
- ☐ NA - Patient was not discharged from an inpatient facility **[If NA, go to *M0200*]****

* At Follow-up, change M0200 to M0230.

DEFINITION:

Identifies whether the patient has recently (within past 14 days) been discharged from an inpatient facility. (Past 14 days encompasses the two-week period immediately preceding the start of care/resumption of care or the first day of the new certification period.)

TIME POINTS ITEM(S) COMPLETED:

Start of care
Resumption of care
Follow-up

RESPONSE—SPECIFIC INSTRUCTIONS:

- Mark all that apply. For example, patient may have been discharged from both a hospital <u>and</u> a rehabilitation facility within the past 14 days.
- Rehabilitation facility is a freestanding rehab hospital or a rehabilitation bed in a rehabilitation distinct part unit of a general acute care hospital.
- A skilled nursing facility means a Medicare certified nursing facility where the patient received a skilled level of care under the Medicare Part A benefit. Determine the following:
  1) Was the patient discharged from a Medicare-certified skilled nursing facility? If so, then:
  2) While in the skilled nursing facility was the patient receiving skilled care under the Medicare Part A benefit? If so, then:
  3) Was the patient receiving skilled care under the Medicare Part A benefit up to 14 days prior to admission to home health care?
  If all three of the above criteria apply, select Response 3. If any of the criteria are not satisfied, but the patient was in some type of nursing facility in the past 14 days, select Response 4.
- Other nursing home includes intermediate care facilities for the mentally retarded (ICF/MR) and nursing facilities (NF).
- If patient has been discharged from a swing-bed hospital, it is necessary to determine whether the patient was occupying a designated hospital bed (Response 1), a skilled nursing bed under Medicare Part A (Response 3), or a nursing bed at a lower level of care or under (Response 4).
- If a patient was discharged from a Long Term Care Hospital, the correct response is 1.

ASSESSMENT STRATEGIES:

Information can be obtained from patient/caregiver or physician's office. When uncertain about the type of facility or whether the facility is an <u>inpatient facility</u>, it may be necessary to check with the facility regarding licensure/designation.

OASIS Implementation Manual
10/03

Figure 31–7 Excerpt from *OASIS Implementation Manual*, Chapter 8, "Item-By-Item Tips" such as allowing for enhanced edit checking and timely quality or reimbursement reporting functions.

Regulatory Requirements for OASIS Data Submission

The conditions of participation stipulate specific time frames for compliance with data locking and submission. Within 7 calendar days of completion of the OASIS assessment, it is required to be "locked," referring to its finalization, with no further changes expected. The assessment file must be submitted to the state no later than the last day of the month following the month the assessment was completed. Agencies may consider submitting files earlier and/or more frequently than required in order to avoid unforeseen crises that might result in delayed submission. Early submission also provides time necessary to allow review of the validation report (a report showing the status of the file and associated individual OASIS assessments being submitted). In the event that the validation report reveals error messages (including fatal file, warning, and fatal record), early submission will allow the agency time to make corrections or to resubmit rejected files.

Strategies to improve OASIS accuracy at the data encoding and transmission phase mirror those of the data collection phase:

- provide effective training for staff with data management roles
- establish a means of evaluating competency of staff involved in all levels of data management tasks
- utilize CMS resources as the guidelines for data processing (Chapter 10 of the *OASIS Implementation Manual* addresses data entry and transmission)

A proactive data quality auditing program will eliminate or minimize the identification of data accuracy problems months later, when the OASIS-based outcomes are used in the OBQI

process. Chapter 12 of the *OASIS Implementation Manual* outlines methods for timely monitoring of OASIS data accuracy.

Special OBQI Impacts Related to Data Processing

Because OBQI reports are generated from OASIS data, subsequent corrections to OASIS data may result in changes to the agency's OBQI reports. This concept has several implications for OBQI. First, agencies should be aware that as OASIS errors are discovered, adherence to prescribed OASIS correction policies will allow the agency to achieve the requirement of "accurate data." This is especially critical when an agency identifies an internal trend related to pervasive misinterpretation or misguidance resulting in extensive miscoding of an item throughout the agency. If this erroneous scoring affects an OASIS item used to generate or risk adjust an outcome measure, the resulting impact on the OBQI report could be substantial. Timely identification and correction of the OASIS data errors may prevent the agency from investing significant agency resources into OBQI activities that are based on invalid outcome report findings. Second, agencies should recognize that apparent changes in outcomes may be due to late or corrected OASIS assessments, rather than due to actual improving or declining outcomes of care. In general, occasional correction of previously submitted assessments will not significantly impact the outcome reports, unless the agency is very small, or unless the agency corrected the same OASIS item(s) on a significant number of OASIS assessments during the report period.

Effects of Delaying an End to an Outcome Episode

Another issue affecting OBQI (related to data collection and transmission) is that data does not appear on an OBQI report until the triggered end of an outcome episode. When a home health discharge or transfer occurs, even if a patient is put "on hold" by the agency, or is expected to return for further care, the end of the outcome episode is triggered and OASIS data from the start of care (SOC) or resumption of care (ROC) will be compared with the OASIS data from the transfer or discharge in order to determine applicable end-result and/or utilization outcomes. Any delay in transferring or discharging the patient will result in a delay in that patient's OASIS data being available to contribute to the agency's outcome report. Additionally, the outcomes will be generated based on the final (transfer or discharge) OASIS scores, so any changes that occur from the last skilled visit until the final data collection may impact the outcome measurement. Two practical examples of this concept apply to payor changes, and practices to extend a patient's home care admission stay.

Payor Changes and OBQI Effects

When a patient's payor source changes from Medicare or Medicaid to private pay, an agency currently has the choice of either making the appropriate changes at the next scheduled OASIS collection time point or completing a discharge assessment and readmit under the new payor. If the agency chooses to discharge and readmit, it will allow the agency to provide a trigger to end the outcome episode at the time when the patient is likely functioning at his best, possibly allowing for the most favorable outcome report presentation. If the agency chooses to continue with the private pay patient under the same admission, then since private pay patients do not currently require data collection, it is possible that this entire episode would be excluded from the agency's outcome reports. Unless the care under the Medicare or Medicaid portion included events to trigger an outcome episode (i.e., a start of care and a transfer), none of the outcomes of care for a patient discharged under private pay would be included in the agency's OASIS-based reports. Agencies should consider the impact of available practice options, in conjunction with the specific discharge practices

and payor change circumstances experienced by the agency.

OBQI Effects of Extending Home Care Lengths of Stay

The onset of Medicare prospective payment to home care in 2000 continues to influence clinical care and utilization practices. One practice that has emerged in some agencies is a conscious effort to lengthen the home care stay. In efforts to minimize financial risk, maximize clinical outcomes, or a combination thereof, some agencies have adopted a practice of providing care until the patient reaches the point at which a home care discharge would have previously been instituted. Now, in efforts to maintain control of the case, the agency maintains an open plan of care and continues with a care plan monitoring approach, often with significantly decreased visit frequency. Assumptions are that this heightened oversight may prevent a decline or exacerbation that would result in a readmission to home care, possibly resulting in a partial episode payment (PEP) adjustment with negative financial implications for the agency. However, the OBQI impact of this practice can be unfavorable for the agency. Again, the patient is likely at his "best" or most optimal level of health and function at the time that he has met his goals or skilled services are no longer required (not to mention the fact that these criteria are triggers to the end of coverage under the Medicare home health benefit). It is possible that over time, his status will decline (even with infrequent home care oversight visits) resulting in a less-favorable outcome presentation when the home care discharge finally occurs, than would have resulted from a discharge of the patient "at his peak." Again, because the contrary could also be true (i.e., the patient could continue to improve after completion of the more intensive plan of care), agencies should analyze their own practice and outcome patterns to determine the most appropriate and desirous approach.

OBQI STEP THREE: OUTCOME REPORT INTERPRETATION

Currently OASIS data is used by CMS to generate several types of outcome reports, each offering unique features to support OBQI or OBQM functions. The OASIS-based reports that support OBQI activities include the risk-adjusted outcome report, the descriptive outcome report, the case mix report, and the patient tally report. Agencies may use these reports to provide an overall comparison of their agency's patient characteristics (case mix report) and outcomes (risk-adjusted and descriptive outcome reports) to the national reference group and to the agency's own profile and performance for a previous time period. In OBQI, the step of outcome report interpretation provides the agency with the global perspective of the agency's comparative performance, in preparation for the next step of OBQI in which the agency will select target outcomes from the report for their OBQI focus.

The Outcome Report Review Team

At each step of the OBQI process, the agency will need to determine exactly which staff will be involved in specific activities, carefully weighing the cost and benefit of decisions regarding each potential participant. Most often, the team that reviews the outcome report also selects the target outcome as a result of their report review. When selecting those who will review the outcome reports, consider the needs of the review. Assure that the team includes representatives that can address the scope of knowledge and operational issues necessary for an effective review. These issues include clinical assessments (including OASIS collection), a degree of history with the agency (someone who can offer anecdotal summaries of changes in care or utilization practices, referral sources, or unique staffing or case mix issues experienced by the agency during the report time period), and a sufficiently broad representation of the pertinent clinical services provided (i.e., nursing, therapies, social work, aide services).

If an agency has experienced chronic understaffing in the area of a particular clinical discipline, for instance occupational therapy (OT), the probability is high that the agency would be tempted to not burden the already scarce OT personnel by suggesting their involvement in these OBQI activities. However, one should consider that a clinically understaffed area *itself* presents a potential area of risk related to clinical outcomes. The OT shortage may be resulting in a conscious or subconscious trend of under-referral for OT services. When OT referrals are made, the shortage of resources may result in underutilization of OT for each patient, either in terms of scope and/or quality of interventions, number of visits, or both. If this OT staffing problem is contributing to unfavorable outcomes for the agency, a clinician best able to identify the related deficiencies would be one knowledgeable in OT-specific assessments, interventions, and care-planning resources. Efficient multidisciplinary representation will offer the agency the best chance at achieving a significant and meaningful focus for OBQI efforts.

Preparing for Outcome Report Review

The OBQI reports are designed to portray the degree of improvement achieved for patients due to the care provided by the agency. It could be perceived as a direct reflection of a provider's competency in their work. For most providers, reviewing a report comparing their performance to their peers brings with it a degree of internalization and emotion—excitement and satisfaction for favorable outcomes, disappointment, frustration, or denial for unfavorable outcomes.

Because these emotional reactions can be powerful, and may present an impediment to OBQI progress, preparing the team for report review should be considered. Prior to the team reviewing their own outcome reports, training should be provided including education on the content and format of the reports, sources for report data, and the use of the report in OBQI. The team should then have the opportunity to review "sample" outcome reports. Fictitious reports and review activities available in the *OBQI Implementation Manual* (www.cms.hhs.gov/oasis) can be used to prepare the team for review of their own agency's reports. In the 2001 CMS-sponsored OBQI Pilot Project, this strategy of pre-review training was used and determined effective in facilitating an efficient actual agency report review.

OBQI STEP FOUR: TARGET OUTCOME SELECTION

The selection of target outcomes presents the first opportunity in the OBQI cycle for the agency to make decisions on how they will utilize OBQI to impact the quality of care for their patients. The goal of the target outcome selection is to determine what the agency's area(s) of focus will be for their OBQI program. Target outcome selection should be based on a list of selection criteria provided in the *OBQI Manual* (see Figure 31–8). The target outcome selection criteria include six factors that provide both a technical screen (i.e., numeric thresholds or relative comparisons) and a subjective screen (i.e., agency's perception of clinical significance and relevance of particular outcome measures to the agency's goals).

These criteria are relatively easy to apply, especially if the selection team has had practice applying the criteria to sample outcome reports. Recognize that in order for the selection team to apply the more "agency-specific" and "subjec-

tive" outcome selection criteria (i.e., *#5 Importance or relevance to your agency's goals*, and *#6 Clinical significance*) the team members will need to be familiar with agency-specific details, including the organization's mission statement, strategic plan/goals, marketing efforts, payor and case mix profiles, and so forth.

Select Descriptive Outcomes Cautiously

The OBQI report contains 41 outcome measures available for target outcome selection. The measures are divided and presented on two reports. The risk-adjusted report includes measures for which some differences in the agency's patients and the reference sample have been "factored out" using outcome-specific, risk-adjustment models. The descriptive report includes measures for which adequate risk-adjustment models have not yet been developed. As risk adjustment models are developed and refined, it is expected that the descriptive outcomes will be transitioned into the risk-adjusted report, eventually eliminating the descriptive report altogether. In the meantime, the *OBQI Implementation Manual* states that agencies are allowed to select a target outcome from either the risk-adjusted or descriptive portions of the OBQI reports, although it is acknowledged that selection of a descriptive outcome will require "some additional care." This essentially refers to the need for the agency to perform a level of "crude" risk adjustment on its own. This might be done by an agency comparing its case-mix profile to that of the reference group, and determining the likeli-

---

Figure 31-8 Target Outcome Selection Criteria

1. Statistically significant outcome differences
2. Larger magnitude of the outcome differences
3. Adequate number of cases
4. The actual significance levels of the differences
5. Importance or relevance to your agency's goals
6. Clinical significance

Source: *OBQI Implementation Manual* 02/2002 version, p. 4.2.

hood that the unfavorable or favorable outcome rate is a reflection of improvement or decline in patient status within the agency's control (i.e., those resulting from care provided or omitted), as opposed to outcome rates that appear favorable or unfavorable simply due to the unique characteristics of the agency's patient mix. Considering the fact that those at CMS and its contractors have yet to achieve adequate models to adjust for risk factors for these descriptive outcomes, it is unlikely that the typical home health agency would have the expertise and resources to achieve this task. Even if an agency were able to perform analyses that provided them with a level of confidence that a true and significant difference between their outcome rate and the reference rate existed, it is possible that between the time the agency starts OBQI with the descriptive target outcome and ends the process 12 months later, the outcome measure may have moved from the descriptive to the risk-adjusted report, adding a variable to the system that would make it difficult to evaluate the impact and effectiveness of the agency's OBQI plan of action.

Consider Specific OASIS Data-Item Issues

After selecting the target outcome and before plunging into the process-of-care investigation, consider specific OASIS data-item issues related to the target outcome selected. Invest some time in reviewing the OASIS item on which your target outcome is calculated. Some OASIS items are fairly insensitive to change, meaning that an agency could realize improvement in their patients, but the type or degree of improvement would not change the OASIS score. In this situation, an agency may be successful at improving patient outcomes, but not specifically the outcomes that are formally captured and reported on the OBQI reports, resulting in a disappointing conclusion to the OBQI experience. An example of how an agency might consider OASIS item-specific issues in target outcome selection is presented in Sidebar 31–1.

Strive for a Positive Experience

When an agency is embarking upon OBQI for the first time, special care should be taken to provide the most opportunities for the agency to have a positive OBQI experience. The field staff hold the key to ongoing collection of quality OASIS data. The results of this OBQI cycle may be the first opportunity for the field nurses and therapists to see first hand how effective OASIS can be in improving the care for the patients they treat. If all the resources directed at accurate data collection, outcome selection and review, and plan of action implementation do not result in a positive change in patient outcomes, it is likely that the agency will lose the buy-in from staff who may not see ongoing commitment to OASIS or OBQI as worthwhile.

As an agency commits to early OBQI efforts, a couple of key strategies can be used to increase the probability of a positive experience.

Select Remediation Versus Reinforcement

As the target outcome selection criteria are applied, the agency is free to choose any outcome (favorable or unfavorable) that meets the outlined criteria. If the agency selects an outcome where their performance is significantly *favorable* to the reference group, then the plan of action would focus on *enhancing* (or reinforcing) the optimal care behaviors that contributed to the favorable outcome. If the agency selects an outcome where their performance is significantly *unfavorable* to the reference group, then the plan of action would focus on *remediating* (or correcting) the faulty or deficient care behaviors that contributed to the unfavorable outcome. Because the margin for change is considerably greater for unfavorable outcomes than it is for favorable outcomes, it is easier to show dramatic improvement when remediating a poor outcome than when enhancing a superior outcome. In fact, some evaluation of agency experience with the OBQI system suggests the possible existence of a "performance-plateau," where superior outcome levels are pragmatically optimal, and subject to insignificant addi-

Sidebar 31–1 Item-Specific Issues in Target Outcome Selection

"Joints R Us" Home Care Agency (JRU) is a recognized leader in its market for its specialty program for knee and hip replacement post-op care. Clinical expertise, carefully designed care protocols, and effective partnering and marketing have resulted in a unique case mix where 75 percent of the agency's cases are status post (S/P) lower extremity arthroplasty. As JRU begins their OBQI process and accesses their OBQI reports, they are shocked and troubled to find a significantly *unfavorable* rate for the outcome of *improvement in ambulation/locomotion*. Prior to OBQI, JRU has measured their "success" with their joint program based on attainment of patient-centered, physician-directed goals, including achievement of:

- specific joint range of motion and strength goals,
- normal wound healing progress,
- effective pain management,
- independence in an effective home exercise program, and
- independence in ADLs, including unassisted ambulation with a walker (which the referring orthopedic surgeons require for 6 weeks post-op).

After the agency gets over the shock of their unfavorable ambulation outcome, the OBQI team begins the formal outcome report analysis and target outcome selection. Due to the unique agency program and case mix, JRU has a hard time even considering any outcome measure *other* than *improvement in ambulation/locomotion* for focus, and it does meet all the target outcome selection criteria. After the agency decides to focus on *improvement in ambulation/locomotion*, the OASIS item M0700 that is used to calculate the outcome measure is examined. The agency realizes that most of their joint replacement patients are admitted using a walker, and requiring assistance to walk on uneven surfaces. Therefore, the majority of the cases are scored as response #1 for M0700 at start of care.

Typically, these patients are discharged "with goals met" in less than 2 weeks. Although they have met all their program goals, including unassisted ambulation, they are still scored a "1" at discharge on M0700, because physician protocols and patient condition require use of an assistive device for 6 weeks post-op. Although the lack of sensitivity demonstrated by this example affects all home care agencies, the impact is intensified for JRU, where factors limiting detection of improvement apply to such a large majority of agency cases (75 percent).

JRU's OBQI team realizes that in order to demonstrate improvement in this outcome measure, the score for M0700 would have to move from a response #1–*"Requires use of a device (e.g., cane, walker) to walk alone* or *requires human supervision or assistance to negotiate stairs or steps or uneven surfaces"* at start of care, to a response #0– *"Able to independently walk on even and uneven surfaces and climb stairs with or without railings (i.e., needs no human assistance or assistive device)"* by discharge. Because this improvement would require the patient to be ambulatory without an assistive device at discharge, care options included earlier discontinuation of supported gait, or a longer home care length of stay. JRU determines that neither of these options represents "better practice" than their current protocols and realizes that due to the issues related to the specific OASIS item, M0700, they could not have a successful OBQI program for this outcome as measured by a change in M0700 from start of care to discharge.

Source: Krulish, L.H. (2002).

tional improvement, regardless of additional care enhancement efforts.

When an agency does select a *favorable* outcome for *reinforcement*, the goal may not necessarily be to *improve* the outcome even more, but merely to maintain a superior or favorable reference group comparison. Although this is still a worthwhile and appropriate perspective, staff often do not see "doing more to get the same outcome" as motivational as when "doing more" produces a "better outcome." Consider a remediation program for the first cycle, and save reinforcement programs for subsequent years, when the commitment and buy-in for OASIS and OBQI is more firmly established.

Stay in Your Comfort Zone . . . For Now

In efforts to assure a positive OBQI experience, do not create a bigger challenge than will be manageable and sustainable. Most agencies have some areas of clinical distinction. Specialty programs or even a single experienced staff member may offer the agency a high level of skill in areas like wound, psychiatric, or cardiac care. Likewise, most agencies have some areas of clinical mediocrity, maybe even incompetence. These areas of weakness may reveal themselves on the agency's outcome reports in ways such as generally poor functional outcomes for an agency with poorly coordinated therapy services. An agency may be aware of an area of clinical weakness, and after viewing the reports, may feel compelled to select a related target outcome. Although this is certainly an acceptable approach, an agency should recognize that it will require simultaneous learning curves for both the OBQI process *and* the unfamiliar clinical practice area(s). Although it is not recommended that areas of improvement opportunity be continually ignored, it is proposed that an agency's initial and future OBQI experiences may benefit if organizational resources are not initially spread so thin as to prevent the agency from gaining a good understanding and commitment to OBQI tasks and concepts. When selecting a target outcome, first-time OBQI agencies may consider staying in their "clinical comfort zone" as a strategy to promote a positive OBQI experience and build a strong foundation for future OBQI efforts.

Focus on a Single Target Outcome

A final and simple approach to promoting a positive initial OBQI experience is to limit the target outcome selection to one quality measure. The *OBQI Implementation Manual* suggests selecting at least one, but no more than three, out-

comes for focus for a 12-month OBQI cycle. Because selecting more than one target outcome will require a sharing of the resources and focus within the organization, it is more likely that in addition to learning OBQI, the various processes-of-care investigation and simultaneous implementation of separate action plans will become complex and possibly confusing to the staff. Once staff have experienced the OBQI process, hopefully with positive and motivating consequences, the agency will have a stronger foundation on which to expand the scope and challenge of future OBQI programs.

OBQI STEP FIVE: PROCESS-OF-CARE INVESTIGATION

The goal of the next step of OBQI—the process-of-care investigation—is to identify opportunities to improve care. For an agency that has selected an unfavorable outcome for remediation, this really means the opportunity to find problems! In keeping with the OBQI philosophy, unless we find problems, we lack identification of the key areas requiring attention and change.

The Should List

To begin this step of OBQI, the care investigation team (usually a relatively small group of five to seven, representing a multidisciplinary perspective) develops a "should list." This is a list of critical care behaviors—including aspects of assessment, intervention, and care planning—that the team believes are vital in achieving the target outcome. For instance, if the target outcome is *improvement in upper body dressing*, the team will compile a list of related care behaviors determined as relevant to achievement of the target outcome. This list is then narrowed down to the most important five to eight care behaviors for the outcome. When developing the should list, the team might utilize established clinical practice standards or guidelines to support their selections and language. A key strategy here is to invest the time into carefully wording the "should-list" behaviors. These care behaviors will be the basis for the chart audits conducted to investigate the agency's care practices. Likely, the chart audits will reveal that one or more of these care behaviors is a problem area for the agency; in which case, the should-list statement can be reworded to form a problem statement. A simple rewording of the problem statement can yield a best practice statement and guide the agency into the last step of OBQI, the plan of action development and implementation. This strategy of encouraging an agency to "think sequentially" (**Should List ➤ Chart Audit Tool ➤ Problem Statement ➤ Best Practice Statement**) when developing their should list is described in Sidebar 31-2.

AVOID TEMPTING CARE REVIEW PITFALLS

As the team reviews charts as part of the process-of-care investigation, they will no doubt reveal two common findings: neither OASIS nor home care providers is perfect. Review of the clinical records will no doubt reveal at least some level of inconsistent or questionable OASIS data collection practices that may relate directly to the OASIS item used to calculate the target outcome. Avoid the "OASIS scapegoat trap." OASIS accuracy concerns should be addressed, but not within or in place of the agency's OBQI program. OASIS-related concerns should be communicated to appropriate agency leadership for inclusion in staff education efforts. Meanwhile, the OBQI team should continue on with the chart audits, focusing the review on the presence or absence of the identified care behaviors that the agency has determined *should* be present.

The revelation that home care providers are not perfect refers to the fact that providers do not always deliver optimal care (and/or the documentation does not always support optimal care). The detection of multiple problems involving clinical performance, coordination of services, and care planning can lead an overzealous performance improvement manager into trying to fix everything at once. Although the notion is commendable, focusing on multiple problems will dilute the focus and resources required for success. It is acceptable to address only a single problem, or if selection of additional problematic clinical actions is desired because the actions are closely related or particularly problematic, the agency may select up to three problems to address in their OBQI program for a given target outcome.

OBQI STEP SIX: PLAN OF ACTION DEVELOPMENT AND IMPLEMENTATION

The final step in the OBQI cycle is development and implementation of a plan of action (POA), based on the agency's problem (or strength) and best practice statements. The POA will serve as the agency's "roadmap" as they implement the best practices that they expect will reinforce or remediate care. Components of the plan of action include identification of:

- quality improvement team members
- target outcome addressed by the plan of action
- goal of the plan (i.e., remediation or reinforcement)
- problem or strength statement
- clinical actions identified as best practices
- intervention actions (the specific activities that will need to occur to carry out the POA; i.e., revision of a clinical form, development of a protocol, staff training, etc.)
- time frames, responsible parties, and monitoring of intervention actions
- plans for evaluating and monitoring compliance with the POA

According to the *OBQI Implementation Manual,* the agency should be implementing the POA within 1 month of accessing the outcome reports. Review of the OBQI pilot project reveals that meeting this objective was a challenge for most of the pilot agencies. Out of the 417

Sidebar 31–2 Utilizing a Sequential Approach to Facilitating the Process-of-Care Investigation Activities

Target Outcome:
Improvement in Bathing

↓

Should List:
For all patients demonstrating an opportunity to improve in bathing, the following care behaviors should occur:
1. When safety recommendations are made related to bathing, follow-up assessment of understanding and compliance (including direct observation of patient/caregiver) occurs until goals are achieved or modified.
2. ...
3. ...
4. ...
5. ...

↓

Chart Audit Tool:

Clinical Actions:	Documentation Present?		Comments:
	YES	NO	
1. When safety recommendations are made related to bathing, follow-up assessment of understanding and compliance (including direct observation of patient/caregiver) occurs until goals are achieved or modified. 2. ...			
3. ...			
4. ...			
5. ...			

↓

Problem Statement:
When safety recommendations are made related to bathing, a follow-up assessment of understanding and compliance (including direct observation of patient/caregiver) does not consistently occur.

↓

Best Practice Statement:
When safety recommendations are made related to bathing, a follow-up assessment of understanding and compliance (including direct observation of patient/caregiver) will be conducted by the case manager (or his/her designee) until goals are achieved or modified.

Source: Krulish, L.H. (2002).

agencies participating in the pilot, 90 percent eventually completed and submitted POAs to the Quality Improvement Organizations (QIOs) running the project. However, in the five states involved in the pilot, the percentage of participating agencies that complied with the 30-day deadline was between 15 percent (New York) and 63 percent (Rhode Island). Early OBQI experience has demonstrated that development of the POA marks a vital step in the survival of the OBQI process for agencies, and the OBQI pilot findings showed that agencies required a considerable degree of encouragement, support, and persistence in order to eventually get over the "POA hurdle." Agencies may find that the QIOs are one such source of needed encouragement and support. CMS has contracted with QIOs in each state to serve as resources to agencies in their OBQI efforts. Contact information for each QIO is available at www.ahqa.org.

Seven Strategies for a Powerful Plan of Action

The following strategies provide guidance to achieve a timely, organized, and effective plan of action development and implementation:

1. *Use clear, specific, and measurable language.* A major pitfall in developing the plan of action is leaving the actions too general and without specific deadlines or accountability by an identified staff member. To avoid any doubt of the expectation, utilize as much clarity as possible. For instance, when two or more staff members are assigned a task, the POA should identify one participant as the "lead," minimizing the chance that each will wait for the other to take charge. Clear and measurable best practice statements will leave no one with questions like: "When an intervention is supposed to occur *every* visit, does this include a home health aide visit?" or "If the best practice represents a clinical action uniquely in the scope of nursing, how will it be met for therapy-only cases?" Careful attention to the wording of statements included in the

plan of action will enhance understanding and compliance with expected actions. An agency can improve the clarity and organization of their POA by utilizing a structured format to develop and record aspects of the plan. An example of such a form is available in the *OBQI Implementation Manual* (2/2002 version, pp. 6.2–6.3).

2. *Keep it simple.* Recognize the purpose and role of the POA. It represents the preparation, training, implementation of best practices, and ongoing monitoring that the OBQI team and field staff will be expected to carry out throughout the remainder of the 12-month OBQI cycle. And both the field staff and management will be expected to sustain their focus and compliance on the POA, in addition to continuing to meet their "usual" job duties.

   Keep the POA simple. Utilize the fewest best practices and intervention actions that will effectively meet your OBQI objectives. Also, recognize that best practices are not always revolutionary or complex. Most care behaviors implemented as best practices by the OBQI pilot agencies represented common, established, and well-accepted clinical practices addressing such activities as guidelines for vital sign monitoring and reporting, standardized pain assessment, or adoption of established clinical parameters to trigger interdisciplinary referrals.

3. *Keep it patient focused.* The overriding goal of OBQI is to improve outcomes that are directly meaningful to home health patients. When developing the POA, focus on aspects of patient care delivery, not the underlying structural components that may only have meaning for the agency. For instance, if OBQI activities reveal inconsistent OASIS-scoring practices within the agency, this is an operational issue that is certainly of concern to the organization. However, it is likely irrelevant to the patient and would not represent a "patient-focused" care behavior. Concentrate on care behaviors representing

assessment practices (i.e., home safety evaluation, nutritional risk assessment), communication or coordination of sevices (i.e., interdisciplinary referrals, patient-related physician contact), and direct interventions (i.e., wound care, diabetic teaching, gait training).

One point to note: Although documentation does not represent a patient-centered care intervention, it does represent a technical activity that can have significant implications in the quality of outcomes a patient achieves. For instance, ineffective documentation and communication of critical directives (i.e., intake restrictions, weight-bearing precautions, or requirements for constant supervision) to the home care team could contribute to otherwise avoidable patient complications. In cases where documentation deficiencies are closely related to patient care delivery, best practice statements may address the more "technical" issue of documentation, along with the associated clinical action or detail to be documented (e.g., Best Practice Statement: For patients with > 1 fall in the past 30 days, the case manager, in communication with the referring physician, will establish patient supervision and assistance requirements, *and document* these requirements on the patient treatment plan.)

4. *Effectively communicate the POA to the staff.* By the time the agency is ready to implement the POA, substantial resources have already been consumed in the foundational activities related to report review, target outcome selection, process-of-care investigation, and POA development. It is possible that the OBQI team is nearing exhaustion just at the time when "the game is about to begin." Because the key to the POA is patient-centered care behaviors, it is the field staff who will be responsible for integrating the new best practices into their day-to-day care. It is likely that most of the field staff have not been actively involved in the OBQI process, and without some thoughtful planning, the critical

POA message may be lost, or perceived as "just another meeting" by invited staff. While sharing the OBQI message and POA with staff through handout materials or a videotape viewing alone may yield disappointing results, it is likely that "just another staff meeting" will be insufficient as well. A combination of several education approaches will likely be required to ensure the agency a good return (i.e., favorable outcomes) on their OBQI investment.

Face-to-face communication of the plan will allow the presenter(s) to evaluate the attentiveness and receptiveness of the participants. Such group meetings also allow for exchange of questions and answers to provide necessary clarification. Written materials to support the information provided will allow staff to reference key points or activities as needed and will benefit visual learners. Videotaping of the session will offer a means for content to be reviewed as needed, either by new hires or by staff members who demonstrate difficulty in complying with the care behaviors as expected.

In order to demonstrate the agency's commitment to OBQI and the importance of this kick-off meeting, the agency should consider ways to differentiate the session from other meetings. Means of differentiation can include a unique location (i.e., restaurant, auditorium), an unusual time (i.e., evening) or a distinctive theme (i.e., pull out those inflatable palm trees that were used for early OASIS training!).

Gain the field staff's buy-in by pointing out how OBQI and the agency's POA are expected to benefit the agency's individual patients. If the target outcome is *emergent care use*, use the OBQI report bar graphs to clearly demonstrate the degree of the agency's unfavorable performance compared to the reference group. Make this further individualized by sharing with the staff examples of the problematic care behaviors that were identified when the patient charts were reviewed. Help the staff share the agency's accountability (e.g., "A significant number of our patients are requiring emergent care, and we believe that our lack of effective and consistent monitoring of wound status may be contributing to this disappointing outcome for our patients.") The presentation should avoid a condemning or punitive tone, but rather reflect a sincere concern for patient well-being and enthusiasm to implement a plan that is expected to fix past care deficiencies. Because staff buy-in is critical to the success of OBQI, thoughtfully plan a presentation that grabs the audience's interest and motivates them to recognize and commit to their crucial involvement in the success of the POA, and eventually OBQI.

5. *Provide quick and ongoing monitoring and communication of best practice compliance.* The plan of action should contain specific details on how the agency will monitor compliance with the new clinical actions or processes that have been selected as best practices. Monitoring should begin soon after the implementation of the POA. Initial monitoring should be intense, possibly including 100 percent record review for presence of the desired care behavior(s) or a joint visit with each staff member to observe their willingness and ability to incorporate the best practice(s) into their care delivery. Because the goal of monitoring is to improve compliance, immediate feedback (both positive and negative) to the involved staff will demonstrate the agency's continued commitment to OBQI and to the expectation of staff accountability for implementing the best practice(s). After an acceptable level of compliance is established, the monitoring level and frequency can be decreased to include a declining percentage of cases for monthly or quarterly review, with feedback to staff.

6. *Maintain high visibility for the best practice(s) and the target outcome.* As the agency continues with day-to-day operations, proactive effort to maintain high visibility for the best practice(s) will ensure that the staff realizes the OBQI initiative is still active in the agency. Without careful promotion, staff may eventually begin to wonder if they are still expected to maintain compliance with the new care behaviors "when our caseloads are so high" or "now that we have a new clinical director."

In addition to promoting the best practice(s), keep the associated target outcome in the forefront as well. This will help maintain staff motivation to comply with the best practice(s), as it directly ties the care behavior(s) to a patient-related outcome that gets measured and evaluated.

Maintaining some focus on the target outcome may also encourage individual clinicians to informally support their care delivery with other care behaviors (e.g., assessments, protocols, or teaching interventions) that they have found successful in achieving the target outcome for their previous patients. This shared focus between the target outcome and the best practice care behavior(s) may prove to be a variation on the current OBQI system that evolves out of agencies' practical application of the OBQI steps.

7. *Avoid the urge to weigh yourself every day.* Once the POA is developed and implemented, members of the OBQI team may display an uncontrollable urge to "weigh themselves every day." This refers to the intense interest in determining if the new care behaviors have made a difference yet in the agency's outcomes. Formal evaluation of the effectiveness of the agency's OBQI efforts will occur at the end of the 12-month OBQI cycle with a formal review of the new OBQI report comparing the agency's current target outcome rate to the agency's previous rate. Monitoring the OBQI reports more frequently may reveal either a lack of significant changes from month to month (that may discourage continued interest in OBQI), or misleading significant changes (either favorable or unfavorable) in the target outcome rate over a short time period, which may be unrelated to the

clinical care provided (i.e., due to seasonal variations in case mix or a batch of corrections to OASIS assessments).

Although monitoring and reporting of compliance with the care behaviors and intervention actions should occur routinely, the overall evaluation of the effectiveness of the entire OBQI plan should be anticipated and reserved for the formal ending of each annual OBQI cycle. The formal evaluation for one OBQI cycle occurs in conjunction with the outcome report review and target outcome selection for the agency's subsequent OBQI cycle. Based on the evaluation findings, the agency may elect to continue with the current best practice(s), revise and re-implement the plan of action for the same target outcome, or change focus to a new target outcome and begin a new process-of-care investigation.

BALANCING OBQI IDEALISM AND HOME CARE REALITY

The *OBQI Implementation Manual* encourages aggressive time frames for OBQI activities. The CMS suggested timeline of 1 month (from accessing the most current outcome reports to implementing the plan of action) is, at least for "first-timer" agencies, proving to be an ambitious schedule. Although agencies have been encouraged to rapidly implement the POA, this is more to ensure that the POA is based on findings from a current outcome report, and less due to the notion that slow POA implementation "cuts into" the 12-month OBQI cycle. The OBQI cycle is completed when the agency is able to access a report representing 12 months of data collected *after* the implementation of the POA. Therefore, due to lag time in outcome re-

port availability after data submission, delays in POA implementation and so forth, a single "annual" OBQI cycle will take more than 12 calendar months. Although some agencies have demonstrated that the 1-month "report to POA" timeline is possible, agencies should be aware of how to evaluate and alter their OBQI activities when the realities of home care do not make the ideal time frames achievable.

When the priority for OBQI gets sidelined (due to an agency crises or lack of focus), progression through the OBQI cycle is slowed or completely halted. When the agency is ready to resume full OBQI activities, it will take a good understanding of the entire OBQI process globally, and of each individual step specifically, to allow the agency to evaluate their OBQI status and determine if they should move ahead, take a step back, or totally start over. (See Sidebar 31–3 for an agency case study demonstrating evaluation and adaptation options for OBQI progression.)

CONCLUSION

The OBQI system should be viewed as a vehicle by which agencies can carry out continuous quality improvement (CQI) activities. Although the steps and processes of OBQI are conceptually established, adaptation and refinement of the system itself is expected. As providers demonstrate the practicality (or impracticality) of current system features, and as the effectiveness (or ineffectiveness) of OBQI in enhancing patient outcomes is studied, it is anticipated that collaborative efforts between CMS, home health agencies, and other interested stakeholders will result in a promising evolution of OBQI.

Sidebar 31–3 Evaluation and Adaptation Options for OBQI Progression: An Agency Case Study

Better Care Home Health Agency (BCHHA) begins their OBQI activities by accessing and reviewing their most recent OBQI reports. Within 3 weeks, they have selected a target outcome for review and have completed chart audits, revealing a care behavior trend that is believed to be contributing to the agency's unfavorable outcome. BCHHA develops a problem statement based on the trend discovered. During the coming weeks, no OBQI activities occur as a result of an unexpected surge in admissions, the exodus of key experienced clinical staff, and an unexpected complaint survey. When the agency is able to resume focus on OBQI, they must determine how to proceed. The agency could access the most recent OBQI reports and determine if the previously selected target outcome still meets the target outcome selection criteria. If it does not, then the agency would need to start again at the outcome report review and select a new tar-

get outcome. If on the new reports the original target outcome still meets the selection criteria, then the agency may proceed ahead with a "mini" process-of-care investigation. Using the same chart auditing criteria as before, the agency could audit a small sample of recent charts to determine if the trend previously identified is still applicable. If it is not, or if a new and more disturbing trend is identified, the agency should proceed with auditing a greater sample of charts and solidifying their problem statement. If the previously discovered trend is supported by the "mini" audit, then the agency could move ahead with their activities to develop their problem statement and best practice statement, and advance to the last step of the OBQI cycle: plan of action development and implementation.

Source: Krulish, L.H. (2002).

REFERENCES

Center for Health Services Research, University of Colorado Health Sciences Center. 2001. OASIS and Outcome-Based Quality Improvement in home health care: Research and demonstration findings, policy implications, and considerations for change. Volume 1: Policy and program overview; Volume 2: Research and technical overview; Volume 3: Research and clinical supporting documentation. Denver, CO: Author.

Cox, M. 2002. Data processing and transmission: The basics. *Home Healthcare Nurse* 20(8): 509–513.

Delmarva Foundation for Medical Care. 2002. Final report: Outcome Based Quality Improvement System Pilot Project. Retrieved from www.cms.hhs.gov/oasis/OBQI_DFMC.pdf (accessed August 5, 2003).

Department of Health and Human Services: Centers for Medicare and Medicaid Services. 1999a. Medicare and Medicaid Programs: 42 CFR Parts 484 and 488: Reporting Outcome and Assessment Information Set (OASIS) data as part of the conditions of participation for home health agencies and comprehensive assessment and use of the OASIS as part of the conditions of participation for home health agencies: Final rules. *Federal Register* 64(15): 3748–3783.

Department of Health and Human Services: Centers for Medicare and Medicaid Services. 1999b. Medicare and Medicaid programs: Mandatory use, collection, encod-

ing, and transmission of Outcome and Assessment Information Set (OASIS) for home health agencies. *Federal Register*, 64(117): 32984–32991.

Department of Health and Human Services, Centers for Medicare and Medicaid Services. 2002. *Outcome and Assessment Information Set Implementation Manual: Implementing OASIS at a home health agency to improve patient outcomes.* Baltimore, MD: Author.

Department of Health and Human Services, Centers for Medicare and Medicaid Services. 2002. *Outcome-Based Quality Improvement (OBQI) Implementation Manual.* Baltimore, MD: Author.

Department of Health and Human Services: Centers for Medicare and Medicaid Services: OASIS Data Submission Specifications (OASIS Correction Policy). 2001, April 20. S&C 01–12. Retrieved from www.cms.hhs.gov/oasis/datasubm.asp (accessed July 21, 2003).

Department of Health and Human Services: Centers for Medicare and Medicaid Services. 2003, February 13. S & C 03-13. Home health survey protocol enhancements (Memorandum). Retrieved from www.cms.hhs.gov/medicaid/survey-cert/sc0313.pdf (accessed August 1, 2003).

Department of Health and Human Services, Centers for Medicare and Medicaid Services. OASIS Web site, www.cms.hhs.gov/oasis (accessed August 1, 2003).

Hittle, D. F., K. S. Crisler, J. M. Beaudry, K. S. Conway, and P. W. Shaughnessy. 2002. OASIS and Outcome-Based Quality Improvement in home health care: Research and demonstration findings, policy implications, and considerations for change. Volume 4: OASIS chronicle and recommendations. Denver, CO: Center for Health Services Research, University of Colorado Health Sciences Center.

Krulish, L. H. 2000. A practical look at outcome enhancement for rehospitalization. *Home Healthcare Nurse* 18(4): 267–274.

Krulish, L. H. 2001. Using OBQI to improve assessment and management of pain. *Home Healthcare Nurse* 19(3): 165–174.

Krulish, L. H. 2002a. *Implementing Outcome-Based Quality Improvement: A hands-on workshop.* Redmond, WA: Home Therapy Services.

Krulish, L. H. 2002b. OBQI and the survey process: An interview with CMS. *Home Healthcare Nurse* 20(9): 574–578.

Krulish, L. H. 2002c. OBQI staff competency tools. *Home Healthcare Nurse* 20(9): 608–614.

Madigan, E. A. 2002. The scientific dimensions of OASIS for home care outcome measurement. *Home Healthcare Nurse* 20(9): 579–583.

Murdock, K. 2002a. Developing and implementing a plan of action to improve care: Practical application. *Home Healthcare Nurse* 20(9): 603–605.

Murdock, K. 2002b. Interpreting outcome reports: Practical application. *Home Healthcare Nurse* 20(8): 523–524.

Murdock, K. 2002c. Selecting target outcomes: Practical application. *Home Healthcare Nurse* 20(8): 529–530.

CHAPTER 32

Benchmarking and Home Health Care

Alexis A. Wilson

Benchmarking is a continuous process of comparison, projection, and implementation. It involves comparing your organization with others, discovering and projecting best trends in practices, and meeting and exceeding the expectations of those watching you. Done correctly, benchmarking will help you to learn from the experiences of others, and it will show you how you are performing in comparison to the best. It will identify your strengths and weaknesses and help you to prioritize your improvement activities. If systematically applied to your operations, the data obtained from benchmarking will also provide you with a corrective action plan. In other words, the data can be used to find where your organization excels and where the problems are that need to be fixed. Benchmarking allows you to set standards, and then to continuously measure performance based on a reference point.

Benchmarks serve as reference points. In the most general terms, a benchmark was originally a sighting point from which measurements could be made or a standard against which others could be measured. In the 1970s, the concept of a benchmark evolved beyond a technical term signifying a reference point (Bogan and English, 1994). The word migrated into the business realm, where it came to signify the measurement process by which to conduct comparisons. In the early 1980s, Xerox Corporation began referring to benchmarking as comparisons with one's primary competitors. They viewed it as a method to continuously measure products, services, and practices against the toughest competitors or those companies recognized as industry leaders. Since then, the benefits of benchmarking have been well recognized in certain industries and operating areas. Benchmarking is a business concept with general management applications for high-level functions such as strategic planning, restructuring, and financial management. In the last several years, benchmarking and benchmarks have become increasingly popular terms in health care. Following Total Quality Management (TQM) and Continuous Quality Improvement (CQI), benchmarking is taking health care to a higher level of quality comparison.

Performance measurement and being compared to other like providers is now an expectation of purchasers, government agencies, consumer groups, and others with a stake in the health care delivery system. Clear demonstrations that performance measurement leads to significant, perhaps cost-saving improvements in care, will mean there is clear evidence that performance information is actually being used by the public to guide decisions about their care. This is a tremendous undertaking that has inherent risks.

Benchmarking is a necessity for organizations engaged in reengineering their processes and systems. Benchmarking helps you to see things differently—or as others outside of the organization may see them. It is a proactive step in assessing what the competition is doing. The primary reason for benchmarking is to help set performance goals above a minimum acceptable value. Another value is that it gives credibility to the goals and objectives of process redesign goals.

Organizations undertake a benchmarking initiative for a number of reasons. Among them are:

- To set challenging but realistic goals
- To define how goals can be accomplished
- To define gaps between the organization's performance and its competitor's performance
- Because improvement is required to stay competitive
- Because the organization is losing market share and needs to turn around
- Because costs are too high
- To find out how the organization measures up against the "best"
- To help management direct the improvement effort
- To uncover emerging technologies or practices.
- To learn from others' experiences
- To provide early warning when the organization is falling behind

BEGINNING TO BENCHMARK

The first step toward benchmarking is a thorough understanding of outcome measurement. The goal is to demonstrate the value of the health care services provided, and in cases where the services do not appear to be valuable, have a reason to try something different. The science of comparative quality measurement poses many conceptual and technical problems, and home care has only recently started using a uniform outcome measurement system. The Outcome and Assessment Information Set (OASIS) was developed by the University of Colorado, under a demonstration grant from CMS (Shaughnessy et al., 2002). OASIS for home care is a group of data elements that rep-

resent core items of a comprehensive assessment of an adult home health patient, and that form the basis for measuring patient outcomes for purposes of outcome-based quality improvement (Institute of Medicine [IOM], 2001). The OASIS was mandated for use in all Medicare-certified home health agencies in 1999, and agencies are required to transmit the OASIS data electronically to their state certifying agencies, typically the state departments of health, who in turn transmit the data to Medicare. It is this data that the CMS will use to create home health report cards similar to what is already a practice for nursing homes (Shaughnessy and Richard, 2002). The thinking is that this data will force agencies to improve upon bad results or risk going out of business. Further, it may profile agencies that provide exemplary care. It also allows consumers to get a view of the type of agencies they might be considering for care.

For health care organizations, one of the best instruments for benchmarking is patient outcome data. Outcomes are an excellent way to compare the effectiveness of services and patient care procedures. It can also be used to determine outcome trends by specific patient population groups, diagnoses, or specific demographic characteristics. Because of external factors that affect health, it is still difficult to attribute a patient or patients' outcomes solely to the actions of a single provider organization, clinician, or department. And, as the patient data are integrated with cost data associated with certain outcome achievement, benchmarking will be possible at an even more detailed level—the outcomes with the costs required to achieve them, which is true benchmarking.

However, it is still premature to claim that benchmarks in home health care have evolved into a "hard science." Home care is just getting started in comparative data analyses. An uncritical reliance on technical adjustments and arbitrary cutoffs said to be statistically significant may produce information that is misleading with respect to the day-to-day decisions that administrators, patients, and families need to make about health care. Comparisons of practitioners, providers, or health care plans on any measures of quality—whether process oriented or outcomes related—risk being wrong, or at least misleading, if they are not viewed with proper adjustments for case mix factors, severity, and/or the presence of other conditions (comorbidity).

ANALYZING THE DATA

Benchmarks of care emerge when someone has the ability to gather meaningful data, compile it, and display results. It also implies knowledge of what the care standards are to achieve an "acceptable" benchmark. The goal of comparative data (or benchmarks) is to provide essential information to health care agencies, patients, referral sources, and payers about the outcomes of home health care provided and the costs to achieve them. Outcomes of care refer to the effects of services provided. Benchmarks refer to a level of care set as a goal to be attained. Internal benchmarks are derived from similar processes or services within an organization; external benchmarks are comparisons with external competitors in the field.

The data you receive in benchmark reports are only as good as the quality of the data collected by the staff. This is the "garbage in, garbage out" adage that is commonly referred to in data processing. Two key concepts critical to understanding data quality are interrater reliability and risk adjustment techniques.

Interrater reliability means that two clinicians will assess the same patient at the same time, using the same tools, the same way. If no interrater reliability exists among staff in an agency, it will not be possible to find any meaningful data relationships, so agencies need to take the time to assess interrater reliability among staff. To do this, each clinician must do her or his assessment privately and independently. For example, two different nurses can independently assess the same patient using the same tools to see if the results they get are the same. Typically, an 80 percent consensus between the clinicians is sufficient. In other words,

8 out of 10 nurses should assess the patient and record the same results for the particular data item or outcome measure. If interrater reliability is low, it means there is little agreement between nurses on the patient score, and more work is needed to help the clinicians reach consensus. Without agreement between raters, the assessments assigned to a patient cannot be assumed to be reliable. If this is the case, consider adding more details or descriptions about how to use the tools and provide case examples.

Risk adjustment, case-mix adjustment, and/or severity of illness are terms that are often used synonymously, and many find them intimidating. The process of risk adjustment basically entails compensating (adjusting) for two or more samples, so that their (adjusted) rates are comparable. Organizations in the past have cited risk adjustment as the culprit that made their agency look bad by saying, "our patients are sicker than the others we were compared to." This argument is increasingly difficult to justify. Although still an imprecise science, risk adjustment techniques have improved steadily (Izzoni, 1997). A risk factor can positively or negatively influence the likelihood of a patient attaining a certain outcome. The most obvious way to adjust for risk factors is to group patients with similar conditions (risk factors). This is called the *stratification method for risk adjustment*. For example, female diabetic patients over 65 years old would be placed into one patient group and those under 65 years into a separate group. The idea is to look at like patients with like characteristics. Patients can be stratified by age, gender, geographic location, diagnosis, or virtually any other characteristic. Other methods encompass more complicated statistical analyses of patient characteristics. For example, prospective payment rates are calculated using a case-mix methodology driven by OASIS data.

The two types of data collected in benchmarking can be quantitative (numbers, ratios, and so on) and qualitative data (word descriptions). Quantitative data is clearly the most common, but qualitative data should not be discounted. In reality, benchmarking strategy should be designed to collect both types of data as opportunities present themselves. Quantitative data can be misleading, and just because an organization has better overall quantitative performance, it does not mean that all the activities within its process are world class. Every data item has strong and weak points. Sometimes qualitative data can help to search out the very best of each part of items being studied, by pointing to particular evaluative descriptions that do not lend themselves to numbers. An excellent example for some patients in health care is the extent to which they felt "cared for" by an organization. The concept of caring is not easily translated to numbers, and yet holds an important ingredient to evaluation. However, in health care in general and the medical research community in particular, acceptance and use of qualitative information will take considerably more time.

Data analysis can be extremely complex. As mentioned previously, issues relating to case mix, risk adjustment, and reliability of the data collected must be taken into consideration because each has a significant impact on the information that outcome reports contain. Although patient outcome data is relatively easy to view on an individual basis, benchmarks provide a comparison, usually by groups, and is more useful. This may be in groups by patient type, outcome type, organization type, or others. Ultimately, you will want the ability to compare yourself on an internal organizational basis as well as on an external basis to others. Essentially, benchmarking has two foci, an internal focus and an external focus.

Internal Focus.   Comparing your own data will always prove interesting. Some ways to accomplish this are to compare lengths of stay by patient type (sex, diagnosis, ZIP code, doctor, etc.). Another interesting comparison is to compare outcome type (health status, independence, etc.) by practitioner. Some primary questions that you will want to ask are: (1) What is a typical patient population profile? and (2) Do less visits mean poorer outcomes? Internal benchmarking involves looking within the organization to determine which areas, functions, or departments

may be performing similar activities and to outline the processes in each area to determine what is most effective and efficient. It is often a good starting point for organizations wishing to engage in benchmarking activities for the first time. Internal benchmarks focus on discrete work processes and operating systems, which in health care include such things as billing, medical records flow, check-in, care delivery, and even strategic planning. This form of benchmarking seeks to identify the most effective operating practices. It should always be considered before any organization looks to the outside. In general, this type of benchmarking is the easiest to conduct because there are usually no confidentiality or security problems to overcome, but it can create some tension due to competition or fear. If an organization can improve a core process by detailing the system (the input) and measuring the results (the output), it can then improve its performance. These performance improvements may be translated to less rehospitalization of patients, higher patient functional status at discharge, or improved short-term financial results.

Comparisons with an internal focus are not as threatening as comparisons to outside groups. Outcomes may be viewed by managers with teams of nurses. Let's say, for example, that your decubitus ulcer population tends to have better wound care outcomes in one geographic area than another. You may see patients in one area become independent in care after only 7 visits, whereas on the other side of town, 10 visits may be provided, wreaking havoc in the cost per case. Having the outcome data makes it easy to go back and look at these groups of patients to discover what (if any) the problem is. Perhaps you will discover that one group lives in a high-rise building where a caretaker assumes care responsibilities in the building. Or, perhaps you will discover that one nurse seems to consistently visit patients long after they should have been discharged.

External Focus.   Beyond looking at trends within your individual organization, benchmarking with other agencies will be both exhilarating and scary. CMS will soon compare data between agencies and use it as a surveillance tool. This is one reason why case-mix and risk-adjustment factors will become increasingly important. Although it is still controversial among providers, public disclosure of reports about your organization is inevitable. When your organization looks good, you will want everyone to see it, but if you look bad, you will need to be able to make corrections. Hopefully, you will have access to internal outcome information well in advance to alert you to any quality or utilization problems before any information becomes public.

For initial comparative reports that you participate in, you may want to be sure that outsiders cannot identify your organization. This is easy enough to accomplish and still provides you with an opportunity to see for yourself how you compare to someone else. Reports should typically show your organization compared to others in the same geographic region and compared to others in the nation. Key questions to begin to answer are: How do you compare with others? What might account for the differences, positive and negative? Can you communicate the data with confidence? If you see some positive data at other organizations, it might behoove you to talk with them to learn how they are achieving such good results. All along the way, the primary issues will be about data integrity and case mix.

Comparative metrics can become useful in sales and marketing. Especially as payers become more interested in the value of services provided (instead of only the costs), your organization will want to provide as much information on outcomes of care compared to the costs to achieve them as possible. External benchmarking enables managers to assess their competitive positions through service or product comparisons. It usually focuses on elements of price, or some other common denominator that is measured among organizations. In business, this is relatively easy. Health care is slightly more complex to benchmark, especially if the effects or outcomes of care are measured, because data collection is more complicated and reliability issues are necessary to consider. External bench-

marking will become increasingly sophisticated as health care identifies common denominators and agrees on their definitions. For example, once functional or health status indicators are agreed to for an apples-to-apples comparison, performance benchmarking will provide useful comparisons about the value of health care services, and not just the cost.

External benchmarking for competitive reasons is still more complex. Some organizations will be apprehensive about this out of concern for patient privacy, or about reverse engineering by others of your organization's best practices. The organizations that look bad will not want others to see their weaknesses, while those that look the best will worry that practice "secrets" could be discovered and used to a competitor's advantage. However, in health care, it is important to remember that benchmarking with a related organization does not necessarily mean you compete for the same customers. A real advantage of the benchmarking process is that it provides insights into how others have become good at what they do. This aspect focuses on discovering how other organizations developed their processes to yield superior performance. At this juncture, you must seek out and analyze the reasons and understand why another organization's processes, methods, or knowledge make their service look superior to yours.

Strategic benchmarking is another form of an external focus. It examines how companies compete. It is seldom industry focused, and instead seeks to identify the winning strategies that have enabled high-performing companies to be successful in their marketplaces. Strategic benchmarking influences the longer term competitive patterns of a company, and the benefits may accrue slowly. Because health care is a relative newcomer to benchmarking, strategic benchmarking is not yet widely used.

Three themes to remember are that benchmarking:

1. Is a systematic way for individuals and teams to learn about processes
2. Makes decisions based on data, not hunches

3. Seeks permanent solutions to problems rather than relying on quick fixes

As you move ahead in outcome measures, benchmarking, and your quality improvement activities, keep these themes at the forefront to help keep you focused.

BUILDING ORGANIZATIONAL CAPACITY

If you stop to think about it, the core of quality improvement is in the outcomes an organization achieves (or does not achieve). If done correctly, benchmark reports can become the driving force for the entire agency. Where you have positive outcomes, the task will be to identify what the process was that drove those outcomes, and how it can be repeated. When the outcomes are not so good, the same procedure holds, but now you are trying to find out what went wrong. Measurement tools, quality standards, and external oversight mechanisms are all important for providing quality home health care, but they do not ensure that all providers will have the capacity to use the measures correctly.

The quest for quality is grounded in awareness of the current needs and future demands of the customer, which in health care is both patients and payers. Business success depends on the company meeting those needs and demands faster, better, and with lower costs than the competition. One of the best ways to achieve success is to benchmark your organization's activities. However, effective use of benchmarks takes work and commitment—it also requires some creativity. To make sense, benchmarks must be relevant to clinical practice and pertinent to home care operations. Combining utilization data with clinical outcomes will be the most revealing way to determine the effects of the care your organization provides. As you collect more information over time, it will become easier to determine best practices and to apply the information to quality improvement activities. It's no secret that if you want your organization to be successful in using benchmarks to improve, the

staff must be invested in the patient outcome measurement process. A recurring problem with measurement initiatives in the past has been a failure to engage clinicians. The staff need to understand why outcome measurement is important, and how it can benefit patients as well as clinical practice.

To get full benefit from clinical data in benchmarking, it is important as an administrator to stop and give thought to "what's in it for me" from the staff's perspective. First, staff need to understand the implications of outcome measurement and the importance of accurate measurement for survival of the organization. Staff need to understand the regulatory as well as the financial implications for the organization. Realistically, the only way to bring the outcome data to life is to show the results of the information that has been collected in benchmark reports and graphs. Staff should receive the reports the agency produces on a regular basis. Ten basic steps to build the capacity of your organization to measure outcomes and successfully benchmark are outlined here:

1. *Be sure that the clinical staff have a common understanding about the data they are collecting. Common data definitions are imperative for apples-to-apples comparisons.* One of the key contributions of the federal mandate that home health agencies collect OASIS data is that it supplies a common set of data and data definitions. For additional indicators, an agency may want to collect (e.g., patient behaviors or other clinical outcomes), step back and think about what the outcomes of care are that are important to your organization and define them so they can be measured consistently. You may choose to start with the OASIS data set first, and then establish common outcome definitions that are more sophisticated and specific to your organization from there. How the data impact your staff and the care they provide will be largely up to the discretion of the managers and administra-

tors of the home health agencies. Do you want to provide reports to the staff by practitioner? Does it make sense to let staff compare their patients' outcomes with other staff? Chances are the answer to these questions is yes.

2. *Organize a system to yield consistent results, no matter who does the measuring.* Systematizing the process is critical. Clearly, the interrater reliability issues are pertinent here, and so is consideration of how to access and manage the data once it is collected. Paper flow will be very important. Systems to consider for managing the data can be as simple as getting the data collection forms safely into the patient's record, scanning the data forms into a computer program for analysis, or entering the forms into a program for analysis.

3. *Provide education.* The answer to most any issue or challenge within an organization is education. Think about the content of staff meetings and consider replacing it with relevant information regarding benchmarks. The teachers will be key. The attitude and presentation of the information about the benefits of quality data for benchmarks will guide the attitude of the staff during implementation. Planning is important at this point, because as you add to clinical documentation and data entry, you need to be thinking about methods to streamline what you are currently doing, or at least to consolidate your efforts.

4. *Use tools, not rules.* How would you feel if someone handed you a dozen forms to fill out at patient admission and discharge and told you, "Here are the new forms Medicare requires; fill them out." In this scenario, the forms become the enemy, and the object is to fill them out as quickly as possible. Again, education is your key to getting staff to understand the importance of outcomes, but they also need to know that they are not alone in the process. The worst possible "outcome" of the data collection process is garbage in, garbage out. Someone at the organization needs to be the cheerleader of outcome measurement and benchmarking, and be available to the staff for joint visits, questions, or merely consoling staff during the adjustment period and beyond.

5. *Integration and more integration.* Integration of outcome measurement tools into the day-to-day clinical operations can be a major challenge. If the expertise is not available to integrate outcome measures into the paperwork, assessments, and care plans, there are some other options to consider. Successful integration of outcome measurement and benchmarking also depends on an integrated effort among the finance and information technology staff. It is wise to sit down with them to discuss what the clinical staff have been asked to do, and outline where you need their help. Time studies may become important to document costs. Revised programming may be necessary to capture the data. Hopefully, this is when you can also discuss third-party software programs to assist with the data collection and reporting or to figure out how your own software (or a new module for your software) will or will not work for electronic data collection and analysis. Some stand-alone programs will integrate utilization and cost data with the clinical outcome data, to provide an in-depth picture of individual and aggregate outcomes and the costs to achieve them.

6. *Allow for clinical judgement.* The staff need to understand how important their role is to meaningful outcome measurement if the benchmarking data is to be accurate and relevant. Their good judgement is imperative to data collection, and they need to be reminded of that. It is also necessary to consider the "gaming" potential in the process of collecting outcome data. When instruments are being

used that depict patient status in categories from bad to good, it is easy to see that it would not take much to consistently rate patients at the worst on admission and at the best upon discharge. To help the staff avoid any potential to falsify information, remind them that it is illegal. As CMS begins to look at the data collected, it will be easy to identify agencies that rate patients uniformly and/or who look too good to be true. Clinicians need to remember that their professional judgement (and reputations) is at stake in assuring that the information collected is accurate and representative of the patients who are being served. In addition, the efforts by the organization will have been wasted if the data collected is falsified.

7. *Ensure clinical applicability.* The quickest way to turn the staff off to the outcome measurement process is if they cannot see the clinical relevance of what they are doing. One way to make outcomes applicable is to integrate the measures into existing documentation forms, which was discussed previously. Another important vehicle to demonstrate clinical relevance is by using the data at staff meetings and in quality improvement meetings. This way, staff are constantly reminded of the importance of the data they collect, and they begin to see the data's usefulness and the impact it can have on improving care. Once staff are tuned into outcome reports on a regular basis, they can set clear performance goals quarter by quarter, or month by month.

8. *Maintain communication.* Above all, once you start the process, stay involved. Communication about the successes and the failures of the data collection, data entry, and data analysis is key. Sit in on quality improvement meetings; perhaps you can point out a solution to a problem or ask a question about the data that had not been thought of before. Talk with staff regularly about their ongoing issues and suc-

cesses. Be sure to document the problems and the progress at meetings. Set time frames for resolving issues, and assign a person to be responsible for sticking to the time frames established. Often, even after problems have been "fixed," they seem to creep back. If one person has responsibility, chances are better the problems really will go away. Help them to create forms and tracking systems to keep on top of their efforts.

9. *Fix obvious problems.* You typically know who represents your staff problems. They will require extra attention and coaching to bring them around to the new way of thinking. Sit with them the first few times as they go through the outcome assessments and discuss the options and selections carefully. If, after time and effort, they continue to have difficulty it is probably a good time to consider an alternate placement

10. *Monitor changes.* Reward yourself and your staff! Celebrate accomplishments and make a big deal of the changes that are successfully implemented. Bulletins, awards, announcements, and recognition are all ways to reward progress and accomplishments. The importance of clinical measurements in benchmarking cannot be overstated.

Benchmarking first is measuring, then comparing. Without quantitative data, it is impossible to fully understand or control your organization. In home health care, benchmarking needs to tell you:

- How much better are patients who received services from you? From your competitors? From others in the industry? Other industries?
- How much did those services cost your organization and the patient? Your competitor's patients?
- How happy were your customers (which today include patients and payers) with

the services they received from you? From your competitors?

- How long did it take to provide the services, and who provided them?

SUCCESS STRATEGIES

The benchmarking process helps you to understand your organization and its practices better, as well as those of your competitors. Benchmarking seeks to find better operating practices in an environment where the pace of change is so rapid that no single organization can ever control or dominate all effective operating practices and good ideas. To be a marketplace leader, one must look outward—as well as inward—for constant improvement and evolution. Identification and adaptation of best practices help an organization avoid being ambushed by unexpected change. A company can accelerate its own rate of improvement by systematically studying others and by comparing its own operations and performance with the best and most effective practices of innovative and successful companies. Benchmarking, therefore, is a pragmatic approach to managing current performance improvement activities and future change.

Very simply, the benchmarking process involves (Wilson and Nathan, 2002):

- Deciding what will be benchmarked
- Defining the items to compare
- Developing measurements to compare
- Defining whether to benchmark internal sites and/or external organizations
- Collecting and analyzing data
- Determining the gap(s) between your data items and the best items
- Developing action plans, targets, and measurement processes
- Updating the benchmarking effort.

Be sure to keep the list of the key measurements you wish to benchmark as simple as possible. Use terms that are common to your industry, like health status, activities of daily living, mortality, rehospitalization, and so forth. Analyze the types of data sources commonly available in your industry or those measurements considered best professional practices. In the beginning phases of benchmarking, do not worry about the confidentiality of the measurements. The important thing is to agree internally on the data items you want to measure, and then to find benchmarking partners outside of your organization. As you compare the benchmarked items to your own, you may find that you are the best, the same, or worse than those you are being compared to. If you are the best, congratulations. If your comparison is negative or the same, an opportunity exists to improve.

The key to any organization's success is to (Wilson and Nathan, 2002):

- Have meaningful measurements to show how well your organization is performing
- Understand how well other organizations can perform similar activities (both competitors and noncompetitors)
- Understand why others perform better than your organization
- Identify any negative gap between your organization and another organization and take effective action to close that gap

Remember, outcomes are the results of the services provided by your organization. Benchmark reports document that. Outcome data will assist you to improve care quality and to integrate permanent solutions of identified problems into daily operations.

REFERENCES

Bogan, C. E., and M. J. English. 1994. *Benchmarking for best practices.* New York:McGraw-Hill.

Institute of Medicine. 2001. *Envisioning the national health care quality report, Executive summary of the Committee on the National Quality Report on Health Care Delivery*, Washington, DC: National Academy Press.

Izzoni, L. (ed.). 1997. *Risk adjustment for measuring healthcare outcomes,* 2nd ed., Chicago, IL: Health Administration Press.

Shaughnessy, P. W., D. F. Hittle, K. S. Crisler, M. C. Powell, A. A. Richard, A. M. Kramer, R. E. Schlenker, J. F.

Steiner, N. S. Donelan-McCall, J. M. Beaudry, K. L. Mulvey-Lawlor, and K. Engle, 2002. Improving patient outcomes of home health care: Findings from two demonstration trials of outcome-based quality improvement. *Journal of the American Geriatrics Society* 50(8): 1354–1364.

Shaughnessy, P. W. and A. A. Richard. 2002. Performance benchmarking: Part 2—Trends in home health care and what's in store for the future. *Caring* 21(11): 20–23 .

Wilson, A. A. and L. Nathan. 2002. Understanding benchmarks. *Home HealthCare Nurse* 21(2): 102–107.

PART V

Management Issues

CHAPTER 33

Administrative Policy and Procedure Manual

Marilyn D. Harris

A policy manual kept current is essential for administration and service delivery of home health care. Merriam-Webster's dictionary (1999, p. 901) defines a policy as

> a definite course or method of action selected from among alternatives and in light of given conditions to guide and determine present and future decisions; a high level overall plan embracing the general goals and acceptable procedures.

Rowland and Rowland (1992) advise that there are three general areas in nursing that require policy formulation: (1) areas in which confusion about the focus of responsibility might result in neglect or malperformance of an act necessary to a patient's welfare, (2) areas pertaining to the protection of patients' and families' rights (e.g., right to privacy and property rights), and (3) areas involving matters of personnel management and welfare. Barnum and Kerfoot (1995) state that a policy is a guideline that has been formalized by administrative authority and directs action to some purpose. Policies should be revised periodically for efficiency, safety, and effectiveness. There are three major components in a policy system: (1) a purpose, (2) a policy rule, and (3) an action directive or procedure. A procedure details the means to be used to achieve the ends specified in the purpose and further delineated in the policy (Barnum and Kerfoot, 1995). Perrow (1979) states that policy rules are necessary in complex organizations because of such things as variability in personnel, clients, and environment. These policies delineate an area of freedom in which a staff member knows when he or she can make a decision. The absence of written policy leaves staff in a position where any decision they make may infringe upon an unstated policy and produce a reprimand.

Before any service is provided, an approved policy must be in place, according to §484.16 of the Medicare conditions of participation (Health Care Financing Administration, 1989, http://www.access.gpo.gov/nara/cfr/). Policies give direction to staff as to what services will be provided under what conditions. Policies also should state what is not provided and the rationale, if appropriate.

POLICY DEVELOPMENT

Multiple levels of agency personnel should be involved in revisions or deletions of policies from an agency's manual as well as in the development of new ones. The development of a policy can take several forms. For one, staff at all levels may identify a need to provide a specific service. This could be done through systematic logging of requests for a service that is not already available through the agency. Information can be gathered from the staff as to the volume of requests for the new service and also as to the rationale. A review of the literature or contact with other agencies that provide the service and their success or failure rate with this service is also beneficial. If the staff initiates the request for a policy, it can be anticipated that some preliminary homework has been done to substantiate the request.

For another, physicians or other referral sources may request that personnel perform a specific service. If the request is initiated from an outside source, staff who are knowledgeable in the specific procedure under discussion should be involved in the development of the policy. For example, pediatric nurse practitioners should be encouraged to give input into development of pediatric-related policies, and nurses with expertise in intravenous administration should be involved with intravenous policies.

Finally, policies can be developed as a result of the internal quality assessment/performance improvement program. Specific areas may be identified through the internal or external review process reports that could benefit from a new or revised policy.

ROLE OF THE PROFESSIONAL ADVISORY COMMITTEE

A professional advisory committee (PAC) is important for the delivery of home health care services for several reasons. For one, the current Medicare conditions of participation (COPs) require a group of professional personnel (i.e., a PAC); for another, a PAC provides an array of professionals who can contribute their expertise to the formation and updating of service-related policies and procedures. Home health care staff at all levels of the organization should be familiar with the PAC and its responsibilities, membership, and manner of operation.

Section 484.16 of the COPs states:

> A group of professional personnel, which includes at least one physician and one registered nurse (preferably a public health nurse), and with appropriate representation from other pro-

fessional disciplines, establishes and annually reviews the agency's policies governing scope of services offered, admission and discharge policies, medical supervision and plans of care, emergency care, clinical records, personnel qualifications, and program evaluation. At least one member of the group is neither an owner nor an employee of the agency.

(a) Standard: Advisory and evaluation function. The group of professional personnel meets frequently to advise the agency on professional issues, to participate in the evaluation of the agency's program, and to assist the agency in maintaining liaison with other health care providers in the community and in the agency's community information program. The meetings are documented by dated minutes.

Because this committee is required to meet frequently enough to carry out its responsibilities, the number of meetings each year will vary with the agency.

At Abington Memorial Hospital Home Care (AMHHC), the PAC is an important advisory committee to the board of trustees and staff. This group of experts has a vital interest in the agency and its services. The committee meets twice a year on a volunteer basis. A subcommittee of the PAC meets on an annual basis to complete the annual program evaluation. This annual report is submitted to the hospital's Professional Affairs Committee, which includes physicians, trustees, and administration, for review, discussion, and approval. It is also shared with the full PAC at the next scheduled meeting. The report is shared with the hospital's board of trustees by the executive vice president/chief operating officer for final approval. A cover sheet that is signed by these two executives, the chair of the PAC, and the executive director is added to the front of the policy and procedure manual each year to verify that the manual has been reviewed and updated to reflect current practice.

POLICY REVIEW PROCEDURE

Policies can be reviewed on an ongoing basis so that all are reviewed annually. Existing clinical service policies should be reviewed by representatives from each discipline to ensure that they are in keeping with current professional standards. Comments and suggestions are then shared with the PAC or board. Other policies, such as admission and discharge criteria and personnel qualifications, should also be reviewed by appropriate committees from the governing body as well as by administrative staff. Still other clinical service policies may need to be reviewed by legal counsel. At other times, an agency may need or want to seek expert advice from an outside consultant, such as an insurance carrier, for related policies.

To make the best use of meeting time and to facilitate approval, copies of proposed policies or changes to existing policies should be mailed to the committee with the agenda before the meeting. If there is an age- or disease-specific policy, it is helpful to have a knowledgeable staff person discuss the change and the rationale with the professional on the committee who has expertise in this area (e.g., chemotherapy policy should be discussed with an oncologist). With this prior knowledge, this individual's support can be beneficial at the time of the meeting.

One important aspect of the development of sound policies is to include professionals and lay personnel with a wide array of expertise in multiple areas of current or projected services. This expertise should be available at the staff, contract, board, and PAC levels. All individuals, whether on a paid or volunteer basis, are interested in the agency they serve and the patients to be served by the agency.

Sound policies are important for several reasons, including risk management, meeting of state and federal regulations, and fulfillment of agency and professional standards. Once these policies are in place, they must be communicated and made available to all levels of personnel in the agency so that compliance is ensured.

APPROVAL PROCESS

The approval process can take several directions, depending on the type of agency and policy. Ultimately, the governing body or individual is responsible for approval. This body may not have the expertise to develop or revise specific policies (e.g., use of infusion pumps). For Medicare-certified agencies, COP 484.16 requires that an agency have a group of professional personnel, many times referred to as a PAC. As noted earlier, the PAC is charged with establishing and reviewing the agency's policies related to scope of services, admission and discharge criteria, clinical records, and other related issues. The PAC should meet frequently enough to fulfill its responsibilities.

After review of the policies by the appropriate committee, recommendations are brought to the governing body for final approval via minutes and discussion by the administrative staff. Board committees and the governing body should meet on a scheduled basis that provides for timely approval of new or revised policies.

Each policy must be dated to reflect the date on which it was initiated, initially approved, and revised. All policies should be reviewed each year. The cover page, as described earlier, verifies that this review process is completed on a timely basis. Previous editions of revised policies should be maintained for future reference.

CONCLUSION

Although the final approval of the agency's policies rests with the governing body or individual, the recommendation for the development of new policies is a team effort. All levels of personnel within a home care agency should share ideas that will keep the agency current and competitive with other home care providers. Finally, approved policies must be communicated to all agency personnel and followed by those to whom they apply. An agency's policy and procedure manual does not belong on the library shelf. It should be readily available to all staff and referred to on a frequent basis by all levels of personnel.

REFERENCES

Barnum, B., and K. Kerfoot. 1995. *The nurse as executive,* 4th ed. Gaithersburg, MD: Aspen.

Health Care Financing Administration. 1989. *Part II. Medicare program. home health agencies: Conditions of participation and reduction in recordkeeping requirements: Interim final rules* (42 CFR Part 484). Washington, DC: Government Printing Office.

Merriam-Webster's Collegiate Dictionary, 10th Edition. 1999. Springfield, MA. Merriam-Webster, Inc.

Perrow, C. 1979. *Complex organizations.* New York: Random House.

Rowland, S., and B. Rowland. 1992. *Nursing administration handbook,* 3rd ed. Gaithersburg, MD: Aspen.

U. S. Government Printing Office. 2002, October. *Code of federal regulations* (42CFR 484.16). Retrieved from the U.S. Government Printing Office via gpo:access: http://www.access.gpo.gov/nara/cfr/ (accessed April 26, 2003).

CHAPTER 34

Discharge Planning

Joann K. Erb

Discharge planning is defined as "the process of activities that involve the patient and a team of individuals from various disciplines working together to facilitate the transition of that patient from one environment to another" (McKeehan, 1981, p. 3). Successful discharge planning requires a thorough understanding of the concepts described in this definition and attention to all these components as a plan is developed. Effective discharge planning is essential to allow hospitals to maintain financial stability and for ensuring continuity of care for the patient.

Discharge planning directly affects the delivery of services by home health agencies. To provide efficient, cost-effective care, home health agencies must have accurate information about the patient's living situation, caregivers, insurance, diagnosis, and plan of care. Equipment and supplies must be available, and patients and families must have received adequate education regarding post-discharge care. Absence of any of these factors compromises continuity of care.

Discharge planning consists of a series of well-defined steps to achieve continuity of care. Use of a decision-making model in this process acknowledges the multidimensional nature of the problem and the impact of a plan on all aspects of the patient–family–provider system. It also encourages involvement of the patient/family in the development of the plan, assists in formulation of reasonable goals, and identifies appropriate outcomes. This process promotes the movement of the patient along the health care system's continuum of care.

HISTORICAL DEVELOPMENT

The health care system in this country continues to be influenced by changes in society and advances in technology. Formal discharge planning programs developed in response to changes in both provision of and payment for health care services as well as changes in illness patterns and social supports for patients.

Before World War I, the sick were traditionally treated at home by the physician and cared for by the family. As medical technology advanced, the hospital became the center of the physician's practice, and the ill were treated primarily in hospitals. The entrance of large numbers of women into the workforce during World War II and a decline in the role of the extended family resulted in decreased availability of the family to care for sick members after hospital discharge. Interest in discharge planning as a method to reduce costs, lower hospital readmissions, and provide the patient with options spurred the development of discharge planning after World War II.

One early example of the interest in discharge planning was the Montefioro Hospital Care Program, the first hospital-based program, established in 1947. This program coupled physician home visits with visiting nurse services to produce a therapeutic environment for patients in their own homes. This program highlighted the need for health care professionals to consider the patient's posthospital situation and develop a plan to extend the benefits of hospitalization after discharge.

The inception of Medicare in 1966 added legislative clout to the development of discharge planning as an essential component of patient care. Hospitals were required to provide some form of discharge planning as a condition of participation.

Implementation of the prospective payment system by the Health Care Financing Administration (HCFA) in 1984 caused heightened interest in discharge planning. No longer could hospitals submit a bill to Medicare at the end of a patient's hospitalization and receive full payment. Hospitals recognized that their financial stability, even their very existence, depended on their ability to care efficiently for patients and prevent unnecessary days of hospitalization.

Since implementation of the diagnosis-related group system, hospitals have focused on the need to control patients' length of stay (LOS) to remain competitive. An institution's discharge planning program became the obvious means to address LOS issues.

Other societal changes that affect discharge planning include increased life expectancy and an increase in chronic illness. The "graying of America" has resulted in an increased number of elderly patients being served by the health care community. In 1994, individuals older than 65 years represented 11 percent of the U.S. population but occupied 40 percent of hospital beds at any given time.

From 1981 to 1994, the average LOS for those older than 65 decreased by 2.2 days, from 10.0 to 7.8 days (National Center for Health Statistics, 1996). By 2001, the average LOS for those older than 65 had decreased even further, to 5.4 days (National Center for Health Statistics, 2003). Because of this decreased LOS and the slower recuperative powers of the elderly, more individuals now require some sort of posthospital care. They must rely on their elderly

spouses and often on aging children to provide assistance and/or care, which may prove inadequate and taxing to the family unit.

"Quicker and sicker" became a widely heard phrase during the period after prospective payment as accusations were made that, to maintain financial security, the health care system was compromising patient welfare by discharging patients too early. As concern grew, Congress responded with legislation aimed at preventing early, unsafe discharge of Medicare patients. Section 9305, Improving Quality of Care with Respect to Part A Services (P.L. 99-509, 1986), required hospital-wide discharge planning services as a condition of Medicare participation.

In June 1988, HCFA published regulations concerning the implementation of this legislation. For hospitals to be in compliance with this legislation, the American Hospital Association recommends the development of policies addressing when to discharge a patient, how to discharge a patient, and how to evaluate a patient's decision-making capability. In general, the focus should be on early identification of patients needing intervention by the discharge planning team, designation of the hospital professionals who are responsible for dealing with potentially difficult discharges, and the general circumstances that must be met to discharge a patient appropriately.

The Joint Commission on Accreditation of Healthcare Organizations (JCAHO) has also increased its emphasis on discharge planning. The 2003 edition of the *Accreditation Manual for Hospitals* (JCAHO, 2003) includes standards that require hospital-wide policies and procedures on discharge planning with emphasis on early identification and intervention for patients with potential discharge problems. In addition, the standards require that hospital policies identify the role of the discharge planner in the initiation and implementation of the discharge plan and the interaction of other health care professionals.

Collaboration of disciplines across the care continuum, inclusion of the patient/family in care planning, and provision of adequate education for the patient/family to meet ongoing health care needs are areas designated by the Joint Commission as essential for hospitals to ensure. Documentation of the discharge plan, including the availability of appropriate services to meet the needs of the patient, must be present in the medical record.

The nursing care standards of the Joint Commission also address the importance of nursing involvement in discharge planning activities. One standard stipulates that assessments, identification of the patient's needs, and discharge planning activities be documented in the medical record. Other standards provide for development of programs and policies that describe how nursing care needs are assessed, evaluated, and met. JCAHO standards now focus attention on how nurses collaborate with other disciplines in planning post-discharge care.

The American Nurses Association's *Standards of Clinical Nursing Practice* (1998) emphasize the importance of discharge planning as an essential component of the nursing process. McKeehan (1981) notes that, when the nursing standards are applied to patient care, discharge planning is inherent in the provision of patient care.

Third-party payers such as health maintenance organizations and preferred provider organizations have recognized discharge planning as a key element in cost containment. Some companies have attempted to assume the discharge planning function for their clients in an effort to ensure that care is provided at the most appropriate and cost-effective level. One potential problem with this system is that hospitals could face liability if the discharge plan developed by the insurer is inadequate or inappropriate. Hospitals are required to ensure that the patient's needs are met, and their ability to accomplish this may be diminished if cost containment is the primary determinant of the discharge plan. In addition, fragmentation and duplication of services may result if hospital staff and insurers are both responsible for arranging follow-up services. The hospital's ability to comply with the JCAHO require-

ment for monitoring quality and appropriateness of the discharge plan may be adversely affected by sharing this responsibility with other parties.

As health care delivery systems have attempted to improve patient care while simultaneously promoting cost-effectiveness, case management has emerged as an innovative model to accomplish these goals. Case management encourages collaboration by coordinating the care provided to the patient by many disciplines across the continuum. Review of the major goals of case management—quality of care, reduced LOS, continuity of care, resource utilization, and cost control—reveals that this model incorporates discharge planning at every level of involvement because the case manager has responsibility for the patient's outcomes over time.

CONCEPTUAL FRAMEWORK FOR DISCHARGE PLANNING

Discharge planning is based on the philosophy that patients are individuals with unique health concerns and have the right to coordinated discharge planning and that hospitals have the responsibility to provide discharge planning as an essential component of patient care. Key concepts include the following:

- a holistic approach to the patient and family and their ongoing involvement in the process
- integration of discharge planning at all points on the continuum of care
- philosophy and objectives of the institution that support the concept of discharge planning
- support and involvement of a multidisciplinary team that includes the physician
- education of health care professionals about available resources and criteria for services

Naylor (1990) notes that discharge planning addresses three crucial areas in health care: (1) access, (2) quality, and (3) cost.

GOALS AND OBJECTIVES OF DISCHARGE PLANNING

The goals and objectives of discharge planning are:

- to help patients return to or improve the level of functioning they experienced before hospitalization
- to ensure continuity of care in the transition from the hospital to the post-hospital environment
- to promote cost-effectiveness and appropriate use of institutional and community resources

The discharge planning process affects not only the patient, but also the hospital and community. Because acute care hospitals are now viewed as only one point on the continuum of care, the discharge planning process has been recognized as an essential element in patient care that contributes to the patient's progress along that continuum.

Because discharge planning affects three systems (patient, institution, and community), each system will have its own expectations.

Patient Expectations

Discharge planning must recognize the individuality of the patient and family and promote the development of a plan of care that recognizes and utilizes the resources of the patient and family. It must accurately identify the patient's needs and develop a plan to ensure continuity of care in the transition from the hospital to the post-hospital environment. Discharge planning must educate the patient and family about the options available and encourage their participation in the decision-making process. It must promote attainment of the patient's maximal potential and personal dignity, and it must assist the patient and family in resuming control of their own welfare and educate them about the resources available to assist in that process.

Institutional Expectations

Discharge planning will promote quality patient care by providing a mechanism to identify a patient's needs and developing a plan to meet them. It will provide for cost-effectiveness by promoting early identification of high-risk patients, timely discharge, and reduction of inappropriate readmissions. The discharge planning process will educate health care professionals as to the structure and function of the process, how that process promotes compliance, and how available community resources are used to meet the needs of the patient. Discharge planning will promote holistic patient care by focusing attention on the impact of illness on the patient/family, and it will promote good public relations by demonstrating the institution's responsiveness to the needs of the patient.

Community Expectations

Discharge planning will provide needed services to individuals who are vulnerable from illness on their return to the community. It will promote use of health resources at the proper level and promote cost-effectiveness. Discharge planning will promote identification and use of community resources and will identify gaps in services and community needs, and it will promote linkages between health care institutions and community agencies.

COMPONENTS OF THE DISCHARGE PLAN

Patient/Family Involvement

The involvement of the patient and family in all aspects of plan development is essential to success. Because discharge planning occurs at a point in a patient's life when he or she is vulnerable, health care professionals must be sensitive to the patient's fears and supportive of his or her needs. Including the patient and family in the planning process demonstrates concern for them and affirms the patient's right and responsibilities for his or her own health. By presenting alternatives and assisting the patient and family in choosing the best option for their situation, discharge planning affirms the dignity of the individual and helps ensure the success of the plan.

The most effective way to do this is by meeting with the patient and family as early as possible in the hospitalization. The discharge planner not only can become aware of the patient's unique situation, but also can be identified as the individual in the hospital who is aware of the patient's post-discharge needs and is committed to providing a means to meet those needs. Early involvement also helps prevent the pre-discharge panic that some families feel as they realize the magnitude of the task ahead.

Family involvement in the planning stage helps identify any area of confusion or conflict and allows for resolution of problems before discharge. Families need to understand what resources, such as home care services or rehabilitation centers, are available and what the family's role in the patient's care will be. Families must have a realistic expectation of the patient's abilities and prognosis, and this requires open communication between the family and health care provider.

MULTIDISCIPLINARY COLLABORATION

Another essential component of the discharge planning process involves multidisciplinary collaboration. The primary physician must take a leadership role in moving patients along the continuum of care. Just as the physician is the gatekeeper for inpatient services, the physician's referral and plan of care are required for post-hospital services. Rehabilitation facilities, long-term care facilities, and home care services all require physician input. Optimally, physicians will know which discharge planner is involved with their patients. For example, many hospitals assign discharge planners to a service or general area, such as orthopedics, oncology, cardiology, or surgery. The benefits of this model are that the discharge planners are aware

of facilities and services for the specialty and are well known to both the physicians and the agencies providing post-discharge care. Ongoing communication with physicians is enhanced by use of a referral form, which can be used to document the ongoing development of the discharge plan. Another efficient method of communication is the use of a computer system with the capability of isolating notes on plan development for easy access by the physician and other involved disciplines.

The importance of involving the primary nurse in discharge planning cannot be overstated. This is the individual who assesses the patient daily, interacts with the family, evaluates the patient's response to teaching, and identifies subtle changes in both patient and family. Part of the discharge planner's role is to educate nurses about requirements for reimbursement, available resources, and the cost of outpatient care. In addition, feedback about the success of past referrals for patients helps ensure continued cooperation. Also important, although less pleasant, is information about plans that did not work—those that resulted in readmission to acute care, a poor patient outcome, or delays in service. These discussions can help pinpoint what, if anything, went wrong and how a similar situation could be handled.

Because of the complexity of a patient's needs, input from disciplines such as physical therapy, occupational therapy, speech therapy, nutrition support, and other departments is often necessary to establish a comprehensive discharge plan. This requires ongoing education of hospital departments as resources and regulations change. As described earlier, computer access to the discharge plan can allow efficient input from involved disciplines.

There has been much discussion in the past as to which discipline should be responsible for discharge planning. Traditionally, this was the responsibility of the social services department. As the need for home care services grew in response to decreased LOS, more nurses became involved to assess skilled care needs and develop a plan for services to meet them. Models of discharge planning are discussed later in this chapter, but it is imperative to state here that both nursing and social services are essential for successful discharge planning. The expertise of both disciplines is required to assist patients and families in achieving their goals. In this era of cost containment, it is imperative that turf issues not be allowed to hinder the discharge planning process. Coordination, collaboration, and communication between these two disciplines are prerequisites for success.

Although multidisciplinary involvement is essential for successful plan development, it may be confusing for the patient and family unless there is a designated person in the role of discharge planner with whom they can communicate in an ongoing manner. Lack of such a designated person can lead families to feel that "no one is in charge." In addition, families as well as patients need support, and this can be provided as the discharge planner involves the family in the development of the discharge plan.

RESOURCES

The availability of key resources will have a profound influence on a patient's discharge plan. If community resources are inadequate to support a patient in his or her own home, other options, such as the patient going to the home of a family member or being transferred to a boarding home, nursing home, or extended care facility, must be considered.

One important community resource for patients returning home after hospitalization is the home health agency (HHA). There has been a dramatic increase in the number of agencies since 1980, resulting in improved access to skilled home care services. New programs, such as 24-hour on-call availability and the ability to care for patients with high-technology needs, including home intravenous therapy and ventilators, have allowed more patients the option of returning home.

Unfortunately, access to unskilled services has not kept pace. Medicare does not cover custodial care, and therefore chronically ill patients with long-term needs cannot receive home-

maker services under Medicare. These are the types of services that many chronically ill, elderly individuals require to remain in their own homes. Availability of low-cost supportive services varies by locality but is generally agreed to be insufficient.

The lack of homemaker services has a dramatic effect on a patient's ability to remain independent and a family's ability to maintain a patient at home. Mundinger (1983) noted that between 25 percent and 50 percent of nursing home patients could be maintained at home with supportive services. This lack of adequate homemaker services may require implementation of a discharge plan that is contrary to patient and family wishes, such as a change in living situation.

The availability of senior transportation services, adult day care, Meals-on-Wheels, hospice, and respite care also influences the discharge plan. Transportation services provide free or low-cost transportation for eligible individuals. Elderly patients who require frequent medical follow-up or outpatient services may not be able to manage if a transportation service is unavailable. Even when senior transit is available, patients may encounter problems. For example, in Pennsylvania, senior transportation services do not cross county lines. If a patient resides in one county and needs to travel to the next county for physician visits or services, the senior transport cannot provide services. Also, not all transport services are equipped to assist physically handicapped individuals, the very group most in need of them.

Adult day care is another service that influences patients' discharge disposition. These programs provide structured, supervised activities for individuals who are unable to be left alone for long periods of time. These programs offer an alternative to institutionalization by providing care during the time when caregivers work. They may provide enough of a respite to caregivers to enable them to continue caring for the individual at home.

Initially, individuals who attended adult day care lost their homebound status and thus were ineligible for home care services. However, Section 507 of the Beneficiary Improvement and Protection Act (DHHS, 2001) amended the homebound requirement for home health services to allow the patient to attend a licensed or certified adult day-care program and still receive services. This change may offer families an option to institutionalization by providing a safe environment for patients while maintaining needed services.

Another supportive service that benefits many elderly individuals is the Meals-on-Wheels program. This program can provide an option to individuals who are unable or unwilling to do their own cooking. Programs vary in style and cost; they may be too expensive for individuals on a limited income, and they may not be able to provide special dietary needs.

The ability of families to care for a terminally ill individual often hinges on the availability of a hospice or palliative care program. These programs offer skilled, Medicare-covered care and supportive services, including volunteers, chaplains, and a multidisciplinary team approach to the care of the dying. The focus is symptom control and support to the patient and family members.

Respite care is the provision of temporary relief to the caregivers of the chronically ill. Some facilities provide short-term inpatient care to allow the family temporary relief of the burden of caring for chronically ill members.

The availability of all these community services influences the development of the discharge plan. An individual who might otherwise be destined for nursing home placement may be able to be maintained at home with community services. Cost is an important consideration, however, because many elderly on fixed incomes may not be able to afford the regular supportive services that they need to stay at home. Because unskilled services are not covered by Medicare but rather are usually funded through state programs, access varies considerably from area to area. Urban areas are more likely to provide a wider range of services than rural areas. It is imperative that discharge planning professionals remain aware of community resources and educate patients, families, and health care providers of their existence.

Thus far, the discussion of resources has focused on services available to patients returning home. Other factors that must be considered during the discharge planning process include availability of rehabilitation centers, skilled nursing facilities, nursing homes, drug and alcohol treatment centers, and vocational training centers. Because acute care institutions are just one point of care on the health care continuum, access to other specialty facilities promotes optimal patient care. Access can be hindered by availability or reimbursement considerations.

Discharge planning professionals must be cognizant not only of the existence of such programs, but also of their financial and medical requirements and must serve as a resource to health care providers.

REGULATIONS

Another essential element that affects the discharge planning process is the regulations affecting the delivery of health care in general and discharge planning in particular. As discussed earlier, Medicare legislation has had a tremendous effect on health care delivery, and regulations initiated for the Medicare population have often been used by other third-party payers. Medicare's influence has not always been positive, however, because Medicare has encouraged the use of a medical model in the care of the elderly when most of the elderly's needs are social or nursing related. To qualify for any unskilled services under Medicare, the elderly must be eligible for skilled services. It is important that professionals involved in discharge planning be active in influencing the development of future legislation and in educating society about the consequences of proposed legislation.

Another regulation that has had an impact on discharge planning is the Balanced Budget Act (BBA) of 1997, Section 4321, *Nondiscrimination in Post Hospital Referral to Home Health Agencies and Other Entities* (U.S. Congress, 1997). This law requires hospitals to provide patients who are referred for home care services with a list of agencies offering the service. The goal is to ensure patient freedom of choice in home care providers.

The law also requires that hospitals list only agencies that had formally applied, and that hospitals could not limit qualified agency providers.

Lastly, this law required that hospitals must notify a patient when there is a financial interest between the hospital and the agency if the patient is referred to that agency.

Zuber (2001) reviewed this legislation from the viewpoint of the home health agency. Because agencies may use coordinators to facilitate the patient's transition from hospital to home care, agencies must ensure that their activities are in compliance with Medicare regulations. The author discussed the differences between discharge planning activities by hospitals and home health coordination, which Medicare defines as the activities to facilitate transfer of a patient from a hospital to a skilled facility or home health agency.

The regulations state that coordination activities by HHAs can occur only after the physician has determined that the patient needs home health services and the agency has been chosen by the patient/family. HHA coordinators must understand that they cannot act as case finders and can only become involved once their agency has been chosen. This will help ensure compliance by HHAs with the Medicare regulations developed to guarantee freedom of choice for patients.

INTEGRATION OF DISCHARGE PLANNING ACTIVITIES

The final element affecting the discharge planning process is the integration of discharge planning activities into all aspects of health care delivery by primary providers. This requires consideration of the significance of illness for patients and families and the need to plan for post-illness care. Physicians in particular, as gatekeepers of the health care system, must recognize that the health care delivery system is a continuum and that a patient's progress along that continuum requires planning and multidis-

ciplinary cooperation that includes the patient and family. As noted earlier, increased use of case management by both hospitals and third-party payers to coordinate care and manage cost has incorporated discharge planning as an essential step in moving the patient along the continuum of care.

RESEARCH RESULTS

Recent research efforts have focused on the elderly as a population that would benefit from specific discharge planning programs, and studies have yielded results significant to all discharge planners. Dugan and Mosel (1992) described a review of medical records for 101 patients aged 75 years or older. One disturbing finding was that 43 patients had no documentation of discharge-planning activities. Equally alarming was the finding that patients living alone were least likely to receive support services after discharge, whereas those living with a spouse were most likely to receive them. This finding supports the idea that, without family to advocate for them, many elders do not get information about possible post-discharge services.

Elderly patients were also the subject of a study by Naylor et al. (1995) that was designed to use the expertise of a gerontologist nurse specialist in the development of a comprehensive discharge plan. The results indicated that the use of this specialist helped reduce the number of rehospitalizations and the cost of post-discharge care in the study period. Results also supported the need for intensive services in the first few weeks after discharge because of the decline in function experienced during hospitalization. These services can prevent costly rehospitalizations, promote good patient outcomes, and reduce costs for the Medicare patient.

Bowles and associates (2002) studied the characteristics of hospitalized older adults not referred for home care services and compared them to patients who did receive a home care referral. Nurses with expertise in discharge planning examined the records of those not referred and found that these patients had many characteristics associated with the need for home care, including age over 70, living alone, impaired activities of daily living (ADLs) ability, and numerous health conditions and medications. More than half had three or more characteristics associated with poor outcomes. In reviewing the records of those not referred for home care, these expert clinicians judged that 97 percent of these patients had unmet needs at discharge and may have benefited from home care. Barriers for inadequate discharge planning included inadequate assessment, fragmentation of the discharge planning process, lack of knowledge, and poor communication. Rehospitalization and decline in health status and ADL ability are some of the adverse outcomes of poor discharge planning. The authors identified the need for improved methods to identify patient characteristics associated with the need for a home care referral and a process to ensure proper plan development.

LeClerc and colleagues (2002) also addressed the consequences of inadequate discharge planning. Their literature review found that current approaches for hospitalized elderly are ineffective, possibly because of the focus on only basic physical and medical needs. Discrepancies between the patient's anticipated needs and actual needs result in plans that "fall short of the mark" (LeClerc et al., 2002).

The reasons for ineffective discharge planning include lack of patient/family involvement and failure to focus on the patient's actual abilities and needs. As a result of unmet physical and emotional needs, patients experience fatigue, decreased mobility, and decreased socialization. The authors urge that discharge planners frankly discuss the recovery process and post-discharge expectations so that patients and families may make realistic decisions about the best discharge plan.

Research has also shown that information needed by home care agencies is often not provided. A study by Anderson and Helms (1993) revealed that pertinent information about the patient and family was frequently omitted in referrals. The results also indicated that the model of discharge planning used did make a difference and that liaison nurses provided the greatest amount of data. Based on the results of a follow-up study, these same investigators (Anderson and Helms, 1995) proposed the adoption of a standardized referral form for all patients referred for post-discharge services that includes nursing, medical, and psychosocial information as well as demographic and financial data.

STEPS IN THE DISCHARGE PLANNING PROCESS

Hedges and associates (1999) describe the steps in discharge planning as assessment, development of the plan, implementation of the plan, and evaluation of outcomes.

Assessment

This process involves identification of patients who will require assistance in planning for post-discharge disposition and evaluation of the patient's medical and nursing needs as well as psychosocial and financial resources.

Because of diagnosis-related groups and the resultant decrease in LOS, this phase of the discharge-planning process has grown in importance. Prompt identification of patients requiring intervention by discharge planners promotes development of a suitable plan and timely discharge.

To accomplish this step effectively, discharge-planning professionals must have open access to all patients. They must be able to screen patients and begin to develop a plan without a physician's order. Screening activities include the use of patient care rounds and high-risk criteria to identify those needing intervention.

High-risk criteria have helped quickly identify patients who may need the involvement of the discharge planner. Some high-risk criteria commonly used in screening are as follows:

- age older than 65 to 70 years
- lives alone or with poor support systems
- life-threatening illness (e.g., cancer, acquired immunodeficiency syndrome)
- conditions requiring a change in lifestyle (e.g., cerebrovascular accident, amputation)

- disease conditions requiring instruction or supervision after discharge (e.g., colostomy, open wound, cardiac or respiratory disease, insulin-dependent diabetes mellitus)
- suspected abuse or neglect
- admitted from nursing home
- multiple readmissions or history of disposition problems.

In an effort to refine further the screening of patients for discharge planning needs, unit-specific criteria have been developed. These include criteria for neurological, surgical, pediatric, and orthopedic units.

The purpose of using high-risk screening criteria is to identify patients quickly and reduce the possibility of patients "falling through the cracks." Even though high-risk criteria are becoming more sophisticated and sensitive, the chance still exists that patients will not be identified. All professional personnel, and nurses in particular, must be alert to identify patients who require discharge planning activities and refer them to the appropriate person in a timely manner.

Tools have also been developed to assist in the identification of patients. These include a screening tool used by primary nurses, a form filled out by the patient or family on admission, and an assessment form completed for patients in the preadmission phase. More and more health care professionals, however, are concerned about the vast amounts of time spent by various disciplines in documentation of the same data. The ideal would be a multidisciplinary assessment form that includes self-reported information from the patient and family that could be used by all disciplines, including the discharge planner, and a form that could follow the patient from one point of service to the next.

Patient care rounds are invaluable in alerting the discharge planner of patients needing intervention who may not be identified by screening alone. An ideal example is a daily meeting involving the discharge planner, social worker, and primary nurses in which every patient on the unit is discussed briefly. This may sound impossible to achieve and would require intensive education of primary nurses about the information needed, but with practice it could be accomplished in a 20-minute session and could be done in walking rounds, with those involved meeting briefly with each primary nurse. In the long run, it is much more efficient than the frantic Friday afternoon phone call concerning the fragile patient suddenly discharged to an unprepared family.

The second part of the assessment involves the evaluation of community resources available to meet the patient's needs. Availability of skilled nursing facilities, rehabilitation centers, nursing homes, and home care services, as well as the patient's eligibility for them, must be identified.

Planning

Once a thorough assessment has been completed, planning can be initiated. The goal should be to return the patient to the least restrictive environment possible to promote the most independent level of functioning. The plan should include short- and long-term goals and reflect a mechanism to adapt the plan to changes in the patient's condition. As discussed earlier, family involvement results in the most successful discharge plan. This is especially true when a patient has been referred for high-technology therapy at home.

Advances in technology and the impetus for early discharge have combined to foster the development of an entire industry devoted to caring for patients with high-technology needs.

Discharge planning for patients needing such technology is discussed in detail in another chapter and will not be detailed in this section. However, a few comments related to discharge planning in these situations are needed. Because of the financial benefits to insurers, many patients and families will be encouraged to accept a plan of this kind. Cost should never be the sole deciding factor in the development of a plan, however. The discharge planner, as a patient advocate, has a responsibility to elicit the family's concerns and make a professional assessment of each family's ability to assume this added responsibility. The family must receive comprehensive instruction about the commitment and responsibilities involved before an informed decision can be made. The family members must also be evaluated for their ability to cope with this added stress. The environment of any patient being considered for high-technology therapy must also be evaluated for safety before the plan is instituted. In addition, there must be a clear understanding of the provider's responsibilities related to these patients. Many companies offer 24-hour coverage for troubleshooting and responding to emergencies. Knowing these resources are available may provide a level of reassurance to patient and family.

Implementation

Implementation of the discharge plan involves making the referral for follow-up care, if needed, and coordinating continuity of care in the transition. For patients who will be receiving home care services, the referral should be made before discharge. Information about the course of hospitalization, the medical and nursing plan of care, medications, and follow-up is essential to the home care agency. If a patient will require complex treatment at home, it may be necessary for the home care nurse to visit the patient in the hospital and educate him or her before discharge. Because this may require time to arrange, a home health agency should be given ample notice of the discharge date. Continuity of care can be ensured only by thorough, timely communication.

Because home care personnel lack access to the medical record, the referral should include as much information as possible about the patient's history and treatment. It is also important to provide families with written information about follow-up services, including the names and telephone numbers of the agencies in-

volved, the type of services and start dates, and the name of a contact in case of problems.

If a patient is to be transferred to another institution, such as a nursing home or rehabilitation center, the initial communication can take place verbally, but a written referral with pertinent information and a copy of the patient's chart should accompany the patient at the time of transfer.

Evaluation

The final stage in the process is the evaluation of the plan for appropriateness and effectiveness. This phase may be more difficult than it appears because it is easy to "forget" patients once they are discharged. For the discharge staff to evaluate the plan, adequate documentation must have occurred. Documentation should be ongoing and should include elements of the plan as they develop. Effective documentation is concise and thorough and outlines the options available and the patient's and family's response and preference. At the time of discharge, a summation note that includes disposition, agencies involved, and services to be provided will facilitate evaluation.

In evaluating the plan, some pertinent factors to consider are as follows:

- Was the plan appropriate for that patient and his or her unique situation?
- Was there adequate coordination with posthospital providers?
- Did the patient and family participate in the plan development, and were they satisfied with the outcome?
- Did the plan provide continuity of care in the transitional period?

For these questions to be answered, data must be collected. Some techniques that can be used in data collection are direct contact with the patient after discharge by means of telephone surveys and written questionnaires, feedback from the agencies providing services after discharge, and ongoing communication with patients, agencies, and physicians. The degree of sophistication utilized depends on the resources available to the discharge planning department. Even departments with limited resources can accomplish the evaluation procedure by using trained volunteers or clerical staff to collect data as long as the selection is random and the sample size is adequate.

DISCHARGE PLANNING MODELS

Numerous organizational models exist for discharge planning programs. There is no perfect model, and the best model for each particular institution depends a great deal on the institution itself. Hospitals are all unique, with different structures and power bases, and the placement of the discharge planning program should be where it will be most successful in that organization. Three of the most common sites for discharge planning departments are the social work department, the nursing department, or a separate department under administration. Wherever the placement, the process must be a multidisciplinary one.

Until recently, social work was traditionally responsible for discharge planning in acute care hospitals. Changes in health care delivery, however, have necessitated an increased understanding of sophisticated medical treatment and the skilled care needs of patients for the development of an effective plan. This requires increased involvement by nursing.

Fullan (1996) describes Abington Memorial Hospital's recent incorporation of team-centered discharge management as the most effective way to permit easy identification of and intervention for patients who require discharge-planning services. Begun in July 1994, this model employs daily scheduled meetings of discharge planning nurses, social workers, and unit nurses to screen newly admitted patients and to discuss care needs of previously identified patients. At the same time that this was occurring in discharge planning, managed care insurers were making increased demands on utilization review, and reviewers were being shifted from Medicare to managed care reviews. Because the discharge-planning nurses had been reviewing most of the Medicare charts because of the hospital's high-risk screening criteria, the decision was made to cross-train these nurses in utilization review. This resulted in reduced duplication; these nurses now perform utilization review and discharge planning for home care services for Medicare patients simultaneously. The form used for case management and discharge planning is shown in Exhibit 34-1.

McKendry and Sherwin (2002) also discussed integration of the utilization review and case management roles and suggested that this approach promoted efficient, timely delivery of quality health care services while reducing redundancy and fragmentation.

Garris (2003) presented an innovative care coordination program developed at the Wilson Medical Center in Wilson, North Carolina. The goal of this program is to improve the management of high-risk, chronically ill patients across the continuum of care. Using a Web-based program, case managers can monitor and manage patients by communicating with patients and providers through the Internet. This communication system allows for better coordination, immediate access to information for all parties, and elimination of duplication of documentation. Wilson's care managers have seen improved care and decreased costs resulting from easier identification of problems leading to better medical management.

This model harnesses the benefits of the Internet to help practitioners improve the quality of care for patients.

QUALITY ASSURANCE IN DISCHARGE PLANNING

Quality assurance can be defined as a process in which standards of care are identified, observed, and measured to ensure the achievement of proper standards; the goal of quality assurance is to make certain that care practices will produce satisfactory patient outcomes.

Quality assurance activities can be viewed as an extension of the evaluation phase of the

Exhibit 34–1 Abington Memorial Hospital Case Management Review/Referral Form

Patient I.D. Label	Ins.	LCD.		D/C
	Tel. #	Date due		

Ins. Ref. # _____

Primary Diagnosis_____ Lives with: _____

Secondary Diagnosis_____ Allergies: _____

_____ P.M.H._____

Procedure/Date _____   _____

_____

ADMISSION REVIEW DATE _____ INITIALS _____ INS. REVIEWER _____

Clinical findings/Studies: _____

_____

_____

_____

_____

_____

_____

_____

Treatment: _____

_____

_____

_____

_____

_____

_____

_____

_____

continues

Exhibit 34–1 continued

HOME CARE REFERRAL

Address change: H.C. Consent: _____

_____   Initial Visit: _____

_____   LMD/Phone# _____

_____   Ht/Wt: _____

Home Services: Nsg ____ PT ____ MSW ____ SP ____ OT ____ HHA ____ HOSPICE _____

CR Assess _____ Med. Teaching _____ Diabetic Teaching _____ Diet Teaching _____

Please see Kardex and/or Discharge Instructions for Discharge Meds.

Specifics: Labs, Wound Care, Ostomy, Foley, etc.: _____

_____

_____

_____

_____

_____

Equipment ordered/from/phone#: _____

_____

_____

_____

_____

_____

Condition on discharge _____

_____

_____

_____

T _____ P _____ R _____ BP _____ Lungs _____

I certify this patient is essentially homebound and requires professional services related to the diagnoses stated above and/or the condition for which the patient was recently hospitalized.

CM _____ Date _____   _____

                                                    Physician's Signature

Source: Courtesy of Abington Memorial Hospital, Abington, Pennsylvania.

discharge planning process because quality assurance activities also focus on the quality and suitability of the discharge plan. Outcome criteria include:

- patient/family satisfaction and compliance with the plan
- appropriateness of the plan and adequacy of information provided by the hospital discharge planner
- quality of the services delivered to the patient by the post-hospital provider

There are other outcomes of interest to the institution that should also be evaluated, such as:

- LOS and decreased discharge delays
- decreased readmissions due to inadequate discharge plans
- improved coordination and efficiency in service delivery and decreased duplication of effort

In addition, quality assurance addresses the process of discharge planning. Examples of criteria that evaluate the process include the following:

- the procedure for timely identification of patients requiring discharge planning activities
- the timeliness of response to referrals for discharge planning
- evidence of patient/family involvement in plan development
- documentation of physician involvement in discharge planning
- documentation of interdisciplinary communication and collaboration
- integration of discharge planning activities into all health care delivery by all disciplines

The objective of a quality assurance plan is to identify areas of deficiencies, make data available to aid in developing solutions to problems, and improve the quality of patient care.

ETHICAL ISSUES IN DISCHARGE PLANNING

Prospective payment for hospitals and diminished community resources have caused changes in health care delivery that can result in ethical dilemmas for discharge planning personnel. As hospitals are pressured to decrease LOS to maintain financial solvency, the frail elderly are increasingly being discharged "quicker and sicker." At the same time, more stringent interpretation of the Medicare home care benefit has resulted in reduction in eligibility for home care services. Tightening restrictions have also decreased the availability of nursing home care under Medicare. The vise is closing, and the victim is the patient.

Concepts such as the inherent dignity of individuals, the right to self-determination, and access to optimal health care may be in conflict with an environment created by prospective payment and inadequate community resources. Discharge-planning professionals, whose practice has been guided by ideals that protect the rights of individuals at a vulnerable period in their lives, are being required to facilitate discharge of patients without having adequate community resources available for post-discharge care.

This is a major stressor for discharge planners as they realize that the plans they have developed are inadequate or only temporary solutions to patients' problems. One common situation is that a frail, chronically ill elderly individual will be hospitalized with an exacerbation of a chronic condition. Because the patient has been acutely ill, he or she often will qualify for short-term home care services. Because Medicare does not cover custodial care, however, once the patient is stabilized, he or she must be discharged from home care services. Discharge planners may make referrals for home care services realizing that these services are short term and that there is inadequate long-term care for the majority of patients who need it.

Another example of an ethical dilemma that discharge planners face is that of a patient being discharged with complex care needs, such as pump-regulated enteral feedings, Hickman catheter, or home ventilator. These patients no longer require hospital-level care and want to return home, but they may not have the necessary support from family or community agencies.

As health maintenance organizations and preferred provider organizations become more interested in discharge planning as a means to control costs, discharge planners may be faced with attempts by providers to implement a discharge plan that is primarily motivated by financial considerations. This will require vigilance by discharge-planning professionals to protect the best interests of the patient. Because these problems are complex, multifaceted solutions must be sought. Community agencies need to be responsive to the needs of complex patients, expand services, and educate staff to care for these patients. Hospitals need to be made aware of limitations in community resources and assist in planning solutions. Families need to have sound education in the care of complex patients and the equipment used by such patients. Most important, discharge planning professionals must join forces and lobby for programs to ensure availability of care to those who need it.

DISCHARGE PLANNING AND THE HOME HEALTH AGENCY

As noted at the start of this chapter, discharge planning has a profound effect on the home health agency. While hospitals and other institutions rely on home care agencies to be the next step in the continuum of care, home care agencies also rely on hospitals, rehabilitation centers, and nursing homes for their very existence. Collaboration between referring institutions and home health agencies is essential to promote optimal patient care. Lack of coordination of services can result in omission or duplication of services. At the heart of interagency collaboration is the referral process.

An incomplete referral results in the HHA attempting to provide quality care without ade-

quate data. Because the patient's well-being depends on the care delivered by the home health agency, it is imperative that discharge planners provide thorough, accurate information at the time of the initial referral.

Discharge planners need feedback on the quality of the plans that they develop and areas that need attention. Home health agencies that maintain close contact with referring institutions can alert discharge planners to problem areas and also to changes in the medical and social conditions of patients referred. This information assists in refining discharge plans if the patient is readmitted.

Referral Sources in Home Health Care

Home health agencies rely on referral sources for their financial survival. There are numerous sources of referrals, the most common being acute care hospitals, managed care organizations, skilled nursing facilities, rehabilitation centers, physicians, and patients themselves. The home care agency must maintain optimum relationships with referral sources in order to be competitive.

The referral is a critical part of the discharge-planning process as the information provided helps ensure continuity in the transition from one area of health care service to another. Referral sources may vary in the amount and quality of information that they can provide about patients, and this can create a challenge to agencies.

An important factor in working with referral sources is the ease of the referral process. Home care agencies must balance the need for complete data with a process that is convenient for referral sources.

The Referral Process

Agencies should have policies and procedures in place to guide the process of accepting patients for service. Agency policies and admission criteria can assist staff in making decisions about whether the agency can safely and adequately provide the needed services. This is especially important in light of the increased demand for high-technology therapies to be provided in the home. If it is determined that a referred patient cannot be appropriately cared for and must be rejected for service, the reasons should be clearly documented on the referral form and the form maintained by the agency. Agency staff may need to access these data later should a question arise about why service was not provided.

Admission or acceptance criteria may vary among home health agencies. However, Medicare provides a general guideline for admission policies, which states, "patients are accepted for treatment on the basis of a reasonable expectation that the patient's medical, nursing, and social needs can be met adequately by the agency in the patient's place of residence" (DHHS, 1989, §484.18). The agency must refer to these guidelines when developing its admission criteria. Also, the criteria for continuation of service and termination of service should logically flow from the criteria for acceptance.

Intake Referral Form

The referral form is designed for initial intake purposes and used by staff for receiving information from an outside source about a prospective client. Although the format may vary by agency, Medicare-certified agencies are subject to federal requirements for clinical records. The record must contain "appropriate identifying information; name of physician; and drug, dietary, treatment, and activity orders, signed and dated clinical and progress notes, copies of summary reports sent to the attending physician, and a discharge summary" (DHHS, 1994, §484.48).

Additional information, such at past medical problems, prognosis, and results of diagnostic studies, improves the ability of the clinical staff to efficiently develop a plan to meet the patients' needs. If the referral source is the patient's family or a community agency, the agency staff will need to communicate with the patient's physician to obtain needed medical information.

Exhibit 34–2 is an example of an intake form used by a hospital-based home care agency.

Rejection of Referrals

If a referral is rejected because the agency cannot meet the needs of the patient or because the patient does not qualify for home care services, there is a risk of alienating the referral source. The agency has the choice of accepting all referrals for evaluation or explaining to the referral source why the patient does not qualify for services. The former approach will expedite discharge of the patient and ease the process for the referral source. However, if a referral is found to be inappropriate after evaluation, it is the responsibility of the agency to advise the patient or family member and to assist them to find other community resources from which needed services could be obtained. This may leave the patient and family in a predicament of having the patient home without anticipated services. If the referral source is a managed care company, the agency will not have this flexibility. It will be the managed care entity that decides the disposition. Discussing the reason that the referral is inappropriate with the referral source provides an opportunity to clarify to the referral source the eligibility requirements and admission criteria of the agency and protects the patient from an inappropriate discharge plan.

Because of the frequently changing interpretation of eligibility for services under third-party payers (and Medicare in particular), it is difficult for referral sources to keep abreast of all home care regulations. Agencies can provide the most current information to those sources as inquiries are made about referrals. An agency that refuses to evaluate a patient for admission to service should give the referral source a reason, such as no skilled services are required, the patient is not homebound, the patient is not in the geographic area serviced by the agency, and the specific services required are not available through that particular agency. Agency managers must clearly define how an inappropriate referral is to be handled. Because confusion on

Exhibit 34–2 Abington Memorial Hospital Home Care Intake Form

---

AMH HOME CARE - REFERRAL INTAKE FORM _____ **RESUMPTION**

TEAM ____   **Patient No.** _____   **Previous Visit** ____ **yes**
____ **no**
                    Pt/family aware of referral ____ **yes** ____ **no**

First Visit _____ **Services: N** ____ **PT** ____ **ST** ____ **OT** ____ **MSW** ____ **HHA** ____

Patient Name: _____   **DOB:** _____

Address: _____

Telephone: _____ **Sex: M   F   District Code:** _____

Emergency Contact/Relation/Phone: _____

Marital: S - M - W - D - O   Lives Alone: Y - N   SS No.: _____

Fee Source:

Primary: _____ _____ _____
            Insurance Co.   ID & Group   Case Manager/Phone #

Secondary: _____ _____
              Insurance Co.   ID & Group

Ins Auth No.: _____ **No. of Visits Approved:** _____ **End date** _____

Referred by: _____ _____
              Name   Phone
Circle Referral Source:

1. **Hospital:** _____ **ADM** _____ **D/C** _____

2. **Rehab:** _____ **ADM** _____ **D/C** _____

3. **SNF:** _____ **ADM** _____ **D/C** _____

4. **N.H.:** _____ **ADM** _____ **D/C** _____

5. **Physician**   6. **Family/Patient**   7. **Ins. Co./Other**

Ordering Physician: _____ **Phone:** _____

Family Physician: _____ **Phone:** _____

Specialist: _____ **Phone:** _____

Diagnosis: **Past Medical History:**

Procedure: _____ **Date:** _____
Medications:
___ **See attached**
___ ✓ **in home**

Exhibit 34–2 continued

Physician's Orders:
___ Hospice
___ Palliative Care
___ High Risk Maternity

RN:
___ CVR assess
___ Med/diet instruction
___ Instruct on reportable s/sx
___ Disease process teaching
___ Wound evaluation
___ Wound care:

PT:
____ HEP
____ Gait training
____ Strengthening
____ Safety evaluation

OT:
____ HEP
____ ADLs
____ Upper body strengthening
____ Safety evaluation

ST:
____ Swallow evaluation

HHA:
____ Personal care

MSW:
___ Long-term planning
___ Community resource assistance

Lab: _____ **Scheduled:** _____

Equipment: _____

High Risk Info:

Gravida ___   Para ___   Ht ___   Wt ___

Lab Results:

Additional Information:

Taken by: _____ **Date:** _____

For Abington Hospital Home Care use only:

Not Admitted:
(circle primary reason)

1. Not Discharged
2. No Skilled Care Required
3. Referred to Homemaker Agency
4. Refused Service
5. Not Homebound

6. Hospitalized
7. Nursing Home Placement
8. Died
9. Unable to Locate
10. Other _____

Ref Intake Form-5/02

Source: Courtesy of Abington Memorial Hospital Home Care

the part of intake personnel will negatively affect the agency, intake policies should be established and communicated clearly to the staff.

Intake Person

As the agency's link to referral sources, the intake position is an important one, because this individual may determine whether a referral source does or does not use the agency again. Factors that can discourage a referral source include a constantly busy telephone signal, being put on hold, constant interruptions when talking with the intake person, and inefficiency of the intake person in obtaining information.

Ideally, the intake person should be a registered nurse because the majority of referrals require home nursing services. This individual must be able to convey a professional understanding of the information given and clarify the requirements for service. Home health agencies are dependent on referrals for survival, and sources of referrals are limited. It is imperative that administrators have systems in place to accept referrals, and collect and maintain referral source data to use as one aspect of the agency's internal evaluation process.

A home health agency must have approved policies and procedures available that address criteria for admission, continuation, and discharge from service. These must be shared with the personnel of the referral sources. The admission criteria should state the types of referrals

that are not appropriate for service and how these referrals will be handled. A positive relationship between the staff of the home health agency and the referral source is one way to generate needed referrals. The end result will benefit the patient, the agency, and the referring source.

CONCLUSION

Discharge planning is a multifaceted process that seeks to promote optimal care for patients in the transition from one point on the health care continuum to another. Prospective payment for hospitals has resulted in increased attention to discharge planning as a means to reduce LOS while promoting optimal patient outcomes.

Multidisciplinary cooperation, communication, and collaboration and the involvement of the patient and family in the development of the discharge plan are key elements in the discharge-planning process. This process consists of four stages: (1) assessment, (2) planning, (3) implementation, and (4) evaluation. Discharge-planning programs need a formal evaluation procedure to identify areas of weakness and develop strategies to improve delivery of services. Discharge planners must educate health care professionals, patients, families, and communities about the services available and the limitations and gaps in service. The referral process must foster communication and collaboration between agencies responsible for optimal patient outcomes.

REFERENCES

American Nurses Association. 1998. *Standards of clinical nursing practice.* Kansas City, MO: ANA.

Anderson, M. A., and L. Helms. 1993. An assessment of discharge planning models. *Orthopedic Nursing* 12: 41–49.

Anderson, M. A., and L. Helms. 1995. Communication between continuing care organizations. *Research in Nursing and Health* 18: 49–57.

Bowles K. H., M. D. Naylor, and J. B. Foust. 2002. Patient characteristics at hospital discharge and a comparison of home care referral decisions. *Journal of the American Geriatrics Society* 50(2): 336–342.

Department of Health and Human Services. 1989. Medicare program, home health agencies: Conditions of participation and reduction in record keeping requirements, interim final rule. *Federal Register*, part 2, 42 CFR, part 484, 54: 33354–33373.

Department of Health and Human Services. 1994. Medicare program, home health agencies: Conditions of participation and home aide supervision, final rule. *Federal Register*, part 409, 413, 418, and 484, 59: 65482–65498.

Department of Health and Human Services. 1999. 1997 summary: National hospital discharge survey. *Advance*

Data 308. Hyattsville, MD: National Center for Health Statistics. Retrieved from *www.cdc.gov/nchs/data/ad/ad308.pdf* (accessed May 26, 2003).

Department of Health and Human Services Health Care Financing Administration. 2001. Clarification of the homebound definition under the Medicare home health benefit. *Program Memorandum Intermediaries Transmittal A-01-21.* February 6, 2001, HCFA Pub. 60A. Retrieved from *http://cms.hhs.gov/manuals/pm_trans/a0121.pdf* (accessed May 28, 2003).

Dugan, J., and L. Mosel. 1992. Patients in acute settings: Which health-care services are provided? *Journal of Gerontological Nursing* 18: 31–35.

Fullan, R. 1996. Team-centered discharge management: On a fast track to performance improvement. *Continuum* 15: 1, 3–9.

Garris, J. 2003. Case study: Building the case for care coordination. *Continuing care.* Retrieved from *www.ccareonline.com/stevens/ccpub.nsf/* (accessed February 18, 2003).

Hedges, G., K. Grimmer, J. Moss, and J. Falco. 1999. Performance indicators for discharge planning: a focused review of the literature. *Australian Journal of Advanced Nursing* 16(4): 20–28.

Joint Commission on Accreditation of Healthcare Organizations. 2003. *Accreditation manual for hospitals.* Chicago: Joint Commission.

LeClerc, C., D. Craig, and J. Wilson. 2002. Falling short of the mark. *Clinical Nursing Research* 21(3): 242–265.

McKeehan, K., ed. 1981. *Continuing care: A multidisciplinary approach to discharge planning.* St. Louis, MO: Mosby.

McKendry, M. J., and J. Sherwin. 2002. Utilization review and case management integration: An idea whose time

had come . . . are you ready? *Case Management* 8(2): 32–35.

Mundinger, M. 1983. *Home care controversy.* Gaithersburg, MD: Aspen.

National Center for Health Statistics. 2003. Health, United States 2003 Table 89. Retrieved from *www.cdc.gov.data/hus/tables/2003/03hus089* (accessed December 15, 2003)

Naylor, M. 1990. Comprehensive discharge planning for the elderly. *Research in Nursing and Health* 13: 327–347.

Naylor, M. D., D. Brooten, R. Campbell, B. S. Jacobson, M. D. Mezey, and M. V. Pauly. 1999. Comprehensive discharge planning and home follow-up of hospitalized elders: A randomized clinical trial. *Journal of the American Medical Association* 281: 613–620.

Naylor, M., D. Brooten, R. Jones, R. Lavezzo-Mourey, M. Mezey. 1995. Comprehensive discharge planning for the hospitalized elderly. *Annuals of Internal Medicine* 120: 999–1006.

Naylor, M. D. and K. M. McCauley. 1999. The effects of a discharge planning and home follow-up intervention on elders hospitalized with common medical and surgical cardiac conditions. *Journal of Cardiovascular Nursing* 14(1): 44–54.

Naylor, M., and E. Shaid. 1991. Content analysis of pre- and post-discharge topics taught to hospitalized elderly by gerontological clinical nurse specialists. *Clinical Nurse Specialist* 5: 111–115.

U.S. Congress. 1997. *Balanced budget act of 1997*, Section 4321. Washington, DC: U.S. Government Printing Office.

Zuber, R. 2001. Home health coordination versus discharge planning: Where is the line? *Home Healthcare Nurse* 19(10): 652–655.

SUGGESTED READING

Adams, C., and D. Blansit. 2001. How the BBA helped agencies get referrals. *Home Healthcare Nurse* 19(7): 652–655.

American Hospital Association. 1974. *Discharge planning for hospitals.* Chicago: AHA.

American Hospital Association. 1984. *Guidelines for Discharge planning.* Chicago: AHA.

American Hospital Association, Society for Hospital Social Work Directors. 1985. *Discharge planning statement.* Chicago: AHA.

Beck, L., et al. 1993. Use of the code of ethics for accountability in discharge planning. *Nursing Forum* 28: 5–12.

Bull, M. 1994a. A discharge planning questionnaire for clinical practice. *Applied Nursing Research* 7: 193–207.

Bull, M. 1994b. Elder's and family members' perspectives in planning for hospital discharge. *Applied Nursing Research* 7: 190–192.

Congdon, J. 1994. Managing the incongruities: The hospital discharge experience for elderly patients, their families, and nurses. *Applied Nursing Research* 7: 125–131.

Haddock, K. 1994. Collaborative discharge planning: Nursing and social service. *Clinical Nurse Specialist* 8: 248–253.

Hansen, J. 1966. *Continuity of nursing care from hospital to home.* New York: National League for Nursing.

Houghton, B. 1994. Discharge planners and cost containment. *Nursing Management* 25: 78–80.

Jackson, M. 1994. Discharge planning: Issues and challenges for gerontological nursing. *Journal of Advanced Nursing* 19: 492–502.

Jones, S., et al. 1995. Changing behaviors: Nurse educators and clinical nurse specialists design a discharge planning program. *Journal of Nursing Staff Development* 11: 291–295.

Lowenstein, A., and P. Hoff. 1994. Discharge planning: Study of staff nurse involvement. *Journal of Nursing Administration* 24: 45–50.

Lucas, M., and L. D. Pancoast. 1988. Referral sources in home health care, *Journal of Nursing Administration* 22 (12): 39–45.

McWilliams, C., and C. Wong. 1994. Keeping it secret: The costs and benefits of nursing's hidden work in discharging patients. *Journal of Advanced Nursing* 19: 152–163.

National Association for Home Care. 1997. *National home care and hospice directory.* Washington, DC: NAHC.

Stiller, A., and H. Brown. 1996. Case management: Implementing the vision. *Nursing Economics* 14: 9–13.

Titker, M., and D. Pettit. 1995. Discharge readiness assessment. *Journal of Cardiovascular Nursing* 4: 64–74.

CHAPTER 35

Strategies to Retain and Attract Quality Staff

Sharon D. Martin and Diane T. Cass

The authors wish to acknowledge Jody Deegan, RN, C for her assistance in the preparation of portions of this chapter.

INTRODUCTION

Many reasons exist for home care administrators to be concerned about strategies to retain and attract quality staff. Two interrelated reasons include the nursing shortage and external/internal forces that impact staff hiring and retention.

Anyone who questions whether we are in a nursing shortage that threatens to worsen in the future need only review the report of the National Center for Health Workforce Analysis that suggests that in 2000 the United States was in a 6 percent registered nurse (RN) shortfall affecting primarily 30 states. By 2020 they estimate 44 states will be affected and the RN shortfall will increase to 29 percent. Exacerbating the situation is the projection that the need for RNs in home care will grow from 130,288 in 2000 to 248,848 in 2020 and "growth in the home health care sector will result in an increase in demand for RNs from 6.5 percent to 9 percent of total RN demand" (National Center for Health Workforce Analysis, 2002, p. 11).

The nursing shortage may create a dearth or absence of qualified applicants entering home care as well as a drain of experienced staff as competitors lure them away with bonuses, promotions, higher wages, or better working conditions. Fewer applicants may place managers in the position of hiring less-qualified candidates or no one at all, resulting in a "damned if you do and damned if you don't" situation. Less-qualified hires may cause stress on both manager and coworker, as they can require more orientation, training, and supervision, both upfront and ongoing. However, holding out for the right candidate can have a devastating impact on existing staff who may need relief from overtime, an excessively large or widespread caseload, or extra off-shifts, holidays, and weekends as home care continues to be a 24/7 operation. The failure to provide such relief can result in staff burnout and resignation, further exacerbating the problem. Unfortunately, the ability to hire "traveling nurses" to temporarily patch a staffing shortage while one seeks the optimal candidate is limited in home care. In addition, the nursing shortage is amplified in many agencies by internal policies or external regulation limiting or excluding the hire of new RN graduates or experienced LPNs, a source of staff for other types of nursing facilities.

Sadly, politics can negatively impact home care. The recent implementation of Medicare prospective payment resulted in a decrease in payments to some agencies and a shift in the length of care and type of patient an agency could serve and still remain solvent. Private insurance, managed care, and state Medicaid programs continue to institute new restrictions for patients to qualify for home care in an effort to cut costs. Of course, paperwork time increases, a part of the job home care nurses dislike. These external forces resulted in some agencies going out of business and others being forced to tighten their belts, some laying off experienced home care nurses. Streamlining became necessary and fewer managers now supervise more employees. Even the increased cost of gasoline places pressure on home care staff as they see more money going into the gas tank while reimbursement for travel plateaus.

Recruitment, hire, and orientation are costly. Luring the best candidates and retaining them is the key to a healthy, functional home care agency. Therefore this chapter offers two strategies for attracting and retaining qualified staff: (1) flextime scheduling and (2) clinical ladders.

This flextime scheduling portion of the chapter describes the experience of a large, private, nonprofit home care agency's development of a flextime policy. A task force was formed to examine current models utilized in business and their suitable application to home health. The task force developed definitions, measurable goals and objectives, and a policy statement and implemented a 3-month, multisite, multidiscipline pilot study with 16 employees flexing. The pilot was evaluated from multiple perspectives. Pretesting and posttesting of all agency employees revealed that flextime was seen as a major benefit to employees by allowing them to better meet personal and family commitments. Evaluation also demonstrated that flextime did not positively or negatively affect productivity or sick time utilization and that the majority of participating employees opted for flexing to earlier work hours.

One strategy cited in the literature for recruiting and retaining valued staff and increasing morale is the use of flexible patterns for scheduling and staffing (French, 1982; Werther, 1983). *Flextime*, also known as *flexitime*, is a work schedule that allows employees some choice of when to start and stop their work day. It provides an opportunity for the person working outside the home to mesh job, family, and

personal responsibilities more easily. It can assist with meeting patient needs for variations in regular caregiving hours. Best of all, in this age of clinical and corporate complexity it is a refreshingly simple concept to implement.

BACKGROUND

The 40-hour work week has been the prevalent schedule of employment for approximately six decades. The Fair Labor Standards Act of 1938, which mandated overtime pay for work over 40 hours, seemed to influence the development of the 5-day, 8-hour work week norm. It was the most obvious schedule to fit the 40-hour mandate, and it has prevailed ever since. Sometime during the 1970s, options to that norm began to be explored (Werther, 1983). At the same time, Poor (1970) spread the idea that the traditional work week was not the only option (Exhibit 35–1).

One of the major social forces encouraging the initiation of flextime is the rise of the dual-career family, in which both husband and wife work. This results in a rise in income with a resultant desire for more leisure time. Also, if children are involved, it becomes inconvenient for parents to work the traditional hours because family obligations may be difficult to satisfy with both parents being unavailable during the same hours. Single-parent families find satisfying family demands even more difficult and need even greater flexibility in the workplace to survive (Perry, 1999).

A second force for change lies in the labor market. Firms have been forced to find innovative ways to attract and retain the staff they need while attempting to keep labor costs down. Flextime stands out as an excellent new benefit that in most cases costs the organization little. In many cases, such as in understaffed hospitals, flextime offers a solution to attracting staff besides costly salary increases. Often, staff who otherwise would have been unable to work at all have returned to the workforce because of creative flextime schedules (Skeler, 1981; Werther, 1983).

Exhibit 35–1 Different Forms of Flextime

- *Staggered hours:* Employees are assigned a variation of regular established work hours.
- *Flextime:* Employees choose a starting and quitting time, stick with that schedule for a period, and work 8 hours a day.
- *Gliding time:* Employees may vary their starting and quitting time daily, but they must still work 8 hours, or another company-set length of time, every day.
- *Variable day:* As long as employees work the number of hours required by the end of the week or month, they can vary the number of hours they work each day.
- *Maxiflex:* Employees may vary their daily hours and do not have to be present for a "core" time on all days.

Courtesy of Sharon D. Martin, MSN, RN, CS.

Source: Data from J. M. Roscow and R. Zager (1983, March/April), "Punch out the Time Clocks," *Harvard Business Review* 61(2): 12–29.

A third force for change is demographics. The baby boom years have passed. The future probably will hold a decreased workforce with decreased unemployment and the competition for the available employees will be greater. Innovative techniques such as flextime may be necessary to attract and retain sufficient staff (Skeler, 1981; Werther, 1983).

Recent research on flexible work arrangements suggests that it is a prized benefit and thus a potent retention and recruitment tool. "A survey by Rutgers University and the University of Connecticut found that workers rate the ability to manage work and family as the most important aspect they look for in a job. Similarly, an online survey commissioned by CareerBuilder found that 87 percent of workers polled were seeking or had sought companies that were flexible, supportive, and understanding of personal and family needs. Jobtrak.com also found similar results among college students and recent graduates when the largest group of respondents (42 percent) said that what they value most when making career decisions was work/life bal-

ance—more than money (26 percnet), advancement potential (23 percent) or location (9 percent)" (Rose, 2001, p. 50).

During a recent hearing concerning health care workforce shortages before the U.S. Senate (February 13, 2001) Brandon Melton, Vice President for Human Resources of the Catholic Health Initiatives organization, outlined the looming crisis. One of the options he discussed to recruit and retain qualified staff was flextime, which he described as family-friendly, a way to "help our employees attain a realistic work-life balance" (p. 6). Finally, several authors discuss the attractiveness of flextime to Generation X employees who value family time and better work–home life balance (Joel, 2002; O'Connor, 2002).

TASK FORCE ON FLEXTIME

The request for flextime, originating from staff, resulted in the formation of a task force composed of administrative and first-line managers. The task force examined models utilized in other business settings to determine their suitable application to the agency and to develop a flextime policy. As mentioned earlier, the task force developed definitions, measurable goals and objectives, and a policy statement and implemented a 3-month, multisite, multidiscipline pilot study with 16 employees. The pilot was evaluated according to criteria established initially by the task force, which included the perspective of the patient, the employee, the supervisor, the team, the payroll department, and administration.

The work of the task force took place through several meetings over a period of 7 months. The task force consisted of one administrator and four first-line managers representing the central and branch offices of the agency. It was believed that the burden of implementation would be at the first-line manager level and therefore that they should have a major role in policy formulation. The task force gathered and disseminated information to staff at team meetings so that there was ongoing staff feedback.

The task force utilized the problem-solving approach in the development of the flextime policy. The first step was the identification of problems and generation of goals. Problems identified were as follows:

- Management time was spent on special requests made by staff.
- Staff desired greater freedom in managing their own time.
- Rigid hours interfered with patient needs and desires.
- Having no nurse available after 4:30 P.M., except the on-call nurse, interfered with physician communication.
- Management reorganization had left down time in the late afternoon for some home health aides.
- With rapid growth and resulting increases in staff, there were problems in accessing telephone lines and sharing office space.

Goals established by the task force provided the direction for developing policy. Goals identified were the following:

- There will always be coverage from 8:00 A.M. to 4:30 P.M. Flextime shall not disrupt the established levels and hours of coverage.
- Productivity will meet or exceed budgeted levels.
- Patient needs and desires will be met.
- There will be decreased management time spent on special requests made by staff.
- Staff satisfaction and morale will increase.
- There will be no lateness and less absenteeism.
- There will be increased capacity to cover cases in other than the 8:00 A.M. to 4:30 P.M. time slot.
- There may be increased opportunity for physician and nurse conferencing to occur.

The next step of the task force was to develop definitions of flextime and core hours and a pol-

icy statement (Exhibit 35–2). The task force's definition of flextime was:

> A work schedule that leaves the standard number of working hours unchanged but allows employees some choice of when to start and stop working within the limitations set by management. There is usually a flexible window at the beginning and end of each day that surrounds a core set of hours when all employees must be present.

THE PILOT PROJECT

Planning

Initial planning involved a literature search and survey of state and out-of-state community health agencies. Information was obtained via a

---

Exhibit 35–2 Flextime Policy

The manager arrives at the decision to approve individual requests for flextime. The day-to-day decisions of a short-term nature, such as alteration of staff schedule to accommodate physician appointments, also fall within the jurisdiction of the manager. This policy, however, is intended to address longer-term alternative work schedules.

Under all circumstances, the patient's and team's needs will be met. Arrangements for supervision of flextime staff are the responsibility of the manager.

Core hours will be 9:30 A.M. to 2:00 P.M., Monday through Friday. The range of visit hours will be 6:00 A.M. to 6:00 P.M.

Starting time governs quitting time each day. Once hours are chosen, they may not be changed without due notice. Anything outside the scope of this policy requires administrative approval.

Source: Courtesy of Sharon D. Martin, MSN, RN, CS.

literature search regarding experience with flextime in the health care setting and a procedure for considering implementing a flextime program (Rosenberg, 1983). One agency surveyed had a formal policy regarding flextime.

Specific objectives for a flextime program were developed. As a result of the flextime program, there would be increased ability to meet patient needs, maintenance of productivity at current budgeted figures, increased staff morale, and decreased or no increased supervisory involvement in managing patient care or program issues as a result of flextime. These objectives were to be utilized in planning and evaluating the pilot as well.

The next step was to determine the feasibility of a flextime program in each of the offices and departments. Each of the managers was responsible for assessing whether a flextime program was feasible in that office or department. The feasibility was based on the function of the office or department as well as on the needs of the staff and community. The flextime program was determined to be feasible by each of the managers. Eligibility criteria for employees were developed based on those of the Cambridge, Massachusetts, Visiting Nurse Association (Exhibit 35–3).

The last step of planning for the pilot project involved developing the evaluation criteria for the pilot. The criteria developed were based upon the objectives and included the perspective of the patient, manager, employee, team, payroll department, and administration.

Implementation

The flextime task force recommended that a 3-month pilot study be done utilizing employees who had indicated an interest in flextime and who met the eligibility criteria. Managers in all offices and departments selected the individuals to participate in the flextime pilot. Five nurses, five home health aides, three outreach workers, two payroll and billing clerks, and one occupational therapist represented each of-

Exhibit 35–3 Eligibility Criteria

- All full-time and part-time regular staff can be considered.
- Staff must have demonstrated themselves to be responsible and independent by meeting expected agency behavior via the performance evaluations.
- Paperwork must be up to date.
- Productivity statistics must meet or exceed expectations.
- Staff must have worked at the agency for at least 6 months.
- The number of individuals participating per team is at the discretion of the manager.
- Award of the flextime benefit is for a period of 6 months.
- Management reserves the right, based on performance and productivity, to require flextime participants to return to a traditional schedule after suitable notification. A 2-week time frame, whenever possible, is the maximum notice time.

Source: Courtesy of Sharon D. Martin, MSN, RN, CS.

fice participating in the pilot. Supervision was accomplished during flexed hours via telephone availability of the manager and the on-call nurse (Table 35–1).

Evaluation

At the end of the third month, an evaluation of the pilot was conducted. Evaluation efforts focused on input from the following areas: the patient, manager, employee, team, payroll department, and administration. Employees kept a log of patients whose visits had been scheduled outside the 8:00 A.M. to 4:30 P.M. workday and submitted a brief narrative statement discussing their experience participating in the pilot. A telephone survey was done by managers to assess patient satisfaction. Individual and team visit statistics were compared with budgeted projections. Increases and decreases in lateness and absenteeism among team members were assessed. Advantages and disadvantages of

Table 35–1 Employees' Adjusted Work Hours, Regular Workday, 8:00 A.M. to 4:30 P.M.

Number of Staff	Flextime Hours
12	7:00–3:30
1	6:30–3:00
2	7:30–4:00
1	8:30–5:00

Source: Courtesy of Sharon D. Martin, MSN, RN, CS.

flextime were elicited from the managers and administration. A presurvey and postsurvey were administered to team members. Increased time spent processing payroll was measured. The task force analyzed the results based upon each of the established objectives.

RESULTS OF THE PILOT PROJECT

The results of the log of patient visits outside the 8:00 A.M. to 4:30 P.M. workday were that many of the staff used the early hours to do their charting rather than make patient visits. The telephone survey of patients indicated only 3 negative responses among 29 patients surveyed. Regarding increased opportunity for physician–nurse conferencing to occur, many staff noted the availability of the physician for consultation in the late afternoon, although most staff were flexing to earlier hours rather than later hours. Results of the pretest and posttest did not reflect an improved ability to meet patient needs. It was believed that the results were skewed, however, because work schedules had always been adjusted temporarily to meet patient needs.

Productivity was maintained at budgeted figures. Productivity and sick time were not affected positively or negatively by flextime. Employees with health problems continued to use sick time; employees with known productivity problems did not improve their performance as a result of flextime. In general, if there were problems with individuals before the pilot study, they remained. If there were no problems, flextime scheduling did not create any new ones.

Survey results reflected increased staff morale. Flextime was valued as a real benefit to pilot participants. Managers indicated difficulties in scheduling team meetings to accommodate various schedules as a disadvantage. Advantages were increased staff morale and increased flexibility to meet patient needs.

The results of the pilot study revealed that the major benefit of flextime was an improved ability of staff to meet family and personal needs and a consequent increase in staff morale. Of those flexing, most chose to flex to earlier hours. Overall, the flextime pilot was successful. The flextime task force recommended approval of the flextime policy, and the board of directors did so.

LIMITATIONS OF THE STUDY

The objectives of the program and the means for determining success or failure of the project should be identified before a flextime study is even attempted (Rosenberg, 1983). Clearly identifying these objectives before implementation allows comparison and a means to determine whether what was planned initially was actually accomplished.

Evaluation criteria established before the study rested heavily upon a prepilot and postpilot questionnaire, which was intended to gauge staff satisfaction and morale. One of the project goals was to increase these two factors among staff. It was never determined by objective measurements whether satisfaction was to be increased among all staff or just among staff utilizing flextime. The pretest and posttest were administered to all staff, however.

Some problems can be identified with this procedure. First, administering the pretest and posttest to everyone may have measured general satisfaction with work rather than response to flextime. Many of the questions reflected factors besides flextime. This was borne out when staff discussed the test. When answering the questions, frequently they were considering events in the office at times not relating to flextime. In addition, Rosenberg (1983) suggests that the pretest and posttest should be administered no sooner than 6 months apart, giving staff enough time to feel as if flextime is the usual state of affairs. Our posttest was administered at a 2-month interval to meet the deadline of a 3-month report on the pilot. This was probably too soon to test any real changes. In fact, when the tests were examined we found that there was little or no difference between the pretest and posttest answers. Because of the broadness of the questions, the fact that the test was given to all employees, and the short time between the administration of the tests, the validity of the results as a means to gauge morale in relation to flextime is questionable.

Another goal of the project was that patients' needs would be better met. From patient responses via telephone or in person, it appears that patients enjoyed the flextime visits. Patients who did not enjoy the earlier visits were rescheduled for visits later in the day.

The third goal of the project, decreased management time spent on special staff requests, was not evaluated by objective criteria. Subjective reports were the sole means of evaluating this goal. A fourth objective, no tardiness and less absenteeism, was only partially measurable. Because starting and stopping times were not measured by a time clock, it was difficult to gauge tardiness. Absenteeism was measurable, however, and no change was found before and after implementation of flextime. The fifth goal, increased capacity to cover cases outside the 8:00 A.M. to 4:30 P.M. time slot, was measured only by subjective reports of staff, patients, and supervisors, all of which were positive. The sixth goal, increased opportunity for physician–nurse conferencing, was not met because the majority of staff flexed to earlier hours. An important factor for consideration is the use of a control group to compare with the experimental group of flextime staff. This would have given valuable comparative information.

EXPERIENCE OVER TIME

Ten years after the initial flextime pilot and policy implementation described above, a literature review gave the surprising result that no articles describing flextime were published in major nursing journals in the 1990s. Although many articles discuss a variety of scheduling options to improve staff retention (Erickson, 1991; Goodroe, 1992; Gowell and Boverie, 1992; Stratton et al., 1992; Sullivan, 1991), none focuses on flextime. Several articles specifically discuss staffing and retention in home care and community health (Ryals, 1991; Sherry, 1994; Whitaker, 1993), but again, none discusses flextime.

Ten years after implementation at the agency, the flextime policy remained intact with the following changes:

- Flexible scheduling has been integrated into the corporate culture. It is no longer viewed as new or different. In fact, it is viewed as peculiar that an organization would not offer something as valuable as flextime to working men and women. It has been a particular benefit in recruiting and retaining staff and in enabling staff to maintain full-time status while meeting personal obligations. Abuses of the system have been rare. A recent survey indicated that approximately 50 percent of professional staff flex in one way or another.

- The policy applies to any agency job description. As direct care staff have flexed, support staff and supervisory staff have followed suit successfully.

- A 4-day, 10-hour schedule has been implemented. This is the most popular flextime mode. Staff nurses report that it is easier to organize their work (e.g., patient visits, phone conferences with physicians, and documentation) within the longer day. This is also the mode most frequently listed by managers as causing the most scheduling difficulties for a team, however. One manager reported asking her team to abandon the 4-day, 10-hour schedule.

- Other creative schedules have been devised, such as three 9-hour days and one 4-hour day or four 9-hour days.

A survey of managers indicated that, although highly valued by staff, flextime was not without its drawbacks. Comments from managers suggested that it could be difficult to keep track of everyone's schedules, to schedule meetings around diverse work times, and to meet deadlines on days when people might not be available. Scheduling problems were most commonly listed as the primary drawback of the policy, occasionally affecting patient coverage and continuity of care. One manager described developing a "buddy system" to solve these problems.

In 2003 the decision was made to limit further entry into the flextime program. No new staff is approved flextime, especially the four 10-hour day option, which proved to be the most troublesome. This is due to a variety of changes in home care.

First, movement into home care prospective payment placed additional stresses on the system. Case management became more important than ever. Patient problems and issues needed immediate resolution. In the past, first-line managers were able to fill in as case managers for nurses absent Monday through Friday. However, streamlining and cost cutting required greater efficiency, and fewer managers now supervise greater numbers of staff. The system could only be stretched so far, and managers recognized that they could no longer effectively fill in for absent staff. Staff who worked four 10-hour days placed the greatest strain on the system.

Second, as home care boomed due to the need to discharge patients quickly from the hospitals and long-term care facilities cut back their admissions due to their own prospective payment stressors, weekend visits in home care increased. Where once weekend admissions were rare, now admissions flow in 7 days per week. As a result, the number of nurses absent Monday through Friday due to compensation time for weekend work has also increased. This decreases the efficiency of the staff's case management Monday through Friday and was determined to be detrimental to patient care.

Nurses absent due to flextime were the added strain that had to go.

Happily, some teams within the agency, such as the psych-mental health nurses, are able to continue flextime without adverse effects on case management due to the unique characteristics of the patients they serve and the decreased need for weekend rotations among this group. Such teams will enjoy continued flextime as long as patient care remains optimal.

As one might expect, the staff was not pleased to give up a very popular benefit that had come to be "expected." However, all recognized the need for optimal patient outcomes as a result of superb case management and the detrimental role flextime seemed to be playing in the nurses' ability to meet that expectation. Some staff gave up the benefit but none resigned due to the change.

However, on a positive note, a modified form of flextime was adopted for those unable to participate in the original program. Opportunities still exist to start early or end late, work longer one day to have a part of another day off for an important appointment, and even to take an entire day with pay to complete community service. This new benefit, 16 hours per year for community service with pay, is a particularly valuable tool for staff with children, as chaperoning a field trip, for example, can qualify as community service. Home care remains extremely flexible when meeting the individual staff person's personal needs for a flexible workweek. The difference is, instead of a recognized weekly flex schedule, staff must now plan ahead and make arrangements with their supervisor on a week-by-week basis.

CONCLUSION

Flextime remains a policy at the agency though in considerably modified form. Some teams can use flextime without adverse effect on case management. Other teams needed to give up the option or move to the modified form. New hires will not be offered the four 10-hour-day option. All staff still enjoy the great flexibility available in week-to-week scheduling. Though considerably changed, the program is still alive and as we move deeper into the nursing shortage, revival of this benefit in its fuller form may become necessary as a powerful recruitment and retention tool.

CLINICAL LADDERS

Clinical ladder programs for nursing have been around for over 30 years. Though initially developed in hospitals, recognition of clinical expertise is important to the nurse in any practice setting including home care. The rewards associated with such a program may be a powerful tool for recruitment and retention, as well as a motivator to improve clinical practice among current staff, though to date no definitive studies have shown that clinical ladders do result in increased recruitment or retention (Buchan, 1997; Schmidt et al., 2003). The absence of such data is not surprising, especially in home care, because there have been few articles published on the implementation of clinical ladders in the home care setting. However, this should not dissuade an agency from implementing a program that recognizes and rewards staff. Therefore, this portion of the chapter describes the experience of a large, private, nonprofit home care agency's development of a clinical ladder program.

Overview

A committee was formed to review the literature, determine who would be eligible, how the program would fit with existing job descriptions, identify the number of levels and criteria for advancement, and write the policy and procedure statements. The program development and implementation process took approximately 2 years. At the end of the initial 2 years, an evaluation of participating staff suggested that they did feel rewarded for professionalism, both intrinsically and financially. The clinical ladder program has remained an integral part of the employee recruitment, reward, and retention

program since its inception over 10 years ago though, like any good program, it has evolved.

Background

Creighton first introduced the idea of a clinical ladder in 1964. Thereafter, the Task Force on Health Manpower, National Commission of Community Health Services (1967) suggested that nurses in the clinical setting should be rewarded for practice excellence through a workplace clinical ladder policy. In the late 1960s, the country was experiencing a nursing shortage in part caused by increased nonnursing duties, inadequate compensation, and lack of professional recognition. The National Commission for the Study of Nursing and Nursing Education (1969), studying the problem of hospital nurse recruitment and retention, determined that career patterns, a system of advancement based on clinical expertise and competence, could be a solution (Lysaught, 1970). Thus, the concept of a clinical ladder was adopted first by hospital rather than community health administrators.

Zimmer published the first article discussing the rationale for clinical ladders in 1972, and the first article describing the implementation of a clinical ladder program in a hospital was published in 1974 (Colavecchio et al., 1974). Since that time, there has been a steady stream of articles published describing clinical ladder programs in a variety of settings, though the majority of reports continue to describe hospital-based programs. The first published report of a clinical ladder program for the home care setting was published in 1990 (Martin and McGuire, 1990).

Early on, the pioneers of clinical ladder programs identified the traditional reward system for nurses, based upon longevity rather than professional expertise, as inadequate. Nurses seeking increased status or pay were forced into management or education, draining talent away from the bedside (Alt and Houston, 1986; Colavecchio et al., 1974; Gassert et al., 1982; Lysaught, 1970; Ulsafer-Van Lanen, 1981). This system also trapped most nurses at one staff level due to the limited number of manager and educator positions available (Sigmon, 1981).

Many authors have identified advantages and disadvantages of clinical ladder programs over the years (Alt and Houston, 1986; French, 1988; McKay, 1986). Some advantages may include improved:

- professional satisfaction
- perception of self, role, and employer
- bedside care
- opportunity for growth and professional advancement

Such a program may also offer increased:

- intrinsic and extrinsic reward for performance and accomplishment
- success of retention and recruitment programs

Disadvantages may include difficulty:

- designing and implementing the program
- defining performance criteria
- staffing units with adequate numbers of staff from each level
- placing new employees on the appropriate level

Unfortunately, clinical ladders may not eliminate the disparity between compensation for clinicians and administrators. There also remains the incongruity of requiring clinical experts to report to and be evaluated by administrators.

Clinical Ladder Task Force

This project began as a result of staff nurse and therapist dissatisfaction with the status quo, a commonly used reimbursement system rewarding all on the same scale despite wide variations in skills, abilities, backgrounds, and educational level. Only seniority within the agency increased pay rate, though at the yearly evaluation monetary consideration was made for either less than or higher than expected performance. No system existed to reward skill or educational development. Sadly, similar systems can be found

today in agencies that have not yet developed alternative reward programs.

The clinical ladder task force was composed of administrators including the chief executive officer and the vice president of program planning (both nonnurses), the vice president of clinical operations (an RN), regional managers (both RNs), the inservice coordinator (an RN), the therapy coordinator (an OTR), and the special services coordinator (an RN). Nursing and therapy staff met with the regional managers and therapy coordinator weekly to provide input and feedback on committee progress. The composition of the task force represented the belief that the clinical ladder program could and should include all clinical staff in the home care agency including RNs, therapists, social workers, and home health aides. The composition of the task force also reflected the top-down management philosophy common in agencies at the time. Today clinical ladder programs have become more common, and shared governance the norm; therefore, a committee to develop such a program would expect to include strong representation from staff, a recommendation consistent with the American Nurses Association report *Career Ladders: An Approach to Professional Productivity and Job Satisfaction* that suggested development of such programs should be "by the nurse, for the nurse" (1984).

A review of the literature revealed no articles describing clinical ladder programs for home care agencies. (As noted earlier, the report of this clinical ladder program, published in 1990, was the first for a home care agency.) Though many reports described programs for hospitals and other health care settings, the criteria used did not neatly meet the needs of the home care setting. The committee thus decided to develop its own behavioral criteria for each level based upon the needs of the agency and the patients it served. Newer clinical ladder programs developed solely for nurses may base development of ladder criteria on the 1984 work of Benner (Froman, 2001; Gustin et al., 1998) or Carper (Schmidt et al., 2003).

After considerable discussion, two decisions were made regarding the ladder's development. First, it should correspond with the current job descriptions and job classification system in order to make the whole project less overwhelming. Second, the ladder would have three levels. The number of levels in a ladder is quite arbitrary depending upon the criteria used to develop the ladder. For example, a ladder based upon Benner's work might have five levels, while a ladder based upon Carper's work might have four. A recent review of ladder programs, albeit in hospitals, found that most use four, but levels varied between one and eight (Buchan, 1997).

Initial clinical ladder development focused upon the RNs as they represented the largest proportion of the total professional workforce at the agency and also because most information available about clinical ladders reflected the RN, therefore making the committee's job a bit easier by building upon published reports. The decision was made to use the existing staff nurse job description, which included criteria commonly found in such job descriptions including skills working in groups, communication, performance of technical nursing skills, knowledge of community resources, professional behavior and development, record keeping and participation in activities such as meetings, and committee work. The existing job description thus became Level I of the Clinical Ladder for RNs. The expectation had always been that RNs new to the agency would be able to at least meet the existing job description criteria by 6 months to 1 year, and we retained that expectation

Designing Clinical Ladders II and III was based upon the beliefs of the committee members that the ladders should be cumulative; that is, a nurse moving to Ladder II should continue to proficiently demonstrate all of the Ladder I criteria, and a nurse moving to Ladder III should continue to proficiently demonstrate all of the Ladder I and II criteria. Members of the committee also valued educational background, years of experience both in home care and in nursing in general, special skills, assumption of special

roles in the agency, and certifications held.

After months of work, the committee, with consistent input and feedback from staff, developed Ladder II (Exhibit 35–4) and Ladder III (Exhibit 35–5). In order to make the clinical ladder program correlate with the existing staff nurse job description, Clinical Ladder II was added as Addendum A and Clinical Ladder III was added as Addendum B.

Additionally, the clinical ladder program needed to correlate with the existing job classification system, a 12-step distribution of all positions in the agency, 1 representing the position requiring the left skill/responsibility and 12 representing the position requiring the greatest skill/responsibility. The staff nurse job description had historically been ranked Job Classification Level 8. Therefore, after development of clinical ladders the Ladder I Staff Nurse Job Description remained at Job Classification Level 8, while Staff Nurse Clinical Ladder II ranked Job Classification Level 9, and Staff Nurse Clinical Ladder III ranked Job Classification Level 10.

This represented a real advance, both monetarily and professionally, for staff nurses as both reimbursement and professional recognition increased as individuals moved into jobs with higher job classifications. In the past the ability to move into higher job classifications had been restricted by the limited number of management positions (e.g., supervisor) or support positions (e.g., in-service coordinator) in existence. The clinical ladder program allowed staff nurses to remain staff nurses while earning greater respect, recognition, and financial reward.

Through discussion within the committee and with staff, the following decisions were made. First, in order to recognize and encourage education, the clinical ladders were designed to allow faster movement through the levels by those nurses with advanced degrees. Second, the specialties chosen to allow progress up the ladder reflected those most important to home care nursing such as skill in home intravenous therapy, chemotherapy, hospice, mental health, and

Exhibit 35–4 Summary of Original Staff Nurse Clinical Ladder II

Ladder II Summary

Applicant must meet all criteria in the following areas:

RN (AD or Diploma):
- Recent, pertinent clinical experience 2¹/₂ years FT* equivalent

BSN:
- Recent, pertinent clinical experience 2 years FT equivalent

MSN:
- Recent, pertinent clinical experience 1 year FT equivalent

PLUS each nurse, regardless of educational background, is required to demonstrate:
- One specialty/role AND certification OR two specialties/roles

In addition to meeting all criteria in Ladder I, the nurse would meet the following:

If a nurse chose a specialty, the following was required:
- Scheduled time to serve as resource to staff.
- Patient visits in specialty as caseload permits.
- One in-service for staff in specialty per year.
- Expectation of self-directed professional development in the specialty.

If a nurse chose the role (physician-oriented caseload), the following was required:
- Meet with physician regularly to review caseload.
- Self-directed development of expertise in the physician's specialty.
- Pre-discharge hospital visits as appropriate for discharge planning.

*FT = full-time employee
Source: Courtesy of Sharon D. Martin, RN, CS.

Exhibit 35–5 Summary of Original Staff Nurse Clinical Ladder III

Ladder III Summary

Candidate must have been successful at Clinical Ladder II for at least 6 months prior to application to Ladder III.

RN (AD or Diploma):
- Recent, pertinent clinical experience 3 years FT* equivalent

BSN:
- Recent, pertinent clinical experience 2¹/₂ years FT equivalent

MSN:
- Recent, pertinent clinical experience 1¹/₂ years FT equivalent

PLUS each nurse, regardless of educational background, is required to demonstrate:
- Two specialties/roles AND certification OR three specialties/roles

In addition to meeting all criteria in Ladders I and II, the nurse must meet the following:
- Present two in-services in specialty for staff per year.
- Participate in community activities related to specialty/role as requested.
- Serve as preceptor as requested.

*FT = full-time employee
Source: Courtesy of Sharon D. Martin, RN, CS

---

infection control. Finally, the role originally available to staff nurses that allowed ladder progress was a physician-oriented caseload; that is, one nurse caring for or coordinating the care of all of the patients of a particular physician, and meeting with that physician regularly to review the caseload.

Certifications from the American Nurses Association (ANA) originally chosen to allow the nurse ladder advancement included general, medical-surgical, gerontological, pediatric, psychiatric and mental health, and basic and advanced community health nurse. In 1991 the American Nurses Credentialing Center (ANCC) became its own corporation, a subsidiary of ANA, and certification opportunities increased. Current certifications offered by the ANCC that may be applicable to the home care setting and advancement in a home care clinical ladder program include community health, gerontology, home health, medical-surgical, pediatric, psychiatric and mental health, case management, perinatal, and many nurse practitioner and clinical specialist certifications, especially those in community health and home health, and the clinical nurse specialist in diabetes management (American Nurses Credentialing Center, 2003).

Nurses that progressed to Clinical Ladder II or III were to meet certain requirements to remain at that level. For example, the nurse at Clinical Ladder II was required to provide one staff in-service per year and to schedule regular time to serve as a clinical resource to staff. At Clinical Ladder III, nurses were to provide two in-services to staff per year and to serve as preceptor as needed. Ladder regression was possible when a nurse did not meet the necessary requirements or continue to demonstrate the criteria from lower ladder criteria.

Following development of the RN Clinical Ladder, similar ladders were developed for the physical therapists (PT) and the occupational therapist (OTR). The plan was to develop ladders for social workers and home health aides as well.

Program Evaluation

Two years after implementation a questionnaire evaluating the clinical ladder program was distributed to 46 RNs, 3 PTs, and 1 OTR with an 84 percent return rate. The results suggested that staff did feel a heightened sense of professionalism from participation in the program and did enjoy increased financial reward without being forced away from direct patient care. Ninety-seven percent of respondents agreed the program should be retained and expanded. Results were less clear in terms of recruitment and retention, however, because most new hires had not been aware of the program when applying, thus stating it did not factor into their decision to take a position. This is not surprising in view of the fact that the program was new, not well advertised, and not stressed during hiring interviews. The staff also suggested the program alone would not cause them to remain employed

at the agency but that other factors integral to home care, such as independence, autonomy, good working conditions, good job hours, and the pay and benefit package, were the deciding factors in continued employment. One might argue that a clinical ladder program reflects good working conditions and factors into the pay and benefit package.

In 2002, 15 years after the original pilot project, the clinical ladders program underwent major renovations based upon the suggestions of staff and first-line managers who felt the original model had functional flaws. Staff (RNs, therapists, and social workers) found that in the new environment of home care prospective payment, where increased productivity and improved patient outcomes are required for agency survival; the requirements of the existing clinical ladder program were difficult to meet. Especially burdensome were the presentation of one or two educational in-services per year and the maintenance of a portfolio demonstrating achievement of the clinical ladder requirements. First-line managers complained that the task of determining that staff did or did not meet clinical ladder requirements fell on them. With fewer managers and more staff reporting to each manager, the job became daunting—yet the ability to determine whether staff met the criteria was particularly important because regression in clinical ladders was possible. As a result, fewer staff participated in the program and cries that, "There are no opportunities for advancement in this agency" increased while first-line managers clamored for reform as well.

A committee, with heavy staff representation, was formed to explore options. After review the committee recommended a complete overhaul of the system. The new system placed all staff nurses in Job Classification 8, but the pay range within that job class was expanded to overlap the old job class pay ranges that had been in Job Classes 8, 9, and 10. Thus the "ceiling" for pay for the staff nurses, therapists, and social workers was raised dramatically such that it overlapped with the pay range for managers. During the change no staff person currently on clinical ladders regressed job class level or suffered loss in hourly pay rate. All new hires now are assigned to Job Class 8.

Next a decision was made to base this professional reward-and-recognition system, renamed the Clinical Advancement Program, upon an existing professional recognition system; that is, national certifications available to nurses, therapists, and social workers. The committee members reasoned that certification was designed to demonstrate professional expertise in a particular area and the recertification process demonstrated maintenance of that expertise. Why not tap into that ready-made system for recognizing and rewarding clinical expertise?

Though most of the certifications available for nurses are through the ANCC, additional certifying bodies are also accepted, such as Diabetic Educator through the American Diabetes Association and Wound, Ostomy, Continence Nurse through the Wound, Ostomy, Continence Certification Board. Interdisciplinary wound management certification as a Certified Wound Specialist is also available through the American Academy of Wound Management. Therapists and social workers also have certification opportunities available through their professional organizations.

Home health aides (HHAs), though originally intended to be included in the clinical ladder program, had not been. Therefore, during the 2002 program redesign HHAs were added. Unfortunately, nationally recognized certification exams could not be found that mirrored the certifications offered to nurses, therapists, and social workers. Thus the agency developed its own rigorous certification examination to be offered to HHAs seeking advancement.

Certification is now the cornerstone of the new Clinical Advancement Program. To encourage participation, the agency pays 100 percent of the cost of both certification and recertification. Staff is not required to pay the agency back if they fail a certification exam. There are no limits to the number of certifications a staff person may hold beyond the natural barrier imposed by clinical practice and the ability to meet the recertification requirements. Staff enjoy a 2 percent raise (in addition to the usual merit and market survey raises) with each certification and recertification. No regression is possible. That is, if a person chooses not to seek recertification, they do not lose the 2 percent initially granted but they do forfeit the additional 2 percent raise they would have gotten with the recertification.

The program serves as a recruitment tool as well. New employees immediately enjoy a 2 percent raise if they have a certification upon hire and enjoy an additional 2 percent at the next recertification, which may be within months.

This elegantly simple program seems to be having the desired effect of keeping the staff at the bedside while encouraging professional development, recognition, and remuneration, as well as serving as a useful recruitment tool. In 2003 over 90 percent of eligible nursing staff had attained certification, and the turnover rate remained extremely low. No complaints regarding excessive expectations or record keeping were heard from staff or managers. The system may be a victim of its own success as the only "problem" identified to date is the reluctance of the staff to move into managerial positions, there no longer being the need to make this shift in order to earn greater pay and professional respect.

CONCLUSION

The clinical ladder program has remained a vital part of the professional life of the staff at the agency. Recent major revisions and reincarnation as the Clinical Advancement Program have only strengthened and simplified it. Today clinical ladder programs are found in many settings including hospitals, long-term care facilities, and home care agencies. Staff has come to recognize and expect clinical ladder opportunities. The design and implementation of programs that recognize and reward professional knowledge, skill, and abilities can serve as the ultimate win-win as agencies enjoy successful recruitment and higher retention.

REFERENCES

Alt, J., and G. Houston. 1986. *Nursing career ladders: A practical manual.* Rockville, MD: Aspen.

American Nurses Association. 1984. *Career ladders: An approach to professional productivity and job satisfaction.* Kansas, MD: Author.

American Nurses Credentialing Center. 2003. Certification catalog. Retrieved from *http://www.nursingworld.org/ancc/certify/cert/catalogs/index.htm* (accessed May 28, 2003).

Benner, P. 1984. *From novice to expert: Excellence and power in clinical nursing practice.* Menlo Park, CA: Addison-Wesley.

Beyers, M. 1998. About improving clinical ladders. *Nursing Management* 29(10): 96.

Buchan, J. 1997. Clinical ladders: The ups and downs. *International Nursing Review* 44(2): 41–46.

Colavecchio, R., B. Tescher, and C. Scalzi. 1974. A clinical ladder for nursing practice. *Journal of Nursing Administration* 4: 54–58.

Erickson, S. 1991. Mother's hours: "Extra" RNs balance the workload. *Nursing Management* 22: 45–46, 48.

French, O. 1988. Clinical ladders for nurses: Expect a resurgence of interest but there will be changes. *Nurse Manager* 19(2): 52–55.

French, W. 1982. *The personnel management process.* Boston: Houghton Mifflin.

Froman, R. 2001. Assessing the credibility of a clinical ladder review process: An interrater reliability study. *Nursing Outlook* 49(1): 27–29.

Gassert, C., C. Holt, and K. Pope, 1982. Building a ladder. *American Journal of Nursing* 82: 1527–1530.

Goodroe, J. 1992. The manager's influence on retention. *Health Care Supervisor* 11: 74–78.

Gowell, Y., and P. Boverie. 1992. Stress and satisfaction as a result of shift and number of hours worked. *Nursing Administration Quarterly* 16: 14–19.

Gustin, T., J. Semler, M. Holcomb, J. Gmeiner, A. Brumberg, P. Martin, and T. Lupo. 1998. A clinical advancement program. *Journal of Nursing Administration* 28(10): 33–39.

Joel, L. 2002. Reflections and projections on nursing. *Nursing Administration Quarterly* 26(5): 11–17.

Lysaught, J. 1970. *An abstract for action.* New York: McGraw-Hill.

Martin, S., and M. McGuire. 1990. A clinical ladder for the community health-care setting. *Journal of Community Health Nursing* 7(4): 189–197.

McKay, J. 1986. Career ladders in nursing: An overview. *Journal of Emergency Nursing* 12: 272–278.

Melton, B. 2001. Hospitals alone can't solve today's health care workforce shortages. *AHA News* 37(8): 6.

National Center for Health Workforce Analysis, U.S. Department of Health and Human Services, Health Resources and Services Administration, Bureau of Health Professions. 2002. Projected supply, demand, and shortages of registered nurses: 2000–2020. Retrieved from *http://bhpr.hrsa.gov/healthworkforce/rnproject/report.htm* (accessed May 22, 2003).

National Commission of Community Health Services. Task force on Health Manpower, (1967). *Health manpower. Action to meet community needs.* Washington, DC: Public Affairs Press.

O'Connor, M. 2002. Nurse leader: Heal thyself. *Nursing Administration Quarterly* 26(2): 69–79.

Perry, P. 1999. 7 ways to tap into a tight labor market. *Materials Management in Health Care* 8(6): 32.

Poor, R. 1970. *4 days, 40 hours, and other forms of rearranged workweek.* Cambridge, MA: Bursk & Poor.

Rose, K. 2001. Workplace flexibility, key to today's staffing: Breaking the workaday mold can lead to staffing success. *Behavioral Health Management* 21(4): 50–54.

Rosenberg, G. 1983. *Issues of the workplace.* Workshop sponsored by the National Council of Alternative Work Patterns, Kennebunkport, ME.

Ryals, S. 1991. Current problems confronting community health services—Part 2. *Aspen's Advisor for Nurse Executives* 6: 8–9.

Schmidt, L., D. Nelson, and L. Godfrey. 2003. A clinical ladder program based on Carper's Fundamental Patterns of Knowing in Nursing. *Journal of Nursing Administration* 33(3): 146–152.

Sherry, D. 1994. Coping with staffing shortages. *Home Healthcare Nurse* 12: 39–42.

Sigmon, P. 1981. Clinical ladders and primary nursing: The wedding of the two. *Nursing Administration Quarterly* 5: 63–67.

Skeler, J. 1981, September 28. Flexible work hours gather momentum. *U.S. News and World Report*, pp. 76–77.

Stratton, T., N. Juhl, J. Dunkin, R. Ludtke, and J. Geller. 1992. Recruitment and retention of registered nurses in rural hospitals and skilled nursing facilities: A comparison of strategies and barriers. *Nursing Administration Quarterly* 16: 49–55.

Sullivan, P. 1991. Common-sense ethics in administrative decision making. *Journal of Nursing Administration* 21: 57–61.

Ulsafer-Van Lanen, J. 1981. Lateral promotion keeps skilled nurses in direct patient care. *Hospitals* 55: 87–90.

Werther, W. 1983. Nontraditional work schedules: Their use in the health care setting. *Health Care Supervisor* 1: 11–20.

Whitaker, R. 1993. A home health agency's operational model utilizing per visit and hourly staff. *Journal of Home Health Care Practice* 5: 38–44.

Worthy, C. 1996. Clinical ladders: Can we afford them? *Nursing Management* 27(9): 33–34.

Zimmer, M. 1972. Rationale for a ladder for clinical advancement in nursing practice. *Journal of Nursing Administration* 2(6): 18–24.

CHAPTER 36

Evaluating Productivity

Lazelle E. Benefield

This chapter discusses the definition of productivity and how productivity is analyzed in home health services. Environmental and staff factors that affect productivity are analyzed, and a procedure to follow to determine staff productivity is suggested. This discussion centers only on how to determine current productivity of staff that provide direct service (i.e., make home visits). Although useful for all providers, this information was originally written for use with professional staff.

Determining current productivity is only one part of a program to measure and improve productivity. How to determine the standard necessary for agency viability, examples of productivity improvement, and how to institute a productivity improvement program in an agency appear in other sources (Benefield, 1996a, 1996b, 1996c; Fry et al., 2004; Homecare Quality Management, 1999).

Productivity is essential to agency viability; therefore, personnel must be both effective and efficient in decision making and clinical practice. A productivity analysis program can assist in monitoring efficiency and enhance the likelihood of providing quality services. Providing quality services involves encouraging staff, who are the agency's most valuable resource, to work toward their potential (i.e., to use the skills they were trained to use). The premise is that monitoring and analyzing productivity will assist staff to use their skills effectively and efficiently.

For an agency to be productive, we must train and retain qualified staff. Staff generally take cues for performance expectations from management, including first-line supervisors and above. When managers have the responsibility and accountability to control many of the factors that affect productivity and organize the work environment to encourage professional growth in staff, the efficiency and quality of services are improved and productivity is increased.

WHAT IS PRODUCTIVITY?

Several assumptions are listed here and form the basis for understanding productivity.

1. Productivity involves more than the balance between nurse hours and cost. Nurse activity, consumer outcomes and perception of quality, and organizational commitment to innovation influence productivity (Lake, 1998).
2. *Productivity* [emphasis added] is the effective implementation of activities in an efficient manner. *Effective care* is defined as the correct action, in the right amount, at the right time. *Efficiency* is the provision of care services without time or material waste (Benefield 1996b, 1996c). "Productivity now includes services, innovation, knowledge, creativity, loyalty, human capital, and more. The measure of

productivity must account for financial performance, operational efficiency, and customer value . . ." (Shamansky, 2002, p. 79).

3. Quality can improve as productivity increases, although many professional staff and managers would initially disagree. The most pressing need in this area involves accurately determining when quality exists and the degree to which the client outcome(s) has been achieved. If we have a clear and measurable method of determining when the outcome has occurred, we can then determine the type of services needed to achieve the outcome.

4. Productivity is an issue in every agency. Many managers incorrectly view productivity improvement as the sole method of improving income generation in an agency. The continued concern over rising health care costs and the need to better evaluate and control factors that improve effectiveness and efficiency have prompted a surge of interest in productivity issues.

5. Productivity evaluation is a greater issue for some agencies than for others, specifically those that use full-time (FT) and part-time (PT) staff. In the past, agency managers with contract staff usually were not concerned with increasing contract staff visitations per unit of time. *Contract staff* are defined as workers who are paid a flat fee per visit. Historically, managers focused on FT/PT staff who were paid a salary for the hours worked and not the visits made. This approach may be changing because many agencies are investigating payment of FT/PT staff on the basis of the number of visits completed.

6. The word *productivity* is usually viewed with some level of discomfort by most staff. One should expect a negative response, either verbally or behaviorally, when the issue is first discussed. Although not necessarily correct, staff often fear an assembly-line approach, staff cutbacks,

and/or unrealistic increases in workload. Staff may believe they must work faster or reduce the quality of care and assume that work cannot be simplified, reorganized, or delegated. Because of the term's negative connotation, all agency personnel require reeducation to understand exactly what productivity is and what it means to the agency.

7. Productivity is a management issue and not exclusively an employee issue. Managers should be directly involved in the process of determining, monitoring, and, if necessary, improving productivity. Other readings provide further detail (Benefield, 1996a, 1996b; Storfjell et al., 1997)

8. *Productivity* is defined as follows:

- output per given input (Kinicki and Williams, 2003)
- the ratio of good and services provided to resources used (Fry et al., 2004)
- "the relationship between the use of resources and the results of that use" (Olson, 1983, p. 46)

The input-output model of productivity is most accurate when measuring productivity in industry (e.g., assembly-line work). In this setting, the number of items or products produced in a given period of time is easy to measure; however, such measurement is difficult in a health service industry. The 1983 Olson definition, "the relationship between the use of resources and the results of that use," was developed to include those in white-collar positions, and best describes productivity in professional positions in the home health care service industry. Productivity in health care measures both the quality and quantity of work done (Sullivan, 1995).

For example, in home care the use of resources may include everything necessary to complete the home visit, known as the product. These resources can include the staff member's time, supplies, agency management time, and other indirect expenses. Historically, the result or output of using these resources is the number of visits, per discipline, per time period. The time period may be 1 day, 1 week, or 1 month. Visits may be separated by type: maternal-child, pediatrics, or hospice; by discipline: registered nurse, therapist, or social worker; and/or by reimbursement method: Medicare, HMO, managed care, grants, with or without prospective or capitation payments. Examples include the following:

- 6 reimbursable visits per RN each day
- 25 pediatric visits per therapist per week
- 120 reimbursable RN visits per week (Monday through Friday, 4 RNs at 30 visits each week, each RN averaging 6 visits per day)
- a predetermined number of visits allowable by type of case, or the average number of visits by type of case/diagnosis

WHAT WE KNOW ABOUT PRODUCTIVITY

What is known about productivity in health care can be summarized as follows:

- Productivity is difficult to measure in a health service industry (Linn and Karsten, 1982; McNeese-Smith, 2001).
- Improving only one area/component of an agency will not affect overall production; assessment must include all areas.
- When evaluating productivity, the agency manager should review the budget for items that account for 80 percent of the expenditures and work on these areas. These expenses most often reflect the cost of personnel.
- Professional productivity does not depend on how fast an employee works but rather on the effective use of time.

Productivity is difficult to measure in a health service industry because of a limited knowledge of what we are measuring. In home health care, the quantity (number) of home visits can be measured, but we are less skilled in measuring and evaluating the quality of the visit. The pro-

vision of the home visit is variable. The interpersonal components of a home visit (e.g., the tasks and behaviors of staff and consumer) are complex and difficult to quantify. The consumer of the service, the client, is variable (Martin et al., 1993) and the client and family unit will demonstrate changing characteristics. No two clients with the same diagnosis will ever demonstrate identical physical, psychosocial, and environmental needs.

The classic work by Linn and Karsten (1982) describe this as an "uncertain product definition," suggesting that it is unclear what the agency is actually trying to produce (visits or health). How much of whatever health is do we wish to produce? The agency's mission statement, such as *service to anyone regardless of ability to pay* or *service to those with the ability to pay*, reflected in the organizational culture and values, may illustrate what the agency is producing: health, visits, or both. In addition to using an agency's mission statement as a guide, managers are assisted in defining health production by insurance companies that define the type and number of services to be reimbursed and by consumers' demands for certain states of health. In other words, agencies provide services that are reimbursable and for which consumers are willing to pay. With little agreement on the range or depth of services, the measurement of productivity in the health services industry is difficult.

Improving only one component of an agency will not affect overall productivity. Productivity improvement involves a systematic assessment of the entire organization rather than just a staffing review. One provider group cannot improve or change productivity unless other components of the system are evaluated. For example, a physical therapist's job tasks may be tied to secretaries who answer the phones and screen calls, to data processing (records may not be transcribed and returned to the therapist for use during the scheduled visit), and to other disciplines. The therapist may be delayed during a home visit in order to supervise a therapy assistant or to meet with an RN regarding the client.

Therefore, we should not expect a change in productivity in one discipline unless productivity improvements occur in all components of the system.

Begin by reviewing the budget for items that account for the majority of the expenses and initially work on these areas. For most home health agencies, the majority of costs are attributed to personnel. This includes staff who deliver the service or product, the home visit, and other personnel whose job it is to support the provider. Managers should evaluate this area first, and then expand to the larger program, other disciplines, and the organization.

Productivity includes the provision of quality care without time or material waste (Benefield, 1996a). In order for staff to provide this type of care, managers should assist staff to identify their professional strengths and skills, refer non-nurse activities to others, and continually focus on whether the task or action being performed is relevant to achieving client outcomes. Productivity is not solely an employee issue. Managers should create the climate and set the pace for effective productivity. Therefore, to embark on a productivity analysis the manager should develop a clear definition of the product—the home visit—assess the entire organization for unnecessary activities, and simplify work processes in order to achieve outcomes.

ANALYZE SERVICE DELIVERY: EFFICIENCY, EFFECTIVENESS, AND EQUITY

Analysis of productivity involves identifying variables that are unique to each agency, including system and specific personnel reviews. Managers gather historical and baseline information first, then embark on a productivity review of personnel. Review personnel productivity, then determine the efficiency, effectiveness, and equity of services provided by the agency as a whole.

Efficiency involves the production of a certain amount of output within a unit of time. An efficiency goal may be to increase the amount of output produced by a given input or to decrease the amount of input (skilled services) required to produce a given output (home visits). An efficient visit is one with minimal time or material waste. In addition to the volume of services, review information about service intensity, such as the complexity level of clients and the case mix of the population served. Case mix may include the type of client, severity of illness, and the service under which clients are admitted. At this stage the degree of agency efficiency may be hard to identify, so list the methods and/or strategies that the agency has used in the past to maintain efficiency. Identify which worked. Examples include incentive pay for completion of additional visits per employee within a set time period and efforts to streamline the admission process.

Effectiveness is the degree to which the process of care delivery was accomplished as intended. Analysis should include an evaluation of whether the correct job function was completed and the level of quality provided. Use staff and management input to determine the expected outputs for the visit. Define which activities and tasks should be completed during the home visit. In addition, use evidence-based guidelines to clarify the standards by which to measure the care given and received. For example, evaluate the activities that should occur during a sequence of home visits for a client with diabetes. Consider what activities should be completed during the home visit(s). The manager should retrieve data to inform these decisions through the agency's quality improvement program. Then the manager can determine a range of expected client responses and, as necessary, use clinical paths or guidelines or other home care quality measures as templates to gauge achievement of client goals.

The *equity* of the service is defined as the distributional effects of a given productivity scheme (Linn and Karsten, 1982); in other words, which population receives the services and whether the services are fairly distributed. The "fair distribution of services" is based on agency philosophy and policy. *Horizontal equity* is how the effects of production are distributed across the population as a whole (e.g., all the types of clients who are served by the agency from their geographic catchment area). *Vertical equity* is how a given production function affects a specific target population. For example, among all the clients who potentially could receive intravenous (IV) therapy, consider whether the agency provides service to all or only a segment of the population.

EVALUATE CURRENT PRODUCTIVITY

To develop productivity standards in an agency, use the following sequence of steps. Select a specific program using one or a group of diagnostic categories or payor types. For the program:

1. Analyze environmental factors that affect productivity.
2. Analyze staff factors that affect productivity.
3. Determine the current productivity of staff.
4. Develop a standard through a management blueprint.

Table 36-1 is an overview of the process detailed here. The process reviews the specific characteristics of the agency's service delivery, including both office and field work, to identify current productivity. The manager should first evaluate efficiency, effectiveness, and equity to determine what productivity standard is needed to maintain agency viability, and then determine whether a productivity *improvement* program is needed to meet the productivity standard.

Although analyzing productivity includes evaluating direct and indirect care activities, as well as financial, consumer, and organizational variables, this chapter is limited to addressing productivity, defined as the number of effective units of home visit service per time period per discipline. This section analyzes environmental and staff factors to determine and evaluate current productivity.

To determine and analyze provider productivity, the manager will evaluate the provision of

Table 36–1 Steps To Develop Productivity Standards

1. Analyze environmental factors that affect productivity.
   - geographic area
   - paperwork
   - technology supports
   - type of program or visit
   - amount and quality of group work
   - staff scheduling
   - percentage of unnecessary activities
   - other
2. Analyze staff factors that affect productivity.
   - experience
   - length of service with agency
   - morale and motivation
   - other
3. Determine the current productivity of staff.
   - Determine baseline data on staff.
   - Collect visit data:
     - type, diagnosis, complexity
     - reimbursement source
     - completed visits
     - travel between visits (time, distance)
     - time spent in direct service, preparation, documentation, other
   - Determine productivity (product number divided by hours of labor).
4. Determine a standard through a management blueprint.

direct client care and staff and environmental factors that affect the provision of services. Analyze environmental and staff factors that contribute to identify areas that hinder and help staff in completing their work.

Analyze Environmental Factors

The manager should respond to the following checklist of questions and include all indirect care factors that affect the staff member's provision of direct client care.

Geographic Area

- Determine, if not already known, the geographic area served by the provider. Is it a densely populated urban area or a sparsely populated rural area?
- Is travel time great? What is the distance between clients in driving time and in miles?
- Do staff physically report in each morning or evening? What is the amount of time allotted to travel to the office?

Paperwork

- Assess which programs generate the most and least paperwork.
- Determine the length of time to admit a client. Which type of client (older, complex diagnosis, particular payer source) requires additional time for documenting the admission?
- Are charts and medical records, either hard copy or electronic, accessible for charting when needed? Is documentation readily retrievable and conducive to multidisciplinary collaboration (Pabst et al., 1996)?
- Are secretaries used for completing all insurance and nondirect care forms?
- Ask the providers where changes can be made to reduce redundancy. For example, do RNs input client assessment data on four different sheets when admitting the client? Are addresses copied on more than one form?

Technology Supports

- Note technology enhancements or challenges in providing direct services to clients (Kelly, 2000).
- Are computer terminals or wireless personal data assistants (hand-held computers) available and used? Are dictaphones used? Are progress notes verbally relayed to the office for transcription?

- If being used, has automated documentation proved helpful to the nurse in documenting compliance with standards (Pabst et al., 1996)?
- Are techniques such as teleconferencing or video-assisted visits being used? Are these effective strategies? Ask staff to identify advantages and challenges (Pabst et al., 1996).

Type of Program or Visit

- List the programs in which the RNs are involved—hospice, pediatrics, high technology, maternal-child health, adult care. Which are high risk due to high volume, complexity, or political factors?
- Does the average visit length differ by type of program? Are different lengths based on severity of client need, reimbursement method, or type of visit; for example, admission, maintenance, screening, or complex (Payne et al., 1998; Storfjell et al., 1997). Review agency policies and practices to determine why particular programs have longer visit times. Repeat the process to evaluate the number of visits by program or case type.
- Which programs do staff consider emotionally draining? Productivity and motivation may decrease as a function of the type of clients cared for; for example, pediatric oncology clients, stroke clients, or clients without family support.
- Which programs do staff shy away from, and why? Are these programs difficult due to client complexity or noncompliance, an unsafe environment, or travel distance?
- Does the financial reimbursement for the service, whether fee-for-service, prospective payment, or capitated fee, influence the visit length and staff hesitancy to complete the home care services? Identify the specific payer plans and their real and perceived influence on visit number and length.

Amount and Quality of Group Work

- List the frequency and duration of educational and administrative meetings. Is a new program or service creating a need for more meetings? Remember that meetings cut into the number of visits possible in a day.

- Are staff returning to the office for informal support? Often, new or inexperienced staff want contact with other staff for technical or moral support. As the complexity of the work increases, the need for peer consultation may also increase. Some agencies require all staff to return to the office at day's end to encourage this peer consultation and to decrease the need for formal team conferences.

Staff Scheduling

Supervisory skill at scheduling staff affects productivity. The number of *expert* managers and staff will influence productivity. Consider these areas:

- How is scheduling done? Are visits planned with geographic proximity in mind? For example, do staff meet each morning, then drive to a distant locale to complete home visits, then return to the office in the evening to check in? When staff must come to the office before beginning visits, they may pass their first client's residence on the way to the office to check in, then retrace the drive to the first client of the day. Perhaps staff can phone in to document when they have begun the day at the first client's home.
- Often a specialty program, such as IV therapy, covers a large geographic area. Are staff expected to cover the entire area or is the care delegated to staff within geographic quadrants?
- Do staff live adjacent to their service area? Are staff purposefully assigned to areas other than where they live? Consider reevaluating this practice.
- Review the assignments that inexperienced and more qualified staff receive. Determine whether differences in assignments reflect differences in the skill level

of staff. Is the novice staff member assigned to a complex client? Is the expert staff member working with clients whom he or she finds unchallenging?

- Assuming a choice of staff within a geographic region, assess how cases are assigned, taking into account an already full caseload, vacations, and other variables specific to the agency. Are staff being effectively assigned?

Percentage of Unnecessary Activities

The manager should review the daily schedule to identify where staff are involved in nondirect care activities that may be better delegated to others (Upenieks, 1998). Follow a staff member for a day and ask him or her to identify redundant activities.

- Answering phones is a major time waster. This is an especially troublesome problem in small agencies that may not provide telephone coverage when the secretary is otherwise occupied. Consider call forwarding to another site, use of an answering service, or a part-time secretary or clerk to cover the busy times, such as early morning or during the lunch hour.
- Do nurses and therapists stock their own bags? Instead, provide staff with a check-off sheet of supplies. This completed sheet can be returned to the office and supplies can be packaged by a paraprofessional or office staff member for pickup the following day.
- Are staff providing services that can be provided by other professional or paraprofessional staff? For example, are therapy staff providing counseling better completed by social workers? Are RNs completing daily care activities that aides are trained to do? Evaluate the degree to which professional staff perform tasks that, although satisfying to the staff, may limit the time they have to provide professional-level interventions that directly impact client outcomes. This is one of the more difficult areas to correct; however,

change in this area will reap major gains in productivity.

Other

What additional agency-specific factors affect the manner in which staff perform their role? Is there a seasonal workload change—are admissions highest in the winter months with slack time in the summer, or just the reverse? Track completed visits by month over the previous 2 years. Identify trends in workload volume or complexity. As needed, modify the number of required full-time positions. When historical trends indicate periods of lower census and visit activity, encourage the use of paid or unpaid employee vacation and compensation time. Many agencies use part-time or contract staff for periods of peak volume.

Analyze Staff Factors

Experience

- Experienced staff should complete more visits per unit of time than inexperienced staff and be more efficient in their use of time. Assuming a similar case mix, are experienced staff visiting more clients than less experienced caregivers? What is the difference in average visit time between experienced and less experienced staff? If visit time is the same, are experienced staff working with complex clients?
- What defines an experienced, effective staff member? A productive staff member may have skills such as:
  - ease in charting
  - greater expertise in assessing client needs, prioritizing, and goal setting
  - the ability to deal with flexibility (the new staff member often complains of having no guidelines)
  - expertise in health assessment
  - expertise in counseling/therapeutic conversations. The staff member is able to avoid overinvolvement in only the social or financial aspects of care and can effectively delegate roles to other professionals. Further definition and discussion of the knowledge and abilities of productive RN staff is detailed elsewhere (Benefield, 1996a).

Length of Service with Agency

Do managers assist new staff to develop expertise in providing effective *and* efficient care? Are prospective staff informed of these expectations in preemployment interviews and during orientation? The manager should require time for an orientation that includes explicit, outcome-focused instruction. Do managers assist new staff in developing expertise in efficiency as well as in the traditional aspects of providing effective home care services? What is the expected orientation time for staff to become fully functional? Determine the point at which you expect a full contribution by staff: 2 months, 6 months, 1 year? After the initial orientation, continuous training is required to maintain up-to-date skills and evidence-based practice.

Morale and Motivation

The manager should identify the morale among staff. What is the level of work readiness and work-related stress (Lynch, 2001)? Consider how the agency management style influences morale (Helge, 2001). Although many variables contribute to changes in morale, the agency's response to the frantic pace of change in the home care industry will affect productivity. Poor management practices will contribute to poor morale and work-related stress, decreases in staff motivation, and decreases in productivity. Carefully analyze the system and program changes within the last 6 to 12 months, then view the managers' responses to the changes and their interaction with staff. The manager should consider whether strategies to improve morale or team building are warranted.

Other

Determine Current Productivity

The manager should assess the current productivity standard in the agency. First, determine whether there is an expected number of home visits per unit of time. In programs with capitation or case rates, the expectation may be a change in functional outcomes within a preselected number of visits. The productivity standard should be unique to each discipline and to each program. The agency variables discussed earlier are unique; therefore, the productivity standard should reflect the unique philosophical and financial characteristics of each agency.

If an agency has a productivity standard in place, staff members must be aware of the standard. RNs may understand the standard of 6 visits per day, averaged to 30 visits per week; however, they may not be clear that these visits must be reimbursable. For example, staff may assume that logging 6 visits per day meets the productivity standard. They may not realize that a visit to a client without the ability to pay and a visit to a client not at home reduce the reimbursable visits from 6 to 4. Therefore, the standard should delineate the visit types; for example, reimbursable and nonreimbursable. Reimbursable visits may include those paid by Medicare, Medicaid, other third-party payers, grants, and donations.

The manager should determine the current productivity of staff, using a computer analysis of information, according to the following guidelines:

1. Determine baseline data (categories) to indicate what defines:
   - an experienced staff member; for example, one with more than 3 years of experience
   - a staff member who is oriented to the agency, such as one with service for more than 3 months
   - contract, PT, and FT staff
2. For a week selected at random, preferably nonvacation and without an unusual number of admissions, determine the following for each staff discipline:
   - basic information: name, discipline, experience level, and type of employment
   - level of effectiveness, ranked as less than, as expected, or greater than expected in skill and effectiveness, of each provider
   - number of visits done in a specific time frame, daily and weekly
   - evaluate the visit/travel log for each employee. Note:
   a. whether the visit was reimbursable or nonreimbursable. Count only reimbursable visits in determining productivity unless otherwise noted by the agency.
   b. whether the visit was completed or the client was not home.
   c. travel distance between visits. Are staff determining the most efficient travel route? Do they drive greater distances than necessary? Is client care mandating early morning or late evening visits? Could another staff member complete these visits?
   d. travel time between visits. Is inner city travel taking as much time as travel to/from a rural area? In other words, should geographic areas be reassigned, or are there extra slow/extra speedy drivers?
   e. visit length, matched with the type and complexity of visit (maternal-child health, adult care).
   f. the type of visit: an admission, a recertification, an emergency, a discharge, or any other type that indicates the expectation of a longer or shorter visit duration.
   g. time spent in other activities, such as telephone calls to physicians or clinic personnel, communication with families, return calls to clients, and gathering supplies. Staff should be completing a travel sheet documenting visits and mileage. This area

can be adapted to include nonvisit time and activities. These might be turned in weekly for the initial productivity review; later, once a month or quarterly reviews should suffice.

3. Use this information, tabulated over a 5-day period, to determine the productivity or output per unit of input for each staff member. Then combine these data by discipline, and/or by program, to determine an overall figure (the number of visits divided by 5 days equals the number of visits per day). Beware of combining figures from dissimilar programs; for example, staff who do postpartum visits may achieve a higher visit rate than those working within the hospice program that may have different expectations. Use the overall productivity figure as a guide and compare it with staff productivity in different programs, in varied geographic areas, and for various employment statuses.

4. Ask these questions when analyzing the information:
   - Are certain geographic areas more difficult to service than others? Are there fewer clients in the area, greater distance between clients, geographically isolated clients, or specific factors such as a bridge or tunnel that cause delays?
   - Which visits take the least and most time? Ask the staff to assist in analysis. They can identify the complexity involved in certain types of visits and identify roadblocks to the provision of care. Managers can then determine whether support services should be used to remove barriers.
   - On the average, does the visit length differ among PT, contract, and FT staff? Are contract staff, who are paid per visit, hurrying through the visit, or are they the most efficient? Note that many agencies pay FT, PT, and contract staff by the visit, so determine whether these data are important for the agency.

Perhaps of greater significance is whether the visit length is different between experienced and new staff.
   - What special circumstances may have skewed or altered the data? Were there increases in sick leave or increases in the number of emergency visits or admissions during the sample week? Was a new computer system implemented during the review period?
   - What do the staff make of the data? Because they provide the day-to-day service and are involved in the complexities of the provision of services, they should be able to describe why the results of the review look as they do.
   - Which staff members are productive? Select staff who are effective and efficient and consistently achieve positive client outcomes without undue time or material waste. These are the most productive staff. What knowledge or abilities do they possess and use on a consistent basis? Interview these staff members to determine how they describe their ability to provide both efficient and effective care. Are productive staff members ones whom managers would easily identify? What characteristics do these staff have; why are they productive? A typical profile of a productive employee is one who is well qualified for the job, highly motivated, has a positive job orientation, and communicates effectively.

THE NEXT STEP: DEVELOPING A PRODUCTIVITY STANDARD

The purpose of this chapter is to provide a method for evaluating the current productivity of all or a segment of the staff who provide direct service to clients. Evaluating staff productivity involves analyzing the environment in which staff work, reviewing the type and quality of staff working in the agency, assessing what is included in a home visit, and having a good idea of what makes a productive staff member in the agency.

The next step is to determine, using fiscal data, the productivity standard necessary to meet expenses and/or generate revenue over expenses. Indirect costs (supplies, overhead, etc.) and direct staff costs are combined to determine the total cost of providing a unit of visit(s) per individual case or per individual nurse. The information is analyzed further to determine (1) the number of visits necessary to cover the cost of agency operation, and (2) the number and/or types of visits necessary to generate a predetermined percentage of revenue over expenses. This is defined as the number of reimbursable visits per staff per unit time and is the threshold standard for a specific program.[1] The standard should be unique to each discipline. For example, therapy visits per day may be different from expected RN visits per day.

Once the current productivity is determined and a productivity standard is developed, evaluate whether there is a need for a productivity *improvement* program. If current productivity does not equal or exceed the standard established for agency viability, then implementing a productivity improvement program is essential. A productivity improvement program includes five dimensions: (1) systematic education of all personnel about the relationship between productivity and agency viability, (2) an assessment of the total operation, (3) adequate staffing and performance measurements, (4) implementation of incentives for increased productivity, and (5) continual evaluation of the productivity standards.

CONCLUSION

The manager should consider the basic assumptions when evaluating productivity. Productivity improvement is not completed in a vacuum. Improving one component of an agency will not increase overall productivity, so consider an agency-wide program. Involve all staff, particularly direct providers, in planning and evaluating the productivity of an agency. Managers hold the key to enhancing productivity through effective coaching and supervision and by creating environments that challenge and motivate staff.

---

[1] Some agencies may determine productivity based on the degree to which a staff member is able to achieve client outcomes and associated quality indicators within a predetermined number of visits and/or total dollar cost.

REFERENCES

Benefield, L. E. 1988. Productivity. In L. Benefield (ed.), *Home health care management.* Englewood Cliffs, NJ: Brady, pp. 164–179. (This chapter was originally published in this text).

Benefield. L. E. 1996a. Component analysis of productivity in home care RNs. *Public Health Nursing* 13(4), 233–243.

Benefield, L. E. 1996b. Productivity in home health care: Assessing nurse effectiveness and efficiency. *Home Healthcare Nurse* 14(9): 699–706.

Benefield, L. E. 1996c. Productivity in home health care: Maintaining and improving nurse productivity. *Home Healthcare Nurse* 14(10): 803–812.

Fry, R. L., C R. Stoner, and R. E. Hattwick. 2004. *Business: An integrative approach,* 3rd ed. Boston: McGraw Hill-Irwin.

Helge, D. 2001. Turning workplace anger and anxiety into peak performance. Strategies for enhancing employee health and productivity. *AAOHN Journal* 49(8): 399–408.

Homecare Quality Management. 1999, February. Case managers increase productivity and efficiency, pp. 17–20.

Kelly, J. 2000, November. Going wireless. *Hospitals and health network,* pp. 65–67.

Kinicki, A., and B. K. Williams. 2003. *Management: A practical approach.* Boston: McGraw-Hill Irwin.

Lake, S. 1998. Applying performance measurement to a nursing service. *Journal of Nursing Administration* 28(3): 3,12.

Linn, N., and S. Karsten. 1982. Managing public health productivity—The art of taming conflict and chaos. *Public Productivity Review* 6(3): 170–183.

Lynch, W. D. 2001. Health affects work, and work affects health. *Business and Health* 19(10): 31–37.

Martin, K., N. Scheet, and M. Stegman. 1993. Home health clients: Characteristics, outcomes of care, and nursing interventions. *American Journal of Public Health* 83(12): 1730–1734.

McNeese-Smith, D. K. 2001. Staff nurse views of their productivity and nonproductivity. *Health Care Management Review* 26(2): 7–19.

Olson, V. 1983. *White collar waste: Gain the productivity edge.* Englewood Cliffs, NJ: Prentice Hall.

Pabst, M.K., J. C. Scherubel, and A. Minnick. 1996. The impact of computerized documentation on nurses' use of time. *Computers in Nursing* 14(1): 25–30.

Payne, S.M., C. P. Thomas, T. Fitzpatrick, M. Abdel-Rahman, and H. Kayne. 1998. Determinants of home health visit length. Results of a multisite prospective study. *Medical Care* 36(10): 1500–1514.

Shamansky, S. L. 2002. Presenteeism . . . or when being there is not being there. Editorial. *Public Health Nursing* 19(2): 79–80.

Storfjell, J. L., C. E. Allen, and C. E. Easley. 1997. Analysis and management of home health nursing caseloads and workloads. *Journal of Nursing Administration* 27(9): 24–33.

Sullivan, M. 1995. *Nursing leadership and management.* Springhouse, PA: Springhouse Corp.

Upenieks, V. V. 1998. Work sampling, assessing nursing efficiency. *Nursing Management* 29(4): 27–29.

BIBLIOGRAPHY

Hassell, I. 2001. Working smarter, not harder. Improving emergency department nurse productivity. *Emergency Nurse* 8(10): 7–8.

Larrabee, S. B. 1999. Benner's novice to expert nursing theory applied to the implementation of laptops in the home care setting. *Home Health Care Management Practice* 11(4): 41–47.

References for Work Improvement Strategies

Hayes, R. 2002, Nov./Dec. How to succeed with process management. *Behavioral Health Management*, pp. 17–20.

Hospital Home Health. 1996, Nov. Total staff productivity up: Tool adds one visit per day. *Hospital Home Health,* pp. 127–130.

Humphrey, C. J. and P. Milone-Nuzzo. 1996. *Orientation to home care nursing.* Gaithersburg, MD: Aspen Publishers, Inc.

Landry, M. T., H. T. Landry, and W. Hebert. 2001. A tool to measure nurse efficiency and value. *Home Healthcare Nurse* 19(7): 445–449.

Sherry, D. 1996. Time management strategies for the new home care nurse. *Home Healthcare Nurse* 14(9): 718–720.

CHAPTER 37

Labor–Management Relations

Jessica S. Eichner

Institutions are often thought to be the bricks and mortar of their buildings, which are easily seen. In reality, people are the institution. If they leave, the institution no longer exists. What is important for any institution, therefore, are the interactions, supports, feelings, frustrations, challenges, and hopes that come from the people who constitute it. The combination of these elements forms the institution's climate (Lockhart and Werther, 1980, p. 103).

The characteristics of the institution's climate influence the relationship between labor and management and affect the effectiveness of the health agency. This climate also influences whether staff feel the need for a union. Administration must therefore be alert to the climate and be aware of and practice ways to enhance a positive relationship with the nursing staff. How management responds to employee needs, requests, and concerns will be a major determinant of the climate; a positive environment will be produced if needs are met. It is a major task for administration to find a "balance between people's needs and organizational needs" (Lockhart and Werther, 1980, p. 132), for such a balance will create and sustain an organization that is effective and vital.

CONCEPTUAL FRAMEWORK

The home health agency should be viewed from a systems theory framework in which both labor and management are seen as vital units of the system. There must be interdependency among the units if the agency is to be effective. The agency as a whole has a need for unity, and each of the units must cooperate with the other. This cooperation will build cohesion among the units, which will enhance the effectiveness of the agency. Labor and management need to view themselves as existing in a partnership in which everyone works for the patient's benefit.

FACTORS INFLUENCING THE LABOR RELATIONS CLIMATE

Many authorities have identified various factors that influence the labor relations climate of an organization and methods for enhancing the positive relationship between labor and management. Zacur (1982) has identified environmental factors, both internal and external, that influence the labor relations climate of certain organizations. Although these organizations were primarily acute care hospitals, it is possible that the same factors would be important in a home health agency. Zacur (1982) identified the following external factors:

- laws such as the 1947 Taft-Hartley Act, which guaranteed the rights of representation and collective bargaining with a nonprofit employer

This chapter is updated from a chapter written by Jessie F. Rohner for the *Handbook of Home Health Care Administration*, 2nd edition (1997).

- professional organizations, such as the American Nurses Association (ANA), which has attempted to improve the economic status of nurses
- the state of the economy, which has put pressure on female employees to request and demand increased salaries and has focused attention on the comparable worth issue
- public sentiment regarding health care professionals

Internal factors identified by Zacur (1982) include the organizational climate, the organization's administrators, the nurses' roles, and the nurses' views.

If the organizational climate is one that tolerates change and new ideas as opposed to being repressive, the labor–management climate may be positive and vital. If administration is parochial in its approach to managing human resources, lacks sensitivity to internal conditions encountered by staff, fails to recognize the professional issues of concern to nurses, and refuses to negotiate or discuss certain issues, the environmental climate will not be healthy and will reduce the effectiveness of the staff.

Another factor affecting the labor relations environment is how decisions are made and policies are determined. If agencies are administered through a bureaucratic organizational structure, and if processes and policies are issued from administration without any participation from caregivers, the environment may be conducive to collective action. Nursing staff cannot be viewed as functionaries at the lower end of the hierarchy without any participation in decision making if their contributions to the attainment of agency goals are to be maximized. Ginzberg (1966) suggested that, because nurses are influenced and affected by conditions in the environment, management needs to maximize opportunities for them to succeed, should carefully match people to jobs, and should provide maximum support to nurses in these positions.

Levitan and associates (1981) indicate that the organizational climate and administration should be secure and certain because uncertainty breeds frustration and dissatisfaction. Another important factor in determining environmental climate is the sense of fairness exhibited or practiced by administration (Gregorich and Long, 1980). Lack of this, perhaps more than any other factor, will promote a sense of collective action.

How nurses view their roles and responsibilities within the organization and how they view the nursing profession will influence the labor relations climate of the organization. These views and perceptions are influenced by factors such as length and type of education. As nurses have received increased education with a more professional orientation, they appear to have become more dissatisfied with an environment that does not acknowledge professional autonomy (Zacur, 1982). Home health nurses need to be involved in decision making regarding patient care, and this must be fostered by administration.

In a study by Meyer (1970), job security, social esteem, autonomy, self-realization, job and salary satisfaction, chance for advancement, membership in state nurses associations, beliefs about union power, and feelings toward authority were some of the variables examined in relationship to nurses' attitudes toward collective action. The following specific variables were found to be significantly related to a positive attitude toward collective action: lack of autonomy, self-realization, and security; low predisposition to submit to authority; low salary satisfaction; and lack of belief that trade union power is too great. Further analysis revealed that, when respondents in the study perceived the organizational climate as more autocratic, their need deficiency scores increased significantly, and mean collective action attitude scores were significantly higher.

Another study by Alutto and Belasco (1972) indicated that those nurses who were most militant and pro-strike were younger nurses with a low feeling of organizational commitment and strong dissatisfaction with their careers. According to Zacur (1982), the primary condition within a hospital that precipitates a nursing militancy or pro-strike attitude is administrators' use of a bureaucratic approach in dealing with human resources and failure to recognize the professional concerns and abilities of the nursing staff. Such a management approach breeds resentment and appears to initiate militant or strike behavior.

Ginzberg (1966) indicates that individuals have a value orientation and a preference system in their work. These are based on needs, goals, and values. Management, therefore, needs to be aware of preference systems and to assist nursing staff in achieving goals and meeting needs within this framework.

Four value orientation categories have been derived empirically and can be used as guidelines by management to identify employee types and their general value orientation (Ginzberg, 1966): (1) individualistic, (2) leadership, (3) social, and (4) ideological. The individualistic type wants to be free from strict direction and interference, choosing to structure his or her own activities while making optimal use of individual capacities in the work setting. The leadership type has an orientation toward building and maintaining relationships with others, having authority over others, directing and leading others, and being more involved in the organizational structure. The basic orientation of the social type is to be a member of a group or team and to be accepted by group members. Individuals of this type strive for group esteem. They have no intention or desire to become "the boss"; they derive satisfaction from the social context of their work. The greatest number of people in the workforce are of this type. The ideological worker is committed to a system of ideals or ideas and has a goal to serve a higher value than meeting personal needs. These individuals seek autonomy not for themselves but for the cause. Although these four types are not mutually exclusive, most individuals exhibit one orientation more strongly, and management could identify this and use it to promote individual well-being and consequently organizational well-being.

Any home health agency that is attempting to promote positive labor–management relations should concentrate on identifying internal and external environmental factors that affect the organizational climate. Attempts should be made to understand the nurses' perceptions, needs, and value orientations so that both individual needs and organizational needs can be planned for and met.

COMMUNICATION AND INTERPERSONAL SKILLS

Communication and interpersonal skills, which are vital to promoting helping relationships, can aid in creating effective labor–management relationships. Scott (1962) proposed that the health of an organization depends upon successful communication, or the imparting of information to all employees. If the home health agency is viewed as a system, then communication can be viewed as a linking process, binding together the various system units (management and labor). Rothstein (1958, p. 34) states:

> Organization presupposes the existence of parts, which considered in their totality, constitute the organization. The parts must interact. Were there no communication between them, there would be no organization but merely a collection of individual elements isolated from each other.

Communication networks should exist in the organization. These networks are decision centers interconnected by channels of communication. A feedback system is crucial for the network because it helps maintain balance among all components of the system. Change can occur, and the system can self-regulate when feedback is received.

Davis (1958) states that communication is the process of passing information and understanding from one person to another. This implies that communication does not occur unless the receiver understands the transmitted information. In organizations, the greater the degree of understanding by the receiver (worker), the more likely the receiver will be to behave and act so that organizational goals are attained (Scott, 1962). Thus communication is viewed as a manager's tool for accomplishing agency goals.

The focus of communication has shifted from being persuasion and conversation oriented to being understanding and negotiation oriented (Cushman, 1980). Talking and discussing provide both labor and management the opportunity to understand and accept diverse points of view and alternative solutions to a problem, which then allows for the successful negotiation of a solution.

For a positive relationship to occur between labor and management, both parties must practice effective sending and receiving skills. Both verbal and nonverbal channels can be used to send messages. The majority of messages are sent without words, however; messages are most often conveyed by body language, facial expressions, gestures and body movements, eye contact, tone of voice, use of silence, and other behaviors. Individuals must constantly be alert to the congruency between their verbal and non-verbal messages. Verbal messages are meant to convey ideas as well as feelings. An important component of verbal messages is asking for re-actions or verbal feedback to ensure that the intent of the words is being understood by those receiving them.

Receiving skills are as critical to effective communication as sending skills. Primary skills in receiving messages are observing behavior and listening actively. An active listening response consists of a feeling component and a content component (Gerrard et al., 1980); the receiver attempts to understand not only what the sender is saying, but also what he or she is feeling. The sender does this by concentrating and asking reflective questions. This aspect of communication indicates interest in the speaker, conveys acceptance, builds trust, and assists the person in developing problem-solving skills. It is important that both labor and management take the time to learn, practice, and participate

in actively listening to each other. Furthermore, effective sending and receiving of messages require that clarification occur. Eliciting feedback from all parties generates understanding between labor and management.

The interpersonal skills of showing respect, empathizing, and developing trust can assist in promoting a positive labor–management relationship. "Showing respect means conveying the attitude that the client has importance, dignity, and respect" (Spradley, 1985, p. 273). Respect should be conveyed by both labor and management through tone of voice, recognition of valuable ideas, and the manner in which people are addressed. Empathizing is a skill that can be used by all individuals to show that they are attempting to understand feelings expressed by others. This skill also encourages the sharing of concerns.

Developing trust is critical if individuals are to work effectively with each other. Management and labor can develop trust for each other by showing acceptance of each other, treating each other as partners, and having open discussions to share feelings. Candid discussions can be part of a labor–management committee approach (discussed later).

Various reasons for communications break-down exist, but most can be traced to the following (Scott, 1962):

- the nature and functions of human language
- purposeful misrepresentation
- the size of the organization
- lack of acceptance
- failure to understand

Distortion and filtering are severe and frequent problems in the communication process. Distortion occurs because messages sent up and down in an organization have to be interpreted by receivers. Because human language is so complex and can be interpreted differently by different individuals, messages can become distorted as they are passed among various individuals. Management can minimize distortion by asking for feedback from receivers to determine whether the content of the message is being interpreted as intended. The existence of social barriers or social distances or a difference in thinking between staff and management can also create distortion. Scott (1962) suggests that most communication breakdowns occur because subordinates do not agree with their bosses about obstacles and problems they are facing. He recommends empathy as one method by which social distances between different levels of employees can be overcome. If managers can project themselves into the framework of the employees, then any messages sent by managers will be more likely to be received and understood by the employees.

Communication breakdown can be caused by deliberate misinterpretation of a message. This occurs primarily in upward communication, when subordinates send to managers the material that they believe will be most accepted. Filtering includes errors of both commission and omission.

As an organization increases in size and complexity, management becomes buried in communication to which response is impossible. Optimum flow of material is necessary if managers are to communicate successfully with staff; thus irrelevant information should be monitored and handled by middle management personnel.

Poor timing and short circuiting are other serious communication problems related to the size and complexity of the organization. Information needs to be released at the appropriate time and received by all employees at the same time or in sequential order. Short circuiting occurs when someone is missed in the communication chain who should have been included. An employee's status may be lowered and angry feelings may result when the employee does not get necessary information at the appropriate time.

Communication breakdowns also occur because staff lack acceptance and understanding of the conveyed information. Even though staff may receive the appropriate material at the right time, they may choose not to accept it for various reasons, such as incongruence in reality between sender and receiver, an ambiguous or unclear message, lack of faith in the sender (low credibility), and incongruence between the content of the message and the receiver's value system. As ambiguity of the message increases, as the credibility of the sender decreases, and as conflict between message content and value system of the receiver increases, the receiver becomes less likely to accept the information (Scott, 1962). These are all affected by the receiver's perception of reality, so that the manager should work first to understand and change the receiver's view of the reality of the situation. Teamwork has been recommended as a mechanism for effectively changing an individual employee's view of reality and thus promoting acceptance of the information.

The last cause of communication breakdown is lack of understanding by receivers who inaccurately translate the symbols used in communication. Scott (1962) suggests that a climate for understanding can be established by management by planning for communication, tailoring the information to fit the employee's frame of reference, and listening to what employees have to say. This last step can be carried out in a nondirective interview between staff and management, which will generate information about needs, complaints, and employee goals. The manager acts as a sounding board only, gathering information that will allow him or her to respond to the needs of staff.

PROBLEM SOLVING

Creative problem solving is another management tool for promoting a healthy labor–management relationship. The use of conceptual models such as an open systems model assists in improving interdepartmental communications (Golightly, 1981). Use of a model serves as a discussion point as information flows from one area to another and discussion occurs among components of the system, between the problem solvers and those who are affected by the solution. This method enhances effective communication, which then facilitates the problem-solving process.

Three levels of problem solving exist in an organization such as a home health agency: the individual process, the group process, and the organizational process, which contains several groups. The normal group approach, the Delphi problem-solving method, and brainstorming can be used by groups to solve problems creatively. Certain factors that affect group problem solving are the problem information held by the group, the extent to which the group accepts that there is a need for action, and the extent of congruence between goals of the individual members and the goals of the group (Vroom and Yetton, 1976).

Organizational problem solving is much more complex than the individual or group process because of the increased number of environmental and personal variables involved. As more individuals are involved, the potential for conflict increases. Objectives for organizational problem solving must be explicit, providing a framework for goal-directed behavior.

Many situations exist in a home health agency that are complex, with many variables interfacing and contributing to the situation. In approaching these situations, it seems appropriate to identify all the contributing factors that interface so that a reasonable problem statement and a solution can be formulated. Figure 37–1 illustrates a model in which all the information is collected, processed, and expanded (Golightly, 1981). Such a model would be useful as labor and management begin to formulate a solution to a complex problem. A systematic gathering of data is done to produce issues, facts, and givens, which are analyzed to formulate problem statements. The middle funnel is inverted to indicate that there are many problem statements rather than just one, and that problem statements may overlap.

As these problem statements are constructed, a people-centeredness approach is emphasized. This approach facilitates change from the manager's perspective and recognizes the contributions of the worker. Management must indicate a willingness to help and to work with the work group. Golightly (1981) indicates that, when

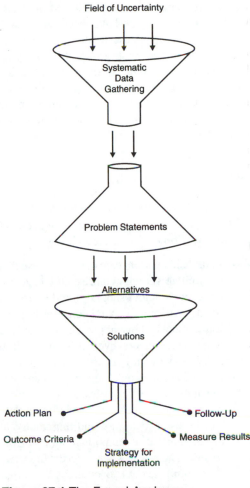

Figure 37-1 The Funnel Analogy.
Source: Reprinted from C. K. Golightly, *Creative Problem Solving for Health Care Professionals*, p. 60, © 1981, Jones and Bartlett Publishers.

management begins to pay attention to the work group, the out-of-balance state begins to change and improve.

After data have been collected and processed, the problem and all its parameters can be defined in small groups. A large group can be divided into smaller groups to address specific issues. Use of such a model with group involvement fosters employee involvement, promotes ownership, and accelerates group acceptance (Golightly, 1981).

After the data have been collected and analyzed and alternatives have been generated, some time should elapse before solutions are recommended. The work group, in identifying the best solution, should consider how a specific solution contributes to the agency objectives, the cost in dollars, the time needed to implement the plan, and the feasibility of the solution (Golightly, 1981).

GENERAL RECOMMENDATIONS

Various authorities have made recommendations on how to promote a positive labor–management relationship. Some of these are as follows:

- Establish a patient care committee. Such a committee should comprise all categories of caregivers and should provide a forum for discussion of general concerns regarding patients. This approach promotes a team concept, creative problem solving, and involvement in decision making.
- Establish some mechanism for recognizing nursing staff's professional contributions. A variety of positive reinforcements can be used to reward and thus motivate organizational commitment and performance. The rewards can range from monetary compensation to citations to verbal recognition only. An important criterion is that the reward be perceived as valuable by the employee, which necessitates that such programs be designed with input from the employees themselves. It seems necessary to define what nurses perceive as professional recognition and how it can be achieved. This would indicate to management what motivational methods to use.
- Encourage a policy of informal staff meetings between nurses and supervisors. Communication can be facilitated during these meetings as input is solicited from nurses and feedback is given regarding the disposition of such suggestions. Critical components of such meetings should be a two-way communication process, the giving of much information and praise, and

an emphasis on positive reinforcement and possibilities rather than constraints (Zacur, 1982).
- Use career counseling to promote professional commitment. Zacur (1982) states that "a long-term developmental approach to staff nurses and their careers can foster organizational commitment and decrease interest in militancy as a means to professional recognition" (p. 76). Administration has a responsibility to ensure that career needs of individuals are maximized, that nurses have the skills and knowledge necessary to perform their jobs, and that they have the opportunity to utilize these skills. This can be accomplished when staff and administration engage in joint planning.
- Provide orientation update sessions. These sessions provide employees with information about current developments and future plans and allow nurses to share their perceptions with management (Gregorich and Long, 1980). Problems can be presented during these sessions, but this is done in a positive, constructive atmosphere.
- Fill front-line supervisory positions with the best possible people and provide education for them to increase their effectiveness. Individuals hired for these positions should demonstrate excellent interpersonal skills, communication skills, and labor relations training. Personal attention should be given by the supervisor to all employees, especially those with great needs. The literature indicates that an organization must meet the needs as perceived by employees, or the union will come along, meet these needs, and win approval of the group (Cangemi et al., 1980). It is suggested that the supervisor's treatment of employees is a critical factor in establishing a positive labor–management climate (Lockhart and Werther, 1980).
- Prepare an employee-oriented publication. Items concerning employees should be incorporated into the publication, along with pictures and praise. Controver-

sial and threatening messages should not be included.

- Support athletic and recreational programs or social events sponsored by employees.
- Design an acceptable suggestion system.
- Develop a plan for rewarding loyal, dedicated employees who have demonstrated commitment to the agency.
- Develop a system to audit and identify feelings, opinions, and needs of employees. This system provides information that can be used to initiate action to meet employee needs and to facilitate movement in accordance with employee goals. Creating a more positive environment requires proactive behavior by management and allows actions to be taken before, not after, a crisis situation occurs. Foster a cooperative environment. "Cooperating is largely a matter of consultation between the two sides" (Werther and Lockhart, 1980, p. 156). Cooperation is sometimes difficult to achieve because both labor and management harbor fears and misconceptions based on past experiences. A cooperative relationship can begin when either side is in a desperate situation and needs help. Favors are given and reciprocation is expected. These requests form the beginning of a cooperative environment. Such an environment can also be initiated by having a formal suggestion plan in which employees can be consulted and encouraged to give suggestions. Jointly sponsored athletic, recreational, and social events provide the opportunity for each side to have a mutually satisfying interaction, to reevaluate opinions of each other, and to build teamwork. For labor–management relations to be positive, adversarial relationships must be abandoned; each side must view the relationship as a cooperative and a helping one, and each side must agree to consult the other before taking action.
- Establish an employee relations program. This program must be perceived as equitable and consistent by staff. This applies

particularly to wages, which must be perceived as satisfactory. If this occurs, the employee relations program and management will have credibility. Nonunionized agencies need to act as though a third party is standing by, judging their actions for fairness and consistency. Agencies should have as part of their employee relations program a philosophy that recognizes the needs of both labor and management. Specific components of such a philosophy include the following (Werther and Lockhart, 1980):

1. Management should recognize staff needs, and all actions should consider these needs.
2. Staff must respect management's need for efficiency and effectiveness.
3. Problem solving should be a joint endeavor between staff and management.
4. Cooperation is the most viable long-term strategy for ensuring agency success.
5. Survival of the agency is paramount.

- Establish a position of employee relations manager. The primary role of such a person would be to act as management's conscience, reminding management of its commitment to an employee relations program. The employee relations manager serves as the expert in resolving employee relations problems, designs two-way communication systems, and assists both parties in utilizing these systems to promote positive interactions and mutual understanding.
- Provide for a formal grievance procedure. "Union leaders stated publicly that the best defense against union organization is an effective grievance procedure" (Gregorich and Long, 1980, p. 109). Having a formal grievance procedure in a nonunion setting provides a mechanism for release of pressure, assurance that employee grievances will be considered, an avenue for communication, and a stimulus for

discovering needs and implementing change. For the grievance procedure to be successful, members of management who have decision-making responsibility in a grievance must be credible, fair, and impartial. Second, employees must have an advocate available to assist in preparing and presenting a grievance. All employees should be encouraged to use the grievance process, without fear of reprisal or being labeled as a troublemaker.

- Establish a labor–management committee. This committee is usually found in an agency that has a collective agreement for the purpose of discussing issues not covered in the collective bargaining process (Hemsworth, 1978).

Such a committee is usually composed of equal numbers of management and nursing personnel. Management can be represented by the executive director, personnel director, nursing manager, or a member of the agency's board. Members of the collective bargaining unit would represent the nurses.

One agency that instituted a labor–management committee discussed the following issues as part of the monthly agendas over a period of 1 year: recruitment of nurses and supervisors; physical plant, including telephone workstations; the need for a nursing support group; charting procedures; agency finances; new services; the agreement with the local hospital; increasing referrals from special hospitals; the employee handbook; and communication patterns. Some time was spent discussing communication patterns. Staff would hear comments made by management that they perceived as derogatory and resulted in angry feelings and low morale. Discussions centered on how to prevent this from happening and how to establish open, candid communication between management and staff.

COLLECTIVE BARGAINING

Another way in which the labor–management environment is influenced is through collective bargaining. Historically, attempts at collective bargaining were met with resistance by nurses who felt it was not professional to withhold services from patients. The conflict of professionalism and unionism existed and prevented nurses from bargaining with employers. However, the trend has changed and unionization is now an acceptable way to ensure that employers recognize and discuss the economic and professional needs of nurses.

The National Labor Relations Act of 1935 was the first piece of social legislation that required employers to engage in collective bargaining with employees. Employees in nonprofit health care organizations, however, were not protected by this federal law to engage in collective bargaining. Not until 1947, when the Taft-Hartley amendment to the National Labor Relations Act was passed, could such employees organize. This legislation enabled health care workers to enter the mainstream of American labor to promote their own professionalism and unity.

The ANA, formed in 1896 as a professional organization committed to quality patient care, approved collective bargaining for nurses in 1946 to assure the public that adequate, high-quality nursing care would be available to all sick people (Kruger, 1961). Thus began an era when collective action was accepted as one way to ensure professionalism. In 1950, however, ANA members approved a policy that no strikes would occur as this would be inconsistent with nurses' professional responsibility to patients. In 1966, the ANA Commission on Economic and General Welfare determined that changes were necessary in the economic security program and rescinded the no strike policy.

During the 1970s, the ANA mounted an aggressive campaign to support the nation's nurses in collective bargaining activities. The numbers of persons covered by collective agreements increased significantly, indicating that the ANA was working to advance the economic and general welfare of nurses.

Hemsworth (1978) outlines what nurses have gained through collective bargaining:

- professional strength through unity
- the legal right to voice concerns for patient care and professional improvement

- the right to contribute to the decision-making process through negotiations
- improved benefits, including job security
- the right to challenge rules through grievance procedures

These gains have been attained primarily through presentation of a unified approach and negotiation.

Although collective bargaining can be viewed as an infringement of management prerogatives and an interference in the employer–employee relationship, nurses have continued to choose such activities as a way to affect employment conditions and to determine and control their practice.

Nurses have been the target of aggressive campaigns by unions and have voted to organize in record numbers. Seeking to reverse the trend of falling union membership, unions have actively reruited service industry workers, the fastest growing portion of the labor force (U.S. Department of Labor, 2003). The Service Employees International Union (SEIU) boasts 110,000 nurse members. Through union representation, nurses and other health care workers seek to outlaw mandatory overtime, to require minimum nurse-to-patient ratios, to improve wages of paraprofessionals, and other advocacy efforts (SEIU, 2003).

Whether employees are represented by a collective bargaining unit or not, employers need to be aware of protections offered them through the National Labor Relations Board (NLRB) that was created by the 1935 Act (U.S.C. Title 29 §§151–169). Section 7 of the act allows employees the right to engage in "concerted activities for the purpose . . . mutual aid or protection." The NLRB has interpreted this section in case law over the years and ruled most recently to extend this right to employees outside the collectively bargained unit. In a 2000 decision with the Epilepsy Foundation of Northeast Ohio (331 NLRB No. 92, 2000), the board ruled that an employee may have a coworker present during an investigatory interview even if they are not represented by a labor union. The NLRB protects concerted activity not only when disciplinary action is expected, but also during the process of organizing. Employees are well advised to consult legal counsel and take steps to be union-free before organizing efforts begin.

CONCLUSION

In a home health agency, management must strive to create a healthy work environment in which labor–management relationships are positive. Management must be sensitive to perceived staff needs and to ways to meet these needs. Programs should be designed to maximize all employee contributions to the program. Both labor and management must work together, using a team approach, effective communication, and problem-solving skills and consulting with each other in an atmosphere of fairness, respect, empathy, and trust. A variety of methods can be used by management to ensure that labor–management relations are positive, that quality patient care is achieved, that employee welfare is maximized, and that organizational goals are met.

REFERENCES

Alutto, J. A., and J. A. Belasco. 1972. *Determinants of attitudinal militancy among nurses and teachers*. Bethesda, MD, ERIC Document Reproduction Service No. ED 063 635.

Cangemi, J. O., L. Clark, and E. Harryman. 1980. Differences between pro-union and pro-company employees. In C. A. Lockhart and W. B. Werther, Jr. (eds.), *Labor relations in nursing*. Wakefield, MA: Nursing Resources.

Cushman, D. 1980. Organizing campaigns: An analysis of management's use of communication techniques, suggestions for union strategy. In R. J. Peters, H. Elkiss, and H. T. Higgins (eds.), *Unionization and the Health Care Industry: Hospital and Nursing Home Employee Union*

Leaders Conference Report, Nov. 29–Dec. 1, 1978 (pp. 24–31). Urbana, IL: University of Illinois.

Davis, K. 1958. *Human relations in business*. New York: McGraw-Hill.

Epilepsy Foundation of Northeast Ohio, 331 NLRB No. 92 (2000).

Gerrard, B. A., W. J. Boniface, and B. H. Love. 1980. *Interpersonal skills for health professionals*. Reston, VA: Reston Hall.

Ginzberg, E. 1966. *The development of human resources*. New York: McGraw-Hill.

Golightly, C. K. 1981. *Creative problem solving for health care professionals*. Gaithersburg, MD: Aspen.

Gregorich, P., and J. W. Long. 1980. Responsive management fosters cooperative environment. In C.A. Lockhart and W. B. Werther, Jr. (eds.), *Labor relations in nursing*. Wakefield, MA: Nursing Resources.

Hemsworth, M. J. 1978. *Nurses in collective bargaining*. Ann Arbor, MI: University Microfilms International.

Kruger, D. H. 1961. Bargaining and the nursing profession. *Monthly Labor Review* 84: 699.

Levitan, S. A., G. L. Mangum, and R. Marshall. 1981. *Human resources and labor markets: Employment and training in the American economy* (3rd ed.). New York: Harper & Row.

Lockhart, C. A., and W. B. Werther, Jr. (eds.). 1980. *Labor relations in nursing*. Wakefield, MA: Nursing Resources.

Meyer, G. D. 1970. *Determinants of collective action attitudes among hospital nurses: An empirical test*. Unpublished doctoral dissertation, University of Iowa.

National Labor Relations Act, Title 29, Chapter 7, Subchapter II, United States Code.

Rothstein, J. 1958. *Communication, organization and science*. Indian Hills, CO: Falcon's Wing.

Scott, W. G. 1962. *Human relations in management: A behavioral science approach*. Homewood, IL: Irwin.

Service Employees International Union, *http://www.seiu .org/health/nurses*. (Accessed June 30, 2003).

Spradley, B. W. 1985. *Community health nursing: Concepts and practice* (2nd ed.). Boston: Little, Brown.

U.S. Department of Labor, Bureau of Labor Statistics, *http:// www.bls.gov/news.release/*. (Accessed January 9, 2004).

Vroom, V. H., and P. W. Yetton. 1976. Leadership and decision making: Basic consideration underlying the normative model. In W. R. Nord (ed.), *Concepts and Controversy in Organizational Behavior* (2nd ed.). Pacific Palisades, CA: Goodyear.

Werther, W. B., Jr., and C. A. Lockhart. 1980. Collective action and cooperation in the health professions. In C. A. Lockhart and W. B. Werther, Jr. (eds.), *Labor Relations in Nursing*. Wakefield, MA: Nursing Resources.

Zacur, S. 1982. *Health care labor relations: The nursing perspective*. Ann Arbor, MI: University Microfilms International.

CHAPTER 38

Human Resource Management

Ann Marie O'Connell

THE HUMAN RESOURCE DEFINED

The value of the human resource to the home health agency directly relates to the importance the agency places on its image as a provider of service to the community. Manufacturers and most service providers depend on quality, pricing, packaging, and the efficiency of their delivery systems to promote their products and services to their customers. Hospital inpatients and outpatients have perceptions based on all their observations and experiences. The home health agency, however, is dependent on the quality of the relationships that exist between caregivers and their patients. Because there is often no other frame of reference for the home care client, the aide, the nurse, the therapist, and other members of the care team assume the identity of the agency itself. The responsibility and accountability are significant and extend well beyond the caregiver's ability to provide a competent level of clinical care. Often, the caregiver is expected to satisfy all the patient's needs, whether these are communicated or not, and is held accountable by the client for doing so. The patient and members of the household may perceive the nurse in stereotypical terms— the selfless Florence Nightingale—committed to service and receiving only intrinsic rewards in return. Whether the agency and its employees are motivated by such humanitarian purposes or not, the agency's success as a service provider is somewhat dependent on the nurse's ability to transform that perception into reality.

The importance of the human resource in home care is significant. The success of the home health agency as an employer is measured by its ability to attract and retain highly skilled and talented individuals for employment. Although the notion that health care attracts altruistic humanitarians who receive their rewards from the services they provide may or may not be true, the health care workers of the 2000s expect their employers to provide the same rewards received by workers in other industries. Today's employees seek and expect income commensurate with the level and scope of their responsibility and benefits that provide security for them and their families. Other priorities include a safe and comfortable working environment, fair and consistent employment policies, equal employment opportunities, free-flowing communication, opportunities for professional growth, and the ability to participate and become involved. Proactive home health employers, and specifically individuals charged with the responsibility of managing the human resource, go farther to create a comfortable and positive employee relations climate. They understand that individuals should give their work 100 percent of their attention to ensure desired agency outcomes.

Discussion and resolution of work-related problems should be encouraged and should take

This chapter is updated from a chapter written by Robert J. Tortorici for the *Handbook of Home Health Care Administration*, 2nd edition (1997).

place in a comfortable, nonthreatening setting to minimize distractions. These encounters are often convened within the human resources department, which proactive employers promote as a confidential staff resource. Many employers supplement this in-house service by offering employee assistance programs (EAPs) through outside contractors to help employees cope with the inevitable demands their personal lives place on their work life.

Perhaps the greatest challenge of home care in the next decade is its extraordinary growth within the largest segment of the U.S. economy: the health care industry. As the Baby Boomer generation ages, the demand for home care services will surely experience exponential growth, yet the national labor force is declining. Health care and home health care must compete aggressively for a larger proportion of a limited human resource, and they must do so at a time when the industry is being pressured to contain costs. The staffing challenge requires a comprehensive, introspective review of the industry's employee management practices as well as aggressive and innovative recruitment and retention strategies. The planning and implementation of such strategies fall within the scope of the human resources department's responsibility.

THE HUMAN RESOURCES DEPARTMENT AND ITS ROLE, GOAL, AND STRUCTURE

Essentially, the human resources administrator and the line manager share responsibility for managing the human resource or, more specifically, for achieving results through the efforts of others. Although the manager's focus is often limited by boundaries of departmental responsibility, the human resources administrator's view is global in scope and spans the entire organization. As a result, the human resources department is positioned appropriately as a management resource and conceptually as the initiator of consistent, proactive "people" policies and practices that enhance the recruitment and retention of staff and ultimately promote the

agency as an employer of choice. Most often the human resources department reports directly to the chief executive officer and appears as a staff (support) rather than a line (operational) function on the organizational chart. As a result, the human resources department does not exist in the chain of command of most employees. It extends its role as a resource beyond the management group to all employees and provides each individual with a safe haven for discussing concerns, issues, and interests that may affect morale. The human resources administrator may help the employee find a solution and may participate with the employee and manager to develop an appropriate action plan. The human resources department exists almost as a consultant to encourage the personal and professional growth of staff and managers, and the human resources administrator of the 2000s will have the expertise to do so.

When each and every employment relationship between employer and employee is perceived as being mutually satisfying, or, in other terms, when each partner in the relationship believes that mutual expectations have been and will continue to be met, the human resources department may close its doors and cease to exist. Such is the goal of every human resources administrator. Is this goal achievable? The answer would clearly be yes if there existed an unlimited financial resource. The reality of the 2000s is the challenge of cost containment, however, a term of particular relevance to the health care industry. Government increases its intervention into health care in response to the public's demand for containment of health care costs, yet the health provider is expected to provide more and better care. This trend has implications for the employee relations climate of the health care employer. The prospect of developing an inventory of employer and employee expectations and a mutual commitment to satisfy such expectations may be an appropriate first step toward the goal. It is clearly necessary for both employer and employee to prioritize their mutual expectations, however, and to develop an action plan within the framework of the organizational planning process. The human resources department should contribute employment policies and programs to the plan after receiving input from staff. To ensure progress, the approach should be comprehensive and should address the broad scope of employee and employer expectations. Typically, the human resources department and its agenda are organized according to the following professional disciplines (Figure 38–1).

Recruitment and Selection

Recruitment and selection involve reaching out into the community and beyond to ensure an adequate supply of qualified candidates for a variety of agency functions. The number of vacancies and the length of time for which positions remain open affect the agency's ability to deliver service. The selection process must ensure that all qualified candidates have an equal opportunity to be considered for employment and that the candidate who offers the best prospect for a mutually successful and satisfying employment relationship is selected. Moreover, an important consideration for human resources department staff is the realization that the impressions of all applicants may affect the agency's image in the community as an employer.

Salary Administration

Whether or not a formal plan and structure exist, the human resources department must ensure fair and equitable pay practices for all employees based on the requirements of the job performed. Therefore, standards should exist that reflect reasonable differences between jobs. Human resources department staff use objective tools for measuring the value of such jobs to the agency. Jobs are then arranged in a hierarchy according to the level and scope of responsibility assigned to each. Salary surveys are conducted among comparable employers to ensure that salary levels are consistent with prevailing rates in the community. In addition, salary practices include mechanisms for staff to achieve

salary growth as they accumulate experience and longevity and perform at required levels.

Benefits

Often grouped with salary administration, benefits administration requires periodic marketplace studies and comparisons to enhance the agency's ability to recruit and retain. The benefit program should be designed to address the specific needs of employees with attention given to cost. Insurance plan premiums are often based on the claims filed by staff. Therefore, cost containment measures and policy provision revisions should be considered to provide the best benefit value for the employer and the employee. Staff surveys should be conducted periodically to determine which benefits staff value the most and if the agency's current options are in alignment with employees' priorities. More and more agencies are adopting a cafeteria-style benefit plan that allocates a dollar amount to each employee with a menu of benefit options from which the employee can pick and choose.

Training

In the health care industry, and likewise in home health care, clinical training is often the responsibility of the professional and paraprofessional departments. The human resources department, however, shares responsibility for ensuring that all employees are adequately trained to perform their job activities. It is also appropriate to provide every employee with an opportunity to develop new skills and to keep them current. Such initiatives may include policies and programs that encourage continuing education for staff, perhaps in traditional educational settings, and financing their participation in seminars and symposia on related topics. The value of providing training programs internally should be emphasized as well because there is usually a wealth of specialized expertise among employees within each home care organization. The internal instructor is able to tailor a program with a specific agency relevance, which participants

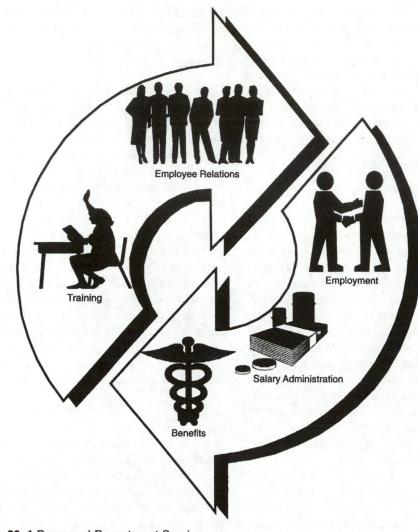

Figure 38–1 Personnel Department Services

may find particularly useful. Human resource–sponsored training programs should be conducted for administrative support and management employees because specialized skills are necessary throughout the agency's operational department. In addition, a fully developed orientation program for all newly hired staff—which introduces them to the agency, its mission, policies, and procedures and gives them an opportunity to meet others—will enhance their ability to adjust to their new environment. It is important to incorporate a presentation by the

agency's president into orientation to acquaint new staff with the agency's leadership and set forth the agency's strategic direction and operational goals.

Employee Relations

The agency's ability to attract and retain highly qualified individuals is linked to the employee relations climate. Although all human resource disciplines have impact, perhaps the most significant measure of an agency's employee relations climate is the effectiveness of its communication network. Unless employee and employer needs and expectations are freely discussed, they cannot be addressed. Periodic forums such as "town" meetings, task forces designed to address a particular issue or problem, and management rounds offer good opportunities for staff to interact with senior management.

The human resources department functions as a forum for communication as well. It also supports managers and staff by helping them find ways to create an atmosphere that supports a free and comfortable flow of information. Of course, effective and meaningful communication is a bilateral process in which the communicator and the receiver accept mutual responsibility for the quality of communication. It is important to note, however, that appropriate and timely action is often necessary after the communication of an employee relations issue. When concerns and problems are communicated but not resolved, they begin to fester, only to affect the employee's comfort level in the employment relationship. Poor morale on the part of one individual can disrupt the morale and effectiveness of the entire team.

Labor Relations

The human resources department is usually responsible for the negotiation of union contracts and for the administration of the agreement while in force. Essentially, the department assumes the role of the employer's agent for such purposes.

Employment Policies and Record Retention

An overwhelming list of federal, state, and municipal laws and regulations guides the human resources administrator, particularly in the employment, salary, and benefit administration and labor relations disciplines (Exhibit 38–1). Whether mandated or not, policies should be organized into a manual or, ideally, into an employee handbook, written in language easily understood by all staff, and distributed to ensure

that every employee has access to it. It is inappropriate to hold individuals accountable for meeting organizational expectations when such expectations have not been communicated effectively. Employment-related laws and regulations also require human resources departments to review and maintain certain documents and information for each employee. In addition, a complete employment history is maintained in the human resources department that is used for a variety of reasons to benefit both employer and employee. The employee, however, should be assured that all such information is kept absolutely confidential and that certain control procedures have been established to ensure the security of such records. It is important to note, however, that an official personnel file should not be in an employee's general correspondence file. Official employment transactions, performance reviews, commendations, and required employment documents should be maintained, and extraneous information should be kept in department files or given to the employee for his or her own personal records. If a legal dispute arises and an employment record is subpoenaed, courts have found that the record a manager keeps on an employee can be considered part of the personnel file, as well as electronic files kept on the employee if the information was used in employment decisions.

Health information about employees must be stored in a separate confidential medical file apart from the employee's personnel file. This includes information attained through pre-employment physicals, workers' compensation injuries, family medical leaves of absence, or health screenings conducted during employment.

THE HUMAN RESOURCES DEPARTMENT STAFF

As mentioned, the human resources department often reports directly to the chief executive officer, and when it does it gives staff the message that senior management places considerable importance on the agency's human resource. Normally the size of the organization, scope of

Exhibit 38–1 Sections of the *Health Care Labor Manual* (vol. 2, Chap. 12; Skoler and Abbott, 2004 (updated quarterly) of Interest to Personnel Department Staff

Topic	Page
Labor–Management Relations Act	12:1
Hazardous Communication	12:31
Labor–Management Reporting and Disclosure Act of 1959, As Amended	12:81
The Equal Employment Opportunity Act of 1972	12:111
Fair Labor Standards Act of 1938	12:135
Age Discrimination in Employment Act	12:173
Public Law No. 72-65	12:181
Occupational Safety and Health Act of 1970	12:187
Public Law No. 73-376	12:217
Extremely Hazardous Substances List and Threshold Planning Quantities; Emergency Planning and Release Notification Requirements	12:219
Health Maintenance Organizations—Employee's Health Benefits Plans	12:230(5)
Nondiscrimination on Basis of Handicap	12:231
Final EEOC Guidelines on Affirmative Action	12:259
Questions and Answers Clarifying Uniform Guidelines on Employee Selection Procedures	12:263
Labor Department Interpretation of Effect on Employee Benefit Plans of Amendments to Age Discrimination in Employment Act	12:273
Restatement and Clarification of NLRB Rules on Election Objectives	12:281
Final EEOC Interpretations: Age Discrimination in Employment Act	12:283
Revised NLRB Procedural Rules	12:287
Final Immigration and Naturalization Reform Rules	12:291
Civil Rights Restoration Act of 1987	12:305
Employee Polygraph Protection Act of 1988	12:309
Drug-Free Workplace Act of 1988	12:315
Interim Final Rules—Drug-Free Workplace Act of 1988	12:317
Guidelines for Federal Workplace Drug Testing Programs	12:337
Americans with Disabilities Act	12:341
Older Workers Benefit Protection Act	12:385
Civil Rights Act of 1991	12:391
Family and Medical Leave Act of 1993	12:405

responsibility, credentials, and qualifications determine the human resources administrator's place on the organization chart. The administrator is usually a generalist with responsibility for all human resources disciplines. It is absolutely essential that the administrator manage the department with sensitivity and flexibility while ensuring fairness and consistency. The individual must have the ability to motivate others, to be empathetic, to place equal value on each employee, and to appreciate the contribution that each makes to the overall mission of the agency. The role also requires exceptionally good judgment and, above all, an ability to communicate effectively. This includes, of course, exceptional listening skills as well.

The human resources administrator is challenged to represent the agency's best interests and to promote its employment policies and programs while also playing the role of advocate for employees. This dual responsibility should not present a conflict to the skilled and effective administrator. A large home health agency may also have specialists, particularly in the area of salary and benefit administration and in recruitment and selection. Support staff are normally responsible for record retention and a variety of administrative and clerical functions.

The individual who has responsibility for meeting and greeting applicants is often the only person who will have the opportunity to leave an applicant with an impression of the agency as an employer. It is obviously important that a person with superior "people" and communication skills be selected, although all members of the department should possess such skills and abilities.

Although there has been much debate about the size of the human resources department, a general rule of thumb is 1 full-time human resources employee for every 100 employees in the organization. Of course, this guideline should be modified to reflect the actual activities assumed by the department, and the talents, abilities, and interests of managers and support staff assigned.

The number of individuals who work in the department cannot predict the quality of the human resources department's outputs, and the cost of the function and its impact on the budget should be a major consideration as well. The notion that the human resources department does not contribute to the bottom line is simply not true. This is especially the case in home health care, where the ability to recruit and retain staff is closely linked to the agency's ability to generate revenue.

FINDING THE RIGHT CANDIDATE FOR EMPLOYMENT

In the late 1980s, health care employers were stunned to discover that their former proportion of the national labor force was no longer available to the health care industry. A nationwide shortage of health care workers, particularly nurses, physical therapists, and home health aides, reached crisis proportions, and health care employers began to experience double-digit vacancy rates with single-digit applicant inquiries. Although the effects were devastating to employers and employees alike, the crisis was a catalyst for positive change. Perhaps the greatest change of all was the industry's realization that health care workers have many of the same needs and expectations as workers in other industries. Employee relations and salary administration practices were revised to accommodate such expectations. As a result, the status of health care workers has escalated in the past decade at a greater rate than it did in the previous 25 to 30 years. Recruitment strategies, once passive, were developed to compete aggressively with those of other industries for a greater share of a limited human resource. The trend is positive, but the momentum must continue because the demand for health care, and particularly home care services, will continue to rise. The proactive recruiter will therefore develop a comprehensive plan that will include initiatives specifically designed to attract candidates who meet job-specific qualifications. The plan will also include an assessment mechanism to provide information about the effectiveness of such initiatives. Of course, the most progressive recruiter will also consider future needs and will target applicants for future consideration.

Advertising

Although advertising is costly, it is often most effective for reaching large numbers of people. There is no magic formula as to the day, frequency, style, or format of the advertisement. Successes and failures, however, could be charted over a period of time and analyzed, thereby providing the recruiter with information that may be useful for future advertising decisions. The look and theme of an ad could enhance or detract from the image that the agency wants to project to the community. It is therefore advisable to consult with advertising experts, perhaps within the agency itself, to find a design that attracts applicants and promotes the agency as a service provider as well. Content should be developed after a careful review of the job description. Presumably, the requirements have been appropriately set, and if so, the ad copy should specifically state required qualifications, salary range, and significant benefits. The goal is to attract as many qualified candidates as possible, but only those who would give the position serious consideration. Although the salary range provides the reader with needed information, a precise salary implies that there is no room for negotiation and should be avoided. Generally, imaginative copy sells. Standard phrases and lead-ins, such as "Large home health agency seeks . . . ," do not project a progressive employer image, and everyone wants to work for a progressive employer.

Professional journals are also effective for certain vacancies, but they are generally used to build an applicant bank for specific programs or departments rather than to fill current vacancies. This venue is particularly appropriate when the number of jobs exceeds the availability of skilled workers. Such periodicals are published infrequently and do not provide an immediate prospect for producing large numbers of candidates quickly.

An even broader approach to advertising may include radio, television, and perhaps mass transit advertising or billboards, particularly for difficult-to-fill positions and when large numbers of staff are required. Such techniques have been used effectively for home health aide recruitment. During nursing shortages, the broadcast media is used extensively to generate interest in the nursing profession. Nonprofit agencies are often able to obtain no-cost public service airtime or low-cost local advertising council assistance in developing their advertising strategies.

Equal employment opportunity employers should draw attention to their interest in minorities and people with disabilities in their employment advertising. Tag lines appear insincere, however. A more innovative approach would be to work such commitments into the main body of the text. Also, advertisements should be placed in publications that have a significant readership among such populations, at least periodically.

Because advertising can be expensive, responsible recruiters will assess the results of all their advertising initiatives on an ongoing basis.

Community Outreach

There are always opportunities for presentations at schools and other community forums. Career days at the secondary school level and college career forums are effective and relatively inexpensive mechanisms for cultivating short- and long-range employment and career prospects. Imaginative recruiters may develop audiovisual presentations that describe employment and career opportunities while subtly promoting the agency as an employer of choice. More important than the presentation itself, however, is the relationship between the recruiter and the school guidance counselor or placement director. These individuals will often refer promising students, recent graduates, or alumni to the agency for consideration. In fact, every recruitment outreach into the community should have as its primary goal the development of a network that will serve the agency as a mega-recruitment resource. Efforts to increase the diversity of your workforce can be helped by developing strong ties to these community agencies. Those agencies that work with individuals returning to the workforce are excellent sources for qualified and eager candidates for employment, as is the state employment service, which is usually more than willing to assist by providing space and candidates for on-site interviewing. Agency-sponsored events, such as job and health fairs, open-house receptions, and on-site seminars, expose participants to other staff members who may be equipped to represent home health care and the agency effectively. They also serve to validate information shared by the recruiter, who is generally expected to accentuate the positives.

Permanent and Temporary Employment Agencies

Temporary employment agencies are excellent sources for satisfying temporary and supplemental staffing needs. A growing trend exists in all industries to utilize temporary agencies for permanent staffing as well and there are advantages in doing so. Although fees tend to be higher than starting salaries for most jobs, the employment agency normally provides and pays for benefits. Generally this represents a savings for the health care employer. The temporary who presumably comes to the employer with the requisite skills becomes acclimated to the health care agency's working environment while satisfying the temporary need. More important, both the employer and the temporary have the unique opportunity to assess each other before entering into a regular and binding employment relationship. Most temporary agencies have buy-out provisions, which essentially permit employers to accept temporaries for regular employment for an additional fee.

Search firms and permanent employment agencies assume advertising and recruitment costs and will produce applicants for employment who have been screened, presumably according to the employer's specifications. Fees for such services are usually a percentage of salary and are somewhat significant. The recruiter must therefore analyze the cost effectiveness of using such a resource. For certain difficult-to-fill positions, or when a confidential search becomes necessary, search firms are often useful. The quality of the service provided by the temporary or permanent referral source, however, should be evaluated according to its track record of referring qualified and talented candidates on a timely basis.

Employee Referrals

Employees are excellent referral sources for highly qualified and talented candidates for employment, and many employers encourage their staff to do so. Many individuals associate with others with similar occupational interests. This recruitment source normally offers a built-in screening mechanism because most individuals will refer people whom they know well and who offer the employer a good prospect for success.

Organizations often develop referral incentive plans that reward employees who refer applicants selected for employment. Generally, there is a requirement that the new hire remain on the job for some months before the bonus is actually paid to the referring employee. Before implementing an employee-referral incentive program, the employer should at least consider the possibility that it may be perceived as a bounty to induce people to work there. To be safe, the human resources department may want to solicit feedback from a representative sampling of employees.

Promotion from Within

The ultimate recruiting pool is the employer's existing staff. A meaningful training and development program, tenure, and experience, and an objective performance assessment system should provide the agency with a mechanism for cultivating and identifying employees within the organization who are ready to step up to higher levels of responsibility. A succession planning process (a schematic of possible replacements for key positions in the organization), a job posting policy, and development programs such as career ladders provide opportunities for upward mobility throughout the organization. The positive impact of a successful promote-from-within policy on the employee relations climate can be enormous, and its value as a cost-effective recruitment tool is as significant. A large percentage of positions filled as promotional opportunities are an indicator of an organization that is well on its way toward becoming an employer of choice.

The goal of an agency's recruitment plan is to locate the candidate for each vacancy who will meet and preferably surpass the agency's expected results. Timeliness is important because vacancies may result in lost revenue and employee dissatisfaction. The selection standard established by the agency should never be compromised. When the applicant flow is insufficient, the recruitment initiative should be adjusted accordingly. Outreach into the community may have to be expanded, a larger geographic area may have to be considered, hiring bonuses may have to be implemented, and multiple recruitment sources may have to be utilized, but the selection standard must remain constant.

SELECTION PROCESS

Everyone has skeletons in his or her work closet. There may be certain events in the past that are not appropriate for an applicant to share with an employment interviewer. Applicants who are skilled at the art of interviewing will provide as many positives as anyone would want to hear while skillfully avoiding negatives. The smart consumer learns as much information about a product as possible before making a purchase. The employer's representative, the interviewer, has the responsibility for learning as much information about the applicant's qualifications as possible before extending a job offer. Thus the object of the interview is to understand both the candidate's strengths and opportunities for growth. Certain preparations should be made to create the right environment for this.

First Impressions

Significant thought and preparation should go into making the right first impression on candidates you want to attract to your agency. Areas to consider include:

- Presenting a good physical environment in the reception area.
- Providing a warm, welcoming atmosphere with a trained receptionist.
- Starting the interview on time; it shows respect for the candidate.
- Putting the candidate at ease; offer a beverage.
- Preparing for the interview; review the applicant's resume prior to appointment; note any gaps in employment, inconsistencies, omissions of fact, and overlapping employment dates that you can review during the interview.

- Knowing the state and federal laws and regulations governing the pre-employment process.
- Developing a series of questions to ask each candidate for the position.
- Planning for a private, attractive area to conduct the interview.
- Arranging the seating to make the candidate comfortable. An interviewer behind a desk can be intimidating, while one seated in close proximity can invite more open conversation.
- Allotting an adequate amount of uninterrupted time to conduct the interview; usually between 45 and 60 minutes for most positions.
- Developing a clear set of criteria that will be used in assessing the candidates.

State and Federal Laws

Every interviewer should be well versed in the variety of state and federal laws and regulations that govern the pre-employment process. Generally, all individuals, including persons with disabilities, who possess bona fide occupational qualifications for a position and are legally permitted to work in the United States must be afforded an equal opportunity for employment consideration. Questions must be carefully constructed to guarantee equal employment opportunity for all who apply. Questions related to one's age, gender, family and/or martial status, religion, race, nationality, pregnancy, health status, and mental health history should be avoided and are likely illegal to ask.

Developing the Interview Tool

Before conducting interviews, develop a series of questions that relate to the competencies needed for the open position. These might include conflict management, customer service, technical knowledge, creativity, and so forth. The questions should probe beyond information already provided on the resume and application form. A particularly effective line of questioning places the applicant in a similar hypothetical

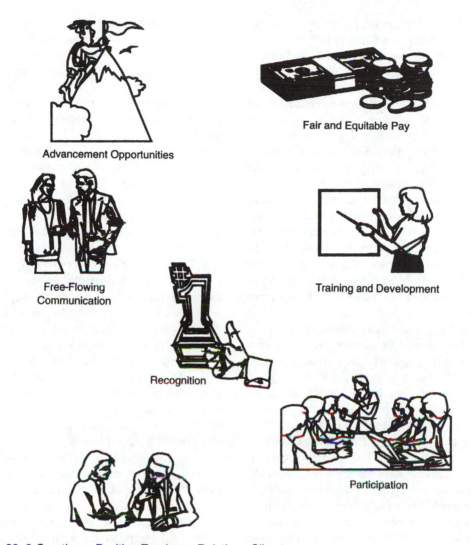

Advancement Opportunities

Fair and Equitable Pay

Free-Flowing
Communication

Training and Development

Recognition

Participation

Figure 38–2 Creating a Positive Employee Relations Climate

work setting. Questions that start "How would you handle . . . ?" produce information that can be evaluated objectively against the requirements of the actual position and work setting. Inquiries that test applicants' proficiency in dealing with difficult and stressful situations and questions that assess their comfort level with the exercise of independent judgment should be considered if, in fact, such issues may be encountered on the job. All questions should be asked in a way to encourage conversation (for example, "Tell me about a particularly stressful situation that you encountered and how you handled it"). On the other hand, leading questions that invite a specific response or a simple yes or no should be avoided.

The Interview

A smile, a firm handshake, and a sincere "Welcome to the XYZ Home Health Agency" are absolutely essential first steps. A good interviewer will recall the anxiety he or she experienced during his or her last interview and will take appropriate steps to put the applicant at ease. Small talk about the weather or about the applicant's trip to the interview site may seem contrived, but extended salutary remarks and perhaps a few minutes of light conversation about something that they have in common can reduce interview jitters. The goal at this point is to establish rapport. Ultimately, the interviewer strives for trust and confidence and tries to convince the applicant that their relationship has evolved into one where a free exchange of information would be to their mutual benefit. This, of course, is true because both the employer and applicant have a vested interest in making the right employment decision, which would not be inappropriate for the applicant to hear.

After these introductory remarks, a limited amount of information about the agency and position should be shared to confirm the applicant's continued interest in the position. Incidentally, asking about an individual's motivation for applying for a job is appropriate, and the response should be weighted heavily. The next part of the interview is fact finding. The object for the interviewer is to gain control of the dialogue and to steer it to those areas of the applicant's work history that are not apparent. To do so, the interviewer should listen and observe and talk only to facilitate the discussion. The more information that the interviewer develops, the better equipped he or she will be to consider the applicant's inventory of positives and negatives and to make an educated employment decision. The applicant, on the other hand, also strives for control and in doing so tries to steer the interviewer's probe away from areas of discomfort and back to the positive attributes of the work history.

Certain techniques are particularly effective for developing additional discussion. Great communicators know how to use body language to solicit additional information. A pause, a gesture that implies interest, and then continued silence imply "keep talking." At the same time,

the interviewer should receive messages from the applicant's body language and should follow up with questions as appropriate. The probe should continue until enough relevant information is accumulated to facilitate an objective decision. Be cautious about filling awkward silences and leading the candidate to the answer you want.

When the interviewer is comfortable that the profile developed is sufficient, the interviewer's role should change. This part of the selection process is devoted to ensuring that the applicant will accept the position if offered and, if not, that he or she will at least speak highly of the agency to others. This is therefore an opportunity for the interviewer to provide specific information about the position and to accentuate the positive aspects of having an employment relationship with the home health agency. An enthusiastic presentation will certainly imply that the agency is an employer of choice.

Although personal interviews should always be conducted before hiring a candidate, telephone interviews for the purpose of screening can be a useful technique when the pool of candidates is large. Telephone interviews can actually provide a more objective assessment of the candidate as they allow you to focus on the individual's responses to your questions more fully. When the position requires a high degree of interaction with multiple departments or is a senior management position in the organization, it may be appropriate for a candidate to be interviewed by a panel of interviewers. In these circumstances, train the panel on the legal aspects of interviewing and work with the panel to develop a consistent set of questions they will ask the candidates. Be cautious about overwhelming the candidate with too many interviewers; three to six panelists is usually the norm.

The Employment Decision

It should be noted that the manager with the vacancy is generally the hiring manager. The human resources department interview is primarily a screening procedure. Presumably, however, the human resources interviewer is the agency's selection expert, and his or her recommendation should be taken seriously. The human resources department is also responsible for ensuring compliance with legal employment obligations and advises the hiring manager accordingly. The hiring manager and the human resources interviewer must ensure that the decision is based on the applicant's skills and abilities as they apply to the specifications of the job. The person selected should also be the individual who offers the best prospect for success. All applicants, however, should receive periodic updates of the status of their applications. When the position is filled, applicants who were interviewed should be contacted, personally if possible, and thanked for their interest. Obviously, close runners-up should not be rejected until the applicant of choice accepts the employment offer.

MAKING A MEANINGFUL EMPLOYMENT OFFER

Regardless of the persuasive skills of the individual making the job offer, the individual in the human resources department responsible for salary administration has the greatest impact on whether the offer will be accepted. The employer, even one that hopes to be an employer of choice, does not have to pay the highest salary in the community, but it does have to set its salary levels according to the market standards that exist for positions with similar requirements and equivalent responsibility. Before developing a wage and salary program, senior management must decide just how competitive the agency's salaries should be. For example, management may decide that salaries in general or salaries for specific positions should be set in the midrange or perhaps in the top 25 percent of local labor market salaries. Management establishes the overall pay philosophy, thereby giving the salary and benefits experts in the human resources department a frame of reference.

To ensure the appeal of an employment offer, wage and salary decisions are based on a thorough and current review of salary ranges and average salaries for similar positions within the employer's recruitment pool. Periodic salary and benefit surveys are published from a variety of local, regional, and national trade and professional organizations. In home health care, state home care associations often provide annual industry surveys, as do the National Association for Home Care and Hospice and the Visiting Nurse Associations of America. These surveys include data on a variety of caregiver and administrative support positions. Also, job descriptions are included to facilitate appropriate comparisons. Although the process is somewhat more complicated, the goal is to compare apples to apples and to ensure that salary levels are set to enhance the agency's ability to fill its vacancies on a timely basis.

Based on the information developed, the compensation specialist can set in-hiring salaries for specific positions and develop ranges that include midpoints and maximum values for each position. Because the base rate is normally paid to individuals with minimal qualifications, decisions are also required about an experienced person's placement on the range. This is a challenge for the salary administrator. In addition, consideration must be given to those who have been in the agency's employ for some time. Thus the job offer for the new hire must be determined precisely to ensure external equity (competitiveness in the community) and internal equity (fairness and consistency within the agency).

A structured wage and salary program also includes a job analysis methodology for arranging positions in a hierarchy according to levels of responsibility and a number of other factors. An objective process is selected from a number of possibilities and is used to determine pay grades. New positions and revised positions should be put through this process as they are created or changed.

Finally, consideration must be given to the method of assuring an employee of ongoing salary growth. Experience and longevity, and perhaps performance, should be compensated. There have been debates about the concept of pay for performance for decades, particularly across the collective bargaining table. The pro argument places a motivational value on a merit increase. The con argument is related to the premise that an objective assessment of performance is unattainable. Regardless of the decision, a wage and salary program must afford staff the opportunity to be paid fairly and commensurate with their responsibility, and it must be perceived as such.

BENEFITS

Benefit costs are on the rise, particularly those that offer medical reimbursement. We are acutely aware of rising health care costs, but workers' compensation premiums represent a staggering expense to employers, particularly those in health care. The good news, however, is that such plans are experience rated and that claims can be controlled with appropriate educational programs and proactive risk management strategies. Risk management committees should be convened to conduct studies of the causes of work-related injuries and illnesses and should be empowered to develop appropriate follow-up plans. Perhaps a staff awareness program that includes training sessions, posters, articles in agency publications, and staff discussion groups would be an appropriate response to a recurring occupational injury. Also, periodic inspections of the workplace to identify and report safety hazards may reduce future occurrences and serve to increase every employee's awareness of such issues. In home care, where significant numbers of employees spend much of their working days driving, representatives of state motor vehicle departments are often willing to conduct on-site driving safety courses. The proactive employer realizes that cost containment of insurance premiums will result in savings that could be applied to other benefit options that better meet the specific needs of the employee population.

EMPLOYEE RELATIONS FOR RETENTION

The first 6 months of employment are the most stressful. This is especially true for caregivers making the transition from acute care to the independent environment of the home health agency. Adequate training and development for all new employees are important, whether on the job or in the classroom. Equally important is the need for the employee to have a mentor, preferably someone other than the manager, who can assume responsibility for providing support and assistance with workplace issues. The manager, however, is the key resource. The new employee's progress should be charted and discussed with the individual on an ongoing basis, and adjustments to this initial training program should be made appropriately. Above all, the manager and every other member of the team should provide encouragement and support. The human resources department plays a special role because the initial employment relationship began there. The members of the human resources department should look for opportunities to interface with the recent hires, even simply to ask how things are going. Periodic progress interviews should take place in personnel, and information shared should be used to make adjustments and interventions on behalf of the newcomer. An orientation presentation for all new employees is an effective mechanism for introducing a group of new employees to the agency and perhaps to the various operational departments as well. Participation on the part of senior staff goes a long way toward placing value on the human resource.

As previously discussed, communication and staff involvement enhance the employee relations environment (Figure 38–2). Programs and practices that promote such efforts serve to improve the climate within the organization. Satisfied employees are only too anxious to talk about their employer in favorable terms to friends and acquaintances, thereby enhancing the agency's community image as well. Finally, the human resources department's role as a staff and management resource should be communicated regularly to staff. Its credibility as a resource will be tested by every employee who visits the department for help and assistance. The human resources department staff must be equipped to handle effectively every employee

issue with sensitivity and expertise and every person as a client with needs and expectations that should be met.

The *Health Care Labor Manual* (Skoler and Abbott, 2004) provides a thorough overview of personnel management topics and is recommended (Exhibit 38–1).

REFERENCE

Skoler, M., and R. Abbott, Jr. 2004. *Health care labor manual* (vol. 2). Gaithersburg, MD: Aspen, Ch. 12:1.

SUGGESTED READING

Belcher, D. 1974. *Compensation administration.* Englewood Cliffs, NJ: PrenticeHall.

Cook, M. 1993. *The human resource yearbook* (1993/94 ed.). Englewood Cliffs, NJ: Prentice Hall.

Henderson, R. 1984. *Performance appraisal* (2nd ed.). Reston, VA: Reston.

Jones, J., W. Murphy, and R. Belton. 1987. *Cases and materials on discrimination in employment* (5th ed.). St. Paul, MN: West.

Morano, R. 1989. *Managing human behavior and development in organizations.* New York: Cummings & Hathaway.

Rothstein, M., A. Knapp, and L. Liebman. 1990. *Employment law—Cases and materials* (2nd ed.). Westbury, NY: Foundation Press.

Tortorici, R. 1988. The nursing shortage . . . crisis or catalyst? *Nurses Network* 2(4): 22–24.

Staff Development in a Home Health Agency

Joan Reynolds Yuan

Nursing is a progressive art, in which to stand still is to go back. A woman who thinks to herself, "Now I am a full nurse, a skilled nurse, I have learnt all there is to be learnt." Take my word for it, she does not know what a nurse is, and never will know. She has gone back already. Progress can never end but with a nurse's life.

—*F. Nightingale* (1914)

The concept of furthering one's education is an age-old one in nursing. Traditionally, it has been an important area in community health agencies. Currently, professional development is vital to the existence of any community or home health agency. In this era of outcome-focused, high-technology/high-touch home care, an extensive knowledge base, sharp technical skills, and appropriate attitudes are necessities for providing quality care to patients, families, and communities; preventing litigation; and remaining in business. With a view to the individual, one considers personal and professional growth, stimulation, motivation, and increasing or maintaining competence. In viewing an agency, one considers the necessity for providing quality care to clients. To accomplish this, a qualified staff must be employed. With advances in theory and technology, education is necessary to ensure understanding and competence. Ongoing education is mandated by regulatory and accrediting bodies such as the Community Health Accreditation Program (CHAP) and the Joint Commission on Accreditation of Healthcare

Organizations (JCAHO). Staff development presents as an important component in the retention of qualified personnel (CHAP, 2002, p. 25). A key factor in the Joint Commission accreditation process appears as standard HR.1: The organization provides development programs for all staff and volunteers (JCAHO, 2002, p. HR-3). The Medicare Conditions of Participation mandate education, as evidenced in these sections:

- Section 484.14: "The administrator . . . employs qualified personnel and ensures adequate staff education and evaluations" (U.S. Government Printing Office, 2002a, p. 565).
- Section 484.30: "The registered nurse . . . participates in in-service programs" (U.S. Government Printing Office, 2002b, p. 571).
- Section 484.32: "The qualified therapist participates in in-service programs" (U.S. Government Printing Office, 2002c, p. 571).
- Section 484.34: "The social worker . . . participates in in-service programs" (U.S. Government Printing Office, 2002d, p. 571).
- Section 484.36: "The home health aide must receive at least twelve hours of in-service training per calendar year" (U.S. Government Printing Office, 2002e, p. 573).

Nursing professional development is a necessity for home health agencies. It plays a critical role in the recruitment and retention of personnel. It has three domains: (1) staff development, (2) continuing education, and (3) academic education (ANA, 2000). Continuing education, learning experiences that contribute to the knowledge, skills, and attitudes of nurses, enhances the quality of health care (ANA, 2000). It can be a dimension of staff development, formal education, a program, or independent study through journals or on the Internet. According to the ANA (2000), nurses pursue academic education for a degree, certificate, or to update knowledge in a specific area. Staff development is "the systematic process of assessment, development, and evaluation that enhances the performance or professional development of health care providers and their continuing competence" (National Nursing Staff Development Organization, 1999, p. 25).

The ANA has developed six standards for nursing professional development (ANA, 2000):

1. Assessment: Information related to the educational needs of the nurse is collected.
2. Diagnosis: Assessment data to determine the target audience and learner needs are analyzed.
3. Identification of educational outcomes: The general purpose and educational objectives for each learning activity are identified.
4. Planning: Collaboration with content experts occurs to facilitate the development of activities to meet the educational objectives of the learners.
5. Implementation: The planned educational activities are implemented.
6. Evaluation: A comprehensive evaluation of the educational offering is conducted.

ROLE AND RESPONSIBILITIES OF THE EDUCATOR

The title of the person responsible for the staff development program will vary from one organization to the next. Such titles may include director of education, nursing supervisor, staff development supervisor, and clinical educator. In this chapter, the person responsible for staff development is referred to as the *educator*. The role of the educator in a home health agency is complex. Responsibilities within the process of staff development include continuing education, in-service education, and orientation of employees. Depending on the size and educational philosophy of the organization, the educator may be responsible for an agency-wide program for all employees. This position requires a blend of educational, clinical, and administrative knowledge and expertise. It is commonly filled by a nurse with a master's degree. This person typically reports to the executive director. The educator may not have line responsibilities, but power is inherent in the role. In many organizations, this person, by virtue of his or her educational background, experience, and knowledge of the organization, has the authority for decision making in the absence of the executive director and the director of professional services.

STAFF DEVELOPMENT: ORIENTATION

Orientation is viewed as the means by which new staff are introduced to the philosophy, goals, policies, procedures, role expectations, physical facilities, and special services in a specific work setting (ANA, 2000, p. 25). Orientation is provided at the time of employment and at other times when changes in roles and responsibilities occur in a specific work setting (p. 5). The educator has the responsibility to orient new employees to the organization as a whole. He or she orients new nursing personnel to the nursing service department. Depending on the structure of the organization, he or she may be responsible for specific orientation to other departments as well. In a general orientation, the new employee is introduced to the physical setting, specific work area, and personnel. The philosophy, purpose, and goals of the organization are addressed. The spirit of the organization is discussed (for example, "This is a team effort;

each job is important to the functioning of the organization. The attitudes of all staff members are important in a service organization, and in this highly competitive era, one must be aware of the treatment of the consumer"). A lesson can be learned by looking at the orientation process at organizations such as Walt Disney World/ Disneyland, where attitudes toward the consumer are of paramount importance. The administrative policies and procedures are reviewed (see Chapter 33). Orientation to the specific job is provided during orientation. Competent and willing preceptors are invaluable in this process. Organizations differ in preceptor responsibilities as well as recognition. In addition to a certificate or luncheon, if the budget allows, a monetary bonus even of $100 is appreciated. Exhibit 39–1 shows a sample orientation form for a nursing department. Clinical policies and procedures are reviewed with the professional staff. In the nursing department, the nurse completes a skills checklist/competency self-assessment form (Exhibit 39-2). This allows for individualization of the orientation program. It enables the educator to identify the learning needs of the new employee, and it enables the new employee to request a review of clinical skills that have not been fully developed. The educator or designee evaluates initial competencies.

Documentation is an area of concentration in the orientation process. Accuracy in documentation is necessary for both quality care and reimbursement purposes. It is important for the educator not only to review the orientee's documentation, but also to make home visits with the new nurse to assess his or her ability to function as a home health nurse and to allow for questions and discussion.

In agencies that are hospital based, opportunities for the transfer of experienced specialized nurses such as maternal child health or intravenous (IV) nurses exist. Orientation to this new position setting is required. Home care's requirements and standards are different from those of the inpatient facility. Home care nursing practice is grounded in evidence-based clinical knowledge and skills within the framework of family, home, and community concepts (ANA, 1999). Caseload management responsibilities and coordination with insurance case managers require orientation. Joint Commission standards are setting-specific. A competent IV nurse could be knowledgeable of the Intravenous Nurses Society (INS) standards but without orientation to the home care setting would have no knowledge of home care standards. Orientation to a new position within the home health agency is another area addressed by the educator. This becomes important as staff nurses move into supervisory positions. Management training can be done in-house or at area institutions. Many consultants are available for this purpose. This is a vulnerable time for the employee, and support in the new role is essential. Documentation of orientation must be provided. This is necessary for both new employees and employees who have changed positions. The employees will sign the orientation forms as well as their job descriptions. These forms will remain in the personnel file.

STAFF DEVELOPMENT: IN-SERVICE EDUCATION

In-service education has been defined in the ANA's *Scope and Standards of Practice for Nursing Professional Development* (2000) as activities designed to assist nurses acquire, maintain, or increase competence in fulfilling their responsibilities to deliver quality health care (p. 6). According to the Joint Commission Standard HR 6, "The organization provides ongoing education, including in-services, training, and other activities" (JCAHO, 2002, p. HR-2). CHAP requires that staff education and training be in accordance with job description requirements and that competencies are assessed (CHAP, 2002, p. 25).

For an in-service program to be viable, it must be backed by the administration. It is the responsibility of the educator to assess the educational needs of the employees. A regularly administered needs assessment tool is helpful. In-service education may be required in several

Exhibit 39–1 Orientation Program

NAME:_____

ORIENTATION START DATE:_____

END DATE OF ORIENTATION:_____ END DATE OF PROBATION:_____ EXTENSION DATE OF PROBATION:_____	DATE EXPLAIN/ DEMO	BY WHOM INITIALS	DATE VERB/DEMO UNDERSTAND	BY WHOM INITIALS
1. ADMINISTRATIVE (By the end of week one):				
A. Agency Structure/Policies:				
1. Introduction				
a. Mission				
b. Philosophy				
c. Organization				
d. Office Personnel & Facilities				
e. Sources of Financial Support				
f. Geographic Area Served				
2. Scope of Services:				
a. Hospice				
b. IV/CHF Team				
c. Maternal/Child Health				
d. WOCN				
e. Psychiatric				
f. Nutrition				
g. MSW				
h. PT/OT/ST				
3. Medical Policies & Standing Orders				
4. Nursing Service Policies				
5. Compliance Program/Code of Conduct				
B. Personnel Issues				
1. Payroll				
2. Schedule				
3. Auto Insurance				
4. Dress Code				
5. Insurance Benefits				
6. Reporting Illness				
7. Staff Inservice/Outside Meetings/Advanced Individual Educational Opportunities				
C. Daysheet				
D. Job Description/Responsibility				
E. Medicare Regulations:				
1. Conditions of Participation				
2. PPS Overview				
3. OASIS Overview				
F. Professional Ethics:				
0 1. Patient/Family Rights				
2. Confidentiality				
G. Regulations Governing HHA:				
1. Type of care				
2. Supervision of Care				
H. Explanation of the role of the supervisor				
I. Policies & Procedures				

Continues

different areas (Barnum and Kerfoot, 1995). Preparatory education such as a physical assessment course may be required. Supplemental education such as management theory may be necessary. Maintenance education for cardiopulmonary resuscitation (CPR) certification, new product orientation, or new procedure orientation many times is indicated. Remedial education for foundational support is another area that is addressed by the educator.

Planning the in-services is the responsibility of the educator with the assistance of the

Exhibit 39–1 Continued

ABINGTON MEMORIAL HOSPITAL HOMECARE ORIENTATION CHECKLIST

NAME:_____

ORIENTATION START DATE:_____

	DATE EXPLAIN/ DEMO	BY WHOM INITIALS	DATE VERB/DEMO UNDERSTAND	BY WHOM INITIALS
J. Community Resources				
K. ATT Language Line				
L. Admission Packet				
M. Weekend/Holiday Schedule				
N. On Call				
O. Chart Review				

Comments:_____
_____
_____
_____

	DATE EXPLAIN/ DEMO	BY WHOM INITIALS	DATE VERB/DEMO UNDERSTAND	BY WHOM INITIALS
II. COMPETENCIES (By the end of week 2): A. CLIA				
B. Skills Lab				
C. Wounds				
D. Nursing Bags: 1. Technique				
2. Supplies: a. bag supplies				
b. billable supplies				
E. Phlebotomy				
F. Computer Communication: 1. Nightly Communication				
2. Demand Communication				
3. Remote Communication (modem)				
4. Serial Communication				
G. Communication: 1. Email				
2. Cell Phone				
3. Voice mail AMH System				
H. Competency Self Assessment				
I. Map Reading.				

Comments:_____
_____
_____
_____

	DATE EXPLAIN/ DEMO	BY WHOM INITIALS	DATE VERB/DEMO UNDERSTAND	BY WHOM INITIALS
III. CLINICAL SKILLS: (By the end of week 10) A. Physical Assessment as per agency policy				
B. High Volume Disease Entities				
C. Nursing Assessment				
D. AHCPR Guidelines				
E. Patient Education Materials				
F. Pressure Ulcer/Wound Care				
G. CHF				
H. Home Visit with Clinical Educator				

Exhibit 39–1 Continued

ABINGTON MEMORIAL HOSPITAL HOMECARE ORIENTATION CHECKLIST

NAME:_____

ORIENTATION START DATE:_____

	DATE EXPLAIN/ DEMO	BY WHOM INITIALS	DATE VERB/DEMO UNDERSTAND	BY WHOM INITIALS
1.Relationship of Nurse to other members of staff: 1. Individual Responsibility				
2. Coordination/Needs of other services				
3. Role as Case Manager				
4. Insurance: a. How to get approval				
b. How to check for approval				
J. Completes Oasis Assessment				
K.Comprehensive Assessment				
L. Case Conference				
M. Schedule: 1. Weekly Card				
2. Planning for the day				
N. Coordination with scheduler				
O. Returning paperwork to supervisor				
P. Assess the need for other services in the home				
Q. Interdisciplinary Conferences				
R. Demonstrate practice of Medicare Conditions of Participation				

Comments:_____

_____

_____

IV. COMPUTER/DOCUMENTATION (by week 12)				
A. Proper Care/Use of Notebook				
1. Battery Care/AC Power Use				
2. Powering ON/OFF, Exiting program properly				
B. Communications				
1. When to communicate				
2. Completes Documentation in designated time frame & transmits appropriately				
C. Clinical Link Program				
1. Email				
2. DOS program/Function keys/Tab key				
3. Episode/Activity/Form				
D. Patient Related Activities				
1. Assigning & "pulling over"				
2. Reviewing chart: View/On file/Complete				
3. Documentation of Patient Chart: a. Daily Visit				
b. Admission				
c. Resumption				
d. Verbal Order				

Continues

Exhibit 39–1 Continued

ABINGTON MEMORIAL HOSPITAL HOMECARE ORIENTATION CHECKLIST

NAME:_____

ORIENTATION START DATE:_____

	DATE EXPLAIN/ DEMO	BY WHOM INITIALS	DATE VERB/DEMO UNDERSTAND	BY WHOM INITIALS
e. Discharge				
f. Transfer				
g. Recertification				
h. Plan of care initiation at SOC				
i. Update & revise POC when necessary				
j. Appropriate Goals at SOC				
k. Individualize Assess, Inter, Teachings to pt needs				
l. Appropriate visit pattern				
m. HA Assessment				
n. HA Supervision: present/nonpresent				

Comments:_____
_____
_____

EVALUATION OF THE ORIENTEE

STRENGTHS   NEEDED IMPROVEMENTS

RECOMMENDED ACTIONS (GOALS)

Orientee Signature _____   Date _____

Initials/Signature   Initials/Signature

interdisciplinary education committee. It is recommended that a long-range 12-month plan be made. This must be flexible, however, because new products, new procedures, and new needs will arise throughout the course of the year. In planning in-services, one must consider the cost of providing the in-service, including the cost of the instructor, the materials, and the time of the staff. It is important to remember that the time staff spend in an in-service must be deducted from the time they spend on reimbursable patient care activities. Consideration must be given to utilizing the least amount of time required to accomplish the task adequately.

The characteristics of the adult learner are another important area for consideration in planning in-services. Adult learning principles have been defined by the ANA (2000) as approaches to adults as learners based on recognition of the individual's autonomy and self-direction, life

Exhibit 39–2 Competency Self-Assessment

NAME: _____   DATE:

COMPETENCY SELF-ASSESSMENT

Using the scale below, please rate each skill according to your knowledge of and/or experience with the competency:

RATING SCALE
1.   I have had no experience with this competency.
2.   I know the basic concepts related to this competency but need review.
3.   I consider myself competent with this skill.

GENERIC COMPETENCIES

	1	2	3	N/A
1. Perform female catheterization				
2. Perform male catheterization				
3. Insert supra-pubic tube				
4. Care of patient with gastrostomy/jejunostomy tube				
5. Insertion of gastrostomy tube				
6. Nasogastric tube placement				
7. Care of the patient with a tube feeding				
8. Auscultation of breath sounds				
9. Perform oropharyngeal/nasopharyngeal suctioning				
10. Care of the patient requiring tracheostomy tube				
11. Insertion of tracheostomy tube				
12. Care of the patient with an ostomy				
13. Perform blood glucose monitoring				
14. Care of the patient with a Jackson-Pratt drain				
15. Perform wound care/dressing changes				
16. Venipuncture				
17. IV catherter insertion				
18. Midline catheter insertion				
19. Post-partum assessment				
20. Newborn/pediatric assessment (inc. PKU & Bilirubin testing)				
21. Psychiatric assessment (inc. Geriatric Depression Scale, Beck Depression Scale & Folstein's Mini-Mental Status Exam)				
* All skills self-assessed as #1 or #2 require review and/or testing in the skills lab.				

experiences, readiness to learn, and problem orientation to learning. Approaches include mutual, respectful collaboration of teachers and learners in assessing, planning, implementing, and evaluating learning (p. 23). Learning activities tend to be experiential and inquiry focused. For example, an in-service on diabetic management would include hands-on experience with a glucose monitoring device.

Creative strategies can be utilized to present mandated maintenance education material such as Occupational and Safety Health Administration (OSHA) programs. This information can be formatted into skits, bingo, or *Jeopardy*-like games (Harris and Yuan, 1994; 1997) to better meet the needs of the adult learner. Resources to consider utilizing for in-services include the agency's staff. An adult nurse practitioner may teach physical assessment. A physical therapist may teach proper body mechanics or chest physical therapy. A social worker may discuss available community resources. Staff attending conferences may have valuable information to share.

Schools of nursing can be another valuable resource. State school extensions may have staff, such as nutritionists, who are available as educational resources. Community resources such as the American Cancer Society can be utilized. Manufacturers of equipment such as colostomy supplies, ventilators, and glucometers are often utilized. Implementation should be carried out in accordance with written policy. The in-service should take place in an appropriate meeting room. If the agency does not have sufficient space, arrangements can be made with a local church, library, or school.

The educator will keep attendance records of the in-services. Individual staff members will maintain educational program records, which will be collected annually and kept in the personnel file. Evaluating educational programs is not an easy task. A written content evaluation is one method. The result of education is an increase in knowledge or skill. The quality assessment/improvement program can be utilized to assess the effects of education on patient care.

STAFF DEVELOPMENT: CONTINUING EDUCATION

One component of staff development is continuing education. In the ANA's *Scope and Standards of Practice for Nursing Professional Development* (2000), continuing education is defined as "systematic professional learning experiences designed to augment the knowledge, skills, and attitudes of nurses and therefore enrich the nurses' contributions to quality health care and their pursuit of professional career goals" (p. 5). The educator controls the budget for the continuing education program. Because funds are not endless, a determination must be made of how much money is allotted for each person. To get as much for the educational dol-

lar as possible, other avenues should be investigated. Affiliating educational institutions may allow a free conference for an agency staff member in exchange for using the agency as a site for student experience. Participation in a planning committee and a cooperative effort with a providing institution can be other ways in which the agency can have staff attend a conference free of charge or at a discounted rate.

In some areas, many continuing education programs are available. Information regarding the continuing education programs can be posted for staff perusal. The individual staff member files a request to attend a conference. Depending on the conference, staffing, and budget, the request is granted or not granted by the educator. Although time off to attend a conference is costly (not to mention the cost of the conference itself), it is usually most helpful for the professional to meet with colleagues from other organizations and to broaden the individual's scope of experience. Attending conferences outside the institution often increases job satisfaction and ultimately may have a positive effect on patient care. It is often valuable to have the individual report the findings from the conference to his or her colleagues. It is important that accurate records be kept. The educator will maintain records of the conferences attended by members of all disciplines. In addition, a record is kept in the personnel folder. In some areas of the country, continuing education programs are not readily available. Independent study and self-learning modules can help fill this void. Continuing education units are available through some nursing journals and Web sites.

ACADEMIC EDUCATION

In this era of high-technology home care and economic restrictions, the need for highly skilled professionals with a broad knowledge base is evident. Many agencies require a bachelor of science in nursing or that a registered nurse be working toward this degree for entry into the organization. The need for specialists in clinical and administrative areas is growing, hence the need for graduate education. Personnel policies should include provisions for furthering one's formal education. This can range from having time off and flexible scheduling to attend classes to taking a leave of absence or a sabbatical. This encompasses undergraduate as well as graduate education. Among the benefits to an organization of utilizing the sabbatical are employee retention, stimulation of employees, development of employee talent, and increased commitment to the organization. The organization must cope with finding temporary replacements and reentry into the organization, however.

Many organizations will maintain a library for staff use. Often, this is the responsibility of the educator. Requests for new books and journals are submitted to the educator. He or she oversees the library budget and maintains adequate records. It is particularly helpful to have a library that includes literature related to community health and home care for staff members who are attending school and doing research.

Education in a community or home health agency is viewed not just as a requirement, but as a necessity and an integral part of an organization concerned about the provision of quality care.

REFERENCES

American Nurses Association. 1999. *Scope and standards of home health nursing practice.* Washington, DC: Author.

American Nurses Association. 2000. *Scope and standards of practice for nursing professional development.* Washington, DC: Author.

Barnum, B., and K. Kerfoot. 1995. *The nurse as executive* (4th ed.). Gaithersburg, MD: Aspen.

The Community Health Accreditation Program, Inc. 2002. *Home health standards of excellence* (Millenium ed). New York: Author.

Harris, M., and J. Yuan. 1994. Oh no, not another handwashing in-service! *Journal of the Society of Gastroenterology Nurse and Associates* 16(6): 269–272.

Harris, M., and J. Yuan. 1997. Creative inservices to meet mandatory education requirements. *Home Healthcare Nurse* 15(8): 573–579.

Joint Commission on Accreditation of Healthcare Organizations. 2002. *2003 Comprehensive accreditation manual for home care.* Oakbrook Terrace, IL: Author.

National Nursing Staff Development Organization. 1999. *Strategic plan 2000.* Pensacola, FL: Author.

Nightingale, F. 1914. *Florence Nightingale to her nurses.* London: Macmillan.

U.S. Government Printing Office. 2002a, October. Code of Federal Regulations (42 CFR 484.14, 565). Retrieved from U.S. Government Printing Office via GPO Access: *http://www.access.gpo.gov/nara/cfr/* (accessed April 26, 2003).

U.S. Government Printing Office. 2002b, October. Code of Federal Regulations (42 CFR 484.30, 571). Retrieved from U.S. Government Printing Office via GPO Access: *http://www.access.gpo.gov/nara/cfr/* (accessed April 26, 2003).

U.S. Government Printing Office. 2002c, October. Code of Federal Regulations (42 CFR 484.32, 571). Retrieved from U.S. Government Printing Office via GPO Access: *http://www.access.gpo.gov/nara/cfr/* (accessed April 26, 2003).

U.S. Government Printing Office. 2002d, October. Code of Federal Regulations (42 CFR 484.34, 571). Retrieved from U.S. Government Printing Office via GPO Access: *http://www.access.gpo.gov/nara/cfr/* (accessed April 26, 2003).

U.S. Government Printing Office. 2002e, October. Code of Federal Regulations (42 CFR 484.36, 573). Retrieved from U.S. Government Printing Office via GPO Access: *http://www.access.gpo.gov/nara/cfr/* (accessed April 26, 2003).

CHAPTER 40

Transitioning Nurses to Home Care

Carolyn J. Humphrey and Paula Milone-Nuzzo

With increasing numbers of patients cared for in their homes, the practice of home care nursing has grown significantly, with the trend promising to increase as Baby Boomers age. The trend toward health care provided in the home coupled with the long-term impact of the nursing crisis has resulted in an increased demand for home care nurses. This has resulted in the transition of nurses from acute settings to the home care organization. What they find upon entering this new practice specialty is not only an adjustment to caring for patients in a different environment, but also the need to acquire many new competencies. More than ever there should be no doubt that home care is *not* just hospital care provided in the home.

The process a nurse must go through to make the move to home care has often been called transitioning to home care nursing. Just as the term *transition* is defined as "a movement, development, or evolution from one form, stage, or style to another" (*Merriam-Webster's Collegiate Dictionary*, 2003), so must nurses who are used to caring for clients in a structured hospital environment transition their skills to a work situation that is both different and unique. It is up to both the nurse and the agency administration to work together to see that this transition is as effective and efficient as possible.

This chapter shares the orientation philosophy and approach that must be in place to have an effective orientation program. By basing practice on the definition of home care nursing

as a comprehensive practice and much different from acute care practice, the stage is set for the affective changes an orientee must make to be successful.

Additionally, the key content areas a nurse *must* master to become an effective home care provider are outlined. Other chapters in this book covering competency evaluation and staff development should be consulted as they are essential for developing a realistic and cost efficient orientation program.

DEFINITION OF HOME CARE NURSING

Home care nursing is a unique field of nursing practice that focuses on caring for an ill client in the home while also providing anticipatory guidance and teaching. Home care's unique goal is to prepare the client for independence in self care. To practice effectively, the nurse requires a synthesis of community health nursing principles with the theory and practice of medical/surgical, maternal/child, pediatric, and behavioral health nursing. Home care nursing is provided to clients experiencing an illness outside the confines of an acute care hospital and integrates caregivers and families within the context of the community to reach the desired outcomes.

Home care nurses care for acutely and chronically ill clients of all ages with a myriad of diseases and conditions. From those who have procedures and treatments to those who wish to live out the final stages of their lives in their homes rather than in an institution, the home care nurse must be competent in many areas. Reflecting this philosophy, the following definition of home care nursing should be used as an orientation framework that will support the new nurse in applying new practices in this important new role:

> Home care nursing is the provision of nursing care to acute, chronically ill and well clients of all ages in their home while integrating community health nursing principles that focus on health promotion, environmental, psychosocial, economic, cultural and personal health factors affecting an individual's and family's health status. (Humphrey and Milone-Nuzzo, 1999, p. 2:2)

Administrators must clearly understand the various ways this definition can be used with clients so that this important role difference can be the basis for the orientation and internalized in all agency operations. The constraints on frequency and duration of home visits under the Medicare Prospective Payment System (PPS) and the current regulatory and economic climate make it increasingly difficult for the nurse to practice this comprehensive role.

To achieve positive patient satisfaction surveys and outcomes, as well as attract and retain the best clinicians, the home care organization must embrace a care philosophy that values and allocates resources to this level of practice. The burden is on the clinical manager to contribute to the agency's philosophy of care and support the role and definition of comprehensive home care nursing, while working to assure this is realistically happening in day-to-day practice.

Currently, third-party payers focus more on medical diagnoses than the comprehensive care needed to achieve long-term health goals and prevent adverse events. If the agency's philosophy is clear in orientation, then the staff nurse and manager can work together in showing how comprehensive care can be both cost and client outcome effective. The foundation for this teamwork is laid during orientation

Many home health agencies require nurses to have at least 1 year of work experience in acute care prior to home care employment. Although this is desirable, it is often not feasible to turn away competent nurses without this experience. It is, however, a better use of resources for managers to thoroughly assess the clinical expertise and competencies of the nurse transitioning from acute care.

Miller and Daley (1996) identified four domains of home care practice, each with varying levels of expertise that managers should recognize as they begin the education process with new nurses. They are as follows:

1. assessing and using physiologic data
2. initiating and monitoring therapeutic interventions
3. assessing and using family and environmental data
4. integrating data, interventions, and context

It is critical for the manager to determine both the clinical practice expertise listed and the caseload management competencies the acute care nurse brings to home care. Building on these strengths during orientation and throughout employment will expedite success.

DIFFERENCES BETWEEN HOSPITAL AND HOME CARE NURSING

Although the application of the nursing process is different when conducted in the patient's home, there are some core practice issues that remain the same. The main one is the use of evidence-based practice.

Evidence-based practice (EBP), defined as "using the best evidence available to guide clinical decision making" leads to quality improvement and positive outcomes (Benefield, 2002). The nurse moving from acute care is likely familiar with protocols, standards, policies, and procedures. With the push for outcome-based quality improvement (OBQI) and the Center for Medicare and Medicaid Services (CMS) Quality Initiative, the process is accelerating. However, many standards and practices approved by national professional groups like the American Diabetes Association (ADA), the American Heart Association (AHA), the Intravenous Nurses Society (INS), the Wound and Ostomy Continence Society (WOCN), and so forth, are applicable to home care.

Because many aspects of home care require skills in addition to knowledge and abilities—conducting an efficient home visit is truly a learned skill—a tendency exists for more experienced nurses to "orient" the new clinician by doing it the way it's always been done. Orientation, scheduled with content that is based on best practices and policies, will eliminate the costs associated with new nurses losing money from "doing it the way we've always done it."

Presenting the Similarities and Differences— Key to Effective Orientation

This section covers some specific areas that nurses find are different when transitioning to home care. These points become the essential core of orientation activities that will help the orientee build on basic knowledge to assimilate the home care nursing role.

Assessment Skills

In the hospital, the nurse focuses on physical and psychological assessment skills for the individual patient cared for in the structured institutional environment. Some acute care nurses who work in specialty areas such as orthopedics or oncology may have more limited assessment skills that focus on a few systems. In home care, the nurse must not only complete physical and psychological assessments, but additionally assess social, economic, environmental, home safety, and family issues that affect the client's care. To accomplish this, the home care nurses must learn how to conduct these assessments efficiently and to determine their impact on the patient's situation.

The nurse transitioning to home care must learn how to complete the necessary paperwork associated with the admission process and comprehensive assessment, the Outcome and As-

sessment Information Set (OASIS) form. The use of a standardized data collection instrument that drives care and reimbursement for services is likely to be a new concept. Discussion of the OASIS data set and sharing a path indicating how the data is used in many agency operations will convey the importance of the clinician in this process.

Autonomy

Even when an acute care institution has a primary nursing system for delivering patient care, acute care nurses care for clients on only one shift (8 to 12 hours). In this situation, there is always another shift, that precedes and succeeds the current shift, meaning that the nurse can delegate to professional colleagues who consider a patient's needs other times in the day.

In home care, the client's 24-hour care must be thoroughly monitored by the primary nurse and documented in the clinical record. This comprehensive care planning requires the home care nurse to plan for care needs 24 hours a day, assure the necessary supplies and medications are available in the home for a duration of time, and consider the support and education the caregivers need until the next visit. In some cases, it requires planning for up to a week between skilled nursing visits.

Time management is a critical attribute for success in home care nursing because each nurse must plan the day efficiently, balancing travel and visit time, professional activities, office work, and paperwork to maximize time. If the orientee has not had previous experience managing several roles and responsibilities simultaneously, often a time management course or specific instruction by the supervisor and the preceptor should be included in the orientation.

Communication with the Physician

The nurse working in an institution interacts with physicians much differently than the home care nurse. There, the physician directly assesses the patient, and opportunities for face-to-face communication and collaborative problem solving occur. Clients receiving home care may not have seen their physician for several days or weeks, and the nurse in the home may never meet or talk directly with the physician unless deviations from the expected occur.

The physician relies on the nurse to make skillful assessments regarding significant changes in the client's condition and communicate them concisely and in a timely manner. This means that the home care nurse must learn how to "paint a picture" of the client over the telephone in less than a minute while suggesting possible causes and interventions. A great learning strategy is to give the orientee a case study. Using a stop watch, practice "calling" a physician in under a minute. The same activity should be done using written communications with the physician.

Determining Frequency and Duration of Care

Discharging a patient from the hospital is a decision made predominantly by the physician, the hospital's utilization review department, and the insurer; rarely does the acute care nurse become involved. From admission, the home care nurse, in collaboration with the physician and any other members of the home care team, use the client's needs and the payment source criteria to determine the *frequency* (how many visits per week) and the *duration* (how many weeks) of care. Needing to communicate with a case manager to receive prior authorization (if applicable) and to ascertain the client's mental and emotional ability to learn the procedure also factor into determining the frequency and duration of care.

Direct Care

The technical skills provided to the client in the hospital center around interpreting laboratory values, monitoring physical reactions to the treatment regimen, overseeing the use of high-technology equipment, and providing hands-on care that focuses on the acutely ill. In the hospital, the nurse is often faced with emergency situations and has the resources of everyone in the institution to assist, if needed.

The focus of home care is on assisting the client to be independent in self care. Although sometimes encountering emergent situations and providing direct care, the clinician is more likely to be teaching clients about their disease process and the best ways to care for themselves. Often, the nurse improvises equipment or suggests the lowest-cost supplies for clients with limited resources.

Additionally, an understanding of how to provide services in a home environment and the roles of other professional and paraprofessional services is critical for the best patient outcomes. Providing direct care involves teaching the client and the caregiver how to perform the procedure or treatment, rather than doing it for them, as might be done in the hospital.

Documentation

The hospital nurse focuses client documentation on highlighting improvement that is being made with an eye to a quick transfer to another level of service or discharge. Many hospitals use charting by exception and record only the patient behaviors that are different from what is expected. Home care uses the chart as the legal documentation of the services provided, so home care documentation is more complex and involved. Home care documentation must focus on the achievement of goals and desired outcomes, as well as the variances experienced by specific patients.

Under the Medicare PPS, organizations are focused on achieving client outcomes in the most efficient ways. To that end, many agencies use critical paths or some kind of preprinted care plans to track the specific care given on each visit with specific patient assessments and interventions noted. This means that the nurse must constantly document the patient's compliance with the overall Medicare home care coverage criteria, and in addition, focus on what outcomes the patient has achieved as well as the ones that remain the focus of future visits.

Home Visiting

Seeing patients in their own environment involves new competencies of visit planning so that all needed supplies and paperwork are ready in the home when the nurse is there. New skills of reading a map, implementing universal precautions in the home setting, and proper bag technique must be learned before a new nurse is able to conduct home visits.

Unlike acute care nursing where the client is a "guest" in the hospital, the home care nurse is a guest in a client's home. This means the nurse must ask before doing things such as washing hands, using the phone, bringing in point-of-care technology, and turning off the television to hear communication and heart sounds better. If the patient refuses, and they rarely do if the request is made with sincere respect for their space and possessions, the nurse may be unable to conduct the visit.

Patient Teaching

No matter how competent the hospital nurse is in teaching clients, payers and regulators demand that clients be discharged from the hospital often before adequate teaching can be completed. The unique function of teaching patients and caregivers in the home is not often fully understood by the new orientee.

When a patient is not acute, the new nurse may ask, "What is there for me to do?" This often means the full role of teaching the patient self care is not totally understood. The orientee must be clear that patient teaching is just as important as technical, hands-on care.

Teaching is a skilled nursing service that is Medicare reimbursable. Whether the patient's insurer is Medicare, managed care, Medicaid, or private insurance, teaching is a valued service because it helps the patient be more self-sufficient. The patient is also able to recognize early signs of problems and how to manage them so that costly interventions such as an emergency room visit or a hospital admission don't occur.

Referral to Community Resources

While in the hospital, the social services department and the discharge planning department primarily assess and coordinate the client's need for external referrals, including home care. As the coordinator of the client's care, the home care nurse is responsible for identifying all needs and ensuring that the client and family have access to resources that can be helpful. A thorough knowledge of local and national community resources, how to access them, and when to collaborate with the agency's social workers result in earlier home care discharge and attainment of short- and long-term outcomes.

Reimbursement

In the hospital, the admission and billing office, in conjunction with the physician, worry about the client's financial information. Although home health agencies have similar departments, the nurse validates and discusses these issues with the client and the family in the home and verifies the client's eligibility for home care services with the physician. Knowing how client care is reimbursed is a unique aspect of home care practice. As service progresses, the nurse may work with an insurance or other case managers in the following areas:

- reporting directly on the goals accomplished and the ones remaining.
- determining the time of discharge based not only on client needs, but also on payer source requirements.
- determining if the patient is eligible for home care services and whether the care provided meets payer-source requirements on a continuing basis.

Safety

In the hospital, workplace safety issues center on institutional Occupational Safety and Health Administration (OSHA) regulations, hospital security, and implementation of internal clinical safety practices such as universal precautions and safety in the parking areas when the nurse leaves work. Home care nurses who visit clients' homes may often be faced with aggressive patients, dangerous neighborhoods, car breakdowns, or other potentially dangerous or violent situations.

OSHA has recently revised guidelines, first developed in 1996, for preventing workplace violence for health care and social service workers (U.S. Dept. of Labor, 2003). This document provides a comprehensive approach to setting up a violence prevention program and gives forms and training suggestions that organizations can use with employees. The nurse transitioning to home care must be aware of how to implement these policies in practice and be able to identify situations that may be potentially dangerous or violent.

Work Environment

In the hospital, the client is always there, usually in the bed or in the room. Everything is familiar and handy for the nurse, who is supported by a myriad of departments such as dietary, laboratory, radiography, pharmacy, laundry, and housekeeping. If something goes wrong, the nurse can call others to assist. In home care, the nurse is always a guest in the client's home and often has to adjust to variations in a client's environment. If present, the family and caregivers should be included in the plan of care and take responsibilities when appropriate. If the client's clinical status has changed, the nurse must rely on clinical assessments and decision-making skills to collaborate with others (such as with the physician via the telephone) and intervene in whatever environment the patient resides.

KEY CONTENT AREAS FOUND IN ORIENTATION

Organization of the Home Care System

The nurse transitioning to home care may be unfamiliar with the larger home care system and with its internal and external influences. Introducing an overview of the various agency personnel; the types of home care agencies; and a description of licensure, certification, and accreditation into the orientation program, the orientee begins with a foundation for understanding the context in which home care nursing is practiced.

Because the nurse transitioning into home care may be familiar with the accreditation process from an institutional perspective, the various roles nurses play in home care accreditation should be clarified. For example, issues that would be appropriate for a state or Joint Commission on Accreditation of Healthcare Organizations' surveyor to discuss with a staff nurse include:

- a review of the process for care and service planning
- the process for coordination between nursing and pharmacy
- interventions used by nurses for medication administration
- the management of hazardous waste in the home

The Specialty of Home Care Nursing

The core of an orientation program should focus on understanding the numerous home care nursing roles and functions such as:

- identification of and referral to community resources
- supervision of paraprofessionals and unlicensed assistive personnel
- delegating to others, including the client's caregivers
- assuming responsibility for the coordination of care
- ensuring continuity of care and client advocacy

The nursing process is a helpful concept to use when teaching about the organized and systematic care that home care provides to clients. Although the nursing process can be applied to all care settings, application of the steps varies from setting to setting. In home care, additional aspects of the nursing process are:

Assessment. The nurse uses expert client-assessment skills because recent physician assessment, access to laboratory values, and other high-technology assessment methods may be unavailable.

Intervention. The intervention phase in home care is heavily focused on patient and family teaching, rather than providing care directly. Because the home care's goal is to assist the client toward independence and self care, the home care nurse must be a skilled teacher.

Evauation. This is the planned comparison of the client's health status with the client-centered outcomes identified in the early stages of care. In home care, ongoing care plan evaluation can help the nurse, in collaboration with the physician, determine when client goals are reached and when home care discharge is appropriate.

The Home Visit

The home visit is the home care nurse's single most important tool. The home care nurse must combine knowledge of the three stages of the home visiting process, with expert clinical and organizational skills and common sense. Several aspects of the home visit should be integrated into orientation for every orientee, whether novice or experienced in other home care settings. These include:

1. *The Three Stages of the Home Visit.* To assure cost-effective and efficient visits are provided, the nurse must master all three home visit stages: (1) the previsit stage, (2) the visit stage, and (3) the post-visit stage. Failure to efficiently plan any of these stages will result in low productivity and increased visit costs.

2. *Bag Technique.* Although often seen as old fashioned, using the nursing bag appropriately, as well as proper hand washing and equipment use and cleaning, is essential to effective patient care. Again, organization and clinical skills are imperative in using the nursing bag in the best way.

3. *Personal Safety in the Home.* Because the nurse is in the community and the privacy of the client's home, the issue of the nurse's personal safety is critically important. An orientation program for a nurse transitioning into home care must include strategies for maintaining personal safety. Such strategies include having available emergency telephone numbers, having information on what to do if the nurse feels unsafe in the home, knowing how to diffuse crisis situations, and knowing policies and procedures for the use of escorts (Durkin and Wilson, 1999; Hunter, 1997).

Infection Control

Infection control in the home is very different from that in the hospital setting. Although the underlying principles and OSHA regulations are often the same, the application of those principles is modified in the community. Compared with the hospital, the home is considered a safer environment for a client. Infection is less of a problem because of the fewer numbers and types of microbes, greater resistance of most people to their own household microbes, and exposure to fewer health care workers (Rhinehart and Friedman, 2004).

However, the home provides some unique challenges that the home care nurse must confront; for example:

- The primary caregiver for the client is usually a relative or friend who is untrained in aseptic technique and infection control measures.

- A client's environment may lack running water or may be extremely disorganized, making it difficult to minimize the risk of infection. The home setting makes it imperative that the home care nurse have the skills to develop creative solutions to infection control problems.

- The familiar red biohazard bags that are seen regularly in the hospital are not used in client homes; rather, trash bags that are disposed of in the general trash are used. Responsibility for disposal of waste often rests with the home care nurse, so a full understanding of the regulations surrounding the disposal of infected waste in the home is important. Families must be trained in the disposal of infected and hazardous waste.

- Additionally, the orientation program must include agency policy and procedures for cleaning contaminated plates as well as eating utensils, linens, bedclothes, and medical equipment used during the home visit. Most of these items can be cleaned in a standard dishwasher or clotheswasher.

The Medicare Home Care Benefit

The hospital nurse transitioning into home care likely is unfamiliar with the many components of the Medicare home care benefit. Because the nurse's judgment of the client's clinical situation is integral to Medicare reimbursement, a thorough knowledge of all Medicare regulations is essential.

1. *Home Care Eligibility.* The coverage criteria a Medicare beneficiary must meet to be eligible for the home care benefit—homebound, require skilled care, have a plan of care signed by a physician, be reasonable and necessary, and services needed part-time and intermittent—are checked by the nurse on each visit.
2. *Skilled Disciplines.* The home care nurse has to apply the concepts of skilled care on every visit. Nursing, physical therapy, and speech therapy are considered stand-alone skilled services whereas occupational therapy, social work, and home health aide services can be provided only if there is a patient need for a skilled service.
3. *Skilled Nursing.* Direct care, teaching based on newly identified needs, skilled observation and assessment, and management and evaluation of the plan of care are patient needs that must be clearly documented for Medicare reimbursement.
4. *OASIS and the Comprehensive Assessment.* In the majority of cases, the nurse is responsible for completing the compre-

hensive assessment that includes the OASIS data set on the first visit and at other periods during the patient's time on service. Selected OASIS items are used for reimbursement through the PPS and additionally through the CMS Quality Initiative. The initiative includes OBQI, the Home Care Compare "report card" initiative that began for home care in October of 2003, for operational and clinical benchmarking on a local, state, and national level. Because OASIS is used in various aspects of the agency's operations, it is a critical aspect of orientation and periodic in-service education programs.

Home Care Documentation

Although nurses in all practice settings are accustomed to the legal and organizational documentation requirements, home care documentation is unique and an essential component of an orientation program. The nurse's documentation serves as the written account of the client's history, status, interventions, and progress toward identified goals. Additionally, it serves as the basis for reimbursement for all third-party payment, and is the key to evaluation of the effectiveness of nursing intervention.

Regardless of whether the client is on managed care, Medicare, in a fee-for-service insurance program, or self pay, the ability to provide nursing services in the home is dependent on the home care nurse's skill in accurately describing what the client's needs are, justifying the skilled care necessary to meet those needs, and describing how the intervention assisted the client in meeting planned goals. The home care nurse must understand and be adept at using the myriad of forms that are unique to home care.

Client Teaching

Client and family teaching is one of the most frequently used interventions of the home care nurse. With the reduction in the number of hospital days for most patients, hospital nurses have little time to teach their patients, so the majority of teaching for self-care must occur in the home following discharge from the hospital.

Just as hospital stays have shortened with the initiation of DRGs in the 1980s, the number of home care visits per episode of care has been reduced as a result of the initiation of home care PPS in 2000. This shortened number of visits mandates that the home care nurse be expert in teaching clients and caregivers how to provide care. Understanding the clients' internal and external motivations, and applying various teaching strategies and independent adult learning approaches allows the nurse to teach in the most efficient and effective manner.

Strategies for Effective Clinical Management

The home care nurse must be an expert in collaborating with others, especially case managers, to provide comprehensive care and assure financial reimbursement. A full discussion of the case management process should be included in an orientation program and include the following:

- a definition of case management
- the role of a case manager
- where case managers are employed
- what case managers expect from a home care agency
- what case managers are concerned about
- how to develop a relationship with a case manager

A full discussion of case management and its role in home care can be found in Chapter 41.

Home Care Nursing Strategies for Success

One of the biggest differences between home care nursing and hospital nursing practice is the home care nurse's degree of autonomy. This independent practice and time with patients and families is what often brings nurses to home care. This positive aspect, however, can become a deterrent if it is not slowly introduced in the orientation program. Because the nurse cannot pass unaccomplished assessments and interventions to the next shift, the nurse new to home care can easily feel overwhelmed by the burden of autonomy. Time, caseload, and stress management strategies should be included in the orientation program as well as the preceptor role in these areas clarified so the orientee can be slowly acclimated to this practice change.

Along with the benefits of independent practice come the isolation and loneliness that new home care nurses often feel. This isolation may result in initial job frustration, with the new nurse quickly returning to an inpatient setting. Given the professional tools discussed previously in a realistic time frame and sharing strategies that allow connection to colleagues and supervisors is the overall goal of the entire orientation program. These strategies may include weekly lunch meetings with other nurses in the agency and attendance at continuing education seminars and case conferences with other professionals involved in the care of a complex client.

Legal and Ethical Aspects of Home Care

Some of the most difficult issues facing home care today are the ethical problems that arise in practice. Changes in the way health care is provided and reimbursed; the large numbers of uninsured individuals and families; changes in the structure of the family; limited resources for all types of care and regulations, such as the Health Insurance Portability and Accountability Act of 1996 (HIPAA); and protecting the rights of the individual all serve to make home care nursing practice increasingly complex. Legal issues in home care are also becoming more pressing.

Home care agencies were often excluded from litigation because they didn't have the deep pockets of hospitals or long-term care facilities. Now that home care is growing and there are large, national chains that have significant financial resources, home care agencies are often included in lawsuits. Knowledge of risk management, fraud, and abuse regulations and the guidelines around abandonment and domestic violence are among the many topics that should be included toward the end of an orientation program.

Specialized Home Care Programs and Services

Many nurses entering home care from the hospital setting are being recruited for their specialized skills. For example, nurses who are wound care experts often transfer to home care to work with clinical staff as a consultant and educator. Specialty cardiac nurses are often recruited to direct a special home care cardiac program. Even though these nurses are specialists, they must learn the basic aspects presented in this chapter to be effective.

All nurses new to home care must understand other clinical programs within and external to the agency including high-technology home care programs such as infusion and telehealthcare, hospice care, psychiatric home care, pediatric, and early newborn discharge programs.

Consider this example: The expert cardiac nurse may be seeing a patient in the home who has severe cardiomyopathy. Instead of being rehabilitated, the client seems to be on a downward progression in his or her illness. The nurse in collaboration with the physician determines that the client is terminal. Without a basic understanding of the criteria for enrollment in hospice care and the benefits afforded the client, the nurse will be unaware of this strategy that might be helpful to the client.

TEACHING STRATEGIES

Although the key content areas are important to an effective orientation program, so too is the way the material is taught. Because the relationship between the new nurse and the home care agency begins during orientation, a poorly planned experience sets a negative tone for the relationship. The teaching strategies incorporated into the orientation program are critical to the learning that takes place and can reduce the

agency investment of time and money. The following teaching strategies are examples that can be integrated into an orientation program:

- *Self-Directed Learning.* This strategy calls upon the learner to read information and accomplish learning activities independently.
- *Clinical Simulation/Documentation Exercises.* These activities use case studies to duplicate common experiences the nurse will find with patients. The learner can practice new skills in a supportive environment and collaborate with other orientees in problem identification and clinical decision making. Additionally, new nurses are given the opportunity to problem solve, question, and develop interventions with the direction of an experienced nurse.
- *Role Play.* By using experienced home care nurses in a role-play situation, the new nurse can learn about complex processes of clinical practice, such as admitting and discharging a patient.
- *Field Trips.* Field trips can be designed to provide a comprehensive understanding of the community and the home care agency. New nurses can be assigned to visit the local senior center or hospice program in the community and then share experiences in a group so everyone benefits from the experience and the information (Humphrey and Milone-Nuzzo, 1999).

CONCLUSION

Acute care nurses can bring a great deal of expertise and a new way of thinking to home health care. There is, however, a body of knowledge specific to the specialty of home care nursing that the acute care nurse must learn before being expected to be an efficient and effective home care practitioner. This chapter has outlined the operational definition of home care nursing that should guide practice, even in the ever-changing health care climate.

The differences between acute care and home care nursing practice as well as orientation content areas have been outlined to assist agencies in developing their own orientation program and competency checklists. Making the transition from acute care to home care is a collaborative effort. Nurses should begin to learn basic home care nursing principles in their educational experience and build upon that knowledge throughout their employment in a home care agency. It is up to the nurse manager and the agency's administration to provide adequate resources to teach the new nurse important content and reinforce the learning throughout the orientation period and beyond.

REFERENCES

Benefield, L. E. 2002. Evidence-based practice: Basic strategies for success. *Home Healthcare Nurse* 20(12): 803–807.

Durkin, N., and C. Wilson. 1999. Simple steps to keep yourself safe. *Home Healthcare Nurse* 17(7): 430–435.

Humphrey, C., and P. Milone-Nuzzo. 1999. *Manual of home care nursing orientation.* Gaithersburg, MD: Aspen.

Hunter, E. 1997. Violence prevention in the home health setting. *Home Healthcare Nurse* 15(6): 403–409.

Merriam-Webster's Collegiate Dictionary, 11th ed. (2003). Springfield, MA: Merriam-Webster.

Miller, M., and B. Daley. 1996. Home health care nursing: There is a difference. *Home Health Care Management and Practice* 8(4): 64–70.

Rhinehart, E., and M. Friedman. 2004. *Infection control in home care*, 2nd ed. Boston, MA: Jones & Bartlett.

U.S. Department of Labor, Occupational Safety and Health Administration. 2003. *Guidelines for preventing workplace violence*, Publication #3148. Washington, DC: Author.

CHAPTER 41

Case Management

Linda A. Billows

Case management has been a hot topic of conversation among home care providers for more than 25 years. The debate has been fueled by a number of factors: the variety of interpretations of what case management is, the concern over duplication of functions already performed by providers, and the use of case management to reduce costs by reducing services. This chapter attempts to bring some clarity to the definition of case management and raises some issues and questions for ongoing discussion.

Because of the interdependence and complexity of the components of health care, one cannot look at case management in isolation. The health care industry has an array of concepts and terms, all of which describe management of and access to health care services. Let's begin by looking at the terms under discussion:

- *Managed care:* The care typically provided by a health maintenance organization designed to enhance cost-effectiveness by eliminating inappropriate service.
- *Managed competition:* A health care theory, largely untested, based on free-market competition. Groups of providers would compete to offer services, and consumers would choose health plans based on which ones offer the best quality for the lowest price.
- *Case management:* As generally interpreted, a term with two contradictory aspects. The first aspect relates to fiscal

management; that is, whether a person falls within policy limits. This has to do with whether people are eligible for a service and what level of payment will be made. The second aspect relates to clinical management, which means a determination of what kind of medical, nursing, or social service intervention is necessary and in the best interest of the client. There was a fairly distinct separation of these functions until the past 10 years or so, when insurance companies, either in their private insurance role or in their role as administrator of Medicare programs, have blurred that separation to control what payers feel is overutilization (Halamandaris, 1990).

The Government Affairs Committee of the National Association of Home Care prepared a white paper on case management approved by the board of the National Association of Home Care in January 1991 that is still relevant today. The following is from that document.

CASE MANAGEMENT DEFINED

There are two fundamentally different types of case management: one performed by providers as an essential part of their care-giving activities, and one that some payers have superimposed on the provider system primarily as a mechanism to control costs. In some cases, both systems are responsible for assessing client needs, developing plans of care, coordinating the various services that clients receive, and carrying out monitoring and quality assurance activities.

COMPONENTS OF CASE MANAGEMENT

The delineation of payer case management functions and provider case management functions are explained below. The functions of a financial manager are as follows:

- *Assessments:* Determining whether the client is eligible under the terms of the payer's program and applying the program's coverage limits
- *Planning:* Validating the home care agency's care plan
- Coordinating benefits where there are two or more payers)
- Defining the payment system
- Conducting program evaluations and provider audits

A payer financial management system should have the following characteristics:

- A proven track record as a fiscal conduit for health and social service programs
- A staff of professionals with home care experience to validate care plans
- An appeals process that is readily accessible to beneficiaries and providers
- An approved cash management plan and/or approved performance bond
- Annual outside performance audits

Provider Case Management

Case management, as practiced in the clinical setting by home care providers, should consist of seven essential functions:

1. *Assessment:* Physical, environmental, psychological, socioeconomic, and eligibility under various third-party programs

2. *Planning:* Care plan development and validation
3. *Coordination:* Interdisciplinary and inter-agency/intraagency
4. *Organization and staffing*
5. *Staffing and resource allocation*
6. *Implementation or care provision:* Implementation of care plans and delivery of service
7. *Evaluation:* Quality assurance measures to ensure that standards of care are met

Care management is done in collaboration with the patient, family, physician, and provider. Given the central role that the care manager plays in determining the effectiveness of the care that is provided, it is essential that the care manager be fully qualified. Care managers should meet the following criteria:

- Employ the interdisciplinary team approach
- Operate as an established legal entity recognized by the state
- Meet all applicable local and state standards
- Carry professional liability insurance
- Have an established and recognized quality assurance program
- Have a proven track record of providing patient care
- Conduct business 24 hours a day, 7 days a week, including all holidays

Additional recommendations include the following:

- All clients do not need case management.
- Case management should be patient driven.
- Patients should choose whether they need case management.
- Case management should promote patient independence.
- Case management should be available to patients of all ages.
- Quality assurance should be a component of any case management function.

Since the initial development of work on case management done in the field of home care, there has been tremendous growth and expansion in the field of case management. Resources now include the Case Management Society of America and the Commission for Case Management Certification. Home care providers must stay abreast of developments in the field of case management as they interact with multiple case managers on a daily basis. Positive working relationship based on a working knowledge of case managers role and perspective can enhance the referral of clients to a home health agency.

The Commission for Case Management Certification (CCMC) defines case management as follows:

> Case management is a collaborative process that assesses, plans, implements, coordinates, monitors, and evaluates the options and services required to meet an individual's health needs, using communication and available resources to promote quality, cost effective outcomes.

The Case Manager's Handbook (Mullahy, 1998) defines a case manager as a person who makes the health care system work, influencing both the quality of the outcome and the cost (p. 9). Managed care and case management are not interchangeable concepts. Managed care is a system of cost-containment programs; case management is a process (p. 5). Discharge planning is the process that assesses a patient's need for treatment after hospitalization in order to help arrange for the necessary services and resources to effect an appropriate and timely discharge (p. 554)

QUALITY ASSURANCE

Quality assurance programs in the case management setting need to start with developing meaningful but accessible measurements of administrative and supervisory activities, comparing program costs with benefits, and monitoring progress toward objectives. The development of

structural aspects of case management may include the following activities:

- A survey of the extent to which qualifications of case managers hired meet job performance expectations
- A review by supervisors of case management, job descriptions, and requirements
- An ongoing review of recruitment activities

Process aspects of case management provide an opportunity to look at how resources are used. The following process activities should be included:

- An evaluation of the effectiveness of pre-service and in-service training provided to case managers.
- The development of norms with the objective of monitoring performance outliers to identify both ineffective case management activities and efficient activities that need to be shared to improve the process.

Outcomes are summary indicators of resource utilization and include efforts such as the following:

- Costing out of care plans (by caseload or by case) in the context of specific case mix factors
- Development of a scale to indicate the level of diversity in care plan services and to determine whether client needs are generally met within a caseload context
- Measurement of client satisfaction and client understanding of the case manager's role

All three of the domains (structure, process, and outcomes) used in the approach by Donabedian (1978, 2003) need to be included for a quality assurance program to address all facets of a service. Additionally, these efforts should be done in light of the need to identify values that are attached to the measurement within each area (Yee, 1990). Is the case manager primarily an advocate or a care accountant? Does the agency respond to client crisis or only to on-going needs after the client has stabilized? To what extent do case managers make care plan and services decisions with others?

TRAINING OF HOME HEALTH AGENCY STAFF

As home health agencies expand their experience in working in the managed care environment, many are including case management training for their staff. The training may include such topics as costing out-of-care plans, case-mix analysis, outcomes, development of industry norms, and so forth. Sharing these training programs with managed care companies and with case managers increases their understanding of the expertise of home health agencies. Home health agencies are broadening their capabilities in outcome data, and these increased capabilities will be extremely useful to agency staff as well as other providers and insurers.

CONCLUSION

Case management and other types of management are being proposed as ways of improving the health care system, yet one has to search far and wide for references to improved client satisfaction. Discussion is focused on cost and impact on providers and insurers, yet there is a lack of clarity about exactly what outcomes can be expected from case management.

- How will case management affect clients?
- How will it improve care?
- What outcomes are expected from a case management system?
- How much will case management cost?
- How much will case management save?
- How will it be monitored?
- Who will be the case manager?
- What is the qualification of the case manager?
- How will duplication be reduced?

As the discussion on all levels continues regarding case management, it will be important for home care providers to continue to be active participants in the debate. Home health agencies may or may not be part of health care systems, but the home health perspective remains unique in any discussion and a vital part of case management from all viewpoints.

REFERENCES

Donabedian, A. 1978. The quality of medical care. In R. H. Ablest (ed.). *Health care regulations, economics, ethics, and practice*. Washington, D.C.: American Association for the Advancement of Science.

Donabedian, A. 2003. *An introduction to quality assurance in health care*. Rashid Bashur (ed.). New York: Oxford University Press.

Halamandaris, V. 1990. The paradox of case management. *Caring* 9: 4–7.

Hoyer, R. 1990. Where are we and where do we go from here? *Caring* 9: 4–12.

Mullahy, Catherine M. (ed.). 1998. *The Case manager's handbook*. Gaithersburg, MD: Aspen Publications.

Yee, D. 1990. Developing a quality assurance program in case management services settings. *Caring* 9: 30–36.

CHAPTER 42

Managed Care

Mary Pat Larsen

In the United States, home care is a dynamic and diverse service industry. More than 7.6 million individuals receive home care provided by approximately 20,000 providers. Annual expenditures for home health care were projected to be approximately $41.3 billion in 2001 (National Association for Home Care and Hospice [NAHC], 2001).

Home care agencies have been providing services to patients for more than a century. Medicare's enactment in 1965 truly accelerated the industry's growth. In 1973 services were extended to certain younger disabled Americans.

Between 1967 and 1985, the number of agencies certified to participate in the Medicare program grew by more than threefold from 1,753 to 5,983 (NAHC, 2001). By the mid-1980s, the number of Medicare-certified agencies leveled off, which was a result of increasing Medicare paperwork and unreliable payment policies. As a result, in 1987, these problems led to a lawsuit brought against the Health Care Financing Administration (HCFA) by a coalition of U.S. Congress members led by Reps. Claude Pepper (D-FL) and Harley Staggers (D-WV), consumer groups, and the National Association for Home Care (NAHC, 2001). The outcome of this lawsuit provided NAHC with the opportunity to participate in rewriting the Medicare home care payment policies. As a result of these revisions, Medicare's annual home care benefit significantly increased, and the number of home care agencies rose to over 10,000 (NAHC, 2001).

However, between 1997 and 2001, there was a 31.5 percent decline in the number of Medicare-certified agencies (down to 7,152) as a result of the Balanced Budget Act (BBA) of 1997 that impacted Medicare home health reimbursement (The Lewin Group, 1999; Medicare Program, 2000).

In 1960, the percentage of the gross national product (GNP) spent on health care was 5.2 percent. In 1992, the percentage of the GNP spent on health care was 14 percent. The rate of growth in health care spending grew 4.8 percent in 1998 and 5.6 percent in 1999. Projected growth in health care spending over the next decade (2000 to 2010) is believed to be fueled in part by rising provider costs and the insurer's inability to negotiate increasing price discounts (Heffler et al., 2001; National Health Expenditures, 2004).

Between fiscal years 1998 and 2000, Medicare spending dropped from $14 billion to $9.1 billion (a 34 percent decrease). No other benefit in the Medicare program experienced proportionate reductions. The main cause of the reduction was the BBA's introduction of the interim payment system (IPS). Essentially the BBA required that reimbursement limits be held to a below-inflation rate of growth by excluding a 2-year period from the home health inflation adjustment.

In addition, payments under IPS were restricted to the lowest of the agency's costs, its per-visit cost limits or its per-beneficiary cost limits. The Lewin Group estimated 90 percent of

Original chapter written by Nina M. Smith.

agencies would have costs that exceeded BBA limits in 1998 by an average of 32 percent assuming no change in Medicare practice patterns.

The BBA directed HCFA to develop a prospective payment system (PPS) for Medicare home health organizations. On October 1, 2000, HCFA implemented home health PPS. The idea behind the move from a modified fee-for-service payment system to a PPS was that by setting a national pay rate, providers would become more efficient in providing care. One indicator that this has become a reality is the HCIS home health data, which reports an average of 73 visits/patient in 1997 decreasing to 42 visits/patient in 2000 (http://www.nahc.org/Consumer/hcstats.html).

Largely in reaction to spiraling costs and drastic changes in Medicare methods of reimbursement, some home health agency survivors have positioned themselves formally (under contract) in the vertical continuum of care by becoming providers for managed care organizations (MCOs).

The number of Americans in some type of managed care arrangement has risen from 15 million individuals in 1984 to greater than 75 million individuals in 1995.

Managed care refers to an overall strategy for containing or minimizing medical care costs, while delivering appropriate medical care. In managed care, enrollees who pay reduced fees to visit their primary care physician (PCP) often cannot visit a specialist without prior authorization from their PCP.

Because the health care industry needed to control and lower costs, managed care became more popular. To contain costs, managed care companies exercise control by denying or limiting coverage, promoting the use of generic drugs, and encouraging prevention and wellness programs and limiting access to certain providers without prior authorization. However, in response, enrollees voiced frustration regarding some limits and as a result preferred provider organization (PPO) and point of service (POS) plans were developed in recent years. These allow enrollees to use both in- and out-of-network physicians and hospitals, although these plans frequently require higher co-pays and deductibles.

Consumers now have more protection with regard to managed care companies as most states have enacted laws concerning managed care such as:

- Forbid financial incentives to physicians who intentionally limit care
- Provide for complaints/appeals of coverage decisions
- Specify when emergency room care is necessary
- Require minimum hospital stays for maternity patients
- Prohibit gag clauses (those clauses that forbid the physician from disparaging the health plan)

Another result of the growth of managed care has been physicians pushing for unionization. Doctors cite a loss in their decision-making authority and a drop in reimbursement from HMOs. As an example, some HMOs specify the number of patients a physician can see in one day and/or deny coverage for certain procedures that are deemed medically necessary by physicians. In some plans, physicians whose expenditures for patients are regarded as too high are dropped from the health plan. Consumers can expect to witness the union movement to continue to gain momentum based on these issues (HIAA and AHCPR, 1995).

The growth and development of managed care shows the change from utilization management and controlling access to the future development of specific, cost-effective services in the least restrictive environments (Exhibit 42–1). MCOs are moving toward constructing organized networks of providers to deliver care in a coherent, integrated, efficient fashion (Sederer and Bennett, 1996)

As plans merge, separate, and grow, they take on characteristics of each other. There are two major types of managed care organizations: payer-based and provider-based. Payer-based organizations include insurance companies,

Exhibit 42–1 Growth And Development of Managed Care

- 1863—Case management was defined through social work systems to coordinate public human services and conserve public funds.
- 1900—Case management started as a part of public health nursing.
- 1929—A rural farmer's cooperative health plan was established in Oklahoma.
- 1929—Two California physicians entered into a prepaid contract to provide comprehensive health care to 2,000 water company employees.
- 1937—The Group Health Association was founded in Washington.
- 1942—The Kaiser-Permanente Medical Care Program was started.
- 1945—After World War II, necessary community services were extended to discharged psychiatric patients.
- 1947—The Health Insurance Plan of Greater New York began.
- 1950—The Hill-Burton Act created a number of community-based regional medical centers.
- 1950s—Employee assistance programs (EAPs) were started as an occupational health service for alcoholics.
- 1951—The Joint Commission on Accreditation of Healthcare Organizations was formed.
- 1954—One of the first independent physician association (IPA) plans was started in California.
- 1963—Community mental health center programs were initiated.
- 1965—Medicaid was established by the federal government to provide health care services to the poor.
- 1965—Medicare was introduced to ensure health care access for the elderly.
- 1965—The Older Americans Act was passed to provide federal funding support for older Americans and the development of the Administration on Aging.
- 1970s—Workers' compensation case management began.
- 1973—Congress passed the HMO act to encourage third-party payers to increase control of medical care delivery and enable managed-

- care plans to increase in numbers and to expand enrollments.
- 1974—The Nixon administration made an attempt to control costs by freezing physician fees.
- 1974—The Employee Retirement Income Security Act (ERISA) allowed self-funded insurance plans to avoid paying premiums and taxes, and to avoid compliance with state-mandated benefits, even though these costs were necessary for insurance companies and managed care plans; it also required that plans and companies provide an explanation of benefits (EOB) statement in the event that a claim was denied and to inform the individual of his or her right for appeal.
- 1979—Seventeen utilization review companies were operating for disability and medical-surgical cases.
- 1979—The National Committee for Quality Assurance (NCQA) was founded by the Group Health Association of America and the American Managed Care and Review Association.
- Early 1980s—Telephonic utilization review for patients with psychiatric and substance abuse problems was started.
- Early 1980s—Preferred provider organizations (PPOs) began to develop.
- 1981—The Omnibus Budget Reconciliation Act (OBRA) was passed to encourage community-based alternatives to provide care to the elderly in lieu of institutional placement.
- 1982—The Tax Equity and Fiscal Responsibility Act (TEFRA) was created to control Medicare costs.
- 1983—DRGs were used as a means for TEFRA control of medical-surgical diagnoses.
- 1985—The Consolidated Omnibus Budget Reconciliation Act (COBRA) was passed to require employers to offer continued health insurance coverage for a certain length of time after the group health insurance had been terminated.
- 1986–1992—Managed behavioral health care companies were carved out of traditional indemnity medical-surgical plans.

Continues

Exhibit 42–1 continued

- 1989—The Physician Payment Review Commission was created to implement legislation that introduced a resource-based fee schedule that limited the amount physicians could charge patients above the fee schedule and volume performance standards.
- 1993—The Health Security Act (HR 3600) was enacted to provide the security of a comprehensive health benefit plan to all Americans that could never be taken away.
- 1994—The Medicare Choice Act was passed to allow Medicare-eligible beneficiaries the

choice of traditional Medicare benefit plans or enrollment in an integrated health plan. •
1996—Congress considered parity for behavioral health programs by carving them back into medical-surgical plans.
- 1988 to the present—Industry consolidation of managed care companies is occurring through mergers and acquisitions to achieve economies of scale and reduce redundant costs.

Source: List reprinted from Blador, R. A. (1996). *Managed Care Made Simple*. Cambridge, MA: Blackwell.

HMOs, PPOs, self-insured employers, third-party administrators (TPAs), and workers' compensation administrators. Provider-based organizations include hospitals, medical groups, home health agencies, and alternate-site companies. The following is a brief description of the types of managed care organizations (Cherney, 1995):

- Insurance companies are difficult to define because they may offer a wide variety of managed care plans, such as an HMO, a PPO, or a hybrid.
- HMOs can be both financiers and providers of health care services that assume all or part of the risks of providing services.
- There are four major types of HMOs plus several hybrid plans:
  1. An independent practice association (IPA) is a separate legal entity formed by physicians for the purpose of contracting with payers. Physicians are contracted by the IPA to provide medical services for a negotiated fee, which is either per capita or fee for service. Physicians retain their individual practices and service IPA patients. This

structure comprises 60 percent of HMO plans.
  2. Staff model HMOs have physicians as employees of the health plan, with a broad range of specialties. The premiums and revenue compensate physicians with salary and incentive programs.
  3. Group model HMOs subcontract for services with multispecialty group practices to provide all or part of the medical services. The health plan compensates the medical group for services at a negotiated rate. Captive group models, recruit and form their own physicians group; independent group models contract with existing, independent multispecialty groups.
  4. Network model HMOs contract with two or more medical practices to provide medical services that are single-specialty medical groups or multi-specialty medical groups. Network physicians can service their own patients as well as the HMO patients.
  5. Other HMO structures include point-of-service (POS) or open-ended plans (care from any willing provider with

higher out-of-pocket expenses), self-insured HMO plans, and any number of other hybrid plans.

- PPOs contract with preferred providers who agree to accept discounts, comply with utilization review guidelines, and assume no financial risk for providing medical services. The incentive to the employee is to use preferred providers to lower their out-of-pocket expenses.
- An exclusive provider organization (EPO) is a type of PPO in which enrollees are covered only for services by network providers.
- Self-insured employers manage their own health care benefits. A company might be a large corporation or a number of small-er, self-insured employers enrolled in a large pool.
- TPAs are local, regional, or national companies responsible for managing health care benefits established by self-insured employers. TPAs are service management providers and do not establish benefits.
- Workers' compensation administrators work with the insurance commissioner in most states to establish workers' compensations benefits and are highly regulated.
- Managed indemnity plans impose utilization review on care delivered by any provider, and providers do not have contracts with the plan.
- Provider-based organizations include hospitals, medical groups, and alternate-site companies that provide care with financial risk.

IMPLICATIONS OF MANAGED CARE IN HOME CARE

Home care markets grew rapidly during the 1980s, and profit margins were at an all-time high. With the introduction of managed care into the home care arena, reimbursements and intensifying competition have affected the many businesses negatively. To ensure operational success, home care companies must begin a strategic analysis of their operations and plan for the future. Agencies that adjust their marketing and operational strategies will be able to position for survival into managed care.

Strategic Planning

Developing a strategic plan is a simple yet difficult process. The steps are simple, but the honesty it takes to review organizational systems comprehensively might be difficult. Using a SWOT (strengths, weaknesses, opportunities, and threats) analysis as a method of review can be an effective tool in honestly recognizing difficulties and strengths. It is important to review current operations, financial status, mix of payer sources, quality, the reputation of the staff, internal and external opportunities and threats, and the impact of change on the organization. Representatives in the process should come from all levels of the agency, and honesty should be encouraged. The administration should realisti- cally assess all aspects of goal setting, objectives, priorities, time frames, methods of achieving results, understanding costs, and implications to agency survival (Good strategic plans, 1993).

CONTRACTING WITH MANAGED CARE ORGANIZATIONS

In a managed care system, the purchaser agrees to pay a premium to the MCO to either provide directly or ensure provision of the most appropriate, cost effective, high quality services to enrollees. These purchasers of managed care may represent various types of organizations, including insurance companies; self-insured employers; federal, state, and county government agencies; and individuals. The MCO's contractual responsibility is to "manage care"; either directly or through subcontracting providers for example home health agencies. A provider delivers purchased services; however, it is not party

to the contract that governs the arrangement between the purchaser and the MCO. The provider
has a separate contract with the MCO.

Maintain an Optimal Bargaining Position/Prepare

In order for a home health agency to gain leverage, they need to understand the degree to which
the MCO views them as central to the provision
of services. The home health agency should assess its own position as well as the MCO's position in the respective marketplace. Learn as
much as possible about the MCO's "track
record." Having knowledge of the MCO's financial stability, structural framework, and administrative record will help the home health
agency gauge the degree to which the MCO is
likely to be rigid or flexible during negotiations.

In most cases, the MCO will present the
provider with a "boilerplate" contract. First and
foremost, examine the critical elements of the
contract:

- Make sure all documents referred to such
  as lists, tables, charts, and any other
  incorporated documents accompany the
  contract.
- Make sure the referenced documents can-
  not be amended or modified without the
  provider's prior approval.
- Ask for a copy of the MCO's contract
  with the purchaser in order to identify any
  requirements that apply because of the
  MCO–provider contract.
- Specify all parties.
- Be certain all definitions are clear and un-
  derstood by all parties.
- Assign obligations or fights.
- Address marketing activities.
- Determine the governing law.
- Determine the full capabilities of the
  provider.
- Delineate covered services.
- Identify standards of care.
- Specify service delivery access.

- Provide for care coordination.
- Determine how referrals are made.
- Consider exclusivity. An exclusivity provision is an agreement by one or both parties to contract exclusively with each
  other. Although the provider may be able
  to negotiate higher rates due to the exclusivity, it may suffer financially if it does
  not receive adequate enrollment. Exclusivity is not generally required in the
  managed care industry and could raise antitrust concerns. Unless there is a clear,
  well-documented business advantage, the
  provider should negotiate to avoid exclusivity provisions and should include a provision stating that the contract does not
  preclude the provider from contracting
  with others.
- Determine how medical necessity and utilization review are accomplished.
- Assess the extent of quality assurance activities.
- Assess the extent of records and reports.
- Determine the limits of stop-loss coverage.
- Understand how coordination of benefits
  is accomplished.
- Determine required copayments.
- Determine limits of insurance coverage.
- Include indemnification clauses.

After reviewing these critical elements, consider
the following (Substance Abuse and Mental
Health Services Administration, 2002):

- What liabilities are created by specific
  provisions?
- Which modifications can the provider not
  afford to proceed with simply because the
  risks are unacceptable?
- How can the proposed modifications be
  drafted so that they reduce provider financial and clinical risk, are equitable to both
  parties, and do not frustrate the essential
  objectives of the MCO?
- Under what conditions should the provider walk away?

Ethics

Although ethics and managed care are not mutually exclusive, it does take a concerted effort to find a collaborative middle ground where care and cost can meet. A number of ethical issues have emerged in response to managed care's growth (Appleby, 1996; Baldor, 1996; Dasco and Dasco, 1996) :

- *Provider–patient relationships*—Mutual trust and cost factors can be at odds.
- *Confidentiality*—The more individuals who have access to medical information, the higher the potential for breach of confidentiality.
- *Universal care*—How do the present system structures provide, at least, minimal care to everyone?
- *Conflicts of interest*—Questions exist as to the role and ownership of services related to the payer, provider, or customer.
- *Clinically appropriate levels of care*—Providers and payers are at odds over patient treatment plans.
- *Contracting*—Leads to questions of incentives and motives for treatment or nontreatment.
- *Rationing of care*—Is it done universally for all or is it only for specific populations?
- *Ethical guidelines*—Identification, education, and awareness are necessary to inform the leaders, the providers, and the public of their responsibilities and methods to address their needs.

Legal and Regulatory Issues

Legal and regulatory issues are changing as fast as managed care can create new problems and stretch the already difficult to interpret laws.

Antireferrals

The Omnibus Budget Reconciliation Act of 1993 (OBRA 1993) extended the prohibitions to cover several additional categories of health services and to include the Medicaid program

(Stark I). Stark I regulations were proposed in March 1992 and completed with final publication in August 1995. Before the final revision was published, the regulations had undergone may changes, were renamed Stark II, and included 11 designated services for which a bill or claim could not be made pursuant to a prohibited referral, with the focus on services provided rather than the entity providing the services. The law also requires that entities providing designated services report ownership information and arrangements to the Department of Health and Human Services (Dasco and Dasco, 1996).

Safe Harbors

Safe harbors provisions are payment practices that would not be subject to criminal prosecution and that would not provide a basis for exclusion from the Medicare program or from the state health care program. In November 1992, the Office of the U.S. Inspector General issued two safe harbor regulations governing managed care activities; they were published in *57 Federal Register* (FR52723), *pp.* 52724–52730, effective immediately. The regulations protect health plans that offer increased coverage or reduced costs to enrollees and protect reductions offered by health care providers to health plans so that neither would be considered illegal remuneration subject to fraud and abuse penalties under the Antikickback statute (Tamborlane, 1993).

Antitrust Issues

Integrated delivery systems—whether horizontal, vertical, or conglomerate—are business relationships that can easily cause antitrust violations if not carefully negotiated. Horizontal integration involves similar businesses that may be direct economic competitors. Conglomerate integration involves businesses that produce unrelated products or services. Price fixing, division of markets, exclusive contracts, and noncompete agreements are the common violations that need to be addressed before contracting (Dasco and Dasco, 1996).

The Future of Managed Care Related to Home Care Populations

According to U.S. Department of Health and Human Services Secretary Tommy Thompson, "One of the biggest fallacies is that (the Administration) is going to force all seniors into HMOs which is not the case," Thompson stated. "There are several proposals on the table right now, but the final decision has not been made."

The George W. Bush administration might not force seniors into managed Medicare plans, but it is clear that MCOs are going to be the centerpiece of the new proposal that includes alternatives to fee-for-service plans. More than half (51 percent) of the health care marketplace currently is enrolled in PPOs, and 18 percent more are in point-of-service plans.

Even Secretary Thompson said, "Prevention and improved disease management programs are the areas we need to focus on the most as we move forward." These, of course, are the key elements that managed care was founded on, and they are not exactly areas of strength.

REFERENCES

Appleby, C. 1996. Ethics and managed care. *Hospitals & Health Networks* 70(13): 20–27.

Baldor, R. A. 1996. *Managed care made simple.* Cambridge, MA: Blackwell, pp. 2–22, 30–32.

Cherney, A. 1995, Sept. Managed care strategies presentation. Walnut Creek, CA: Western Medical Services.

Dasco, S. T., and C. C. Dasco. 1996. *Managed care answer book: 1996 supplement.* Gaithersburg, MD: Aspen.

Freeman, M. C., and T. Trabin. 1994. *Managed behavioral healthcare: History, models, key issues, and future course.* Washington, DC: U.S. Dept. of Health and Human Services and U.S. Center for Mental Health Services, pp. 9–17.

Good strategic plans will guide you to success in managed care market. 1993. *Managed Home Care Report* 2(5): 2–3.

Health Care Financing Administration. National Health Expenditures Projections: 2000–2010. Available at *www.hcfa.gov* (accessed February 10, 2004).

Heffler S., K. Levit, S. Smith, and C. Smith. 2001, March/April. Health spending growth up in 1999: Faster growth expected In the future, *Health Affairs* 20(2).

The Lewin Group. 1999, August 11. *An impact analysis for home health agencies of the Medicare home health interim payment system of the 1997 Balanced Budget Act.* Washington, DC: National Association for Home Care.

McCue, Michael T. 2003, March. It's time for all Americans to play follow the leader. *Managed Healthcare Executive* 114: 76–80.

Medicare program: Prospective payment system for home health agencies. 2000, July 3. *Federal Register* 65(128): 41128–41214.

"HIAA and AHCPR join forces to help consumers choose and use managed care plans." (press release, August 28, 1995)

National Association for Home Care and Hospice. 2001, Nov. Basic statistics about home care. Available at *http://www.nahc.org/Consumer/hcstats.html* (accessed December 2003).

Sederer, L. I., and M. J. Bennett. 1996. Managed mental health care in the United States: A status report. *Administration and Policy in Mental Health* 23(4): 289–305.

Substance Abuse and Mental Health Services Administration. 2002, Aug. 17. Managed care contracting. Available at http://www.samhsa.gov (accessed June 5, 2003).

Tamborlane, T. A. 1993, June. Managed care: New legal challenges. *Caring:* 62–65.

CHAPTER 43

Community-Based Long-Term Care: Preparing for a New Role

Pearl B. Graub and Emily Amerman

Directing health or social service organizations in an era of rampant change and heightened competition challenges managers' every waking moment. As government and private payers shift costs, tighten reimbursement, and experiment with prospective payment and capitation, the truism that "form follows finance" is brought home anew. Reimbursement policy and economic incentives have a profound impact on the delivery of service by home health care providers and indeed by all providers. More than ever before, our vision of service delivery must not be limited by current regulatory parameters.

A tremendous demographic and cultural shift has been occurring, one that will have a major effect on home health care. The number and proportion of older Americans are increasing dramatically. As a result of increased longevity and a low birthrate, one in five people will be older than 75 in the year 2020. People over the age of 75 are more likely than younger persons to experience chronic illnesses and other disabling conditions that interfere with their ability to function independently. They are more likely to be at risk of living in a nursing home or to be in need of ongoing health and social services. This surge in numbers of disabled older people, coupled with shortened acute care stays, means an increasing emphasis on long-term care. The demand for long-term care services has led policy makers and providers to respond with incremental and noteworthy changes. Ultimately, home health agencies will provide greater and

greater proportions of service to patients with needs outside those currently defined as "skilled care."

The combination of increasing demand for long-term care and the interest by governments and private payers in substituting long-term home care for institutional care when clinically and economically feasible bodes well for home health agencies. The growth in demand for community-based long-term care will create both an opportunity and a challenge for home health agencies in the next decade. Since 1982, home health agencies in Philadelphia have had the opportunity to collaborate in community-based long-term care. This chapter describes the Pennsylvania model of home and community-based long-term care as it is operationalized in Philadelphia and the critical role home health providers play. To place the model in context, current trends in long-term care policy and practice are outlined. The chapter concludes with observations and recommendations to assist home health administrators in planning and competing for involvement in community-based long-term programs.

LONG-TERM CARE DEFINED

For decades "long-term care" referred to a place or a facility where chronically ill, old people were cared for until they died. The reality is that for every older person in an intermediate or skilled care facility, there are at least two people who look the same who live in the community. Thus, approximately 5 percent of those over age 65 are in a nursing home at any one time; another 10 percent who need comparable levels of long-term care are at home. The fact that the largest provider of long-term care services is the American family is finally coming to light. Studies continually affirm that *most* long-term care is performed by family caregivers, despite myths to the contrary. However, families need help caring for their loved ones and that need contributes to an ever-increasing demand for long-term care services.

More recent definitions of long-term care refer to a systematic plan of care provided over an indefinite time period to chronically ill, functionally disabled adults, most of whom are old. Because many older people have multiple health and social service needs, and because they may not remain medically stable, long-term care must cut across service delivery systems (health, mental health, and aging) as well as across service settings and levels of care. Long-term care consumers may need acute care, restorative care, extended rehabilitation, maintenance or custodial care, and/or support and hospice care. They may need institutional care or they may be cared for at home. Their *level of care* no longer automatically determines their *locus of care*. The goal of long-term care is to promote the highest level of independent functioning possible in the least restrictive setting while attending to the consumer's preferences and ensuring his or her safety.

CURRENT POLICY AND PROGRAM TRENDS

The rapid increase in the number of persons needing long-term care and the corresponding rise in Medicaid expenditures (and Medicare to a lesser degree) has led state and federal policy makers to set in motion a dramatic shift from institutional to community-based long-term care. Some states have placed moratoria on the building of new long-term care facilities; many have discouraged the growth of nursing home beds in other ways. As states shift dollars to programs designed to prevent or delay placement, Medicaid expenditures for community-based alternatives to nursing home care have grown substantially. The Commonwealth of Pennsylvania, for example, expects 40 percent of the Medicaid long-term care beds in the state to be in community-based long-term care by 2008.

Financial incentives, aligned with consumer preference for community-based care, have offered a powerful inducement for the development of a range of long-term care options in the community. The notion of community-based long-term care is not new. For the past 30 years, the Health Care Financing Administration (now the Centers for Medicare and Medicaid Services, or CMS) has been experimenting with community-based models of care for older adults at risk of institutionalization. In the mid-1980s, the federal government financed a nationwide study of the viability of in-home long-term care called The National Long-Term Care Channeling Demonstration. They also studied the feasibility of health maintenance organizations (HMOs) with long-term care benefits added, called social health maintenance organizations (SHMOs). A variety of other experiments targeting specific populations or disease management strategies have been funded, such as the Medicare Alzheimer's program. However, in the last decade, two programs have emerged as the most widely replicated models of community-based long-term care, the Home and Community Based Services (HCBS) programs, and the Program of All-Inclusive Care for the Elderly (PACE).

The Home and Community Based Services program gives states the option of using federal Medicaid waivers to move money targeted to publicly funded nursing home care to community-based long-term care, as long as the population served meets the clinical and financial eligibility criteria for a nursing facility. Administered by the state Medicaid agency, HCBS programs are generally operated by local Area Agencies on Aging (AAAs) or by long-term care providers. In these programs, a subset of people identified as nursing home eligible have the option of care at home, assisted by a care manager and an array of supportive services. HCBS consumers are offered a wide range of providers from whom to receive services and are involved in a process of continuous quality assessment of those providers. Home health care is a key service in this model, assisting with ongoing interdisciplinary assessment and chronic disease management.

PACE, modeled after its San Francisco–based parent, On Lok, is a fully capitated system of acute and long-term care for frail elders in the community. PACE offers the full spectrum of community-based long-term care services, as well as primary and specialty medical care, medications, hospital, home care and nursing home care, and palliative care when necessary. PACE receives a single monthly payment for each person in the program from Medicaid and Medicare, and offers an individualized plan of care based on the person's needs and preferences. Once a demonstration program, PACE is now a type of Medicare-managed care provider (established by Congress in 1997). The focal point of care is an enhanced adult day health center that participants attend from 1 to 5 days weekly, where their care plan is developed and managed by an interdisciplinary team consisting of a geriatrician, nurse, social worker, physical therapist, occupational therapist, speech and recreational therapist, nutritionist, personal care aide, and driver. The goal of PACE is to maximize quality of life by promoting independence and reducing unnecessary hospital and nursing home use. In contrast to HCBS, most PACE services are provided directly by the interdisciplinary team and PACE staff, with a select network of contracted providers.

Both HCBS and PACE participants must meet the financial and clinical eligibility criteria for a Medicaid long-term care bed. In Pennsylvania, the Area Agencies on Aging serve as the gatekeepers to long-term care, screening applicants, and providing preadmission assessment to determine a level of care and recommend a locus of care. Hallmarks of both HCBS and PACE are that they are responsive to the consumer's desire to remain as independent as possible living at home, and that the cost of services is lower than the cost of a state-subsidized nursing home bed.

Nationwide, the majority of community-based long-term care programs rely on two principal components: *care management*, which includes comprehensive assessment, development of a plan of care, implementing the care plan (providing and arranging for services), ongoing follow-up and monitoring, and periodic formal reassessment of the person' needs; and *care,* which is the provision of a range of intervention and services that may include home health, personal care and homemaker service, home-delivered meals, adult day health care, transportation, emergency response systems, durable medical equipment and assistive devices, heavy cleaning, home repairs, legal services, financial management, pastoral counseling, primary medical care, palliative care, and others.

Support to caregivers, in the form of caregiver assessment, education, training, peer support, and various kinds of respite, has become an integral part of community-based long-term care to bolster this silent, unpaid workforce. In fact, a federal Family Caregiver Support Program was initiated in recent years, offering a subsidy and services specifically aimed at prolonging the efforts of families caring for loved ones at home.

Pennsylvania continues to pursue integrated models of care, breaking down barriers between systems and levels of care to offer a flexible menu of options rather than separate silos of care. An example of this is the effort to combine HCBS and Domiciliary Care (adult foster care).

Several additional trends warrant mentioning. First, the crucial role of the direct caregiver in long-term care has finally gained national attention, as has recognition of the current and future *direct care workforce shortage.* As baby boomers begin to need long-term care over the next 50 years, the workforce shortage will be multiplied exponentially. Major steps must be taken to develop not only a new focus on the direct care worker that embraces respect, excellent training, and attractive wage and benefit packages, but also a new culture of long-term care. That new culture celebrates the autonomy, dignity and privacy of the consumer, assures their right to make decisions about their care, offers care at home or in home-like environs, and fully integrates the direct care worker on the care team as a consumer advocate and a keen observer of their well-being. Policy makers, foundations, and providers are presently promoting direct-care initiatives and long-term care culture change efforts.

A second trend is *consumer cost sharing* for services in state and local programs serving people over-income for fully subsidized care. The challenge in cost-sharing policy is to implement systems that are fair to the consumer, streamlined and simple, offer rights of appeal, and keep the cost below the revenue generated. A third trend, evolving from the disabilities community, is *personal assistant services*, which offer consumers in community-based long-term care programs the option of hiring, directing, and supervising their own personal assistant. The consumer defines the parameters of the job and is granted the resources and freedom to purchase and arrange the service.

Another significant development over the last 20 years is the proliferation and evolution of private long-term care insurance. There are now over 120 policies available, most of which cover both institutional and in-home long-term care. About nine policies corner the market. As the insured become beneficiaries, they will need home health care and an array of other services. Long-term care expenses, including home care, are now tax deductible, thanks to the Health Insurance Reform Act of 1996.

Practical experience and a review of the literature confirm that nursing and social work are the two professional disciplines most appropriate to direct community-based long-term care. The interrelationships among medical history, active medical problem, health status, functional capacity, cognitive status, emotional well-being, family relationships, and the physical environment are complex and demand the knowledge and skills of both nursing and social work. At its best, community-based long-term care engages consumers, families, professionals, and paraprofessionals in prevention, rehabilitation, maintenance, and management of chronic diseases and conditions. Nurses or social workers may be selected to be care managers; the best service delivery models use both nurses and social workers, and some use interdisciplinary teams.

THE AREA AGENCY ON AGING: A PARTNER IN SERVICE DELIVERY

Area Agencies on Aging (AAAs) were mandated by the Older Americans Act of 1965. Numbering more than 600, they form a nationwide network of planning and service agencies focused on the well-being of older citizens. Their major responsibilities include planning, advocacy, program development, and the prudent purchase of services. AAAs prepare an annual area plan delineating demographic trends, projected service needs, gaps in service, and priorities for program development and service delivery in their planning and service area. Each year, a fixed allocation of federal and state money, derived from several funding streams, is made to each AAA, with which the AAA is to carry out its plan. AAAs fund a wide array of services for older people, including senior center nutrition and recreation programs; health screening and promotion programs; and services to homebound people, such as home delivered meals, homemaker services, and chore services. In their role as advocate for older people, AAAs often fund employment programs, legal services, and public education programs on issues relating to aging. AAAs also may host a nursing home ombudsman.

In their role as a prudent purchaser, AAAs develop specific program standards and specifications for services. Because they are not usually direct service providers, they endeavor to create and encourage a climate of healthy competition among providers. At one time, some AAAs selected service providers on a competitive basis so that all potential providers in the service area would have the opportunity to seek public funding to deliver services to AAA consumers. Providers were selected on the basis of written proposals, price, in-person presentations, and other criteria. This process promoted a high quality of care and simultaneously kept prices down.

With the rapid increase in Medicaid expenditures for long-term care, states are becoming increasingly interested in establishing AAAs' capacity to serve as gatekeeper, conserving resources by ensuring that the most needy people are served and directed to resources prudently. The AAA is viewed by policy makers as a logical choice for gatekeeper because of its mission of advocacy for older adults and its experience in assessing need and allocating resources effectively. At one time, AAAs were thought to be exempt from the financial incentives provider agencies have to prescribe their particular service and to prescribe it in amounts and ways that increase revenue but decrease burden and expense. In the early days of the AAA network, AAAs commonly allocated blocks of funds to homemaker agencies, for example, and permitted those agencies to identify needy consumers and prescribe service. AAAs found that providers tended to serve fewer consumers with larger blocks of service than judged necessary by the AAA. However, AAAs too, in becoming providers of community-based long-term care services, must monitor themselves to assure that they do not succumb to viewing consumers' needs in terms of the solutions they have readily available, whether or not other approaches to care may be better. On the other hand, control of consumer assessment and care plan development by care managers employed by the AAA has led to an increase in the number of consumers served, an increase in the choices of delivery patterns, and a reduction in average consumer cost.

AAAs then become the point of access to publicly financed service and, in the minds of some policy makers, are in a position to control that access consistent with larger policy goals. In some states, the AAA network is the basis for the expansion of publicly funded, community-based long-term care benefits. The Philadelphia AAA is an example of this model.

The Philadelphia Model

The AAA for Philadelphia County is the Philadelphia Corporation for Aging (PCA). In 1982, PCA hosted and administered the Philadelphia Channeling Project, part of the National Long-Term Care Channeling Demonstration. This national demonstration examined the efficacy of community-based long-term care, assessment, care management, an array of selected services, and the impact on outcomes for participants. Following the demonstration, the Pennsylvania Department of Aging (PDA) adopted the model and expanded it to other counties within Pennsylvania between 1985 and 1990. This program, Community Care Options (CCO) administered in Philadelphia by PCA, was supported by Pennsylvania state lottery funds to maintain a population of very frail adults in their own homes. In 1990, Pennsylvania committed lottery funds for this program to go statewide and changed its name to the Options Program, which continues today.

In 1995, the Pennsylvania Department of Public Welfare (DPW) followed many other states in seeking Home and Community Based Services (Medicaid waiver) for older adults from HCFA (now CMS). Medicaid is a federal/state matching program, and the Pennsylvania match is 53 percent federal government and 47 percent state government funds. DPW administers the program through the PDA and the AAAs; it is known as the PDA Waiver. The PDA Waiver program was initiated in Philadelphia and then expanded across the state. As in the Options Program, consumers have to be clinically eligible for a nursing facility; however, they must also be financially eligible for Medicaid (nursing home grant).

In 2001, Pennsylvania implemented the "Bridge" Program for individuals clinically eligible for a nursing facility at Medicaid-income levels, but with assets up to $40,000 above Medicaid allowable assets. The goal was to serve the near-eligible, assisting them to spend down into full eligibility for the PDA Medicaid Waiver. Funds for this program were allocated from the nationwide Tobacco Settlement Fund.

To be eligible for PCA's community-based services—Options, Waiver, or Bridge—each consumer must be assessed by PCA's preadmission assessment program and judged to be eligible for nursing home care but be able to be cared for at home. Care at home is feasible because of willing family caregivers and the availability of an enriched array of health and social service support through these programs. These community programs provide care management as well as home health care, homemaker services, home-delivered meals, adult day care, chore service, mental health evaluation and counseling, transportation, respite care, emergency response systems, and many other related services.

A PCA assessor, in consultation with other involved disciplines, conducts a comprehensive multidimensional assessment of the consumer's medical history, current health, functioning, mental status, emotional well-being, environment, social supports, and resources (personal, social, and financial). A careful assessment of caregiving efforts by informal supports is included and reflected in the individually tailored care plan. In conjunction with the consumer, the care manager determines the type, amount, scope, duration, and pattern of delivery of the service to be provided. All care plans are shared with the primary care physician. Care managers are vested with responsibility for orchestrating all services noted on the care plan and monitoring the consumer's overall care. At regular intervals, care managers reassess the needs of their consumers and caregivers, and monitor the performance of service providers.

Care managers purchase service on behalf of the consumers on their caseload in accordance with the specific tasks and schedule in the care plan. Every day a consumer is on the active caseload, funds are encumbered with which to purchase services. Care managers can spend up to 80 percent of the daily Medicaid reimbursement rate for a nursing home bed. In 2003, this was about $97.00 daily (Pennsylvania Department of Public Welfare, www.dpw.state.pa.us). Care managers for Options are responsible for maintaining their aggregate caseload cost at or below the 80 percent cap. They are permitted to shift funds between consumers as long as the total caseload expenditure is below cap. For the PDA Waiver, it is an individual cap of 80 percent. This ability to treat consumers differentially has a powerful effect on care manager behavior. Care managers allocate resources with caution, recognizing that preserving a cushion of dollars permits them to respond more fully if a consumer temporarily needs more intensive, and therefore costlier, service. Care managers have strong incentives both to serve and to conserve. They quickly become prudent purchasers of service on behalf of their consumers and invariably keep their caseload expenditure level below the cap. This occurs despite the fact that some of their consumers may be using resources temporarily at twice the level of the cap.

In addition to planning, authorizing, and orchestrating service delivery for consumers, care managers perform functions historically associated with social casework. While they encourage and facilitate medical follow-up and compliance with health care regimens, they also counsel consumers and families. They negotiate with them about caregiving tasks. They provide short-term, problem-oriented counseling. They arrange access to entitlements, housing, and protective and legal services when necessary. They serve as a general source of information and as a "one-stop shopping" resource for questions or problems facing consumers and their families. Their job responsibilities suggest strongly to us that social work is a necessary prerequisite for the job of care manager.

Care management staff of the Options, Bridge, or Waiver Programs consist of 96 social workers organized in 16 teams of 6 care managers. Given the number and complexity of health problems faced by our consumers, nurses could also be an intelligent choice for care managers, but PCA selects the more generalist social workers for line staff, choosing to employ community health nurses at the supervisory level. Nursing expertise is critical and must be easily available. Each team of social workers has a social worker supervisor and a nursing consultant. The nursing consultants are responsible for adding nursing perspective to clinical decision making and to the overall program design and operation. They review assessments and make recommendations concerning individual consumer needs. They educate service providers as to the goals and objectives of the program and conduct orientation sessions for health subcontractors. They assist in development of contract specifications for health services and in monitoring the performance of health care providers. They identify training needs of care managers in the area of health care assessment and service delivery, and they provide or arrange training. The nurses essentially define the relationship between care managers and home health providers. The Pennsylvania Department of Aging mandated several years ago that medically frail consumers being served by the Medicaid Waiver program must be receiving a monitoring visit from a nurse consultant at least quarterly.

The provision of health and social services by multiple organizations usually involves end-to-end relationships, as when a discharging hospital refers for home health care and then home health care discharges to a social service agency, or parallel service delivery without collaboration, as when one agency provides counseling and another provides medical transportation. Interactive collaborative relationships between different providers are atypical, but in the provision of long-term care they are a necessity.

Analysis of service utilization by consumers of care management programs shows that the principal expenditure is for personal care service. As would be expected, community-based long-term care consumers need high levels of personal care (bathing, grooming, and toileting) and home support (shopping, cooking and cleaning). At any time, about 95 percent of these consumers are receiving personal care service. The second most frequently used service is nursing care. Approximately, half of the consumers are in receipt of nursing at any one time. All other directly controlled services are utilized at comparatively much lower rates. By far, the critical professional dyad is the social work care manager and the provider's home health nurse. Although all service providers must seek prior authorization from the care manager to initiate or change the delivery of service to a consumer, in the case of home health services, care managers exercise administrative authority over service provision while relying heavily on the clinical judgment of the nurse or other home health professional. Care managers rely on the home health nurses for frequent updates on consumer condition and guidance on plans of care. The experience of reporting to care managers is a new one for home health nurses, but the level of conflict between care managers and home health providers has been surprisingly low from the outset. Nurses sometimes find the need to get prior authorization to visit cumbersome, but care manager involvement has its benefits, too.

Several other aspects of the care manager and community health nurse collaboration should be highlighted. The capitated approach to financing care and the care manager control over spending creates cost consciousness among providers as well. In this model, home health professionals become sensitized to the economic consequences of providing service. For example, nurses who are aware of the cost of consumable medical supplies use them in a way that is different from that of their colleagues who are not attending to cost. Providers become conscious of the cost of the care they are giving and assist care managers in their efforts to be prudent, recognizing that unused resources are available for use when necessary later on. Another benefit is that when nurses identify consumer needs in the normal course of their duties that they or their agency are unable to meet, they can contact the care manager and immediately enlist a powerful ally in addressing those needs. Last, but no less important, providing ongoing care to long-term care consumers is physically and emotionally exhausting. Home health nurses have the assurance they are not solely responsible for the welfare of their patient; they can readily share their clinical and emotional burden with their care manager colleague. Joint home visiting, case conferencing, and peer support have strengthened service delivery in many difficult case situations.

BECOMING A LONG-TERM CARE PROVIDER: OBSERVATIONS AND RECOMMENDATIONS

From 1977 to 1995, PCA selected providers by using a competitive bidding process. Home health providers were competitively selected from 1982 to 1995, at first annually and then every 3 years, with annual performance audits and price negotiations. PCA received proposals from many home health agencies, experienced a wide range of provider behavior, and worked closely with many different home health subcontractors. The selection process used by PCA included a written proposal, an oral presentation, submission of references, and a weighted list of criteria by which judgments were made that resulted in the selection decision. With the tightening of budgets, price became an increasing concern. Selection decisions revolved around factors such as demonstrated experience in home health care delivery, history and reputation of the agency, current patient census (Medicare and others), past performance, conceptual understanding of the long-term care program and the special characteristics of service delivery in long-term care, the longevity and experience of nursing and rehabilitation staff, and responsiveness as a prospective subcontractor.

In 1995, the system changed. The Pennsylvania Department of Public Welfare and Department of Aging, influenced by the disabilities community, promoted greater consumer involvement and choice within the service culture and therefore an expanded pool of providers. Having a larger number of providers allows consumers more options for care. Consumers select

the agency of their choice and participate in the development of their care plan. For the Medicaid Waiver, any agency that "qualifies" may be enrolled by Medicaid and then certified to provide Medicaid Waiver services. For the Options and Bridge programs, contracts are developed. To qualify, an agency must:

1. Be licensed—Home Health, Medicare certified
2. Disclose qualifications of the agency staff
3. Disclose the composition of the agency board of directors
4. Have professional liability insurance
5. Be a corporation registered with the IRS and have a state Employer Identification Number
6. Submit their last tax audit report
7. Have documentation of Joint Commission on Accreditation of Healthcare Organizations certification (if applicable)

The differences between long-term care and skilled care are important to understand before entering into a contract. Nurses need to be liberated from the limitations imposed by prospective payment. Long-term care is different from skilled care in several significant ways. Rather than focus on diagnosis and treatment of medical problems, long-term care assumes comorbidities and management of chronic conditions with some degree of permanent (if not progressive) disability. Long-term care is therefore principally concerned with functioning and the way a person lives and operates within his or her environment. Ideally, long-term care services create a supportive environment within which a functionally disabled person can live as independently as possible. A second difference between long-term care and skilled care is apparent when analyzing the tasks involved in the care. Eighty percent to 90 percent of long-term care in nursing homes, for example, is either personal care or tasks such as laundry and housekeeping, provided by paraprofessionals. The role of the physician is secondary. What is needed is organization, coordination, and supervision of paraprofessionals. *Physicians are crit-*

ical to the provision of long-term care but are not central.

A final difference between long-term care and skilled care that must be clearly understood is the nature of the clinical problems presented and the characteristics of the consumers served. Although PCA serves consumers ranging in age from 18 to 103 years, the vast majority are older than 80. Although many need skilled care intermittently, such as expert wound care, incontinence evaluation and training, infusion therapies, or medication teaching, often the number of visits they are allowed by the insurer is extremely limited. About 20 percent of the nursing care provided is custodial; the care manager can authorize continued nursing visits to monitor skin integrity, ensure proper medication administration, support families with tube feedings and other technical caregiving tasks, and ensure that small functional gains are maintained. Some professionals, by focus or personality, prefer to tackle reversible or unambiguous problems. Most long-term care consumers suffer from multiple chronic conditions or impairments. At a minimum, the professionals who serve them must be able to tolerate ambiguity, comparatively small gains, and the eventual decline of most of their patients. Professionals do best who are mature, thrive on complex problems, appreciate small signs of progress, and enjoy extended relationships with their patients. Home health agencies serving long-term care patients will need to take this into account as they select and train personnel.

Community-based long-term care operates with an ideology to which home health providers must be oriented. "Skilled care," which triggers Medicare reimbursement, is reimbursable when there is rehabilitative or restorative types of potential. "Chronic" care or maintenance is non-Medicare reimbursable, yet Options, Bridge, or Waiver may provide this service. Nursing, physical therapy, occupational therapy, or speech therapy may be utilized preventatively.

Good agencies are rightfully proud of their track records, and past performance is an important ingredient to their selection by consumers. PCA monitors the quality of provider agencies, and the results of these administrative and clinical audits and consumer satisfaction surveys are reflected on a provider "report card." When making a selection, consumers consult the most current provider report card and choose based on quality, price, proximity to their home, and so forth. At the other end of the same continuum are organizations that have developed as temporary staffing agencies. Typically proprietary, they have a comparatively less-developed vision of good service and agency mission as a community caregiver. They often present a posture that communicates, "We will be happy to serve you in any way you require, as long as you pay us." The motivation of these organizations is clear and their flexibility is appreciated, but their apparent lack of internal performance standards shakes confidence.

New financing arrangements, combined with the special nature of long-term care patients' needs, are propelling home health agencies into highly interactive relationships with gatekeepers and other providers. This too requires a conscious commitment and careful orchestration of effort to achieve success. In the Philadelphia model, it is the AAA that identifies eligible consumers, assesses them for service need, develops the care plan, and then arranges for the provision of home health care as part of a larger care plan that the AAA controls. When long-term care benefits are financed by payers such as long-term care insurers, PACE programs, or Medicare HMOs with expanded care benefits, a similar gatekeeping and allocation function is likely to exist outside the home health provider. Many home health agencies have gained experience in contracting with HMOs to serve enrollees in their Medicare risk plans. As such, participating home health agencies have two consumers when before they only had one. They must serve their patients but also serve the needs of the organization that has overall care management responsibility. Thus concomitant with the development of this new long-term care market, there may be a diminishing of previously enjoyed autonomy on the part of the home health provider.

Two questions for agencies contemplating the provision of long-term care are: Will they be able to grasp the complexities of the new enterprise and perform the clinically and administratively challenging tasks required? Will they strike an adequate balance between dedication to an agency mission and performance and productivity standards, and a position of flexibility and openness to new ideas and program requirements? In our experience in working with agencies of different identities—voluntary, religious, and proprietary—that balance has been struck successfully.

The outstanding need in community-based long-term care is integration of financing and service delivery across systems. The adage "form follows finance" speaks to the root of the problem. Acute care hospitals, rehabilitative care agencies, mental health centers, AAAs, housing, HMOs, and so forth may each have oversight and gatekeeping responsibility over one aspect of a consumer's care. There is little coordination and much duplication. On behalf of consumers, providers of all kinds must advocate for integrated funding and provision of care. Tighter budgets necessitate a change in this direction. The growing demand and need for community-based long-term care services will drive development of integrated, flexible systems designed to work for the consumer, the provider and the payer.

PART VI

Financial Issues

CHAPTER 44

Understanding the Exposures of Home Health Care: An Insurance Primer

Brian M. Block

There is an essential need for those who administer or manage home health care organizations to protect the present and future financial security of their businesses. Those who have been in the field for any length of time know the home health care organizations that have failed. Some of the failures include organizations with poor fiscal and reimbursement planning, lack of accreditation, and poor human resource practices; organizations that are too narrowly defined in scope and wind up working with too few referral sources or are too focused on one patient type (which becomes extinct in the reimbursement community); and those that do not cooperatively work with the continuum of other services and organizations necessary for the comprehensive care of their patient cohorts. Each of these examples of failure, as well as many others, unfortunately and typically represents a slow occurrence that takes place over years of struggling to continue to provide essential clinical services.

The insurance question that must be asked is: What are the risks inherent in doing business as a home health care organization? Even if the myriad of reasons for failure are planned for, monitored, and controlled, an allegation of or substantiated negligent act filed against the professional home health care staff and therefore the organization can, in a very short time, create a decline in the public and professional community's opinion of the organization and can precipitate a financial disaster that will probably force the organization to close its doors.

A home health care organization must transfer and then actively control its risk of loss. Insurance provides for security from unforeseen events that cannot be controlled by other means. Insurance is necessary to protect an organization from a loss or losses that cannot be anticipated or afforded. Risk management is the primary mechanism and process through which the home health care organization can control the chance and uncertainty of loss. Risk management involves a group of active techniques that evaluates and monitors an organization's exposures. Exposures are defined as the possible events, conditions, or employee or consumer behaviors that can cause a loss. These activities are integral to the home health care organization's strategic plan, and must be focused to reduce the probability of a loss actually occurring and to assist the home health care organization's return to usual and customary operations should a loss occur.

The goal of this chapter is to introduce the reader to the basic principles of insurance and the types of coverage available, to describe what exposures are present in home health care, and to discuss some techniques for risk management.

TYPES OF INSURANCE

Insurance is the transfer of risk from one party to another for a price through a legal contract that spells out the terms, perils covered, and exclusions. Overall, certain factors and/or conditions must be present for an insurance contract. These include an insurable interest, the ability to predict losses, the ability to predict the monetary value of the losses, and a certainty that the losses are accidental or unplanned. An insurable interest, in simple terms, implies that a tangible asset exists. Assets may include a wide variety of elemental components, such as employees, owned property or vehicles, or the care, custody, and control of the physical and emotional well-being of consumers. In addition and to meet these criteria, any insurance company or carrier must have enough experience with the home health care industry in order to be interested in it as a class of business with whom to do business.

Experience with the industry would imply a sufficiently large number of insured organizations so that an understanding of home health care operations, exposures, and losses can be anticipated and trended by insurance industry monitors—and the insurance industry monitors consider the type, scope, and monetary value of losses, which may be expressed in cumulative terms or by a loss ratio. The loss ratio is determined by dividing the monetary value of losses for a specific type of coverage by the premium paid for that specific type of coverage. Insurance is also based on the principle of indemnity; that is, following a loss, placing the insured in the same financial position that existed before the loss occurred. Insurance protects the assets or financial stake in the property or casualty to be covered.

Losses must be unplanned or accidental; organizations must not cause losses to occur, the loss ratio must not exceed certain profitability standards, and the frequency of small losses and near misses must not create a "big accident waiting to happen" suspicion about the home health care organization's insurability. Carriers recognize that the probability of most losses can be lowered through an active program of risk management.

Home health care organizations are responsible for minimizing their exposures and for complying with the standards of local, state, and federal regulatory and accrediting bodies that define the safe operation of their business. Home health care organizations should consider the purchase of insurance for the following insurable interests and exposures: owned and leased property and contents; easily transportable equipment such as computers; professional and general liability; liability for the directors and officers of the corporation including employment practices; automobile/commercial vehicle, including nonowned auto coverage; workers' compensation; crime; and excess or umbrella coverage.

Property

Property insurance provides security from losses related to the direct physical loss or damage to covered property. *Property* is defined as a building or dwelling, and includes all permanently installed indoor and outdoor fixtures, machinery and equipment, and other personal property used to maintain the building; business property contents such as furniture; and personal property of others in the care, custody, and control of the organization.

Home health care organizations minimally should make sure that their policy insures against fire, lightning, internal explosion, volcanic action, vandalism, sinkhole collapse, and sprinkler leakage. Important other coverage includes loss of business income; damage due to the weight of ice, snow, and sleet; damage due to glass breakage; and damage due to collapse. Organizations in geographic areas where there is a high risk of flood or earthquake should consider this additional coverage as well. Home health care organizations should work closely with their insurance agent or broker to make sure that the proper perils are covered by insurance.

Home health care organizations may not need the entire extent of coverage available. The business office space may be within a singular building that is leased or rented or may be a suite of offices within a larger complex of offices. In either case, the property exposure would be the actual business furnishings owned by the organization; any personal property of others in the care, custody, and control of the organization; and other building and property exposures agreed to by the organization and spelled out in the lease agreement. The lease agreement will probably include a requirement that the landlord must be an additional insured on the insurance policy of the home health care organization, and may require that the home health care organization indemnify and hold harmless the landlord for certain exposures, perils, or loss. Be sure to have the corporate attorney review any and all lease agreements. Insurance policies protecting the home health care organization's property exposures usually include a type of coverage called a *blanket*, and may indemnify against either the actual cash value or replacement cost of property should a loss occur. Actual cash value is based on the principle of depreciation; replacement cost is based on what it would cost in today's market to replace the loss.

Property exposures for home health care organizations are managed through good basic business practices. If the organization stores medical supplies (including pharmaceuticals) or consumer medical information or charts, however, the organization's exposure increases. The agent or broker securing insurance for the organization should be aware of all risks when placing coverage.

Liability

Liability is defined as the failure of an individual or organization to exercise the proper degree of care required of an average person in that particular situation. The principle driving this definition is that of negligence. *Negligence* is a wrong committed by one person or organization against another. It is an improper action that causes bodily injury or property damage and that is or may be perceived as in the care, custody, and/or control of the negligent party. Therefore, a home health care organization's liability exposure may also be present because of an accidental occur-

rence or adverse incident. All employees, contracted professional staff, and the organization itself may be held legally responsible for any action that leads to the bodily injury or property damage of others.

Liability insurance covers both the financial obligations resultant to the injured person's claim and the cost of legal defense. It covers any necessary tangible restitution as well as any potential award for pain and suffering. There are two types of liability insurance available: occurrence and claims made. Both types of policies provide a home health care organization insurance for bodily injury or property damage to others. The occurrence type or form of liability insurance furnishes coverage during the policy period regardless of when a claim is reported and filed with the carrier by the insured. The claims-made form of liability insurance furnishes coverage only for claims that are reported or filed during the policy period or within 60 days of the policy's expiration, and only when the date of alleged negligence occurred after a retroactive date. The retroactive date defines the specific date when the policy actually begins.

Home health care organizations have a vicarious liability as well. This means that the organization itself may be held liable for any negligent act committed in the performance of assigned duties or on behalf of the organization by employees or contracted professional staff.

Liability of Directors and Officers

Directors and officers of any corporation are defined by the organization's bylaws and usually include the members of the board of directors and may encompass administrative/senior management employees such as the chief executive officer, the chief operations officer, and the chief financial officer. These individuals can be held liable, or have an exposure, for any and all activities of the home health care organization. Liability insurance for directors and officers provides coverage for the identified individuals who commit wrongful acts such as error, neglect, or breach of duty. Examples of wrongful acts include fiduciary malfeasance and misfeasance, failure to adequately supervise professional activities, and employment practices. Employment practice exposures comprise violations of Title VII of the Civil Rights Act such as discrimination, improper hiring practices, wrongful termination, and manifesting a hostile workplace including sexual harassment.

It is the responsibility of the board of directors and officers of a home health care organization to ensure that recognized standards of care are followed, that staff have earned appropriate academic degrees and hold proper licensure to do their job, and that the environment within which business is conducted is free from defects that might cause bodily injury or physical damage to others. These basic principles apply whether professional staff are employees of the organization or are performing duties for the organization on a contractual basis.

General Liability

General liability coverage provides insurance for bodily injury or property damage to clients' families, vendors, visitors, or others not employed by the home health care organization caused by perils within the organization's premises or resulting from its business operations. General liability coverage also includes protection from a claim that is the result of an accusation of libel, slander, or invasion of privacy, as well as medical payments for bodily injury. General liability exposures faced by home health care organizations are centered primarily on the premises from which the operation is directed. Examples are failure to remove ice from the entryway to the building, failure to post notice of a wet floor, failure to repair expediently or to remove dangerous physical-plant problems (for example, wet ceiling tile) that then results in injury to others. Fire legal liability is also a possible exposure.

It is essential for the home health care organization to check its lease or business complex agreement about the extent of their liability to these exposures. It is necessary to strictly enforce policies about emergency procedures regarding smoke and/or fire, expedient physical-plant repairs, and removal of hazards and perils due to seasonal variations.

Professional Liability

Professional liability insurance protects professionals or an organization's professional staff who fail to meet the standards of skill and care generally accepted for that profession or occupation. The protection afforded by this coverage includes both direct injury or harm and indirect injury or harm (emotional trauma, pain, and suffering). An individual, the legal guardian of an individual, or an individual's estate may file a claim. Professional liability also includes the failure of any professional with regard to "duty to report" or "duty to warn."

Home health care organizations are faced with exceptional professional liability exposures. Two essential questions should be asked:

1. Are the professional staff credentialed and trained and supervised properly for the performance of all aspects of their duties? This implies the certainty of competence in the performance of the employee's duties.
2. Are the duties performed under the direct order of a professional legally and medically authorized to order such duties?

Even if the home health care organization contracts for the services of any or all professionals, the organization itself is liable for the professional activities performed. Contractual professional staff should be included in the organization's professional liability coverage as contingent employees. The home health care organization should require all contractual employees to purchase their own professional liability insurance policy to a minimum of at least $1 million, and the organization should be named an additional insured on each contract employee's policy.

Umbrella Liability

An umbrella policy provides insurance for liability claims when an award for damages is in excess of the limits of the underlying insurance policies that are in force, such as the general and/or professional liability policy. The umbrella policy may add excess limits to the directors and officers and commercial vehicle liability coverage as well, and should be purchased with this in mind. There are multiple limits of insurance that apply to underlying liability coverage; however, the two major limits to consider are the per-occurrence and the aggregate limit amounts. The occurrence limit is the dollar amount the carrier will pay for a single, individual claim. The aggregate limit is the maximum amount an insurer will pay for all covered losses during the policy period. When limits are reached, additional coverage is provided through the purchase of an umbrella or excess policy. Home health care organizations should purchase an umbrella policy to provide coverage in the event of a catastrophic or shock loss, such as a wrongful death.

Automobile/Vehicle

There are two different forms of insurance that compose an automobile policy. Both include property and casualty coverage as they relate to commercial vehicles. The property section of the commercial vehicle package policy protects an insured from loss due to comprehensive or collision damage and is specific to an insured's vehicle(s). The vehicles that are covered must be scheduled (i.e., listed specifically). *Collision* is defined as a direct and/or accidental loss that results when two vehicles collide, when the vehicle collides with another object, or when the vehicle is upset (overturned).

Comprehensive coverage is defined as the direct and/or accidental damage to an insured's vehicle from anything other than collision. For example, hitting or being hit by a deer is a comprehensive coverage. Protection from economic loss due to negligent ownership (failure to repair bad brakes), poor maintenance, or negligent use of an insured vehicle is provided in the liability section of an automobile policy. As with all liability coverage, this protection is designed to

cover damages that an insured is legally obliged to pay as a result of bodily injury or property damage to others as a result of a vehicular accident.

A business auto coverage policy is necessary for home health care organizations. For example, if the organization owns a fleet of vehicles, coverage would be essential in order to conduct business. If the organization requires that professional staff drive their own vehicles in order to conduct business, however, the business auto coverage policy would specify coverage for nonowned autos only. Nonowned autos may, depending on the carrier, be added as an endorsement to the general liability section of an organization's commercial policy. This is also true for hired autos (i.e., any vehicles hired, leased, rented, or borrowed and used for business purposes). Nonowned auto coverage only provides protection to the home health care organization for the negligent act of the driver. It does not protect the driver or provide coverage for repairs to their damaged vehicle. The insurance policy purchased by the vehicle's owner should respond to the use of insurance to repair a damaged vehicle regardless of collision or comprehensive circumstances.

The use of nonowned autos raises an additional exposure for home health care organizations. Whenever a vehicle is used on behalf of a home health care organization in the course of business, the organization has a responsibility to ensure that the vehicle is properly registered (and, if applicable, inspected) and that the driver of the vehicle is licensed and insured. It is best to make sure that the organization's policies and procedures incorporate the aforementioned points and that all staff is properly educated.

Workers' Compensation

Most states have promulgated compulsory laws that require employers to provide coverage for employee work-related injuries and for employer protection against common lawsuits that may be brought by employees (or their survivors) to recover damages from job-related injuries. The following applies to those states that mandate workers' compensation insurance. All injuries sustained by an employee arising out of and in the course of employment are covered. Additionally, occupational diseases specific to a particular trade or occupation are covered. Workers' compensation insurance provides cash (a portion of wages), medical benefits, and rehabilitation for injured employees. It doesn't matter who, why, or what caused the injury to occur and as such is considered a no-fault or single remedy coverage.

Workers' compensation insurance implies that employers should provide as safe a work environment as can be maintained, given the scope of the organization, and that employees should be integral to the maintenance of the worksite. Furthermore, employers must consider their return-to-work and modified-duty policies. Also, employees must be informed of their workers' compensation rights and their duties should an injury occur.

It is strongly suggested that organizations establish a safety committee, contract for the assistance of a workers' compensation loss control expert to assess an organization's exposures (and to make recommendations), and educate their employees regarding safe work practices. Although carriers recognize that a zero employee injury policy is impossible, all organizations can improve their safety record continually.

Home health care organizations have distinct workers' compensation exposures. The nature of the work may demand lifting and transferring consumers, entering buildings and dwellings that may not be in the best repair, physical activities with clients, and performing duties with individuals who may be less than cooperative. For organizations that provide injections, there is always the risk of needle sticks and exposure to communicable diseases. Home health care employees are potentially exposed to bloodborne and airborne pathogens on a regular basis. For this reason, as well as others, a strong education program related to safety procedures and potential risks is necessary; even the basics (e.g., universal precautions, proper lifting techniques) need to be reviewed at least yearly with the most experienced employees. Organizations that contract for professional staff through another organization or agency also hold a responsibility to ensure that the employing organization or agency has workers' compensation insurance that covers their employees on the home health care organization's worksites. As a risk management tool, transfer of risk is an important consideration.

Crime

Very simply, crime insurance protects an insured from burglary, robbery, theft, forgery, mysterious disappearance, extortion, and computer fraud. Although crime insurance does not cover dishonest acts committed by the insured (see the section entitled Liability of Directors and Officers), coverage is extended to all employees, a custodian of the insured's property, a messenger transporting an insured's property (including money and securities) from one location to another, and individuals watching over or guarding an insured's property. Coverage should be purchased to protect the home health care organization that is recipient payee of consumers' benefits such as social security payments, housing allowances, and the like as well.

There may be a loss due to typical crime exposures (robbery, burglary, etc.); however, some primary exposures for home health care organizations are employee dishonesty, forgery, or alteration (particularly of client records) and mysterious disappearances of equipment, supplies, or medicines. The single best method for controlling these exposures is focused on the organization's record-keeping procedures, including the location of client records (and the method of checking them in and out) and supplies allocated. An occasional field check of activities is strongly recommended.

Transportable Equipment

Inland marine coverage is insurance to protect a home health care organization's easily transportable property (e.g., computers). The home health care organization needs to consider that an investment made in electronic data processing, including computer hardware and software, is an insurable interest and can be covered by an inland marine policy form, an electronic data processing floater, or may be covered through the business property policy.

RISK MANAGEMENT

The exposures of home health care organizations have been touched upon in each section of this chapter. As the field continues to mature, there will be additional exposures not already mentioned; however, there are some good basic principles of risk management to consider. *Risk management* is the processes and strategies applied by management that minimize an organization's exposure to potential loss. Risk management activities focus on the corporate culture necessary to develop, carry out, and coordinate activities; it involves all levels of the organization, centers on employee behavior, and is an essential ingredient in an organization's quality improvement plan.

A good risk management program includes 11 components, and behind each of the components is the focus on exposure, near misses, and actual loss. The home health care organization should consider a 5-year retrospective analysis of near misses and actual loss, trend here and now near misses and losses, and actively be involved with hazard identification and accident investigation. Zero tolerance for avoidable losses should be built into the home health care organization's human resources policies and management practices.

The following are the 11 suggested components of a risk management program:

1. an accident prevention and safety mission statement developed and understood by the directors and officers and staff at all levels in the organization
2. annual organization-wide loss control strategic planning, with, at a minimum, quarterly ongoing analysis of goal attainment
3. a quality improvement or quality insurance plan that considers hazard identification, and an analysis of trends that is developed and monitored by direct authority within the organization
4. solid employee practices driven by employee competency, including screening and hiring, orientation, annual performance evaluations, staff development, and employee supervision
5. consumer satisfaction analyses, including an evaluation of the organization's primary customers, referral sources, and the community within which the organization does business
6. a safety committee that monitors the mechanical and physical plant, infection control, and holds regularly planned disaster drills
7. a mechanism to ensure inventory control and minimize employee theft
8. a system minimally to oversee transportation issues and to review annually all policies and procedures
9. a workers' compensation review, including return-to-work/modified-duty policy and loss analysis
10. an active training program that focuses on risk management issues
11. a plan to have all facets of the risk management program linked to administrative planning and decision making

PURCHASING INSURANCE

Home health care organizations should evaluate carefully their exposures, develop and actively pursue loss control/risk management activities, and assess carefully their insurance needs. It is important that home health care organizations earnestly consider working with an insurance agent or broker who can understand the unique aspects of their business. Home health care organizations should purchase insurance coverage to match their risks. The types of insurance described here can be put together into one commercial package policy when only one insurance company writes all coverage. Some carriers will have a better form (coverage within the policy itself) for a particular type of coverage, however, and then the home health care organization could purchase their policies from several companies. This too is an issue to discuss with the organization's broker or agent. Remember that the single goal in purchasing insurance is to provide proper coverage for the organization's unique needs.

CONCLUSION

This chapter has purposefully outlined the possible exposures of home health care organizations through a delineation of the various types of insurance coverage available and provided descriptions of how those might apply to home health care organizations.

CHAPTER 45

Budgeting for Home Health Agencies

Vern A. Peterschmidt

A budget is a combination of a look back at your historical performance, a review of your current operations, and an analysis of all the related components for the purpose of developing a road map that will lead you to a planned successful conclusion. The steps that must be followed are spelled out in the budget document. This is the road map that, if followed, should ensure your future success.

ROAD MAP

You must first understand where you have been and why you have been there. Being aware of how the road map changed over the years is critical to understanding your opportunities that lay ahead. External sources are many times the driving forces that affect your internal operations. You must understand those external sources, which could include dealing with nursing shortages or major changes in the Medicare payment system. The budget document will reflect your understanding of industry, your own operation, and the planning required in establishing and achieving your stated goals.

To understand where you have been, you must accumulate both historical and current data in a format that is consistent from year to year, accurate, timely, and understandable by the management, owners, and members of the board of directors of the agency. This involves an ongoing approach in evaluating your operations. Identifying your opportunities and realiz-

ing your concerns is a function of understanding all aspects of your business.

Several major components must be analyzed in establishing an appropriate budget process.

Patients and Clients

The number of patients necessary to meet the revenue projections for the budgeted period must be identified. Your Medicare and like type service patients are the core source when identifying revenue. Maintaining or expanding your patient volume is critical in reaching your stated revenue goals. Your hourly, private pay, hospice, and various waiver program revenues are all based on patient or client volume. With some waiver programs, the state identifies the available clients; otherwise, the agency is responsible for projecting its own patient volume. Patient volume is number one in maintaining patient revenue. Patients are generated from a solid and consistent referral base.

Referral Base

The agency must be aware of its referral sources; identify the major admitters including physicians, hospitals, and other sources; and identify situations that could affect referrals in a positive or negative way. Potential changes of personnel at the physician's office, physicians retiring, new physicians in the marketplace, new hospital discharge planners or changes in hospital policies, and agency staff changes are all factors that must be taken into account when projecting Medicare or other patient volume. An increase or decrease in the competition in the same patient service area will also be a factor in maintaining or expanding an agency's patient base. Expanding the types of services offered should enlarge the referral sources. Specializing in disease management such as cardiology or diabetes would have a positive effect on the agency's referral base. Positive and continuous communications with the various referral sources must be maintained. Knowing your market share is critical in determining your agency's growth potential. Monitoring your client or hourly services is critical because various state-funded programs often change both the eligibility criteria and the payment amount based on available funding sources.

Patient Volume

Once the referral base is established an analysis should be made of the current and historical patient volume. A 12- to 18-month review of your patient volume would be appropriate with the following areas identified.

- Identify patient volume by referral source starting with the largest volume admitter.
- Identify payer base (Medicare, Medicaid, insurance, charity, etc.) by referral source.
- Identify the staffing requirements based on type of patients and related nursing, therapy, and aide visit requirements.
- Analyze the current staffing level and capabilities and determine if improved staff efficiency can cover any increase in patient volume.
- Determine that there is available qualified staff that can be hired on either a full-time, hourly, or per-visit basis, if additional staff is required to meet projected demand.
- Realize that under Medicare, there are financial winners and losers. An increase in patient volume resulting in additional losses would be inappropriate. However,

accepting a certain volume of patients that produces a loss would be appropriate if an overall increase in the agency's manageable and profitable patients or clients is possible.
- Understand that a major change in the Medicare regulatory requirements could affect patient eligibility or services. Such a change could also affect patient referrals, volume, visits, and payment levels. Changes in insurance contracts, hospice payment levels, and state waiver programs would affect utilization. A conservative approach to the budgetary effect of potential regulatory and other changes should be applied when projecting patient volume, visits, and payments. Industry publications are a good source in projecting changes in major payer contracts such as Medicare.

Payer Sources

The amount of anticipated revenue will be a breakeven point in establishing the expense area of your budget. Understanding your payer sources is critical in projecting an accurate revenue amount. There are numerous payer sources, with each payer having specific regulations and rules to follow and rate formulas and pay structures to understand and maintain. Agencies must have the power to obtain the data from their existing accounting and statistical systems in order to develop that revenue road map that will guide them though the revenue portion of their budgeting process.

MEDICARE

The major payment change in Medicare occurred when we left the cost-based system for the Prospective Payment System (PPS). PPS requires a business approach in order to maintain and hopefully improve an agency's financial and clinical outcomes. An understanding of the components that drive the payments and net revenues is the budgetary issue that must be addressed.

Episodes

The patient volume will determine the number of episodes that will be projected in the agency's budgeted period. Along with projecting the number of patients, an agency's recertification percentage must be established. The percentage of recertifications is identified by dividing the number of patients into the number of episodes for a specific period (Exhibit 45–1).

If an agency has a 1.4 episodes per patient ratio, this would indicate that 40 percent of the Medicare patients required a second episode. Therefore, projecting episodes is obtained by multiplying the number of estimated patients by the recertification percentage (Exhibit 45–2).

Episodes are the building blocks for identifying the Medicare revenues and associated costs and determining the Medicare-related profit or loss. Tracking your patients over the last 18 months along with your episodes will identify both the consistency in your monthly patient referrals and your recertification ratio.

Benchmarks

Once your historical data is reviewed and analyzed, an agency-specific benchmark can be set for targeting the number of patients, episodes, visits per episode, case mix, and recertification ratio for the budgeted period. You will also be able to monitor your own benchmarks against regional and national benchmarks. Benchmarks are the indicators that an agency will attempt to follow to reach their budgeted or projected goals. Benchmarks or projected outcomes are established through a complete understanding of an agency's own operation. Similar regional and national benchmarks can then be compared against agency data to better understand one's own agency compared against the competition and industry standards. Having the operational data of your peer organizations available will assist your agency in setting realistic and competitive goals.

Case Mix

Case mix is the indicator for tracking the intensity of the services required for a Medicare patient. The higher the case mix, the more intense the service and normally the higher number of visits. Understanding the process for calculating an agency's specific case mix is critical in identifying budgeted Medicare revenues and costs (Exhibit 45–3). The following is a method for identifying case mix.

Full episodes and related payments are only used in calculating the average Medicare payment per episode because including low-utilization payment adjustments (LUPAs), partial episode payments (PEPs), and significant change in conditions (SCICs) would distort the average episode payment and subsequent case mix.

The agency-specific standard payment rate is an area-specific rate that takes into account that area's wage-labor factor. All Medicare-certified agencies in a given service area will have the same standard payment rate. Although Medicare should normally increase the standard PPS episode payment rate based on inflationary factors, the area-specific labor factor can be unpredictable and can often have a negative effect on the agency's specific episode payment rate.

Medicare Payments

Once the case mix is determined, the Medicare revenue can be determined by taking the projected Medicare patients times the recertification ratio times the estimated average Medicare payment per episode (Exhibit 45–4).

Because not all Medicare episodes are full episodes, the budgeted Medicare revenue must be reduced by the revenue associated with those episodes that would not be full episodes, such as LUPAs, PEPs, and so forth. An agency's paid end-of-episode report for the historical period should be obtained from either in-house records or the fiscal intermediary. From these reports, an adjustment or contractual allowance percentage can be determined. Full-episode revenue would normally need to be reduced by 10 to 15 percent (Exhibit 45–5).

Because the allowance percentage is based on historical data, considerations should be given as to the possible changes that could occur in the

Exhibit 45–1 Method to Determine an Agency's Recertification Percentage

Historical Data	
Number of Episodes	1,960
Number of Patients	1,400
Episodes per Patient Ratio	1.4

Exhibit 45–3 Process for Calculating an Agency's Specific Case Mix

Historical Data	
Total Full Episode Payments	$4,900,000
Number of Full Episodes	1,960
Average Payment per Episode	$2,500
Agency-Specific Std. Payment Rate	2,200
Case Mix	1.136

budgeted period. A change in the percentages of LUPAs or outliers would affect this allowance percentage. In the budget process, the Medicare exceptions to the full episodes should be reviewed for reasonableness. Understanding the reasons for an agency's LUPAs, outliers, PEPs, and SCICs will help to improve the overall management of the Medicare patients and payments and should reduce your agency's allowance percentage.

Visits

Under the Medicare PPS payment system, visits should be calculated on a per-episode basis. Although visits are not a factor in determining the revenues for the majority of the PPS episodes, visits do relate to costs, and therefore visit volume will determine the level of profit or loss per episode.

Average number of visits per episode is one of the major indicators that requires continuous monitoring. A high number of visits per episode would normally indicate reduced profits or even losses. Visits per episode should track somewhat with case mix. The lower the case mix the fewer

Exhibit 45–2 Method to Project Estimated Episodes

Budget Period	
Estimated Patients	1,500
Recertification Ratio	1.4
Budgeted Period	
Estimated Episodes	2,100

visits, with the higher case mix episodes requiring more visits. An agency should always be aware as to where they stand concerning their average visits per episode with regional and national averages. Estimating visits per episode should be a major component in determining direct patient care salaries (Exhibit 45–6).

Exhibit 45–7 is an example of the calculation for determining Medicare visits. A visit distribution calculation will also need to be determined for Medicaid, insurance, and other types patients.

MEDICAID

Budgeting for Medicaid revenues is dependent on the form of payment within your state Medicaid program. Some states are still on a cost-based system with the lower of a payment ceiling or actual costs as the basis for reimbursement. The per-visit ceiling is often based on the current Medicare LUPAs per-discipline rates. With per-visit costs on the rise due to the reduced number of visits throughout the industry, the per-visit ceiling limits become the actual per-visit payments.

Under a Medicaid fee-per-visit payment arrangement, an agency must again be aware of the fee structure and budget revenues based on historical experience, allowable funding under the state Medicaid plan, projected number of Medicaid patients, and the associated visits. While many Medicaid arrangements may not cover the full cost of their services, the payments normally will cover the agency's incremental or direct

Exhibit 45–4 Method to Determine Medicare Revenue

Budgeted Period		
Medicare Patients		1,500
Recertification Ratio		1.4
Estimated Episodes		2,100
Current Payment per Episode	$2,500	
Estimated Percentage Increase (%)	3.2	
Adjusted Episode Payment	$2,580	$2,580
Budgeted Medicare Revenue		$5,418,000
Allowance Percentage (%)	10	
Medicare Revenue Adjustment @ 10%		541,800
Adjusted Budgeted Medicare Revenue		$4,876,200

costs. An agency's per-discipline incremental cost per visit should be identified during the budget process.

INSURANCE

Most insurance coverage for home health services is on a negotiated fee-per-visit basis. The major concern with insurance coverage is the number of various insurance carriers and tracking the various payment arrangements. When budgeting for insurance coverage, an agency must track the visits and payments by major insurance carrier. These major players could represent 60 to 80 percent of insurance cases.

Exhibit 45–5 Calculation for Determining the Allowance Percentage Using Historical Paid Episode Data

Historical Period	
All Episodes	1,960
Average Payment—Full Episodes Only	$2,500
Projected Full Payment	$4,900,000
Actual PPS Payments	$4,410,000
Difference	$490,000
Allowance Percentage (%)	10

Estimating the number of visits and associated payment rates for these carriers, plus estimating the visits and revenues for the other insurance carriers, is necessary to accurately identify visits and revenues for insurance-related services.

CHARITY

Not-for-profit agencies can be funded for certain charity and no-pay services. These services should be budgeted because such community funding can be limited to a gross cap. It is also appropriate for all agencies to budget for charity care in order to understand the cost associated with these services. Charity or low paying patients are at times a necessary cost of doing business. Accepting these patients will frequently open the door for other full paying or Medicare patients.

SALARY COSTS

Salary and related costs are the major operational costs of a home health agency. Identifying the full-time equivalents (FTEs) required to meet the projected visit complement is a critical step in preparing the salary and related cost portion of the expense budget (Exhibit 45–8).

Exhibit 45–6 Method to Estimate Visits per Episode

Total Episodes		2,100		
	% of Episodes	Episodes	Visits per Episode	Est. Visits
Full	90	1,890	15	28,350
LUPA	8	168	2	336
Outlier	2	42	60	2,520
Total	100	2,100		31,206

In addition to the direct patient care FTEs, the agency must factor in the FTEs for the case managers or other clinical directors and supervisors. Depending on how the agency is organized, the individuals who are assigned to open a case require additional time and could affect the per-diem visit calculation. The direct patient care salary cost should include a detailed listing by each employee by discipline including the additional positions that may be required.

A similar schedule of patients, visits, and FTEs must be calculated for the salary cost associated with the non-Medicare visits. Because these like-type visits require reduced paperwork and related documentation, the productivity for such visits should be greater than similar

Exhibit 45–7 Calculation for Determining Medicare Visits

Visit Distribution		
	%	Visits
SNC	45	14,043
PT	30	9,362
OT	2	624
ST	2	624
MSW	1	312
HHA	20	6,241
Total	100	31,206

Medicare visits. A detailed listing of direct patient care employees, by discipline, for the combination of Medicare- and Medicare-type services should support the budgeted salary and fringe benefit costs. Salaries should also be identified by the hourly rate by employee.

Contract personnel should be identified along with the full-time nursing and other clinical positions. Contracting for clinical staff is necessary to fill the gaps in the staffing requirements due to changes in patient or visit utilization.

Based on the historical and projected staffing requirements of the organization, the detail schedule of employee-by-employee budgeted salaries and fringe benefit costs must include all administrative positions. The possibility of consolidating administrative responsibilities should always be considered. Outsourcing of certain administrative functions should also be considered if such outsourcing would decrease costs and improve efficiency.

FRINGE BENEFITS

The cost associated with fringe benefits will be based on the combination of the number of full-time employees and the anticipated cost of the fringe benefit package offered to the employees. A review of the fringe benefit package should be made each year to determine if the agency can afford the same level of benefits. Also, a compari-

Exhibit 45–8 Method to Determine Direct Patient Care FTEs

Paid Hours	2,080
Less: PTO Hours	<200>
Administrative Hours	<144>
Direct Patient Care Hours	1,736
Days Available for Patient Care	217

FTE Calculation—Medicare

	Visits	Visits per Diem	No. of Days Required	Days per FTE	FTE
SNC	14,043	5.0	2,809	217	13.0
PT	9,362	5.0	1,872	217	8.2
OT	624	5.0	125	217	.6
ST	624	5.0	125	217	.6
MSW	312	3.0	104	217	.5
AIDE	6,241	6.0	1,040	217	4.8
Total	31,206		6,075		27.7

son of an agency's benefit package with peer organizations would be helpful. Verification of the costs of the components of the fringe benefit package applicable for the budget period must be made. In certain situations, part-time or contract personnel may be appropriate in place of full-time staff. This will assist in controlling excessive fringe benefit costs.

OTHER COST ITEMS

The remaining operating costs include those administrative overhead costs and other costs associated with the visit disciplines and other programs. These costs must be shown in detail as indicated in your chart of accounts. An item-by-item historical review of these costs is necessary to fully understand their significance and overall reasonableness. Such costs can range from computer services and leased equipment to cell phone and utility costs. Projected routine (nonbillable) supplies and nonroutine (billable)

supply costs must be identified separately for Medicare purposes.

CAPITAL

A separate capital budget must be completed. Depending on available cash and capital requirements, a decision must be made regarding whether to lease or purchase required equipment and computer hardware. Capital purchases will require calculation of depreciation and additional cost for the purchase of maintenance agreements. Obsolescence is a factor that must be taken into account in considering a purchase versus a lease.

CONCLUSION

The difference between budgeted and actual revenue and costs should be monitored on a continuous basis, normally monthly. Unexpected changes in budget assumptions due to unrealized or unpredictable changes in major revenue or cost factors will require adjusting the budget results. These changes could occur during the budget period. Competition for qualified nursing personnel and retroactive adjustments to third-party payment arrangements would also require mid-term budget corrections.

A well thought-out and documented budget will be the road map that, if followed, will allow an agency to meet projected targets or benchmarks and achieve financial success.

CHAPTER 46

Reimbursement

Patricia A. Sevast

Home care expenditures for the federal government have grown significantly over the years with costs to the government estimated to exceed $45 billion dollars in the next few years. These costs grew from $3.3 billion in 1990 to over $18 billion in 1997 (Centers for Medicare and Medicaid [CMS], 2003a). Although this growth was spurred, in part, by the federal government and other insurances seeking alternate ways to hold down inpatient costs, the biggest push has come from managed care's efforts to provide cost-effective care and reduce inpatient stays. Managed care organizations (MCOs) have supported special programs such as short stay maternal-child programs followed by home care visits and other disease management programs.

Managed care's influence has also been felt in home care. In states with high managed care programs, home care visit utilization has been reduced significantly, sometimes half of Medicare visit utilization. The effect has been lower utilization and higher costs.

Home care agencies have instituted many new programs and technologies to manage utilization for managed care. These include intravenous infusion (IV) care, new birth services, pharmaceuticals, durable medical equipment (DME), adult day care, and wound care specialists, among others. In many cases, "primary" agencies obtain exclusive contracts with insurance carriers and contract for wide geographic coverage of staffing. The primary agency will provide a central point for intake and coordination of care, billing, and communication with the case management coordinators within the insurance company. Technology continues to perform a greater role in home care. Services requiring sophisticated equipment can now be provided in the home. Applications, such as new methods of wound care, allow care to be home based.

Over the years, the ownership of home health agencies (HHAs) has changed. HHAs started out as independent agencies, government health departments, or visiting nurse associations (VNAs). CMS reported that during the period of growth between 1985 and 1997, the number of certified agencies grew from 5,983 to 10,444. Hospital-based programs grew from 1,277 to 2,634 (Table 46-1).

Following the implementation of the Medicare Prospective Payment System (PPS), agency participation in Medicare dropped to 7,152 in 2000, the lowest since 1994. Changes in reimbursement, government efforts in fraud and abuse investigation, and mergers and acquisitions all played a role in the changing picture of the home health industry. Many individual agencies became parts of regional chains, with smaller chains merging into large industry chains. Hospital-based agencies and VNAs have consolidated into components of integrated delivery systems to acquire contracts. Consolidation at this level has been somewhat forced over the last several years by fierce competition and a focus on cost reduction. Hospitals first entered the market with expectations of engaging in money-making ventures, but now the goal is "positioning" the agency in a way that will

Table 46–1 Number of Medicare-Certified Home Care Agencies, by Auspice, for Selected Years, 1967–2000

| | Freestanding Agencies | | | | | | Facility-Based Agencies | | | |
Year	VNA	COMB	PUB	PROP	PNP	OTH	HOSP	REHAB	SNF	TOTAL
1967	549	93	939	0	0	39	133	0	0	1,753
1975	525	46	1,228	47	0	109	273	9	5	2,242
1980	515	63	1,260	186	484	40	359	8	9	2,924
1985	514	59	1,205	1,943	832	4	1,277	20	129	5,983
1990	474	47	985	1,884	710	0	1,486	8	101	5,695
1991	476	41	941	1,970	701	0	1,537	9	105	5,780
1992	530	52	1,083	1,962	637	28	1,623	3	86	6,004
1993	594	46	1,196	2,146	558	41	1,809	1	106	6,497
1994	586	45	1,146	2,892	597	48	2,081	3	123	7,521
1995	575	40	1,182	3,951	667	65	2,470	4	166	9,120
1996	576	34	1,177	4,658	695	58	2,634	4	191	10,027
1997	553	33	1,149	5,024	715	65	2,698	3	204	10,444
1998	460	35	968	3,414	610	69	2,356	2	166	8,080
1999	452	35	918	3,192	621	65	2,300	1	163	7,747
2000	436	31	909	2,863	560	56	2,151	1	150	7,152

VNA: Visiting nurse associations are freestanding, voluntary, nonprofit organizations governed by a board of directors and usually financed by tax-deductible contributions as well as by earnings.

COMB: Combination agencies are combined government and voluntary agencies. These agencies are sometimes included with counts for VNAs.

PUB: Public agencies are government agencies operated by a state, county, city, or other unit of local government having a major responsibility for preventing disease and for community health education.

PROP: Proprietary agencies are freestanding, for-profit home care agencies.

PNP: Private not-for-profit agencies are freestanding and privately developed, governed, and owned non-

profit home care agencies. These agencies were not counted separately prior to 1980.

OTH: Other freestanding agencies that do not fit one of the categories for freestanding agencies listed.

HOSP: Hospital-based agencies are operating units or departments of a hospital. Agencies that have working arrangements with a hospital, or perhaps are even owned by a hospital but operated as separate entities, are classified as freestanding agencies under one of the listed categories.

REHAB: Refers to agencies based in rehabilitation facilities.

SNF: Refers to agencies based in skilled nursing facilities.

Source: HCFA, Center for Information Systems, Health Standards and Quality Bureau, February 2001. Also in *Basic Statistics about Home Care 2001* (November 2001). Washington, DC. National Association for Home Care.

---

allow it to secure MCO contracts and/or be part of a system that will minimize patients leaving the system, control referrals, and provide less-expensive alternatives. Over the years, hospitals and managed care programs have learned to move patients through the system with more

control of treatment and utilization; this has proved the strength of the affiliated or owned agencies in surviving Medicare restrictions in payment methodologies. Securing a solid referral base is key to success in maintaining control of volume and cost within the agency.

This chapter covers current reimbursement trends for home health services with a concentration on Medicare because Medicare still pays for a substantial portion of home care services. This chapter concentrates on basic aspects of current Medicare reimbursement and addresses recent changes implemented by CMS. Medicare has been most restrictive in determining eligibility for coverage. Coverage is determined by the Social Security law, CMS, and fiscal intermediary interpretation of coverage regulations.

OVERVIEW

Major changes in recent years with the implementation of prospective payment models in several provider areas have been driven by shortages in the Medicare trust funds and efforts of managed care to reduce costs. Successful cost reductions by managed care have been the basis for Medicare's goals of controlling costs and utilization.

Efforts to introduce a prospective payment system for home care were introduced in the 1980s and demonstration projects were funded into the 1990s. Congressional activity regarding PPS was increased as a result of increased patient and visit utilization. As indicated earlier, expenditures grew from $3.3 billion in 1990 to $18 billion in 1997. Visits per patient grew from 27 in 1989, to 60 in 1994, and to 72 in 1995. Fraud and abuse efforts on the part of CMS (then the Health Care Financing Administration, HCFA) through a program known as Operation Restore Trust revealed a 40 percent rate of overutilization in home care. Industry leaders claim that these figures were overstated, but the numbers encouraged Congress to hasten reimbursement reform.

The federal government provides home health care, or funding for such services, under a variety of programs created by the Social Security Act, including Medicare (Title XVIII) and Medicaid (Title XIX) and other special programs. These programs provide funding for specific services. Medicare was enacted July 1, 1965, and became effective on July 1, 1966. Medicare is a two-part program commonly referred to as Part A and Part B. Under Part A, Medicare beneficiaries receive insurance coverage for inpatient hospitalization, skilled nursing facility care, hospice, and some home care visits. In addition to Part A coverage, beneficiaries may purchase, for a monthly fee, supplemental insurance for Part B coverage. The monthly premium is determined by a formula set forth in the law. Part B covers physician services, pathology services, outpatient services, laboratory services, equipment, home care, and other services. Most services under Part B are covered at 80 percent of reasonable and customary charges, a fee schedule, or prospective payment, following an annual deductible. Following passage of the Balanced Budget Act of 1997, home care is funded by both Part A and Part B. For services under Part B, there are no current coinsurances or deductibles, although Congress has considered these annually. Industry efforts have succeeded in defeating these proposed legislative changes.

Medicare is an entitlement program with benefits offered to persons who are at least 65 years of age and eligible for Social Security retirement benefits, who are younger that 65 but have been eligible for Social Security for at least 2 years as a result of a disability, or who have end-stage renal disease. There are six types of services that are considered reimbursable under home health benefits: (1) skilled nursing, (2) home health aide service, (3) physical therapy, (4) speech therapy, (5) occupational therapy, and (6) medical social work.

ELIGIBILITY

In order for care to be covered by Medicare, eligibility and coverage requirements must be met. Eligibility requirements include a valid Medicare number; care provided under a physician signed plan of treatment; homebound; and the need for intermittent skilled nursing, physical therapy, or speech therapy. (Occupational therapy does not qualify a patient for initial coverage, but can qualify a patient for continued coverage.) In eligibility criteria, intermittent means at least one visit every 60 days or not daily for more than 3 weeks unless a reasonable end point is identified.

Medical social work and home health aide services are considered to be nonqualifying services. These services can be provided only as long as the patient meets eligibility requirements for home care (Exhibits 46–1 and 46–2).

Care provided by professional staff is usually referred to as "skilled." Skilled nursing care is rendered by a licensed nurse. Skilled nursing care includes, but is not limited to, observation and assessment; teaching; administration of injections; and direct care interventions, such as wound care. Under the general category of nursing, but deemed "unskilled," are home health aide services. These usually include personal care services and may also be an extension of therapy services. Nursing care must be "part-time and intermittent." This phrase, an often discussed and contested element of the coverage definition, has been defined to mean less that 8 hours a day, inclusive of nursing and home health aide care delivered.

Home care services may be provided only in the patient's home or place of residence unless the patient meets special criteria for provision of outpatient services in the home. These outpatient services are reimbursed fee-for-service and are not covered under prospective payment at this time.

To be considered homebound, the patient must be unable to regularly leave the home without considerable and taxing effort. This does not mean that the patient can never leave the home, but the clinical record must document functional limitations that indicate that the patient cannot regularly leave home without assistance.

The Medicare Conditions of Participation (COPs) in section 484.18 (DHHS, 2000) and the Medicare Home Health Agency manual (HIM 11) in sections 201.6, 204.1, 204.2, 204.3, and 204.5, both address the issue of physician orders. Because home health benefits are covered only if the beneficiary is provided care under the plan of treatment signed by the physician, this issue is significant in that failure to comply with

physician orders can lead to payment denial under reimbursement regulations and survey deficiencies under state survey.

For PPS, all physician orders for services provided during the episode must be signed prior to submission of the final claim. Orders must be obtained at the beginning of the episode when the plan of treatment is established, and any modifications to the plan that occur during the 60-day episode must be written on verbal orders and signed by the physician. The plan of treatment established at the beginning of each episode is required to be documented on the CMS Form 485. The 485, as it is commonly referred to as, is an official form, or software-generated format, defined by CMS in the COPs and Medicare coverage manual (HIM 11) (CMS, 2003a). Each box on the 485 is defined and used to document the disciplines ordered, visit frequency and duration, and clinical interventions for each discipline. A new 485 is generated for each 60-day episode. Modifications or changes to the plan of treatment during the episode, also known as verbal orders, are documented on forms developed by the individual agency.

Prior to PPS, agencies submitted one claim per month for services provided. Billing regulations required that all orders pertaining to care during the month be signed prior to submission of a claim.

In developing PPS, CMS wanted to avoid cash flow problems and developed the concept of the Request for Anticipated Payment (RAP). For billing purposes, a RAP is not considered a claim and is not subject to signed physician order requirements. A final claim, submitted at the end of an episode, does have to comply with signed physician order requirements.

The home health PPS billing process was designed by CMS to have two steps, RAP and final claim. Following the start of a case or beginning of an episode, the agency can submit the RAP. The final claim is submitted following the end of the episode or discharge date, whichever is sooner. There should be only one request for anticipated payment (RAP) filed with the Medicare intermediary for each episode. If the final claim is not filed in a timely manner, Medicare takes

Exhibit 46–1 Home Health Benefit Overview and Admission Screening Tool

Home Health Benefit Overview and Admission Screening Tool
Venue: Skilled care under a Medicare Certified Home Health Agency

Medicare as Primary Payer	Key Factors and Alert Points
Technical Coverage	Enrolled in Part A OR Part B of Medicare. No pre-hospitalization requirements. Patient remains under the care of a **physician who will sign the Plan of Treatment** (form 485) and be responsible for ongoing care of the patient.
Clinical Coverage/Qualifiers	1) Patient must be **homebound**. 2) Patient must need **skilled** services of a Registered Nurse, Physical Therapist, or Speech Therapist to initiate care. Occupational Therapy, Medical Social Work, and home health aide considered dependent services. These services can be provided as long as qualifying services is covered. Occupational Therapy may continue as a qualifying service once a RN, PT, or ST has initiated care. 3) Services must be **intermittent** – at least one visit every 60 days; RN/aide services do not exceed 35 hours a week; RN visits not daily (7 days a week) for more that 21 days, unless there is a reasonable end-point. 4) Services are **reasonable and necessary** to meet the medical needs of the patient as ordered on the plan of care. Skilled services include, but are not limited to observation and assessment during acute or unstable periods; teaching activities; administration of IM or IV medications; extensive wound care; administration of treatments; establishment and monitoring of treatment or therapeutic exercise programs; and other skilled interventions.
Reimbursement Driver	Since 10/1/2001, payment is based on the Home Health Prospective Payment System. Payment is based on a 60 day episode of care, unless 4 or fewer visits made in episode, then the agency is paid a per visit payment. The episode payment rate is established by the scoring of 23 questions in the Outcome and Assessment Information Set (OASIS). OASIS is collected and scored at Start of Care, Recertification (prior to end of 60 day episode), and resumption of care (following hospital stay during 60 day episode). Episode rates may be prorated based on readmission to agency, transfers between agencies and changes in the patient's condition during the episode. Limited outlier payments. Elements used in scoring include selected clinical, functional, and utilization criteria. Projected use of 10 therapy (physical, speech, and/or occupational) significantly increases reimbursement.
Benefit Limitations	Unlimited episodes are covered as long as coverage criteria are met.
Unique Payer Requirements	1. Physician certification on admission and recertification (every 60 days). Signed verbal orders needed to cover changes. 2. Claims subject to medical review, known as ADR's (Additional Documentation Requests). Denials issued after medical review.
OIG Focus: Potential Fraud and Abuse Related to Case Management	1. Billing for services when the patient is not homebound; services are not necessary; visits are excessive and made only to exceed therapy or low visit threshold; visits not made (fraud); visits made without physician's orders; services not provided when needed. 2. Improper OASIS and or ICD-9-CM coding to increase reimbursement. 3. High cost patients are not afforded services needed.
Case Management Priorities in Pre-Admission Evaluation	Patient must meet Medicare/agency admission and eligibility criteria, including safe and adequate home environment. Caregiver availability/willingness/ability often an issue in determining appropriate level of care.
Other Payment Rules Impacting Case Management	1) Consolidated billing under home health PPS includes payment in episode rate for all supplies and outpatient therapy services, does not include DME. 2) Early discharge/transfer rule (reduced hospital payment for discharge prior to the geometric mean for 10 targeted DRGs).
Managed Care	Acceptance, Restrictions and Opportunities
	Possible contract arrangements include fee-for-service, capitated, or discounted rates. Pre-authorization usually required. Opportunities for increased revenue through contracts for types of visits, including costly admission visits or visits of excessive time. Many managed care plans do not have homebound requirement. Potential ability to carve out costly supplies for separate payment. OASIS data collection required of all aduld patients, except maternity services.

Exhibit 46–2 Admission Screening and Utilization Management Record

Admission Screening and Utilization Management Record

Patient: _____   **Anticipated Admit Date:** _____   From: _____

Prior Functional Level: Assisted Living   Home with Home Health (for) _____
Independent/home   Home with in-home care (family)   LTC Facility/limited Assistance

Estimated LOS: _____   Anticipated discharge planning needs: _____

Relevant Diagnoses: _____
For the following DRGs, early discharge/transfer to SNU, HH, Acute Rehab, LTAC impacts acute payment: 14, 113, 209, 210, 211, 236, 263, 264, 429, 483

3-day qualifying stay: _____ to _____   OR Prior hospital or SNF stay within prior 30 days ending: _____

SNF days remaining: ___as of ___/___/2001   Skilled qualifier(s) _____

Utilization and Assessment Information

Item/Service	PTA (✓) Date(s) Expected duration if a current treatment
IV Therapy	*
TPN Continuous Tube Feeding	*
Ventilator	*
Chemotherapy	*
Transfusion	*
Tracheostomy	**(recent)** *
Infection: **VRE MRSA** **Wound UTI URI** **Other:** _____	* Describe infection site, type and duration of antibiotic therapy. * *Indicates a level of service or treatment characteristic that may qualify for LTAC if LOS is anticipated to be 21 days or longer.*
Diagnostic Services Planned After Transfer?	
Ultrasound	
Scan/MRI	
Doppler	
Endoscopy	
Other	
Intake History Recent weight loss of ___ # in ___ days Recent weight loss of ___ # in ___ months Must be fed Nausea/vomiting	
Wound Care Simple Complex	Stage III-IV pressure ulcer Condition requires intensive treatment? Yes* No Postoperative wound care Condition requires intensive treatment? Yes* No Stasis ulcer * *Patient may be a candidate for LTAC*
Depression (new diagnosis)	
Fever	
Pain Management	
PT OT Speech Projected duration:	Condition requires frequent medical supervision? Yes* No Requires/can tolerate up to 3 hours of therapy per day? Yes* No Significant practical improvement expected? Yes* No Significant progress/tolerance level for therapy demonstrated in acute? Yes* No * *Patient may be a candidate for Acute Rehab*
ADL Self-Performance Bed Mobility: Physical help 1 2 Transfer: Physical help 1 2 lift Eating: Physical help Aspiration Risk Toilet Use: Physical help 1 2	Prior functional level in ADLs (if known): Bed Mobility: Independent Physical help 1 2 Transfer: Independent Physical help 1 2 lift Eating: Independent Physical help Aspiration Risk Toilet Use: Independent Physical help 1 2

Source: Courtesy of Patricia A. Sevast

back the amount paid for the RAP (auto-cancellation) and a new RAP needs to be filed. Final claims should be submitted on time to avoid this costly problem and relieve cash flow delays.

Each agency needs to have an established system to ensure that:

- Orders are written.
- Orders are complete.
- Orders are sent to the physician.
- Signed orders are received.
- A system is in place to communicate with the billing department.

Many agencies can use their software vendor for all or part of these criteria. The HIM 11 indicates that all changes to the plan of treatment must be covered by verbal orders and that all orders must be signed prior to billing.

Coverage of care and claims processing of home health claims responsibility has been contracted through regional fiscal intermediaries (FI). FIs are insurance companies that contract with CMS to process claims, monitor coverage requirements, and have audit responsibilities for the agencies assigned to them.

PROSPECTIVE PAYMENT

From the inception of Medicare until October 1, 2000, Medicare reimbursed home health agencies the lower of cost or charges for their services. Claims were submitted on a monthly basis to the FI. Visits and supplies were listed, claims processed and paid, and each agency submitted an annual cost report at the end of the year to determine final settled payment.

Prior to October 1, 2000, Medicare reimbursed providers of home health reasonable cost of the performing services up to predetermined per-visit cost limitations excluding certain non-allowable costs. Such a system did not foster operational efficiency within agencies, and was believed by HCFA (now CMS) to result in excessive visits to Medicare beneficiaries. Throughout the early to mid-1990s, costs for the Medicare home health benefit increased significantly. Prompted by several high profile fraud cases and spiraling costs, changes in the Medicare home health payment system were set in motion.

The Balanced Budget Act of 1997 (BBA of 1997), the Omnibus Consolidated and Emergency Supplemental Appropriations Act of 1999 (OCESAA), and the Balanced Budget Refinement Act of 1999 (BBRA) established the framework for a transition to a PPS. Medicare established an Interim Payment System (IPS) during the period of transition from cost reimbursement to PPS. IPS resulted in per-beneficiary cost limitations and reductions in existing per-visit cost limitations to significantly reduce cost to the Medicare program during the transition.

As established in the proposed rule (October 28, 1999) and refined in the final rule (July 3, 2000), new requirements were established for home health PPS. PPS was effective for claims with dates of service on or after October 1, 2000. Under PPS, Medicare pays home health agencies a predetermined base payment adjusted for health condition and care needs of the beneficiary. The initial standard episode payment was $2,115.30. This amount was increased for episodes ending on or after April 1, 2001, to $2,161.84, and episodes ending on or after October 1, 2001, to $2,274.17. Standard episode rates were increased for each subsequent year to $2,159.39 effective October 1, 2002, and $2,235.65 effective October 1, 2003. The payment is also adjusted for geographic differences in wages for HHAs across the country. The adjustment for health condition, or clinical characteristics, and service needs of the beneficiary is referred to as the *case mix adjustment*. The home health PPS provides HHAs with payments for each 60-day episode of care for each beneficiary. If a beneficiary is still eligible for care after the end of the first episode, a second episode can begin; there are no limits to the number of episodes a beneficiary can receive as long as Medicare eligibility is maintained. The episode payment includes reimbursement for all visits made to the beneficiary, supplies, and outpatient therapy received in an outpatient setting while the beneficiary is receiving care under a home health episode.

Criteria for Medicare coverage continue to include:

- Valid Medicare number
- Homebound
- Under the care of a physician
- Order for services
- Skilled
- Reasonable and necessary
- Intermittent

The home health PPS is composed of several main features used to calculate payment rates and methods, which include:

A. Split Percentage Payment Approach—Under this system, for an initial episode, an agency receives an initial payment of 60 percent of the case mix and wage-adjusted 60-day episode rate as soon as it notifies the fiscal intermediary of an admission. A final 40 percent payment is made at the close of the 60-day episode. For subsequent episodes, the initial percentage payment is 50 percent and the final payment is 50 percent.

B. Request for Anticipated Payment (RAP)—This is the formal request made by the home health agency to the intermediary for the initial percentage payment. This is not a claim and is not subject to the requirement that the physician sign the plan of care before the agency bills the RAP. However, the RAP must be based on a physician's verbal order or a referral prescribing detail orders for the services to be rendered that is signed and dated by the physician. If a verbal order is received to initiate services, an attestation relating to the physician's orders by the registered nurse or therapist responsible for furnishing or supervising the care is documented by the signature and date entry in box 23 of CMS Form 485.

C. Case-Mix Methodology—The case-mix system uses selected data elements from the Outcome and Assessment Information Set (OASIS) assessment instrument and an additional data element measuring receipt of therapy services of at least 10 visits. The data elements are organized into three dimensions: (1) clinical severity factors, (2) functional severity factors, and (3) service utilization factors. Each of these influences the case mix. There are four clinical severity levels, five functional severity levels, and four service utilization severity levels. As a result, there are 80 ($4 \times 5 \times 4$) possible combinations of severity across the three dimensions. Each combination defines one of the 80 groups (Home Health Resource Group or HHRG) in the case-mix system. Each of these HHRGs corresponds to a different payment rate.

D. Partial Episode Payment (PEP)—The partial episode payment is an adjustment to a full episodic payment based on certain events. The first example of a PEP adjustment would occur if a beneficiary elected to transfer to another home health agency during the 60-day episode. The second case would be if a beneficiary is discharged and returns to the same home health agency during the 60-day episode. Patients who elect to enter a Medicare-managed care program during their home health episode are subject to a PEP adjustment.

E. Low-Utilization Payment Adjustment (LUPA)—A LUPA is for beneficiaries whose episode consists of four or fewer visits. These episodes are paid at a standard service-specific per-visit amount, labor adjusted, multiplied by the number of visits actually provided during the episode. These rates are adjusted annually and are published in the *Federal Register* with the adjusted episode rate.

F. Significant Change in Condition (SCIC)—A SCIC adjustment occurs when a beneficiary experiences a significant change in condition during the 60-day episode not envisioned in the original physician's plan of care and original case-mix assignment. Payment is prorated based on days served in each segment of the episode.

G. Outlier Payments—Additional payments are made to the 60-day case-mix adjusted episode for beneficiaries who incur unusually large costs. The additional payment is based on a relatively complex formula and includes a fixed dollar amount loss.

BILLING

Most home health agencies use a software program to bill for services to Medicare. Those agencies without a billing software package use the FISS (Fiscal Intermediary Shared System) to perform direct data entry of claims. Effective October 16, 2003, HIPAA's (the Health Insurance Portability and Accountability Act) standard transaction and code set regulations require all health care providers to bill electronically for services. Features of commercial software programs include, at a minimum, charge entry, billing, development of the plan of treatment, and management of accounts receivable. Many programs include modules for data entry of OASIS. Electronic entry and transmission of OASIS data is required for transmission to the state OASIS data repository and to obtain the PPS Health Insurance Prospective Payment System (HIPPS) code for billing. Patient admissions and visits are usually documented in the patient clinical chart and then data is entered or transmitted into the system. OASIS assessments required for Medicare PPS patients are completed by the home care providers using the system. Completed and reviewed OASIS assessments are generated from the system and transmitted to the state for subsequent processing by Medicare, as well as to the agency billing system. The billing system uses the admission, visit, and OASIS assessment data to create claims for electronic submission to the Medicare Fiscal Intermediary for payment. Remittance advices are then received from the Fiscal Intermediary and payments are posted to the agency system or, if there were problems with the claim, adjustments are made and the claim is resubmitted.

The Medicare Prospective Payment System method of home health reimbursement was implemented on October 1, 2000, and the information systems changes required for support of PPS by the systems were extensive. Software vendors had to modify their software to provide PPS functionality as well as developing an interface with the state system to electronically receive OASIS assessment scoring data.

PPS ISSUES

High therapy utilization scoring is a problem throughout the home health industry under PPS. Some agencies score all episodes that have at least one therapy open as a high therapy utilization episode because Medicare will automatically downcode the score if the actual therapy visits do not reach 10. If the agency does not score the episode as high therapy utilization and the actual number of therapy visits does reach 10, Medicare will not automatically upcode the episode and therefore will not pay the higher amount unless the claim is resubmitted.

Many home care agencies have experienced problems associated with answering M0825, commonly known as the *therapy threshold question*. Many other agencies across the country have erred on the side of answering this question positively, resulting in overpayments and overstatements of revenue and accounts receivable. These bills have been automatically downcoded by the fiscal intermediary with the submission of the final claim.

COST REPORTS

With the implementation of PPS, agencies are no longer reimbursed based on a cost report settlement. Learning from previous experience with hospice, where no costs were initially required, CMS continues to require the annual submission of a cost report. The cost report will provide needed data related to agencies' costs in order for CMS to monitor the agencies' costs for future reimbursement analysis.

CLINICAL OASIS SCORING

As stated earlier, OASIS documentation and the selected answers to 23 of the OASIS items form the basis for home health Medicare PPS reimbursement (Table 46–2). The clinician's understanding of the OASIS items, along with the total documentation of the comprehensive assessment, is the basis for payment. The OASIS items are explained in the OASIS manual, specifically Chapter 8, OASIS Items in Detail. Based on the scoring methodology, inaccurate OASIS answers can lead to errors in payment, most significantly, undercoding or upcoding. Undercoding will lead to case-mix weights with lower reimbursement than appropriate to the patient's condition; upcoding leads to higher reimbursement than appropriate. Accurate assessment is essential to compliance with both coverage regulations and the Conditions of Participation and survey issues.

DIAGNOSIS CODING

Diagnosis coding, selection of the appropriate and accurate ICD-9CM code for home health patients, has become a critical issue under PPS. In the past, Medicare coverage regulations required the clinician to identify the primary and secondary diagnoses and codes for inclusion on the Form 485. These codes were also placed on the Uniform Billing (UB)-92 for billing. Medicare regulations have been changed to specify that the diagnoses codes listed on the clinician's OASIS assessment must agree with the codes listed on the plan of treatment (Form 485) sent to the physician and the UB-92.

Under cost reimbursement and medical review, these were not often correct, although valid codes were required for billing. Under PPS, the primary diagnosis and, in certain manifestation code situations, the secondary diagnosis is significant. Primary diagnosis and secondary diagnosis are specific OASIS items included in case-mix weight scoring. Selection of primary diagnosis (M0230) and in some cases secondary diagnosis (M0240) can raise the clinical domain score from C0 to C1 or C2, resulting in increased payment per episode of an average of $100 to $450. CMS and the intermediaries have placed this OASIS item high on the list of items at risk for fraud and abuse.

Medicare billing regulations and conditions of participation require that all diagnoses related to the plan of treatment be included on the Form 485.

SIGNIFICANT CHANGE IN CONDITION

The PPS final rule specifies certain situations where adjustments to payment will be made. One such adjustment is the Significant Change in Condition (SCIC). Originally designed to allow for increased payment in cases where the patient's condition changes unexpectedly, the formulas developed by CMS rarely provide additional payment. The prorated payment is computed based on days of service before and after the change. A SCIC adjustment must be reported if the change in condition and resumption of care assessment results in a lower case-mix weight. The agency has the option not to report a SCIC if the case-mix weight is higher but the payment has been reduced due to the formula used.

THERAPY THRESHOLD

In the analysis of data used to establish the PPS case-mix weights and payments, CMS indicated that high therapy use was an indicator of overall increased utilization of services by home health agencies. In the final rule, CMS established that 10 combined (physical therapy/occupational therapy/speech therapy) therapy visits would be used to establish the threshold for high therapy cases. The pre-existing OASIS data elements did not include any OASIS question that addressed this issue. As a result, a new OASIS question, M0825, was established. M0825 asks: "Therapy Need: Does the care plan of the Medicare payment period for which this assessment will define a case mix group indicate a need for therapy (physical, occupational, or speech therapy) that meets the threshold for a Medicare high-therapy case-mix group?" The available answers are "Yes," "No," and "Not applicable." If the clinician answers "Yes," then four points are added to the calculation of the service domain section of the HHRG. The result is a service utilization score of S2 or S3, and a calculated increase in episode payment of an average of $1,850. The HIPPS code on the RAP initiates the first payment to the agency. When the final claim is submitted to the intermediary,

Table 46–2 Home Health Resource Group Case-Mix Classification Decision Tree Logic

Clinical Severity Domain

OASIS+ Item	Description	Value	Scoring
M0230/M0240	Primary home care diagnosis (or initial secondary diagnosis ONLY for selected ICD-9 manifestation codes)	—credit only the single highest value: If Orthopedic diagnostic group (DG)*, add 11 to score If Diabetes DG*, add 17 to score If Neurological DG*, add 20 to score	Min = 0-7 Low = 8-19 Mod = 20-40 High = 41+
M0250	IV/Infusion/ Parenteral/value: Enteral therapies	—credit only the single highest value: If box 1, add 14 to score If box 2, add 20 to score If box 3, add 24 to score	
M0390	Vision	If box 1 or 2, add 6 to score	
M0420	Pain	If box 2 or 3, add 5 to score	
M0440	Wound/Lesion	If box 1 and M0230 is Burn/Trauma DG*, add 21 to score	
M0450	Multiple pressure ulcers	If 2 or more stage 3 or 4 pressure ulcers, add 17 to score	
M0460	Most problematic pressure ulcer stage	If box 1 or 2, add 15 to score If box 3 or 4, add 36 to score	
M0476	Stasis ulcer status	If box 2, add 14 to score If box 3, add 22 to score	
M0488	Surgical wound status	If box 2, add 7 to score If box 3, add 15 to score	
M0490	Dyspnea	If box 2, 3, or 4, add 5 to score	
M0530	Urinary incontinence	If box 1 or 2, add 6 to score	
M0540	Bowel incontinence	If box 2–5, add 9 to score	
M0550	Bowel ostomy	If box 1 or 2, add 10 to score	
M0610	Behavioral problems	If box 1–6, add 3 to score	

*Refer to the National Center for Health Statistics, International Classification of Diseases, 9th Edition, Clinical Modification (ICD9-CM) codes included in each diagnosis group (DG).

Functional status domain

OASIS+ Item	Description	Value	Scoring
M0650 (current) M0660 (current)	Dressing	If M0650 = box 1, 2, or 3 Or } add 4 to score M0660 = box 1, 2, or 3	Min = 0–2 Low = 3–15 Mod = 16–23
M0670 (current)	Bathing	If box 2, 3, 4, or 5 add 8 to score	High = 24–29
M0680 (current)	Toileting	If box 2–4, add 3 to score	Max = 30+

Continues

Table 46-2 *(Continued)*

Functional status domain

OASIS+ Item	Description	Value	Scoring
M0690 (current)	Transferring	If box 1, add 3 to score If box 2–5, add 6 to score	
M0700 (current)	Locomotion	If box 1 or 2, add 6 to score If box 3–5, add 9 to score	

Service utilization domain

OASIS+ Item	Description	Value	Scoring
M0175—line 1	No Hospital discharge past 14 days	If box 1 IS BLANK, add 1 to score	Min = 0–2
M0175—line 2 or 3	Inpatient rehab/SNF discharge past 14 days	If box 2 or 3, add 2 to score	Low = 3
M0825	10 or more therapy.	If yes, add 4 to score visits.	Mod = 4–6 High = 7

Source: Federal Register, July 3, 2000, Washington, DC, p. 41194.

the intermediary Pricer software counts the therapy visits that are reported on the claim. If the Pricer software counts at least 10 therapy visits, the full episode payment is made. If less than 10 therapy visits are on the claim, the software automatically downcodes the HIPPS code to what the code would have been if M0825 had been answered "No," and recalculates the payment.

The agency payment is recalculated and shown on the remittance advice as the lower HIPPS code and dollar amount. The Pricer software only works to the intermediary's advantage; that is, the software will not automatically upcode the HIPPS code to a higher payment if the agency originally answered "No" and did provide 10 or more therapy visits. The agency must cancel the claim, re-enter the OASIS, obtain a new HIPPS code, and rebill, sending a new RAP and final claim for the episode.

OASIS DATA COLLECTION AND SCORING

Under PPS, reimbursement is based on the case-mix weight assigned to the patient's 60-day episode of care. The case-mix weight, or

HHRG, is determined by scoring the patient at the time of admission or reassessment at 60-day intervals. The score is based on 23 OASIS data items integrated into the assessment process.

OASIS was originally developed by CMS and was the basis for the planned implementation of Outcome Based Quality Improvement (OBQI). CMS had planned to use OASIS for outcome measurement as far back as March 1997 when the proposed changes to the COPs included reference to OASIS and OBQI implementation. Later, CMS decided to use the OASIS data elements to develop the case-mix system for home health PPS. The OASIS regulations, published in the *Federal Register* on January 25, 1999, revise the Medicare Conditions of Participation for home health agencies. The OASIS requirements were to be implemented in February 1999, but were delayed due to privacy issues and went into effect in July 1999. This provided home health agencies with just over 1 year of experience with OASIS prior to the implementation of PPS.

The OASIS regulations required home health agencies to incorporate the OASIS items as developed by CMS into the patient assessment process. For OBQI purposes, the data is transmitted to the state for later processing of OASIS case-mix reports, adverse event reports, and later in 2003, risk-adjusted outcome reports. The OASIS data collection process is also used as the basis for determining the home health agency's PPS case-mix category for reimbursement. The software system used by an agency for OASIS transmission also calculates the case-mix score and converts the score to a HIPPS code for billing.

CMS has published an OASIS manual that contains all of the requirements for OASIS data collection and reporting.

HHRG/HIPPS CODE ASSIGNMENT

The Medicare PPS billing requirements, as developed by CMS and published by the fiscal intermediaries and included in training materials, indicate that the HHRG (case-mix weight) determined by the calculation of the OASIS scoring process must be translated to the HIPPS code, be accurate, and be placed on the RAP and final claim. The HIPPS code on the RAP must be the same as the HIPPS code on the final claim unless a SCIC has occurred and the SCIC HIPPS code is listed on the claim on a different line, with a corresponding date of assessment.

The OASIS regulation and OASIS manual require that all OASIS questions required for the reason for assessment (RFA M0100) be answered, carefully following indicated skip patterns.

MEDICAL REVIEW

As part of their contracting responsibilities, the fiscal intermediaries are responsible for claims processing and monitoring for compliance. Fiscal intermediaries have developed systems and edits within the processes to identify high-risk claims. Through a process of random and targeted review, the intermediaries identify claims for review. Medical review staff makes coverage determinations based on clinical record documentation.

In response to claims entering the FISS, the intermediary sends to the home health agency a request for additional documentation (ADR). The agency is required to respond to the ADR within 35 days of issuance. Intermediary review staff obtain the clinical record and billing claims information. The record is reviewed for compliance with eligibility and coverage standards, including support for OASIS scoring, visit utilization, and physician's orders. Coverage denials can be made related to any area of eligibility requirements. Denials for lack of support of OASIS scoring may result in reduced payment in the form of lower HHRG payments. Denial of visits for lack of orders, skill, or medical necessity may result in no change in reimbursement or reduction in episode payment if the denial brings the total number of visits to a LUPA episode or lowers the number of therapy visits to below the therapy threshold.

Providers have the right to appeal denials if liability is attached. If the denial is medical in nature, the patient can appeal or assign representation to the provider to appeal. The appeal or Request for Reconsideration must be filed within 60 days of the initial determination. This appeal is reviewed at the intermediary level by medical staff separate from staff that made the initial claim determination. If the denial is overturned, payment is made. If the denial is upheld, the provider has 6 months to file a request for an administrative law judge review. At this time, the appeals process is under revision. The proposed rules may provide a longer appeal time period and insert a review level at the first level of appeal.

CONCLUSION

Major changes in recent years with the implementation of the PPS models in several provider areas have been driven by shortages in the Medicare trust funds and efforts of managed care to reduce costs. Successful cost reductions by managed care organizations have been the basis for Medicare's goals of controlling costs and utilization. The implementation of the Medicare PPS in 2000 changed the method of reimbursement to providers of home health care services. Home health care administrators and staff must be cognizant of the main features and methods used to calculate payment rates as well as all other issues related to the current PPS method of reimbursement.

REFERENCES

Centers for Medicare and Medicaid Services. 2003a. *CMS health care industry market update.* http://cms.hhs.gov/reports/hcimu/

Centers for Medicare and Medicaid Services. 2003b. *HIM 11 home health agency manual.* Washington, DC, p. 41194.

Department of Health and Human Services. 2000. *Federal Register code of federal regulations* (Title 42) Parts 409, 410, 411, 413, 424, and 484 Medicare Program; Prospective Payment System for Home Health Agencies; Final Rule.

Department of Health and Human Services. 2003. *Code of federal regulations* (Title 42) Section 405.1801 et seq. Washington, DC: U.S. Government Printing Office.

BIBLIOGRAPHY

Cahaba Government Benefits Administration. 2003. *Medicare reference guide for home health agencies.* Des Moines, IA: Author.

National Association for Home Care. 2001. *Basic statistics for home care 2001.* Washington, DC: Author.

CHAPTER 47

How to Read, Interpret, and Understand Financial Statements

D. Scott Detar

Financial statements used by administrators of home health organizations vary from organization to organization. Home health organizations may be nonprofit or commercial enterprises operating for profit. Depending on the organization, financial reports may be on a cash or accrual basis. This chapter approaches the reading and understanding of a home health organization's financial statement from the perspective of a nonprofit organization. Many of the interpretations, ratios, and conclusions are the same regardless of the type of enterprise (nonprofit or for profit). Where there are differences, they are noted and explained. This chapter assumes that accrual basis financial statements are prepared.

CASH BASIS OR ACCRUAL BASIS

Cash basis accounting simply means recording only those transactions when cash is received and disbursed. There is no attempt to record receivables for service rendered or payables for amounts owed by the organization. Many small nonprofit organizations use the cash basis of accounting during the year, principally because it is the most simple method of record keeping. The cash basis method of accounting is merely the recording of the activity in the organization's checkbook.

As organizations grow in size, however, there is a need to see not only a more accurate, but also a more complete picture of their financial results on a regular basis (i.e., monthly, quarterly, or annually). Organizations will use the accrual basis of accounting to record transactions during the accounting period. The accrual basis requires organizations to record transactions resulting from the receipt and disbursement of cash as well as amounts owed them for services rendered and the amounts they owe for goods and services. The underlying accounting principle used in recording accrual basis transactions is to match revenue earned during the accounting period to expenses incurred to generate that revenue for the same accounting period.

Many administrators or executives of organizations, whether nonprofit or commercial enterprises, operate using the cash basis theory. They understand what is going into the bank and what is coming out of the bank. These same administrators or executives many times mistakenly believe that the accrual basis is more complicated. In fact, accrual basis statements can be quite easy to read. A thorough understanding of the financial statements will assist the administrator in his or her ability to make informed day-to-day operational decisions. The informed administrator each month should be reviewing four financial statements and at least one schedule of statistics.

The first statement is the income statement, or, for nonprofit organizations, the statement of revenue and expenses for the period under review. The second statement is the balance sheet, listing all assets and liabilities at the end of the period. The third statement, the statement of functional expenses, allocates expenses by program. The fourth statement, the statement of cash flows, is a meaningful and integral part of the financial picture relating the accrual basis to the cash basis. The schedule of statistics needs to be available and reviewed in conjunction with these four financial statements for the administrator to be properly informed. This chapter discusses how to read and interpret each of the four financial statements.

SCHEDULE OF STATISTICS

A thorough understanding of home health agency financial statements involves a careful review and understanding of the basic statistics or data used to generate the financial statements. Three basic statistical essentials are described here.

Visits

For all accounting periods shown, the number of visits should also be reported. Visit reporting should include current reporting periods, year to date reporting periods, and budgeted periods. Visits should be detailed by fee source (the payer) and also by discipline (the type of service, e.g., nursing, therapies, etc.). Many home health agencies also provide hours in addition to or in lieu of visit data.

Personnel

Employee statistics for the period reported on are the number of employees (full and part time)

in each service area calculated in terms of a full-time equivalent (FTE). FTE equates all full- and part-time employees into a common denominator for employment. This statistic should be available for service areas (nursing, therapies, etc.) as well as administrative departments.

Accounts Receivable Aging Percentages

Accounts receivable aging percentages by pay source must always be presented when reviewing balance sheets and income statements. The aging columns should be labeled as current (0 to 30 days), 30 to 60 days, 60 to 90 days, 90 to 120 days, and more than 120 days. Aging is usually based on the month in which services were performed.

Analyzing statistics along with financial statements is likely to have an immediate impact on the administrator's understanding of an agency's operations, but their longer-term benefits may have even greater value. As third-party payers move toward capitation as a method of reimbursing health care service providers, the pressure on those providers to control costs per capita is sure to increase. That's when an even closer look at the numbers—revenue per visit, personnel cost per visit, and the like—will make a critical difference in an agency's financial success.

INCOME STATEMENT

The income statement details revenue and expenses during the accounting period reported. In Exhibit 47–1, the accounting periods shown are 2003 and 2002. Revenue, or the fees billed for the home health visits and services provided to patients, is reflected in the period the services were provided by agency personnel. Revenue is generally reported net of any contractual allowances or reserves for uncollectibles. Revenue is the dollar equivalent of service agency individuals (nurses, therapists, etc.) provided patients during the period.

In the example, the administrator should ask the question, "Why did revenue increase by $528,000?" This can be answered by reviewing

Exhibit 47–1 Home Health Agency Statement of Revenue, Expenses, and Changes in Fund Balances: Years Ended December 31, 2003, and December 31, 2002

	2003	*2002*
REVENUE		
Nursing and related service fees	$1,823,146	$1,294,811
Investment and other income	10,207	10,590
TOTAL REVENUE	1,833,353	1,305,401
EXPENSES		
Program services	1,459,188	990,221
Administrative	511,123	417,562
TOTAL EXPENSES	1,970,311	1,407,783
LOSS FROM OPERATIONS	(136,958)	(102,382)
NONOPERATING INCOME		
United Way appropriation	78,290	76,000
Municipal appropriations	57,250	59,330
Grant	17,588	—
Contributions and bequests	33,434	45,350
Total Nonoperating Income	186,562	180,680
Revenue and Income in Excess of Expenses	49,604	78,298
Fund Balances at Beginning of Year	452,039	373,741
Fund Balances at End of Year	$501,643	$452,039

the visit activity for each of the two accounting periods included in the schedule of statistics. Normally, published financial statements do not present visit activity for the accounting period. As an administrator, however, you should request visit activity as an integral part of the financial statements your controller provides you on a monthly and year-to-date basis. Increases in service fee revenue should be consistent with increases in service volume measured in visits or hours. If the change in revenue is not proportional to the change in service volume, then other factors, such as rate increases or a large bad debt reserve adjustment, should be investigated.

Expenses are reflected, as noted, in terms of program services and administrative expenses. Program service expenses represent the direct cost of providing visits and services to patients during the accounting period. Program service expenses generally include salaries and contract services for personnel, payroll taxes, benefits, transportation, and other related direct costs of providing service. These expenses, over time, should remain fairly constant as a percentage of revenue. As with service volume, there is a general expectation that program service expenses change in the same relationship as revenue changes from accounting period to period. Program service expenses that increase faster than revenue may be an indication of inefficiency in productivity (simply stated, people doing fewer visits for the same or more dollars) or general overspending in nonpersonnel areas. In addition, it may also be an indication that the agency needs to increase its revenue rates to keep up with the inflationary cost of providing service. Increasing individual rates for visits may not be easy with managed care fixed-price contracts becoming the norm for an agency.

Administrative expenses typically are the fixed expenses necessary to handle the agency's day-to-day operations. This category generally includes administrative and clerical personnel salaries and related payroll taxes and benefits, occupancy expenses, office operation, legal and professional expenses, professional dues, publications, public relations, and any other related expenses. These expenses do not increase significantly from year to year unless there are changes in the fixed operations, such as a new facility, more people, or a significant change in visit volume. When one compares the expenses on a month-to-month basis, there should be small or insignificant variations each month. When making long-term comparisons, increases in the level of administrative expenses that are in excess of the local inflation rate and are not accompanied by significant increases in the level of administrative services may indicate a lack of control over spending and should be addressed immediately.

The term *operating income (loss)* indicates whether the organization is charging enough fees for the services provided to cover the cost of delivering services and managing the operation. Income is a positive number and mathematically indicates that fees are greater than costs. (Loss) is a negative and indicates that fees are less than costs. Typically a nonprofit organization reports an operating loss. Generally, the operating loss is planned, and the planned loss is covered by other items of income or support included under the title "nonoperating income." The for-profit service provider does not usually report an operating loss. If the organization is reporting several successive periods of losses, the cash flow statement (explained later) must be reviewed fully to determine how the organization is paying for the losses.

Nonoperating income generally reflects the results of fund-raising activities conducted by the nonprofit organization during the accounting period. Typically in this category, you may expect support from individual or corporate contributions, federated fund-raising organizations (e.g., the United Way), or local municipal governments supporting general purpose services or objectives. A review of this category for several

years offers a basic understanding about the level of independent (board) fund-raising activity compared with that of the administrative staff. Administrative fund-raising typically results in United Way or municipal support and grants for specific programs.

In reviewing the income statement, the administrator will learn how much revenue was generated for the accounting period, how much it cost to generate the revenue, whether the agency made a surplus, and whether it received any contributions during the period. However, for an accurate understanding of the organization, the administrator should not look at the income statement alone. This is only one part, and reading and understanding it must be interrelated with the other financial statements.

BALANCE SHEET

The income statement provides the administrator an indication of what happened during the accounting period. The balance sheet provides the administrator with a picture of the financial health of the agency at a point in time. The financial health is gauged by the relationship of total cash and receivables to the amount of liabilities and debt. A large amount of cash with a low amount of receivables indicates that the organization is collecting its receivables on a regular and frequent basis. A small cash balance with a large amount of receivables and a large amount of liabilities may indicate that the organization is unable to collect its receivables in a timely manner. The administrator should review the aging of accounts receivable in conjunction with the review of cash, accounts receivable, and liabilities.

The balance sheet is a financial statement that must balance. The amount of the assets owned by the organization must equal the amount of liabilities owed by the organization plus the equity. In comparison, the income statement does not balance but provides the results of operations.

In analyzing a balance sheet (see Exhibit 47–2), there are several key ratios of which the

Exhibit 47–2 Home Health Agency, Balance Sheet: December 31, 2003, and December 31, 2002

	2003	2002
ASSETS		
Cash	$170,768	$251,398
Accounts receivable, net of allowance for doubtful accounts of $66,300 (2003) and $43,000 (2002)	252,254	136,501
Interfund receivable	—	341
Prepaid expenses	9,319	6,365
TOTAL CURRENT ASSETS	432,341	394,605
Land, building, and equipment, at cost, less accumulated depreciation	262,718	139,899
TOTAL ASSETS	$695,059	$534,504
LIABILITIES AND FUND BALANCES		
LIABILITIES		
Notes payable	$ 9,007	$ 13,384
Deferred grant	75,892	5,260
Interfund payable	—	341
Accounts payable and accrued expenses	108,517	63,480
TOTAL CURRENT LIABILITIES	193,416	82,465
FUND BALANCES	501,643	452,039
TOTAL LIABILITIES	$695,059	$534,504

administrator should be aware in order to understand the organization. First is the current ratio, which equals the total current assets divided by total liabilities. Current assets consist of cash, accounts receivable, and inventory. Current liabilities consist of accounts payable, accrued expenses, and the amount of debt the organization must repay in the 12 months after the close of the accounting period. This ratio provides the administrator with a benchmark of the amount of assets readily available to liquidate the liabilities. In the example in Exhibit 47–2, current assets divided by current liabilities equals a current ratio for this organization of 2.24. Usually any ratio above 1.5 to 1.0 indicates better than average financial health. The larger the ratio, the better the health of the organization.

A second basic ratio is working capital. Working capital quantifies available liquidity.

Working capital is the excess of current assets over current liabilities, theoretically an amount that can be turned readily into cash. In Exhibit 47–2, working capital is current assets minus the current liabilities, which equals a working capital of $238,925.

Our particular example indicates a significant amount of working capital and a high current ratio. A closer look at the components, however, may yield slightly different results. Both of these indicators measure liquidity, the amount of liquid assets available to cover current liabilities. The example organization has a deferred grant. The deferred grant represents a cash grant provided to cover certain designated expenses for a particular program. It is deferred because the grant funds were not spent in the reporting accounting period and will be spent or refunded in a succeeding accounting period. If one reduces both current assets and current liabilities by the amount of the deferred grant, the current ratio and amount of working capital are 3.04 and $238,925, respectively. These amounts are still high for a home health agency.

Another area to analyze is the change in and the level of accounts receivable. Accounts receivable should be analyzed in conjunction with service fee revenue, the change in units of service or visits, and the accounts receivable aging listed on the schedule of statistics. First, how does the amount of accounts receivable at the balance sheet date compare with total service fee revenue for the accounting period? Or, how much of the revenue billed during the accounting period has not been collected as of the balance sheet date? In the example agency, 13.8 percent of the period's revenue is receivable. Is 13.8 percent meaningful? The 13.8 percent may be more meaningful if reflected in terms of days accounts receivable are outstanding. How many days does this represent? Is this an improvement over last year, or are collections slower? These are among the questions to be asked.

To determine the number of days of service revenue in accounts receivable, a simple equation is used:

$$\frac{\text{Total amount of accounts receivable}}{\text{Total revenue} \div \text{the number of days in the accounting period.}}$$

where accounts receivable represents the total amount as of the balance sheet date, total revenue is the total billed for services for the accounting period, and number of days represents the number of days in the accounting period. In the example agency, this number is 50. For the prior year, it is 38. Now one year can be compared with the previous year. We know the period-end receivables represent more days of revenue than the previous period. We do not know the cause. The administrator must investigate reasons, such as above-average billing in the last 2 months of the year or a general slowdown in collections, or a combination.

Another common financial ratio used to analyze accounts receivable is turnover. Turnover is the number of times accounts receivable are col-

lected during the accounting period. A high turnover number indicates quick collections, and a low turnover number indicates slow collections. To calculate turnover, simply divide the days in the accounting period as calculated above by the number of days in accounts receivables. In our example, 365/50 equals 7.3 times. This compares with 9.6 times the previous year. If the turnover ratio is decreasing from period to period, this is a strong indication of a deterioration in collections. The reasons need to be investigated further and corrective action put into place immediately.

Generally, the type of pay source will determine the number of days and the turnover. Insurance companies, Medicare, and other third-party payers often pay no more quickly than 60 days after billing, which may be 90 days after service. This payment time frame will cause the days in accounts receivable and turn-over to be closer to 90 and 4 times, respectively. Typically, home health organizations have turnover ratios in a range of 3.0 to 4.0. Any turnover number lower than 3.0 indicates serious cash flow problems and the inability of the agency to regularly pay current expenses in a timely manner.

The last major ratio on the balance sheet is fund balance or equity. This category indicates the amount of investment in the organization. Equity is usually compared with total debt to determine a relationship between the amount of investment by the owner and the amount of investment by creditors. In a nonprofit organization, the owner is replaced by the board or the community benefiting from the services provided. Generally, a financially sound organization maintains a ratio of debt to equity no worse than 1:1. In a labor-intensive service business, debt compared with equity should not be lower than 1:1. If not, the organization may experience shortages of cash from time to time.

In conclusion, the balance sheet is a snapshot. Look at its details. Compare it with prior years. What are the trends? Often, trends provide an indication of what is around the corner in the next accounting period.

FUNCTIONAL EXPENSES

The statement of functional expenses (see Exhibit 47–3) details expenses for the accounting period by type of expense (i.e., salaries, benefits, taxes, etc.) in the program service and administrative areas. The statement should be reviewed and analyzed in conjunction with the income statement, and the visits and FTEs in the schedule of statistics for each accounting period presented. The statement of functional expenses

will provide information to answer questions concerning a fluctuation between accounting periods (e.g., Why are salaries higher? Why did transportation expense more than double?). The schedule of visits for each accounting period will assist in this review and in answering those questions.

Additionally, there are certain basic relationships that should be consistent from period to period. Payroll taxes and employee benefits are expense categories that should remain consistent when expressed as a percentage of salaries. Transportation expense generally changes in direct proportion to any changes in visits provided. Occupancy expense (e.g., building costs,

Exhibit 47–3 Home Health Agency Statement of Functional Expenses: Years Ended December 31, 2003, and December 31, 2002

	Program Services	Administrative	Total Expenses 2003	Total Expenses 2002
Salaries	$959,804	$314,293	$1,274,097	$833,684
Employee benefits	153,167	59,894	213,061	137,941
Payroll taxes	76,138	28,186	104,324	72,135
Total Employee Compensation	1,189,109	402,373	1,591,482	1,043,760
Professional fees and contract service payments	177,398	35,112	212,510	187,964
Clinic expenses	2,074	—	2,074	2,273
Supplies	19,130	10,429	29,559	24,041
Telephone	—	10,510	10,510	8,912
Postage and shipping	—	7,700	7,700	5,862
Occupancy	9,457	14,563	24,020	22,176
Local transportation	52,636	2,110	54,746	32,674
Conferences, conventions, and meetings	1,437	5,144	6,581	4,965
Printing and publications	—	6,276	6,276	4,863
Membership dues	—	5,930	5,930	4,843
Interest expense	—	1,529	1,529	1,411
Total Expenses before Depreciation	1,451,241	501,676	1,952,917	1,343,744
Depreciation of land, building, and equipment	7,947	9,447	17,394	14,039
Total Expenses	$1,459,188	$511,123	$1,970,311	$1,357,783

maintenance, and insurance other than health and workers' compensation) is usually predictable and generally does not vary from accounting period to accounting period, except in cases of major repairs.

The functional expense statement also will provide the administrator with information on a program basis. The administrator will note the direct cost of each program. Administrative cost also may be allocated to each program to reflect the real cost of the program or service. The programs should be compared with the same programs in prior accounting periods for variances.

An interesting and informative analysis pertaining to the functional expense statement is to review the direct expense categories (salaries, payroll taxes, benefits, contract services, transportation) in relationship to visits. This analysis can be performed on both a total agency basis and an individual program basis. In addition to reviewing direct expenses in relation to visits, the direct expenses should be reviewed in relation to FTEs.

Experience shows that administrative expenses generally are consistent from period to period. If visits are increasing over time, program service costs should increase, but the administrative or indirect costs should remain fairly flat. There is a visit volume level in every organization at which another administrative function or person may be required. When additional administrative personnel are hired, administrative costs could change by a percentage usually greater than the percentage change in visit volume.

In summary, the functional expense statement is used to review consistent spending patterns from accounting period to accounting period, to verify that spending bears some consistent relationship to the level of service provided, and to review expenses on a program basis, all in conjunction with the schedule of statistics.

CASH FLOWS

The statement of cash flows provides a reconciliation of net income reported on the accrual basis to the change in cash for the accounting period. The statement reports cash flow from operations, cash flow from the purchase of fixed assets, and cash flow from financing activities. The statement answers the question, "Where did the profit go?" or "What did the organization do with the profit?"

In the example agency statement in Exhibit 47–4, the reader will note that net income for the year of $49,604 resulted in cash provided by operating activities totaling $63,960. In examining the components resulting in positive operational cash flow, note that three items changed significantly: accounts receivable, deferred grant, and accounts payable. These are line items on the balance sheet with significant variance from the prior year. The positive operational cash flow is a result, however, of the agency receiving a grant and not spending the entire amount in the accounting period.

What did the organization do with the $63,960 of cash provided by operations? The statement tells us the organization made its regular debt service payments on a note payable and purchased fixed assets. In this example, the cost of the fixed assets purchased exceeded the cash flow from operations, and beginning year cash was required to purchase the assets. Therefore, the informed analyst may conclude that fixed assets were purchased by $63,000 of deferred grant funds and $77,000 of the organization's cash reserves.

This statement completes the link between the balance sheet and the income statement. Some financial analysts choose to review this statement first when analyzing operations. Regardless of the order of review, the statement of cash flows is a necessity to give a full understanding of the agency during the reporting period.

CONCLUSION

To fully understand a financial statement, notes should accompany the statement. The notes should be read and analyzed in conjunction with statistics and ratios. Many times the notes

Exhibit 47–4 Home Health Agency Statement of Cash Flows: Years Ended December 31, 2003, and December 31, 2002

	2003	*2002*
Cash Flows from Operating Activities		
Revenue and income in excess of expenses	$ 49,604	$ 78,298
Adjustments to reconcile revenue and income in excess of expenses to net cash provided by operating activities		
Depreciation	17,394	14,039
(Increase) decrease in:		
Accounts receivable	(115,412)	(17,873)
Prepaid expenses	(2,954)	(1,559)
Increase (decrease) in:		
Deferred grant	70,632	(432)
Accounts payable and accrued expenses	44,696	4,949
Net Cash Provided by Operating Activities	63,960	77,422
Cash Flows from Investing Activities		
Purchase of fixed assets	(140,213)	(11,281)
Cash Flows from Financing Activities		
Principal payments on note payable	(4,377)	(3,651)
Net Increase (Decrease) in Cash	(80,630)	62,490
Cash Beginning of Year	251,398	188,908
Cash End of Year	$170,768	$251,398

provide information that may answer questions or explain hidden liabilities and obligations or one-time transactions significantly affecting relationships.

This chapter only scratches the surface of financial statement interpretation. It gives administrators a basis for understanding the financial statements provided by their financial departments. Many administrators receive more information and detail than is explained here. You should sit down and review with your controller certain basics and attempt to build from there. Look at the information supplied with a skeptical eye. Ask questions. Look at relationships. This will provide the basis for informed, educated decisions.

CHAPTER 48

Mangement Information Systems

Kristy Wright and Brian Thomas

THE EVOLUTION OF MANAGING INFORMATION

The days of managing all but extremely small amounts of data by hand or even on a spreadsheet are long gone. Methods of data acquisition, its use, and sheer volume of material continue to increase at a speed that can be disabling to the administrator who wants to make the best decisions for the home health agency (HHA). In addition, the advent of the Medicare Prospective Payment System (PPS) and emerging disease management programs has propelled the industry into a world dependent on its ability to manage its information.

Management information systems (MISs) have evolved from processing large amounts of data in order to create compilations of information into organized reports to fashioning and using meaningful management tools that pull data from multiple sources, analyze its interrelatedness, and predict outcomes for the future. In the current health care environment, an administrator making decisions without effective information management tools puts the home care agency at risk for financial loss, poor clinical outcomes, and poor competitive advantage. In addition, the movement to point of care solutions has created a new level of access to information for the care staff and created a new age of care-giving tools.

USING INFORMATION TO MANAGE THE ORGANIZATION

The current information needs of a home care organization vary from agency to agency. Few, if any, agencies are not automated in some form. Generally, however, the decision faced by HHAs is to what level the sophistication should be expanded and at what cost. Although reasons to move to more sophisticated MISs may be subtle, the basis for automation should be evaluated by considering the current and future needs of the HHA.

Although home health agency administrators define the needs of their agencies based on differences in growth, size, and corporate structure, there are similar information needs shared by all agencies including:

1. *Measurement of clinical outcomes.* This need is in response to internal organization improvement activities, Outcomes Based Quality Improvement (OBQI) requirements, adverse events monitoring, state and national home care report cards, accreditation standards, and requirements from third-party payors.
2. *Measurement of financial performance.* Survival under PPS and the ability to effectively negotiate managed care contracts requires measuring current and predicting future financial performance of

the organization. PPS has also made it necessary to integrate clinical and financial activities into single management information tools. The entire process of care including referrals, direct care activities, supplies, supporting activities, and billing and tracking receivables must now be monitored and controlled in real time to assure the financial success of the HHA.

3. *Strategic planning.* Probably one of the most critical activities of an administrator, strategic planning has become more and more dependent on the ability to utilize available data to analyze trends, predict future performance and related organization needs, and test the what-ifs of a new strategy.

4. *Effective resource management.* This is a two-fold issue for most organizations. First, HHAs need to be able to measure current resource utilization (whether it be human resources, overhead resources, or other tangibles) and prepare for future resource requirements. Second, computerization and use of technology itself leads to better utilization of resources, especially human resources. The time savings realized can be significant and apparent through increased productivity, decreased overhead, and improved cash flow.

TYPES OF INFORMATION SYSTEMS AVAILABLE IN THE HOME CARE MARKET

Back Office Systems. These are MISs that provide support to all "office-based" operations including referral management, quality improvement processes, and physician relationship management. In addition, the back-office systems generally provide overall financial management including billing, accounts receivable, and cost management.

Point-of-Care Systems. These systems enable access to the clinical record including the admission process, OASIS data collection, care planning, and overall clinical care management

facilitating the use of patient history and clinical information as a care-giving tool.

Report Technology. This is perhaps the most important part of any MIS. Report technology provides the agency with quick access to review both financial and clinical data to effectively manage the organization.

Outcomes Measurement Systems. These are most frequently obtained through a vendor separate from the point of care/back office system vendor. The types of outcomes measurements may include not only clinical, but also financial, and are benchmarked against other HHAs in a defined geography or demography.

Preparing Your Organization

Several steps exist to prepare your organization for selection and implementation of a new or upgraded management information system. It is essential to review your strategic business plan and not only determine the information needs implied by the plan, but also evaluate how the plan might change with the improved availability of data driven information. What kind(s) of technology is or will be required? What uses does the organization have for information? How will the organization's information needs change over the next 5 years? What technology is currently in place in the organization?

A thorough review of existing information technology within the organization is the next logical step. It is important to know what is already in place and how effective it has been in managing information. A thorough accounting of what will no longer be used or required and what parts of your existing systems will need to be integrated or interfaced with a new system can serve as the basis for your search criteria.

Another step that should not be overlooked is a review of the current technology experience of the various staff who will use the new information system. It is important to consider not only the hands-on users, but also the support staff who must educate others and maintain the system and the staff (including management) who will rely on the system's information output.

A review of the financial resources of the organization will determine the amount and level of information technology that can be purchased. Preparing the organization to assume the initial and ongoing costs may require structured timing of implementation, delaying other projects and expenses, and seeking funding or financing.

Finally, preparing other stakeholders who will not be directly involved in the complex process of selection and implementation or the use of the information technology will help the whole process go more smoothly. It is important for everyone to realize that some projects not related to the information system will be put on hold and resources (including support personnel) will be directed toward this major endeavor. Organization-wide support and cooperation will be needed to minimize complications during implementation.

SELECTING THE RIGHT INFORMATION SYSTEM FOR THE ORGANIZATION

The selection of an appropriate information system is one of the most important financial decisions an HHA must make—not just the amount paid to the vendor who sold the system to the HHA, but more important, the internal costs for development, setup, training, and data entry. As difficult as this decision may be, the goal is to computerize with the most flexible and upgradable system available.

When one is making the decision to implement an information system, software should be selected first, and then the compatible hardware should be selected. The most common mistake for the first-time buyer is selecting hardware first, or when upgrading, limiting the selection process because of the desire to reuse as much of the existing hardware as possible. Only if the HHA has a preselected platform should hardware be one of the initial parameters of the selection.

The decision of whether to use consultants in selecting an information system is dependent on several factors. The obvious would seem to be the availability of financing to pay for outside consulting assistance. If, however, the organization does not possess the needed expertise and experience internally to prepare the organization and design a selection process, the cost/benefit of consultants must be evaluated. Making the wrong selection has far-reaching implications and costs that can literally destroy an organization.

Whether you choose a consultant approach or design your own selection process, the steps that should be taken are:

1. *Convene a core selection committee.* Members of the committee should be representative of that staff who will be involved in the final decision of which information system will be purchased. Representatives on the committee should include administration, finance, billing, information systems or technology (IS or IT), and clinical staff who will be using the system. Although several committee members may continue as part of the implementation team, keep in mind that this committee's primary responsibility is to *select* the right system.

2. *Develop preliminary selection criteria.* This is the first assignment of the selection committee. Criteria at this point should be high-level critical indicators and should also be flexible. The selection criteria will be refined and expanded later in the process (Exhibit 48-1). It is also important to segregate your selection criteria into required features, desired features, and luxury items. This will be a beneficial tool once you discover that no vendor or product has all the things that you want.

3. *Select vendors for consideration.* There are many resources (publications and Internet) available that list software vendors and describe the basics of their products. An intentioned review of these resources will produce a preliminary list of possible vendor choices. You can also meet representatives of the many different vendors at both state and national home care conferences. A simple mailed request for infor-

Exhibit 48–1 Selection Criteria

Selection Criteria
[SAMPLE]

_____ Single data base
_____ Maturity of product
_____ Size/resources of company
_____ Commitment to development and support
_____ Financial stability of company
_____ Commitment to home care
_____ Windows based
_____ Applicability to all services/companies
_____ "Vision" of company re: IT, IS & HMC
_____ PPS data tracking capabilities
_____ Ease of use for field staff
_____ Facilitation of billing (timeliness, tracking, etc.)
_____ Availability of and flexibility in designing and changing reports
_____ Value over the life of the system (considering not only initial purchase price but also future customization, development and maintenance costs)
_____ New staff orientation requirements
_____ Migration from current system
_____ Meets OASIS criteria
_____ Flexibility in user interface design and database security
_____ Database independence
_____ Maintenance/upgrade requirements
_____ Level of support
_____ Cost

Source: Courtesy of VNA, Western Pennsylvania, Butler, Pennsylvania.

---

mation (RFI) will produce enough material to narrow the choices to a much more manageable number. This list should contain no more than 10 vendors. At this point, a more comprehensive request for proposal (RFP) is in order. In your RFP, include information about your organization, your information needs (current and future), current systems being used, required/desired/luxury features, financial constraints, and any other pertinent information related to your particular situation. From the proposals received, a small group of four to six semi-finalists should be chosen.

4. *Gather information.* This is the most intensive step in the selection process and focuses on gathering much more specific information from each of the semi-finalist vendors. Information can be obtained in a number of ways including software functionality demonstrations at your site (demos), site visits to vendor headquarters, visiting vendors at trade shows, talking to others who are using the system, and visiting other sites where the software is in use. It is important to determine which functionalities are in general use versus in beta testing or not even released for testing. Nothing throws an implementation off more than finding out midway through that a particular function is not actually available yet. It is helpful to develop evaluation tools to assist in comparing and

Exhibit 48–2 Evaluation for Software Demo

Evaluation for Software Demo

Product Name:_____ Date:_____

Components being evaluated   ☐ Billing/Financial   ☐ Clinical   ☐ Scheduling

1.   This product is easy/intuitive to use: (please circle)
     strongly disagree   disagree   neither agree or disagree   agree   strongly agree

2.   This product's functionality is equal to or better than our current product. (please circle)
     strongly disagree   disagree   neither agree or disagree   agree   strongly agree

3.   Identify strengths of this product:

    _____

    _____

    _____

    _____

    _____

    _____

4.   Identify weaknesses of this product:

    _____

    _____

    _____

    _____

    _____

    _____

5.   Additional Comments:

    _____

    _____

    _____

    _____

    _____

    _____

Source: Courtesy of VNA, Western Pennsylvania, Butler, Pennsylvania.

---

contrasting different vendors (Exhibit 48-2). At this point, the list of vendors should be pared to two or three finalists.

5.   *Finalize your selection criteria.* This is the time to go back to your selection criteria and revise the list based on what you've learned during information gathering. It is not unusual to find that no single vendor or product meets all your needs and frequently there are several criteria that no vendor or product satisfies. Be realistic in your final criteria and come to consensus within the core committee.

6.   *Make selection based on objective information.* If the information gathering step is the most intensive, the final selection will be the most emotional. Individual members of the core selection group will, by now, have their favorites. To avoid a selection being made based on whoever is

Exhibit 48–3 Home Care Software Vendor Selection Tool

Home Care Software Vendor Selection Tool
Developed by VNA, Western Pennsylvania

STEP ONE: Develop list of desired criteria for software

This may be done through brainstorming or by having individuals list their desired criteria. It is important that the list be limited to no more than 15 items. This can be done by eliminating duplicative items, combining like items or eliminating items that are not clearly described. Do not eliminate an item just because only one or two members of the group think it is important. Examples of items you might identify include:

> Cost
> Functionality
> Ease of clinical note
> Availability of user group

STEP TWO: Rate criteria

Have each member of the group (individually) order the criteria from least important to most important with 1 being least important up to the total number of criteria. For example, if you had 15 criteria, number 1 would be the least important and number 15 would be the most important. The above list might look like this:

> 2 Cost
> 4 Functionality
> 3 Ease of clinical note
> 1 Availability of user group

If there are 10 people on the selection committee, you should have 10 lists of ordered criteria at the completion of this step.

STEP THREE: Total scores for criteria

Add all the order ratings for each criteria to come up with a total score for that criteria. For example, if you had 3 members on the committee and the first criteria (let's say "cost") received a 2, a 3, and a 4, the total score for "cost" would be 9 (2+3+4). Repeat for each criteria.

In our example, the results might be:

> Costs 9
> Functionality 10
> Ease of clinical note 9
> Availability of user group 4

STEP FOUR: Calculate weights for each criteria

1

continues

Exhibit 48–3 continued

<u>First,</u> calculate the highest score possible for any criteria:
Total number of criteria multiplied by the total number of committee members
In our example, the highest score for a criteria would be 12 (4 criteria times 3 members).
Keep in mind that there might not be a criteria that actually gets the highest score. To get
that score, everyone in the group would have to rate the criteria as the most important.

<u>Second,</u> calculate the weighted multiplier:
100/highest score possible - weighted multiplier (round to nearest whole number)

In our example, the weighted multiplier would be 8 (100/12 = 8.3)

<u>Third,</u> weight each criteria using the following formula:
total score of criteria multiplied by the weighted multiplier

In our example, the weights would be:

Cost = 72 (9 X 8)
Functionality = 80 (10 X 8)
Ease of clinical note = 72 (9 X 8)
Availability of user group = 32 (4 X 8)

Note: The leader of the selection committee should perform these calculations and <u>not</u> share the
results with the group at this point to avoid influencing the next steps.

STEP FIVE: Apply criteria to each vendor finalist

This method works best when evaluating two vendor finalists. It can be used for three, but
becomes too cumbersome for more than three.

As a group activity, determine which vendor <u>best</u> meets each criteria. This doesn't necessarily
mean that one vendor meets the criteria completely and the other doesn't meet it at all that
would be just too easy!). Just decide which one does the best at meeting the criteria. If it is
impossible to choose one vendor over the other on a criteria, give credit to each vendor. Be
careful to avoid doing this with too many of the criteria. Also, do not give partial credit to
vendors. In other words, do not give 3/4 credit to one vendor and 1/4 to the other. They either
both get the whole credit or none at all.

In our example, it might look like this

Criteria	Vendor A	Vendor B
Cost	X	

2

continues

Exhibit 48–3 continued

Functionality		X
Clinical note		X
User group	X	

STEP SIX: Calculate scores for each vendor

Apply weighted scores to each criteria/vendor. For example:

Criteria	Vendor A	Vendor B
Cost	X 72	
Functionality		X 80
Clinical note		X 72
User group	X 32	
TOTAL	105	152

Clearly, Vendor B would be the committee's choice.

Source: Courtesy of VNA, Western Pennsylvania, Butler, Pennsylvania.

the most vocal or influential member of the committee, an objective-weighted tool should be utilized to make the final selection decision (Exhibit 48-3).

7. *Finalize a contractual agreement.* Finalizing a contract should be left to the experts. This has become a very specialized field of contract law, and you should seek out an attorney who has experience in the area of technology. The benefit of employing an attorney to review an information systems contract (which is usually supplied by the vendor) far outways the cost.

8. *Create a partnership.* By the end of the selection process, the chosen vendor characteristics should complement the characteristics of the HHA. Both organizations should share similar business cultures, work ethics, and visions of the future.

There should also be an atmosphere of mutual respect, win-win attitudes, and open communication. The final selection is only the beginning of a long relationship between the HHA and vendor. The going will be much easier if both organizations enter into the relationship as partners who share in each other's successes. Once that relationship is in place, it is equally important to continue to develop the relationship and be willing to share and participate in each other's success.

HOME TELE-MONITORING SYSTEMS

Home tele-monitoring is a burgeoning market in the home care industry. It is the newest form of information systems providing information on the patient's condition rather than the HHA's performance and outcomes. Making the decision to invest in home tele-monitoring technology can be difficult in the best situations. The financial investment is significant, the risks can be high, and the need to achieve a positive return is critical to future success. In spite of the risks, this relatively new technology in home care holds the promise of redefining the industry. A growing body of research indicates that the outcomes being realized with the use of home tele-monitoring are extremely promising.

In order to ensure that your outcomes are as good as or better than the reported results, you must design a strategy before you begin choosing the type of technology that will support the implementation of any strategic plan. The worst possible decision is to invest in home tele-monitoring because "everyone else is doing it and we can't be left behind."

The key question to ask is: "What problems are we trying to solve?" Each organization experiences a unique set of business and clinical challenges depending on structure, size, available resources (including human), and patient demographics. Even common industry challenges are shaded by individual organization characteristics, and the combinations of specific issues are endless.

Two of the more frequently encountered concerns, especially under PPS, include the number of visits per episode and the rising cost per visit. In addition, a nursing shortage nearing crisis level is making it more and more difficult to sustain the patient volume needed to survive. Add to that conundrum increased competition, and the need for additional revenue streams and you're facing a true business dilemma.

Clinically, positive outcomes have become the measure by which home care is evaluated. Not only is CMS measuring and reporting home care outcomes, but also managed care organizations are demanding proven outcome reports from their home care providers. Even if the demand weren't there, most of us are motivated by a mission to keep people living independently in their homes.

Whatever the combination of these challenges you are facing or additional concerns you have, they should drive your home tele-monitoring plan. Not until you have fully explored the obstacles before you can you wisely choose the best implementation process and system that will result in positive financial and clinical outcomes.

As mentioned, the financial investment in fully implementing a home tele-monitoring program can be significant. The monitors are obviously the greatest single expenditure, but, depending on the type of monitoring system chosen, several other costs must be considered. Peripheral devices (i.e., pro-time, blood glucose, EKG, cameras, etc.) are frequently not included with the monitor itself. In addition to the monitors that are placed in the patient's home, there may also be a central or base monitoring unit that resides at the home care organization that must be purchased along with software license fees.

Several ongoing or repeating costs can also be incurred such as transmission fees, monitor or base station repairs, and software upgrades. The most frequently overlooked ongoing cost is staff who will install the monitors and educate patients, perform video visits, review incoming monitor readings, assess the need for clinical follow-up, and troubleshoot problems (both technical and clinical).

Once you've evaluated your business and clinical needs and determined the amount of capital that you are able to invest, a specific system can be chosen that will provide the greatest returns on your investment. Although the technology is still in its infancy and only a limited number of vendors are offering monitoring systems, there is still an adequate number of choices and the market is growing daily.

A key decision to make is whether you need all video monitors, all nonvideo monitors, or a combination. Video monitors allow remote face-to-face contact with the patient and visualization of patient condition and care processes, but they still require a clinician to make each "tele-visit." The time constraints for the clinician may limit the number of patient monitoring contacts that can be made. Another consideration with video monitors is the quality of the transmission in your particular geographic area. Monitors without videos do not permit the visualization of the patient but also do not require a clinician to make a tele-visit. In both cases, a clinician is required to assess the monitor readings; however, a single clinician can handle more patients on the nonvideo monitors. Patients using nonvideo monitors are frequently monitored on a daily basis and may be monitored several times a day without requiring a clinician contact.

The transmission capabilities of the monitors are also a deciding factor. Many rural areas do not have the quality of phone lines to handle transmission of video and sometimes even data adequately. Newer technology is adding satellite transmission or Internet capability. Whichever you choose, a trial run from more rural areas is highly recommended.

Standard monitoring features and the availability of optional peripherals directly impact clinical and financial outcomes. For example, one of the most frequently monitored patient conditions is congestive heart failure. If the plan is to make this a cornerstone of your program, the availability (and preferably a standard feature) of pulse oximetry and weight scales going beyond the normal 250 lbs. limit is critical to the success of your program.

Finally, as in choosing any other vendor, the level of technical support, education, and commitment to your program from the vendor can make or break the outcomes of your plan.

CONCLUSION

All home health agencies have similar information needs that include measuring clinical outcomes and measurement of financial performance, strategic planning, and effective resource management. These needs vary based on the difference in growth, size, and corporate structure of an agency. It is important that administrators prepare the staff of their agencies for the selection and implementation of a new or upgraded MIS to decrease the risk for financial loss, poor clinical outcomes, and poor competitive advantage in the 21st century.

PART VII

Legal/Ethical/Political Issues

CHAPTER 49

Legal Issues of Concern to Home Care Providers

Ann P. Sherwin

INTRODUCTION

Home care providers come in a variety of forms and types. Providers may include the various business forms of sole proprietorships, partnerships, limited partnerships, corporations, and limited liability companies. Home care providers hold a variety of tax statuses that may be for profit, not for profit, or charitable.

The types of home care providers include but are not necessarily limited to home health agencies, visiting nurse associations, durable medical equipment companies, infusion care or high-technology companies, diagnostic testing companies, medical supply companies, hospices, specialized service agencies, private duty nursing services, homemaker–home health aide services, and companion services.

The laws of an individual state govern and may limit the organizational forms, tax status, and types of home care providers who are authorized to operate within that particular state. The state may require that the home care provider qualify to provide services through the state's registration, certificate of need, licensure, certification, and/or accreditation laws.

Failure to meet these minimum threshold legal requirements of the individual state law may prevent a home care provider from lawfully operating within that particular state.

Even after the home care provider has met the state's legal requirements for operation within a state, a number of evolving legal issues are likely to continue to affect the practices of the home care provider.

This chapter on legal matters in home care highlights a number of legal issues affecting home care providers in their business dealings and in the provision of health care and health-related services.

ANTITRUST

Antitrust is activity that restricts trade and discourages free competition in the marketplace. The general purpose of both state and federal antitrust laws is to promote and maintain free and fair competition in the marketplace. The federal antitrust statutes are the Sherman Act, the Clayton Act, the Federal Trade Commission Act, and the Robinson Patman Act. The provisions of these laws prohibit certain artificial business manipulations such as the unfair competitive practices of group boycotts, dividing up the marketplace, exerting undue monopolistic practices, illegally tying products, and price fixing. The antitrust provisions basically prohibit an agency from agreeing with or conspiring with its competitors not to compete and from competing unfairly. The business practices of health care providers have come under increased scrutiny by the Federal Trade Commission for activities that may have an anticompetitive effect in the health care marketplace.

Mergers, joint venture activities, and other combinations engaged in by a wide variety of health care providers have exposed the health care industry to examination for possible antitrust violations.

This increased scrutiny should be of great concern to the health care community. A judgment or finding of a violation of the antitrust laws against a home care provider poses great risk. In addition to a court order halting the illegal antitrust activity cited as the violation, the violator is exposed to high penalties. Moreover, private parties who successfully prosecute an antitrust violation against a business may recover triple monetary damages and attorneys' fees in amounts that can be staggering and fatal to that business's viability. In a Florida case, the court determined that the intent of a joint venture between a hospital and a durable medical equipment company and the manner in which it was implemented were anticompetitive. A $2.3 million dollar jury verdict in the case was upheld on appeal to the Eleventh Circuit Court of Appeals.[1]

CORPORATE LIABILITY OF PROVIDERS

There are a number of legal theories of liability under which a health care company may be found liable to other parties. These legal theories are breach of contract, agency, respondent superior, ostensible agency, and the evolving theory of corporate negligence.

A breach of contract requires that a contract exist between the parties whereby an offer is made, acceptance is given, and some form of consideration is given to bind the contract. This may involve an activity between the patient and a home care agency whereby the home care provider offers certain services to the patient, the patient agrees to accept the services, and the consideration to the contract is the agreement of payment for the services. A patient may have a cause of action for breach of contract against the home care provider if services were not provided as agreed to, such as if the program's marketing materials promised certain high-quality services and the provider did not deliver the quality or scope of services promised in its agreement.

The principle of respondent superior is that employers are liable for the acts of their employees when employees act within the scope of their employment. It is also known as the master and servant rule in that the master is deemed to be responsible for the acts of his or her servants.

Theories of vicarious liability hold a health care company/provider indirectly liable for the action and omissions of its employees, agents, and ostensible agents. Ostensible agents are those persons who act with the apparent authority of the health care provider, in that the health care provider holds out these agents and/or persons as employees, and the public would have no reason not to consider these persons as agents or employees of the health care provider. This theory of negligence requires that the patient look to the health care provider rather than the individual health care practitioner for care, and that the health care provider hold out the practitioner as its own employee. This holding out or appearance occurs when a health care provider acts or omits to act in some way that leads the patient to a reasonable belief that she or he is being treated by the health care provider and/or one of its employees.

A number of courts have created a direct legal duty owed to the patient by the health care provider as an additional duty to the already established legal duty held by each individual health care practitioner to his or her patients. This new theory of liability is a departure from the notion that a corporation could not be directly liable for the negligence of health care practitioners because corporations are prohibited from practicing medicine and from practicing under any individual health care practitioner's individual professional license. This prohibition, also known as a prohibition against the corporate practice of medicine, has now evolved into a direct duty to patients under a new theory of corporate negligence. This direct duty and/or theory of corporate negligence reflects a growing appreciation on the part of the courts and of consumers that health care providers play an increasing role in the selection of health care practitioners on behalf of the consumer. Evidence of this increased role of the health care provider is found in the selection of health care practitioners as employees and independent contractors for the patient. Of special note are health maintenance organizations and preferred provider organizations and their duties in their selection of health care service providers and health care practitioners made available to the consumer. The duty owed to the patient under this theory of corporate negligence is measured in activities such as the selection of the health care practitioner, the credentialing and recredentialing of staff, the supervision of the quality of care rendered, and the verification of skills, training, and retraining required to maintain optimal levels and reasonable standards in the provision of health care services as promised to the consumer by the health care company/provider.

TORTS AND CIVIL LIABILITY

A home health care provider can be liable for damages if it is found to have committed a tort. A tort is a wrongful act or injury committed by one person against another. The types of torts are defined and governed by the laws of each particular state.

Intentional torts require the intent to commit harm; that is, an actual, conscious desire on the part of one person to harm the other. Examples of intentional torts include an intentional act to commit harm, battery, the intentional infliction of emotional distress, fraud or willful concealment, and misrepresentation or deceit.

A battery is an intentional touching without permission or consent. No harm need occur to the patient for a finding of battery to be lodged against a health care provider. Patients have successfully sued health care providers for battery where treatments to their person were provided without their consent.

Fraud is defined as a concealment or misrepresentation of a material fact that induces a patient's reliance. When a patient reasonably relies on a home care provider's misrepresentations and then suffers damages as a result of that reliance, the patient has a cause of action in negligence against the provider.

Intentional infliction of emotional distress is usually defined as outrageous conduct that results in physical and emotional harm to an injured party. Its finding by the court involves activities by a party that are in themselves sufficiently outrageous to warrant a separate tort of intending to cause the other party emotional distress.

Negligence is behavior that falls below the legal standards defined to protect people from harm or the lack of due care that a reasonable person would be expected to exercise in given circumstances. To determine negligence, a court examines whether the wrongdoer knew or should have known how to act in the circumstances, and whether the wrongdoer did not take reasonable precautions or did not act in a way to avoid or prevent harm and injury to the patient. In other words, the home care provider is held to a standard of care, defined as the reasonable standard under which home care providers generally operate in order to provide safe, reasonable care that protects patients. If the home care provider's actions or inactions fall below this reasonable standard of care and harm to the patient results, the provider is guilty of negligence.

In any tort, the injured party must show a causal relationship between the wrongdoer's conduct and the resulting damage to the injured party. As such, the injured party or patient must show that the home care provider engaged in conduct that involved a foreseeable risk of harm to the patient, and the injury resulted from this action or omission on the part of the home care provider.

Damages in such circumstances may be either compensatory or punitive. Compensatory damages are those that compensate the injured party for loss of earnings, diminution of earning capacity, medical and other expenses, and pain and suffering. Punitive damages are punishment damages. Punitive damages may be awarded where the wrongdoer's conduct is sufficiently outrageous to warrant punishment beyond the simple compensation of the injured party for actual damages. Punitive awards are often made in cases of willful and negligent behavior where the wrongdoer knew of the danger and willfully acted to harm the injured party or willfully failed to act, knowing that likelihood of harm was great.

Criminal liability covers prosecution by a state or by the federal government against a home care provider who commits an act that is specifically punishable under the law.

State laws may require that certain serious adverse patient events regardless of their cause must be reported to licensure or health department authorities. This is in conformance with some states' affirmative requirements for the reporting by health care workers of suspected abuse and neglect of the elderly, children, and special at-risk persons.

FRAUD AND ABUSE

The federal laws under the Social Security Act and its amendments established the health insurance programs that we know as Medicare and Medicaid.[2] Medicare is a federal program that provides health insurance for the benefit of the elderly and disabled as well as other programs for dialysis patients. Medicaid is a state-administered program designed to help needy citizens pay for medical expenses. Medicaid is funded jointly by the federal government and by each state, and serves impoverished individuals who are aged, blind, or disabled, or members of families with dependent children. States are responsible for setting standards for reimbursement and claims processing through the adoption of regulations and the development of policy within federal guidelines according to an individual state plan.

The Medicare statute authorizes the Secretary of Health and Human Services (HHS) to admin-ister the Medicare program to pay for health benefits for the elderly and disabled. This responsibility has been delegated by the secretary to the Administrator of the Health Care Financing Administration (HCFA), renamed and now known as the Centers for Medicare and Medicaid Services (CMS). The CMS promulgates rules, regulations, and guidelines for the Medicare program and enters into contracts with private organizations to assist in program administration. These organizations are known as fiscal intermediaries under Medicare Part A and as carriers under Medicare Part B.

Additions to the Medicare law under the Social Security Act, known as the fraud and abuse amendments at 42 U.S.C. Section 1395nn, provide for prohibitions and penalties with respect to certain abusive and fraudulent activities in the Medicare and Medicaid programs.[3] The most basic prohibitions under the fraud and abuse amendments are those making it a crime for a provider to knowingly or willfully make false or fraudulent claims; concealing or failing to disclose certain information; soliciting, receiving, or offering to pay a remuneration in return for referring an individual to another for the furnishing of any item or services; or knowingly and willfully making a false statement of material facts with respect to the conditions of operation in a hospital, skilled nursing facility, or home health agency.

The CMS has delegated the responsibility for investigating fraud and abuse in the federal health insurance program to the Office of the Inspector General (OIG). The OIG has independent authority to sanction providers who have violated the fraud and abuse laws. Additionally the OIG works with the U.S. Department of Justice, the Federal Bureau of Investigation (FBI), the state Medicaid Fraud Control Units (MFCUs), and the intermediaries to combat abusive and fraudulent activities within the Medicare and Medicaid health insurance programs.

The Social Security law provides that fraud and abuse of the Medicare and Medicaid programs or their beneficiaries may result in criminal, civil, or administrative actions against the perpetrators. The civil money penalty provisions of the fraud and abuse amendments authorize the OIG to assess fines and penalties in thousands of dollars for each false item claimed against the Medicare and Medicaid program. The OIG may also impose civil and administrative sanctions in the form of program exclusions or monetary penalties on individuals and entities for engaging in fraud and abuse of the Medicare and Medicaid programs and/or their beneficiaries.

In addition, the Medicare and Medicaid Patient and Program Protection Act, Public Law 1900–93, provides for a wide range of authorities to exclude individuals and entities from Medicare and Medicaid programs. Exclusions are typically made for conviction of fraud against a private health insurer, obstruction of an investigation, controlled substance abuse, and the revocation or surrender of a health license. Program exclusion is mandatory and lasts for a minimum period of 5 years for those convicted of program-related crimes or patient abuse.

The OIG typically refers cases for criminal prosecution to the U.S. Department of Justice, which may enlist the services of the FBI in its prosecution and investigation of the matter.

MFCUs are responsible for investigating fraud in the Medicaid program. MFCUs receive funds from the OIG. The MFCUs prosecute persons charged with defrauding the Medicaid programs and those charged with patient abuse and neglect.

Many activities may trigger an investigation of a provider by the OIG including but not limited to special areas of focused review for all providers; variation in numbers of visits or number of denials; inaccurate, inadequate, or missing documentation; complaints; and news publications.

Investigators may contact the provider directly or circumvent the provider and attempt to question employees, contractors, or suppliers, all without notice to the provider. The investigators' demeanor may vary from friendliness to hostility. They may act in a manner that causes division and dissension in your company. In any event, unless you are under arrest, an investigator has no duty to be completely up front with you or to inform you of your basic legal rights. You as an individual are expected to know your rights under the U.S. Constitution and the Bill of Rights.

Under all circumstances, any investigation of your company is serious business. Even the threat of an investigation can have a chilling effect on your business and employees. As such, you must take any and all inquiries and investigations about your home care business seriously. If you have any indication that you or your company may be the focus of an investigation or that your employees may have been contacted by an investigator, you should always consult with your attorney. If you do not have an attorney, you should seek counsel immediately.

In the event that your company is served with a search warrant or is informed that it is the target of a criminal investigation, you must contact an attorney to preserve and protect your rights, even if you insist that you are not guilty of any wrongdoing. Failure to protect your rights during an investigation can be evidence of a waiver of those rights for the duration of the investigation and proceedings. Therefore, it is imperative that you act quickly to protect and preserve your rights and the rights of your company.

If you are required to provide certain documents and business records as the result of a valid subpoena or official court order for such documents, then you should keep copies of, and a record of, all documents supplied to the authorities. Keep a record of all contacts with investigators whether formal or informal of which you have knowledge, including a listing of the persons who were present and the content of the contact or meeting. There is no such thing as an informal meeting during an investigation. Do not be lulled into a feeling of false security. Investigators are typically required to set forth a description of their meeting and contact in a written report to their superiors. As such, the formal report of investigation is made and written in the words of the investigators, which may vary with what you consider to be an accurate transcript of the events and commentary made during the meeting or contact.

Keep your attorney involved in all phases of your contacts. Beware of meeting informally with investigators in a way in which you may unintentionally waive your rights. You should resist feeling pressured to answer before you are prepared to discuss the issues. It is important to think out a plan of action for your home care business and your staff. Your plan might include education of your staff to defuse confusion and allay employee fears and concerns, identification of a central contact person to handle all questions and inquiries about your home care business, creation of a central distribution person for all documents released or provided to authorities, and development of a plan for dealing with the press.

A part of this process that you eventually must confront is the business decision of whether to litigate the matter or to attempt to reach a settlement of the alleged violation. The downside risks of damage to your business, reputation, and the expense of litigation should be examined carefully by you in counsel with your attorney. Issues of collateral enforcement activities and reporting by investigators to other federal agencies, state certification, licensure and private accreditation bodies and the resultant effect on your business must be considered in your decision on how to best proceed in the matter. If a settlement agreement is reached and litigation is avoided, certain provisions such as releases and confidentiality agreements should be included in the settlement agreement as a continued protection for your health care business.

It is of utmost importance to your home care business to keep up to date with whatever is the current focus of the Office of the Inspector General (OIG) in looking at fraud and abuse issues. Additionally, the OIG issues General Advisory Opinions and Fraud and Abuse Advice wherein the OIG alerts providers to situations it may deem abusive or fraudulent. It is in your best interest to be aware of what the most recent advisories note and to make sure your business is in compliance with current OIG thinking. You may find your business activities are completely in line with regulations or that they may be considered outside program requirements. This guidance should assist you to correct and/or confirm the compliance of your business practices.

DECISION MAKING, PRIVACY, AND INFORMED CONSENT

Every individual has the right to consent to treatment and the right to refuse treatment. The legal basis for consent and refusals of consent originates from the constitutional right to privacy and the common law right to be free from bodily intrusion. The right to privacy is not an absolute right, however, as each state holds countervailing interests that must be taken into consideration when individuals make decisions to withhold or refuse to consent to treatment for others or for themselves.

Generally speaking, consent can be express or implied. Expressed consent is by either written or spoken direct words. Written consent is evidenced by a signed consent form. Internal agency policy, state law, and licensure, certification and/or accreditation standards determine which procedures require a person's written consent. Implied consent is consent evidenced by the person's conduct. For example, a patient holding out his or her arm for a nurse to take a blood pressure reading is a form of implied consent. Consent may also be implied by the law in emergency situations when the patient is unconscious and relatives cannot be reached and immediate treatment is required to prevent serious bodily damage or to save the person's life. Public policy favors the preservation of life and recognizes that in emergency situations, requiring health care workers to wait would do more harm to the patient and that in such situations health care workers should take immediate actions to save and preserve a life.

For a consent to be valid, it must be informed. The doctrine of informed consent arises from each individual's right to self-determination. The law provides that each patient has the right to be free from bodily intrusion, and to decide what will or will not be done to his or her own body. The law of informed consent requires that a physician must disclose information about a medical procedure or treatment to the patient so that the patient can weigh and consider the information prior to making a decision. Generally, the courts have found that the physician's duty to inform the patient is nondelegable to other health care providers, and that the physician has the duty to disclose information about medical procedures to the patient and obtain the patient's informed consent. For a consent to be valid, the patient must be of sound mind and consent voluntarily. Ideally, disclosure of information about a treatment or procedure should be given in advance of the treatment, so that the patient has time to reach a considered decision and so that allegations of coercion are avoided.

A failure to obtain the informed consent of a patient is a form of negligence, also known as malpractice. A legally valid informed consent is one given by the patient after information about the treatment or procedure is given to the patient. The information disclosed to the patient for a valid consent includes the diagnosis and condition of the patient, the purpose and nature of the proposed treatment, material risks and adverse reactions to treatment, the probability of success of the treatment, alternative treatments, and the prognosis if treatment is not given. Courts usually hold physicians to a reasonable patient standard of disclosure. The reasonable patient standard of disclosure requires that the physician disclose those risks that are material to the patient's decision making process. For example, the risk of a hysterectomy would be material to a woman of childbearing age in her decision whether to consent to or refuse a particular course of treatment or procedure.

Just as every person has the right to consent to treatment, every person has a similar right to refuse treatment. The right to be free from bod-ily intrusion and the right to self-determination derived from the constitutional right to privacy are essential rights owned by each individual. Competing with these individual rights, however, are the countervailing interests of the state. These countervailing state interests are the preservation of life, the prevention of suicide, the protection of third parties, and the safeguarding of the integrity of the medical profession. When a court determines that a patient's right to privacy outweighs the countervailing state's interest in a specific patient's circumstance, then the court will probably uphold the patient's decision to refuse treatment.

Individuals enjoy privacy rights in their health care and treatment. Persons with certain diagnoses, such as patients with a diagnosis of Acquired Immune Deficiency Syndrome (AIDS), may own an increased measure of protection in a number of states where statutory-specific protections to safeguard the patient's privacy have been put into law. Federal law protects the disclosure of the name, diagnosis, and treatment of patients undergoing treatment in federally assisted drug rehabilitation programs. The intent of these laws is usually twofold: to encourage treatment and to protect the privacy and confidentiality of the persons seeking treatment.

Privacy in the contents of medical records is deemed to be a right owned by the individual person unless proper authorization for the release of information is given by the individual. The patient's privilege and privacy rights in his or her communications and the relationship between the physician and patient has been a privilege long recognized by the courts. The patient may also own other legally recognized privileges in his or her relationship with health care providers, and these privileges are usually determined under a state's own laws and statutes.

In April 2003, health care providers were required to comply with the Standards for Privacy of Individually Identifiable Healthcare Information under the Health Insurance Portability and Accountability Act (HIPAA) of 1996.[57] The Department of Health and Human Services (HHS) issued the Privacy Rule and the Office for Civil Rights (OCR) has been given the authority to implement and enforce it.

The purpose of the law is to promote the standardization of health care transactions and safeguard health care information. HIPAA includes guidelines for the electronic transmission, use, and disclosure of health care information, specifically, protected health care information (PHI) by covered entities. PHI is individually identifiable health information that is transmitted or maintained in electronic or any other form or medium. Covered entities include health plans, health care clearinghouses, and health care providers who transmit health information electronically in connection with a standard transaction. Covered entities must comply with all HIPAA regulations as standard transactions on code sets, privacy, and security. HIPAA contains requirements for patient consent, authorization, uses, as well as PHI disclosures for treatment, payment, and healthcare operations. The rules confer certain rights on individuals including rights to access and amend health information and to obtain a record of when and why their PHI was shared with others for certain purposes. Specific physical and technical security safeguards to electronic systems are required. Additionally, HIPAA contains requirements for notice to and assurances from external associates such as business contractors.

Violations of HIPAA requirements may result in penalties including civil monetary penalties, criminal penalties, and exclusion from Medicare. Further requirements under HIPAA are likely, and with the danger of penalties attached to HIPAA, it is imperative that the home care provider stay up to date on HIPAA's requirements as a part of program compliance.

ADVANCE DIRECTIVES

Advance directives are documents within which patients direct the kind of health care they would or would not want and/or appoint someone to make health care decisions on their behalf if they are unable to make the decisions for themselves. Advance directives are typically called living wills or health care powers of attorney. The Patient Self Determination Act (PSDA) was passed by Congress in 1990 and focused on an adult's right to refuse life-sustaining treatment and gave force to patients' rights to accept or refuse medical treatment and to state laws regarding these rights.[4]

The PSDA is an effort to allow each person an opportunity to control his or her future in the event of incapacity and the acknowledgment and response to the less often discussed issue that the past practices of life "at any cost" and even against a person's own wishes is partly responsible for the exorbitant cost of aggressive care and treatment during the last weeks of life, that such care is generally futile and not expected to improve the quality or length of a patient's life, and that many patients, if capable to decide, would refuse such care or not choose it for themselves.

State laws within which these rights are described include, but may not be limited to, durable powers of attorney, living will acts, health care powers of attorney, and surrogate decision-maker laws. The PSDA applies to all health care institutions receiving Medicare or Medicaid funds, and compliance with the PSDA is incorporated into Medicare and Medicaid provider agreements as a requirement for reimbursement.[5] The PSDA requires the care provider agency to:[6]

- Provide written information to each adult patient on admission (inpatient facilities), enrollment (HMOs), and at first receipt of care (hospices and home health or personal care agencies). The information provided must describe the individual's legal rights under state law to accept or refuse medical care and to write advance directives for incorporation into his or her medical record.
- Maintain written policies and procedures regarding advance directives and provide written information to the patients about those policies.
- Document in the patient's medical record whether the individual has executed an advance directive.

- Ensure compliance with state law requirements regarding advance directives.
- Provide, either independently or with other like institutions, for education for the staff and community on issues concerning advance directives.

Information provided to the patients should include a description of how the individual state's law handles continuation or withdrawal of treatment from incompetent patients who have not executed advance directives.

Patients are presented with advance directive information on the first visit. Due to the numerous documents signed and the limitation on time for staff to explain the directives and the capacity of patients to understand the directives, some patients do not appreciate the importance of the advance directive. Educational efforts directed toward patients should help to correct these deficiencies. Written information or brochures explaining the meaning of the advance directive and its purpose for the individual can be given to the patient so that it may be reviewed and reflected upon within the individual patient's time frame. Materials should be written in plain language, to be easily understood by the patient. Materials should be available in the language of the patient or given via interpreters, and personnel should be available to disseminate information via appropriate means to the disabled and impaired.

A follow-up telephone call or provision of an address to write to for additional information or guidance would be helpful to some patients and families. Agency staff should be educated about advance directives so that they may easily explain the directives to a patient and answer basic questions about directives. An individual in the organization should be designated as the resource person for staff and patients for further information on advance directives.

Patients requiring specialized or further assistance should be referred to appropriate resources such as their own attorney or the local bar association.

Any patient or family member or caregiver presenting a purported valid legal paper that authorizes a health care power of attorney, durable power of attorney, guardianship, surrogacy, or similar document should be referred to the agency's designated advance directives person, so that the authenticity and legal effect of the documents may be verified and included in the medical record. Any conflicts, discrepancies, or questionable validity in the existence of or content of an advance directive document, whether it is originated by staff, patient, family, or outside parties, should be referred to the designated advance directive person for investigation and resolution. In cases of unresolved problems or questions with directives that will affect your staff and the care rendered, you need to consult your company's attorney for specific advice in the individual case.

It is important that all staff be aware that, as with any medical directive, an advance directive may be changed or withdrawn by the competent patient at any time and by any means, and that a patient may refuse to execute an advance directive. Additionally, staff should be reassured that generally states and courts protect health care providers who act *in good faith* in reliance on a valid advance directive.

State law governs the effect and interpretation of advance directives. Because these state laws are ever-evolving on the subject of advance directives, and a multiplicity of legal documents that have the effect of an advance directive may be present for a patient, your staff and company should have access to a designated advance directives resource person or contact in order to resolve questions and educate staff on the effect of an advance directive document in the care and treatment of a particular patient.

LABOR AND EMPLOYMENT ISSUES

Recent areas of concern for home care providers in labor matters are the wrongful termination of employees, negligent hiring and supervision of staff, and characterizations of workers in an employee versus independent contractor status.

The wrongful termination of employment is a matter of increased litigation in employment law.

The common law recognizes that most employers and employees enjoy a relationship defined as employment-at-will, meaning essentially that either party may terminate the relationship for any reason, at any time. Due to certain federal regulatory and state law requirements, employers have increasingly utilized employee handbooks to define and describe the expectations of the employment relationship with employees. Courts in many states are increasingly taking the view that employee handbooks are evidence of, and may constitute proof that, the employment-at-will relationship is ended or modified and that a contract of employment exists between the employee and employer.

Employment contracts confer certain duties, rights, and privileges upon employees and duties upon an employer that were not necessarily contemplated in the employment relationship and that are not required in an employment-at-will relationship. An example of this may be a formal, written disciplinary procedure agreed to be followed prior to any termination of employment status. Employees are increasingly invoking the existence of an employment contract when an employee handbook is utilized in a company. Home care providers should be especially diligent in reviewing their employee handbooks to include certain provisions such as a disclaimer or language indicating that the handbook is not a contract and that the handbook does not intend to alter the employment-at-will relationship between the parties. Employers should be cautious about provisions that may infer that employees hold greater rights than were intended in the employment relationship.

Negligent hiring and supervision practices should be an area of great concern to home care providers. The increase in the number of home care personnel assisting a patient in the less controlled environment of the patient's home, and an increased examination of the home care industry in its self-monitoring of home care activities, will probably cause a heightened scrutiny as to which factors constitute reasonable hiring practices in the home care industry. Medical equipment drivers and delivery persons, health care professionals, home health aides, companions, infusion care company personnel, medical diagnostic testing personnel, and a variety of health care–related workers are entering into the privacy of the patient's home. With this reality in mind, a number of states currently require pre-employment criminal record checks for all employees who provide patient care services in the home. Certain states may limit the criminal record check to home care personnel who provide patient care services to children, the elderly, or persons defined as at special risk for harm from mistreatment or abuse. Some continue to foster the belief that federal regulations should require all home care agencies receiving Medicare funds to conduct criminal background checks before hiring home care workers.

Courts have recognized that health care providers and facilities that provide health care services hold a duty to protect the patients for whom they care and to whom they render health care services. This minimum protection on hiring employees comes into play in the activities of screening applicants for patient care positions; verification of valid, current, and appropriate licensure or certification for the position sought; and diligent verification of employment and personnel references as to the appropriate character and demeanor of the applicant in patient care service activities.

Negligent supervision of staff is another factor and risk in employment litigation. Current federal regulations requiring supervision of home health aides should assist to minimize findings of negligence in matters involving this category of employee. A number of states have implemented similar protective laws to require supervision of nonlicensed professionals providing health care and health care–related services to patients at home.

A continuing issue for home care providers in many states is the characterization of workers performing work for the home care providers in the status of independent contractors versus employees. Such characterizations may carry serious tax and labor policy implications for your business. Employees are workers whose wages are subject to withholding taxes at federal, state, and, in some cases, local levels. Employee status causes the employer to both withhold and contribute to federal taxes, Social Security, state workers' compensation funds, state unemployment, and similar programs enacted for the security and benefit of employees. These programs are additional costs to all employers for their employees. Employers are exempt from providing such benefits and treatment to independent contractors.

The home care industry has typically utilized the services of certain workers such as physical therapists, speech therapists, and occupational therapists on a per-visit basis under contract. A controversy continues as to whether these categories of workers may be classified as independent contractors rather than employees. The main issue is that employer and employee status is usually defined by control and direction by the employer over the employee. Conflicts in interpretation occur, because for many home care providers, the provider is required to have a measure of control over such workers, and yet in industry practice and according to this worker group's own professional licensure statutes, these workers have traditionally acted and been treated as independent contractors.

Although it may seem advantageous to your agency to classify a worker as an independent contractor and avoid certain employer responsibilities, such a misclassification may result in major costs, penalties, fines, and liabilities to your company.

Labor matters of these types will continue to confront the home care industry as new types of workers and responsibilities to those workers and to consumers evolve in the health and home care service industry.

Matters and legal requirements dealing with immigration issues for foreign healthcare workers and any evolving requirements related to homeland security matters are potential areas for new laws to which the homecare business must keep alert and informed.

AMERICANS WITH DISABILITIES ACT

The Americans with Disabilities Act (ADA) gives rights and protections to individuals with disabilities to the same extent that they are presently provided to individuals on the basis of race, sex, national origin, and religion.[7] It prohibits discrimination against workers with disabilities in all aspects of employment and requires access of disabled persons to public transportation and public accommodations.[8]

In developing the ADA, Congress made note that approximately 43 million Americans have one or more physical or mental disabilities and that such persons are routinely discriminated against solely because of their disabilities.[9] An increased and more favorable integration of individuals with disabilities into society is a major goal of the ADA.

Under Title I of the ADA, employers with 15 or more employees may not discriminate against a qualified individual with a disability because of the disability of such individual, in regard to job application procedures; the hiring, job assignment, advancement, or discharge of employees; employee compensation or fringe benefits; job training; and other terms, conditions, and privileges of employment.[10] An employer must provide reasonable accommodations for disabled workers, unless that would impose an undue hardship on the employer.[11] Only employees and applicants who are qualified individuals with disabilities are protected.[12]

The term disability means: (1) a physical or mental impairment that substantially limits one or more of the major life activities of an individual; or (2) having a record of such impairment; or (3) being regarded as having a substantially limiting impairment.[13] In determining whether a condition is a disability one must consider the unique characteristics of each applicant or employee on a case-by-case basis. The term *qualified person with a disability* means an individual with a disability who meets the skill, experience, education, and other job-related requirements of a position held or desired, and who, with or without reasonable accommodation, can perform the essential functions of such positions.[14] The identification of the essential function of each job is the key to ensuring compliance with the ADA, because the duty to employ individuals and provide reasonable accommodations, job standards, and medical examinations each relate to the essential function of the job. Essential functions are primary job duties that are intrinsic to the employment position, rather than marginal or peripheral functions that are incidental to the performance of primary job functions.[15]

A major standard of the ADA is the requirement for employers to provide reasonable accommodations that do not involve an undue hardship on the employer so that qualified persons with disabilities can perform the essential functions of jobs.[16] Reasonable accommodations also demand that the employer make equally available all services and programs provided in connection with employment, such as wellness programs, cafeterias, counseling services, and transportation. Reasonable accommodations may include, but are not limited to making existing facilities used by employees readily accessible to and usable by persons with disabilities; job restructuring; modifying work schedules; reassignment to a vacant position; acquiring or modifying equipment or devices; adjusting or modifying examination, training materials, or work policies; providing qualified readers or interpreters; and other similar accommodations.[17] Tax credits and deductions are available for some of these costs.

Employers are required to make a good faith effort to find a reasonable means of accommodation. Consultation with federal, state, or local rehabilitation and disability organizations familiar with the needs of disabled workers may provide useful input into the determination of a reasonable accommodation. Employers should prepare a written record to document the efforts taken, sources consulted, options considered, potential costs of available accommodations, and the resulting decision.

The most significant element of Title I of the ADA concerns the employment application process and determination of final hiring, promotion, or termination decisions. Employers are prohibited from utilizing any procedure or taking any action, in the process of screening applicants and during the hiring process, that could have a discriminatory effect against a qualified individual with a disability.[18] Many job applications have historically included questions regarding applicant disabilities, hospitalizations, or illnesses. It is recommended that employers review all job application forms and eliminate questions about physical or mental disabilities.

In order to establish that the disabled status of an applicant or employee was not a factor in the employment-related decision, employers should base all employment decisions on clearly articulated job criteria. In addition, the specific reasons for all adverse decisions, including all medical evidence, accommodations considered, and the reasons for rejecting such accommodations should be clearly documented in writing in the employer's personnel files.

The ADA has established prohibitions against discrimination in application and hiring that encompass a general prohibition as to the use of medical examinations and inquiries into whether a person has a disability. However, in certain circumstances medical examinations are permitted, such as when job related and consistent with business necessity or when required by federal, state, or local law.[19] In all situations, strict confidentiality of the medical examination results is required and the information regarding such exams should be kept in a separate file from the personnel file.[20] When medical exams are performed as a condition of employment, the company should ensure that all of the ADA conditions are met, such as that the exam is a post-offer exam, that the physician performing the exam has been provided a written job description for each position sought, and that such physician has specified if there are essential tasks that the individual cannot safely perform without undue risk of harm to him- or herself or others.

Individuals with contagious diseases such as hepatitis, tuberculosis, AIDS, or HIV infection are considered disabled under the ADA.[21] An employer is permitted to limit the job opportunities of individuals with an infectious disease only if it can demonstrate that the infectious disease constitutes a significant risk to the health or safety of others; that is, a direct threat that cannot be eliminated by reasonable accommodation.[22] If an individual poses a direct threat as the result of a disability, the employer must determine whether a reasonable accommodation would either eliminate the risk or reduce it to an acceptable level. Actions taken against individuals because of a belief that they may communicate an infectious disease to others cannot be based on fears, stereotypes, or generalizations. The Centers for Disease Control (CDC) guidelines state that HIV-infected health care workers who adhere to universal precautions and who do not perform invasive exposure-prone procedures pose no threat of HIV transmission to their patients.[23]

An employee or applicant currently engaging in the illegal use of drugs is not entitled to ADA protection because such individuals are not included in the definition of qualified individual with a disability.[24] Alcoholism is considered a disability under the ADA, and alcoholics are protected from discrimination unless the alcoholism interferes with the individual's ability to work or poses a threat to the property or safety of others. Reasonable accommodation requires health care providers to employ former drug addicts or alcoholics for most health care positions. Nevertheless, employers are permitted under the ADA to:[25]

- Prohibit the use of alcohol or illegal drugs at the workplace by all employees
- Prohibit employees from being under the influence of illegal drugs at the workplace
- Require employees to follow the requirements of the Drug-Free Workplace Act of 1988
- Require employees to meet the job-related requirements established by federal regulatory agencies regarding drugs and alcohol
- Hold a drug user or alcoholic to the same qualification standards for employment or

job performance and behavior to which they hold other individuals, even if any unsatisfactory performance or behavior is related to the drug use or alcoholism of such individual

Reasonable accommodation of the alcoholic employee and former drug-addicted employee qualified for the position may include access to substance abuse rehabilitation programs and leaves of absence for treatment.[26]

The ADA neither requires nor prohibits drug testing by employers to determine illegal drug use.[27] The ADA permits employers to adopt or administer reasonable policies or procedures, including but not limited to drug testing, to ensure that employees or applicants are not currently using illegal drugs. Drug testing is not considered a medical examination subject to the limitation of the ADA, and the ADA permits employers to conduct drug testing of job applicants and employees and make employment decisions from the results of those tests.[28] However, employers must be careful that drug testing does not violate state or local laws or patient confidentiality laws.

Your company must post notices issued by the Equal Employment Opportunity Commission (EEOC) that inform applicants and employees of the provisions of the ADA.[29] Such notices should be posted conspicuously on the employer's premises, including personnel offices and other places where applicants and employees are likely to see them, such as the cafeteria, staff meeting room, and so forth. Such notices must be made available in various formats so that persons with impaired vision and other disabilities are notified of the ADA requirements. Your company might also include information about ADA obligations in job application forms, job vacancy notices, and personnel manuals. Employers must retain employment records and job applications for at least 1 year for ADA purposes and for longer periods under certain state laws and for other federal regulatory purposes.[30]

Title III of the ADA prohibits discrimination based on disability in the full and equal enjoyment of the goods, services, facilities, privileges, advantages, or accommodations of any place of accommodation by any person who owns, leases (or leases to), or operates a place of public accommodation.[31]

A public accommodation is described as a privately owned establishment that makes its services, goods, or programs available to the public.[32] The public accommodation requirements apply to all types of health care facilities including home health agencies and to all areas in such companies such as lobbies, restrooms, parking areas, and the like. In order to assist a disabled person to experience full and equal enjoyment of a facility, places of public accommodation may be required to:[33]

- Modify eligibility criteria policies or practices that have the effect of discriminating against or excluding people with disabilities
- Remove architectural barriers that restrict accessibility and communications
- Supply auxiliary aids and services
- Provide transportation services on an equal basis

Health care providers and insurers may need to increase office accessibility by installing ramps, establishing accessible parking spaces, enlarging the office's physical entrance, rearranging furniture, and widening doors or modifying other spaces to facilitate wheelchair access or movement.[34] Bathrooms must also be accessible to disabled persons, and modifications may include installation of grab bars, rearrangement of partitions, mirrors, and towel dispensers, and raised toilet seats.[35] If your company has limited funds, the rules prioritize the order in which existing barriers should be removed:[36]

1. Measures that will enable individuals with disabilities to physically enter a place of public accommodation
2. Measures that provide access to those areas of a place of accommodation where goods and services are made available to the public

3. Measures to provide access to restroom facilities
4. Any other changes necessary to remove barriers

The ADA does not require that alterations be made to existing facilities. It does require that if alterations are undertaken that could affect the facility's usability, those alterations must, to the maximum extent feasible, make the altered portions of the facility readily accessible to and usable by persons with disabilities.[37] New facility construction must be designed and constructed so the facilities are readily accessible to and usable by persons with disabilities, unless it is structurally impracticable to do so.[38]

Public accommodations are required to provide auxiliary aids and services to enable a person with a disability to use the available goods and services, unless to do so would fundamentally alter the program or would constitute an undue burden.[39] The term auxiliary aids and services includes methods of making aurally or visually delivered materials available to individuals with visual or hearing impairment, and the acquisition or modification of equipment or devices for disabled persons.[40] Auxiliary aids and services include:[41]

- Qualified interpreters or other effective methods of making aurally delivered materials available to individuals with hearing impairments
- Qualified readers, taped texts, or other effective methods of making visually delivered materials available to individuals with visual impairments
- Acquisition or modification of equipment or devices
- Other similar services and actions

The ADA specifically provides in regulations that landlords and tenants are jointly responsible for public accommodation requirements; however, the responsibility for and the cost of compliance with the ADA may be allocated in the leases.[42] As such, your company should review its facility leases and amend them to include necessary changes where appropriate. Your company may claim certain tax deductions for removing architectural, transportation, or communication barriers in your physical plant and company property.[43] In addition, eligible small businesses may take a tax credit for accommodations made to comply with the ADA.[44]

The ADA, and many state and local laws, require health care providers to treat all disabled persons, including those with AIDS or HIV infection. Because AIDS and HIV infection and other infectious diseases are considered disabilities under the ADA, health care providers are prohibited from denying treatment to any patient because he or she has AIDS, HIV infection, or some other infectious disease.[45]

In *Glanz v. Vernick*, a patient was refused treatment due to his HIV infection.[46] The patient sued under Section 504 of the Rehabilitation Act, and the health care facility was found liable for the health care worker's discrimination under the theory of respondent superior. The court based its decision on the fact that although the treatment of AIDS- or HIV-infected persons posed a minimal risk of infection, that risk was so small that a refusal to treat was legally insupportable.

The ADA gives the health care provider a duty to communicate with all patients who have impaired hearing, vision, or speech.[47] It is very important that all patients understand the nature and risks attendant to medical treatment. Appropriate auxiliary aids must be furnished where needed to ensure effective communication. The examples provided in the ADA regulations note that an interpreter, rather than a written summary, may be necessary to communicate in an effective manner to persons with hearing, vision, or speech disabilities.[48] The ADA also requires that interpreters be qualified to provide interpretive services and be able to interpret effectively, accurately, and impartially both receptively and expressively, using any necessary specialized vocabulary.[49]

As a limitation on the public accommodation requirements, your company is not required to provide services to individuals who pose a direct threat to the health or safety of others.[50] If your company concludes that a disabled person poses a direct threat, such that he or she is violent or acts in a threatening manner, that person may be denied the services of the public accommodation.[51] Additionally, your company may deny access of accommodation to current illegal drug users.[52]

Many questions remain as to the effect and extent of rights and responsibilities under the ADA. The federal courts and the EEOC hear discrimination complaints and lawsuits under the law, and questions will likely be answered on a case-by-case basis. However, this does not mean you should wait to comply with the law. It is imperative that you seek counsel when a question arises as to compliance with the ADA that you are unable to resolve easily on review of the regulations and your own internal procedures. Due to the substantial legal remedies afforded injured persons under the ADA, it is in your company's best interest to carefully document your attempts to comply with the ADA and to seek counsel when further advice is needed. The ADA provides harmed persons with substantial legal remedies and so imposes new and increased liability risks on health care providers, employers, and public accommodations. A plethora of questions remain on the extent of a disabled worker's rights and the limitations of an employer's or public accommodation's responsibilities under the ADA.

Your company should develop its own policies and procedures to comply with the ADA and state and local laws. Legal counsel should be sought for advice in particular circumstances and to assist in developing undue hardship and business necessity defenses where a reasonable accommodation cannot readily be provided. Relevant federal, state, and local laws should be reviewed, and administrative and supervisory staff and all personnel should be educated as to their responsibilities and rights under the various nondiscrimination laws in their multiple roles as employer, employee, and care provider.

TAX MATTERS

Increasingly, the tax-exempt status of health care providers is being challenged by a variety of sources. These sources of challenge are at the municipal, city, county, state, and federal levels. Pressure on governments to secure revenues through tax funding has caused the authorities to closely examine the tax-exempt status of both nonprofit and tax-exempt 501(c)(3) charitable health care providers. In addition, the taxing authorities are taking a closer look at health care providers due to reasons such as the diversification of health care providers into lines of business and business ventures viewed as unrelated and/or in contradiction with the provider's articles of incorporation, charter, and/or mission, and the fact that a number of health care providers are earning surplus revenues and/or are operating in ways that are divergent and inconsistent with their original charitable purposes.

Tax matters of concern to home care providers may also arise in the accounting methods on which the tax treatment of certain transactions are predicated on Medicare cost accounting and allocation principles. The Internal Revenue Service (IRS) has cautioned health care providers that the IRS's method of accounting and definitions of certain transactions for tax purposes vary from those utilized in the federal health insurance program known as Medicare. These differences in tax interpretation and characterization must be carefully considered by home care providers in managing the business affairs of their home care companies.

ENVIRONMENTAL ISSUES

Environmental issues are of great legal concern for all health care providers. The increased complexity of treatment modalities, pharmaceuticals, supplies, and equipment utilized in the home environment equates with ever-increasing issues of how to deal with the waste and environmental results associated with such treatments and materials.

The Occupational Safety and Health Administration (OSHA), under the authority of the Department of Labor, is the federal agency vested with the responsibility of developing and enforcing regulations and developing guidelines that encourage and cause employers to create and maintain safe workplace environments for employees.

OSHA has become increasingly active in the monitoring of the activities of health care providers in their actions for protecting health care workers. For example, OSHA issued instructional guidelines from its Office of Occupational Medicine, Directorate of Technical Support, entitled *Work Practice Guidelines for Personnel Dealing with Cytotoxic (Antineoplastic) Drugs*.[53] This instructional publication outlines practical precautions recommended for health care providers involved in the handling, preparation, administration, and disposal of antineoplastic agents. The main thrust of the publication is the protection of the health care worker and the environment from the unknown long-term effects and hazards of new drugs and technologies that health care providers may utilize in their everyday work. Similarly, in February 1990 OSHA issued a revised instruction CPL 2-2.44B from its Office of Health Compliance Assistance, *Enforcement Procedures for Occupational Exposure to Hepatitis B Virus (HBV) and Human Immunodeficiency Virus (HIV)*.[54] This instruction provides standards for the management and treatment of health care workers potentially exposed to HBV and HIV. Essentially, the standards require that employees at substantial risk of contacting body fluids must be offered hepatitis B vaccinations free of charge by employers and that employers must report any needlestick requiring medical treatment. OSHA acts to protect health care workers by the enforcement of such standards through site inspection, citations, and fines.

Noncompliance with OSHA standards may also result in collateral enforcement activities adverse to a home care provider by the licensure, certification, and accreditation bodies whose approval is a basic legal requirement for the continued operation of the home care provider.

Other worker protection laws, such as the federal and state employee right to know laws requiring posted notices to employees of workplace exposures to known hazardous chemicals and agents, govern all employers, including home health care providers.

The U.S. Environmental Protection Agency (EPA) is also concerned with the risks that new technologies may present in the uncontrolled disposal of medical waste, infectious waste, hazardous waste, and contaminated supplies such as needles and sharps from a patient's home.

In an effort to educate home care personnel and patients about such hazards, in January 1990, the EPA issued a pamphlet entitled *Disposal Tips for Home Health Care—Educating Your Patients,* as an instruction to home care personnel in their disposal practices of medical waste from the home.[55] Similar efforts and legislation are occurring at the state level in an effort to regulate waste created in the care and treatment of patients in their homes. In a number of states, past laws that excluded home health agencies and various home care providers as generators or producers of medical, infectious, or hazardous waste are now including home care providers in their state's legal definition of a producer of these wastes. This new designation is likely to subject home care providers to a plethora of regulatory and reporting requirements. Such trends are likely to continue in the future and shall subject home care providers to even greater scrutiny and requirements under state environmental protection and waste management laws.

These issues should be of great concern to home care providers in that these environmental and worker protection requirements expose the provider to greater accountability and increased exposure for liability if it fails to comply with the regulatory standards. Environmental claims are typical exclusions in most policies of insurance, and as such, the liability exposure for home care providers is one that cannot be easily protected against by a policy of insurance. Moreover, many state environmental laws are strict liability laws that provide that if the home care company is found to have violated the environmental law, then it must pay the mandated fines and costs of cleanup or correction. Under strict liability laws, it is usually irrelevant whether the violator knew of or intended to cause the violation. All that is necessary is a finding that the violation occurred and that the home care company/provider was the violator. Environmental damage claims and fines and the costs of cleanup can be astronomical. As such, it is crucial that home care providers pay serious attention to the development of environmental laws in their communities and at both state and federal levels of government.

WHAT TO CONSIDER IN SELECTING AN ATTORNEY

"One cool judgment is worth a thousand hasty counsels. The thing to be supplied is light, not heat."[56] Perhaps we should best look to the words of President Woodrow Wilson in his address on preparedness given in Pittsburgh, Pennsylvania, on January 29, 1916, for words of inspiration in your considerations of what to look for in selecting an attorney to assist you with legal matters and matters of concern to you in your home care business.

It has been evident that employer/employee disputes, conflicts with government agencies and regulators, consumer concerns, and litigation are beginning to confront, and are of increasing concern to, home care providers. In these and similar matters, your health care business may require the services of an attorney.

The key to a productive relationship with an attorney is personal compatibility. You must be able to speak openly, freely, and candidly with this individual. As a general business counselor, you should look for an attorney who offers guidance, suggests alternatives to proposed actions, and anticipates, thereby preventing legal problems.

Legal expertise and judgment are key attributes to seek in an attorney. A lawyer should have a working knowledge of the laws and regulations that affect your business.

Legal expertise in the matters in which an attorney will likely be involved is of increasing importance for health care providers in the ever more regulated service industry of home care. However, home care providers are similar to all companies in that they face a growing complexity of business and legal issues that demand technical knowledge. Certain areas of your business that may require special attention include pension planning, complex tax matters, securities issues, labor matters, and patent and trade secret protection.

With this perspective in mind, a health care organization should seek out an attorney who concentrates his or her practice in the health care industry, and in particular in the representation of home care service and product providers. Securing the services of an attorney who concentrates his or her legal practice in health care matters may assist you to avoid the recurring time delay and frustration of educating your attorney about what that thing is that you and your company do.

Alternately, you may seek references from your accountant and banker or from other companies in the home care industry. Your trade associations may be helpful in assisting you to secure appropriate counsel. In any event, you should feel free to ask the attorney for a number of client references and check them out. The American Bar Association, the lawyer referral service of the local bar association, the National Health Lawyer's Association, the American Association of Nurse Attorneys, and the American Academy of Hospital Attorneys are just a few of the many organizations that may be able to direct you to attorney members who concentrate their legal practice in health care matters or in a related area of concern to your company.

Due to both the litigious and the regulatory nature of health care services, for specific matters it may be in your company's best interests to seek out experienced attorneys in special matters (e.g., malpractice defense litigators in negligence matters and criminal defense attorneys in fraud and abuse matters).

If your current general counsel is an attorney experienced in health care matters, your counsel will probably seek out these attorney specialists when it is in your company's best interests to do so. Many policies of insurance for liability require that your company utilize the insurance company's counsel in matters of defense under the policy of insurance or risk the possibility of no insurance coverage of the matter and nonpayment of attorney fees under the policy of insurance.

In any event, your company's general counsel should be experienced in home care provider matters related to your specific home care business. An experienced health care attorney is able to recognize when it is imperative for you to retain an attorney with experience in specialized matters. For example, as just mentioned, due to the legal criminal procedural issues that may occur at a certain juncture in a fraud and abuse investigation, your health care attorney may suggest the retention of the additional legal services of an experienced criminal defense attorney in order to best proceed in protecting your rights and those of your home care company. Protecting your company's legal position and putting you and your company in the best possible legal position should be the goal for you and your attorney in such matters.

ENDNOTES

1. *Key Enterprises of Delaware, Inc. v. Venice Hosp.* 919 F.2d 1550 (11th Cir. 1990), vacated and reh'g en banc granted 979, F.2d 806 (11th Cir. 1992).

2. U.S.C.A. 42 § 1395 et seq.

3. 42 U.S.C. § 1395nn.

4. The Patient Self Determination Act of 1990, Pub. L. No. 101–508, 105 Stat. 1388-44-115, 42 C.F.R. § 489.100–104.

5. 42 CFR § 489.100–104.

6. 42 CFR § 489.102.

7. 42 U.S.C.A. §§ 12101–12117.

8. 42 U.S.C.A. §§ 12111–12117, 12141–12189.

9. 42 U.S.C.A. § 12101(a).

10. 42 U.S.C.A. § 12112(a).

11. 42 U.S.C.A. § 12112(b)(5)(A).

12. 42 U.S.C.A. § 12112(a).

13. 42 U.S.C.A. § 12102(2).

14. 29 CFR § 1630.2(m).

15. 29 CFR § 1630.29(n)(1).

16. 29 CFR § 1630.2(o).

17. 29 CFR § 1630.2(o)(2).

18. 29 CFR § 1630.10.

19. 42 U.S.C.A. § 12112(d)(4)(B).

20. 29 CFR § 1630.14(d)(1).

21. 28 CFR § 36.104.

22. 28 CFR § 36.208.

23. Centers for Disease Control. (July 12, 1991). *Recommendations for Preventing Transmission of Human Immunodeficiency Virus and Hepatitis B Virus to Patients During Exposure-Prone Invasive Procedures,* 40 MMWR1, 3.

24. 29 CFR § 1630.3(a).

25. 29 CFR § 1630.16(b).

26. *Rogers v. Lehman,* 869 F.2d 253(4th Cir. 1989).

27. 42 U.S.C.A. § 12114(d)(2).

28. 42 U.S.C.A. § 12114(d)(1)–(2), 29 C.F.R. § 1630, App.

29. 42 U.S.C.A. § 12115.

30. 29 CFR § 1602.

31. 28 CFR § 36.201(a).

32. 28 CFR § 36.104.

33. 28 CFR §§ 36.302–310.

34. 28 CFR § 36.304(b).

35. 28 CFR § 36.304(b).

36. 28 CFR § 36.304(c).

37. 28 CFR § 36.402(a).

38. 28 CFR § 36.40–407.

39. 28 CFR § 36.303(a).

40. 28 CFR § 36.303(a).

41. 28 CFR § 36.303(b).

42. 28 CFR § 36.201(b).

43. I.R.C., 26 U.S.C.S. § 190.

44. I.R.C. § 44. (1992). *Disabled Access Credit,* 1992 U.S. Master Tax Guide, CCH, 1338, 1991.

45. 28 CFR § 36.104.

46. 756 F. Supp. 632 (D. Mass. 1991).

47. 28 CFR § 36.309.

48. 28 CFR § 36.309.

49. 28 CFR § 36.303, 28 C.F.R. §36.309.

50. 28 CFR § 36.208(a).

51. 28 CFR § 36.208(b), (c).

52. 28 CFR § 36.209.

53. Occupational Safety and Health Administration. (1986). *Work Practice Guidelines for Personnel Dealing with Cytotoxic (Antineoplastic) Drugs* (OSHA Publication No. 8–11). Washington, DC: OSHA.

54. Occupational Safety and Health Administration. (1990). *Enforcement Procedures for Occupational Exposure to Hepatitis B Virus (HBV) and Human Immunodeficiency Virus (HIV).* Washington, DC: OSHA.

55. Environmental Protection Agency. (1990). *Disposal Tips for Home Health Care—Educating Your Patients* (EPA Publication No. EPA/530-SW-90-014A). Washington, DC: EPA.

56. Wilson, W. (1981). *The Papers of Woodrow Wilson* (A. S. Link, ed.). Washington, DC: Library of Congress.

57. Pub. L. No. 104-191, §§ 261–4, 42 U.S.C.§ 1320d–1329d-8; 42 § U.S.C. 1320d-2, Title 45 C.F.R. Part 160, 45 C.F.R. Part 164.

CHAPTER 50

Understanding the Basics of Home Health Compliance

Deborah A. Randall

I. INTRODUCTION: WHY COMPLIANCE PLANS AND COMPLIANCE PROGRAMS?

The first major reason to establish a working and effective compliance plan is as insurance against the possibility of significant errors occurring in the operations of a home health entity, causing adverse economic events and possible regulatory and sanction actions by governmental agencies, third-party insurers, and private parties. The second reason for organized compliance plans is to demonstrate the proper intentions of a health provider when confronted with the possibility of an investigation by a governmental organization; that is, looking for indicators of intentional or reckless attitudes toward laws and regulations on behalf of the health provider. When the home health provider can offer firm evidence of its established intentions to routinely review, address, and improve important areas of functioning that are subject to legal controls and have a monetary or quality of care impact on payers and customers, many governmental authorities will take these efforts into account in their recommendations of possible further investigations, potential prosecutions, and penalty demands.

A third positive reason for establishing an effective compliance program is to present the home health provider's best business characteristics when it is being assessed in the commercial world, where it must compete for the

contracts and affiliations that will increase its market position, look for networking opportunities, or show its top value if and when it may be the subject of an acquisition consideration by others.

II. THE GOVERNMENTAL ORGANIZATIONS INVOLVED IN COMPLIANCE AND HOME HEALTH AGENCIES

The home health agency (HHA) that wants to be at the top of its form in dealing with the compliance landscape needs to know about the agencies of government that have a role in investigations, audits, legal proceedings, and penalty recommendations. The following sketches introduce the players and their general areas of emphasis.

A. The Office of the Inspector General

The Office of the Inspector General (OIG) is part of the federal Department of Health and Human Services, which has its headquarters in Washington, D.C., and has numerous regional offices. The Inspector General is an individual appointed to be independent of the Secretary of Health and Human Services and whose office has responsibilities to review areas where fraud, abuse, or waste may reduce the nation's funds to provide the health and welfare services that the Social Security Act in the Medicare and Medicaid Programs makes available for qualified Medicare beneficiaries and Medicaid recipients eligible under the states' plans. The OIG staff conducts studies of aspects of the health industry and of its administration by the Department of Health and Human Services. OIG also investigates and brings legal actions against companies and individuals who OIG believes are engaged in fraud and abuse. OIG issues both alerts, which are indications of OIG concern about industry practices and developments, and advisory opinions, which are responses to individual inquiries as to whether certain identified practices would provide a basis for action by the OIG under the antikickback sections of the federal law. Additionally, the OIG publishes "guidances" with regard to the establishment of effective compliance programs by industry sectors. The OIG guidance on effective home health agency compliance programs was published in final form (after circulation for comments by any interested reader of the *Federal Register* draft version) in August 1998. It identified numerous risk factors (some of which might not truly be "illegal" in the view of nongovernmental advisers but all of which are important to note in compliance planning).

The OIG's staff, who are lawyers, auditors, and other trained professionals including investigators, conduct their own investigations and also collaborate with the Department of Justice through its U.S. attorneys offices in each of the 50 states. In dealing with the OIG, health providers should always contact their experienced health counsel before agreeing to speak even informally with the OIG, including with OIG staff who may be conducting an industry-focused study or evaluation, and not a focused investigation based on the possibility of a violation of law. Although it is important for the OIG to have accurate, realistic information about how the home health industry works, there are no protections against the OIG's taking information noted in a general inquiry into a company-focused investigation, should something "come up" in the review. On the other hand, the OIG has many legal tools at its command because of powers Congress has given the

office (and money, through the HIPAA fraud sections from 1996). Under regulations, if the OIG presents a home health agency (HHA) with a written list of documents it wishes to review and these are not otherwise protected by law, the HHA has 24 hours to respond with the documents (or work out through counsel how they will be produced). No such regulation exists to compel a person to talk to the OIG, absent a subpoena properly executed. In certain cases, an HHA's health attorney may approach the OIG's office to provide a limited amount of information by interview. Because the OIG's office collaborates with the Department of Justice on criminal cases (the "kickback" statute is a criminal law, for example), it is very important to know what legal rights protect an individual and a company when an investigation is underway.

Finally, the OIG's staff take action on the "exclusion" of an individual or company from participation in the Medicare and Medicaid programs through mandatory actions (which result from convictions under certain laws) or "discretionary" actions (which follow the OIG's assessment of whether the exclusion should be put in place). An exclusion prevents the individual or company from participating in any federally funded program—which means much more than simply Medicare or Medicaid—but those two are the "death sentence" for many who wish to have a job or professional career in the health field. Furthermore, if an individual or company is excluded, another provider cannot hire that person or entity in a capacity relating to services that will be billed to Medicare or Medicaid without that billing being illegal. As a result, many health attorneys negotiating with OIG strive to deal with infractions through monetary penalties (bad as that may be), rather than allow their clients to be "excluded" because their livelihood in their fields would end.

B. The Federal Bureau of Investigation

The Federal Bureau of Investigation (FBI) supports the Department of Justice in criminal investigations. It is not mandatory for a health company employee to speak with an FBI agent, and HHAs should accurately inform their employees of their rights with regard to these and other inquiries such as from the OIG. On the other hand, it is essential that the HHA never direct the employee (or contractor) to stonewall, lie, alter documentation, or withhold information at the agency's direction, because this could be grounds for criminal charges of obstructing justice. If an employee is named in a valid subpoena, he or she needs assistance of counsel and that lawyer will explain those rare (but important) circumstances under which an employee would be advised to assert constitutional protections against testifying.

C. The Medicaid Fraud Control Units

The Medicaid Fraud Control Units (MFUCUs) exist at the state level to investigate civil and, in some states, criminal matters; to recommend actions; and to assist in prosecutions with the attorneys general of the states. In some states, the MFUCUs have units at the county level. The MFUCUs are the primary agencies concerned with activities that result in fraud and abuse directed at Medicaid funds. However, the states and the federal government are partners in the funding of Medicaid programs, and thus there is a continued federal concern and coordination with the states. In the home health field, this collaboration intensified greatly as a result of reviews of home health operations during the mid-1990s known as Operation Restore Trust. The federal–state proportions of Medicaid program funding vary, and the Medicaid state plans also vary as to which optional or waiver programs a state may have instituted in the home health area. In some states, particularly vulnerable patient populations, such as children, AIDS patients, the frail elderly, and traumatic brain injury patients in assisted living facilities or group homes, are in Medicaid waiver programs, so that the notion of Medicaid "abuse" may be clearly connected with quality of care concerns. Additionally, some states' programs in the personal care area provide for home attendant and 24-hour live-in programs including, in some circumstances, individuals (rather than companies) who are directly engaged by the patient who is the Medicaid recipient. The MFUCU may be concerned in such settings with the possibility of abuse of the system by the patient (who may not be entitled to the extensive services being provided), or abuse toward the patient by a paraprofessional.

D. Fiscal Intermediaries

Federal fiscal intermediaries (FIs) are contractor organizations engaged by the Medicare program to perform medical review of submitted claims and to audit cost reports of Medicare-certified HHAs. Although Medicare home health reimbursement converted in October 2000 to a largely per-episode fixed-rate system from a per-cost, visit-based reimbursement subject to cost limits, Medicare-cost report submission is still mandatory and requires application of cost-reporting principles found in regulations and in the Provider Reimbursement Manual, HIM-15. FIs must scrutinize claims filed by HHAs for suitability of the payment rate applied against the diagnostic and functional profile described by the HHA's staff visiting the patient. The FI will also look for patterns and practices suggesting errors, intentional up-coding, or routine submission of high reimbursement predicted codes (through the requests for anticipated payments [RAPs] that are 60 percent of the total payment for the episode) that are subsequently reduced if the final claim shows a lesser number of therapy visits, for example. FIs perform medical reviews of the documentation supporting select claims, and may place HHAs on focused review if the claims patterns trip compliance screens (which are confidential and not available to providers).

The Medicare cost report audit performed by the FI results in a "settlement" in which the as-filed cost report may be adjusted for simple errors, for misallocation of costs among what are called reimbursable cost centers and nonreimbursable activities and cost centers, and to remove costs the HHA may have claimed as appropriate but for which the FI finds Medicare will not pay any part of the costs. These include marketing, fundraising, personal items, luxury items, alcoholic beverages, educational seminars and travel unrelated to the home health field, the "profit margin" in charges to an HHA from a related organization or individual, interest expense from a related party loan, and other costs not considered "reasonable and necessary" by the FI. Cost reports from the year 2000 are still being audited by FIs in 2003. Once settled, the cost reports may be "re-opened" by the FIs for additional adjustment within the 3 years following the date of the settlement. Cost report submissions, workpapers, and substantiating provider accounts that look fraudulent to FIs may be brought to the attention of outside program integrity units, or directly to the OIG.

E. Program Integrity Contractors

Program integrity (PI) contractors were established in 2002 to be external organizations, separate from FIs, that would investigate and assess evidence of problematic claims or reporting by providers. These organizations are alerted by the FIs if a provider initiates a substantial repayment action by communicating to the FI a provider error and submitting a check for the provider's calculated overpayment. These organizations use sophisticated computer software and analytic strategies to identify evidence of fraud and abuse in claims submissions. If HHAs have unusual patterns of billing at very high reimbursement episode rates or home health resource groups (HHRGs) under the home health prospective payment system (PPS), or if there were patterns of visits or disciplines that seemed to "scam" some aspect of PPS billing, one may assume the PI contractors will be tracking these cases.

F. State Survey and Certification Agencies

The state agencies are contracted to the Medicare program to establish an organizational framework to survey providers participating in Medicare and also do "validating" surveys when

independent accreditation organizations such as the Joint Commission on Accreditation of Healthcare Organizations (JCAHO) and the Community Healthcare Accreditation Program (CHAP) do the continuing survey work for HHAs admitted into the Medicare program. State survey agencies are required to train their staff on the Medicare Conditions of Participation (COPs), found at Title 42 of the Code of Federal Regulations, Part 484; to follow the survey protocols and Interpretive Guidelines to the Medicare State Operations Manual; to do chart reviews; and to make home visits of HHAs. This includes a sample of all patients and not merely Medicare patients in the "skilled intermittent" home care program of a home health agency. If an agency has divisions that do other kinds of work—for example, personal attendant or hospice—those will be separated off from, and not be subject to, the federal home health survey. They might, however, be surveyed on state licensure grounds or under different COPs; for example, for hospice.

State survey agencies are on the front line for COP compliance efforts and are often critical in recent years, having been the subject of negative reviews by the General Accounting Office as lax in fulfilling their survey responsibilities. State survey agencies are also looking for irregularities in nursing documentation, the absence of evidence of a visit, or the skimpiness of visits that could suggest under-serving of patients. They survey for document alterations such as whiteouts, for the provision of services without recorded physician orders, for failure to have adequately credentialed staff, and for evidence of patient abuse. State survey agencies are also responsible for determining whether there is adequate supervision in branch offices, and for recommending (or not) the certification of such branches to the Medicare CMS Regional Offices that grant the status necessary for an HHA to bill services provided through those offices. Finally, state survey offices receive the encrypted transmissions of the CMS Outcome and Assessment Information Set (OASIS) documents and survey HHAs for the adequacy of that recordation against the content of the medical record. Like the state MFUCUs, the state survey and certification agencies have played an expanded role since the Operation Restore Trust reviews of HHAs in the mid-1990s. There also is a significant amount of information that routinely is exchanged among the state agency, the MFUCU, the FI, and OIG.

III. COMPLIANCE AND THE LAWS

All HHAs must have an appreciation of the laws that apply to their functioning, especially in relation to the governmental agencies they bill. HHAs participating in Medicare and Medicaid already are required to comply with the COPs and any state licensure provisions (which are not repeated here). The following six areas of law have particular relevance for the fraud and abuse compliance of HHAs. Other laws, such as in the areas of labor and employment, OSHA, tax and corporate securities, real estate, and certificate of need are extremely vital to all home health agencies but are beyond the scope of this chapter. The laws applicable to privacy and the Health Insurance Portability and Accountability Act (HIPAA) are discussed in another chapter of this book.

A. False Claims

False Claims Acts may be either civil or criminal; the federal system contains both. When a law is criminal, the level of proof that a prosecutor must meet in prosecuting the case to a jury or to a judge is the "beyond a reasonable doubt" phrase that many nonlawyers have heard—even if they have not themselves served as jurors. Simply stated, this is an extremely high level of proof a case must meet. The penalties for the defendant may also potentially be extreme and definitely dramatic: large fines and/or imprisonment. A central part of criminal cases usually is "intent" on the part of a person or a business entity to have engaged in the conduct that was violative of the law. With criminal false claims cases, the billing for services or the submission of a cost report (among other actions) is al-

legedly with the intention to submit something false. An example could be an HHA that sends in claims for a person whom the agency knows was not provided the number of visits listed on the final claim to the Medicare program—perhaps because the visits are invented, or perhaps because the Medicare number is real but the person was not actually admitted. Also potentially criminal would be providing and billing for services that were known not to be medically necessary; for example, more physical therapy services than the patient's condition warranted, in order to reach the 10 or more therapy visit level for PPS. That level significantly raises the amount an HHA is paid under the HHRG rates. A false cost report claim could intentionally list costs as "reimbursable" when the agency executives knew that these costs were clearly nonreimbursable—personal items for the family of executives of the corporation, for example.

Civil false claims acts authorize the government and sometimes private parties to recover monetary penalties and multiple damages from persons who "knowingly" submit false or fraudulent claims or statements in support of claims. The federal False Claims Act (FCA) is the law most HHA managers should focus upon in the billing area, because it contains the "whistleblower" provisions rewarding individuals who are the original source of information leading to successful federal cases against Medicare providers. These cases are also referred to as "qui tam" [pronounced "qwee" or "key tahm"] cases. Under the FCA, a claim may be false because (1) it is intentionally submitted and known to be false, (2) it is submitted with "reckless disregard" for whether it is true or accurate, or (3) it is submitted with "intentional ignorance" on the part of those responsible for the submission as to whether it is true or accurate. Because the monetary penalties are both a multiplier of three times the amount deemed "false" and an $11,000 penalty per claim (which could be the individual beneficiaries in an HHA's submission or perhaps a line item error within the claim), FCA cases may go from an error base in the thousands of dollars to a penalty in the multiple millions. Most cases are settled with the government, because it may be impossible for the provider to undertake the uncertainty of a court case and the catastrophic effect of the full penalty liability and remain fiscally viable. The amount of reward to the whistleblower can also be in the millions, which provides an obvious incentive to undertake these cases. The initial phases go on without the provider's knowledge, because the submission to the court is "under seal" at the court while the early investigation is under way. Sometimes the first a provider is aware of the matter is when a staff member tells management that he or she has been approached for an interview by the OIG, the FBI, or the whistleblower's attorney. Sometimes the government subpoenas the provider, demanding extensive document production. There are parallel state FCA laws in most states.

B.   Mail and Wire Fraud; False Statements

Another basis for a federal criminal action might be the use of mail or phones to file false claims. The mail or wire fraud case could be based on electronic billing or cost report submission, or the fraudulent back-up documentation sent to the government when the FI makes a request for further substantiation for claims. Similarly, a provider could be accused of making false statements under another federal law. These could be untrue verbal statements or responses prepared in writing when questions are posed by the FI; it could be the alteration of clinical notes by nurses or therapists. There is a different, criminal law prohibiting the submission of false claims with criminal intent in the Medicare or state health programs. This charge can be added to the total along with the criminal FCA; for example, to make "counts" in a criminal indictment issued by a grand jury.

C.   Failing to Disclose Overpayments

If a provider finds that it has received payments to which it is not entitled, and the provider knowingly conceals or fails to disclose to the FI that fact and the reason for that overpayment, such actions could be deemed criminal under another provision of the federal law. Potentially, this action could range from being paid twice for a claim to failing to inform the FI of a known error on the cost report that favored the provider. This provision of the law has not been utilized much by the federal prosecutors, but it is actually one of the simplest to understand from an ethical standpoint. If you have money you do not deserve, you have to pay it back. There are some Medicare regulations that address unknown errors in favor of a provider when they are first discovered 4 or more years after payment. In some situations, the Medicare regulations state "without-fault" payments can be retained. The Medicare Prescription Drug, Improvement and Modernization Act of 2003 contains provisions for nonpenalty adjustments for minor mistakes in billing. Consult knowledgeable health counsel immediately if your organization thinks it may be in a circumstance where it is holding funds that seem to be duplicate or "windfall" payments.

D.   Antikickback Laws

The Medicare and Medicaid antikickback statutes are another area of the law in which the basic legal concepts and implementing compliance measures are extremely important. The law is complex and you will need to have assistance of counsel in creating or reviewing certain business relationships, including relationships with patients. The antikickback law addresses referrals and the arranging for referrals, and states that it is illegal to provide or receive anything of value (called a "remuneration") whether it is in cash or in "kind," with the intent of referring, arranging for referrals, or recommending a referral for services or items that ultimately the Medicare or Medicaid program will pay. These statutes set Medicare and Medicaid in a different world than virtually all other businesses and industries, where favors, gifts, entertainment, cross-referral arrangements, rewards for "loyalty," and such are part of the business environment. However, Congress has been clear that it feels Medicare and Medicaid programs can be corrupted through such arrangements because they can distort professional judgment, reduce patient choice, lead to excessive and thus abusive services, and prevent excellent and cost-effective providers from competing in the marketplace of medical services, equipment, and supplies.

Because the antikickback statutes have a broad definition and criminal penalties, they have proved difficult to administer and interpret from both the government and the providers' side. One question has been whether any desire for referrals in establishing a relationship taints the entire effort even if there are other, acceptable bases for the relationship. In the famous Greber case,[1] where physicians were provided an opportunity to earn a fee in reading the reports of cardiac monitoring by a specialist to whom they referred, the court's opinion stated that even if one of the reasons for an arrangement was to induce referrals, it could be a criminal matter. The OIG also has been zealous in interpreting the statutes and regulations. However, Congress required the creation of "safe harbor" regulations that set out the situations in which no legal action would be taken against persons who may have arrangements that on a technical level appear to involve the statutes. *At a minimum,* HHAs need to have their contracts, leases, vendor arrangements, independent contractor and physician relationships, liaison positions involving hospitals or other institutional providers, marketing activities, fundraising solicitations, charitable and reduced payment procedures, "complimentary" screenings, and other activities reviewed carefully by home health counsel in light of the antikickback laws.

Congress also required the OIG to address the confusion about the antikickback laws with advisory opinions. These are responses to individual inquiries about activities that may appear to implicate the antikickback statutes. When the OIG advisory opinion favors an arrangement, the clearance only pertains to that particular person or company. However, the opinions have proven to be useful guidances. One of the more recent advisory opinions involving home health concerned the question of whether circumstances suggested "inducements" to beneficiaries to "self-refer" (a prohibited referral covered by the statute) to a particular Medicare HHA. OIG found that providing Medicare beneficiaries a medical alert device and the response services for free, although a technical violation of the statute, was acceptable because (1) the government had endorsed in the PPS system for home health agencies a flexibility in the identification and delivery of services for the fixed episodic payment, (2) the CMS had supported many kinds of telemedicine, (3) the service was not advertised, and (4) it was provided selectively after the HHA assessed the patient for need. (See the OIG Advisory Opinion Number 03-04.) Sometimes OIG's other guidances create confusion or contradictory advice to their official opinions. For example, during the summer of 2002, OIG issued a guidance with regard to Medicare beneficiary inducements. In that issuance, OIG stated that items of insignificant value such as pens, pencils, coffee mugs, and so forth, which were of $10 or less in value per gift or $50 per beneficiary per year, would not be considered kickbacks. The implication, of course, is that items or services above that level could cause scrutiny by OIG.

E. "Stark" Laws

The "Stark" laws are amendments to the Social Security Act that govern the relationships that physicians can have, or are prohibited from having, with other components of the health industry or other entities. Again, this is an exceedingly complex area of law, and health counsel advice is strongly urged. In the second Stark law enacted by Congress, physicians were barred from virtually all ownership of "designated health services" of which home health is one (other services included physical therapy and parenteral and enteral nutrition, which are areas where some HHAs also have business lines). Nonownership financial arrangements between physicians and HHAs are legally secure only when they are described in a written contract that follows particular criteria set out in the regulations that the CMS publishes. Although HHAs are not required to have medical directors, Medicare-certified HHAs must have professional advisory committees under the COPs, and physician participation is included. Additionally, some HHAs feel that for quality of care purposes and to strengthen the communication with attending physicians whose patients the HHA is serving, physician consultants or directors are important. If such physicians are compensated by the HHA, their relationship must fit the Stark regulatory requirements: The arrangement must be in writing, must be for at least a year in duration, must be at fair market value and commercially reasonable, and must not vary in compensation based upon volume. Originally, OIG took the position that a physician contract must refer to specific times and days on which a physician will serve if the contract is not a full-time arrangement. Practically, that is not reasonable in the world of physician services, and CMS has delayed issuance of certain parts of the Stark rules because of this issue. The contract can never be dependent upon the volume or number of referrals the physician herself or himself makes to the company.

Whenever an HHA establishes an arrangement with what could be a referral source, it is necessary to document the basis for "fair market value"; it is not simply what the physician or company demands. The HHA should have documented, independent indications of how it established that the financial terms were reasonable in light of the exterior market for services: The OIG will expect that this is independent of the proximity to the referral potential itself, even when it is not part of the negotiation (and cannot be). The HHA must also be able to defend why that particular arrangement is necessary in the first place. This analysis is particularly crucial when, for example, an HHA wishes to establish a charting station at an institutional provider location, or wishes to compensate a physician for services when that physician has served on a voluntary basis in the past.

F. Civil Money Penalties

The Civil Money Penalties (CMP) provisions of the Social Security Act authorize the Inspector General of the Department of Health and Human Services (DHHS) to impose civil money penalties and assessments and to exclude persons and companies through administrative proceedings (that is, tried first before a DHHS administrative law judge rather than before a civil court federal judge). The basis for OIG action includes that a provider knew or should have known that services were not provided as claimed or were false or fraudulent, that the provider knowingly charged the Medicare fees substantially in excess of those billed other payers, that the provider's under-serving the patient constituted a serious quality concern, or that the provider knowingly charged for medically unnecessary services. Penalties under CMP are up to three times the remuneration and $10,000 for each line item or service. Up-coding under Medicare home health PPS could be a basis for CMPs. CMPs are available for cases of false or fraudulent claims in all federal health care programs except federal employee health benefit plans.

IV. THE ESSENTIAL ELEMENTS OF AN EFFECTIVE COMPLIANCE PLAN

Although the degree of formality of a compliance plan depends on the size and complexity of the HHA organization, there are certain essential elements that, in addition to an appropriate employee manual and rigorous policies and procedures, set out the framework for making compliance "work." The protections of an effective compliance plan initially stemmed from their use in addressing sentencing under criminal laws. An effective compliance plan could persuade a judge to lessen or vary a sentence when there was room for a span or spectrum of punishment. When OIG issued its guidance for HHAs' compliance programs in 1998,[2] the OIG reviewed the different functional areas for such plans and suggested areas of "risk" for HHAs.

Sometimes those "risks" were interpretations that OIG had never directed for public comment or analysis through the rulemaking procedures that providers are entitled to under the federal Administrative Procedure Act. Certainly some OIG interpretations had not been litigated through the government's bringing either a civil or criminal case focused upon such an issue.

A.   Compliance Standards and Procedures

An HHA's compliance plan must have standards and procedures that are "a clearly delineated commitment to compliance by the home health agency's senior management and its divisions including affiliated providers operating under the home health agency's control and other health professionals . . . with an emphasis on preventing fraud and abuse," according to the OIG guidance.[3] This means an HHA needs a code of conduct and an articulation of what the ethical bases are for the business function. The HHA also needs to direct its employees to avoid behaviors and attitudes that are dishonest; abusive of the public trust; fraudulent or abusive procedures with regard to documentation, billing, or interactions with the public and governmental agencies; and out of compliance with known standards for quality and licensure and certification. The HHA must link its operational procedures to its compliance mission, and distribute these materials throughout its organization in order for the concept of compliance to be live and not on a shelf, unread and ignored.

B.   Steps to Prevent and Detect Offenses

An HHA's compliance plan must lay out how it will identify the areas of function within the organization, as it pertains to the field of home health services, that may be vulnerable in light of the manner in which the home health industry functions. This is what makes it essential to tailor a compliance plan to the specific organization, and what makes expertise in the home health field so essential from a review and auditing perspective.

C.   Compliance Oversight

A compliance officer must be appointed who has the authority and the characteristics likely to make the compliance function successful. The individual must be ranked at a high level of personnel within the organization and have sufficient independence of function that he or she could report past the highest executive employee, directly to the governing body, should there be evidence of compliance failures at the top of the organization.

Essential qualities in a compliance officer include excellent communication skills, an established knowledge base in the relevant regulations (or ability to learn rapidly), unimpeachable integrity, an approachable nature, and the capacity to engender confidence of the senior management of the company. Although some large HHAs have hired compliance officers from outside the company, most HHAs have looked within, and many have compliance officers who also function in other company roles. Many organizations create a compliance committee that includes those with operational expertise in clinical, finance, accounting, and other areas and who can support the compliance officer. Most compliance experts recommend that the compliance officer be empowered to exercise considerable autonomy, and that this include identifying at an early stage of an internal investigation the need for an outside counsel's review of the facts and responses. The OIG has signaled its disapproval of naming the CEO, CFO, or inside counsel to the post of compliance officer, because of the inherent conflict between establishing or defending policy and investigating whether errors have been generated because of executive mismanagement or misdirection. The OIG in April 2003 described the following as primary responsibilities for a compliance officer:

- overseeing and monitoring implementation of the compliance program
- reporting on a regular basis to the company's board of directors, CEO, or president, and compliance committee (if

applicable) on compliance matters and assisting these individuals or groups to establish methods to reduce the company's vulnerability to fraud and abuse

- periodically revising the compliance program, as appropriate, to respond to changes in the company's needs and applicable federal health care program requirements, identified weakness in the compliance program, or identified systemic patterns of noncompliance
- developing, coordinating, and participating in a multifaceted educational and training program that focuses on the elements of the compliance program, and seeking to ensure that all affected employees and management understand and comply with pertinent federal and state standards
- coordinating personnel issues with the company's human resource/personnel office to ensure the exclusion lists have been checked
- assisting the company's internal auditors in coordinating internal compliance review and monitoring activities
- reviewing and, where appropriate, acting in response to reports of noncompliance brought to his or her attention from all sources
- independently investigating and acting on matters related to compliance
- participating with the company's health counsel in the appropriate reporting of any self-discovered violations of federal health care program requirements
- continuing the momentum and, as appropriate, revision or expansion of the compliance program after the initials years of implementation[4]

The compliance plan of an HHA must be reviewed by and endorsed by the governing body of that organization in order for it to have relevance when a governmental agency conducts an investigation or suggests it may take action against a provider. A board of directors' resolution to initiate compliance planning, the documentation in the board minutes of its review of the written product from the compliance officer, and periodic reports on its compliance program implementation are all important.

D. Screening Employees

One of the essential elements of a compliance plan is an effective method for screening individuals for histories of, or tendencies to engage in, illegal activities. This means HHAs need to utilize background checks and reviews for criminal records, within the limits of state employment law. The HHA must also screen vendor companies and new and current employees against the OIG exclusion list and the other available federal program exclusion lists. The OIG list is available and downloadable from the OIG Web site, www.oig.hhs.gov. Many HHAs do not realize that the obligation for this screening is for their present employee base, not merely new hires. Additionally, the review should be annual (this can be by groups or by employee hire date) to maintain a reasonable confidence that there have not been new occurrences of exclusion of employees. The application for employment can include a certification that the potential employee has not been excluded from the Medicare or Medicaid programs; if that application proves to be false, swift response is available to the HHA.

The implication of exclusion of an individual is at least twofold. First, the HHA as a Medicare provider is barred by federal law from billing claims if the agency has employed an excluded person in the area of business directly related to the providing and billing of Medicare services (a broadly interpreted definition). Second, the individual presents a potential concern with regard to compliance monitoring even if he or she is engaged in activities unrelated to the barrier to billing. If an HHA should find it has inadvertently violated this statutory provision, health counsel can assist in approaching the appropriate authorities for resolution of the matter. Recently, an FI attempted to require an HHA to certify at the time of a cost-report audit by the FI that the HHA had screened against the OIG exclusion list and not billed any claims in the year under review (the claims being part of the cost report data). This requirement was not part of any regulation nor was the form the FI presented approved by the Office of Management and Budget (OMB). Consequently the HHA was directed to refuse, politely, and counsel had the senior audit manager of the FI agree the "requirement" did not have CMS backing. It is very important that providers not "certify" facts when the requirement is not mandated by law.

E. Communicating and Training about Compliance in the HHA

The compliance plan of an HHA will be lifeless if there is not sufficient training on what compliance is, what the standards and practices are, what new requirements may have issued from the payer world (assuming the issuances are accurate), and how an employee can raise an issue appropriately and know action will be taken. Some providers train their employees initially on the compliance plan and then it falls out of view. This will provide virtually no protection should an investigation result in the HHA being under scrutiny. The government wants to know how a company can prove it did not recklessly disregard or intentionally ignore a potential problem. Therefore, training needs to be ongoing and the occasions recorded; the best training includes focused work for documentation and billing areas of the company. The training documents need to be thoroughly understandable. Annual training should be mandatory, and special training is necessary if there are agency errors of significance or new developments affecting HHAs. Compliance training highlights should be included in regular staff and supervisory meetings, so that the communication is constant, natural, consistent, and the "real deal," not a "big deal." Periodically, an HHA may choose to have an outside expert provide training; this is particularly appropriate for training of the board of directors. In light of the guidance

issued in March 2003 by the OIG and the American Health Lawyers Association about responsibilities of boards of directors (both for profit and not for profit), board involvement in the effectiveness of compliance necessitates board comprehension of the full impact of the responsibilities.

F. Monitoring and Auditing

Monitoring and auditing are the heart of an effective compliance program. The OIG guidances recommend an initial baseline audit by trained and knowledgeable counsel and consultants from outside the agency. When an HHA chooses to use health counsel on a consultative basis, or to do "check-up" audits later in the implementation of the compliance program, this review can also have important protective value for the company. The baselines, whether externally or internally conducted, can identify the HHA-specific areas of vulnerability and the need for emphasis. Materials reviewed include, but are not limited to:

1. corporate organization and structure
2. corporate-related organizations; for example, home infusion, DME, management companies, holding companies, subsidiaries, and hospital affiliates
3. contracts (including leases) with independent contractors, managed care organizations, physicians, referral sources, and vendors
4. position descriptions
5. policy and procedure manuals with particular focus on trouble areas in home care
6. employee manuals
7. orientations and training manuals
8. financial statements including any quarterly reports to the FIs
9. cost reports, settlements, and notices of program reimbursement
10. internal and external audit reports and management letters
11. correspondence with the FI in other areas, such as additional development requests (ADRs)

12. survey and accreditation reviews
13. outcome-based quality improvement reports and adverse event reports
14. correspondence concerning other governmental audits or inquiries
15. information concerning grievances (patient and employee)
16. history of legal actions against the company (if any)

Subsequent regular audits from within the HHA should be coupled with a confidential reporting mechanism through which an employee may report concerns without threat of retaliation or punishment (other than for abuse of the system). A hotline, preferably maintained internally, is a common mechanism. Although some agencies note that the hotline is silent much of the time after the initiation of the compliance program, this author feels that may indicate training is insufficient and the articulation of responsibilities of everyone in the functioning of the organization may be inadequately understood. The hotline is a mechanism for suggestions and concerns, not just the reporting of potential fraud. In performing the actual internal audits, compliance officers need audit tools, a prioritization method, a schedule including reports to the executives and governing body, and guidance for when the results of an audit suggest a further investigation is necessary and when that should be conducted by counsel to preserve the confidentiality of the results from governmental document requests or inquiry.

G. Enforcement

Enforcement must be effective all the way up the ladder of responsibility within an organization. If it is not appropriate, measured, and responsive, the compliance program will lack credibility within the ranks of the organization. Unenforced policies signal to the government investigators that a compliance program is unlikely to be serving as a deterrent to improper behavior, and the associated value of the compliance structure in dissuading the government from pursuing a case or reducing a penalty is

lost. Feedback is essential to the individual who has brought a legitimate concern to the attention of the compliance officer. With response and feedback, many potential whistleblowers recognize that the company is ethical and determined to do the right thing, and this strengthens the resolve of the employee to support and protect the agency rather than threaten it by a qui tam lawsuit.

IV. HOT TOPICS IN HOME HEALTH COMPLIANCE REVIEWS

Although the landscape will, of course, change both for the individual HHA and for the industry, there are areas that need particular focus in today's regulatory atmosphere. Several of these are addressed here; many more also deserve attention.

A. Failure to Provide Quality Care

The home health industry has historically been blessed with not only a good and close rapport with the patients it serves, but also the good fortune of few incidents of poor quality delivery. With the advent of PPS reimbursement methodologies, the industry moved from a posture where it got paid its costs but could not officially and legitimately make a profit (return on equity was removed from the Medicare cost-based reimbursement by Congress prior to PPS). Under PPS, the home health industry has moved to the possibility of positive profit return, thus there is an incentive to conserve resources, encourage independence in the patient at the earlier stages rather than provide extra visits, and structure the service mix to the diagnosis and functional level—with positive reimbursement consequences when the per-episode payment exceeds cost. A similar restructuring of approach accompanied the institution of DRGs for hospitals and the elimination of cost-based reimbursement in all but the specialty hospital areas of pediatrics and psychiatric services. (Out-patient hospital payments, rehabilitation hospitals and units, and long-term care hospitals have all moved in recent times to a PPS model.)

Now HHAs must self-audit for quality of care indicators lest they be accused of underserving patients. The Medicare program plans to publish and publicize, on an individual and statewide basis, the relative successes of HHAs in improving certain functional limitations of patients. An eight-state demonstration program was initiated May 1, 2003, and the entire 50 states moved to this outcome review and publication as of November 2003. One must assume that the OIG, the state survey agencies, the FIs, and the contractor program integrity companies are being charged to identify patterns of underservice. Such cases might be deemed "false claims" by the government, because a certified HHA that bills for Medicare patients states that it is in compliance with Medicare rules and the provisions of the participation agreement the provider has with the Medicare program. A Medicare provider is prohibited from discriminating against a patient because of the payment source and also in asserting (the government would argue) that the claim sent was for good quality care. If the patient is intentionally underserved with a negative outcome, the legal case might be made that the value of the service was below "value." Such cases have been successfully brought under the False Claims Act in the nursing home industry when there have been exceedingly poor quality services and bad outcomes.

B.   Up-coding

Home health has not had coding-accuracy-to-billing compliance issues in the past because a visit was of a single value for a given discipline. With PPS, it is possible for an unscrupulous HHA employee to either exaggerate the patient's clinical profile in the OASIS or knowingly assign more therapy services than is medically necessary, or both. Such actions would affect the payment rate per episode, as would the deliberate failure to record a significant change in condition (SCIC). A SCIC breaks the episode into parts, and in virtually all cases lowers the reim-

bursement dramatically. It is clear that FIs are screening for OASIS/coding irregularities and are down-coding cases for a variety of reasons. FIs can also see patterns of initial high-therapy visit estimates, followed by agencies' failing to "make" the 10 therapy threshold. HHAs should be doing their own sample draws of claims to check accuracy of coding by all responsible individuals with the agency.

C.   Hospital Referrals to Owned or Controlled Home Health Providers and Suppliers

The Medicare portion of the Social Security Act, in Section 1802, contains a patient "freedom-of-choice" provision that allows a patient to choose any qualified (in the case of home health, this would mean certified) provider as the care deliverer. In the Balanced Budget Act of 1997, Section 4321, Congress enhanced the ability of patients to make informed choices about the availability of post-hospitalization care by adding a a reference to post-hospital referral to home health agencies and other entities in the Social Security Act's requirements for a hospital's discharge planning function. Beginning 90 days after the August 5, 1997, enactment of the act, hospital discharge planners were to:[5]

1. inform the patient of the availability of home health services through individuals and entities that participate in the Medicare program and that serve the area in which the patient resides and that request to be listed by the hospital as available
2. not specify or otherwise limit the qualified provider that may provide post-hospital home health services
3. identify (in a form and manner specified by the secretary) any entity to whom the individual is referred in which the hospital has a disclosable financial interest (as specified by the secretary . . .) or which has such an interest in the hospital

In December 19, 1997, draft regulations, HCFA (now CMS) noted:

> The process of making a choice includes being provided options to make an informed and confident decision. Hospital [sic] providing a list of available Medicare-certified home health agencies will assist patients in making such decisions. *Although a hospital is free to design the list's format, the list is neither a recommendation nor endorsement by the hospital of any particular home health agency's quality of care.*[6]

In a November 2002 regulation, CMS stated:

> [T]he information made available . . . would serve to ensure that the financial interests between hospitals, HHAs and other entities do not lead to program integrity abuses such as steering certain patients (for example, healthier patients) to certain HHAs (for example, hospital-owned).[7]

These referrals from hospital parent to HHA subsidiary/department remain a hot spot for HHA compliance if the HHA is collaborating with the hospital in any hospital actions to taint the choice process. This might occur through undue influence by the hospital or by the manipulating of referrals to independent HHAs—for example, by sending only the least profitable cases or the charity cases to such HHAs. Although the antitrust laws are beyond the scope of this chapter, HHA compliance officers and CEOs should also understand that there are market conditions under which an independent HHA might make a credible argument that a hospital is attempting to monopolize the market by directing its referrals only to its owned subsidiaries. Such a case would be strengthened if the hospital were engaged in "predatory" practices such as failing to honor a patient's initial request for an independent HHA.

D.   Sham "Joint Ventures"

Over the years, many health lawyers have seen providers attracted to the possibility of a "joint venture" in which an existing health care company—often a durable medical equipment (DME) provider—will approach an HHA and offer it the opportunity for a joint venture. These ventures may be designed to serve the same geographic area that the DME company already serves, the offer may require little capitalization from the HHA (or hospital), and the existing DME company becomes the "manager" and runs the new business including providing the inventory and employees. Frequently, the existing DME company will offer discounts on the supplies and equipment from its own store or inventory so that the proposed joint venture has the prospect of attractive profits in the spread between the acquisition cost for the materials and the fee schedule paid by Medicare, Medicaid, or third-party insurers.

In April 2003, the OIG published an alert warning that some joint ventures may be regarded as shams set up to direct kickbacks to the provider which refers, and thus are illegal under the civil and criminal laws. (See Appendix 50C.) When such arrangements vary the payout based on the referral volume, they certainly are a risky and potentially illegal arrangement. In reviewing the HHA contracts and structures, a compliance officer may find a long-standing relationship with a DME company and wonder about its legality. Any true joint ventures must be reviewed by health counsel skilled in HHAs, supplier and provider operations, and the fraud and abuse laws. The OIG seems to suggest that if the question you ask is "Is this too good to be true?", the answer may be "Yes, and it's trouble." However, ventures can exist outside the boundaries of the safe harbor for joint ventures and still not violate the statute.

E.   Physician Orders

There are numerous compliance issues associated with physician orders; only a few will be mentioned here. When medical records do not contain written and signed verbal orders to verify changes HHA staff make in the manner in which services are delivered, the impact may be one of both quality and timing. For example, an agency that bills without a system in place to review that orders were received and signed could subject itself to overpayment exposure. Some HHAs have billing software systems that permit "holding" bills until a flag is dropped when the signed order arrives, and the bill is then electronically transmitted. The failure of an agency to use such tools where available could risk a false claims suit from an aggressive prosecutor who might argue the failure constituted intentional ignorance about the suitability of a claim for payment. Quality of care is implicated in the appearance of nurses taking steps in treatment without proper collaboration with physicians, even in states where the nurse practice act is broadly written and interpreted.

CONCLUSION

Home health agencies benefit from the review that accompanies the proper implementation of a compliance program and will be more protected from error, investigation, and penalties from governmental regulators and prosecutors. Ignoring such benefits is not a wise business decision. That said, a compliance program must be effective, utilized, updated, and reviewed at all levels including the governing body. Absent that commitment, the protections a compliance program affords will be greatly diminished and the intentions of the managers of the company could be called into question in any governmental probe.

ENDNOTES

1. *United States v. Greber,* 760 Fed.2d 68 (3d Cir. 1985).
2. 62 Federal Register 42410 (8/7/98).
3. Ibid., at 42413.
4. Extract from Office of the Inspector General, Department of Health and Human Services, *Compliance Program Guidance for Pharmaceutical Manufacturers*, April 2003, pp. 40–42. Also published at 68 *Federal Register* 23731 (May 5, 2003). As this goes to print, this is the most recent issuance of compliance guidance from the OIG, and each issuance has shown the evolution of the government's concept of the compliance officer's role.
5. Balanced Budget Act of 1997, Section 4321 "Non-discrimination in post-hospital referral to home health agencies and other entities." Although the section title suggested these provisions would go beyond HHAs, the text of the act only referred to HHAs.
6. 62 *Federal Register* at 66743, emphasis added.
7. 67 Federal Register 70373 at 70375 (November 22, 2002).

APPENDIX 50A

DEPARTMENT OF HEALTH & HUMAN SERVICES   Office of Inspector General

Washington, D.C. 20201

[We redact certain identifying information and certain potentially privileged, confidential, or proprietary information associated with the individual or entity, unless otherwise approved by the requestor.]

Issued: **February 3, 2003**

Posted: **February 12, 2003**

[name and address redacted]

Re: OIG Advisory Opinion No. 03-4

Dear [name redacted]:

We are writing in response to your request for an advisory opinion concerning a proposed program to provide free medical-alert pagers and pager monitoring service to homebound patients during the period that they are receiving your company's home health services (the "Benefit"). Specifically, you have inquired whether the Benefit would constitute grounds for the imposition of sanctions under the civil monetary penalty ("CMP") provision for violations of the prohibition against inducements to beneficiaries under section 1128A(a)(5) of the Social Security Act (the "Act"), as well as under the CMP and exclusion authorities at sections 1128A(a)(7) and 1128(b)(7) of the Act, respectively, as these sections relate to the commission of acts described in the anti-kickback statute, section 1128B(b) of the Act.

You have certified that all of the information provided in your request letter, including all supplementary information, is true and correct and constitutes a complete description of the material facts regarding the Benefit.

In issuing this opinion, we have relied solely on the facts and information presented to us. We have not undertaken any independent investigation of such information. This opinion is limited to the facts presented. If material facts have not been disclosed or have been misrepresented, this opinion is without force and effect.

Based on the facts certified in your request for an advisory opinion and supplemental submissions, we conclude that the Benefit would not constitute grounds for the imposition of civil monetary penalties under section 1128A(a)(5) of the Act, and, while the Benefit could potentially generate prohibited remuneration under the anti-kickback statute (if the requisite intent to induce or reward referrals of federal health care program business were present), the Office of Inspector General ("OIG") would not impose administrative sanctions on [Company S] in connection with the Benefit under sections 1128(b)(7) or 1128A(a)(7) of the Act (as those sections relate to the commission of acts described in section 1128B(b) of the Act).

This opinion is limited to the Benefit and, therefore, we express no opinion about any ancillary agreements or arrangements disclosed or referenced in your request letter or supplemental submissions.

This opinion may not be relied on by any persons other than [Company S], the requestor of this opinion, and is further qualified as set out in Part IV below and in 42 C.F.R. Part 1008.

I.   FACTUAL BACKGROUND

[Company S] (the "Requestor") is a for-profit provider of home health care services. Its patients are covered by private insurers and federal health care programs, including Medicaid and Medicare. The Requestor proposes to provide the Benefit to homebound patients during the period that they are receiving its home health services. The provision of free medical-alert pagers and pager monitoring service to the Requestor's homebound patients will facilitate a rapid response to those who have fallen, are injured, or otherwise need emergency assistance, thereby forestalling the need for more expensive care and services. The Requestor estimates that the retail value of the Benefit would be between $20 to $30 monthly and $240 and $360 per year. The Requestor initially plans to provide the Benefit through a third-party service, but eventually will provide the service itself.

II.   LEGAL ANALYSIS

The provision of free services to patients covered by Medicare and Medicaid implicates section 1128A(a)(5) of the Act, enacted as part of the Health Insurance Portability and Accountability Act of 1996. Section 1128A(a)(5) of the Act prohibits a person from offering or transferring remuneration to a beneficiary that such person knows or should know is likely to influence the beneficiary to order from a particular provider, practitioner, or supplier items or services for which payment may be made by Medicare o Medicaid. Violations are punishable by CMPs.

For purposes of section 1128A(a)(5), "remuneration" includes transfers of items or services for free or for other than fair market value. <u>See</u> section 1128A(i)(6) of the Act. For purposes of enforcement, the OIG has set a threshold of $10 per item and $50 in the aggregate, per patient, per year. Items or services valued in excess of this threshold implicate the statute. No statutory exception applies to the Benefit.

Standing alone, the Benefit would implicate section 1128A(a)(5) of the Act. Notwithstanding, in this instance, the Centers for Medicare and Medicaid Services (CMS) – construing congressional intent in 42 U.S.C. 1395fff(e)(1) – has provided that, as part of the benefits for which payment may be made by Medicare, a home health agency "may adopt telehealth technologies that it believes promote efficiencies or improve quality of care," HIM 201.13, although the use of such technologies may not substitute for services ordered by a physician. By ensuring prompt emergency assistance and potentially forestalling the need for more expensive care and services, the provision of the Benefit is reasonably related to the delivery of home health services and to the fostering of efficiency and quality of care. Given CMS' express encouragement of innovative telehealth technologies in the delivery of home health care, we conclude that the provision of the Benefit by the Requestor in the context of home health services would not be an impermissible inducement under section 1128A(a)(5) of the Act.

III.   CONCLUSION

Based on the facts certified in your request for an advisory opinion and supplemental submissions, we conclude that the Benefit would not constitute grounds for the imposition of civil monetary penalties under section 1128A(a)(5) of the Act, and, while the Benefit could potentially generate prohibited remuneration under the anti-kickback statute (if the requisite intent to induce or reward referrals of federal health care program business were present), the OIG would not impose administrative sanctions on [Company S] in connection with the Benefit under sections 1128(b)(7) or 1128A(a)(7) of the Act (as those sections relate to the commission of acts described in section 1128B(b) of the Act).

IV.   LIMITATIONS

The limitations applicable to this opinion include the following:

- This advisory opinion is issued only to [Company S], the requestor of this opinion. This advisory opinion has no application, and cannot be relied upon, by any other individual or entity.

- This advisory opinion may not be introduced into evidence in any matter involving an entity or individual that is not a requestor to this opinion.

- This advisory opinion is applicable only to the statutory provisions specifically noted above. No opinion is expressed or implied herein with respect to the application of any other federal, state, or local statute, rule, regulation, ordinance, or other law that may be applicable to the Benefit, including, without limitation, the physician self-referral law, section 1877 of the Act.

- This advisory opinion will not bind or obligate any agency other than the U.S. Department of Health and Human Services.

- This advisory opinion is limited in scope to the specific arrangement described in this letter and has no applicability to other arrangements, even those which appear similar in nature or scope.

- No opinion is expressed herein regarding the liability of any party under the False Claims Act or other legal authorities for any improper billing, claims submission, cost reporting, or related conduct.

This opinion is also subject to any additional limitations set forth at 42 C.F.R. Part 1008.

The OIG will not proceed against [Company S] with respect to any action that is part of the Benefit taken in good faith reliance upon this advisory opinion as long as all of the material facts have been fully, completely, and accurately presented, and the Benefit in practice comports with the information provided. The OIG reserves the right to reconsider the questions and issues raised in this advisory opinion and, where the public interest requires, rescind, modify, or terminate this opinion. In the event that this advisory opinion is modified or terminated, the OIG will not proceed against [Company S] with respect to any action taken in good faith reliance upon this advisory opinion, where all of the relevant facts were fully, completely, and accurately presented and where such action was promptly discontinued upon notification of the modification or termination of this advisory opinion. An advisory opinion may be rescinded only if the relevant and material facts have not been fully, completely, and accurately disclosed to the OIG.

Sincerely,

/s/

Lewis Morris
Chief Counsel to the Inspector General

Appendix 50B

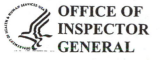

**OFFICE OF
INSPECTOR
GENERAL**

SPECIAL ADVISORY BULLETIN

OFFERING GIFTS AND OTHER INDUCEMENTS
TO BENEFICIARIES

August 2002

Introduction

Under section 1128A(a)(5) of the Social Security Act (the Act), enacted as part of Health Insurance Portability and Accountability Act of 1996 (HIPAA), a person who offers or transfers to a Medicare or Medicaid beneficiary any remuneration that the person knows or should know is likely to influence the beneficiary's selection of a particular provider, practitioner, or supplier of Medicare or Medicaid payable items or services may be liable for civil money penalties (CMPs) of up to $10,000 for each wrongful act. For purposes of section 1128A(a)(5) of the Act, the statute defines "remuneration" to include, without limitation, waivers of copayments and deductible amounts (or any part thereof) and transfers of items or services for free or for other than fair market value. (See section 1128A(i)(6) of the Act.) The statute and implementing regulations contain a limited number of exceptions. (See section 1128A(i)(6) of the Act; 42 CFR 1003.101.)

Offering valuable gifts to beneficiaries to influence their choice of a Medicare or Medicaid provider[1] raises cost and quality concerns. Providers may have an economic incentive to offset the additional costs attributable to the giveaway by providing unnecessary services or by substituting cheaper or lower quality services. The use of giveaways to attract business also favors large providers with greater financial resources for such activities, disadvantaging smaller providers and businesses.

The Office of Inspector General (OIG) is responsible for enforcing section 1128A(a)(5) through administrative remedies. Given the broad language of the prohibition and the number of marketing practices potentially affected, this Bulletin is intended to alert the health care industry as to the scope of acceptable practices. To that end, this Bulletin

---

[1] For convenience, in this Special Advisory Bulletin, the term "provider" includes practitioners and suppliers, as defined in 42 CFR 400.202.

such an arrangement is the American Kidney Fund's program to assist needy patients with end stage renal disease with funds donated by dialysis providers, including paying for their supplemental medical insurance premiums. (See, e.g., OIG Advisory Opinion No. 97-1 and No. 02-1.)

Elements of the Prohibition

Remuneration. Section 1128A(a)(5) of the Act prohibits the offering or transfer of "remuneration". The term "remuneration" has a well-established meaning in the context of various health care fraud and abuse statutes. Generally, it has been interpreted broadly to include "anything of value." The definition of "remuneration" for purposes of section 1128A(a)(5) – which includes waivers of coinsurance and deductible amounts, and transfers of items or services for free or for other than fair market value – affirms this broad reading. (See section 1128A(i)(6).) The use of the term "remuneration" implicitly recognizes that virtually any good or service has a monetary value.[3]

The definition of "remuneration" in section 1128A(i)(6) contains five specific exceptions:

- Non-routine, unadvertised waivers of copayments or deductible amounts based on individualized determinations of financial need or exhaustion of reasonable collection efforts. Paying the premiums for a beneficiary's Medicare Part B or supplemental insurance is not protected by this exception.

- Properly disclosed differentials in a health insurance plan's copayments or deductibles. This exception covers incentives that are part of a health plan design, such as lower plan copayments for using preferred providers, mail order pharmacies, or generic drugs. Waivers of Medicare or Medicaid copayments are not protected by this exception.

- Incentives to promote the delivery of preventive care. Preventive care is defined in 42 CFR 1003.101 to mean items and services that (i) are covered by Medicare or Medicaid and (ii) are either pre-natal or post-natal well-baby services or are services described in the Guide to Clinical Preventive Services published by the U.S. Preventive Services Task Force (available online at http://odphp.osphs.dhhs.gov/pubs/guidecps). Such incentives may not be in the form of cash or cash equivalents and may not be disproportionate to the value of the preventive care provided. (See 42 CFR 1003.101; 65 FR 24400 and 24409.)

---

[3] Some services, such as companionship provided by volunteers, have psychological, rather than monetary value. (See, e.g., OIG Advisory Opinion No. 00-3.)

3

hardships that chronic medical conditions can cause for beneficiaries, there is no meaningful basis under the statute for exempting valuable gifts based on a beneficiary's medical condition or the condition's severity. Moreover, providers have a greater incentive to offer gifts to chronically ill beneficiaries who are likely to generate substantially more business than other beneficiaries.

Similarly, there is no meaningful statutory basis for a broad exemption based on the financial need of a category of patients. The statute specifically applies the prohibition to the Medicaid program – a program that is available only to financially needy persons. The inclusion of Medicaid within the prohibition demonstrates Congress' conclusion that categorical financial need is not a sufficient basis for permitting valuable gifts. This conclusion is supported by the statute's specific exception for non-routine waivers of copayments and deductibles based on individual financial need. If Congress intended a broad exception for financially needy persons, it is unlikely that it would have expressly included the Medicaid program within the prohibition and then created such a narrow exception.

Provider, Practitioner, or Supplier. Section 1128A(a)(5) of the Act applies to incentives to select particular providers, practitioners, or suppliers. As noted in the regulations, the OIG has interpreted this element to exclude health plans that offer incentives to Medicare and Medicaid beneficiaries to enroll in a plan. (See 65 FR 24400 and 24407.) However, incentives provided to influence an already enrolled beneficiary to select a particular provider, practitioner, or supplier within the plan are subject to the statutory proscription (other than copayment differentials that are part of a health plan design). Id. In addition, the OIG does not believe that drug manufacturers are "providers, practitioners, or suppliers" for the limited purposes of section 1128A(a)(5), unless the drug manufacturers also own or operate, directly or indirectly, pharmacies, pharmacy benefits management companies, or other entities that file claims for payment under the Medicare or Medicaid programs.

Additional Regulatory Considerations

Congress has authorized the OIG to create regulatory exceptions to section 1128A(a)(5) of the Act and to issue advisory opinions to protect acceptable arrangements. (See sections 1128A(i)(6)(B) and 1128D(b)(2)(A) of the Act.) While the OIG has considered numerous arrangements involving the provision of various free goods and services to beneficiaries, for the following reasons the OIG has concluded that any additional exceptions will likely be few in number and narrow in scope:

- Any exception will create the activity that the statute prohibits – namely, competing for business by giving remuneration to Medicare and Medicaid beneficiaries. Moreover, competition will not only result in providers matching a competitor's offer, but inevitably will trigger ever more valuable

5

Finally, the OIG reiterates that nothing in section 1128A(a)(5) prevents an independent entity, such as a patient advocacy group, from providing free or other valuable services or remuneration to financially needy beneficiaries, even if the benefits are funded by providers, so long as the independent entity makes an independent determination of need and the beneficiary's receipt of the remuneration does not depend, directly or indirectly, on the beneficiary's use of any particular provider. The OIG has approved several such arrangements through the advisory opinion process, including the American Kidney Fund's program to assist needy patients with end stage renal disease with funds donated by dialysis providers. (See, e.g., OIG Advisory Opinion No. 97-1 and No. 02-1.)

Conclusion

Congress has broadly prohibited offering remuneration to Medicare and Medicaid beneficiaries, subject to limited, well-defined exceptions. To the extent that providers have programs in place that do not meet any exception, the OIG, in exercising its enforcement discretion, will take into consideration whether the providers terminate prohibited programs expeditiously following publication of this Bulletin.

The Office of Inspector General (OIG) was established at the Department of Health and Human Services by Congress in 1976 to identify and eliminate fraud, abuse, and waste in the Department's programs and to promote efficiency and economy in departmental operations. The OIG carries out this mission through a nationwide program of audits, investigations, and inspections.

The Fraud and Abuse Control Program, established by the Health Insurance Portability and Accountability Act of 1996 (HIPAA), authorized the OIG to provide guidance to the health care industry to prevent fraud and abuse and to promote the highest level of ethical and lawful conduct. To further these goals, the OIG issues Special Advisory Bulletins about industry practices or arrangements that potentially implicate the fraud and abuse authorities subject to enforcement by the OIG.

7

APPENDIX 50C

ATTACHMENT 1.—LIST OF SUDs KNOWN TO BE REPROCESSED OR CONSIDERED FOR REPROCESSING—Continued

	Medical specialty	Device type	Regulation No.	Class	Product code	Risk [1,2,3,3*]	Critical/semi-critical/non-critical	Premarket exempt
227 ..	Surgery	Scissor Tips	878.4800, 884.4520, 874.4420	I	LRW, HDK, HDJ, JZB, KBD	2	C	Y
228 ..	Surgery	Laser Fiber Delivery Systems	878.4810 874.4500 886.4390 884.4550 886.4690	II	GEX EWG LLW HQF HHR HQB	1	C	N

1 = low risk according to RPS
2 = moderate risk according to RPS
3 = high risk according to RPS
3* = high risk due to neurological use

Dated: April 23, 2003.

Jeffrey Shuren,

Assistant Commissioner for Policy.

[FR Doc. 03–10413 Filed 4–23–03; 5:03 pm]

BILLING CODE 4160–01–P

DEPARTMENT OF HEALTH AND HUMAN SERVICES

Office of Inspector General

Publication of OIG Special Advisory Bulletin on Contractual Joint Ventures

AGENCY: Office of Inspector General (OIG), HHS.

ACTION: Notice.

SUMMARY: The OIG periodically develops and issues guidance, including Special Advisory Bulletins, to alert and inform the health care industry about potential problems or areas of special interest. This **Federal Register** notice sets forth the recently issued OIG Special Advisory Bulletin addressing certain contractual joint venture arrangements.

FOR FURTHER INFORMATION CONTACT: Vicki Robinson or Joel Schaer, Office of Counsel to the Inspector General, (202) 619–0335.

SUPPLEMENTARY INFORMATION:

Special Advisory Bulletin: Contractual Joint Ventures (April 2003)

Introduction

This Special Advisory Bulletin addresses certain complex contractual arrangements for the provision of items and services previously identified as suspect in our 1989 Special Fraud Alert on Joint Venture Arrangements.[1] While

[1] The 1989 Special Fraud Alert was reprinted in the **Federal Register** in 1994. *See* 59 FR 65372 (December 19, 1994). The Special Fraud Alert is

much of the discussion in the 1989 Special Fraud Alert focused on investor referrals to newly formed entities, we observed that:

[t]he Office of Inspector General has become aware of a proliferation of arrangements between those in a position to refer business, such as physicians, and those providing items or services for which Medicare or Medicaid pays. Some examples of the items or services provided in these arrangements include clinical diagnostic laboratory services, durable medical equipment (DME), and other diagnostic services. Sometimes these deals are called "joint ventures." *A joint venture may take a variety of forms: it may be a contractual arrangement between two or more parties to cooperate in providing services, or it may involve the creation of a new legal entity by the parties, such as a limited partnership or closely held corporation, to provide such services.* (Emphasis added.)

Notwithstanding that caution, the Office of Inspector General (OIG) is concerned that contractual joint venture arrangements are proliferating.[2]

A. Questionable Contractual Arrangements

The federal anti-kickback statute, section 1128B(b) of the Social Security Act (the Act), prohibits knowingly and willfully soliciting, receiving, offering, or paying anything of value to induce referrals of items or services payable by a federal health care program. Kickbacks

also available on our Web page at *http://oig.hhs.gov/fraud/docs/alertsandbulletins/121994.html.*

[2] The kinds of contractual arrangements addressed in this Special Advisory Bulletin are sometimes referred to as "joint ventures" or "contractual joint ventures" or may be referenced by other terminology. For purposes of the analysis set forth in this Bulletin, a "joint venture" is any common enterprise with mutual economic benefit. The application of this Bulletin is not limited to "joint ventures" that meet technical qualifications under applicable state or common law.

are harmful because they can (1) distort medical decision-making, (2) cause overutilization, (3) increase costs to the federal health care programs, and (4) result in unfair competition by freezing out competitors unwilling to pay kickbacks. Both parties to an impermissible kickback transaction may be liable. Violation of the statute constitutes a felony punishable by a maximum fine of $25,000, imprisonment up to 5 years, or both. The OIG may also initiate administrative proceedings to exclude persons from the federal health care programs or to impose civil money penalties for kickback violations under sections 1128(b)(7) and 1128A(a)(7) of the Act.

This Special Advisory Bulletin focuses on questionable contractual arrangements where a health care provider in one line of business (hereafter referred to as the "Owner") expands into a related health care business by contracting with an existing provider of a related item or service (hereafter referred to as the "Manager/Supplier") to provide the new item or service to the Owner's existing patient population, including federal health care program patients. The Manager/Supplier not only manages the new line of business, but may also supply it with inventory, employees, space, billing, and other services. In other words, the Owner contracts out substantially the entire operation of the related line of business to the Manager/Supplier—otherwise a potential competitor—receiving in return the profits of the business as remuneration for its federal program referrals.

Some examples of potentially problematic contractual arrangements include the following:

• A hospital establishes a subsidiary to provide DME. The new subsidiary enters into a contract with an existing DME company to operate the new subsidiary and to provide the new subsidiary with DME inventory. The existing DME company already provides DME services comparable to those provided by the new hospital DME subsidiary and bills insurers and patients for them.

• A DME company sells nebulizers to federal health care beneficiaries. A mail order pharmacy suggests that the DME company form its own mail order pharmacy to provide nebulizer drugs. Through a management agreement, the mail order pharmacy runs the DME company's pharmacy, providing personnel, equipment, and space. The existing mail order pharmacy also sells all nebulizer drugs to the DME company's pharmacy for its inventory.

• A group of nephrologists establishes a wholly-owned company to provide home dialysis supplies to their dialysis patients. The new company contracts with an existing supplier of home dialysis supplies to operate the new company and provide all goods and services to the new company.

These problematic arrangements typically exhibit certain common elements. First, the Owner expands into a related line of business, which is dependent on referrals from, or other business generated by, the Owner's existing business.[3] The new business line may be organized as a part of the existing entity or as a separate subsidiary. Typically, the new business primarily serves the Owner's existing patient base.

Second, the Owner neither operates the new business itself nor commits substantial financial, capital, or human resources to the venture. Instead, it contracts out substantially all the operations of the new business. The Manager/Supplier typically agrees to provide not only management services, but also a range of other services, such as the inventory necessary to run the business, office and health care personnel, billing support, and space. While the Manager/Supplier essentially operates the business, the billing of insurers and patients is done in the name of the Owner. In many cases, the contractual arrangements result in either

---

[3] The Owner's referrals may be direct or indirect and may include not only ordering or purchasing goods or services, but also "arranging for" or "recommending" goods and services. *See* section 1128B(b) of the Act. For example, a hospital may generate business for a DME company, notwithstanding that orders for specific DME items must be signed by a physician who may or may not be a hospital employee.

practical or legal exclusivity for the Manager/Supplier through inclusion of non-competition provisions or restrictions on access. While the contract terms of these arrangements may appear to place the Owner at financial risk, the Owner's actual business risk is minimal because of the Owner's ability to influence substantial referrals to the new business.

Third, the Manager/Supplier is an established provider of the same services as the Owner's new line of business. In other words, absent the contractual arrangement, the Manager/Supplier would be a competitor of the new line of business, providing items and services in its own right, billing insurers and patients in its own name, and collecting reimbursement.

Fourth, the Owner and the Manager/Supplier share in the economic benefit of the Owner's new business. The Manager/Supplier takes its share in the form of payments under the various contracts with the Owner; the Owner receives its share in the form of the residual profit from the new business.

Fifth, aggregate payments to the Manager/Supplier typically vary with the value or volume of business generated for the new business by the Owner. While in some arrangements certain payments are fixed (for example, the management fee), other payments, such as payments for goods and services supplied by the Manager/Supplier, will vary based on the number of goods and services provided. In other words, the aggregate payment to the Manager/Supplier from the whole arrangement will vary with referrals from the Owner. Likewise, the Owner's payments, that is, the difference between the net revenues from the new business and its expenses (including payments to the Manager/Supplier), also vary based on the Owner's referrals to the new business. Through these contractual payments, the parties are able to share the profits of the new line of business.

B. Safe Harbor Protection May Be Unavailable

Under the kickback statute, a number of statutory and regulatory "safe harbors" immunize certain arrangements that might otherwise violate the anti-kickback statute. (*See* 42 U.S.C. 1320a-7b(b)(3); 42 CFR 1001.952.) To qualify for safe harbor protection, an arrangement must fit squarely in one of these safe harbor provisions. Some parties attempt to carve otherwise problematic contracting arrangements into several different contracts for discrete items or services (*e.g.*, a management contract, a vendor contract, and a staffing contract), and

then qualify each separate contract for protection under a "safe harbor." Such efforts may be ineffectual and leave the parties subject to prosecution for the following reasons.

First, many of these questionable joint venture arrangements involve contracts pursuant to which the Manager/Suppliers agree to sell items and services to the Owners at a discounted price. However, where a discount is given as part of an overarching business arrangement, it cannot qualify for protection under the discount safe harbor. Simply put, the discount safe harbor does not protect—and has never protected—prices offered by a seller to a buyer in connection with a common enterprise. To be protected under the discount safe harbor, a price reduction must be based on an arms length transaction. (*See* 42 CFR 1001.952(h) under which "the term *discount* means a reduction in the amount a buyer * * * is charged for an item or service based on an arms-length transaction."). As we expressly stated in the preamble to the 1991 safe harbor regulations, the provision of items or services to a joint venture by a participant in the venture is not an "arms length" transaction:

> Another problem exists where an entity, which is both a provider and supplier of items or services and joint venture partner with referring physicians, makes discounts to the joint venture as a way to share its profits with the physician partners. Very often this entity furnishes items or services to the joint venture, and also acts as the joint venture's general partner or provides management services to the joint venture. * * * *These arrangements are not arms length transactions where the joint venture shops around for the best price on a good or service. Rather it has entered into a collusive arrangement with a particular provider or supplier of items or services that seeks to share its profits with referring physician partners. [We did] * * * not intend to protect these types of transactions which are sometimes made to appear as "discounts" * * ** (Emphasis added) (*See* 56 FR 35977; July 29, 1991).

In short, a discount is not based on arms length transaction if it is provided by a seller to a purchaser in connection with a common venture, regardless of whether the venture is memorialized in separate contracts.

Second, even if the various contracts could fit in one or more safe harbors, they would only protect the remuneration flowing from the Owner to the Manager/Supplier for actual services rendered. In the contractual arrangements that are the subject of this Bulletin, however, the illegal remuneration is often the difference between the money paid by the Owner to the Manager/Supplier and the

23150   **Federal Register** / Vol. 68, No. 83 / Wednesday, April 30, 2003 / Notices

reimbursement received from the federal health care programs. By agreeing effectively to provide services it could otherwise provide in its own right for less than the available reimbursement, the Manager/Supplier is providing the Owner with the opportunity to generate a fee and a profit. The opportunity to generate a fee is itself remuneration that may implicate the anti-kickback statute.

C. Indicia of a Suspect Contractual Joint Venture

To help identify the suspect contractual joint ventures that are the focus of this Special Advisory Bulletin, we describe below some characteristics, which, taken separately or together, potentially indicate a prohibited arrangement. This list is illustrative, not exhaustive.

New Line of Business. The Owner typically seeks to expand into a health care service that can be provided to the Owner's existing patients. As illustrated in Part A, examples include, but are not limited to, hospitals expanding into DME services, DME companies expanding into the nebulizer pharmacy business, or nephrologists expanding into the home dialysis supply business.[4]

Captive Referral Base. The newly-created business predominantly or exclusively serves the Owner's existing patient base (or patients under the control or influence of the Owner). The Owner typically does not intend to expand the business to serve new customers (*i.e.*, customers not already served in its main business) and, therefore, makes no or few *bona fide* efforts to do so.

Little or No Bona Fide Business Risk. The Owner's primary contribution to the venture is referrals; it makes little or no financial or other investment in the business, delegating the entire operation to the Manager/Supplier, while retaining profits generated from its captive referral base. Residual business risks, such as nonpayment for services, are relatively ascertainable based on historical activity.

Status of the Manager/Supplier. The Manager/Supplier is a would-be competitor of the Owner's new line of business and would normally compete for the captive referrals. It has the capacity to provide virtually identical services in its own right and bill insurers and patients for them in its own name.

Scope of Services Provided by the Manager/Supplier. The Manager/

Supplier provides all, or many, of the following key services:
• Day-to-day management;
• Billing services;
• Equipment;
• Personnel and related services;
• Office space;
• Training;
• Health care items, supplies, and services.[5]

In general, the greater the scope of services provided by the Manager/Supplier, the greater the likelihood that the arrangement is a contractual joint venture.

Remuneration. The practical effect of the arrangement, viewed in its entirety, is to provide the Owner the opportunity to bill insurers and patients for business otherwise provided by the Manager/Supplier. The remuneration from the venture to the Owner (*i.e.*, the profits of the venture) takes into account the value and volume of business the Owner generates.

Exclusivity. The parties may agree to a non-compete clause, barring the Owner from providing items or services to any patients other than those coming from Owner and/or barring the Manager/Supplier from providing services in its own right to the Owner's patients.

As noted above, these factors are illustrative, not exhaustive. The presence or absence of any one of these factors is not determinative of whether a particular arrangement is suspect. As indicated, this Special Advisory Bulletin is not intended to describe the entire universe of suspect contractual joint ventures. This Bulletin focuses on arrangements where substantially all of the operations of a new line of business are contracted out to a would-be competitor. Arrangements involving the delegation of fewer than substantially all services, or delegation to a party not otherwise in a position to bill for the identical services, may also raise concerns under the anti-kickback statute, depending on the circumstances.

The Office of Inspector General (OIG) was established at the Department of Health and Human Services by Congress in 1976 to identify and eliminate fraud, abuse, and waste in the department's programs and to promote efficiency and economy in departmental operations. The OIG carries out this mission through a nationwide program of audits, investigations, and inspections.

---

[5] The Manager/Supplier may also provide marketing services, although in many instances no such services are required since the Owner generates substantially all of the venture's business from its existing patient base.

The Fraud and Abuse Control Program, established by the Health Insurance Portability and Accountability Act of 1996 (HIPAA), authorized the OIG to provide guidance to the health care industry to prevent fraud and abuse and to promote the highest level of ethical and lawful conduct. To further these goals, the OIG issues Special Advisory Bulletins about industry practices or arrangements that potentially implicate the fraud and abuse authorities subject to enforcement by the OIG.

Dated: March 27, 2003.

Dennis J. Duquette,
Acting Principal Deputy Inspector General.
[FR Doc. 03–10626 Filed 4–29–03; 8:45 am]
BILLING CODE 4150–01–P

DEPARTMENT OF HEALTH AND HUMAN SERVICES

National Institutes of Health

Proposed Collection; Comment Request; National Institute of Diabetes and Digestive and Kidney Diseases Information Clearinghouses Customer Satisfaction Survey

SUMMARY: In compliance with the requirement of Section 3506(c)(2)(A) of the Paperwork Reduction Act of 1995 to provide opportunity for public comment on proposed data collection projects, the National Institute of Diabetes and Digestive and Kidney Diseases (NIDDK), the National Institutes of Health (NIH), will publish periodic summaries of proposed projects to be submitted to the Office of Management (OMB) for review and approval.

Proposed Collection

Title: NIDDK Information Clearinghouses Customer Satisfaction Survey. *Type of Information Request:* EXTENSION. The OMB control number 0925–0480 expires July 31, 2003. *Need and Use of Information Collection:* NIDDK is conducting a survey to evaluate the efficiency and effectiveness of services provided by NIDDK's three information clearinghouses: National Diabetes Information Clearinghouse, National Digestive Diseases Information Clearinghouse, National Kidney and Urologic Diseases Information Clearinghouse. The survey responds to Executive Order 12862, "Setting Customer Service Standards," which requires agencies and departments to identify and survey their "customers to determine the kind and quality of service they want and their level of satisfaction with existing service." *Frequency of Response:* On occasion.

---

[4] These examples are illustrative only. This list is not intended to suggest that other analogous ventures are not equally suspect.

CHAPTER 51

The HIPAA Standards for Privacy
of Individually Identifiable
Health Information

Larri A. Short.

In 1996, Congress enacted the Health Insurance Portability and Accountability Act (HIPAA).[1] This law was designed to ensure that individuals would be free to change jobs without losing their access to group health insurance coverage because they (or a family member) have a serious medical condition. In addition, the law created a self-regenerating revenue pool to fund the war against fraud in federally funded health care programs and a tough new set of offenses tailored to the needs of prosecutors intent upon rooting out fraud and abuse in both commercial and federal health care programs.

Although the title of the legislation does not reflect this initiative, HIPAA also included provisions, under the heading of Administrative Simplification, that were intended to "improve the efficiency and effectiveness of the heath care system, by encouraging the development of a health information system through the establishment of standards and requirements for the electronic submission of certain health information."[2] These provisions were structured to foster computerization of the common administrative and financial transactions that underlie the relationships between health care providers and suppliers and their payers and those between employers and the health plans that cover their employees.

To this end, the HIPAA Administrative Simplification provisions mandate the development of national identifiers for employers,[3] health plans,[4] providers,[5] and individuals[6] and the adoption of standard transactions and code sets for:

- Health claims or equivalent encounter information
- Coordination of benefits
- Health care payment and remittance advices
- Health claim status assessments
- Health plan eligibility determinations
- Referral certifications and authorizations
- Health claims attachments
- Enrollment and disenrollment in a health plan
- Health plan premium payments
- First reports of injury[7]

Just as importantly, the Administrative Simplification provisions require health plans to accept any transactions submitted to them electronically so long as the electronic submission is in the standard format and uses the standard code sets and identifiers. Although HIPAA allows providers and employers to decide for themselves whether to use electronic transactions, it mandates that any providers or employers who choose to do so must use the standard formats, code sets, and identifiers. Subsequent legislation has, however, changed this construct somewhat for many providers and suppliers that bill Medicare.

The standard transactions promulgated by the Department of Health and Human Services (DHHS) in August 2000 as the first step in the implementation of Administrative Simplification originally were slated to become effective on October 16, 2002. Because it appeared that significant numbers of providers and health plans, including many state Medicaid programs, would not be able to meet this statutorily mandated deadline, Congress enacted the Administrative Simplification Compliance Act (ASCA)[8] at the end of 2001.

ASCA permitted all entities subject to the Administrative Simplification provisions of HIPAA to apply for a 1-year extension to the original October 2002 deadline for implementing standard transactions. Significantly, ASCA also made billing Medicare electronically a condition of payment as of October 16, 2003, for all providers (e.g., hospitals, home health agencies, hospices, and skilled nursing facilities) with 25 or more full-time equivalent employees and for all physicians and suppliers (e.g., home medical equipment suppliers and infusion therapy companies) with 10 or more full-time equivalent employees.

In addition to providing authority for regulations establishing standards and code set requirements for electronic transactions, HIPAA's Administrative Simplification subtitle also instructs DHHS to develop security standards designed to ensure the confidentiality, integrity, and accessibility of computerized data used to support the operation of the health care system. DHHS published the security regulations in final form on February 20, 2003.[9] They become effective April 21, 2005.

The security regulations establish scalable, technology-neutral requirements. They will obligate all health care providers and health plans subject to the HIPAA Administrative Simplification provisions to implement reasonable and appropriate administrative, physical, and technical safeguards to ensure the integrity and confidentiality of electronic health information at rest and in transit, to minimize the risk of unauthorized data use, and to protect against reasonably anticipated threats or hazards to data security. In addition, the security rules mandate that providers analyze their systems for security risks and develop and document policies to address specific vulnerabilities prior to the rule's compliance date. Providers then will have to keep their security policies current with technological developments.

Congress, in an unusual move, incorporated another provision in the HIPAA Administrative Simplification subtitle, directing itself to enact legislation to protect the privacy of individually identifiable health information by August 1999.[10] Congress also instructed DHHS to promulgate privacy regulations if it failed to enact a health information privacy law within the specified time frame.

As had been the case in the past when Congress had considered federal medical records privacy legislation, neither the House nor the Senate was able to reach a consensus on the best approach to the issue by the 1999 deadline. As a result, DHHS issued privacy regulations applicable to the same entities subject to the transactions and security regulations implementing other provisions of the HIPAA Administrative Simplification subtitle. The Standards for Privacy of Individually Identifiable Health Information were published as a final rule at the close of the Clinton administration on December 28, 2000,[11] and amended by the George W. Bush administration to correct operational problems and to address certain philosophical concerns on August 14, 2002.[12] Because of ASCA, the privacy standards were the first of the HIPAA Administrative Simplification regulations to take general effect. Compliance was first required on April 14, 2003, for all organizations subject to the rule except small health plans.[13] Such plans had until April 14, 2004, to come into compliance.

The privacy rule is by far the most controversial of the suite of interlocking regulations that have been developed to implement the HIPAA Administrative Simplification provisions. The controversy stems in part from the fact that the privacy standards may be fairly characterized as both overinclusive and underinclusive.

The privacy standards are overinclusive because they govern how health information in any format—electronic, paper, or oral—must be handled, notwithstanding that the regulations are authorized by a statute that is intended to foster *electronic* data interchange.

The privacy standards are underinclusive because they are limited in scope. Although it is true that the HIPAA privacy rule is the first federal law addressing medical records privacy, the rule only establishes a federal floor of privacy protections. More stringent state laws will continue to control. Furthermore, the privacy standards do not reach all individuals and entities that routinely hold or have access to individually identifiable health information in today's society. Rather, the standards only regulate various components of the health care delivery system. Once health information has been shared with organizations outside that sphere, such as employers, life insurance companies, or drug and device manufacturers, the protections afforded under HIPAA no longer apply.

The privacy standards are also controversial because they, like the health care delivery system they are intended to regulate, are complicated. As a result, implementing the rules will likely be expensive. Moreover, the complex requirements seem antithetical to a goal of *simplification*. Finally, the privacy standards are controversial because they require cultural changes in the delivery of health care. Health care professionals have always operated under professional standards of conduct that strictly prohibit the sharing of patient data with those outside the health care delivery system without patient consent. Not surprisingly, these professionals question the need to regulate their handling of health information *inside* the health care system. However, the HIPAA privacy rule does just that and, in so doing, will force everyone involved in the delivery of care to rethink how they behave on a daily basis.

To assist in grappling with the demands of the HIPAA privacy standards, this chapter explains the requirements of those regulations as they apply to a typical home health agency or hospice. Less attention is given to issues, such as the rule's implications for research, that do not

concern the majority of home care and hospice providers. The discussion focuses first on the interplay between the HIPAA privacy rules and state laws that have heretofore been the sole rules governing the privacy of medical records. The HIPAA requirements specifying how health care providers should handle individually identifiable patient health information are addressed next. The discussion then turns to the individual privacy rights created by HIPAA and the implications of those rights for agency operations. A review of the regulation's requirements for a privacy compliance program as well as a discussion of the implications of HIPAA for providers that offer health insurance as a fringe benefit follows. The chapter closes with a discussion of DHHS's planned approach for enforcement.

INTERPLAY BETWEEN FEDERAL AND STATE HEALTH INFORMATION PRIVACY LAWS

Even though, as a general rule, HIPAA Administrative Simplification provisions preempt contrary provisions of state law,[14] agencies must recognize that implementation of the federal privacy standards will not result in a completely uniform approach to health information privacy across the United States. As a result, organizations operating home health agencies or hospices in multiple states will have to continue to administer programs subject to different requirements in different jurisdictions.

By their terms, the HIPAA privacy standards do not preempt any provision of state law that "provides for the reporting of disease or injury, child abuse, birth, or death, or for the conduct of public health surveillance, investigation, or intervention,"[15] nor do the standards preempt any provision of state law that "requires a health plan to report, or to provide access to, information for the purpose of management audits, financial audits, program monitoring and evaluation, or the licensure or certification of facilities or individuals."[16]

The federal privacy standards also allow state governments—but not private individuals or organizations—to seek determinations from DHHS that HIPAA does not preempt provisions of state law that are necessary:

- To prevent fraud and abuse in the provision of or payment for health care
- To permit appropriate regulation of insurance and health plans
- To accommodate state data collection initiatives addressing health care delivery or costs
- To serve a compelling need related to public health, safety, or welfare that outweighs any required intrusion into individual privacy[17]

Accordingly, even home health agencies and hospices that operate in only one state will find that they must grapple with the problem of incomplete federal preemption. The HIPAA privacy standards, by their own terms, do not preempt any contrary provision of state law that "relates to the privacy of individually identifiable health information and is more stringent than a standard, requirement, or implementation specification" under HIPAA.[18] Although the federal regulations define both "relates to the privacy of individually identifiable health information"[19] and "more stringent,"[20] HIPAA does not assign the task of deciding whether federal or state law controls to DHHS or to state authorities. Rather, it leaves the task to the organizations that are subject to the rules.

Because they fall outside the ambit of privacy laws, state laws that relate to mental competency and to qualifications as a personal representative (including those that define the rights of unemancipated minor children) will continue to control when agencies face decisions that turn on such requirements.

This chapter will, of necessity, only discuss the privacy requirements under the federal privacy standards. Agencies must overlay state law privacy requirements that continue to have effect under HIPAA's preemption provisions. This overlay will come into play most prominently when agencies consider issues such as their continued use of written consents to handle health information for purposes of treatment, payment, or health care operations; their procedures for dealing with disclosures of information for public policy purposes; and their policies for using and releasing health information that relates to stigmatizing conditions, such as AIDS/HIV or other sexually transmitted diseases, mental health problems, alcohol and substance abuse, or health information that relates to genetic make-up. Agencies must reflect controlling state laws in the notice of privacy practices mandated by HIPAA as well as in their policies and procedures for day-to-day operations.

Agencies looking for resources to assist them with their own analysis of preemption issues can find summaries of state privacy laws prepared by the Health Privacy Project at Georgetown University at www.healthprivacy.org. Those summaries also include Web addresses for statutes and regulations posted by state governments.

Home health agencies and hospices looking for detailed privacy preemption analyses prepared by others should contact their state associations or the state hospital association and/or bar association. In many jurisdictions, these organizations have developed crosswalks of the HIPAA privacy standards to state privacy laws that include conclusions about which provisions of state law continue to control. Agencies will often find that analyses prepared by state professional associations are available free of charge or at nominal costs. In a few states, the department of health or the attorney general's office has prepared an official state analysis documenting which state laws and regulations will continue to be enforced against organizations subject to the HIPAA privacy standards. Where these types of analyses have been prepared, they should be available for download on state Web sites. Agencies must look for state-prepared analyses after the April 14, 2003, compliance date under federal law, because many jurisdictions will develop and revise their analyses as they develop more experience with HIPAA.

AGENCY HANDLING OF INDIVIDUALLY IDENTIFIABLE PATIENT HEALTH INFORMATION

The HIPAA privacy standards for handling identifiable health information may be summarized in a single sentence: *Covered entities may not use or disclose protected health information except as required or permitted by the regulation.* This simple statement provides a structure for an organized discussion of the privacy rule's information handling requirements. Perhaps more importantly, it illustrates that to understand the HIPAA privacy standards, it is essential first to pay close attention to the rule's definitions. There are several key defined terms in this basic statement of the privacy rule's information handling requirements.

Key Definitions

Covered Entities

By statute, all of the regulations promulgated to implement Administrative Simplification, including the privacy standards, apply only to "covered entities." There are three categories of covered entities:

1. Health care clearinghouses
2. Health plans
3. Health care providers that transmit individually identifiable health information electronically in connection with a HIPAA standard transaction

Health Care Clearinghouses. Health care clearinghouses are defined in the HIPAA regulations[21] as organizations that translate health care transactions containing nonstandard data elements or structured in nonstandard formats into HIPAA standard electronic transactions. Clearinghouses can also provide translation services that run the other way, converting HIPAA standard transactions into alternative formats that are more compatible with an organization's needs. Billing services are the most common type of clearinghouse familiar to home health agencies and hospices.

Home health providers and hospices with 25 or more full-time equivalent employees and smaller agencies that wanted to take advantage of the quicker turnaround on electronic claims began billing Medicare electronically using the HIPAA standard transactions and code sets on October 16, 2003. Other payers that invested heavily in HIPAA upgrades to their computer systems, such as state Medicaid programs and commercial insurers that have heretofore required community-based providers to submit paper claims, also began insisting upon electronic billing using the HIPAA standard transactions. Agencies that are not ready to submit standard transactions electronically will need to turn to clearinghouses to achieve compliance. They should expect to have to pay a clearinghouse on a per-transaction basis.

In planning for compliance, agencies need to recognize that there is more to submitting HIPAA standard transactions electronically than having HIPAA-compliant billing software or retaining a HIPAA-compliant clearinghouse. The standard transaction that will replace the electronic UB-92—the X 12N 837 institutional claim—can require data elements not currently used for home health and hospice billing. To be adequately prepared for the conversion to HIPAA electronic standard transactions, agencies must ensure that they routinely collect all of the required information and organize the information collected in ways that are compatible with efficient operations. Crosswalks are available online to help agencies plan any necessary form and process revisions.[22]

Clearinghouses cannot resolve *missing* data issues. Prudent agencies revised their forms and processes well in advance of the October 16, 2003, deadline to avoid potential problems with missing data if pre-October 16, 2003, claims must be resubmitted after the HIPAA standard transactions compliance date. The Centers for Medicare and Medicaid Services (CMS) has indicated some willingness to consider the use of some gap fillers but has stated that providers will still be expected to make a "reasonable effort" to obtain missing data elements before filing re-bills. Providers should watch intermediary bulletins for instructions. Although many Medic-aid programs and commercial carriers may follow Medicare's lead, it remains to be seen how accommodating they will be with respect to missing data on post-October 16 re-bills.

Health Plans.   Health plans include individual insurance policies and group health policies that provide or pay for medical care.[23] Medical care is, in turn, defined to mean diagnosis, care, mitigation, treatment, or prevention of disease or injury affecting any structure, or function of the body as well as transportation for and essential to medical care.[24]

Health plans subject to HIPAA Administrative Simplification[25] include Medicare, Medicare + Choice, Medicaid, SCHIP, CHAMPUS/Tricare, federal employee health benefit plans, commercial health insurance plans, health maintenance organizations, multi-employer welfare benefit plans, long-term care policies (excluding nursing home fixed-indemnity policies), and most health plans provided under the auspices of the Employee Retirement Income Security Act (ERISA), regardless of whether the ERISA plan is fully insured or self-insured. The only ERISA plans that escape the reach of HIPAA are those that have fewer than 50 participants *and* that are administered entirely by the sponsoring employer without assistance from a third-party administrator.

Some insurance policies that provide coverage for health care services are expressly excluded from the reach of the HIPAA Administrative Simplification regulations. They include insurance plans that have traditionally been regulated by state insurance commissions as property and casualty policies, such as workers' compensation plans, accident and disability income protection plans, automobile liability insurance, and credit insurance.

The definition of a health plan under the HIPAA regulations is important to home health agencies and hospices. All health plans subject to the HIPAA rules are obligated to accept and process all HIPAA standard electronic transactions submitted to them by any health care provider or supplier after October 16, 2003. No plan will be able to require community-based providers to use paper claims. Moreover, because of the standardization of electronic data interchange processes that is at the heart of HIPAA, agencies will be able to bill all of their payers electronically using essentially the same processes.[26] This fact should eventually permit many home health agencies and hospices to reduce the number of employers tasked with processing non-Medicare claims. Once all the start-up problems have been resolved by both the agency and the plans, it also should significantly improve cash flow from those plans that required paper billing.

The definition of a health plan is also important because many home health agencies and hospices that offer health insurance coverage as an employee benefit will find that they have obligations under HIPAA Administrative Simplification related to their operation of a health plan as well as their status as regulated health care providers.

Certain Health Care Providers.   The HIPAA privacy standards do not apply to all health care providers. Instead, they reach only those providers that bill their payers electronically or engage with their payers in other electronic data interchanges (e.g., eligibility checks, referral certifications, and authorizations) that were converted to HIPAA standard transactions in October 2003.[27]

Home health agencies and hospices that are small enough to avoid the requirement to bill Medicare electronically (i.e., fewer than 25 full-time equivalent employees) do not have to comply with the privacy rule unless they voluntarily decide to bill Medicare electronically or are required to bill another payer electronically to receive payment. Private duty agencies that always bill their patients instead of their patients' payers will not be subject to the rule either. Because faxes, e-mail, and electronic funds transfers do not constitute HIPAA standard electronic transactions, using these tools will not transform a provider that otherwise does not engage in electronic data interchange into a covered health care provider subject to the HIPAA privacy standards.

It can also be important to consider the type of services that an organization provides before deciding whether the operation qualifies as a covered health care provider subject to the privacy standards. Any provider, physician, practitioner, or supplier, as those terms are defined for Medicare purposes, is a health care provider under HIPAA. So too is "any person or organization who furnishes, bills, or is paid for health care in the normal course of business."[28] Although the definition of health care is expansive,[29] it does not reach every type of service that community-based providers offer. Home care agencies that specialize in the provision of chore and housekeeping services or that offer only companion services will not meet the definition of a health care provider regardless of whether they are able to bill some payers electronically for that care using standard transactions. They, therefore, do not have to comply with the HIPAA privacy standards.

Special Categories of Covered Entities. The privacy standards also provide two ways for certain covered entities to band together and act as one unified covered entity rather than as multiple independent covered entities. They are called *organized health care arrangements* and *affiliated covered entities*. Both of these options have relevance to certain home health agencies and hospices.

Organized health care arrangements are made up of different types of covered health care providers that: (1) hold themselves out to the public as a joint arrangement and (2) participate in integrated utilization review or quality assessment programs or are paid for services collectively under the same shared-risk arrangements.[30] Hospital-based home health agencies and hospices fit into this special category. As a result, the privacy standards permit, but do not require, such agencies and their hospitals to: (1) use a joint notice of their privacy practices, (2) have combined privacy policies and procedures and a common privacy officer, and (3) share identifiable patient information among themselves to carry out treatment, payment, and

health care operations functions. The joint privacy notice must identify the various care delivery sites and covered entities that make up the organized health care arrangement, and it must stipulate that the component entities share patient data freely.

Affiliated covered entities[31] are legally separate covered entities that are under common ownership or control.[32] As long as the individual covered entities formally designate themselves in writing as an affiliated covered entity and maintain that documentation for 6 years from when it is last effective, they may act as a single organization for privacy standards purposes.[33] Obviously, this option is open to home health agencies or hospices that are members of chain organizations. It also is available to sister companies (e.g., a commonly owned or controlled home health agency and hospice or a commonly owned or controlled Medicare-certified home health agency and noncertified home care agency).

The privacy standards also provide for "hybrid entities."[34] These are organizations that: (1) are involved in business activities that include both covered and noncovered functions, (2) formally delineate their covered function components in writing and maintain the documentation for 6 years after it is no longer effective, and (3) erect firewalls between the covered and noncovered components to effectively contain individually identifiable health information within the covered component. Provided a hybrid entity takes these steps, it in essence only has to apply the requirements of the privacy standards to its designated covered function components.[35]

Those home health agencies that operate lines of business that do not meet the definition of a health care provider (e.g., chore and housekeeper services, companion services, Lifeline services, transportation services) may want to consider using the hybrid entity option to limit their obligations under the HIPAA privacy rules. Agencies considering this option should realize, however, that they will have to have a written authorization from a patient receiving home health or hospice services before they can share individually identifiable information about that patient with divisions involved in noncovered functions.

Use and Disclosure

The basic statement of the information handling requirements of the privacy standards makes it clear that the regulations govern both a covered entity's use and its disclosures of protected health information (PHI). Not surprisingly, both "use" and "disclosure" are defined terms under HIPAA.[36] Use refers to how identifiable health information moves around within a covered entity organization. Disclosure refers to the movement of information from a covered entity to a separate organization, which may or may not be another covered entity.

When a home health agency nurse talks to a physical therapist employed by the same agency about a patient that they have in common or a hospice interdisciplinary team meets to review patient status, those are uses of protected health information under the HIPAA privacy rule. When a home health nurse calls a patient's physician, who is in private practice in the town where the agency is based, to talk about a need for a change in the patient's plan of care, that conversation would be a disclosure under the HIPAA privacy rule. The same would be true when a hospice nurse calls a funeral director to make arrangements for a patient who has died.

Protected Health Information

The strictures of the privacy standards apply to PHI, which is also a defined term.[37] From the perspective of a health care provider, PHI is individually identifiable *patient* health information transmitted or maintained in any form— electronic or paper. Because PHI is information and not records, the term even reaches oral exchanges of patient data. Home health agencies and hospices routinely have PHI in both their medical records and their billing records.

Records Relating to Decedents.   Importantly, particularly from the perspective of hospice providers, the privacy rule requirements governing the use or disclosure of PHI apply to decedent PHI in the same way they apply to PHI that pertains to patients who are still alive.[38]

Records Relating to Employees. Health records that providers hold, in their role as employer, about their employees (e.g., physical examination reports, TB test results, and immunization records needed to comply with state licensing requirements, reports on job-related injuries or illnesses need to comply with applicable occupational safety and health laws or for workers' compensation purposes) are, by definition, not PHI subject to HIPAA requirements.[39]

De-Identified Information.   The privacy standards only regulate the handling of PHI. Therefore, covered entities may avoid having to deal with the standards' requirements if they de-identify information before using or disclosing it for purposes other than the de-identification process.[40] Information only qualifies as de-identified if there is no reasonable basis to believe that identification of the subject would be possible using modern data-mining techniques. Taking off name, contact information, Social Security number, HIC number, and medical record number is not enough.

The privacy standards stipulate that information may be considered de-identified if an expert certifies that enough data elements have been removed considering the circumstances of the contemplated use or disclosure. Absent an expert certification, covered entities must remove a long list of data elements to avoid privacy rule obligations. Specifically, those elements include: (1) name, (2) address except the first three digits of the ZIP code, (3) dates of birth, death, admission, discharge, and so forth, (4) phone number, (5) fax number, (6) e-mail address, (7) URLs and Internet Protocol address numbers, (8) biometric identifiers (e.g., fingerprints, voice prints, retinal scans), (9) Social

Security number, (10) medical record number, (11) health plan numbers, (12) account numbers, (13) certification/license numbers, (14) license plate numbers, (15) device identifiers and serial numbers, and (16) full-face photographs and comparable images.

For those home health and hospice providers using paper medical records systems and even for many of those using electronic records, removal of all these data elements from each and every page of an individual's medical or billing record would be prohibitively burdensome, particularly if multiple records need to be sanitized. As a result, for these organizations, the only viable way to avoid the burdens of the privacy rule through de-identification will be to limit uses and disclosures to data aggregated from the records of numerous individuals.

Limited Data Sets.   Because ZIP codes and various dates are often essential for research, the privacy standards also provide for the creation of "limited data sets" that contain these data elements but none of the other elements that must be removed to create de-identified data under the safe harbor approach. Technically, limited data sets are still PHI, but they may be used for research, public health purposes, and healthcare operations—but not any other purposes—without restrictions as long as the recipient of the limited data set signs a data use agreement promising, among other things, not to attempt to re-identify the data, specifying how and by whom the information will be used and agreeing not to use it for any other purpose.[41]

Required Disclosures of Patient PHI

Generally speaking, the privacy standards do not obligate home health agencies and hospices to disclose PHI. There are two exceptions to this general rule.[42] First, with a few limited exceptions,[43] patients must be given access to their own medical and billing records. Second, an agency must make patient records available to the government so that the DHHS Office of Civil Rights can assess the agency's compliance

with the privacy standards or the Centers for Medicare and Medicaid Services can determine whether the agency is in compliance with the transactions standards and, once they become effective, the security standards. It is not necessary for agencies to seek permission from the patient, or the patient's representative in the context of an incompetent adult, a minor, or a decedent, before records are released to the agencies that have been tasked with enforcement of the HIPAA Administrative Simplification provisions.

Permitted Uses and Disclosures of Patient PHI

As a general rule, home health agencies and hospices need permission to use or disclose PHI. The type of permission required varies, depending upon the circumstances. Most of the time, the permission will be regulatory. In a few instances, it will come from the patient in the form of an oral agreement, an inferred agreement, or a passed up opportunity to object. In all other situations, the patient will have to authorize the proposed use or disclosure in writing.

Regulatory Permission to Use and Disclose PHI

The privacy rule allows covered entities to use and disclose PHI for purposes of treatment, payment, and health care operations without obtaining oral or written permission from the patient, on the assumption that patients impliedly consent to such uses when they seek care or insurance coverage for health care services. The standards also permit, but do not require, covered entities to make certain public policy uses and disclosures of PHI without permission from the patient in situations where DHHS has determined that the public's interest in the data should outweigh the individual's privacy rights. Finally, because DHHS recognizes the common good that can come from fund-raising activities undertaken by health care provider organizations such as hospices, the standards also permit limited use of PHI for such purposes without patient permission.

Uses and Disclosures for Treatment, Payment, and Health Care Operations. Under the privacy standards, home health agencies and hospices, as well as all other covered health care providers, are allowed to use PHI without obtaining permission from the patient to treat their patients, to seek payment for treatment rendered, and to carry out all the functions necessary to properly operate their business.[44] That said, the standards expressly give agencies the discretion to seek written consents from patients to use or disclose their PHI for purposes of treatment,[45] payment,[46] and/or health care operations[47] if state laws demand or if, in the professional judgment of agency management, such a practice is desirable.[48] Because of the provision making the use of written consents related to treatment, payment, and operations (TPO) optional, agencies wishing to continue current practices or to use up old admissions forms that contain consents to release records to Medicare and/or other payers may do so.

Home health agencies and hospices have direct treatment relationships with their patients.[49] Home medical equipment (HME) companies have direct treatment relationships when they are billing payers for patient care but not when they are supplying goods to home health agencies and hospice that are reimbursed under the consolidated payment provisions of home health PPS or the per diem payments made to hospices. Whenever community-based providers or suppliers have direct treatment relationships with their patients, they must give (or if the contact is by mail or overnight delivery service, mail) the patients a copy of their notice of privacy practices[50] no later than the first date of service on or after April 14, 2003 (or the day after a service is delivered by mail).

Except in emergency situations, providers and suppliers having direct treatment relationships with their patients also must make a "good faith effort" to obtain a written acknowledgment from the patient that he or she received the privacy notice.[51] The acknowledgment requirement applies regardless of whether the agency has decided to obtain written consents to use and disclose PHI for TPO.

The privacy standards permit agencies that are part of an organized health care arrangement to rely upon a joint privacy notice given to a patient earlier by the hospital. Similarly, agencies in an affiliated covered entity do not have to redistribute notices to patients who received them earlier when they were admitted by a different member of the affiliated group. Prudent agencies will ignore this option. They will instead elect to incorporate the distribution of their then-current privacy notice and the request for an acknowledgment into their admissions process. This approach protects against failing to give a notice and seek an acknowledgment from patients who are community referrals. It also avoids the administrative burden of tracking whether a patient received the notice earlier, either from the agency itself, from another member of the organized health care arrangement, or from another provider in an affiliated covered entity of which the agency is a part.

The privacy standards do not specify any particular form for the acknowledgment of receipt of privacy practices so long as the acknowledgement is signed or initialed by the patient or the patient's representative. Agencies are free to develop any system that works well for them within the confines of their normal admissions processes. They do not have to keep a signed copy of the privacy notice that was given to the patient. Most home health agencies and hospices are including a separate acknowledgment line or box somewhere on the admissions form that the patient is asked to sign.

If, for any reason, a patient refuses to sign the acknowledgment upon request, it is sufficient for the admitting nurse or therapist requesting the signature to document the efforts made to get the acknowledgment, the patient's refusal to sign, and any explanation the patient gave for the refusal. That documentation should be signed and dated by the nurse or therapist. The same procedures apply when truck drivers deliver goods for which HME vendors will bill the patient or the patient's payer. The privacy standards do *not* require agencies to deny care to patients who refuse to sign an acknowledgment.

When HME vendors ship supplies or equipment by mail or overnight delivery service, it is sufficient for them to include a copy of their privacy notice along with a tear sheet or separate form which they ask the patient to mail back acknowledging receipt of the notice. No additional follow-up efforts on the part of the vendor are required if the patient does not comply with the request to return the acknowledgment. The rule also does not obligate the vendor to supply the patient with a postage-paid card or envelope for the acknowledgment.

Because of the way treatment is defined in the privacy standards, covered health care providers are always free to disclose PHI about their patients to other health care providers that are or will be involved in the patient's treatment without getting a written authorization from the patient. The HIPAA privacy rules are not intended to interfere with the provision of quality health care services to patients. As a result, the definition of treatment contemplates that covered providers may need to consult with other providers about a patient's care or refer patients to other providers for additional services. Accordingly, the privacy standards permit the sharing of PHI to accomplish these tasks without the need for obtaining a written authorization from the patient.[52]

The privacy standards also allow covered entities to disclose PHI for the payment purposes of *another* health care provider, regardless of whether that provider is a covered entity, without obtaining a written authorization from the patient.[53] For example, home health agencies or hospices could provide clinical laboratories asked to perform blood tests on their Medicare patients with information about the diagnoses that precipitated the test requests because the labs must bill Medicare directly and they often must include diagnosis codes on their claims to get paid. When a home health patient is admitted for emergency care, the hospital may tell the

agency why the admission occurred because the agency needs the information to complete the OASIS transfer assessment and, ultimately, to get paid.

Finally, the standards let covered entities disclose PHI for some, but not all, health care operations of *another* covered entity without seeking authorization from the patient.[54] Specifically, such disclosures are permitted when the covered entity receiving the PHI will use the data for: (1) quality assurance purposes, (2) population-based health improvement initiatives, (3) case management, (4) care coordination, (5) training programs, or (6) fraud and abuse detection or compliance activities. Importantly, the shared PHI must relate to a patient with which the covered entity receiving the information has or had a relationship, the disclosed PHI must be relevant to that relationship, and the disclosed PHI must be the minimum amount of information needed by the recipient to accomplish the purpose of the disclosure. Home health agencies and hospices holding managed care contracts that require quality assurance reporting may find this provision of the law particularly useful.

Uses and Disclosures for Public Policy Purposes. Numerous situations exist where a disclosure of PHI without patient permission would be appropriate from a public policy perspective. Accordingly, the privacy standards contain provisions that allow covered entities discretion to use or disclose PHI without patient authorization, or even oral permission, so long as only the minimum amount of information necessary to accomplish the purpose is released, the identify and authority of the recipient of the shared information is properly verified, and other specified situationally specific safeguards are followed.[55] The list of permitted public policy disclosures includes:

- Uses and disclosures required by law[56]
- Uses and disclosures for public health activities[57]
  1. Reporting of births, deaths, infectious diseases, and so forth

2. Reporting of child abuse
3. Reporting of adverse events, product defects, required product tracking information, or post-marketing surveillance information associated with FDA-regulated products
4. Reporting to employers for workplace medical surveillance purposes, about a work-related illness or injury or to facilitate compliance with regulations of the Occupational Safety and Health or Mine Safety and Health Administrations

- Disclosures about adult victims of abuse, neglect, or domestic violence[58]
- Uses and disclosures for health oversight activities, including audits, surveys, licensing, and civil, administrative, or criminal investigations[59]
- Disclosures for judicial and administrative proceedings[60]
- Disclosures for law enforcement purposes[61]
- Uses and disclosures about decedents[62]
  1. Reporting to coroners and medical examiners
  2. Contacting funeral directors
- Uses and disclosures for cadaveric organ, eye, or tissue donation purposes[63]
- Uses and disclosures for research purposes[64]
- Uses and disclosures to avert a serious threat to health or safety[65]
- Uses and disclosures for specialized government functions[66]
  1. Military and veterans activities
  2. National security and intelligence activities
  3. Protective services for the U.S. president and others
  4. U.S. Department of State medical suitability determinations
  5. Correctional institutions and other law enforcement custodial situations
- Disclosures for workers' compensation[67]

The privacy standards' public policy exceptions do not, in and of themselves, obligate home health agencies and hospice to disclose information. They only provide a mechanism for making disclosures that may be mandated or permitted by other laws or that may simply be desirable from a public policy perspective without obtaining permission from the patient.

The first of the public policy disclosure provisions permits home health agencies and hospices to use or disclose PHI without patient permission when some other law requires the disclosure. Agencies wishing to rely on this provision of the privacy rule in lieu of obtaining a written authorization from the patient must recognize that the provision only protects PHI disclosures that are *required* by law, not those that are merely permitted by law.[68] With the exception of that caveat, there are no other safeguards that must be met to take advantage of this particular public policy provision.

The provision allowing disclosures of PHI when the release is required by law arguably subsumes most of the other public policy releases permitted, without benefit of patient permission, under the privacy standards. Agencies should not be misled into relying on this fact, however. The drafters of the privacy standards included other more-specific public policy situations so that more detailed safeguards consistent with the purpose of each use or disclosure could be built into the regulations.

Agencies wishing to rely on the privacy rule's public policy provisions should always select the most relevant of the provisions and follow that provision's privacy-safeguard dictates. If agencies find the safeguards in an applicable public policy provision too burdensome, they have the option under HIPAA of getting a written authorization from the patient prior to any disclosure of PHI. In addition, agencies must recognize that the HIPAA Administrative Simplification regulations do not preempt more stringent state laws affecting medical records privacy.[69] As a result, state-law requirements that may impose additional safeguard obligations must be considered when decisions are made about disclosures for public policy purposes.

Home health and hospice providers will probably have occasion to rely on several of the other HIPAA public policy provisions. A discussion of those most likely to be of interest to the typical agency follows. Readers considering public policy disclosures not included in this discussion should refer to the HIPAA regulations themselves. Readers also must be ever mindful of the need to factor in state law requirements that continue to apply under the HIPAA preemption provisions.

Because of the provision covering public health activities, agencies may, among other things, report deaths, infectious diseases, and child abuse to local public health authorities and file Med-Watch forms with the FDA without patient permission. Agencies may also report elder abuse, neglect, or domestic violence but only if, and to the extent that, the disclosure is required by law, if the victim agrees, or if the disclosure is *expressly* required by state statute or regulation *and* the agency believes, in the exercise of professional judgment, that the disclosure is necessary to prevent serious harm. Under most circumstances, agencies that make such reports also must promptly inform the subject of the report that the report has been or will be made.[70]

The public policy provision permitting disclosures for health care oversight means that agencies have no HIPAA-related excuse for stopping Medicare surveyors from reviewing patient charts. The same applies with respect to auditors from the fiscal intermediary tasked with reviewing cost reports. Responses to program integrity requests for records for postpayment review also are allowed under this provision without patient permission. Because the health care oversight provisions only permit disclosures to governmental oversight agencies, organizations that are accredited by the Joint Commission on Accreditation of Healthcare Organizations (JCAHO) or the Community Health Accreditation Program (CHAP) must execute business associate agreements[71] with their accrediting organization and treat the accrediting body's review of patient records as a matter of health care operations.

Agencies will still be allowed to respond to civil subpoenas without patient permission using the public policy exception for judicial and administrative proceedings. Some agencies may find that their current policies for subpoena responses do not tract the safeguards built into the HIPAA provisions. There are no restrictions on an agency's ability to release documents in response to a court order or to a subpoena, discovery request, or other lawful process that is backed by a court order. When agencies receive subpoenas or discovery requests in civil cases without an accompanying court order—as they often do when malpractice actions are being planned or personal injury cases are being pursued—they may find that the simplest and safest course is to obtain a written HIPAA-compliant authorization from the subject of the PHI prior to responding. When such authorizations are prepared and submitted by plaintiff's attorneys, prudent agencies also will insist that the patient's signature be notarized. Otherwise, to make the disclosure without an authorization, agencies must receive "satisfactory assurances," in the form of a written statement and supporting documentation,[72] from the party seeking the information that reasonable efforts have been made to: (1) notify the individual who is the subject of the PHI of the request or (2) obtain a "qualified protective order"[73] from the court with jurisdiction over the dispute underlying the discovery request. Absent such assurances or an authorization, the agency itself must make reasonable efforts to notify the individual or to seek a protective order.

As is the case with surveys, HIPAA also fails to provide an avenue to escape program integrity investigations or other investigations of billing improprieties. Simply put, the privacy standards' public policy provision dealing with law enforcement allows agencies to release records without patient permission when they are presented with search warrants, grand jury subpoenas, civil investigative demands, or the like.

Hospices will be particularly relieved to know that they may disclose PHI to funeral directors, consistent with applicable state and local laws, as necessary to carry out their duties. Such information may be disclosed prior to, and in reasonable anticipation of, the individual's death as well as after the fact. For patients who wish to be organ donors, hospices may also contact organ and tissue banks to facilitate donations. Similarly, agencies may share PHI with coroners and medical examiners for purposes of identifying a deceased person, determining cause of death, or performing other duties authorized by law.

Whenever PHI is disclosed pursuant to a public policy provision, covered entities must log the disclosures so that each disclosure can be accounted for in accordance with the privacy standards' individual rights requirements.[74] To ensure that no more than the minimum amount of information necessary is released[75] in accordance with the public policy safeguard requirements applicable under HIPAA, to ensure that state law requirements not preempted by HIPAA are followed, and to capture the information needed to properly account for such disclosures, it will be important for home health agencies and hospices to centralize control over public policy disclosures. The person or persons assigned this responsibility will need to have clinical credentials to make the appropriate minimum necessary decisions and to exercise professional judgment when that is a required element of an applicable safeguard. In addition, agencies focused on risk management will document each step taken to comply with the safeguards in the applicable public policy provision whenever they make a disclosure in reliance upon such a provision in lieu of obtaining a patient authorization.

Uses and Disclosures for Fund-Raising. Under the privacy standards, agencies may use, or allow a business associate or a related foundation to use, demographic and date of service patient data—but not other types of PHI, such as diagnosis—to raise funds *for their own benefit* from patients and their families.[76] Regardless of how fund-raising contacts are made, agencies must ensure that written materials related to the initiative describe how the recipient of the solicitation may opt out of receiving any future fund-raising communications. This requirement means that agencies must establish systems to record opt-out requests and make reasonable efforts to ensure that they are honored. In addition, providers that anticipate conducting fund-raising campaigns must include a provision in their notice of privacy practices stating that PHI may be used for that purpose.

Uses and Disclosures Based on Oral or Inferred Permission or a Decision Not to Object

Discussions with Home Caregivers. Fortunately, for home and community-based providers, the privacy standards recognize that there will be times when health care providers need to share PHI with a patient's family member, other relative, or close personal friend because that individual is involved in the patient's care or in paying for the patient's care.[77]

When the patient is present and capable of making health care decisions, the privacy standards permit agency personnel to talk with a patient's caregiver based on: (1) the patient's oral agreement to the conversation, (2) a reasonable inference drawn from the circumstances, or (3) the patient's decision to pass up an opportunity to object to the conversation.[78] If a field nurse wants to teach a patient's daughter about the patient's medication regime, the nurse may ask the patient for permission. The nurse may proceed with the conversation with the daughter if the patient affirmatively agrees, if the patient responds by calling her daughter into the room, or if the patient does not object when the nurse asks the daughter to join them for the discussion. Although the privacy standards do not require providers to document that appropriate patient permission was obtained, prudent agencies will train their staff to note in the medical record discussions with caregivers involving PHI along with information about the type of permission obtained from the patient prior to any such discussion.

When a patient is not present, an agency cannot offer him or her the opportunity to agree or object to a disclosure of PHI to a home caregiver or a relative or friend otherwise involved in the patient's care. Nonetheless, agency staff may talk to a patient's caregivers if, in the exercise of professional judgment, they believe it is in the best interest of the patient and the conversation includes only PHI that is directly relevant to the person's involvement in the patient's health care.[79] Obviously, it is prudent to document such discussions.

The privacy rule provision allowing caregiver conversations when the patient is not present may be most relevant to home health agencies and hospices in the context of telephone calls from family members placed to the agency office. Although agencies may respond to these calls applying the applicable safeguards for discussions with caregivers when a patient is not present, they need to develop reasonable procedures for verifying the caller's identity.[80] Because the privacy rule is a performance standard, it leaves the details of an appropriate verification process to covered entities. Some agencies may elect to ask the caller to give the last four digits of the patient's Social Security number or some similar type of not so commonly known information. Others may decide it is more reasonable to assign their patients identification numbers or passwords and to speak on the telephone only with callers who can provide the code.

As an added precaution, agencies should consider asking patients, as part of the admissions process, for a list of people to whom the agency may speak with on the phone. To be maximally protective, this list should take the form of a HIPAA-compliant authorization that details not only the individuals to whom the agency may speak, but also the types of PHI the agency may share. Of course, this approach does not obviate the need for adequate verification procedures.

The rules governing caregiver discussions when patients are not present apply when the patient is physically present but not mentally competent to make health care decision. HIPAA does not speak to the definition of mental competence. Rather, it simply assumes that providers will follow applicable state laws governing competency decisions.

Facility Directories. Although the provisions of the privacy standards dealing with facility directories have more relevance to hospitals, hospices that run inpatient facilities are bound by the same rules. Basically, facilities are allowed to compile facility directories that include patient names, locations within the facility, general descriptions of patients' conditions that do not communicate specific medical information (e.g., good, fair, serious, critical), and religious affiliation so long as the facility informs the patient of the directory on admission and provides the patient or the patient's representative with the opportunity to object, in whole or in part, to being included in the directory.[81] Directory information may be disclosed to members of the clergy and, with the exception of religious affiliation, to the general public. Special rules govern the operation of directories when patients are admitted under emergency circumstances.

Disaster Relief. Home health agencies may play an important part in emergency response and/or disaster relief efforts in certain communities. When agencies become involved in this type of activity, the privacy standards permit them to disclose information about a victim's location, general condition, or death to public and private organizations such as the Red Cross involved in coordinating the disaster relief effort. When it is possible, victims should be asked for oral permission to list them with the disaster relief agency.

Uses and Disclosures Requiring Written Authorization

Under HIPAA, home health agencies and hospices must obtain written authorizations from patients for any use or disclosure of PHI that does not qualify for regulatory permission or for permission based on an oral agreement or a passed up opportunity to object. Although it is unlikely that home health agencies and hospices hold such documents, authorizations also must be obtained for all *uses* of psychotherapy notes[82] by anyone other than the originator or students working with the originator. In addition, authorizations are needed before PHI may be used or disclosed for marketing purposes. HIPAA prohibits health care providers from conditioning treatment on an individual's decision to sign a privacy authorization requested by the provider.

Form of Authorization.   All HIPAA-compliant authorizations must be drafted in plain language and, unless they are combined with an informed consent to participate in a clinical trial, they must be visually and organizationally separate from other documents.[83] Although the privacy standards do not prescribe a specific format, they do stipulate the data elements that must be included in a valid authorization.[84] Those elements include (1) a description of the PHI to be used or shared that identifies the information in a specific and meaningful fashion, (2) the identity of the person or class of persons authorized to make the requested use or disclosure, (3) the identity of the person or class of persons authorized to receive disclosed information, (4) a description of the purpose of the use or disclosure,[85] (5) an expiration date or event,[86] (6) a statement explaining the individual's right to revoke the authorization, (7) a statement explaining the covered entity's ability or inability, under the privacy standards, to condition treatment, payment, health plan enrollment, or eligibility on the individual's willingness to sign the authorization, (8) a statement explaining the potential for information disclosed pursuant to the authorization to be redisclosed without benefit of the protections of the privacy standards, and (9) a signature and date. If an authorization is executed to permit a health care provider to use or disclose PHI for marketing purposes, the authorization also must indicate whether the provider is being paid for the marketing initiative. Whenever an agency asks a patient to sign an authorization, it must give the patient a copy of the signed form. An example of a HIPAA-compliant authorization form is presented in Figure 51–1.

Home health agencies and hospices do not have to insist that authorizations be on an agency-supplied form. An authorization presented in letter format or on a form developed by a third party, such as a plaintiff's attorney, is acceptable as long as the authorization contains all of the necessary elements. Prudent agencies will, however, establish procedures for verifying the completeness of all authorizations before they release records. Those procedures should include steps to ensure that what otherwise appears to be a valid authorization has not expired. They also should involve verifying that the patient's instructions are being carefully followed both with respect to the scope and the recipient of the released PHI.

Revocation of Authorization.   A patient may revoke a privacy authorization at any time as long as the revocation is in writing. A sample form that may be used for revocations is presented in Figure 51–2. Revocations are not effective to the extent that an agency has taken action in reliance on a valid authorization. The right to revoke authorizations imposes an additional tracking burden on covered entities. Agencies must develop systems to match up requests to revoke authorizations with authorizations themselves, either physically or through appropriate database systems, so that PHI will not inadvertently be used or disclosed inappropriately.

Authority of Personal Representatives.   Personal representatives may sign and revoke authorizations under the privacy standards because, in all regards, they stand in the patient's shoes for purposes of administrative simplification.[87] As is the case with competency, the privacy standards do not define acceptable personal representatives. Rather, the regulations defer to state law by extending state-law rights to make health care decisions to include the right to make privacy decisions about associated PHI.

Generally speaking, for adults or emancipated minors, acceptable personal representatives are individuals who have legal authority to make health care decisions for an individual because they are the individual's court-appointed guardian or they hold the individual's health care power of attorney. Legal authority to act on

Section A: Must be completed for all authorizations

I hereby authorize the use or disclosure of my individually identifiable health information as described below. I understand that this authorization is voluntary. I understand that if the organization authorized to receive the information is not a health plan or health care provider, the released information may no longer be protected by federal privacy regulations.

Patient Name: _____   ID Number: _____

Persons/organizations providing information: Persons/organizations using or receiving information:
_____   _____
_____   _____

Specific description of information (including date(s), if relevant):
_____
_____

Description of <u>each</u> purpose of authorized use or disclosure:
_____
_____

(Note: "At request of [patient's name]" is sufficient when patient initiates authorization and elects not to provide a more detailed statement of purpose.)

Expiration Date
This authorization will expire on ____/____/____ (DD/MM/YR) or on the occurrence of the following event:
_____

Revocation
This authorization may be revoked at any time by notifying [Provider Name] in writing at _____
_____. If I revoke this authorization,
I understand that it will not have any effect on actions [Provider Name] took before it received the revocation.

Section B: Must be completed if health care provider or health plan requested the authorization or authorization is for research

1. Health care provider or health plan must complete the following:
   a. Will provider or health plan receive financial or in-kind compensation in exchange for using or disclosing the health information described above?   Yes ____   No ____
2. Patient must complete the following:
   a. I understand that I may see and copy the information described on this form if I ask for it, and that I get a copy of this form after I sign it.   Initials_____
   b. I understand that, in most situations, my health care provider will treat me regardless of whether I sign this authorization. If the purpose of the authorization is to allow research-related treatment, I understand I will not be able to get that treatment without signing this form.   Initials _____
   c. I understand that a health plan may condition enrollment or eligibility for benefits on my signing an authorization releasing requested medical records other than psychotherapy notes prior to my enrollment in the plan. However, once I am enrolled, the plan may not refuse to pay for my care, adjust my eligibility for benefits or remove me from the plan if I refuse to sign an authorization.   Initials _____

_____   _____
Signature of patient or patient's representative   Date
Printed name of patient's representative: _____
Relationship to the patient: _____
_____   _____
Witness   Date

* YOU MAY REFUSE TO SIGN THIS AUTHORIZATION *

Figure 51–1   Sample Authorization Form for Use or Disclosure of Information

[Use Agency Letterhead]

I wish to revoke an authorization given earlier for certain uses and disclosures of health information.

Patient Name_____   Date_____

Address_____   DOB_____

_____   SSN_____

☐ Check here if you have attached a copy of the authorization being revoked

☐ Check here to identify the authorization you are revoking by describing it below

     1. *Description of information authorized for use or disclosure:* _____

     _____

     _____

     2. *Description of each purpose of the requested use or disclosure:* _____

     _____

     _____

     3. *Date the authorization was signed:* _____

_____ ***[Initials of patient or guardian]*** I understand that the uses or disclosures of health information that already have been made based upon the original authorization cannot be taken back.

_____   _____

Signature of Patient or Guardian*   Date

_____

Print Name of Patient or Guardian

* If this revocation is being signed by an individual's personal representative, please indicate the basis for the representative's authority:_____
_____(e.g., state law, court order, etc.)

Figure 51–2   Sample HIPAA Authorization Revocation Form

behalf of decedents usually falls to the executor of the decedent's estate or to the next of kin. For unemancipated minors, the child's parent or guardian is usually recognized as the child's personal representative unless state law: (1) expressly gives the minor control, (2) permits the parent to cede control to the child and the parent has done so, or (3) gives a health care provider discretion to determine whether the child or the parent should make a health care decision.

Record Retention Requirements. Authorizations must be maintained for at least 6 years from the date that they are *last* effective. Similarly, authorization revocations must be held 6 years from their effective date.

Marketing. Marketing involves communications about a product or service that encourages the recipient of the communication to buy or use the product of service. Importantly, communications such as newsletters and health fairs that promote health in a general manner do not qualify as marketing activities under the privacy standards.[88]

Home health agencies and hospices must obtain written authorizations from their patients before they use or disclose PHI for marketing purposes unless the agency presents the marketing proposal during a face-to-face encounter with the patient or the marketing involves the distribution of promotional gifts of nominal value, such as key chains with the agency logo.[89]

In addition, the privacy standards definition of marketing is so narrow that it also allows for certain activities that many would consider "marketing" under the common use of the term. Specifically, the following activities are carved out of the definition of marketing:

- Communications describing a health-related product or service that is offered by the agency
- Communications about the patient's individual treatment needs, including contacts to remind patients of appointments
- Communications for case management or care coordination purposes or to direct the patient to or recommend to the patient alternative treatments, therapies, health care providers, or settings of care[90]

Under the marketing carve-out provisions, agencies are free to contact patients, former patients, and patients' family members to promote all of the agency's lines of business. Medicare-certified home health agencies that also offer private duty and/or chore services, operate Meals on Wheels and/or community transportation programs, or distribute emergency call systems under the same corporate umbrella should consider taking advantage of this option. The privacy rule even permits agencies to be paid to carry out marketing campaigns for products that they sell by the product vendors as long as the agency does not outsource the mailings to or share, in any other way, with the vendor the names and addresses of the patients being contacted.[91]

Certified agencies that have spun off the provision of ancillary products and services into sister companies because of Outcome and Assessment Information Set (OASIS) considerations do not have the same flexibility to promote their sister company's services. That said, such agencies can take advantage of the exception permitting marketing without patient authorization during face-to-face encounters. This exception allows nurses to alert patients to support products and services available from sister organizations. Prudent agencies will ask patients who express interest in obtaining services from a sister organization to contact the company directly or they will obtain a written authorization allowing the nurse to make the contact.

Agencies that anticipate using PHI without an authorization for marketing purposes under the face-to-face exception or for activities that have been carved out of the definition of marketing must state their intentions to do so clearly in their notice of privacy practice. Most home health agencies and hospices will need to state that they sometimes contact patients to confirm scheduled visits and/or visit times.

The Minimum Necessary Requirement

Many privacy advocates consider the privacy standards' minimum necessary requirement to be the heart and soul of the regulation. Most of the cultural changes that health care providers will experience because of the implementation of the privacy standards will stem from the combined effects of the minimum necessary requirement with the regulation of PHI uses.

The minimum necessary requirement obligates covered entities to take reasonable steps to limit their uses, disclosures of, or request for PHI to the minimum amount of information necessary to accomplish the intended purpose.[92] This requirement applies to oral communications as well as written or electronic communications. In fact, it applies to all uses or disclosures of PHI except for:

- Disclosures of or requests for PHI for treatment

- Disclosures of PHI to the individual who is the subject of the information
- Uses or disclosures of PHI made pursuant to an authorization
- Disclosures of PHI to DHHS for purposes of privacy standards enforcement
- Disclosures of PHI required by the standard transactions
- Uses or disclosure of PHI required by other laws[93]

The exception to the application of the minimum necessary requirement for treatment-related disclosures is extremely important. It allows a complete medical record to move with the patient as the patient moves through the continuum of care. Many complaints filed with the authorities charged with enforcement of the privacy standards in the months immediately after the standards became effective in April 2003 suggest that some health care providers may be withholding PHI from downstream treatment providers because of unfounded concerns about liability under HIPAA. If agencies experience difficulty obtaining discharge summaries and necessary medical records from local hospitals, they should refer the hospital's counsel to the provision at 45 C.F.R. § 164.502(b)(2)(i) excepting disclosures between health care providers for treatment purposes from the minimum necessary requirement, to the provisions at 45 C.F.R. § 164.506(c)(2) allowing disclosures for another provider's payment purposes, and to the frequently asked questions posted at http://www.hhs.gov/ocr/hipaa. If this fails, providers may wish to consider contacting the DHHS Office of Civil Rights to seek help educating the hospital.

Routine Uses of PHI. In most situations, the privacy standards do not obligate health care providers to make case-by-case determinations of what constitutes the minimum amount of information necessary.[94] Rather, for routine uses of PHI, providers are required to establish role-based information access systems. To do this, providers must first ask who needs PHI to do

their job, what PHI each job class needs, and what restriction, if any, should be placed on access rights assigned to any given job class. They then must establish systems through policies and procedures to impose reasonable limits on PHI access. Those policies and procedures must expressly state when the entire medical record may be used. It is also important for agencies to remember that PHI is found in both medical records and billing records. Policies and procedures for implementing the privacy standards' minimum necessary rule must address both types of records.

Agencies may find it helpful to build from the job descriptions they already have to identify classes of individuals and to document permitted records access. Because the standard of compliance is a reasonableness one, agencies may take into account whether they use paper or electronic medical records, the demands of their current service delivery models, the size and resources of the agency, their ability to configure systems to limit access based on roles, the practicality of reorganizing systems, and other such factors when they design policies and procedures to implement a role-based access system for routine uses of PHI. Agencies should network at state association meetings and conferences about approaches being taken to implement the minimum necessary requirement because determinations of compliance with reasonableness standards inevitably involve peer comparisons on the part of enforcement authorities and courts.

For example, a small to mid-sized agency using paper medical records, a teamed service delivery model, and electronic billing processes may conclude that managers, supervisors, and quality assurance staff need access to the complete medical and billing record of all agency patients but that field nurses and therapists need access to the complete medical records only of those patients they are routinely assigned to visit. Home health aide access may be limited to the care plans prepared for the patients to which they are assigned and to their own field notes. Intake specialists may only need access to referral forms, hospital discharge summaries, and information required to complete the agency's intake form, and billing staff may need access only to audit sheets containing claims information prepared by nurse reviewers tasked with checking charts and coding information to ensure that all eligibility, coverage, and technical requirements for billing have been met. Weekend and call nurses may be granted access to summary status information routinely left on a telephone tree about on-service patients and to their own notes.

Routine Disclosures of and Requests for PHI. Agencies will also need to develop policies and procedures specifying protocols for complying with the minimum necessary requirement when *routine disclosures of or requests for* PHI are made. Routine disclosures may be treatment related (e.g., submissions of 485s to physicians for signature, calls to physicians about patient care needs, contacts with HME companies to order supplies and durable medical equipment [DME], calls to pharmacies to arrange medication refills, care summaries sent to hospitals or hospices to which patients are discharged), payment related (e.g., negotiations with prior authorization staff and care coordinators at managed care payers, responses to Additional Development Requests [ADRs]), or operations related (e.g., data submissions to cost report accountants, communications with attorneys handling a malpractice case). They also may involve disclosures required by public policy considerations (e.g., reports of infectious diseases and deaths filed with public health agencies, dealings with surveyors). The same applies to routine requests by the agency for information from other treatment providers, payers, or public health authorities.

Nonroutine Uses, Disclosures of, or Requests for PHI. The minimum necessary requirement obligates agencies to make case-by-case determinations whenever nonroutine uses, disclosures, or requests for PHI are involved. To meet this requirement, agencies must develop poli-

cies and procedures that specify the criteria to be used to make the minimum necessary call and that assign responsibility—ideally by job class(es)—for the various types of uses, disclosures, and requests that may occur. Prudent agencies will assign personnel with clinical expertise to make such case-by-case calls and they will develop procedures for documenting how and by whom such decisions were made.

Responsibility for the Minimum Necessary Decision. The privacy standards recognize that tensions may develop over what constitutes the minimum amount of necessary information when covered entities must share PHI with outside organizations. The inevitable question is who has the ultimate authority to decide what is needed—the entity called upon to disclose PHI or the entity requesting the information? The privacy standards answer the question by granting the final authority to the covered entity releasing the PHI. That said, the standards also permit covered entities to rely upon the judgment of the requester, so long as it seems reasonable under the circumstances, if the requestor is:

- A public official asking for information under one of the privacy standards' public policy provisions
- Another covered entity (including health plans)
- A nonhealth care professional (accountant, lawyer, etc.) providing services to the covered entity
- A researcher working with the approval of an institutional review board or a privacy board[95]

Agencies should remember that the minimum necessary requirement is not intended to impede patient care. Application of the requirement must always be consistent with professional judgment and standards.

Documentation Requirements. Agencies must retain copies of the policies and procedures development to meet their obligations under the privacy standards; the minimum necessary requirement is for 6 years from the date the policy was last effective. Because of the privacy standards documentation requirements, agencies are well-advised to include version numbers, effective dates, and revision dates on all HIPAA policies.

Incidental Disclosures

Fortunately, the privacy standards expressly state that incidental uses and disclosures of PHI will not be considered violations of the regulation if:

- The use or disclosure occurs as a by-product of an otherwise permitted use or disclosure.
- The use or disclosure is limited in nature.
- Minimum necessary requirements are being met.
- Reasonable safeguards have been taken.[96]

Most of the examples that DHHS has provided of incidental disclosures are more applicable to the hospital or the physician office setting than they are to home care.[97] Nonetheless, a review of these examples should provide agencies with a sense of the reach of the incidental disclosure provision. According to DHHS, disclosures of PHI that occur when information is overheard by hospital visitors, other patients, or staff when nurses are coordinating patient care at a nursing station, when care providers are talking with patients in their rooms, when presentations are made during rounds, or when patient names are called in physician waiting rooms may qualify as an incident disclosure. So too may PHI seen by visitors, patients, or staff because of the use of sign-in sheets, bedside charts, X-ray light boards, and patient care signs. The key is always that the PHI disclosures must be secondary to uses or disclosures made consistent with the provider's minimum necessary policies. They also must occur despite the provider's implementation of reasonable administrative, physical, and technical safeguards designed to prevent unintended access to PHI. Analogous situations occur in home care when family members and visitors overhear discussions with patients in their bedrooms, when home charts or aide care plans are left in the possession of home health patients, or when "Do Not Resuscitate" signs must be posted over a patient's bed in accordance with local laws to alert EMS personnel to the patient's wishes.

To illustrate the distinction between permissible incidental disclosures and secondary disclosures that would constitute a violation of the privacy rule, consider the following example.

> A small hospice is holding an interdisciplinary team (IDT) meeting in the back room of its two-room office. The room is normally off limits to the public. The copy machine repairperson needs to work on a nearby machine during the meeting. Any PHI the repairperson overhears will be a permissible incidental disclosure as long as the participants in the meeting are all authorized to access the information being discussed under the hospice's role-based access policies, the team has been alerted to the presence of the outsider by the receptionist who showed him to the machine and, perhaps, by the visitor's badge that he is wearing, and the team members are speaking in low voices, avoiding the use of full names whenever possible. In contrast, any PHI that the repairperson overhears after the IDT meeting breaks up because a nurse and a therapist are gossiping about the mother of a mutual friend who was assigned to the nurse but not being seen by the therapist would not qualify because the discussion between the nurse and the therapist was not a permissible one under the hospice's minimum necessary policies.

Business Associates

Outsourcing of care delivery, administrative, and financial functions is a common practice in the health care industry. So too is the retention of professionals, such as accountants, coding consultants, and attorneys, needed to assist with certain routine, often recurring, business needs of providers and health plans. Although organizations called upon to provide these services frequently need access to PHI to do their jobs, they do not usually meet the definition of covered entities under the HIPAA Administrative Simplification provisions. When this is true, DHHS has no statutory authority under HIPAA to regulate them directly under the privacy standards.

Nonetheless, DHHS determined that the privacy standards would be ineffective if they failed to impose appropriate limits on the PHI handling practices of outsource vendors and professionals involved in the operation of today's health care system. Therefore, DHHS decided to do indirectly what it could not do directly. Specifically, it mandated that covered entities must impose appropriate privacy requirements by written agreement on all organizations performing services for or on their behalf involving the use or disclosure of PHI. The standards expressly extend the requirement of business associate (BA) agreements to organizations providing legal, actuarial, accounting, consulting, data aggregation, management, administrative, accreditation, or financial services if the provision of those services requires access to PHI.

Terms of Business Associate Agreements. Acceptable BA agreements must have termination provisions that allow agencies to end the arrangement whenever they become aware that a business associate has violated a material term of the contract and has failed to cure the breach to the agency's satisfaction. In addition, the BA agreement must:

1. Establish permitted and required uses and disclosures of PHI by the business associ-

ate. Those uses may include proper management and administration of the business associate as well as uses and disclosures consistent with the purposes underlying the agency's retention of the organization.
2. Prohibit the business associate from using or disclosing PHI in a way that would violate the privacy standards if done by the agency.
3. Prohibit the business associate from using or disclosing PHI other than as permitted or required by the contract or as required by law.
4. Require the business associate to implement appropriate safeguards to prevent uses or disclosures of PHI not permitted by the contract.
5. Require the business associate to report to the agency inappropriate uses or disclosures of PHI of which it becomes aware.
6. Require the business associate to bind any subcontractors given access to the agency's PHI to the same requirements.
7. Require the business associate to cooperate with the agency as necessary to allow the agency to honor patients' rights of access, amendment, and accounting.
8. Require the business associate to make its internal practices, books, and records related to the use and disclosure of the agency's PHI available to DHHS for purposes of determining the agency's compliance with HIPAA.
9. Require the business associate to return or destroy agency PHI at the termination of the contract if feasible or, if not feasible, to continue to protect the PHI in accordance with contract terms.[98]

Sample BA contract provisions are included as an appendix to the preamble of the final privacy standards.[99]

The final security standards will require agencies to impose additional requirements on business associates. Specifically, by April 21, 2005, agency BA agreements must obligate contractors to implement administrative, physical, and technical safeguards sufficient to reasonably and appropriately protect the confidentiality, integrity, and availability of any PHI that the business associate creates, receives, maintains, or transmits electronically on behalf of the agency. The agreements also must require business associates to bind their subcontractors to the same obligations. Finally, BA agreements compliant with the security rule must demand that agencies be informed of any security incident experienced by the business associate or its subcontractors involving or potentially involving agency PHI.[100]

Who Is and Who Is Not a Business Associate. Common home health agency and hospice business associates include: (1) members of the agencies' professional advisory committees, (2) medical directors of home health agencies retained to provide policy direction and administrative services, not direct patient care, (3) billing companies, (4) management companies, (5) coding consultants, compliance consultants, accountants, and lawyers who use PHI to do their jobs, (6) JCAHO and CHAP, (7) copying services, (8) microfilming services, (9) transcription services, (10) answering services, (11) software and hardware vendors with PHI access during troubleshooting work, (12) off-site record storage facilities where the vendor has physical control of the stored records, and (13) shredding services that process agency documents containing PHI off site.

Arrangements with staffing companies and with other covered health care providers for staffing purposes also create BA relationships. For example, a Medicare-certified home health agency that contracts with a private duty agency for home health aide staffing services must treat the private duty company as a business associate because employees of the private duty agency will be privy to certain certified agency PHI, but the private duty agency will not, itself, have a treatment relationship with the patient. The same applies when agencies contract with hospitals for a therapist because the hospital therapist will have access to agency PHI even though the hospital itself will not be treating the agency patient.

Despite the lengthy list of common agency business associates, there are many common situations in which agencies are not required to have BA agreements with organizations that have access to the PHI of their patients. Mere conduits do not have to be treated as business associates. In other words, no need exists for agencies to attempt to negotiate BA contracts with the post office, overnight courier services, or their telecommunications vendors.

Financial institutions like banks and credit card vendors are not usually required to be treated as business associates either. That said, banks providing lock box services that require them to process explanations of medical benefits from payers should be asked to sign a BA agreement.

Organizations that do not require PHI to do their jobs but that have incidental contact with agency PHI do not have to be treated as business associates. Landlords with rights to access and inspect leased premises, cleaning services not tasked with shredding PHI-containing documents, and maintenance service providers like plumbers and copying machine repairpersons admitted to agency offices in accordance with policies and procedures designed to properly limit their access to PHI to incidental exposures fall into this category. Researchers using agency data in accordance with applicable provisions of the privacy standards are not business associates; neither are other members of an organized health care arrangement or an affiliated covered entity to which an agency belongs.

Agencies do not need BA agreements with their patients' payers. In other words, BA agreements with CMS, fiscal intermediaries, state Medicaid programs, state community-based waiver programs, health maintenance organizations, and other managed care organizations with which agencies hold preferred provider contracts or commercial insurers are not necessary so long as the only relationship between the agency and the payer is a provider-payer one. A

BA agreement would be needed if an agency were to hire the local Blue Cross affiliate to serve as a third-party administrator for its self-insured health plan because that relationship falls outside the provider-payer rubric.

Agencies also do not need BA agreements to share PHI with other health care providers or suppliers that are treating agency patients.[101] In other words, no BA contracts are called for with community physicians overseeing the care of agency patients, nor do agencies need agreements with acute-care hospitals, rehabilitation hospitals, or skilled nursing facilities that refer them patients on discharge. Similarly, they do not have to worry about having contracts with providers to whom they refer patients on discharge.

The BA analysis can become more complex, however, when home health agencies and hospices have relationships with other providers and suppliers for underarrangement products or services to be furnished to patients while they are on service at the agency. When a home health agency arranges for one of its patients to receive outpatient physical therapy services that require the use of immobile equipment at a local hospital, the hospital would not be a business associate because it would be admitting the patient to its outpatient department and providing a direct treatment service to the patient in its own right. The home health agency would merely be paying for the hospital service under consolidated billing. The same analysis applies when a hospice contracts with a pharmacy to dispense pain medicines or with an ambulance service to provide transportation needed by its patients.

The analysis is different when home health agencies and hospices buy medical supplies from a local HME vendor that must be given PHI to deliver the supplies to the patient's home. This difference results because of a nuance in the definition of health care, which only reaches the provision of products that are dispensed pursuant to a physician's prescription.[102] If vendor-delivered supplies are sold to a home health agency because they are covered under consoli-

dated billing or to a hospice because they are covered under the hospice per diem and if the supplies are of a type that do not have to dispensed by the HME company pursuant to a physician's prescription that the HME vendor holds in its records, then the provision of the supplies does not conform to the definition of health care and is, therefore, also not treatment. Accordingly, the supplier is not functioning as a treatment provider to the patient in its own right. As such, the supplier must be treated as a business associate of the agency. In contrast, if the vendor provides an agency patient with DME that must be billed to Medicare under Part B or with a prescription drug and, as a result, the vendor must receive a physician order, then the vendor is acting as a health care provider furnishing treatment in its own right. No BA agreement is required.

The arrangements between hospices and nursing facilities can be particularly difficult to analyze because both entities are clearly treating the patient in their own right and, in that sense, are not business associates. However, to the extent that a hospice contracts with a nursing facility for any noncore services or supplies, it may well be creating a BA relationship akin to that with a staffing agency or an HME vendor that does not need its own physician orders for the supplies delivered to agency patients.

Another complicated BA analysis turns on the fact that the privacy standards do not require covered entities to have BA agreements with members of their workforce.[103] As is the case with many privacy standard requirements, understanding this provision requires attention to the regulation's definitions. The privacy standards define workforce to mean "employees, volunteers, trainees, and other persons whose conduct, in the performance of work for a covered entity, is under the direct control of such entity, whether or not they are paid by the covered entity."[104] This definition of workforce certainly could be read to imply that home health agencies and hospices do not need to treat professionals like therapists and social workers that often work as 1099-contractors under per visit or per diem arrangements as business associates. The same applies with respect to volunteers who are a required part of every Medicare-certified hospice's care delivery team and are deemed to be employees for purposes of the hospice conditions of participation.[105]

A review of DHHS's discussion of the workforce definition in the preamble to the privacy standards strongly suggests, however, that taking this tack may not represent the best approach from a compliance or risk management perspective. Specifically, DHHS notes that independent contractors should only be viewed as workforce members, and thus excepted from the BA contract provisions, if "the assigned work station of the persons under contract is on the covered entities [sic] premises and such persons perform a substantial proportion of their activities at that location."[106] This situation is contrary to the working arrangements that agencies have with independent contract professionals and paraprofessionals and with many hospice volunteers. Further, in discussing the need for BA agreements with volunteers, the preamble states that when volunteers

> ... work on the premises of the covered entity, the covered entity may choose to treat them as members of the covered entity's workforce or as business associates.... If the volunteer performs its work off-site and needs protected health information, a business associate arrangement *will be required*. In this instance, where protected health information leaves the premises of the covered entity, privacy concerns are heightened and it is reasonable to require an agreement to protect the information."[107] (emphasis added)

Given this discussion, prudent agencies should integrate BA provisions into their contracts with per diem or per-visit professionals and paraprofessionals. Home health providers that ignore this admonition could fall victim to overly zealous Medicare surveyors who could cite the absence of BA provisions in the written agreements that agencies are required to have with their contractors[108] as deficiencies under the conditions of participation on medical records confidentiality and on compliance with applicable federal, state, and local privacy laws.[109] They also could find themselves facing a complaint-triggered view by DHHS Office of Civil Rights authorities tipped off to the BA violation by the survey team.

The same approach seems prudent in the hospice context with respect to contract employees even though the hospice conditions of participation currently contain less clear-cut privacy provisions. In addition, because virtually all hospices routinely ask their volunteers to sign confidentiality agreements, they should strengthen those letter agreements to incorporate privacy rule BA requirements where applicable, recognizing, of course, that hospice volunteers will not hold the type of records that necessitate them ever being asked to participate in records access, records amendment, or the accounting processes. If nothing else, this approach should serve to reenforce the importance of patient privacy rights with volunteers who may not be as attuned to the potential impact privacy indiscretions could have on an agency's reputation in the community or its exposure to enforcement actions and private litigation for privacy violations in an environment becoming increasingly more focused on personal privacy issues.

Compliance Deadline for Having Business Associate Agreements in Place. An agency that had an existing *written* contract with a business associate as of October 15, 2002, and that did not open that contract to renegotiate any terms prior to April 14, 2003, is permitted to operate under that agreement without updating it until April 14, 2004, or until the contract is renewed or modified, whichever is sooner.[110] Despite this transition provision, agencies were required to be in a position to honor patients' individual rights as of April 14, 2003. Because of this, prudent agencies updated their contracts by April

2003 with those business associates holding medical or billing records critical to patients wishing to exercise their rights to access or amend PHI as well as with those business associates engaged in activities that carry an accounting obligation. Because the transition provisions were inapplicable to oral contracts, all agencies should have entered into compliant BA agreements by April 2003 with business associates previously retained on the basis of an oral arrangement. Answering services often fell into this category.

Agencies that have elected to take advantage of the BA extension period should consider negotiating provisions into those yet to be signed BA agreements designed to address their security rule obligations. If vendors balk at including requirements to address a rule that does not become effective until 2005, the contract can be drafted to make the security requirements executory provisions that become effective on the security rule compliance date.

Business Associate Liability Issues.   Under the privacy standards themselves, agencies are not entirely responsible or liable for the actions of their business associates. Moreover, agencies have no duty to monitor or oversee the means by which their business associates carry out privacy safeguards or the extent to which BAs abide by the privacy requirements of their contracts. That said, agencies are expected "to investigate when they receive complaints or other information that contain substantial and credible evidence of violations"[111] by a business associate. When an investigation reveals a material breach of the BA agreement, agencies must take reasonable steps to cure the breach and to mitigate, to the extent practicable, any harmful effects stemming from an impermissible use or disclosure of PHI by the business associate. Absent cure, covered entities must terminate their contract with the BA, if feasible, or, if termination is not feasible, report the situation to DHHS.[112] Agencies contemplating reporting a business associate to DHHS should recognize that, because they, not the business associate, are a covered entity, they are

really reporting themselves. In discussing the concept of infeasibility, the preamble to the privacy standards observes that a covered entity may not "choose to continue the contract with a noncompliant business associate merely because it is more convenient or less costly than contracts with other potential business associates."[113]

Despite the approach taken under the privacy standards, covered entities will undoubtedly be named as defendants when patients bring lawsuits for privacy violations regardless of whether they or their business associates were responsible for the conduct at issue. The health bar expects patients to attack covered entities for BA breaches using contract law theories in those jurisdiction where patients would be seen as third-party beneficiaries of the BA agreement.

Because the privacy standards arguably create a new, higher standard of care, it may be easier than it has been historically for patients who can prove damages to prevail in tort actions for invasion of privacy. Agencies should expect to be found jointly and severally liable if the conduct underlying a successful suit was committed by their business associates. In addition, agencies should recognize that plaintiffs may be able to use state consumer protection laws to attack organizations that distribute misleading notices of privacy practices or that agree to special privacy accommodations but fail to follow through or have their business associates follow through. Agencies must take care to ensure that their business associates are aware of their privacy practices. They also must implement effective systems for alerting BAs to any agreements they make to adjust their privacy practices to meet individual patient needs.

To address these liability risks, agencies should build adequate for-cause termination provisions into all of their BA contracts. Moreover, they should include provisions requiring BAs to report to them promptly, not just actual breaches of the BA agreement, but also any complaints the BA receives about privacy issues. Thought should be given to including indemnification provisions and privacy practice audit rights in BA agreements as well. In addition, where practical, agencies should consider including staff from their business associates in privacy training sessions.

INDIVIDUAL PRIVACY RIGHTS

In addition to specifying how covered entities may use and disclose PHI, the privacy standards establish a number of patient rights. Some of these rights expand upon rights, such as the right to inspect and copy medical records, that have long been available to patients in many states, merely making those rights the law throughout the country. Other of the HIPAA privacy rights, such as the right to receive an accounting of disclosures made for certain purposes that fall outside the realm of TPO, are currently unheard of and will force agencies to develop potentially burdensome new systems to ensure compliance.

In addition to detailing patients' privacy rights, the standards establish timelines for compliance. In many instances, they also set forth allowable grounds for denying a patient's request and establish due-process procedures that agencies must follow when a patient disagrees with an agency decision not to honor a patient request.

Prudent agencies will develop and implement well-thought-out individual rights policies and procedures because failures in this area will be readily apparent to patients and their families. Perhaps more importantly, perceived failures may leave patients thinking that their only recourse is filing a complaint with DHHS.[114] Such policies should, of course, comply with the detailed requirements of the privacy standards. Perhaps more importantly, however, policies should be designed to ensure that patients and their families understand the limits of the agency's obligations under the applicable HIPAA individual rights provision and the reasoning behind any agency decision that runs counter to their request.

Right to Receive a Notice of Privacy Practices

With the exception of inmates, the privacy standards guarantee patients the right to receive from home health agencies and hospices a paper copy of a notice detailing the provider's privacy practices.[115] These notices describe an agency's privacy practices, define the agency's privacy obligations, and explain the patient's privacy rights and how they may be exercised.

Notice Form and Content

The privacy standards spell out the categories of information that must be included in a compliant notice of privacy practices. They do not, however, specify the form that the notice must take beyond requiring that the notice be written in plain language. Agencies are free to design their notices to coordinate with their standard admissions package. Those using admissions booklets will undoubtedly want to use a different format than those using folders containing loose forms and brochures. Despite the temptation to condense the privacy notice as much as possible, agencies should consider their patients' ability to read small type when they design their notices.

The regulations specify that the notice must begin with the statement:

> THIS NOTICE DESCRIBES HOW MEDICAL INFORMATION ABOUT YOU MAY BE USED AND DISCLOSED AND HOW YOU CAN GET ACCESS TO THIS INFORMATION. PLEASE REVIEW IT CAREFULLY.

In addition, the notice must:

- Describe the agency's intended uses and disclosures of PHI. The description must include examples of uses for purposes of treatment, payment, and health care operations. It also should explain the agency's practices with respect to business associates as well as its practices for sharing information with family members and in-home caregivers.

- Describe each of the public policy situations in which the agency may be called upon to release PHI without the patient's consent. Agencies that choose to leave out some of the permitted public policy provisions will have to get a written authorization if they are ever faced with the need to make one of the omitted disclosures.
- If applicable, state that the agency will use PHI for fund-raising.
- If applicable, state that the agency will use PHI for those purposes carved out of the definition of marketing, including, if applicable, providing telephone appointment reminders.
- State that all other uses or disclosures of PHI require the agency to obtain a written authorization from the patient and explain that authorizations are revocable.
- Describe the patient's privacy rights and provide a brief description of how to exercise those rights. If the agency will require written requests for records access, amendments, or accounting, the notice should so indicate. The description must address the right to:

1. Request restrictions on certain uses and disclosures of PHI and indicate that the agency is not required to agree to requested restrictions
2. Receive confidential communications
3. Inspect and copy PHI
4. Request amendments to PHI
5. Receive an accounting
6. Receive a paper copy of the notice of privacy practices

- State that the agency is required by law to maintain the privacy of PHI and to provide individuals with notice of its legal duties and privacy practices with respect to PHI.
- State that the agency is required to abide by the terms of its then-current notice of privacy practices.

- State that the agency reserves the right to change privacy practices at any time. Agencies that fail to include this statement are obligated to apply each version of their privacy practices to PHI created or received during the time period when a particular version was in effect.
- Describe the procedures for filing complaints about the agency's privacy practices with DHHS and with the agency and state that individuals will not be retaliated against for complaining
- Identify by name or title and telephone number, the person or office to contact for further information about the agency's privacy practices.
- Carry an effective date. Prudent agencies will also include a version number so that they can establish with certainty which notice of privacy practice was in effect at any given time.[116]

Although the privacy standards do not address the issue, agencies should consider including a statement in their notice of privacy practices alerting patients to the fact that the agency owns its medical and billing records. The privacy standards merely give patients a degree of control over the information in those records.

Other Notice Considerations

DHHS permits agencies to prepare summaries of their notices of privacy practices.[117] Agencies that elect to do so must, nonetheless, distribute copies of their entire notice along with the summary. Agencies concerned about the difficulty of getting patients to sign acknowledgments without being given time to read the entire notice of privacy practices may want to take advantage of such a layered notice.

Members of an organized health care arrangement, which typically would include hospital-based or hospital-affiliated home health agencies or hospice, are permitted, but not required to use a joint notice of privacy practices.[118] Joint notices must name the various covered entities that are subject to the notice and detail all care delivery sites subject to the joint notice. Joint notices also should explain that all members of the organized health care arrangement will share PHI freely for TPO. Many hospital-based or affiliated agencies may prefer to use their agency-specific notices tailored to address issues, such a home charts, that are unique to home care.

Acknowledgments

As discussed earlier, except in emergencies, agencies must make a good faith effort to obtain a signed acknowledgment from patients that they were given the notice of privacy practice.[119] The acknowledgment can take any form convenient to the agency. If a patient refuses to sign, then agencies must document efforts to obtain the signature and provide an explanation of why those efforts were unsuccessful.

Distribution of Privacy Notices

Agencies were required to distribute paper copies of their notices of privacy practices to all patients on service as of April 14, 2003. This distribution was to occur on or before the first visit on or after the April 14 compliance date. Agencies also must provide a notice to newly admitted patients no later than the date of the first home visit.[120] Technically, notices do not have to be given to patients who have received a copy from the agency previously and are being readmitted for another episode of care. Similarly, new notices do not have to be given to patients who received a joint notice from another member of an agency's organized health care arrangement prior to being discharged to home care. That said, agencies are well-advised to incorporate copies of their then-current notice and forms for obtaining an acknowledgment of notice receipt into their standard admissions package. Taking this tack ensures that hospital-based agencies handle community referrals compliantly and, probably more importantly, it eliminates the need to track whether a particular individual has ever received a privacy notice and, if they have, whether it was the current version.

The privacy standards also require agencies to post a copy of their current notice of privacy practices in their reception area and, if they have a Web site, to post the notice there as well. Finally, agencies must make copies of their notice available upon request to anyone—patient or not—who requests a copy.[121]

Revisions to Privacy Notices

Agencies must revise their notice of privacy practices whenever they make material changes to their practices for handling PHI or honoring individual rights.[122] Except when required by law, a material change to any term of the notice may not be implemented prior to the effective date of the notice reflecting that change. Agencies must distribute the revised notice to new admissions and obtain acknowledgments of receipt. They do not, however, have to distribute copies of the revised notice to patients who are on service at the time of the change or obtain new acknowledgments from them.[123] Rather, it is sufficient to post the new version and to make the revised version available to on-service patients upon request.

Copies of notices of privacy practices must be retained for 6 years from the date they were last effective and copies of acknowledgments must be kept for 6 years from the date they were signed.[124]

Privacy-Related Admissions Issues

Agencies should recognize that, under the privacy standards, the acknowledgment of privacy practices is not an acknowledgment that the patient has read the privacy notice or that the patient understands the notice. Rather, it is merely an acknowledgment that the patient received a copy of the notice. Given the current length of admissions visits, agencies should consider developing scripts for admissions staff to facilitate delivery of the notice of privacy practices in a way that recognizes both the time constraints facing staff and the problem patients may have with information overload. Perhaps admitting nurses could suggest that the patient read the summary, leaving the body of the notice for review after the visit. If no summary is provided, the nurse could ask the patient to read the notice later and call the contact person on the notice to review questions. At a minimum, however, admissions personnel should touch on, if relevant, the patient's role in protecting home records and the agency's practices for sharing information with home caregivers and other family members.

Right to Request Accommodations and Confidential Communications

The privacy standards allow patients to request that agencies restrict their practices for using and disclosing PHI to better suit the patient's needs.[125] Agencies are not required to agree to any such requested restrictions, but if they do, they are bound to the agreement until the patient requests or permits termination of the agreement in writing, agrees orally to terminate the agreement and that agreement is documented in the record, or the agency informs the patient in writing that it is terminating the agreed-upon restriction.[126]

Because any agreement to a patient request for a change in an agency's normal privacy practices binds the agency, admissions staff must understand the limits of their authority to grant such requests. Prudent agencies will not permit field staff to agree to requested changes in privacy practices. If staff are permitted to acquiesce to certain types of patient requests for special accommodations, agencies must implement procedures to ensure that the changes are effectuated. Agencies should recognize that patients disappointed because of a failure to honor promises of special privacy treatment are the most likely to file a complaint with DHHS. Furthermore, such complaints could trigger a privacy enforcement action.

Agencies must accommodate reasonable requests from patients to receive confidential communications about clinical or billing matters at an alternate address or by an alternate means.[127] Although agencies may require such requests to be submitted in writing, they are not

permitted to ask for an explanation of why the request is being made.

Admissions and office staff alike must be trained in procedures for documenting patient requests to receive, or not receive, communications of PHI by specific means or in specific ways (e.g., requests not to leave messages on an answering machine, requests to have bills sent to a relative, etc.) and for ensuring that reasonable request are honored. Adding space on admissions forms for this type of information would be a good place to start.

Right to Inspect and Copy PHI

With certain limited exceptions, the privacy standards give patients a right to inspect and copy PHI about themselves held by an agency or an agency's business associate as long as the PHI is in a designated record set.[128] Medical records and billing records are, by definition, designated record sets.[129] So too are enrollment, payment, claims adjudication, and case or medical management record systems maintained by or for a health plan.[130] Although it would not be common at the typical home health agency, it is conceivable that some home health agencies and hospices may hold PHI in other types of designated record sets that qualify as such under the term's catchall definition of "a group of records . . . used, in whole or in part, . . . to make decisions about individuals."[131] Each agency should review its recordkeeping systems to determine whether it holds any unusual designated record sets that must be searched when access requests are filed by patients or their personal representatives.

A patient's right to inspect and copy PHI applies as long as an agency retains its medical and/or billing records regardless of whether those records are held on site or at an off-site storage facility. Likewise, the estate or next of kin of a decedent may exercise the decedent's access rights for as long as the agency has the records.

Requests to access PHI must be granted or denied within 30 calendar days of the request for records held on site and within 60 days for records stored off site.[132] If an agency experiences difficulty meeting these timelines, it may qualify for a single 30-day extension period, provided it notifies the patient in writing of the need for more time, explaining both the reason for the delay and giving a projected date when the requested records will be available for inspection and copying.

Only three types of PHI are completely exempt from the HIPAA provisions on records access. They are psychotherapy notes; information compiled in reasonable anticipation of, or for use in, litigation; and certain PHI protected from disclosure under the Clinical Laboratory Improvements Amendments of 1988 (CLIA).[133] Agencies holding these types of PHI should consider organizing their records in ways that make it easy to segregate the information that should not be released in response to requests to inspect and/or copy records.

Agencies may grant access requests in whole or in part for PHI that is not exempt from review. They may deny a patient access to PHI if some or all of the services at issue were provided for a correctional institution, if the records involve ongoing research and the patient agreed to forego access on trial enrollment, if the information is protected by the Privacy Act,[134] or if the PHI was obtained under a promise of confidentiality and release of the requested PHI would likely identify the source of the data. When access requests are denied for any of these reasons, the denial is not subject to review.[135]

Agencies also may deny access to all or part of a patient's records on grounds that are subject to review.[136] These reviewable grounds include denials based on the belief that allowing the patient to see the requested PHI is likely to endanger the patient or another person or that the information references another person and the release of the PHI is likely to result in harm to that person. Agencies may also prohibit personal representatives from reviewing a patient's records if the representative's review, in the judgment of a licensed health care professional, would be likely to cause harm to the patient.

Whenever access is denied for a reviewable reason, the written denial notice given the requestor must state the reason for the denial and include information about how to ask for a de novo review of the decision from an agency employee or volunteer who is a licensed health care professional and who was *not* involved in the original denial decision. The decision of the reviewer will be final.[137] Agencies that wish to be well prepared if they face a DHHS inspection triggered by a complaint about a failure to provide full access will also document precisely what PHI has been withheld and why.

Written policies and procedures on records access care mandatory.[138] In those policies, agencies should specify who, by job title, will be responsible for reviewing and processing access requests initially and who, again by job title, will handle access denial review duties. Prudent agencies will not involve their privacy officer in either of these tasks so that patients will feel they have an avenue for complaints about adverse access decisions without resorting to calls to DHHS. Access policies must also identify the agency's designated record sets. Copies of these policies should be retained for 6 years from when they are last effective.

The privacy rule provisions on PHI access allow patients to both inspect and copy their records. If patients are willing to accept copies of their records in response to an access request, agencies may respond to the request by providing the copy. However, if patients want to see the original medical record or to look at the computer screens containing billing information to ensure that they are reviewing the records in their entirety or to avoid having to pay any copying fees, then agencies must oblige the inspection request.[139] To protect the integrity of records from the agency's perspective, procedures should require an agency employee to be present while the patient is reviewing any original record.

Agencies may charge cost-based copying fees that include both the cost of duplicating and the value of employee time spent making the copy. Agencies may also bill patients for the actual cost of postage if the patient asks that the record be mailed. The privacy standards do not allow agencies to charge patients a fee for assembling the records for review, although they do permit such charges if copies must be made and sent to third parties pursuant to a signed authorization from the patient submitted by the third party.[140] The privacy standards themselves do not specify dollar and cents limits on copying fees. Many state laws, which will continue to apply under the preemption provisions of the HIPAA Administrative Simplification provisions, do set such fees.

The privacy standards also permit, but do not require, agencies to prepare summaries of records for patients who are willing to accept them in lieu of reviewing request records.[141] Agencies may charge patients for the time required to prepare such summaries as long as they advise patients of the charge in advance.[142]

Prudent agencies will require access requests to be presented in writing. They will also develop tracking systems for access requests to ensure that records are provided in a timely manner. Procedures for collecting records in response to access requests must ensure that, when appropriate, charts are assembled from different episodes of care and that records are obtained from business associates, agency branch offices, and all relevant affiliated covered entities or organized health care arrangement members. Agencies that keep the original medication log in a home chart also will have to retrieve the log to respond properly to a request for access to all PHI for a patient who is still on service. A form that agencies may use to record access requests and to track agency responses is provided in Figure 51–3.

Right to Request an Amendment

Patients also have a right to ask home health agencies and hospices to amend PHI contained in designated record sets.[143] This right applies as long as the agency holds the records. Agencies are *not* required to honor every amendment request. Moreover, when appropriate, they may accept or deny amendment requests in whole or in part.

Agencies are not required to make a requested amendment if the challenged information was not created by the agency.[144] For example, if the problematic PHI is in a discharge summary received from a local hospital or a clinical lab report, the agency should refer the requestor to the provider that originated the record. If that provider allows the amendment request, the agency will receive a correction from the provider in due course.[145] The agency will then be obligated, under the privacy standards, to integrate the noticed correction into its records. Not surprisingly, the duty to incorporate corrections applies whenever agencies receive notices about PHI amendments from other providers or payers.[146]

Agencies also are not required to make changes to PHI that would be ineligible for inspection and copying pursuant to a patient request for access.[147] Removing this subset of PHI from the totality of data subject to amendment requests seems logical because patients have no way of knowing about a potential problem with data they have no right to see.

Most importantly, agencies are not required to make amendments to information that they deem to be accurate and complete.[148] Given this, prudent agencies will establish amendment policies and procedures that assign health care professionals to the task of assessing amendment requests. Although there is no requirement under the privacy standards for a review of denied amendment requests, agencies should consider the merits of incorporating such a process into their procedures from a risk management perspective in an effort to satisfy patients who are upset about decisions not to delete statements from the medical record like "patient was noncompliant" or "patient was belligerent." Again, it is advisable not to involve the privacy officer in the amendment process so that dissatisfied patients have an avenue for complaints other than DHHS. Regardless of the nature of the amendment policies an agency decides to adopt, those polices should be memorialized in writing and maintained for at least 6 years from their last effective date.

[Use Agency Letterhead]

Patient Name_____   Date_____

Date of Birth_____   Telephone _____

Social Security No._____

Please provide access to health information in the following records:

☐   Medical Records
☐   Billing Records
☐   Other_____

Description of Information _____
_____
_____(e.g., type of information, date ranges, etc.).

Please provide the information in the following way:

☐   On-site review of record(s)
☐   Paper copy of record(s)
☐   Electronic copy of record [*Only include this option if agency has ability to provide electronic copies of medical and billing records*]

☐   Check this box to have copies of the records mailed [*if applicable,* or e-mailed] to you _____
[*If applicable under agency's policies*] I understand that I will be charged a reasonable copying of **[insert number]** cents per page for hard copies of my records and postage if I request that my records be mailed.

_____   _____
Signature of Patient or Guardian*   Date

_____
Print Name of Patient or Guardian

**If this request is being signed by an individual's personal representative, please state the basis for the representative's authority:_____
_____
_____(e.g., state law, court order, etc.).

Figure 51–3   Sample Request for Access to Health Information

continues

FOR USE BY AGENCY

Copy of completed form is to be sent to requester within 30 days of request for records located on-site and within 60 days if the relevant records are in storage off-site.

Access granted:

Date records were reviewed or mailed:_____

Access denied:

The following reasons for denial of access are *not* subject to review. Check any that apply:

☐   Requested information is psychotherapy notes.
☐   Requested information was complied in anticipation of litigation.
☐   Requested information is subject to or exempt from the Clinical Laboratory Improvement Amendments of 1988.
☐   Services discussed in the requested records were provided on behalf of a correctional institution.
☐   Requested information involves research that is still ongoing and patient agreed to the denial under such circumstance.
☐   Requested information is subject to the Privacy Act.
☐   Requested information was obtained under a promise of confidentiality and access likely to reveal the source of the information.

The following reasons for denial of access are subject to review upon request. Check any that apply:

☐   Requested information is likely to endanger the life or physical safety of the subject of the information or another person
☐   Requested information references another person and access is likely to cause substantial harm to that person
☐   Access was requested by a personal representative and granting access to the representative is likely to cause substantial harm to the subject of the information or another person

Figure 51–3   continued

Requests to amend PHI must be granted or denied within 60 calendar days of the request.[149] If an agency experiences difficulty deciding how to respond to a particular request, it may qualify for a single 30-day extension period, provided it notifies the patient in writing of the need for more time, explaining the reason for the delay and giving a projected date when the amendment decision will be reached. A form that agencies may use to track the processing of amendment requests is presented in Figure 51–4.

Patients must be notified in writing if their amendment request has been denied. The notice should explain the basis for the denial and outline the follow-up options available to the patient.[150]

If patients disagree with a decision to deny an amendment request, they may ask the agency to attach their amendment request to the record whenever the challenged information is disclosed. Alternatively, they may ask to have a statement of disagreement outlining their views included in the record. Agencies are permitted to add rebuttal statements as well. Agencies must

FOR USE BY PATIENT WHEN ACCESS IS DENIED BASED ON A REVIEWABLE REASON:

I wish to request a review of **[insert agency name]**'s denial of my request for access to my health information.

_____   _____
Signature of Patient or Guardian*   Date

_____   _____
Print Name of Patient or Guardian   Social Security Number

**If this request is being signed by an individual's personal representative, please state the basis for   the   authority:_____
_____ (e.g., state law, court order, etc.).

FOR USE BY AGENCY WHEN REVIEW OF ACCESS DENIAL IS REQUESTED

Name and title of the licensed healthcare provider designated as the reviewing official for **[insert agency name]**._____
[Insert agency name] will abide by the decision of designated reviewing official. That decisions is as follows:

- ☐   Requested access granted
- ☐   Requested access denied *[circle one]* in whole or in part.

If access is denied to only part of the requested information, specify the information that may be _provided: _____

_____
_____
_____
_____

As the designated reviewing official for **[insert agency name]**, I certify that I was not involved in the original decision to deny access to the requested health information.

_____   _____
Signature and Title of Reviewer   Date

_____
Print Signature and Title of Reviewer

Figure 51–3   continued

---

devise a system for highlighting information that has been subject to an amendment request so that any linked statements of disagreement and rebuttal can be routinely copied and sent with the challenged information whenever a disclosure of that information is necessary. Agencies also need to think carefully about how they will integrate statements of disagreement and necessary rebuttals into their billing records.

If agencies agree to an amendment, any changes in their records should be made in accordance with professional standards. Agencies that accept an amendment request must notify the patient in writing of their decision. They must also

[Use Agency Letterhead]

Patient Name_____   Date_____

Address_____   Date of Birth_____

_____   SSN_____

I am requesting a change in the information contained in (check all that apply):

    ☐   Medical record
    ☐   Billing record
    ☐   Other (please describe) _____

I am asking for this change because I believe the information, described in the section below,

    ☐   Is inaccurate
    ☐   Pertains to someone other than me
    ☐   Is not relevant to my health care or payment for services
    ☐   Other (please describe) _____

The information I believe should be changed is described below (please give date of the entry or report and suggested change).

Below are the names and addresses of persons or companies you should notify if my Request for Amendment is granted:

_____   _____
Signature of Patient or Guardian*   Date

_____
Print Name of Patient or Guardian

*If this request is being signed by an individual's personal representative, please indicate the basis for the representative's
authority:_____
_____(e.g., state law, court order, etc.)

Figure 51–4 Sample Request for Amendment of Health Information

inform persons identified by the patient as needing revised information.[151] In addition, agencies must tell other organizations, including business associates, to whom they have transferred the incorrect information *if* it is likely that the outside organization has or may rely on the erroneous data. This admonition extends to payers that have relied on the erroneous information to determine payment rates. Accordingly, agencies need to establish procedures for assessing the billing implications of all accepted amendment requests. Failure to refund overpayments when amendments are processed could put agencies at risk under various health care fraud and abuse laws.

No specified timeline exists for completing amendment notifications other than a privacy rule requirement that it be done in a reasonable period.[152] Prudent agencies will inform other health care providers promptly to minimize the risk of tort liability that could accrue if a patient were injured because of another provider's reliance upon erroneous information. Similarly, to mitigate risk under applicable fraud and abuse laws, agencies will deal expeditiously with payers due refunds attributable to an error discovered through the amendment process.

Right to an Accounting

Although no health care provider in the country has ever been asked to provide such information in the past, the privacy standards obligate agencies to furnish any patient who asks with a listing of certain disclosures of the patient's PHI made over the prior 6 years.[153] PHI released prior to April 14, 2003, is exempt. Fortunately, there is no duty to account for any *uses* of PHI within the agency, nor is there a duty to account for disclosures made for purposes of TPO, disclosures made pursuant to a written authorization, or disclosures that occurred because an agency honored a patient's request to access his or her own records. No log of limited data set releases is required either. In addition, PHI discussed with caregivers pursuant to an oral agreement is exempt from the accounting requirement as is PHI released in other situations where an oral agreement or an opportunity to object is sufficient permission for the disclosure. Finally, agencies do not have to account for incidental disclosures or disclosures made pursuant to the public policy provisions relating to national security or correctional facilities. There are also provisions that force agencies to temporarily refrain from accounting for certain disclosures made to health oversight agencies or law enforcement officials and that, thereby, impose certain tracking requirements on agencies as well.[154]

Despite the long list of disclosures excluded, the accounting requirement will be extremely burdensome for many agencies because it reaches most record releases under the public policy exceptions.[155] Agencies will have to be prepared to tell patients who inquire whether their records have been selected for review by a Medicare surveyor or whether a public health report about elder abuse or a communicable disease or a MedWatch report has been filed about them. The accountings will also have to detail record releases to HHS for purposes of assessing compliance with the privacy standards as well as releases pursuant to civil subpoenas and to document productions in fraud investigations. In addition, disclosures to or by business associates for purposes other than TPO will have to be logged. Such disclosures include those involving business associate data uses related to fundraising.

Although the privacy standards do not require agencies to notify patients of recognized violations of the rules, accountings must list any known accidental or intentional disclosures that do not qualify as incidental disclosures. Agencies could expect to learn about such disclosures because of reports made under the terms of BA agreements or because of recognized security breaches.

With a few exceptions, accountings must include:

1. Date of the disclosure
2. Name and, if known, the address of the person or organization that received the PHI
3. Brief description of PHI
4. Brief statement of the purpose of disclosure[156]

There are special rules intended to mitigate the burden of accountings when records are made available for research purposes or when multiple disclosures of PHI are make to the same person or entity over a period of time for a single purpose.[157]

Requests for accountings, like requests for amendments, must be acted on or denied within 60 calendar days of the request. If an agency experiences difficulty pulling together a requested accounting, it may qualify for a single 30-day extension period, provided it notifies the patient in writing of the need for more time, explaining both the reason for the delay and giving a projected date when the amendment decision will be reached. See Figure 51–5 for a form suitable for tracking accounting requests and agency responses to them.

Agencies must provide one free accounting per year to any patient who asks.[158] Agencies may impose a reasonable, cost-based fee if a patient requests additional accountings as long as they inform the patient of the fee in advance and allow the patient to withdraw the request to avoid the fee. In addition, agencies must maintain a copy of all accountings given to patients for 6 years.[159]

As is the case with records access and amendments, the accounting right requires agencies to establish policies and procedures for tracking requests and responding in a timely manner. Those policies must specify, by title or job class, the individual(s) who will be responsible for receiving and processing accounting requests.[160] There are no requirements under the privacy standards for the credentials of personnel assigned responsibility for preparing accountings. Effective accounting policies also must address the procedures agencies will use to centralize public policy releases and establish systems to capture the data needed to assemble an accounting when asked to do so.[161] As with all other policies and procedures developed to meet privacy rule requirements, the accounting policy must be maintained for 6 years after it is last effective.

THE PRIVACY COMPLIANCE PROGRAM

The privacy standards require home health agencies and hospices to establish a privacy compliance program structured along the lines of the voluntary regulatory compliance programs that many agencies have adopted to address risks under health care fraud and abuse laws. As part of this program, agencies must appoint a privacy officer to be responsible for the overall implementation and operation of the agency's HIPAA privacy compliance efforts. The privacy officer must be thoroughly familiar with the privacy standards themselves and with other guidance documents disseminated by regulatory authorities so that he or she can serve as the agency's privacy resource and speak with authority to patients and family members who raise privacy issues. Being the privacy officer does not have to be a full-time job. Rather, the demands on the privacy officer's time will be determined by the size and nature of the agency's operations.

Agencies must update existing policies and procedures to address privacy issues and, where necessary, develop new policies to meet the rule's demands. Agencies also must have procedures in place to ensure that policies are updated and revised as necessary and appropriate to comply with changes in the law[162] and in agency operations. All material changes in policies and procedures must be reflected in revisions to an agency's notice of privacy practices.[163] Policies and procedures underlying implementation of the privacy standards must be maintained for 6 years from their creation or their last effective date, whichever is later.[164]

Effective implementation of an agency's privacy compliance program will, of course, require training (and periodic retraining) of agency personnel in privacy procedures.[165] Orientation training programs will have to be revamped to address privacy too. Agencies also should consider whether it would be prudent to invite certain business associates to initial and ongoing privacy training presentations. As is the case with regulatory compliance programs, management will be responsible for setting the tone needed to ensure that a culture of privacy continues to characterize day-to-day operations.

Not surprisingly, the privacy standards mandate that agencies institute procedures for disciplining members of their workforces who fail to follow the agency's privacy policies.[166] Any sanctions imposed for privacy infractions must be documented. It only makes sense to use personnel records for this purpose and to integrate privacy compliance with other disciplinary procedures typically administered by personnel responsible for human resources management.

[Use Agency Letterhead]

Patient Name _____   Date_____

Address _____   Date of Birth _____

_____   SSN _____

INFORMATION REQUESTED

Please provide an accounting of disclosures of health information made by **[insert agency name]** and its business associates from _____ to _____.
I understand that I cannot ask for records going back more than six years. Also, I understand that the practice does not have to list any disclosures made before April 14, 2003.

[Optional Section] **FEES**

There is no charge for the first accounting requested in a 12 month period. I understand that I will be charged $_____ for each additional accounting that I request within a 12 month period.

    ☐   This accounting is free.

    ☐   The fee for this accounting is $_____

_____   Date _____
Signature of Patient or Guardian*

_____
Print Name of Patient or Guardian

* If this request is being signed by an individual's personal representative, please indicate the basis for the representative's authority_____
_____ (e.g., state law, court order, etc.)

Figure 51–5   Sample Request for HIPAA Accounting of Disclosures of Health Information

---

Agencies must establish procedures for accepting complaints about their privacy practices. Those procedures must accommodate complaints that come from patients, patients' families, *and* employees and they must provide that the agency will not intimidate or retaliate against anyone who files a complaint.[167] Agencies must maintain complaint logs, investigate every complaint, and document its disposition.[168] Whenever a complaint reveals a privacy compliance problem, agencies should implement corrective actions plans. Those plans must include steps to mitigate, to the extent practicable, any harmful effect of an identified privacy rule infraction.[169] When appropriate, they also should include recommendations for appropriate disciplinary actions and for modifications to agency policies and procedures designed to prevent future problems of a similar nature.

Last, but certainly not least, the privacy standards require agencies to put in place appropriate administrative, technical, and physical safeguards to protect the privacy of PHI. The privacy rule explains this obligation by saying that agencies must take steps to "reasonably safeguard protected health information from any intentional or unintentional use or disclosure that is in violation of the standards . . . [and] to limit incidental uses or disclosures made pursuant to an otherwise permitted or required use or disclosure."[170] This requirement has become known as the "mini-security rule" buried inside the privacy rule.

The privacy rule's security requirement should spur agencies to rethink many aspects of their everyday operations with an eye toward adjusting behaviors in practical ways to increase the privacy of patient-specific health information. Agencies should be asking themselves a long list of questions about their operations like those that follow. This list is meant to be illustrative only. Agencies undoubtedly will be able to recognize additional areas of concern simply by walking through their offices and thinking through their field operations.

The office is a good place to start. Does the agency have a policy for escorting visitors (including repairpersons) whenever they must be allowed in areas other than reception? Are visitors badges required?

Has the agency located or oriented its fax machines, copiers, and computers in ways that limit access to PHI, both with respect to agency visitors and agency staff itself? Does the agency have procedures in place to ensure that fax cover sheets with appropriate warnings are used routinely and that fax numbers are appropriately verified before communications containing PHI are sent? Are incoming faxes picked up quickly? Are originals always removed from the copier?

Must medical records be checked out of a centralized records room that is staffed during the day and locked at night? Are records routinely returned to the records room when they are no longer being used? Does the agency have clean desk policies that obligate staff to put records containing PHI in locked drawers or the records room when they leave for the day? Are staff instructed to turn pages over if they must leave their desks briefly during the day? Are covered in-boxes used, particularly for the receipt of field notes? Is shredding the norm for papers containing PHI? Are there provisions for ensuring that management records and computer runs containing PHI are properly filed, not left in piles on the floor?

Agencies should ask themselves security questions about their computer system issues as well. Does everyone who uses a computer—whether in the office or in the field—have their own password that is appropriately robust and kept secret? Do screen savers pop up after a limited period of computer inactivity and are passwords needed to reactive the computer? Are passwords required to boot up laptops and handheld devices used in the field? Are offices always locked after hours? Does the agency have policies governing e-mailing of PHI? Does everyone know them and abide by them?

Home health agencies and hospices also have to think about privacy issues associated with the use and handling of field charts. Does the staff store field charts in the trunks of their cars, out of site, when they are in transit? Does the staff only take that one patient's chart into a patient's home? Does the agency provide field staff with record containers that can be locked while in the car trunk and when nurses and therapists take charts home to work on them at night? Is the staff prohibited from keeping copies of notes and storing them in their homes?

Home records are still permissible under the privacy standards, but agencies should use a format—a folder or envelope, perhaps—that conceals the contents from casual observers. Patients also should be explicitly informed about their responsibility for safeguarding the chart. Do field charts contain the minimum possible amount of PHI? How does the agency deal with the home chart on discharge?

Oral communications in the field can raise privacy issues too. Does the agency prohibit staff from making phone calls from a patient's home when the subject of the call is a different patient? What are the rules about using cell phones or pay phones in public places?

As is the case with the minimum necessary rule, the privacy rule's mini-security provision is a performance standard. Compliance will be judged using a reasonableness standard, which is a facts-and-circumstance test that eventually takes into account the actions of an agency's peers. Agencies should look to their state associations as a good forum for information about appropriate approaches to privacy rule security compliance. Agencies should expect Medicare surveyors to be more interested in these types of issues in the future and should endeavor to share their survey experiences to help other providers in the community better understand evolving expectations about privacy safeguards.

Prudent agencies will not delay working through the risk assessment processes required under the security standards; neither will they delay upgrading their security processes. Despite the fact that the compliance date for the security rule is April 21, 2005, it seems inevitable that the dictates of that rule will color expectations for compliance with the mini-security provision under the privacy standards as time goes by.

One element of an effective fraud and abuse compliance program recommended by the DHHS Office of Inspector General is conspicuously absent from the administrative requirements of the privacy standards. Specifically, the standards impose no direct duty on providers to establish privacy-focused internal monitoring and auditing programs. In recognition of the fact that privacy must become central to the culture of health care under HIPAA, prudent providers will incorporate privacy into existing fraud and abuse compliance initiatives or ongoing quality assurance programs.

HOME HEALTH AGENCIES AND HOSPICES AS EMPLOYERS

Home health agencies and hospices often qualify as two types of covered entities under the HIPAA Administrative Simplification rules. First and foremost, most are covered entity health care providers that must protect the confidentiality of PHI in accordance with the privacy standards, conform their billing practices to the requirements of the standard transactions and code set rule, and, eventually, implement adequate security measures to guard patient data that is held and moved electronically. Those agencies that offer health insurance coverage to their employees as a fringe benefit may also be health plans that must conform to HIPAA's demands.

Handling Group Health Plan PHI

The HIPAA Administrative Simplification provisions define ERISA-covered group health benefits programs as health plans if the plan has 50 or more participants *or* if the day-to-day operations of the plan are handled by a third-party administrator.[171] Both fully insured plans and self-insured ERISA plans are subject to HIPAA. Given these definitions, many of the health plans that agencies have established for their employees will be covered health plans under HIPAA. The compliance obligations that agencies face because of this will depend on the size of the health plan and the manner in which the plan is operated.

Some health plans operated by home health agencies and hospices probably qualify as small health plans, meaning that they have annual receipts of less than $5 million.[172] DHHS has interpreted this definition to mean, for insured plans, that premiums for the plan's last fiscal year were $5 million or less and, for self-insured plans, that claims, excluding stop-loss premiums, were $5 million or less. Being a small plan is significant in that such plans have an extra year, until April 14, 2004, to come into compliance with the privacy standards. They will also have an extra year of grace with respect to security rule compliance. Unfortunately, the same is not true for the small health plan compliance deadline with the transactions standard. Small plans and large plans that filed for ASCA extension were all required to begin accepting and sending standard transactions by October 16, 2003.

Agencies with fully insured health plans can avoid taking on privacy standards plan compliance obligations if they limit the health information that they allow the insurer to release to them in their role as plan sponsor to: (1) data on which employees are enrolled in the plan and (2) summary claims information that is used only to obtain premium bids or to modify, amend, or terminate the group health plan.[173] Because plan participants will receive privacy notices from the insurer or HMO, the agencies operating fully insured ERISA plans also are excused from the obligation to distribute notices of privacy practices.[174]

Agencies that insist upon receiving more than summary health data about employees enrolled in the group health plans they sponsor—regardless of whether those plans are insured or self-insured—will have to amend their ERISA plan documents to incorporate provisions to:

- Establish the permitted and required uses and disclosures of PHI that the agency may make
- Provide that the group health plan will disclose PHI to the agency only upon receipt of a written certification that the plan documents have been amended to incorporate the following provisions and that the agency as the plan sponsor agrees to:

  1. Not use or further disclose plan PHI other than as permitted or required by the plan documents or as required by law
  2. Ensure that any subcontractor to whom the agency provides PHI agrees to the same restrictions and conditions applicable to the agency
  3. Not use or disclose the information for

employment-related actions and decisions or in connection with any other benefit or employee benefit plan sponsored by the agency

4. Report to the group health plan any inappropriate uses or disclosures of plan PHI of which it becomes aware
5. Make available PHI in accordance with the privacy standards' access rules
6. Honor the privacy standards' amendment provisions
7. Make available information for required accountings
8. Make information on agency internal practices, books, and records relating to plan PHI available to DHHS for purposes of determining plan compliance with the privacy standards
9. If feasible, return or destroy all PHI received from the group health plan when it is no longer needed for the purpose for which disclosure was made and, if such return or destruction is not feasible, limit further uses and disclosures to those purposes that make the return or destruction infeasible
10. Ensure that adequate separation is maintained

- Provide for adequate separation between the group health plan and the agency. To this end, the plan documents must:

  1. Describe those agency employees or job classes to be given access to plan PHI
  2. Restrict the uses of plan PHI by these employees to plan administration functions (payment or operations) that the agency handles for the group health plan
  3. Provide an effective mechanism for resolving issues of noncompliance by agency employees[175]

In addition, fully insured group health plans that share more than summary health data with the sponsor of the plan under the rules just outlined must also maintain a notice of privacy practices and make that notice available to plan participants upon request.[176] Self-insured plans that share PHI with the plan sponsor must distribute notices of privacy practices no later than the compliance date for the health plan, thereafter at the time of enrollment, and within 60 days of a material revision to the notice. No less frequently than every 3 years, the plan also must notify current enrollees of the availability of the notice and how to obtain a copy.[177] Fortunately, given the way that most health plans and their third-party administrators currently maintain records, the privacy standards do not require plans to send notices to dependents covered under the plan. Rather, it is sufficient if the notice is addressed only to the named insured.[178]

Although many agencies with fully insured health plans historically have received too much employee data to qualify for exemption from significant privacy rule duties, a significant number have rethought, or are rethinking if they have a small plan 2004 compliance date, their need for the extra data in light of the administrative burdens that will attach to receiving it. Similarly, many agencies with self-insured plans are reconsidering whether they would be better off to move back to a fully insured option. Regardless of the approach they take, home health agencies and hospices should not ignore their roles as covered health plans under the privacy standards. The risks of noncompliance are just as great for plans as they are for providers.

Handling Employee Health Records

Most agencies maintain substantial amounts of health information about their employees in personnel files. The information often is needed to establish compliance with licensing and certification requirements, OSHA regulations, or local public health reporting requirements. Because this data is carved out of the definition of PHI,[179] employee health information is not protected by the privacy standards. Other rules on medical records privacy, such as those under the Americans with Disabilities Act, may apply. In many ways, however, the regulations that govern the handling of most employee health information are less stringent than the HIPAA privacy rules applicable to patient or health plan data. Agencies interested in building a lasting culture of privacy should consider voluntarily tightening up their management of employee health information. Otherwise, they may find it more difficult to convince staff of the importance of burdensome tasks required to comply with HIPAA's patient-focused and enrollee-focused privacy dictates.

ENFORCEMENT

Direct Enforcement Under HIPAA

The HIPAA statute itself details penalties that are applicable to covered entities that violate regulations promulgated to implement all aspects of the law, including the privacy standards.[180] The statute stipulates general penalties for failure to comply with the requirements of the statute and its implementing regulations. Those penalties are limited to "a penalty of not more than $100 for each such violation, except that the total amount imposed . . . for all violations of an identical requirement or prohibition during a calendar year may not exceed $25,000."[181] Because no regulations implementing the substantive provisions of the Administrative Simplification enforcement provisions have been published yet, even in proposed form,[182] the potential monetary import of the statute remains unclear. In essence, the answer will turn on how DHHS defines "violations of an identical requirement."

Not withstanding that uncertainty, it is clear that the imposition of civil monetary penalties is supposed to be a penalty of last resort. The statute prohibits fining covered entities if they did not know and, with reasonable diligence, would not have known that they were violating the law. This provision provides some protection from the wrongdoing of business associates. It also provides covered entities some protection for that period after a rule becomes effective while enforcement authorities are still developing and disseminating interpretations of ambiguous sections of the regulations. In addition, the statute stipulates that no penalty may be imposed if a compliance failure was due to reasonable cause and not willful neglect so long as the covered entity addresses the problem in accordance with a corrective action plan and schedule agreed to with the enforcement authorities.

DHHS has assigned responsibility, under the these general penalty provisions, for enforcing the privacy standards to the DHHS Office of Civil Rights. CMS has been given similar authority with respect to the transactions standards and the security standards. Both offices have announced that they intend to approach enforcement through outreach and education and to use civil penalties as a last resort.

The HIPAA statute also provides for the imposition of criminal penalties of not more than $50,000, imprisonment of not more than 1 year, or both, if a person knowingly and in violation of the regulations implementing HIPAA Administrative Simplification obtains PHI or discloses PHI to another person. If the offense is committed under false pretenses, the fine increases to a maximum of $100,000 and the possible jail term to 5 years. If the offense is committed with the intent to sell, transfer, or use PHI for commercial advantage, personal gain, or malicious harm, the perpetrator may be fined up to $250,000, imprisoned for up to 10 years, or both.[183] The U.S. Department of Justice is tasked with enforcing Administrative Simplification criminal penalties. The law also states expressly that no violation may be prosecuted both civilly and criminally.[184]

Privacy Enforcement Under State Law

Until recently, state medical records privacy laws have included weak penalties or have relied exclusively on sanctions under professional licensing laws. As a result, they were rarely enforced. That may be changing in large part because many state legislatures, spurred on by identity theft concerns, increasing public focus on financial and health privacy, and the HIPAA preemption provisions, have updated and strengthened their medical records privacy laws, sometimes with an eye also toward closing perceived loopholes in HIPAA.

No privacy right of action exists under HIPAA. Health care providers should, nonetheless, expect to see civil suits in state courts raising privacy issues when there is an egregious breach involving the disclosure of numerous patients' PHI. Simply put, such cases may look attractive to the class action plaintiff's bar. Plaintiffs likely will use a variety of legal theories such as breach of contract where state law supports the notion that the patient is a third-party beneficiary of a business associate contract; invasion of privacy based on the contention that the HIPAA privacy standards create a new, higher standard of care in the community; and even violation of consumer protection laws which arguably prohibit making false and misleading statements in a notice of privacy practices.

Indirect Enforcement Under Medicare Rules

Although CMS has instructed state survey agencies not to take on HIPAA enforcement tasks at this time, Medicare-certified home health agencies and hospices should, nonetheless, expect privacy requirements under the applicable conditions of participation to receive added attention. Ultimately, it is conceivable that surveyors will help define industry standards with respect to the privacy rule's minimum necessary requirement and its demands for administrative and physical safeguards.

Finally, the individual rights provisions under the privacy standards potentially expose home health agencies and hospices—along with all other healthcare providers—to another round of heightened fraud and abuse enforcement as patients call the fraud hotline or, worse yet, file whistle blower suits under the False Claims Act because they misunderstand information that they see in their medical records.

ENDNOTES

1. Public Law 104-191, August 21, 1996, U.S.C.C.110 Stat.1936. Available online at *http://aspe.hhs.gov /admnsimp/pl104191.htm.*

2. Public Law. 104-191, Title II, Subtitle F, U.S.C.C. 110 Stat. 1935, 2021 (codified at Soc. Sec. Act § 1171-79, U.S.C. §1320d - 1320d-8).

3. 67 Fed. Reg. 38009 (May 31, 2002) (codified at 45 C.F.R. Parts 162.605 and 162.610). See *www. cms.hhs.gov/hipaa/hipaa2/regulations/identifiers/ default.asp*

4. Under development; no projected completion date. See *www.cms.hhs.gov/hipaa/hipaa2/identifiers/default .asp.*

5. Proposed rule published May 7, 1988. See *www.cms.hhs.gov/hipaa/hipaa2/regulations/ identifiers/default.asp* for copy. According to DHHS semi-annual regulatory agenda dated Dec. 22, 2003, final rules, expected to be issued in Dec. 2003, have been delayed.

6. The national standard for individuals has been put on hold because of privacy concerns.

7. Proposed standards for claims attachments and first reports of injury have not yet been published.

   A final rule promulgating the remainder of the standards was published at 65 *Fed. Reg.* 50312 (August 17, 2000). Final amendments to this rule were published at 67 *Fed. Reg.* 38044 (May 31, 2002). Copies of the standard transactions regulations along with the implementation guidelines explaining the use of the standards and the applicable required code sets may be found at *http://www.cms.hhs.gov/hipaa/ hipaa2/regulations/transactions/default.asp.*

8. Pub. Law 107-105 (Dec. 27, 2001), 115 Stat. 1003. Available also at *www.cms.hhs.gov/hipaa/hipaa2/ regulations/asca/asca.pdf.*

9. 68 *Fed. Reg.* 8833 (Feb. 20, 2003). Available also at *www.cms.hhs.gov/hipaa/hipaa2.*

10. Public Law 104-191, § 264(c)(1), U.S.C.C. 110 Stat. 1936, 2033.

11. 65 *Fed. Reg.* 82461 (Dec. 28, 2000). See *www .hhs.gov/ocr/hipaa.*

12. 67 *Fed. Reg.* 53181 (Aug. 14, 2002). See *www .hhs.gov/ocr/hipaa.*

13. A small health plan has annual receipts of $5 million a year or less. 45 C.F.R. § 160.103. DHHS has interpreted this definition to mean paid insurance premiums of $5 million or less for insured plans or paid claims, excluding stop-loss premiums, of $5 million or less for self-insured plans during one plan's last full fiscal year. See *www.cms.hhs.gov/hipaa/hipaa2/ default.asp,* Frequently Asked Questions.

14. 45 C.F.R. § 160.202.

15. 45 C.F.R. §160.203(c).

16. 45 C.F.R. § 160.203(d).

17. 45 C.F.R. § 160.203(a).

18. 45 C.F.R. § 160.203(b).

19. According to 45 C.F.R. § 160.202, "relates to the privacy of individually identifiable health information" means that "the state law has the specific purpose of protecting the privacy of health information or affects the privacy of health information in a direct, clear, and substantial way."

20. According to 45 C.F.R. § 160.202, more stringent means, in the context of a provision-by-provision comparison of a state law and the requirements of the HIPAA privacy standards, a state law that meets one or more of the following criteria:

    1. With respect to a use or disclosure, the state law prohibits or restricts the use or disclosure in circumstances under which HIPAA would permit it, except if the disclosure is required by HIPAA to allow DHHS to assess compliance or the disclosure is to the individual who is the subject of the health information.

    2. With respect to the rights of an individual who is the subject of the health information, the state law permits greater rights of access or amendment than does HIPAA.

    3. With respect to information to be provided to an individual who is the subject of the health information about a use, disclosure, right, or remedy, the state law provides the greater amount of information.

    4. With respect to the form, substance, or need for express legal permission from an individual who is the subject of the health information, the state law provides requirements that narrow the scope or duration, increase the privacy protections afforded, or reduce the coercive effect of the circumstances surrounding the express legal permission.

    5. With respect to recordkeeping or requirements relating to accounting of disclosures, the state law provides for the retention or reporting of more detailed information or for a longer duration.

    6. With respect to any other matter, the state law provides greater privacy protection for the individual who is the subject of the health information.

21. 45 C.F.R. § 160.103.

22. See *www.afehct.org/aspire.asp* or *www.uhin.com/ standards/1_to_standards/02-A_UB92-STD6.pdf.*

23. 45 C.F.R. § 160.103.

24. 42 U.S.C. 300gg-91(a)(2).

25. See *www.cms.hhs.gov/hipaa/hipaa2* for a decision tree tool that may be used to determine whether a particular insurance plan qualifies as a covered entity health plan subject to regulation under the HIPAA Administrative Simplification rules.

26. Implementation specifications for the X 12N 837 institutional claim form that will replace the UB-92 define the code sets that must be used to complete the claim. The use of local codes by state Medicaid programs will be eliminated. That said, the X 12N 837 does contain mandatory, situational, and optional data elements. Accordingly, providers should expect commercial carriers to issue what are being called *companion guides* explaining their expectations for the submission of situational and optional data elements. Medicare and Medicaid will publish provider bulletins containing the same type of information.

    Because HIPAA requires all health plans, including the federal government plans, to accept standard electronic transactions regardless of whether the transaction contains data elements that the plan does not want, providers, in theory, should be able to use identical processes to bill all payers so long as they are willing to determine which of their payers has the most demanding requirements and prepare all claims containing those data elements.

27. 45 C.F.R. § 160.103. *Also see www.cms.hhs.gov /hipaa/hipaa2* for a decision tree tool that may be used to determine whether a particular organization qualifies as a covered health care provider subject to regulation under the HIPAA Administrative Simplification rules.

28. 45 C.F.R. § 160.103.

29. According to 45 C.F.R. § 160.103, "Health care means care, services, or supplies related to the health of an individual. Health care includes, but is not limited to the following: (1) Preventive, diagnostic, therapeutic, rehabilitative, maintenance, or palliative care, and counseling, service, assessment, or procedure with respect to the physical or mental condition, or functional status, of an individual or that affects the structure or function of the body; and (2) Sale or dispensing of a drug, device, equipment, or other item in accordance with a prescription."

30. 45 C.F.R. § 160.103.

31. 45 C.F.R. § 164.504(d)(1).

32. Common ownership of two or more organizations exists for purposes of the privacy standards if a single individual or organization owns 5 percent or more of each. 45 C.F.R. § 164.504(a). Common control of two or more organizations exists if a single individual or organization has the power significantly to influence or direct the actions or policies of each. *Id.*

33. Chains with home offices that are legally separate companies and that do not qualify as a health care provider must treat the home office as a business associate.

34. 45 C.F.R. § 164.103.

35. 45 C.F.R. § 164.504(a)–(c).

36. 45 C.F.R. § 160.103.

37. 45 C.F.R. §160.103.

38. 45 C.F.R. § 164.502(f).

39. 45 C.F.R. § 164.501.

40. 45 C.F.R. § 164.502(d)

41. 45 C.F.R. § 164.514(e).

42. 45 C.F.R. § 164.502(a)(2).

43. Psychotherapy notes, information compiled in anticipation of litigation, and information protected by the Clinical Laboratory Improvements Amendments of 1988. 45 C.F.R. § 164.524.

44. 45 C.F.R. § 164.506.

45. Treatment is defined at 45 C.F.R. § 164.501 to mean "the provision, coordination, or management of health care and related services by one or more health care providers, including the coordination or management of health care by a health care provider with a third party; consultation between health care providers relating to a patient; or the referral of a patient for health care from one health care provider to another." This definition is broad enough to permit hospitals to provide home health agencies and hospices with discharge summaries and other needed medical records when they refer a patient without obtaining a written authorization from the patient being referred. It also permits agencies to discuss a patient with their attending physician; refer home health patients to adult day care centers, skilled nursing facilities, hospices, and so forth; and provide discharge summaries and other needed medical records to the next health provider in the patient's continuum of care, again without obtaining a written authorization from the patient.

46. Payment is defined at 45 C.F.R. § 164.501. The definition of payment activities permits agencies to: (1) seek determinations of eligibility, coverage, or medical necessity; (2) submit information to payers required to obtain pre-, concurrent, or retrospective certifications and authorizations; (3) bill and manage their claims; (4) undertake collection activities; and (5) report name, address, date of birth, Social Security number, payment history, account number, and agency identifying information to consumer reporting agencies.

47. Health care operations is defined at 45 C.F.R. § 164.501. It consists of: (1) quality assessment and improvement activities, including outcomes evaluation and development of clinical guidelines and protocols; (2) case management and care coordination; (3) contacting health care providers and patients with

information about treatment alternatives; (4) reviewing the competence or qualifications of health care professionals; (5) conducting training programs with students or trainees; (6) accreditation, certification, licensing, and credentialing activities; (7) conducting or arranging for medical review, legal services, and auditing functions, including fraud and abuse detection and compliance programs; (8) business planning and development, including cost-management and formulary development and administration; (9) customer service activities that do not result in disclosure of PHI; (10) resolution of internal grievances; (11) sale, transfer, merger, or consolidation of all or part of a covered entity with another covered entity or an entity that, following the transaction, will become a covered entity and the due diligence related to such a transaction; and (12) other similar business management and general administrative activities.

48. 45 C.F.R. § 164.506(b).
49. 45 C.F.R. § 164.501.
50. Privacy notices are discussed in detail under a later section of this chapter entitled "Individual Privacy Rights."
51. 45 C.F.R. § 164.520(c)(2).
52. 45 C.F.R. § 164.506(c)(2).
53. 45 C.F.R. § 164.506(c)(3).
54. 45 C.F.R. § 164.506(c)(4).
55. 45 C.F.R. § 164.512.
56. 45 C.F.R. § 164.512(a).
57. 45 C.F.R. § 164.512(b).
58. 45 C.F.R. § 164.512(c).
59. 45 C.F.R. § 164.512(d).
60. 45 C.F.R. § 164.512(e).
61. 45 C.F.R. § 164.512(f).
62. 45 C.F.R. § 164.512(g).
63. 45 C.F.R. § 164.512(h).
64. 45 C.F.R. § 164.512(i).
65. 45 C.F.R. § 164.512(j).
66. 45 C.F.R. § 164.512(k).
67. 45 C.F.R. § 164.512(l).
68. "Required by law" is defined at 45 C.F.R. § 164.103.
69. HIPAA's preemption provisions are discussed in more detail earlier in this chapter.
70. 45 C.F.R. § 164.512(c)(1) and (2).
71. See later for a detailed discussion of privacy rule requirements relating to business associates.
72. 45 C.F.R. § 164.512(e)(1)(iii) and (iv).
73. 45 C.F.R. § 164.512(e)(1)(v).
74. The requirements for accounting for certain disclosures are discussed in substantial detail later in the section entitled "Individual Privacy Rights."

Agencies that elect to obtain an authorization whenever possible rather than rely upon the public policy provisions of the privacy standards can minimize the administrative burden of the accounting requirement because PHI disclosures made pursuant to an authorization do not have to be logged in the required accountings.

75. See later for a detailed discussion of the privacy standards minimum necessary requirement.
76. 45 C.F.R. § 164.514(f).
77. 45 C.F.R. § 164.510.
78. 45 C.F.R. § 164.510(b)(2).
79. 45 C.F.R. § 164.510(b)(3).
80. 45 C.F.R. § 164.514(h).
81. 45 C.F.R. § 164.510(a).
82. Psychotherapy notes mean notes recorded "by a health care provider who is a mental health professional documenting or analyzing the contents of conversation during a private counseling session or a group, joint, or family counseling session and that are separated from the rest of the individual's medical record. Psychotherapy notes exclude medication prescription and monitoring, counseling session start and stop times, the modalities and frequencies of treatment furnished, results of clinical tests, and any summary of the following items: diagnosis, functional status, the treatment plan, symptoms, prognosis, and progress to date" 45 C.F.R. § 164.501.
83. The privacy standards do not address an agency's obligations to provide privacy notices, authorization forms, and so forth in languages other than English. Agencies should assume that they have the same obligations under the Civil Rights laws with respect to HIPAA forms as they do with other forms and patient communications.
84. 45 C.F.R. § 164.508.
85. If the patient initiated the authorization and does not wish to reveal the purpose of a requested release of PHI, it is sufficient for the authorization to state the purpose as "at the request of the individual." 45 C.F.R. § 164.508(c)(1)(iv).
86. The statement "end of the research study," "none," or similar language is sufficient if the authorization is for research that includes the creation and maintenance of a research database or repository. 45 C.F.R. § 164.508(c)(1)(v).
87. 45 C.F.R. § 164.502(g).
88. 67 *Fed. Reg.* 53181, 53189 (August 14, 2002).
89. 45 C.F.R. § 164.508(a)(3).
90. 45 C.F.R. § 164.501.
91. Agencies should be mindful of the fraud and abuse implications of such arrangements under federal and state anti-kickback statutes and should seek advice from competent legal counsel to ensure that arrange-

ments with vendors are structured to avoid undue risk.

92. 45 C.F.R. § 164.502(b)(1).

93. 45 C.F.R. § 164.502(b)(2).

94. 45 C.F.R. § 164.514(d).

95. 45 C.F.R. § 164.514(b)(3)(iii).

96. 45 C.F.R. § 164.502(a)(1)(iii).

97. See *OCR Guidance Explaining Significant Aspects of the Privacy Rule,* pp. 15–20 (Dec. 4, 2002) at *www.hhs.gov/ocr/hipaa/privacy.html.*

98. 45 C.F.R. § 164.504(e).

99. 67 *Fed. Reg.* 53181, 53264-66 (August 14, 2002).

100. 45 C.F.R. § 164.314.

101. 45 C.F.R. § 164.502(e)(1)(ii)(A).

102. 45 C.F.R. § 160.103.

103. 45 C.F.R. § 160.163.

104. 45 C.F.R. § 160.103.

105. 42 C.F.R. § 418.70.

106. 65 *Fed. Reg.* 82461, 82480 (Dec. 28, 2000).

107. 65 *Fed. Reg.* 82461, 82645 (Dec. 28, 2000).

108. See 42 C.F.R. § 484.14(f).

109. See 42 C.F.R. §§ 484.10(d) and 484.12(a).

110. 45 C.F.R. § 164.532(d).

111. 65 *Fed. Reg.* 82462, 82505 (Dec. 28, 2000).

112. 45 C.F.R. § 164.504(e)(1). See also *ORC Guidance Explaining Significant Aspects of the Privacy Rule,* pp. 33–53 (Dec. 4, 2002) at *www.hhs.gov/ocr/hipaa/privacy.html.*

113. 65 *Fed. Reg.* 824561, 82645 (Dec. 28, 2000).

114. DHHS has posted a form and other information for consumers about filing complaints on the World Wide Web at *www.hhs.gov/ocr/privacy/howtofile.htm.*

115. 45 C.F.R. § 164.520(a).

116. 45 C.F.R. § 164.520(b).

117. See *OCR Guidance Explaining Significant Aspects of the Privacy Rule,* pp. 103–113 (Dec. 4, 2002) at *www.hhs.gov.ocr/hipaa/privacy.html.*

118. 45 C.F.R. § 164.520(d).

119. 45 C.F.R. § 164.520(c)(2)(ii).

120. 45 C.F.R. § 164.520(c)(2)(i).

121. 45 C.F.R. § 164.520(c)(2)(iii).

122. 45 C.F.R. § 164.522(b)(3).

123. 45 C.F.R. § 164.520(c)(2)(iv).

124. 45 C.F.R. § 164.520(e).

125. 45 C.F.R. § 164.522(a)(1).

126. 45 C.F.R. § 164.522(a)(2).

127. 45 C.F.R. § 164.522(b).

128. 45 C.F.R. § 164.524.

129. 45 C.F.R. § 164.501.

130. Ibid.

131. Ibid.

132. 45 C.F.R. § 164.524(b)(2).

133. 45 C.F.R. § 164.524(a)(1). See also 42 U.S.C. § 263a and 42 C.F.R. 493(a)(2) for discussion of CLIA.

134. Only applicable to organizations that are part of a federal government department or agency.

135. 45 C.F.R. § 164.524(a)(2).

136. 45 C.F.R. § 164.524(a)(3).

137. 45 C.F.R. §§ 164.524(a)(4) and 164.524(d).

138. 45 C.F.R. § 164.524(e).

139. 45 C.F.R. §§ 164.524(b) and 164.524(c).

140. 45 C.F.R. § 164.524(c)(4)(i) and (ii).

141. 45 C.F.R. § 524(c)(2)(ii).

142. 45 C.F.R. § 164.524(c)(4)(iii).

143. 45 C.F.R. § 164.526(a)(1).

144. 45 C.F.R. § 164.526(a)(2)(i).

145. 45 C.F.R. § 164.526(c)(3).

146. 45 C.F.R. § 164.526(e).

147. 45 C.F.R. § 164.526(a)(2)(ii) and (iii).

148. 45 C.F.R. § 164.526(a)(2)(iv).

149. 45 C.F.R. § 164.526(b)(2).

150. 45 C.F.R. § 164.526(d).

151. 45 C.F.R. § 164.526(c).

152. 45 C.F.R. § 164.526(c)(3).

153. 45 C.F.R. § 164.528(a).

154. See 45 C.F.R. § 164.528(a)(2) for details.

155. See 45 C.F.R. § 512 and discussion earlier in this chapter on public policy disclosures.

156. 45 C.F.R. § 164.528(b)(1) and (2).

157. 45 C.F.R. § 164.528(b)(3) and (4).

158. 45 C.F.R. § 164.528(c)(2).

159. 45 C.F.R. § 164.528(d)(2).

160. 45 C.F.R. § 164.528(d)(3).

161. See earlier discussion on public policy disclosures for more details.

162. 45 C.F.R. § 164.528(i).

163. See earlier discussion on "Rights to a Notice of Privacy Practices" for more details.

164. 45 C.F.R. § 164.530(j).

165. 45 C.F.R. § 164.530(b).

166. 45 C.F.R. § 164.530(e).

167. 45 C.F.R. § 164.530(g).

168. 45 C.F.R. § 164.530(d).

169. 45 C.F.R. § 164.530(f).

170. 45 C.F.R. § 164.530(c).

171. 45 C.F.R. § 160.103 and 42 U.S.C. § 300gg-91(a)(2).

172. 45 C.F.R. § 160.103.

173. 45 C.F.R. § 160.504(f)(1).

174. 45 C.F.R. § 160.508(a)(2).

175. 45 C.F.R. § 160.504(f)(2) and (3).

176. 45 C.F.R. § 160.520(a)(2).

177. 45 C.F.R. § 160.520(c)(1).

178. 45 C.F.R. § 160.520(c)(1)(iii).

179. 45 C.F.R. § 160.103.

180. Pub. L. 104-91, 110 Stat. 1936, 2029 (codified at 42 U.S.C. §§ 1320d-5 and 1320d-6).

181. 42 U.S.C. § 1320d-5.

182. DHHS has published a proposed rule on enforcement procedures, but not substantive enforcement issues. 68 *Fed. Reg.* 18895 (April 17, 2003).

183. 42 U.S.C. § 1320d-6.

184. 42 U.S.C. § 1320d-5(b)(1).

CHAPTER 52

Ethical Practice in the Daily Service to Home Care Clients, Their Families, and the Community

Julie K. Tennant

First Quarter: No ethical issues reported.
Second Quarter: No ethical issues reported.
Third Quarter: No ethical issues reported.
Fourth Quarter: No ethical issues reported.
—*Professional Advisory Committee*
Annual Report

What this professional advisory committee is really saying is not that they have no ethical issues to address, but, rather, that they have not recognized and addressed any of the ethical issues that their company and clinicians have encountered.

GETTING EXCITED ABOUT BIOETHICS

Bioethics is more than the esoteric discussion of the moral play, it is real-life dilemmas that affect everyday decision making in home care.

Many times ethical issues are thought of as those life-and-death accounts printed in the newspapers: withdrawing life support from a brain-dead victim, discontinuing a feeding tube from a terminally ill client, or seeking treatment for children when parents wish to withhold it for religious reasons. However, in home care, because there is such a close relationship with the clients and their caregivers, the ethical issues encountered by clinicians are most frequently those of daily living and growing old. Can it really be true that the company reporting no ethical issues for an entire year heard none of the following statements discussed within its company, by its staff, or by family members?

"I think ethical issues in home care are about deciding if a feeding tube should be withdrawn from a terminally ill client or withdrawing life support from a lingering severely brain injured trauma victim. I don't see a patient falling repeatedly and insisting upon staying home with only the assistance of her elderly husband as an ethical issue."

Nurse manager in a home care company

"I don't know why I feel so compelled to keep visiting this lady. I have tried every method I know to ensure safe self-administration of her medications. I keep going to visit her even though I have so many other clients in need of my help."

Oncology nurse clinical specialist in a home care company

"We don't involve the client's family in ethical discussions. They aren't members of the health care team."

Ethics committee member in a home health company

"I can't decide which is best, visiting more often or using more expensive dressings."

Registered nurse providing care to a home health client

"We had a professional ethicist come to do an in-service last year. It was not interesting for the staff. We learned very little from her and I don't think our money was well spent."

Administrator in a home care company

"That daughter keeps pulling out her mother's urinary catheter. I think she really wants her to be in the hospital with a urinary tract infection."

Registered nurse providing care to a home care client

Each of these statements confirms the existence and the importance of ethics in managing home care. Behind each statement is an ethical dilemma confronting the speaker, a dilemma that needs to be investigated, addressed, and resolved in the planning and delivering of home care. Recognition of these dilemmas as ethical issues and discussion of possible resolutions may permit more effective treatment, may affect family support, may address life safety concerns, and may bring to light other situations that impact or sometimes undermine an effective care team plan. How the practitioner and the company address ethical issues is a clear indication of the completeness and adequacy of the care planning as a whole. It represents the difference between the excellent and the adequate.

As indicated in the real-life examples just noted, often the first step in addressing ethical issues is to recognize them. This requires both training and organizational support. The practitioner needs to have an understanding of bioethics, how it is defined, and how to recognize situations and issues that would benefit from investigation. Then the practitioner needs to have the willingness to address the issue, gather information, and bring that information to a bioethics advisory committee or other company organization to seek support, understanding, and resolution to the dilemma being confronted. Although the support organization is often in place in the form of a bioethics advisory committee or a professional advisory group, the ability to recognize ethical dilemmas

and the willingness to bring these dilemmas forward is frequently a shortcoming.

An excellent reference for teaching bioethics and developing an understanding of its elements can be found in *Principles of Biomedical Ethics* (Beauchamp and Childress, 2001) Now in its fifth edition, Beauchamp and Childress (2001) have provided what one of its critics, Gordon, describes as a ". . . reasonable and workable framework to help understand the factors that are often at play when ethical decision making is undertaken" (Gordon, 2002, p. 322). This framework, which Gordon alludes to, is built around four principles described by Beauchamp and Childress as (1) autonomy, (2) beneficence, (3) nonmaleficence, and (4) justice (Beauchamp and Childress, 2001). These four principles have been so widely accepted in the field of biomedical ethics that authors such as Gallagher and associates writing about ethical dilemmas in home care case management reference them only as " . . . four main themes in relation to ethical concerns and dilemmas" (Gallagher et al., 2002, p. 85). This broad acceptance is probably based upon the premise that use of these principles helps to bring down barriers to recognition and to bring understanding to the underlying ethical issues. As Gillon describes the four principles approach, " . . . it seems to cut across national, cultural, religious, political and philosophical divisions and to provide a common set of prima facie moral commitments, a common moral language and a common moral-analytic framework for biomedical ethics" (Gillon, 1995, p. 323). Clearly, from the real life examples given, there is a need within home care for such a common moral language and a way to recognize, understand, address, and have an impact on ethical issues that occur daily.

GETTING STARTED: THE FOUR PRINCIPLES APPROACH

Education with a goal of clear understanding of the Beauchamp and Childress (2001) framework and their four principles can be used as a foundation for an effective bioethics program. The first of these principles is autonomy.

Autonomy is self-rule or self-governance. Beauchamp and Childress expand on this to define the traits of the autonomous person ". . . which include capacities of self-governance, such as understanding, reasoning deliberating, and independent choosing" (Beauchamp and Childress, 2001, p. 58). The moral rules attached to this principle by the authors are (p. 65):

1. Tell the truth.
2. Respect the privacy of others.
3. Protect confidential information.
4. Obtain consent for interventions with patients.
5. When asked, help others make important decisions

A concept closely tied to autonomy in health and home care is competence in decision making. Beauchamp and Childress conclude that "patients or subjects are competent to make a decision if they have the capacity to understand the material information, to make a judgment about the information in light of their values, to intend a certain outcome, and to communicate freely their wishes to caregivers or investigators" (Beauchamp and Childress, 2001, p. 71). They qualify this definition by adding: "Sometimes a competent person who is generally able to select means appropriate to reach his or her goals will act incompetently in a particular circumstance" (Beauchamp and Childress, 2001, p. 71).

Consider the example given earlier involving the elderly couple. This is a real-life case in which the wife had, as reported by the home health aide, been to the hospital three times over the weekend because of falls. The client had suffered multiple cuts requiring suturing and bruises. The husband also reported that she had fallen several times in addition to the hospital trips and that he had struggled to get her back to the bed or chair. The client insisted each time that she wished to be home with her husband. Clearly, she was making an autonomous choice to remain in her own home. However, was she competent in this situation to intend a certain outcome and to select means appropriate to reach her goals? By insisting upon staying

home, was she really selecting the goals of safety and belonging with her familiar surroundings and with her husband? Were there other family members and were they aware of this couple's circumstance? Could the client's goals be reached by a safer means?

Nonmaleficence is the second principle. It is, simply stated, the " . . . obligation not to inflict harm on others" (Beauchamp and Childress, 2001, p. 113). Beauchamp and Childress further define this concept by stating, "The principle of nonmaleficence does not imply the maintenance of biological life, nor does it require the initiation or continuation of treatment without regard to the patient's pain, suffering, and discomfort" (Beauchamp and Childress, 2001, p. 135). The moral rules attached to this principle by the authors are (p. 117):

1. Do not kill.
2. Do not cause pain or suffering.
3. Do not incapacitate.
4. Do not cause offense.
5. Do not deprive others of the goods of life.

The case mentioned previously involving the oncology nurse clinical specialist was documented in the minutes of a home health company bioethics committee. The story that the nurse told about the client was that she had been asked by the client's case manager to visit and assess the client's pain and the effectiveness of her pain management. The client was 50+ years old, had a cancer diagnosis, lived alone in a garden apartment, had an estranged son living in the area, and had been an accountant involved in many community activities prior to her illness. The oncology nurse visited, and in consultation with the physician, instructed the client in some adjustments to her pain management regime. As a part of this instruction, the nurse assisted the patient in organizing her medications in a pill organizer.

She revisited 2 days later to check on the effectiveness of the changes and on the client's ability to manage her medication safely. The nurse found that the client reported no improvement in her pain and the carefully organized medications of 2 days ago were now all mixed up in a bowl in the bathroom. The client could not explain this and expressed a great need for this nurse to return. The nurse devised what she felt was truly a safe method for the safe self-administration of the medications and scheduled another appointment with the client. This specialty nurse was concerned that her frequent visits to this client were impacting her ability to visit other clients in need of her attention. She was also concerned that her advice about medication administration might lead to potential harm to the client.

She revisited. On this day, the client's medications were in a plastic bag in the freezer. The client had no explanation for this. The nurse suggested having the son or a neighbor involved in organizing the medications. The client insisted that she was capable of this with the nurse's help and refused to involve the others. The nurse revisited. This time she had to search for the medications and found them in a suitcase under the bed. The client had no explanation but felt with the nurse's help, she would be safe with her medications from this time forward. The nurse scheduled another appointment and asked to bring the case to the bioethics committee. She was out of ideas. The nurse's principle concern was that she had proposed a plan for use of a pill organizer and a change in the pain medicine regime that now appeared to be potentially harmful, because the patient was unable to follow the new plan, an issue of nonmaleficence.

As a member of the bioethics advisory committee, a home health aide asked the simple question, "Who else visits with this lady?" This home health aide understood what Gillett described in his essay on "Reasoning in Bioethics": " . . . intuitions . . . are grounded in relationships of belonging, being nurtured, loving, and being loved, which rank among the most important of the bases of human survival" (Gillett, 2003, p. 246). The committee asked the nurse if she observed any other signs of incapacity such as clothing warn in an unusual way. The answer was no. After a roundtable discussion, the committee suggested the nurse revisit and ask the client if she were rearranging her medications in order to influence the nurse to visit more frequently.

The nurse did this and the client's response was, "Of course, I was wondering how long it would take for you to figure it out." With the client's permission, a volunteer friendly visitor began coming to her home weekly. As with most attempts to identify an issue as specific to one ethical principle or another, this case involved the nurse's concern about causing the client no harm and it involved other principles that follow, as well.

The third principle is **beneficence**. Beneficence is best described in the New Testament parable of the Good Samaritan. Here the Good Samaritan met an injured man on the road to Jericho. He "had compassion, and went to him and bound up his wounds . . . brought him to an inn, and took care of him" (St. Luke, *NRSV* 10:30–36). This is what Beauchamp and Childress (2001) describe as positive beneficence: " . . . positive obligations to others" (p. 167). They divide beneficence into two principles: (1) positive beneficence and (2) utility. Utility is defined as requiring " . . . that agents balance benefits and drawbacks to produce the best overall results" (Beauchamp and Childress, 2001, p. 165). Their moral rules of obligation for beneficence are (p. 167):

1. Protect and defend the rights of others.
2. Prevent harm from occurring to others.
3. Remove conditions that will cause harm to others.
4. Help persons with disabilities.
5. Rescue persons in danger.

The everyday example of the nurse providing care to a home care client and trying to make a decision, in consultation with the physician, about which is best, visiting more frequently or using a more expensive treatment, is familiar to all involved in home care. This is daily practice of the ethical principle of utilitarian beneficence. Since the dominance of managed care and the introduction of the Medicare prospective payment system, clinical decision makers in home health are struggling with what Brock (2000) describes as problems for prioritization efforts in his discussion of the bioethics agenda. Advocates for a strong bioethics presence in home health-recognize the complexity of these decisions for clinicians and the need for a forum for discussion within a bioethics advisory committee.

Justice, or more specifically, distributive justice is the fourth principle described by Beauchamp and Childress. Distributive justice "refers to fair, equitable, and appropriate distribution determined by justified norms that structure the terms of social cooperation. Its scope includes policies that allot diverse benefits and burdens, such as property, resources, taxation, privileges, and opportunities" (Beauchamp and Childress, 2001, p. 226). The authors suggest the following as valid material principles of distributive justice (p. 228):

1. To each person an equal share
2. To each person according to need
3. To each person according to effort
4. To each person according to contribution
5. To each person according to merit
6. To each person according to free-market exchanges.

"That daughter keeps pulling out her mother's urinary catheter. I think she really wants her to be in the hospital with a urinary tract infection." This was a comment the author heard while knocking on the door of a client and her daughter's home during an observation visit. Entering the home, it was obvious that the 50-year-old daughter was angry with the nurse. The daughter explained that her mother had been uncomfortable early in the morning and she (the daughter) could not irrigate the catheter. She had decided to remove the catheter rather than have her mother remain uncomfortable. The nurse responded by saying that this had happened several times in the past and that every effort had been made to emphasize the need for the daughter to call the nurse when the catheter became occluded.

While the nurse was preparing for her visit and procedures, the author took the opportunity to speak with the daughter. It was revealed that this daughter had sole responsibility for her mother's care for over 4 years. When asked what she did for fun, the daughter said, "I never have any fun." Asked about family support, she said, "I have three brothers around here and one who lives in another state." When asked if her brothers helped with her mother's care, she said, "No, they would never think of it." Asked if she had thought of requesting their help, she said, "No, but I told one he didn't have to go fishing so often." It seems that Jecker (2002) writing about justice and family care giving was writing about this overwhelmed daughter. In her paper, Jecker talks about the duty of justice to act as the caregivers for frail, elderly parents and how this burden of care giving falls disproportionately on women (Jecker, 2002, p. 121):

> Surely there is something wrong with this picture. . . . The language of justice and rights . . . bears relevance to the family in at least two distinct ways. First, justice divides the burdens of caring fairly among family members. It rejects imposing burdens disproportionately on one group within the family. Second, justice protects personal projects and plans central to people's lives and identities. It establishes moral limits to infringing on activities that impart crucial meaning to individuals' lives or constitute a central part of individuals' identities.

The nurse did not realize that this daughter had had no relief from the burden of care giving for 4 years, and she did not realize the impact this had on the success of her plan for the client's care. Taking this case to a bioethics committee meeting with the goal of complete and accurate care planning could make the difference between excellent and merely adequate home care.

GETTING EDUCATED: A WORLD OF RESOURCES

It seems improbable that a home care company can serve clients for an entire year without encountering an overwhelmed caregiver, an elderly couple trying to remain independent long after it is safe to do so, or professional staff working to decide where to focus their efforts. Clearly, recognition of an ethical dilemma seems to be the beginning of the ethics process for home care.

Recognition demands education. In the real-life examples referenced here, the administrator did not feel the professional ethicist had given her staff the information they needed to be effective in recognizing ethical dilemmas. Professional ethicists can be an effective source of information to a home care company. They introduce the vocabulary of ethics and provide a framework for analyzing dilemmas. They empower the staff to share their stories of concern about their practice and their clients. They provide the company with advice about structuring policies related to bioethics and forming a bioethics advisory committee, and they can serve as an ongoing professional resource.

Other educational resources include university bioethics centers and ethics networks. Home care companies can contract with universities for student ethicists just as they contract for student nurses, therapists, and pharmacists. Universities can also serve as a resource for employees seeking more information about bioethics, and their libraries and classes can provide up-to-date information to bioethics committees.

There are ethics networks for more than a dozen states and more than 20 regional and metropolitan areas of the United States. They can be located by accessing the World Wide Web. The networks serve to bring information about bioethics from the region to the reader. One Internet search engine lists 9,052 individual resources when searching for bioethics networks. Among these are invaluable resources such as the Joseph and Rose Kennedy Institute of Ethics at Georgetown University in Washington, D.C. These resources can provide a form of continuing education to members of a bioethics committee and to clinicians serving patients. Examples of articles that can be obtained through these and other Internet resources include "Taking Care of One's Own: Justice and

Family Care Giving" by Jecker (2002); "Ethical Challenges in End-of-Life Therapies in the Elderly" by Gordon (2002); and "Ethical Dilemmas in Home Care Case Management" by Gallagher et al. (2002).

GETTING STARTED: THE BIOETHICS ADVISORY COMMITTEE

The work of the bioethics advisory committee begins with the creation of its philosophy, purpose statement, and bylaws. Home care companies may decide to form a separate entity with the sole purpose of addressing ethical issues or may include this function in the work of a professional advisory committee.

The philosophy statement of a bioethics advisory committee is a focused reflection of the company's general philosophy or mission statement. Companies may have an egalitarian view in which it is recognized that everyone should receive an equal distribution of health care. They may hold a utilitarian or consequence-based view, which believes that the right act is the one that produces the best overall result, with equal consideration given to all of the persons or groups involved. Other companies may subscribe to the libertarian view, accepting that distribution of health care is best left to the free market (Beauchamp and Childress, 2001).

Included in the philosophy statement may be the scope of responsibility of the committee. It may focus the committee solely on ethical dilemmas in patient care. It may include professional ethics or the professional obligations of providers. The company may wish to extend the work of the advisory committee to include business ethics, although this is less common. However, many companies include in their philosophy statements a charge to consider the relevant needs and interests of the company and of society at large.

The purpose guidelines for bioethics advisory committees outline the group's functions and almost universally emphasize an advisory focus. Groups usually have their work directed toward providing a forum for discussion of ethical dilemmas presented by clinicians and by clients and their families. Emphasis may also be given to providing support, guidance, and affirmation to clinicians, clients, and families.

Bioethics advisory committees are frequently charged with advising the company in the development of new policies and in the review of existing policies. Examples of policies reviewed with a focus on bioethics include informed consent, assessment of patient decision-making capacity, clinician safety, do-not-resuscitate orders, uncompensated care, research participation, client rights and responsibilities, and corporate or organizational compliance.

Members of the bioethics advisory group have the responsibility to educate themselves, staff members, clients and their families, and the community concerning bioethical issues. They serve as an expert resource on the topic of bioethics for these groups. As previously reviewed, the source of the committee member education can be a professional ethicist, a university ethics center, or an agent within the company acting as a trainer with the support of printed materials.

The structure of a bioethics advisory committee varies with the organization. Membership representing the full scope of services of the organization, a community member, clergy, and administration can provide insightful depth and balance of understanding for complex bioethical issues. The case involving the oncology clinical nurse specialist reviewed earlier demonstrated that the home health aide was an invaluable member of the bioethics committee. She brought to this committee's deliberations cultural, economic, and social diversity. The community and clergy members serve to remind the clinical members that the client is a member of a family and a community.

Members usually serve a 2-year term with an option to serve another term. Attendance and educational requirements are outlined in the policy. They may include one out-of-company educational experience annually or participation at a bioethics network meeting and regular attendance at committee meetings. Members are generally appointed by the committee chair using as a guide open positions within the committee, with an eye on keeping representation from the organization balanced and upon interests of the individual.

Selection of the committee chair may be based upon educational preparation, experience, willingness to serve, and availability. The chair is generally appointed by administration and serves one term. Continuing education requirements for the chair usually exceed those of members, requiring attendance at additional seminars, network meetings, and the like. The chair's responsibilities include developing the meeting agenda, notifying members of meetings, distribution of educational materials and opportunities to members, and documenting the work of the committee. The chair also serves as an ambassador for the committee, getting the word out and building trust among company members in the advisory function of the bioethics committee.

Meetings are regularly scheduled, monthly or more frequently if needed, with additional opportunities for emergency consultation. Regular monthly meetings may include an educational component and a case presentation. Examples of educational presentations include religious perspectives on bioethical decisions, creating an ethical practice environment, and balancing client need and resources. Members or outside speakers can provide the committee with these and other educational experiences.

Case presentation begins with case finding. As with our earlier examples, clinicians and their leaders may not recognize an ethical dilemma within a case. A key to success in case finding is balanced representation from the entire company on the bioethics advisory committee. Advisory committee members hear hallway conversations, participate in case conferences, conduct record reviews, and collaborate in care planning. They can help colleagues identify ethical dilemmas and encourage them to bring a case to the advisory committee. Frequently, clinicians are reluctant to bring their case to an advisory committee because they fear they do not know the language of bioethics or they may be found negligent by a group of their peers in their management of a case.

Clinicians can receive guidance for their case presentations from the committee chair or members. Clients' names or identifiers are removed from any written or spoken communications, allowing complete confidentiality. They can be identified as Mr. X or Mrs. Y. The clinician is asked to tell the story of the client including a brief medical history and the plan of care, the client's view, the family's view, and his or her view of the dilemma. There is no need for the clinician to identify the ethical issue as one of justice, beneficence, nonmaleficence, or autonomy. As has been demonstrated from our review of cases, these are infrequently isolated issues. Cases usually involve more than one dilemma such as balancing the client's right to choose with available resources or the need to do the right thing for the client and not overburden the family caregivers. Frequently, clinicians who have presented a case more than once to a bioethics advisory committee seek to identify the ethical dilemmas involved and to learn the language of bioethics.

Planned ethical consultations involving the entire membership of the committee can follow a prescribed format. A clinician, client, or family member may present cases. This may include a written profile of the case together with an oral presentation by the individual bringing the case. Following this, members of the committee may seek clarification from the presenter and will engage in discussion of the situation. They will bring the discussion to a focus on the ethical dilemmas, usually seeking to place them within the structure of the four principles approach. Following this, the committee will discuss with the presenter possible resolutions to the dilemma, keeping in mind the charge to support and affirm the clinician. Ethics advisory committees usually adhere to the "two-cents rule": everyone gets the opportunity to put their "two cents worth" of input into the conversation. This allows each member of the advisory committee a formal opportunity to contribute to the discussion of the dilemma and of possible resolutions. Using this rule ensures that a broad representation of opinions are heard. The goal of a planned ethical consultation is to provide the care team members, client, and family with possible resolutions to identifiable ethical dilemmas and to affirm the work of the care team members and the contributions of the client and the family. Follow-up to a consultation may include a written summary of the response of the client and family to an offered solution to the dilemma.

Emergency consultations involve case situations that cannot wait for a regularly scheduled meeting of the bioethics advisory committee. The elderly lady living with her husband and in danger of further injuring herself from falls is an example, mentioned earlier, of a case in need of emergency consultation. This consultation would most likely involve the clinician, three to four advisory committee members that included the chair or an administrator, the client's physician, the client and her husband, and their extended family, if possible, all with the client's permission. The consultation would probably take place in the client's home. Identifying a consultation as an emergency consultation is usually the responsibility of the committee chair or an administrator familiar with the work of the bioethics advisory committee.

GETTING THE WORD OUT: BUILDING TRUST

As with anything else of value, building trust in the work of a bioethics advisory committee takes time. It requires solid education of the committee members, expert guidance of the chair, commitment of the organization, and assignment of value by participants. With each case consultation, the word will go out that the client, their family, and the care team benefited from interaction with the advisory committee. One of the most frequently heard comments by clinicians following a presentation to an advisory committee is: "I don't know why I waited so long to bring this case to this committee!" This is affirmation that the bioethics advisory committee has had an impact on the care of clients, the support of clinicians, and the work of the client's family and the community.

SUMMARY

The attention to bioethics within a home care company is required by accrediting bodies such as the Community Health Accreditation Program and The Joint Commission on Accreditation for Healthcare Organizations and by the Medicare Conditions of Participation. How a home care company defines this attention to ethical practice has been the focus of this chapter. Using the "four principles approach" authored by Beauchamp and Childress, a framework for studying and applying the principles of bioethics has been presented. These principles include autonomy, beneficence, nonmaleficence, and justice. Each principle has been defined using a real-life case example. These examples are intentionally not those of life-and-death situations, but rather, everyday occurrences in home health care. They are meant to emphasize the importance of ethical practice in the care of every client by every clinician every day. They are also intended to enhance awareness among home health administrators of the importance of committing resources to the development of bioethics advisory committees, to educating committee members and care team members in identification of bioethical dilemmas, and to including the community in the process.

Specifics involving the development of a bioethics advisory program have been presented. These include the focused philosophy of a bioethics program as an extension of the philosophy of the total organization; the bylaws, membership, and structure of a bioethics advisory committee; and the format for planned ethical consultation and emergency consultation. Attention has been given to educating committee members and company employees on the importance of bioethics, the identification of bioethical issues, and case finding. The goal of this chapter reflects the goal of a planned bioethical case consultation; that is, to " . . . provide the care team members, client, and family with possible resolutions to identifiable ethical dilemmas and to affirm the work of the care team and the contributions of the client and the family."

REFERENCES

Beauchamp, T. L., and J. F. Childress. 2001. *Principles of biomedical ethics* (5th ed.). New York: Oxford University Press.

Brock, D. 2000. Broadening the bioethics agenda. *Kennedy Institute of Ethics Journal* 10(1): 21–38.

Gallagher, E., D. Alcock, E. Diem, D. Angus, and J. Medves. 2002. Ethical dilemmas in home care case management. *Journal of Healthcare Management* 47(2): 85–97.

Gillett, G. 2003. Reasoning in bioethics. *Bioethics* 17(3): 243–260.

Gillon, R. 1995, Dec. Defending "the four principles" approach to biomedical ethics. *Journal of Medical Ethics* 21(6): 323–325.

Gordon, M. 2002. Ethical challenges in end-of-life therapies in the elderly. *Drugs Aging 2002* 19(5): 321–329.

Jecker, N. 2002. Taking care of one's own: Justice and family care giving. *Theoretical Medicine* 23: 117– 133

New Revised Standard Version Bible. 1989. Division of Christian Education of the National Churches of Christ in the U.S.A.

CHAPTER 53

Participating in the Political Process

Kathleen Carlson Mebus and Barbara Kovalcin Piskor

Government's influence on professional practice, quality health care, and agency administration increases with each passing year. Federal, state, and local laws and regulations impact the day-to-day operations of your agency. Examples abound from federal Medicare legislation that is important for home health reimbursement to state laws that govern licensure of agencies and discipline-specific practice, to local zoning ordinances that may regulate building occupancy and biohazard disposal. Knowledge of these statutory and regulatory mandates is crucial. It is also crucial to know how to influence statutory and regulatory decision making.

The effective home health administrator needs to develop positive relationships with political leaders at all levels of government and have, at least, a basic knowledge of law making (legislative branch of government), law enforcement (executive branch of government), and law interpretation (judicial branch of government). Laws, regulations, and judicial decisions are the elements of public policy, some of which can be influenced by interest groups (Kingdon, 1995). This chapter will present information on the political process so that the home health administrator can communicate effectively and strategically with leaders who develop legislation, promulgate regulations, and make judicial decisions.

Revolutionary changes have occurred in health care delivery in recent years. Modified reimbursement mechanisms, increased con-

sumer expectations, and workforce shortages have converged to require astute, quick responses including legislative action. From a professional and organizational perspective, an administrator has the responsibility to participate in the political process—proactively and reactively.

Proactive behavior includes:

- Registering to vote and voting
- Networking with colleagues
- Gaining knowledge
- Building relationships with legislative leaders

Reactive behavior includes:

- Individual and group response to proposed legislation
- Litigation/judicial decisions
- Political action

PROACTIVE BEHAVIOR

Registering to Vote and Voting

One of your most important proactive behaviors is to register to vote *and* to vote. Voter registration became easier when Congress enacted the National Voter Registration Act of 1993 (also known as the NVRA and the Motor Voter Act), 42 U.S.C. 1973gg-5(a), (b). The NVRA was enacted "to enhance voting opportunities for every American and to remove the vestiges of discrimination which have historically resulted in lower voter registration rates of minorities and persons with disabilities. The NVRA has brought new voices to the political process by making it easier for all Americans to exercise their fundamental right to vote." States now use their motor vehicle and drivers' license system, mail-in registration forms, as well as, in some states, the Internet for voter registration. To investigate voter registration further, contact the state entity charged with election activities. In many local areas, county boards of elections are charged with this responsibility. Additionally, there is a national database called VOTE SMART that can be accessed for information on each state. Contact it via the World Wide Web at http://www.vote-smart.org or phone 1.888.VOTE-SMART. Project Vote Smart is a nonpartisan, nonprofit organization devoted to providing information on voting, issues, and candidates.

A voter has special standing in a legislator's district. They are the power that puts elected officials into office and can likewise remove them from office. As a result, elected officials are dependant on voters for their continued privilege to hold office. It is important to note that voting records are public information and show whether you voted in a particular election, but not how you voted. Although elected officials represent everyone living in a defined population, they listen first to active voters. You can compare voters and nonvoters to members of an organization. Those who are members influence the policies that are established even though the outcome benefits a larger population. Those who are nonmembers may benefit from the ultimate outcome, but they have no voice in developing and implementing the agenda.

Encouraging voter registration and voting among your staff and consumers is also important. Voter registration campaigns promote good citizenship and do not jeopardize the tax-exempt status of 501(c)(3) organizations. The registration campaign cannot be linked to voting for particular candidates; it must be nonpartisan. Many agencies include voter registration information in newsletters that are read by staff and consumers. "How to obtain an absentee ballot" makes for an interesting article and can be particularly relevant for homebound consumers. There is nothing more effective than including the statement "I am a registered voter in your district" when writing to legislators.

As a first step, you should learn the names of federal, state, and local officials where you live and the names of those who represent the service area of the agency. Simply providing ZIP code information or telephone number at the VOTE SMART Web site will yield state and federal legislators' names as well as relevant contact information.

Networking with Colleagues

When a legislative crisis at local, state, or federal levels threatens access to care, action must be taken immediately to protect the ability of health care providers to deliver services. There is no time to search out political allies when legislative or regulatory actions are pressing. Home health administrators, therefore, should develop active networks of support before crisis situations evolve.

Trade and professional organizations undertake the constant scanning of the political environment essential to influencing the political process as well as understanding the bigger picture. Membership in your professional organization and/or trade association is the best way for you to routinely obtain health care legislative information, to quickly network with other home health administrators, and to influence public policy. Most of these organizations dedicate staff to reviewing, analyzing, and monitoring legislative action and most identify government relations as a priority activity. Organizations relay useful information to their members via newsletters, journals, and Web sites.

Lobbying activity by members of a group, commonly referred to as advocacy efforts by nonprofit organizations, is often referred to as "grassroots lobbying." There are two definitions one must take into account when lobbying for 501(c)(3) agencies or organizations. The Federal

Tax Code definition of grassroots lobbying activities and the lobbying activities of a membership group as a whole are different. The Federal Tax Code, 42 U.S.C. § 4911(d)(1)(A), defines grassroots lobbying as "any attempt to influence any legislation through an attempt to affect the opinions of the general public or a segment thereof." In the exception list, however, it notes that influencing legislation with respect to an organization does not include communication between the organization and its bona fide members with respect to legislation or proposed legislation. Lobbying activities must also be germane to the accomplishment of the organization's exempt purpose. "Grassroots" is the term professional and trade organizations use when referring to their membership. It is important to remember the differences because a tax-exempt entity can lose exempt status by using the public to lobby for its issue. There are fewer restrictions on lobbying activities than political activities allowed and disallowed for tax-exempt entities. For further information you can contact your legal counsel or accountant as well as http://www.not-for-profit.org, http://www.independentsector.org, and http://www.irs.gov/charities.

Every home health administrator eventually becomes a grassroots lobbyist from the perspective of lobbying through a professional trade or membership organization or by the agency director and the employees advocating at the local level of health care policy making. In either case, learning the fine points from experienced colleagues is helpful. You can also take advantage of mentoring programs offered by professional and/or trade organizations. Additionally, there are workshops at state and national meetings, lobbying skills seminars, guides to state legislative lobbying, and workbooks available from firms specializing in training the neophyte. With the host of resources available lobbying becomes second nature with little effort.

Participation in coalitions is one technique common to the lobbying community. Coalitions are made up of dissimilar organizations acting together to address a common issue. This requires organizations and individuals to put aside their differences while work is focused on one theme only. Success requires a basic set of guiding principles that all participants agree will direct the activities of the group and level-headed discussions to keep the process moving until the goal is reached. Coalitions are most effective when they are short lived, focused, and energetic. The differing interests of the coalition members provide a broad base of support by increasing visibility and awareness beyond what a single organization can provide.

Gaining Knowledge

Home health administrators stay current because their day-to-day work includes reading provider bulletins, journals, newsletters, and trade publications whose primary focus is to report changes in provider responsibilities, clinical updates, quality, and efficiency. It is also necessary, however, to supplement this reading with public policy focused material. Although the federal government and each state have developed Web sites that include links to proposed legislation and basic information about the legislative process, these sources do not provide the political implications of the proposals. Accessing legislative and regulatory information is not difficult; reducing it to proportions that are meaningful to your responsibilities as an agency leader, however, can be overwhelming.

Most professional and trade organizations serve this purpose by filtering the abundant material to prevent overload and perusal of unnecessary information. Of utmost importance is the analysis of proposals and their impact on the industry. Information about legislative issues and arguments for or against particular proposals also can be found in newsletters written specifically to address upcoming legislative activity, in dedicated sections of trade and professional journals, and on Web sites for trade and professional organizations. Educational institutions, political parties, and foundations are other sources that can be easily accessed on the Internet (Exhibit 53–1).

Exhibit 53–1 Quick Reference Contact Information

INFORMATION	CONTACT	DESCRIPTION
State-based legislation, legislators, and legislative process	**Examples:** **http://www.legis.state.(Insert State Postal abbrev.).us;** **http://www.legis.state.ga.us** **http://www.legis.state.pa.us**	Most states use a variation on this Web address. Examples are for Georgia and Pennsylvania.
Federal legislation/bills, members, and process	**http://www.house.gov** **http://www.senate.gov**	U.S. House of Representatives U.S. Senate Having the specific number of a bill is helpful in a search.
Federal legislation	**http://thomas.loc.gov**	Key reference on bills, voting records, and committees.
Voting, presidential candidates, key votes, legislator contact information	**http://www.vote-smart.org** **1.888.VOTE-SMART** **(1.888.868.3762)**	Project Vote Smart . A nonprofit, nonpartisan organization.
Local, state, and federal issues with local contacts	**http://www.lwv.org**	League of Women Voters. A nonprofit, nonpartisan organization.
Proposed/final regulations, government publications	**http://www.access.gpo.gov** **http://www.pabulletin.com**	*Federal Register, Congressional Record* Similar publications for state legislative activities.
Gateway to governmental information including federal, state, local, and tribal agencies	**http://www.firstgov.gov** **http://www.whitehouse.gov**	Federal government's official Web portal.
Public policy	**Examples:** **http://www.urban.org** **http://www.heathpolicy.ucla.edu**	Urban Institute University of California, Los Angeles
Practice issues with legislative links	**Examples:** **http://www.nursingworld.org** **http://www.apta.org** **http://www.aota.org**	Professional organizations such as American Nurses Association, American Physical Therapy Association, American Occupational Therapy Association
State-specific issues with some federal content and/or links	**Examples:** **http://www.pahomecare.org** **http://www.tahc.org**	Trade organizations such as Pennsylvania Homecare Association, Texas Association for Home Care
General federal contact information	**1.202.224.3121**	U.S. Capitol switchboard
Selected governmental agencies	**http://www.hhs.gov** **http://www.cdc.gov** **http://www.nih.gov**	Health and Human Services, Centers for Disease Control and Prevention, National Institutes of Health

Search engines such as http://www.google.com and http://www.yahoo.com are extremely helpful. A brief descriptor will identify many resources with direct links to the document.

A hard copy of federal legislation and proposed regulations can be secured through your legislator or by writing/calling:

Senate Document Room	House Document Room
SH-B04 Hart Senate Office Building	H2-B18 HOB Annex II
Washington, DC 20510	Washington, DC 20515
Phone: 1.202.224.7860	Phone: 1.202.226.5200

Similar resources are available from each state, though many jurisdictions are referring callers to Internet sources.

Understanding the Legislative Process

Another step in the development of political and legislative awareness is to learn or review where legislative decision making occurs and the timing of votes. Knowing the difference in this process among the various levels of government is important. If you understand the process, you can take appropriate and quick action. For example, after months of inaction on a particular bill, reaction may be required within 24 hours. Your interest and participation in this process can influence the outcomes of decisions that affect public policy for the entire population of a state or nation.

Local Government

Depending on the nature of your agency's services, local government may be your primary focus. For example, when an agency serves more than one county, you might find a county with its own health department reluctant to provide financial support to an outside visiting nurse association. On the other hand, another county may find it less costly to support community agencies delivering health care services and provide funding for specific programs.

Political subdivisions such as townships or wards are concerned about accessibility of public buildings by the handicapped, low-income housing, or transportation of the elderly. Whatever the subject, involvement with groups studying issues that impact other areas of health care identifies the home health administrator as a citizen concerned for the total health of the community. Some communities have community health partnerships where business and others join forces to understand the community's needs and develop plans to address the most pressing needs. Such issues bear a direct relationship to problems faced by home health agency clientele. Your agency may be targeted to solve a particular problem and your input during the planning stages helps the community understand the limits of your resources.

One approach to increasing your visibility at the local level is to host or sponsor joint luncheons or affairs for county commissioners and state or federal legislators. Although the emphasis may be national issues or state issues, the local impact of such meetings is of great importance. County officials frequently take advantage of these forums to raise pertinent questions on your behalf. Additionally, this provides legislators who sponsor health care proposals the opportunity to explain their legislation and update the group on any pending action. An occasion such as this can reinforce the legislators' involvement in and support of health care issues. The legislator not only provides the public with information, but also is viewed by colleagues as a knowledgeable resource on health care. If your agency is sponsoring the event, remember to showcase the issue rather than the legislator to avoid the appearance of partisan politics.

It should be apparent after interacting with elected officials that your issues and their issues may not share the same priority. The home health administrator needs to investigate an elected official's special interests to develop creative attention-getting approaches for health issues. For example, if an elected official is concerned about a segment of the population, perhaps an underserved minority, place emphasis on how proposed legislation will affect that group. By arranging to have your elected official accompany your staff on a home visit, you can create a graphic impression of the legislation's impact.

How often your agency is asked to participate in county-appointed task forces or study groups is a gauge for evaluating your effectiveness in a community's political process. You will be one of the first invited if you have been accepted as a knowledgeable and politically astute individual who has an investment in the community.

States and Federal Government

All 50 states have an established process for creating laws. The constitution of the state outlines the required steps to introduce, consider, and pass legislation. Each state has its own distinct system of checks and balances to protect the individual rights of its citizens. You can usually obtain pamphlets outlining your state's system from your elected state officials or by accessing this information on states' Web sites. The federal government has Web sites for the House and Senate that include the basic legislative process for Congress. Although it is not necessary to learn all the intricate maneuvers, it is important to understand the time elements and processes involved in passing legislation. For example, the committee that the bill is referred to can be crucial to its success. Your communication with the chairperson of the committee and its members can be as influential as your contacts with your legislator.

In any given legislative session, more proposals are developed than any one person or special interest group can follow. Several thousand bills are introduced in the House of Representatives and Senate each year. These bills address many subject areas such as taxes, appropriations, licensing laws, access to health care, sunset of government agencies, insurance changes, and health care reform. When issues arise that affect your special interest, you need to understand what prompted a legislative proposal. The background information you need about a particular piece of legislation can usually be obtained from a professional or trade association. You can alert the legislator of your interest by asking for a copy of the bill or research a state's Web site that has direct links for copies of legislation. However, before you communicate a position, try to anticipate the legislator or staff's questions and be prepared to answer them or offer to obtain the information they need. Once again, follow-up is essential.

Your role in the legislative process as a member of a trade or professional organization is to follow through with association directives for legislative action. Your role as the director of an agency is to seek ways to protect or further your agency's interests. Occasionally, an association position does not meet your agency's needs. When this situation occurs, contact your professional or trade association to make sure you understand its position. Associations frequently evaluate legislation based on the broadest application of a proposal to its entire membership. If, in your judgment, you cannot support the association's position, do not take any action unless the position specifically jeopardizes your agency. It is imperative that you work through your association, not your legislator, to resolve any differences. Dissension in a group is certain death to a proposal. Work with people who have the same interests as you and are willing to listen to your views.

Regulatory Process

Most laws, once enacted, have implementation and enforcement provisions vested in a state authority, the executive branch of government. Enacted legislation rarely has the specifics needed to guide its implementation (Longest, 1996). Rules and regulations are subsequently promulgated to outline how the government will implement and enforce the law. From your experience with Medicare Conditions of Participation, state regulations governing licensure laws, and Occupational Safety and Health Administration (OSHA) blood-borne pathogen regulations, to name a few, you can see how regulations influence care delivery on a day-to-day basis.

State governments have various methods for proposing these rules. Some follow an orderly process; others have no specific requirements. In a few states, regulations are merely guidelines, but in others, they carry legal implications. Regulations may affect the delivery of home health services to a greater extent than the original law; therefore, determine what legal standing regulations have in your state. This determination directs your next course of action. Whether you provide written comments, appear before a regulatory agency or seek court action you need to understand the process.

Frequently, the regulatory process provides for public input. If so, this is an excellent opportunity for you, as a provider, to influence how government oversees the health care delivery system. You can exert influence by actively responding when given the opportunity to see draft language in advance or through participation in advisory groups sharing their expertise on how the regulations would affect their environment. Once again, start with statewide trade or professional organizations if you are affiliated with one that regularly follows legislative and regulatory activities. Significant groundwork and legal opinions may already have been obtained. If, on the other hand, you find that little or no work has been accomplished by these organizations, volunteer to serve on a committee to address the regulatory issue. You can also offer to serve as a resource to the regulating agency because of your expertise in the area being regulated. If public comments are requested, respond within the required deadline and send copies to your legislators. Legislators can sometimes be influential with the agency issuing the regulations. Also send copies of all correspondence to your national or state organizations to assist the associations in monitoring how much membership activity is taking place.

If you are not affiliated with an organization or your issue is not a priority for that organization, network with others who share your concerns. A quality document can be produced for submission to the regulating agency by group effort. Although it is usually beneficial for administrators to respond individually, there are times when a group effort has greater impact. Coalitions can be as important in the regulatory process as in the legislative process.

As an individual, you can apply the same strategies used by national and state associations. By contacting the government agency or the individual within the agency who is responsible for issuing the regulations, you can express your interest in the development of the regulations. You may have the opportunity to affect the early draft of the regulations. Some government agencies, however, prefer no outside involvement until an initial draft has been prepared, although written recommendations with a rationale prior to publication may be appreciated and cause the agency to consider the practicality of the rule. When public input is sought, you should respond with documentation supporting your position.

Building Relationships with Legislative Leaders

Personal Contact

In assessing the political environment, the home health administrator should strive to identify who influences decision making within the local community and the state legislature. Developing lasting relationships with these key political figures is paramount. Your goal is to know the legislators and be known by them. Relationships at the federal level are more difficult because of the large constituency each congressperson and senator represents, and local congressional offices may not be convenient to your location. It is important to communicate with all officials periodically, however, because you may need their help. Use your agency board members to identify key political players within the community. Board members, through past community activities, may already have relationships with politicians. By involving board members and/or professional advisory committee members, you not only save time, but also increase their involvement in problem solving for the agency. Agency staff can also be helpful in identifying which politicians have been helpful in the past.

Office Visits

Once you have identified your elected officials, make your initial contact via a letter of introduction. Next, make an appointment to visit their local office. This may seem daunting, but in fact it is easily accomplished by simply calling their office. Prior to your first meeting, take the opportunity to send a letter introducing yourself as the agency director. If possible, investigate their voting record on health issues and their committee membership.

While visiting the legislator, a short presentation about your agency, its mission, and the service area it covers gives you an entree to find out how the legislator makes decisions about health care and who they use as resources when they have a question about health care. Many legislators have family members who themselves are health care professionals. This may not be to your advantage because the legislator will rely on them for information. Where a legislator gets health care information is important for you to know. This knowledge gives you a clue for how to approach issues in the future.

Don't be disappointed if your meeting is not with the legislator. Many legislators have key staff members who assist with health care issues, and meetings with them can be just as beneficial. Always treat the staff with the same courtesy that you would extend to the policymaker. You are dependant on staff for access in the future.

Your legislator probably serves on several committees. Issues that come before these committees are of particular interest to him or her. Because legislators focus on committee responsibilities, it is impossible for them to be experts in every field, but the expectation is that they will have information available to them. You can volunteer to become their home health resource. You may be uncomfortable at the first visit, but you are likely to find a responsive legislator who knows that health care affects every constituent. Follow-up on your part is essential to developing a meaningful relationship. Being recognized by the legislator and the staff as someone who benefits their constituency and likewise benefits them makes them more likely to respond when you need help. Ask if a staff member handles health care issues. If so, that person becomes your conduit.

A follow-up thank you to the legislator and the staff member is not only gracious, but also keeps your name and home health on their radar screen. Some additional hints:

- Maintain regular contact with your legislator and his or her office. Routine communication builds rapport.
- Place officials and staff on your mailing list for a newsletter or periodically send them event news from your agency.
- Offer the legislator an opportunity to spend a "day with staff" making home visits to his constituents. This makes home health tangible for legislators and increases their understanding of your environment.
- Provide a photo opportunity with publication in your newsletter. This is a way to showcase your elected official's involvement with the agency.

These activities create a positive framework from which to continue contacts with legislators. When you write or call about an urgent vote or ask them to sponsor a specific bill, they will remember your efforts. Get to know legislators by finding others who have had experience with them. Share your initial reactions but reserve judgment until you compare your experiences to theirs. Ask how others have been successful in their encounters.

There are opportunities to meet legislators at any function where elected officials are present such as local chamber of commerce meetings, ribbon-cutting ceremonies, and town meetings. Make every effort to be introduced by someone who is known to the legislator. This contact becomes a bridge for later communications. The key is to develop a lasting relationship with the legislator. You may have an occasion to meet the legislator at a social function. By all means take advantage of the opportunity to be introduced by the host or hostess. A short note acknowledging the introduction should follow. Follow-up builds recognition. You don't want to miss opportunities to advance your position the next time you see the legislator because he or she is not familiar with your name.

Capitol Visits

Visits to legislators' home offices are usually in a relaxed atmosphere with attentive staff. A visit to the capitol, in your state or in Washington, D.C., is valuable. You are able to see, first hand, legislative and political processes in play. The staff is different, the environment is stiffer, and the activity more hectic. Just as you want your legislators to understand home health, you owe it to the legislators to understand their environment.

Capitol visits are usually time limited and can be complicated by activities not controlled by the legislator or his staff; however, a legislator will always see a constituent, especially a constituent who is known to him. There may be an important floor vote at the exact time of your appointment. You, the visitor, have to be flexible. Time constraints necessitate being prepared with a crisp message and a direct request. You may have only a brief 10 minutes to make your point. This is when the homework you have done in the district pays off. You may be the last person to speak to the legislator prior to a vote on the issue that concerns you.

The contrast between the district and capitol offices can be striking and intimidating. A legislator knows when you make a special effort to discuss your concern at his capitol office that the issue is of utmost importance to you. Your legislator and his or her seniority in the assembly can help you move an issue to the front of the legislative agenda. Whether the legislator is in the majority or minority, whether they are a committee chair, hold a caucus position, or are a respected orator makes a difference in how much influence they can exert.

One lobbying and networking activity is for members of an organization or a coalition of organizations to develop a "Day at the Capitol" event. When preplanned and well executed, these events provide media exposure for your issue. The difficulty is assuring that a critical mass of an organization's membership will be available on a particular date. Typically there will be a briefing on the issues prior to visits with individual legislators. Afterwards, the group may meet again to discuss the responses they received or a response form might be provided for feedback to the organizers. This information gathering assists with planning the professional and trade organization's next step to securing an outcome that benefits the membership. Whether the issue is health or business related, your participation shows commitment to the issue and provides you with the opportunity to hear how others promote your cause. Facts alone are not necessarily convincing, but conviction and dedication to a cause signals the legislator that you will stay the course until the job gets done.

When interacting with legislators and their staff, it is imperative not to be confrontational. From a legislator's perspective, your issue may not warrant pressing other legislators from the same party to vote one way or the other if he or she has a major bill up for a vote the same day. However, the next time you approach the legislator he or she will remember any bad behavior on your part. This may seem obvious, but it bears mentioning because the relationship has to be maintained in order for you to effect any change in public policy to benefit home health. You can always follow up with a letter expressing your disappointment with the legislator's decision not to support your position. Your legislator may not be able to support you on an issue but could be very helpful at another time.

Be knowledgeable about current home health issues that are facing the House or Senate chamber. Make sure you understand the differences between state and federal officials, legislation, and/or regulations. Addressing a state official as "Congressperson" is a clue that you are not knowledgeable and you immediately lose credibility. The title of "Senator" or "Representative" is appropriate.

Your trade association, both national and state, can be of assistance with issue briefs. Many organizations develop fact sheets with "talking points" specific to the issue for use at these visits. The information function is a key mechanism of interest group's influence with policymakers (Longest, 1996). If there are a number of you visiting at the same time, appoint a spokesperson for the group and have individuals give examples of how the proposed legislation affects their agency. Use this opportunity to integrate information about the benefits of home care and about your specific agency. Those issues that directly impact your ability to deliver services should be paramount among legislative issues facing your agency.

REACTIVE BEHAVIORS

Individual and Group Response to Proposed Legislation

The Need for Quick Action

When legislation is pending, your actions are usually reactions. Although the time from the introduction of legislation to passage is generally long—sometimes spanning years—there are times when quick strategic moves are required. Knowing who to contact and when to contact them improves the success rate for your desired outcomes.

Unless you subscribe to a daily legislative service, you will have to depend on your trade or professional association to alert you when to communicate with your legislator. Associations have professional staff who are called lobbyists or government relations' specialists who track the daily activities of the legislature, and they advise members when action is imminent. Instant notification via telephone or e-mail is used when issues are at a critical point in the legislative or regulatory process. Because time can be limited when responding to crises, organizations now use Web site reference links and listservers. For example, members of an organization will receive an e-mail providing information about a legislative committee's call for a vote with the specific action to be taken. When immediate action is requested, telephone calls, faxes, and e-mail are the best use of your time. However, when there is enough time to send a personal letter, it has the greatest impact of all.

Committee Action

Action on issues becomes urgent when certain deadlines approach. The first time-sensitive action is required when a committee has scheduled a vote on a specific proposal. Sometimes public notice is required prior to a committee meeting, but it can be as short as a 24-hour notice. Committees can vote bills up or down or amend bills to satisfy a special interest group such as home health. Initially communications are directed to the legislators serving on the committee reviewing the bill. Your legislator may not be a part of this deliberation if he or she does not serve on the committee. If this is the case, you should communicate with the chairperson of the committee. Even though your legislator may not serve on the committee, his or her influence among members of his or her party may strengthen your position. Therefore, keep your own legislator apprised of your concern because the bill will come before the entire assembly for a vote.

Floor Action

After committee action the bill is ready for review by the entire assembly of House or Senate members. The general rule is that a legislative body has 3 days to review the proposal. While the proposal is before the legislature for action, there is opportunity for further amendments, and this is the time that the caucuses (private meetings of the respective political parties) discuss bills. You may be directed to take action when a bill is ready for debate by the House or Senate.

When either the full House or Senate has approved a bill, the process begins anew in the opposite chamber. Committee action, action before the entire chamber, and final approval are again required. You have the same opportunities for input as you did in the chamber of origin. The time lag between steps in the process can be very short or it can be extended by adjournments, holidays, and elections. Your legislator's office can be helpful if they know you have a particular interest in a bill. You can ask to be contacted when action occurs.

For the specific legislative process in your state, review the state constitution or contact your trade or professional organization. Some states such as Maryland have action limited to a 90-day session, and Nebraska has only one legislative body. Web pages have become the mode of transmission for legislative information. You can access your state's proposed bills online as well as information about your legislators and their staff. The text of the bill is retrievable and the status of a bill is usually listed.

Public Hearings

Public hearings may be part of your state's process to give proposed legislation as much exposure as possible. Differences can be aired, and as a result of the hearing, negotiated compromises may be achieved. Input at this stage is critical. If you plan to testify and have never testified before a legislative committee, it is advisable to learn the committee members' positions on the issue before the hearing. Call the committee members' offices and ask if the legislator has taken a position. Legislators on opposing sides of an issue can become aggressive in their questioning, particularly when an audience is present. It is important to remember that the hearing's purpose is to address the issue, not the position of an individual legislator. Some states require written testimony while others hold general discussions. You can ask staff for the procedure particular to your state. Remember to avoid technical jargon common to your environment, use plain examples, be courteous, and never knowingly give incorrect information. If you are questioned and do not have the available information, it's perfectly acceptable to inform the legislator that you will be happy to obtain the information and forward it to them.

Policy making is not limited to data and statistics. Stories are the real power of public hearings. The media are particularly attentive to human-interest stories, and sometimes focus more on the anecdote than the issue. Just as one well-documented case study can spur further research, we would expect that contextually appropriate stories might aid policy makers in their decision making. Unfortunately, untrue or unproven stories told before large audiences can negatively impact policy decisions. Seasoned legislators are guided by stories but instinctively ask questions to determine the impact of proposals on both those supporting and those opposing the issue.

In the values versus data debate, McDonough (2001) states "anecdotes help to signal problems with existing programs and policies that have been unrecognized or insufficiently understood." He shares the concept from Deborah Stone's *Policy Paradox* (1997) that challenges the concept of policy making as simply a scientific exercise in data analysis. Therefore, when considering policy differences that are grounded in divergent value structures, empirical research rarely helps un-less and until participants allow for those value differences (McDonough, 2001). This is the essence of party politics. Use narrative carefully and only to illustrate what happens to individuals or groups as a result of the proposed change to law or regulation.

If written testimony is required, it is usually beneficial to summarize your points rather than read from the prepared statement. This gives the panel an opportunity to ask questions rather than just listen to a presentation. You can also correct information that may have been delivered by other participants. Public hearings can be held throughout a state that gives a special interest group the opportunity to have its position restated several times. Repetition of your message from multiple sources is beneficial. Actual case experience can be illustrated more completely when legislators visit different communities throughout a state.

TIPS FOR COMMUNICATING WITH YOUR ELECTED OFFICIALS

Letter Writing, E-Mails, and Telephone Calls

Be consistent, concise, and credible. It is helpful in communicating with your legislator to include the following: the bill number, the committee or subcommittee to which the bill has been assigned, your position, a rationale or supporting example, and a specific request for support or opposition.

The following is a list of essential items to include when you are writing a letter to a legislator:

- the proper address (frequently letters never reach their intended destination because of incorrect addresses).

  The proper salutation (although "The Honorable" is appropriate for the address, it is not appropriate within the letter; "Dear Senator/Representative/Assembly Representative" is correct for state-level officials, "Dear Senator/Congressman or Congresswoman" is correct for federal officials)

- the issue (include bill number when referring to legislation)
- a summary of what the bill proposes
- your position with rationale (use clear, concise, credible facts)
- specific examples of how the legislation, regulations, or policies affect you and the delivery of client services in the legislator's district
- the action you wish the legislators to take
- your address within the letter itself, not just on the envelope

The most difficult task in writing to a policy maker is to keep the message limited to one page. Because there are numerous interest groups pursuing legislative action, communications longer than a single page lose the interest of the reader.

Large interest groups frequently use petitions and postcards as a means of generating support among their members. Mass communication shows that someone is interested enough to generate lots of paper, but does not necessarily sway the position of a legislator. Most petitions and postcards do not have a return addresses on them and as such have little value to the legislator. Legislators are likely to respond to the interest group rather than the individuals who sent the cards. This tactic may be used when an issue

has become highly controversial and the opposing sides are trying to impress legislators by showing how many of their members they can motivate and activate. Numbers are important to legislators when correspondence comes from voters within their districts. As few as five well-written letters that express the writers' concerns far outweigh the nondescript messages of petitions and postcards.

E-mail is still evolving as a tool for influencing legislators. Just as a form letter or petition has lesser value than a thoughtful letter, so too e-mail can evoke little response unless it is thoughtful *and* a street address is given in the body of the e-mail. Return e-mail addresses do not indicate where in the state a particular individual lives. No legislator will spend time answering communications they cannot verify as coming from their constituents. Frequently, the first response you receive will be a form e-mail acknowledging receipt of your communication. Your concerns may be addressed later with appropriate follow-up from the legislator's office.

Now more than ever, the speed of communication has been impacted by technology. Organizations can reach every member requesting immediate action on an issue. Memos to legislative staff and elected officials can be generated via the Web; a barrage of e-mail can cripple a legislator's computers. Use this tool to your advantage by not abusing it. Although state and federal information is Web-accessible, legislators hesitate to use this technology for regular communication. With the proliferation of companies specializing in Web technology, we may see a dramatic change in how elected officials use the Internet to their advantage.

Once a bill progresses to final passage and a vote is imminent, there is insufficient time for the U.S. Postal Service to deliver a letter. Facsimiles are appropriate for actions occurring during the next 48 hours. If an action is to occur within 24 hours, telephone contacts and e-mails are of greater value.

Telephone calls should be scripted in order to take maximum advantage of 2 to 3 minutes on a single issue. Start by identifying yourself as a constituent, give no more than three bulleted points supporting your position, and ask the legislator to cast a vote supporting your position on the issue. If the legislator knows you, there may be an opportunity for dialogue on the issue. If you can't speak directly to the legislator, ask for the staff person who is handling the issue. Calls are generally logged. A well-timed call may tip the balance in your direction if a legislator does not have a firm position on the issue.

A sample message outline for a telephone communication is:

My name is Evelyn Jones. I am the administrator for XYZ Home Health Agency. I, and most of my staff and patients, reside in your district.

Please support Senate Bill___. The bill provides increased reimbursement for home care visits. If care is not provided in the home, many residents will need to be admitted to nursing homes in order to receive care. Many elderly can be adequately cared for at home and at less cost.

Please vote yes. Thank you.

It is appropriate to follow through after an action has occurred. A thank-you note to officials who supported your position is always appreciated. If the legislator votes in opposition to your position, you have several options in your communication—ask for the legislator's rationale or agree to disagree, restating your position. This follow-up correspondence keeps the lines of communication open between you and the legislator. The goal is to maintain a working relationship with the official.

LITIGATION/JUDICIAL DECISIONS

The judicial system functions as a "check and balance" to the legislative and executive branches of the government, and the role of the judiciary is interpretive. The judge or court actually looks at the words in a law and determines what is meant by how it is written. Rulings of the courts set precedent for succeeding cases involving the same law. Interpretation takes into account intent only to the extent of the words used to craft the law. If there is a negative result on an industry or profession, a change in the law may be necessary. There is ongoing debate as to whether litigation should be used to shape public policy. It is considered a reactive strategy (Jacobson and Soliman, 2002). Challenges to existing policies, alteration of the implementation of policies, and stimulating new policies are frequently the goal of litigation by special interest groups (Longest, 1996). The courts can issue declaratory judgments when approached to clarify the meaning of laws. They can issue injunctions to cease and desist actions when there is probable harm to the group requesting court intervention, or the court can rule invalid laws of state governments when determined to be unconstitutional. All of these outcomes set the stage for changes to or outright repeal of laws and regulations.

The judicial system has sometimes been used to address provision of care issues. When current regulations are interfering with care delivery and there is little likelihood of legislative success, litigation may be the only alternative. It can be expensive but effective. Trade and professional organizations lend support to each other by filing friend of the court, *amicus curiae,* briefs when their interests might be harmed or served by the outcome of the case.

As an example, one case that had monumental impact for home health occurred because there were varied interpretations from fiscal intermediaries about coverage. A national class action suit, *Dugan v. Brown,* was initiated in 1987 to challenge what was perceived, at that time, as the dismantling of the Medicare home health benefit. Many home health agencies, combined with the National Association for Home Care and Congressman Harley Staggers (D-WV) to challenge the Department of Health and Human Services. The lawsuit, sometimes referred to as the "Staggers lawsuit," resulted in the revision of the Medicare coverage standards (Legal Advocacy, 2003). Even today, the coverage of daily visits to Medicare beneficiaries owes its recognition to this successful lawsuit.

POLITICAL ACTION

The objective of political action is to gain access to people rather than access to information about legislative and regulatory proposals. There is, however, a natural affinity between the people we elect and the work they do. Although political action activities are generally reactive, trying to influence elections to further support your mission, they can also be classified as proactive when open seats occur and there is an opportunity to elect someone who supports your agency prior to being elected.

Political action should be considered separately from the legislative process. Political action is people oriented rather than issue oriented. It deals with the direct efforts of an individual or group to affect the outcome of an election to public office. Most often, political action efforts are translated into raising and expending financial contributions to run political campaigns. In addition to dollars, anything of value, such as personal services, a loan of property, or gifts of stationery, can be considered efforts to affect the outcome of an election. States' laws vary concerning the amount of control they impose on campaign financing. In some states, corporate donations are not permitted, while in others they are. Limits on financial contributions to candidates vary from state to state and at the federal level.

Because the purpose of political action is to affect the outcome of an election, before you make personal financial contributions, you must carefully evaluate how you are perceived in the community. Although you would contribute as an individual, your public prominence may link you to your agency. As an agency administrator, you must be clear on both state and federal laws before becoming directly involved in any political activities, particularly because these activities are under close scrutiny for abuse and excessive influence. You as an individual are not restricted from engaging in political action, including making financial contributions to a candidate's campaign. The Hatch Act, 5U.S.C. §§ 7321–7326, regulates federal employees' political activity, and specific state laws may re-

strict state employees. At the federal level and in most states, campaign records are open to public scrutiny. As an administrator, you need to weigh carefully the value of having your name appear in these records even though you contributed as an individual citizen.

The neophyte is advised to work through organized groups, such as political action committees (PACs) of state and national organizations. If you have worked with a legislator for longer than 6 months, you are in a position to evaluate how well that legislator responds to you and the issues affecting your agency. Your input can assist PACs in their evaluations of candidates because PACs solicit information from many sources to determine who warrants financial support or endorsement.

As a rule of thumb, PACs consider seniority, committee chairships, party position, committee membership, and financial need in determining whom to support. It follows, then, that the majority of financial contributions are given to incumbent candidates. Frequently, small health-related PACs overlook legislators who do not serve on health care committees or who do not hold party seniority. Nevertheless, you can usually request a PAC to review a particular legislator or candidate with accompanying documentation of how the individual supports your issues.

Involvement with a state or national PAC does not negate your opportunity to work with a specific legislator or elected official. If you are personally active in party politics and clearly identified in the community as an agency director, then you should consider ways to identify yourself as a private citizen to offset any potential political backlash for your agency. As a private citizen, you may assess a candidate's commitment and make a personal contribution to the campaign fund. Agencies designated as 501(c)(3), however, are prohibited from making donations to political campaigns. A nonprofit agency's tax status would be jeopardized by direct political contributions.

General fundraisers for political parties provide an opportunity for the administrator as an individual to participate in political action without endorsing specific individuals. When attending political functions, make certain that the candidates know you are there. A follow-up letter commenting on the success of the event gives you yet another opportunity to point out your participation.

CONCLUSION

Many federal, state, and local laws and regulations have a direct impact on the ability of a home health agency to provide care. Sometimes larger issues obscure the fact that proposed changes will decrease available funding. An agency, therefore, needs many information resources to keep abreast of the constant changes.

Sometimes issues being considered are so crucial that the staff and board members of an agency should take the initiative to contact their legislators. To assist these individuals who are not involved in government issues on a day-to-day basis, it might be necessary to circulate a legislative fact sheet stating the problem, the alternative, and the expected outcomes. Agency directors should understand lobbying restrictions, which prohibit influencing the public, placed on tax-exempt organizations before they embark on any assertive campaign.

Although it should be obvious that there are many nuances in dealing with the players in the legislative-regulatory arena, the final impact is related to your ability to communicate. Individual letters are far more effective in influencing lawmakers than petitions or form letters. At key times, telephone and e-mail contacts are even more effective. Whatever the mode of communication, it should be clear, concise, and credible. The elected official should be clear about your position on the issue. The same communication techniques are appropriate for all levels of elected officials. If you communicate with federal legislators, you should send a copy to your state officials. Copying legislators within a congressional district creates the potential to generate a chain of support for your position. As you become more involved in the process, information sharing between you and your elected official will be mutual.

The best communication tool for all citizens, and yet the most frequently ignored one, is the power of the individual vote. Voting is your final evaluation of the overall effectiveness of an elected official in responding to you as a concerned citizen or a professional health care provider with a special interest. Although you cannot expect an elected official to support your position 100 percent of the time, you have the right to expect a knowledgeable response to your inquiries as well as the official's rationale for his or her vote.

Home health administrators have known for years how to generate community support. Because communications and networking are common activities for any agency director, it is not difficult to expand this activity to include the politicians and key elected officials in your community. Be aware that they, too, have a role to play in the future of your organization.

REFERENCES

Jacobson, P. D. and S. Soliman. 2002. Litigation as public health policy: Theory or reality. *The Journal of Law, Medicine & Ethics* 30(2): 224–238.

Kingdon, J. M. 1995. *Agendas, alternatives, and public policies,* 2nd ed. New York: Harper Collins College Publishers, Chapter 3.

Legal Advocacy. n.d. *The National Association for Home Care.* Retrieved from *http://www.nahc.org/CHCL/chcl.html* (accessed March 24, 2003).

Longest Jr., B. B. 1996. *Seeking strategic advantage through health policy analysis.* Chicago: Health Administration Press, Chapters 5 and 6.

Mc Donough, J. E. 2001. Using and misusing anecdote in policy making. *Health Affairs* 20: 207–212.

Stone, D. A. 1997. *Policy paradox: The art of political decision making.* New York: W.W. Norton.

PART VIII

Strategic Planning/Marketing/ Survival Issues

CHAPTER 54

Strategic Planning

Edward R. Balotsky and David B. Smith

INTRODUCTION

Strategic planning is difficult, rewarding, and essential for organizations. It shapes the way an organization changes so that it can better accomplish its goals and more effectively adapt to environmental pressures. Organizational change is inevitable, but even the most effective strategic planning may not always control the way an organization changes. Successful home health agencies, so dependent on third-party payment regulations and referrals from potential competitors, are like the champion downhill skier, a little out of control.

The men's downhill races in the 1976 Winter Olympics changed the strategies of racers. Franz Klammer seemed "out of control" for the entire run. Yet, he won the Olympic gold medal. Up until Klammer's run, the prevailing thinking among downhill racers was that the winner of a race would be the one who was in the best condition, had the best technique, and skied just this side of the edge of losing control. The thinking changed. To win one now had to ski on the other side of the edge of losing control. In 1976, Klammer was the only one (of truly world-class skiers) who skied out of control. Because every other top skier was trying to ski just short of losing control and since Klammer was lucky, he won easily. Now all the top skiers, perhaps 15 or 20 of them, are skiing out of control, and on any given day it is largely natural selection stemming from factors beyond the skiers' control

that determines who wins. During any run, there are many blind variations in the form of ruts, bumps, human error, and so forth that are beyond the control of the skiers at the speed they are now going. The skier who skis most out of control and is luckiest in avoiding falling will win. Because there are so many good skiers skiing "out of control," the odds are excellent that one of them will always take enough risks and manage enough miraculous recoveries to beat the under-control skier (McKelvey, 1982).

The top skiers made a strategic choice: They chose to go for the gold rather than the less-risky strategy of good, average performance. Organizations can make risky strategic choices that aim for market dominance or more conservative ones that aim for average performance. The rapid technological, regulatory, and competitive changes in the home health care market, however, make almost any strategy a risky one. Strategic planning helps make those choices and controls their implementation.

No matter what choices are made, successful strategic planning must move at the speed of the winning downhill skier. Such planning is not a special set of procedures, a committee structure, a set of statistical projection techniques, or a document that can be produced by a consultant for the right price. It involves an understanding of how organizations change and the use of that knowledge to shape changes in an organization that will, as much as possible, ensure its success. The first section describes how organizations change; the second, how strategic planning can help shape those changes; the third, how to develop strategic planning capacity; and the final section, pitfalls to avoid in the strategic planning process.

HOW ORGANIZATIONS CHANGE

Organizations resist change because it is stressful and disruptive. Figure 54-1 summarizes the process by which changes take place in organizations. An organization must adapt effectively to its environment to succeed. When it fails to achieve at least the minimum performance needed for survival, it looks for ways to turn things around. Change involves risk. The larger the change, the greater the cost and disruption and, consequently, the greater the risk. As a result, most organizations attempt to turn things around by making modest adjustments that involve incremental change for the organization. If modest changes fail, an organization searches for more drastic solutions. That search will progress through four distinct phases.

Phase I—Manipulation of the Environment

Organizations invest effort in getting others to change rather than changing themselves. One tries to change the reimbursement policies, influence the granting of certificates of need to restrict competition, or change consumer patterns of utilization. If such efforts are successful, the organization does not have to change at all. Home health agencies and the associations that represent them fight such battles.

The proliferation of health care marketing reflects this concern with reshaping the environment. Many organizations equate a marketing focus with an advertising campaign designed to increase market share; their scarce resources would be better spent in changing their organizational structure or tailoring the mix of services provided to rapidly respond to market demands. As suggested in Chapter 55, successful marketing is not an isolated activity; rather, it is an integral part of the more extensive

process of strategic planning and organizational change.

Most providers of health services have recognized the limits of environmental manipulation. The acute care hospital experience with the shift from retrospective to prospective payment is well documented, particularly the drastic reduction in average length of stay (ALOS) and total admissions and the increase in the case-mix index. In dealing with these changes, hospitals have resorted to drastic solutions that have directly affected the character and structure of their own organizations.

The result of environmental manipulation need not be negative, however. Home health care is uniquely positioned to be a "winner" in the prospective payment wars. The growth of managed care has reversed home care's traditional role as a residual set of services provided only after other institutional interventions to one that is in the forefront of market-driven reform (Benjamin, 1993). The result has been a dramatic increase in the utilization of home care programs as providers reacted to reduced revenues by shuffling patients through less intensive treatment regimes. Between 1980 and 1993, Medicare home care visits increased from 22,428 to 184,397 and expenditures climbed by 175 percent (Lumsdon, 1994a). During the 1990s, home care was the fastest-growing sector in the health care industry (Taylor, 2002), with total expenditures rising to $32.4 billion in 2000 (CMS, 2002). An estimated 2.5 million Medicare beneficiaries received home health services in 2002 (Medicare acts, 2002). The environment for home care providers is predicted to be far from tranquil, however, as the expected consolidation among providers, regulatory and reimbursement changes highlighted by the Balanced Budget Act of 1997, the development of outcomes-based performance standards, and the rise of disease management programs (CMS, 2002; Leavenworth, 1995; Shriver, 1996) continue to challenge industry participants. Shortell and associates' (2000) prediction of health care systems emphasizing primary and home-base care has also materialized (Binstock, 2002).

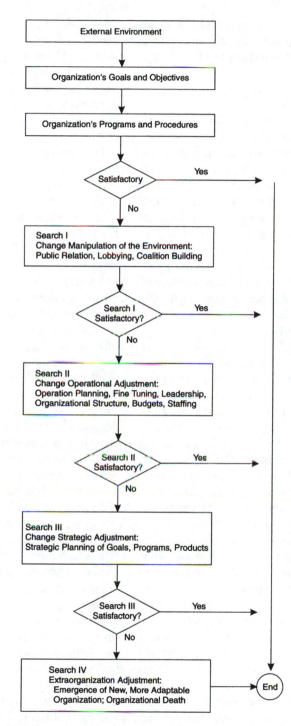

Figure 54-1 Organizational Response to Problems in the Environment.
Source: Used with permission from *The White Labyrinth: A Guide to the Health Care System,* 2nd ed., by David Barton Smith and Arnold D. Kaluzny. Chicago: Health Administration Press, 1986.

The home health care "winners" will be those organizations that proactively influence these key environmental stakeholders and trends.

Phase II—Operational Adjustment

If environmental manipulation fails to ensure adequate performance, then an organization will attempt to address the immediate operational issues. Revenue shortfalls have produced chronic staff and budget reductions (Stoil, 2003). The administrator may be fired and new leadership brought in to help turn things around. In some cases, this is a poor substitute for more fundamental changes that are needed. Operational adjustments can improve efficiency and quality of services. Such efforts absorb most of the time of management. Yet, no matter how well performed, these activities alone will not ensure success, or even survival.

The home health care sector is not static. As indicated in Figure 54-2, products or services have a life cycle. It is perhaps most useful to think of home care as a market rather than as a discrete product. That market existed long before the emergence of the modern hospital around 1920 (Starr, 1982) and will continue regardless of hospital structural changes. Home care products and services, however, have changed dramatically. Some, such as the remote monitoring of vital signs, are in the embryonic and growth stages. Others, such as managed care systems (capitation case management, preferred provider organizations, and health maintenance organizations [HMOs]), have entered the more competitive growth and shake-out stages of the life cycle. Other products, such as the more familiar packaged array of fee-for-service home health services, have reached maturity, where growth in net income is restrained by both competition and restriction of third-party payment. Home care organizations must continually scan the environment, as major change in an environmental variable can decrease, accelerate, or reverse a product's position on the life cycle. The more traditional private duty nursing services that were in the de-

cline stage of the life cycle, for example, have gained a significant life extension through the shift in Medicare payment toward subacute care. Third-party payment, technological and regulatory changes, and access to capital will continue to affect both the actual home health care products delivered and the organizations that provide them.

Fragmentation remains a characteristic of the industry. Although large for-profit companies exist, the majority of the industry is composed of thousands of small independent regional and local providers. In 2001, independent agencies represented 52 percent of the market; chain, government, and church-owned facilities represented 30 percent, 15 percent, and 3 percent, respectively (CMS, 2002). In 1994, 35 percent of hospitals offered a home care product, but the growth of these programs flattened and consolidation began as regulation, reimbursement changes, and alternative providers impacted the market (Burns, 1995). Not surprisingly, managed care organizations are shaping the structure of home care delivery. Case management groups, such as the National Preferred Provider Network (NPPN), are developing home care networks in response to increases in home care costs (Marshall, 1996). Size and critical mass are now crucial barometers of home care success (Trans Healthcare, 2003). These networks are contracting with home care providers capable of servicing large, defined geographic markets with a broad line of product diversification. The selected providers are expected to offer the benefits of economy of scale and clout in negotiating with suppliers, as well as the willingness to share any cost reductions with their clients (McNamee and Schiller, 1994; Snyder, 1995). In response, free-standing home care agencies are using horizontal and vertical networking of all types, including home care HMOs, in an attempt to provide what has become "one-stop shopping" for everything outside the acute care setting (Lumsdon, 1994b). Home health merger and acquisition (M&A) activity remains a consistent but maturing strategic response; after peaking at 137 transactions in 1997, 83, 63, 31,

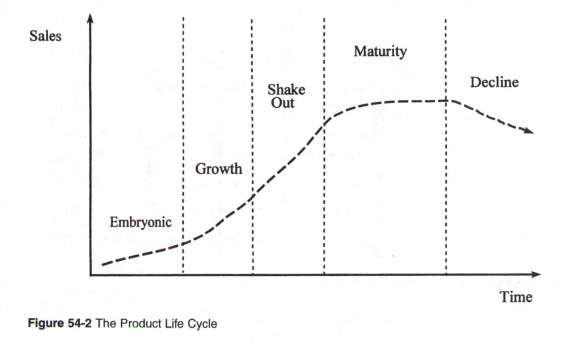

Figure 54-2 The Product Life Cycle

28, and 28 mergers occurred from 1998 through 2002, respectively (By the Numbers, 2002; Hoppszallern, 2002). Insurance companies are pursuing similar strategies, including the development of internal case management, as a method to control home care expenditures (Koco, 1994). Concentrating on efficiency and quality alone, then, may not stave off the erosion of the traditional home health agency's share of health care expenditures in the face of these emerging vertically integrated hospital systems of community care, or HMOs and other emerging permutations of insurance and service organizations.

Phase III—Strategic Adjustment

A strategic adjustment involves changing goals, programs, and products to better respond to regulatory or market pressures and to adopt new products in the introduction and growth phase of their life cycle. This is not an easy thing for organizations, particularly when staff have strong professional identities, yet the capacity to engage effectively in such adjustments will determine the ability of an organization to survive. Working effectively at this level and changing products and services to adapt to shifts in regulatory or market pressures is the acid test of effective strategic management.

It is often useful to think of products as separate and distinct from the medical specialty or allied health occupational group services that form the traditional building blocks of health services organizations. The product line management approach attempts to identify a single center of accountability for financial and quality of care issues. This is a logical extension of the matrix-type organizational structure illustrated in Figure 54-3. The traditional approach is to divide an organization into major specialty areas. In Figure 54-3, these areas are the vertical columns (nursing, billing, etc.). The products are the horizontal rows. This particular hypothetical home care agency or company has defined four products: (1) a home hospice service,

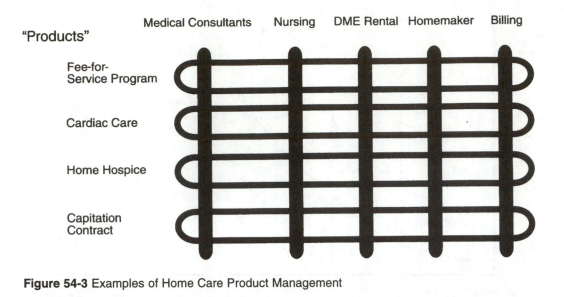

Figure 54-3 Examples of Home Care Product Management

(2) a conventional fee-for-service program, (3) a highly specialized posthospitalization cardiac care program, and (4) a special capitation subcontract with an HMO. Although a good deal of overlap exists in the kinds of services offered by each of these products (medical consultants, nursing, durable medical equipment rental, etc.), it is often advantageous, particularly in a competitive environment, to manage them separately; that is, organize the home care agency by rows (products) rather than columns. This may lead to better cost and quality control as well as more responsiveness to the needs and demands of a special segment of the market.

Defining the products of a home care program may seem like belaboring the obvious. Sometimes, however, it's not that obvious. Products may be defined by geographical boundaries, third-party markets, or medical specialty. There are also three basic additional ways health care products or services can be redefined, as illustrated in Figure 54-4. First, the time commitment during an illness episode can be either narrowed or widened. One can focus on a narrow time during posthospitalization or view the service or product as one involving a more extensive time commitment. The latter would imply a commitment to serving the chronically ill and providing long-term maintenance and rehabilitative services. Second, the nature of the services can either be restricted to more narrow technical services or expanded to include broader social-psychological support services. The broader definition of the product, for example, might involve the development of social and recreational services. Conversely, the more narrow definition might simply include rental of specific pieces of durable medical equipment.

The relative attractiveness of these alternatives, however, depends on how specific services are bundled for payment. Arrangements for payment can be negotiated with third parties or the client for each specific service rendered, either by illness episode or admission (a prospective payment system) or by the person covered (HMO). The bundling of services for payment, of course, defines the time commitment and breadth of services that will be provided. The movement from a fee-for-service payment system to ones where third parties shift risk onto providers has required a fundamental

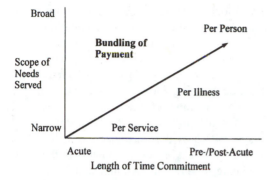

Figure 54-4 Alternative Definitions of Product

change in orientation. A strong financial position for a provider is facilitated under such payment arrangements not by providing a high volume of relatively costly and complex services, but by reducing the volume of costly services and substituting less costly treatments. Health care providers are scrambling to adjust to the shift in bundling of acute care services into payments for illness episodes and bundling based on capitation arrangements. The ripple effect of these shifts in financing has forced fundamental redefinitions of most health services products as well as the organizational structures and relationships in which services are delivered. A positive outcome for home care providers has been the recognition of home care services as a competitive necessity in the prospective payment environment (O'Donnell, 1993) because the home setting is attractive to managed care payers as a less-costly alternative to institutionalized care. Many home care organizations are meeting this challenge/opportunity by restructuring to offer a full line of home care products rather than single service offerings such as home infusion or nursing care services (Lumsdon, 1994a).

Phase IV—Extraorganizational Adjustment

If none of these searches is effective, an organization either dies or is transformed into a completely different entity. The hospital industry is a prime example of both outcomes. Between 1983, the inaugural year of the Medicare prospective payment system (PPS), and 1991, 505 U.S. acute care hospitals closed (Burda, 1992). M&A activity accelerated during the 1990s. In 1994 and 1995 alone, 20 percent of U.S. community hospitals changed ownership (Lutz, 1995). Another 910 transactions occurred between 1996 and 2002 (Fong, 2003; Hoppszallern, 2002). The latter part of the 1990s witnessed the beginning of a variety of hybrid multi-institutional, multiservice, community-based health care structures that acquired providers at an accelerating rate in order to develop regional integrated delivery systems (IDS) (Coile, 1995). By 2001, 2,260 hospitals were IDS members while another 1,341 facilities participated in a network; thus 73.4 percent of the nation's stock of 4,908 community hospitals were involved in the multi-institutional setting (By the Numbers, 2002).

From Vertical to Virtual Integration

Most IDSs construct their systems through horizontal and vertical integration. This is the traditional strategy that equates the accumulation and ownership of capital, labor, and equipment with competitive advantage. However, with the emergence of global competition, and the resultant downsizing, reengineering, and reduced organizational slack, many organizations do not have sufficient capital to invest in new technology, products, or markets (Welles, 1995). At the same time, knowledge has become more important than labor and is more accessible via information technology. In this environment, few assets remain such for long. Businesses have responded by outsourcing functions previously performed in-house. In the process, vertical integration is rapidly being supplemented by a new paradigm, "virtual integration."

Virtual integration is a temporary network of independent organizations linked by information technology to share knowledge, skills, costs, and access to each other's markets (Byrne et al., 1993). Participants contribute their core competencies in a combination of talents that allows the rapid exploitation of a specific opportunity. A virtually integrated structure is a strategic collaboration in which common ownership of assets is replaced by contractual arrangements (Goldsmith, 1995). The main advantage of this approach is the ability to efficiently harness separately existing resources without the capital requirements associated with in-house production of all services. The major drawback of virtual integration is the loss of control that occurs without a central entity that can force compliance among multiple organizational structures (Clark, 1995). Thus, the decision facing managers is the trade-off between the financial incentives for virtual integration and the control possible in the vertically integrated organization. The result has been a continuum of integration in which few organizations outsource all functions. Rather, a middle ground is taken in which functions essential to unique competencies are produced internally, while less essential needs are acquired from the marketplace (Chesbrough and Teece, 1996).

Health care ventures have been no exception to this overall pattern. The newest health care organizations involve institutional providers, physicians, and payers that have linked in various organizational structures in response to managed care pressures. For example, the terms "virtual hospital" and "hospital without walls" have been used to describe coordinated health care services provided outside their traditional structures (Pallarito, 1996). The appeal of these virtual structures is simple: Vertical integration in health care has proven to be expensive and extremely cumbersome to manage. Some describe health care's experience with vertical integration as a "costly mistake" (Goldsmith, 1994), citing the obsolescence of assets acquired by such integration as not creating the best value for health care buyers.

The virtual network model of the future may already be operating. In California, individual physicians are creating linkages through membership in giant medical groups and independent practice associations (IPAs). These evolving structures control access to extremely large blocks of patients, giving these groups real market power in negotiating capitation rates with managed care organizations. There is IDS or hospital ownership in some cases, but the majority of the medical groups and IPAs remain independent, using short-term contracts as the dominant method of maintaining an optimal provider network. As a result, hospitals and other health providers have been forced into the role of "price-taking subcontractors in the managed care food chain" (Robinson and Casalino, 1996, p. 16).

The California experience bodes well for the home health care organization. The deemphasis of hospital-based care under full-risk capitation is well documented, as is the positive impact on home health utilization. Managed care has matured into a product line that has shifted from a hospital to a home-based focus point (Goldsmith et al., 1995). For the home care provider, the value-added argument for contracting with dominant managed care groups is compelling: These groups provide access to larger patient blocks than is possible for the unaffiliated home health agency, and providers can do so in an efficient, economical manner while maintaining the autonomy of the agency (Robinson, 1996). Given this environment, home health care organizations have become attractive partners for these emerging virtually integrated networks of providers. Home health agencies, however, must create virtual organizations of their own that they can provide unified packages of cost-effective services across broad geographic areas that include the entire market areas of managed care plans.

HOW STRATEGIC PLANNING SHAPES CHANGE IN ORGANIZATIONS

Effective strategic planning radically alters the natural process of organizational change. Its focus is on change rather than the maintenance of the status quo, viewing the stages of organizational change not as places to go only in desperation, but as inevitable steps in an ongoing process of organizational development. Strategic planning transforms what is essentially a passive, often unconscious, reactive mechanism of organizational change into a self-conscious, proactive, future-oriented process. At each stage in the process of organizational change outlined in Figure 54-1, effective strategic planning anticipates the questions, develops answers, and makes choices. Those choices are based on an assessment of the external environment, a refined sense of the mission and goals of the organization, and a knowledge of the key issues in each of the four phases of organizational development.

Assessment of the External Environment

The *strategic process* is the search for the optimal fit between the internal strengths of an organization and external opportunities, while solving external threats and internal weaknesses. Intelligence is critical to the strategy process. What do we know and what do we need to know to position ourselves strategically? What trends in payment and regulation of the health care industry will affect home health care services? What changes in the population and economics will shape demand for home health services? The population of those over 75 is growing rapidly, and the relative wealth of this population segment appears to be growing. Household size is decreasing as well. Also, the popularity of mass-market, homogeneous products appears to be waning, as consumers are seeking more alternative product choices. For home health services, these trends represent distinct opportunities for attracting new market share.

Everyone remotely involved in the health sector is engaged in environmental assessment. Porter (1991) believes that intensity of rivalry within an industry must be an organization's first priority and lists five key factors that environmental assessments should consider:

1. The potential of an attractive and growing market invites greater competition.

2. One needs to know what new entrants to the market are likely, and what position existing competitors are likely to take.

3. The threat exists of potential substitute products or services that will affect the competitive environment; for example, the growth and development of hospice programs, subacute care units in hospitals, life care communities, HMOs, and the return of the physician or nonphysician practitioner home visit can all affect home health care service demand.

4. Greater competition will in turn increase the bargaining power of customers.

5. Greater competition will also increase the bargaining power of suppliers, who in the home health market are largely composed of the staffing resources necessary for the actual provision of care.

Wheelen and Hunger (2004) add a sixth issue to the mix: the level of stakeholder power in a market. The market share of managed care organizations, the state-level regulatory climate, and business coalition activity will all affect the strategic choices that a home care organization can consider. The importance of the environmental assessment cannot be overstated, as the future viability of the home care provider will depend upon the accuracy of this analysis.

Clarifying Goals and Objectives

Goals and objectives have to represent a good deal more than financial ratios and utilization and budget projections. There is a fine line between organizational autism, which ignores the environment, and organizational emptiness, which ignores any internal vision and is preoccupied with short-run market demand. Either extreme will destroy the organization. Strategic planning involves a wide scope of vision and a long-term perspective. One needs to articulate the special vision of the organization that helps to impose order upon the chaotic signals of the environment. It also helps to give a sense of cohesiveness and common purpose to those involved in ensuring the success of the organization.

Identifying Strategy in Each Phase of Organizational Change

At each phase of organizational change, the question becomes not what action can alleviate the immediate problem, but what can be done to ensure the overall effectiveness of the organization's strategy in achieving its vision. Questions such as the following need to be asked and answered.

> **Phase I, Environmental Manipulation:** How can the market be shaped and the regulatory climate influenced to better assure organizational success?
>
> **Phase II, Operational Adjustment:** What changes to current activities can be made to improve the organization's strategic position?
>
> **Phase III, Strategic Adjustment:** What choices are available in new goals or products? On the basis of internal experience, what are the organization's core competencies, and are these competencies being utilized to the best competitive advantage of the organization?
>
> **Phase IV, Extraorganizational Adjustment:** What new organizational forms are possible? Which forms should be pursued? Should the organization compete with others or form coalitions?

Answers to such questions form the framework for the strategic plans of an organization, linking immediate operational issues to efforts for the active creation of a future for the organization. The ultimate consideration for the home care organization is the development of a structure that will build and maintain the distinctive competencies of the organization.

STEPS IN DEVELOPING STRATEGIC PLANNING CAPACITY

Many detailed outlines of the specific actions and steps involved in an overall strategic planning process exist (Hax and Majluf, 1996; Mintzberg et al., 2003; Wheelen and Hunger, 2004). Others have concentrated on health care as a unique industry (Coddington et al., 2001; Drazen and Metzger, 1998; Ginter et al., 2002; Shortell et al., 2000) or have supplied case studies of strategic planning in health care that help put flesh on the abstractions (Dubbs, 2002; Full, 2001; Guo, 2002; Horak, 1998). In simplest terms, however, the strategic planning process can be reduced to four critical steps.

Commit the Resources to Do It Right

Strategic planning is least likely to be done by those who need it the most. Administrators faced with rapid change in their environment as well as increasing competition have difficulty stepping back from the immediate day-to-day crises they face. The result has been the use of in-house planning staffs or consultants external to the organization to dictate strategic direction to those individuals most responsible for the success or failure of the planning process. Although these groups can play a key role in facilitating the planning process, the most critical resource that has to be committed is the time of key decision makers within an organization. Initially, several full days may be needed to clarify and reach agreement on the process, as well as follow-up sessions necessary to help reinforce and further clarify the process. If effective, this strategic planning format becomes embedded in the decision-making routines of the organization and is no longer perceived by executives as "something else I have to find time for." There is also a need either to build the internal staff support or to contract out for the development of the information base to "feed" the strategic planning process. The level of effort and cost of these information-gathering activities will depend on the size and complexity of the organization, the size and complexity of the market and regulatory environment with which the organization must deal, and the level of detail and degree of certainty that the managers involved determine are necessary to make strategic decisions. Just as with the time commitments of top managers, the initial cost will be relatively high; however, as such information gathering gets built into the daily operations of the organization, these maintenance costs will decline.

Pick the Right Participants

Strategic planning must be done by the key decision makers in an organization. It is not something, such as a certificate-of-need application or a required long-range planning document, that can be delegated to either a staff person or a consultant. The top managers in an organization are responsible not only for strategy formulation, but also for making the strategy work. It is thus the responsibility of the chief executive officer to pick the individuals who will be involved in the strategic planning process. These individuals need to have a working knowledge of the organization and the intellectual ability to think strategically, rather than parochially or defensively, about their own special concerns. The basic work group should include no fewer than 3 and no more than 12 individuals. It need not include all those who hold the key formal organization positions on the board, medical staff, and administration, but should be designed to ensure, as much as possible, the support of all those groups needed to implement whatever strategic plans are developed.

Provide an Effective Link between Operational and Strategic Planning

Strategic planning operates in the gray area between the broad ends espoused in the organization's mission statement and the overall direction and the specific means incorporated in the operational plans of department heads and middle managers. Those operational plans include operating budgets, staffing, construction and capital equipment, and program and marketing plans. The strategic document needs to be translated into operational plans. This conversion requires the bottom-up participation of those responsible for these operational areas in the creation, implementation, and evaluation of strategy efforts.

Strategic plans that emerge insulated from any understanding of operational difficulties are doomed to failure. The strategic planning process for several for-profit hospital chains in the 1980s, for example, developed the concept of incorporating an in-house HMO into the product mix. Strategically, it was brilliant. Operationally, it almost proved disastrous because of the failure to consider the potential competitive impact upon the existing base of admitting physicians. Eventually, these chains were forced to divest their HMO products in order to maintain the good graces of their physician stakeholders. Similar anecdotes of the gaps between strategy and operations abound, illustrating the need for a regular dialogue between operational and strategic planning.

An effective dialogue between strategic and operational planning can take place through well-designed joint operational and strategic planning sessions. These sessions can also be built into the day-to-day review and consultation process between top and operational managers. The goal is to provide the opportunity for operational managers to shape strategies as well as their implementation.

Develop an Orderly Process for Accomplishing the Tasks

There are many ways that the essential tasks of strategic planning can be accomplished. The method used is not critical; what is important is that the process is well understood by and acceptable to the key participants and proceeds in an orderly manner. The opportunity for more open-ended, chaotic brainstorming and free association should not be excluded but must take place within a formal structure so that the ideas can be subjected to critical appraisal and put to work. Regardless of the method employed, the following steps should be included in the strategic planning process:

Step 1: Assess current situation. Collect information and evaluate the organization's present strategic position. Assess potential future opportunities and threats.

Step 2: Revise objectives. Set new objectives based upon the assessment in Step 1.

Step 3: Generate and evaluate strategy alternatives. Explore alternatives in all four phases of organizational change in light of their potential to achieve the desired objectives.

Step 4: Select the best strategies. Within the four phases of organizational change, make choices. The choices should have the benefit of review by operational managers as well as the support of the governing body.

Step 5: Develop detailed plans for the selected strategies. Provide opportunities for input from operational managers or, if this is a new venture for the organization, from outside consultants.

Step 6: Implement the plans. Delegate responsibility to a manager and those involved in each plan's operation.

Step 7: Monitor performance. Timing is important. Regularly review to determine whether the strategies are accomplishing their intended objectives. Make midcourse corrections as necessary.

Step 8: Update the organization's situation, using this information as input for the next regularly scheduled strategic planning cycle.

PITFALLS TO AVOID IN THE STRATEGIC PLANNING PROCESS

The strategic planning process requires no small investment of an organization's scarce material, time, and human resources. The end product, the planning document, represents a competitive advantage that can be an invaluable blueprint for guiding an organization toward the accomplishment of its goals. Yet, many well-developed, appropriate strategic plans are never implemented. The reasons why the planning process fails have been thoroughly discussed in the literature (Clark and Boissoneau, 1995; Dervitsiotis, 2002; Hoffman, 2002; Press, 2001; Ward, 2003; Whelan and Sisson, 1993) but can be summarized as four pitfalls that, if not avoided, virtually doom any planning activities.

The Strategy Rests in the Mind of the CEO

The best strategic plan is worthless if it exists primarily in the mind of the chief executive officer (CEO). Successful planning must be characterized by frequent, bilateral communication among the key organizational members charged with the implementation of the plan. Too many CEOs fail to take their vision from the implicit to the explicit level or develop strategy without input from other important players. Equally important, strategy must be viewed as an internally generated product, not just the recommendations of an outside consultant. A strategic plan developed in isolation will result in an underutilized and misunderstood document that may hinder rather than support the organizational mission.

The Strategic Plan Is Not Complete

Sound strategic planning must consider all pertinent issues affecting an organization's outcomes. The value of including all personnel involved with plan implementation now becomes more obvious; a broad set of opinions should facilitate the identification and consideration of potential results that may occur after strategies are operational. Information-gathering efforts should provide supporting documentation in this evaluation process. It is impossible to anticipate every contingency, but the validity of any planning activity is directly linked to the thoroughness of the endeavor.

The Planning Process Is Biased

Many strategic plans are predisposed to failure because of an organization's internal environment. Strategic potential may never be realized due to premature budgeting that establishes operating budgets prior to strategy decisions. The political climate within the organization must be controlled so that power struggles, the ability to take risks, and the tendency for people to avoid change do not circumvent the implementation effort. Employee reward systems, either financial or personal, should be linked to the process. In short, an internal environment not geared toward meaningful strategic planning will hinder a successful outcome.

Strategic Plans Are Not Monitored

Follow-up is crucial to the strategic planning process. Too many strategies are initiated but never evaluated until the next formal planning period. As a result, planning becomes meaningless to organizational members because there is no feedback or concern shown regarding the value or success of the plan nor are modifications made to bring unsuccessful activities into line. To maximize the impact of the planning process, strategies must be monitored regularly during the lifetime of each planning period.

CONCLUSION

This brief summary may suggest that the process of strategic planning is easy and obvious. It is neither. Some readers may conclude that they are already doing it. That is probably correct. The key question is not whether organizations should do strategic planning, but how well it is done and whether the process can be improved. Many tools and techniques can be applied to strategic planning. There is no end to the information that could be collected, analyzed, and utilized in such a process. What improves the process in one setting may be ineffective in another. Strategic planning is a process for bringing about organizational change and growth. Like the process of individual change and growth, it is very personal and individualized: You learn by doing it. Organizations that have the most successful strategic planning are motivated to engage in it not so much by grim survival pressures but by the uniquely human drive to grow and to become all that they are capable of becoming. This motivation is particularly evident in health care organizations, which have social responsibilities that may be stronger than mere survival goals (Liedtka, 1992). To paraphrase Rene Dubois's conclusion in his classic work *Mirage of Health:*

> The earth has never been a Garden of Eden but a Valley of Decision where resilience is essential to survival . . . To grow in the midst of dangers is the fate of the human race, because it is the law of the spirit. (Dubois, 1959, pp. 281–282)

REFERENCES

Benjamin, A. 1993. An historical perspective on home care policy. *The Milbank Quarterly* 71: 129–166.

Binstock, R. 2002. What's ahead for 2003? *Nursing Homes Long Term Care Management* 51: 21–24.

Burda, D. 1992. Hospital closings drop for third straight year. *Modern Healthcare* 22: 2.

Burns, J. 1995. More consolidation on the home front. *Modern Healthcare* 25: 86–90.

By the Numbers '02. 2002. *Modern Healthcare.* Available at *www.modernhealthcare.com/docs/ByTheNumbers 2002.pdf* Accessed May 13, 2003.

Byrne, J., R. Brandt, and O. Port. 1993. The virtual corporation. *Business Week* 3304: 98–102.

Centers for Medicare and Medicaid Services. 2002. Health care industry market update: Home health. Available at *www.cms.hhs.gov/reports/hcimu/hcimu-06282002.pdf* Accessed May 13, 2003.

Chesbrough, H., and D. Teece. 1996. When is virtual virtuous? *Harvard Business Review* 74: 65–73.

Clark, B. and R. Boissoneau. 1995. Strategic planning and the health care supervisor. *Health Care Supervisor* 14: 1–10.

Clark, C. 1995. Planning along the continuum of care. *Healthcare Financial Management* 49: 20–24.

Coddington, D., K. Moore, and E. Fischer. 2001. *Strategies for the new health care marketplace: Managing the convergence of consumerism and technology.* San Francisco: Jossey-Bass.

Coile, R. 1995. Assessing healthcare market trends and capital needs: 1996–2000. *Healthcare Financial Management* 49: 60–65.

Dervitsiotis, K. 2002. The importance of conversations-for-action for effective strategic management. *Total Quality Management* 13: 1087–1098.

Drazen, E. and J. Metzger. 1998. *Strategies for integrated health care: Emerging practices in information management and cross-continuum care.* San Francisco: Jossey-Bass.

Dubbs, N. 2002. Organizational design consistency: The PennCARE and Henry Ford Health System experiences. *Journal of Healthcare Management* 47: 307–319.

Dubois, R. 1959. *Mirage of health.* New York: Harper and Row.

Fong, T. 2003. Consolidation squabble. *Modern Healthcare* 33: 7.

Full, J. 2001. Physician recruitment strategies for a rural hospital. *Journal of Healthcare Management* 46: 277–282.

Ginter, P., L. Swayne, and W. Duncan. 2002. *Strategic management of healthcare organizations,* 4th ed. Malden, MA: Blackwell.

Goldsmith, J. 1994. The illusive logic of integration. *Healthcare Forum* 37: 26–31.

Goldsmith, J. 1995. It's time for virtual integration. *Hospitals & Health Networks* 69: 11.

Goldsmith, J., M. Goran, and J. Nackel. 1995. Managed care comes of age. *Healthcare Forum* 38: 14–24.

Guo, K. 2002. Roles of managers in academic health centers: Strategies for the managed care environment. *The Health Care Manager* 20: 43–58.

Hax, A., and N. Majluf. 1996. *The strategy concept and process: A pragmatic approach,* 2nd ed. Englewood Cliffs: Prentice Hall.

Hoffman, R. 2002. Strategic planning: Lessons learned from a big-business district. *Technology & Learning* 22: 26–34.

Hoppszallern, S. 2002. Mergers + acquisitions. *Hospitals & Health Networks* 76: 51–56.

Horak, B. 1998. Strategic positioning: A case study in governance and management. *Journal of Healthcare Management* 43: 527–540.

Koco, L. 1994. AMEX brings managed care to LTC. *National Underwriter, Life & Health* 98: 37, 50.

Leavenworth, G. 1995. Trends in home health care. *Business & Health* 13: 55.

Liedtka, J. 1992. Formulating hospital strategy: Moving beyond a market mentality. *Health Care Management Review* 17: 21–26.

Lumsdon, K. 1994a. No place like home. *Hospitals & Health Networks* 68: 44–52.

Lumsdon, K. 1994b. Home care prepares to catch wave of managed care contracting. *Hospitals & Health Networks* 68: 58.

Lutz, S. 1995. 1995: A record year for hospital deals. *Modern Healthcare* 25: 43–52.

Marshall, J. 1996. EPO network. *Managed Healthcare* 26: 31–32.

McKelvey, B. 1982. *Organizational systematics, taxonomy, evolution and classification.* Berkeley: University of California Press.

McNamee, M. and Z. Schiller. 1994. Prepping for radical surgery. *Business Week* 3353: 97.

Medicare acts to protect coverage for homebound beneficiaries. 2002. *Health Care Financing Review* 24: 193–194.

Mintzberg, H., J. Lampel, J. Quinn, and S. Ghoshal. 2003. *The strategy process,* 4th ed. Upper Saddle River, NJ: Prentice Hall.

O'Donnell, K. 1993. Home care shaping up as competitive necessity. *Modern Healthcare* 23: 34–36.

Pallarito, K. 1996. Virtual healthcare. *Modern Healthcare* 26: 42–47.

Porter, M. 1991. Toward a dynamic theory of strategy. *Strategic Management Journal* 12: 95–117.

Press, C. 2001. Why strategies fail. *Health Forum Journal* 44: 26–31.

Robinson, J. 1996. The dynamics and limits of corporate growth in health care. *Health Affairs* 15: 155–169.

Robinson, J., and L. Casalino. 1996. Vertical integration and organizational networks in health care. *Health Affairs* 15: 7–22.

Shortell, S., R. Gillies, D. Anderson, K. Erickson, and J. Mitchel. 2000. *Remaking health care in America: The evolution of organized delivery systems,* 2nd ed. San Francisco: Jossey-Bass.

Shriver, K. 1996. Bumpy road ahead for post-acute providers. *Modern Healthcare* 26: 44.

Snyder, K. 1995. Home care marriages. *Drug Topics* 139: 44–46.

Starr, P. 1982. *The social transformation of American medicine.* New York: Basic.

Stoil, M. 2003. Legislative prospects are dim. *Nursing Homes Long Term Care Management* 52: 6–7.

Taylor, M. 2002. Home health cleanup working. *Modern Healthcare* 32: 20.

Trans Healthcare acquires bankrupt rival: Deal more than doubles company's size. 2003. *Health Care Strategic Management* 21: 4.

Ward, D. 2003. Strategic planning at ACE. *Presidency* 6: 18–23.

Welles, E. 1995. The awakening. *Inc.* 17: 23–24.

Wheelen, T., and J. Hunger. 2004. *Strategic management and business policy,* 9th ed. Upper Saddle River, NJ: Prentice Hall.

Whelan J., and J. Sisson. 1993. How to realize the promise of strategic planning. *The Journal of Business Strategy* 14: 31–36.

CHAPTER 55

Marketing: An Overview

Karen L. Carney

Marketing is a journey; it is the path an organization takes to move toward its strategic business objectives. It encourages an organization to understand how it relates to its environment and to identify what relationships it needs to make the trip. As in any journey, there are several steps that contribute to its success: analysis of the environment, preparation and planning, implementation, evaluation of progress, and adaptation to remain on course.

This chapter will explore marketing and how home care providers can harness the power of marketing to move their agencies along the path toward their marketing goals.

WHAT MARKETING IS AND ISN'T

Marketing is not a discrete function. It is a way of doing business that cannot be separated from the organization's overall journey. Each individual within a home care agency has a marketing role, though it is not always a consciously accepted role. Internal operations and all the functions that constitute the agency's capabilities combine to create the agency's product, which is an integral component of the agency's marketing. That means every staff member affects the product and thereby the marketing. Expensive marketing materials and promotional promises are worthless if they are not backed by the day-to-day actions that create the agency's true product. Home care providers must foster a marketing mindset among all staff, helping them understand how they contribute to the agency's success at meeting customers' needs.

Some home care providers believe they have achieved continued growth without investing in "marketing." The truth is that they have been involved in marketing all along, any time they reached out to potential or existing customers to understand the customers' needs and helped customers understand the benefits of their agency's capabilities. For years, many agencies have relied on this informal marketing. They had a good product that satisfied customers' needs and therefore was in demand. However, without a structured environmental analysis and concerted effort to regularly assess and satisfy customers' needs, this informal marketing cannot sustain any home care provider as the market changes.

To be successful, marketing demands an organized approach. The home care organization's goals must be clearly delineated and its marketplace surveyed to determine the best actions for reaching those goals. To take a trip, one first must know the destination. What are the options for traveling there—by car, by plane, by ship? What obstacles or barriers must be overcome to arrive there—immunizations, up-to-date passports, and so forth? What is the climate like? Does the terrain consist of rugged mountains or urban pavement? What clothes and how much money should be brought as resources? Is there a better time of year to visit? What types of facilities such as hotels and restaurants exist? All these questions make a difference, because there is always more than one option for reaching a specific destination. Marketing for home care works in a similar manner.

Agencies must have a good sense of their own marketplace and what is happening in their environment. Is the market growing with managed care or already saturated? Is it dominated by a few health care systems or fairly fragmented with a high level of competition? Who dominates the home care market and what services do they provide? The choices one makes for a marketing plan depend on the answers gained from this early analysis.

Based on the goals that have been set and the terrain that must be covered, the home care provider then maps a route for arriving at its goals. What marketing steps are necessary? How can the agency solve problems for its various customers and make itself indispensable? Supplies, equipment, and resources must match the terrain to be covered and be used on a consistent and continual basis to repeatedly present the agency's capabilities to its various customers in a manner that appeals to them.

A primary tool for any marketing effort is the marketing plan, which serves as the road map. It focuses a home care organization's limited resources in a structured effort to reach specific milestones. An effective marketing plan creates an integrated array of outreach activities that build on previous efforts to move an agency ever closer to its goals. Because every home care organization is different, each one's marketing plan will be different as well.

Marketing relies heavily on the principles of communication that foster the exchange of information and ideas as well as products and services. A critical component of marketing is the understanding of the customer. With that knowledge, home care providers can shape their products and marketing messages and efforts to appeal to the customer's needs and goals. The marketing process is cyclical, repeating itself as the home care provider continually seeks information to understand the customer and adjusts its products and marketing efforts.

Unfortunately, marketing is a concept that has had a troubled history in health care. Often perceived as sales, marketing has been denigrated as somehow robbing the compassion from health care and elevating concerns for money over the concerns for the patient.

In reality, marketing is the sum of any activities that help a home care organization align its goals, needs, and interests with its customers' goals, needs, and interests. By doing this, home care organizations position themselves as partners to their customers, providing services and resources that help the customers achieve their goals. Marketing is a long-term process that must continually repeat itself. Even home care providers that achieve success must reinvent that success the next year, and so on.

THE ROLE OF MARKETING IN HOME CARE

Traditionally, organized marketing has been avoided by home care providers for several reasons. Even just 20 years ago, there was little competition in home care. Most agencies served distinct territories with little overlap. As the Medicare program grew as a payer source, more agencies, especially proprietary home care providers, appeared in many markets. When the Health Care Financing Administration (now called the Centers for Medicare and Medicaid Services, CMS) initiated the Medicare diagnosis-related groups (DRGs) for inpatient acute care in the early 1980s, home care utilization boomed. The DRGs created an incentive for hospitals to decrease hospital lengths of stays. Home care became the natural next step for hospital patients who were sent home earlier in their recuperation. Areas without certificate of need requirements experienced tremendous expansion in the number of home care providers, while existing agencies experienced double-digit growth throughout the late 1980s into the early 1990s.

At the same time, managed care became a more dominant force in the health care industry. Managed care focused on the price and value of health care services, causing many providers to rethink their approach to positioning their agencies in the marketplace. Managed care also brought a greater emphasis on accountability— what exactly is a home care agency providing when it accepts a new patient? How many visits will be provided and for how long? What outcomes will be achieved and efficiencies gained? Home care agencies needed to answer those questions, providing data and information such as critical pathways that outlined more definitively the parameters of the service they provide.

These market occurrences—increasing competition and managed care—have increasingly encouraged home care providers to adopt a more structured approach to marketing. With the advent of a Medicare prospective payment system, home care providers should check the Medicare regulations as well as with their accountants to determine what impact marketing activities will have on their cost report and financial viability.

Marketing has also been a taboo subject for many agencies due to staff resistance. Clinical staff typically balk at marketing and its sales connotations. In practice, however, marketing is similar to the clinical assessments home care staff perform. When staff visit new patients, they don't try to "sell" them an intravenous the patients don't need. Instead, the staff asks a series of questions, assessing the patients' conditions as well as their situations. Based on that assessment, staff develop a treatment plan that is adjusted as the patients progress toward their goals. Marketing works in the same way.

Despite the home care industry's reluctance to embrace it, marketing remains an essential element for home care providers that want to build their business success. Marketing takes the organization's mission and strategic business goals and translates them into the marketing steps needed to realize those goals. A structured marketing effort brings a home care agency numerous benefits:

- *Focused effort.* A marketing plan captures the energy of the organization and focuses it on achieving its goals. Decisions can be

made as to where to invest time and energy because the goals have been established. With a clear marketing plan, everyone in the organization can work toward the same goal. Resources can be interwoven and applied toward a common goal, multiplying the impact of the resources.
- *Consistency and cohesiveness.* A marketing plan unites the organization in striving for the same goals, ensuring that all actions and messages are geared toward those endpoints. Marketing messages presented to customers are consistent and therefore complement one another.
- *Strategic growth.* A structured marketing effort helps steer the organization in the directions of its goals, attaining growth in specific areas and product line capabilities. As opportunities arise, an agency can quickly determine if the opportunities are consistent with its goals, and based on that, whether it should pursue the opportunities.
- *Advantageous use of resources.* Every organization has limited resources. A structured marketing effort helps a home care provider use its resources efficiently in the areas that will help it achieve its goals.
- *Ongoing customer feedback.* A key element in every organized marketing effort is the gathering of feedback, data, and information from customers. Although the mechanisms for attaining that feedback may vary, the purposes don't. Feedback enables an agency to adapt and evolve its marketing efforts, responding to the inevitable changes in the marketplace.

How then can home care providers harness this power of marketing to craft a road map that will lead them to their business goals?

THE MARKET ANALYSIS

All marketing planning starts with analysis. Few home care providers can afford to stand still in the current health care marketplace. A constant stream of decisions to be made exists, from whom to partner with to which contracts to pursue. A market analysis pulls together market intelligence in a cohesive, organized format to narrow an agency's options and identify the most advantageous paths to follow. It helps an agency determine where it currently stands and identifies landmarks and milestones that will help the agency travel to its future destination.

A good market analysis does not have to be expensive, though it is usually time consuming. Questions form the most basic level of analysis. Good questions generate good information, but few home care providers have practiced the art of asking questions. Consider how many times home care staff interact with customers, potential customers, vendors, and other market sources on any typical day. If those staff were armed with questions, they could help their agency fill in the gaps of its market intelligence. For example, if an agency is considering launching a new pediatric asthma program, it can encourage staff to ask questions such as: "How are children with asthma currently cared for? What other home care providers have a special pediatric asthma program? What sets those asthma programs apart? What kinds of problems occur in managing the care of children with asthma?" The answers can be jotted down and returned to the agency for inclusion in the overall market analysis that will help shape the agency's final development of its pediatric asthma program.

The goal is to ask questions that can't be answered with a yes or no. However, the most critical step in the questioning approach is to capture the answers in black and white, whether in a database, on paper, or with an index card system. Too often the information remains in a staff member's head where it cannot be combined with feedback from other sources and cannot be retained if that individual changes positions or leaves the company.

The market analysis can be directed toward the development of a specific program such as the example of a pediatric asthma program, or it can provide a market overview for the agency's entire operations. In the past, comprehensive market analyses were done every 2 to 3 years. In today's rapidly changing health care market, it is better to perform one at least annually and to continuously monitor the market during the year for any significant alterations that might occur in the meantime.

Competitive analysis. A competitive analysis identifies competitors, surveying their strengths and weaknesses. Gather feedback from customers and potential customers to evaluate how the agency compares. Some factors about competitors to assess include annual patient volume, referral sources, payer mix, competitive advantages, market share, market relationships, market position, weaknesses, financial viability, service record, and profile of capabilities.

A competitive analysis also should review more than just other home care providers. Competition for home care patients can stem from subacute or transitional care units, outpatient clinics, rehabilitation facilities, skilled nursing facilities, and physician offices. What are these providers offering and how does it compare to what the home care agency can provide? The same types of information gathered for competing agencies should be collected for these providers as well as to help the home care organization understand more fully how it fits into the overall health care market.

Internal analysis. An internal analysis should assess the agency's strengths, weaknesses, opportunities, and threats (a SWOT analysis). Information should be included on the agency's payer mix and its patients' demographics, including diagnoses, patient volume, and visit utilization. The home care provider needs to assess its agency's identity, financial viability, and relationships with other providers and organizations. The analysis also should answer: Where do current referrals come from and where is there potential for more referrals? Once a list of current and potential referral sources is compiled, rank the referral sources by priority based on their referral potential, revenue generated by each referral, patient demographics, and openness to new or expanded home care resources. The ranking creates a tier of customer priorities, highlighting their potential for generating business. The ranking is an individualized decision that is determined by each agency. In one agency, a new multigroup practice of physicians that has an alliance with the hospital where the home care agency is based may be a top priority. For another agency in the same market, that physician practice may be a lower priority precisely because it has an established relationship with a home care provider that may be difficult to penetrate.

Customer analysis. Agencies need to identify their customers, who can range from consumers and patients to payers, physicians, legislators, and other local community organizations (see Exhibit 55-1). The ability to understand customers individually and to respond to their specific needs will substantially affect the agency's marketing success. For example, consumers are not physicians and do not require, or desire, the same types of marketing messages. Individual customers are seeking different assurances and information about how the home care provider solves their problems or serves their needs. The home care provider's job is to help each customer understand "What does home care mean to me?" and "How does it help me?" At the same time, the home care agency needs to gather information on how the customers perceive home care and the agency. It should collect information on their needs, issues, goals, and life stages (i.e., retiring, starting families, etc.) as well as their demographics and disease incidence rates.

In addition to customer information, the analysis should provide information on a variety of factors (see Exhibit 55-2) that will help paint a picture of the current marketplace.

Agencies can gather this market analysis information in several ways. The first step should be to tap existing knowledge among staff members. Staff encounter a broad array of market intelligence daily but often aren't aware that management wants it. At the same time, staff can be encouraged to make every encounter more valuable through the use of effective questioning techniques. By asking a series of focused questions, over time the staff can uncover qualitative information that can help shape the agency's marketing strategy.

Numerous other sources of market intelligence exist: competitors' Medicare cost reports, research studies, Medicare program statistics, national health care statistics from various companies as well as the National Center for Health Statistics, the U.S. Census, literature searches via online databases, local newspapers and magazines (including help wanted ads), trade publications, division of health and human services for each state, division of insurance for each state, national associations (e.g., American Heart Association) and self-help groups.

The central focus of the market assessment phase should be to identify problems and uncover unmet needs. These problems become opportunities for savvy home care providers. Take a situation where the assessment uncovers a high incidence of pediatric asthma that is causing repeated emergency hospitalizations. A home care provider could partner with a local hospital and area pediatricians to develop a clinical pathway that transcends various health care settings to more effectively manage the care of children with asthma, reducing the need for unplanned hospitalizations, decreasing the incidence of complications, improving the patients' quality of life, and reducing the cost of caring for those children. The pediatric asthma program would be attractive to managed care organizations and other payers who are struggling to reduce the costs of caring for that specific population. Other options would be to hire staff with special training in respiratory care or partner with a home medical equipment provider to offer a package of specialized asthma capabilities. It could be that the home care provider already has specialized pediatric asthma capabilities. The assessment then may help uncover why those services haven't been fully utilized.

The analysis will also give the provider a base of information on which to forecast demand for specific sets of services.

Exhibit 55-1 Key Customer Audiences for Home Care

- Assisted living facilities: administrators, social workers, clinical staff
- Community organizations: administrators
- Consumers
- Continuing care retirement communities: administrators, social workers, clinical staff
- Donors
- Hospital administrators
- Hospital discharge planners/case managers
- Industry associations
- Investors
- Legislators, local government officials
- Local businesses: owners, human resource directors
- Media representatives
- Patients and families
- Payers/managed care organizations: case managers, contract managers, provider relations directors
- Physicians
- Regulatory officials
- Senior centers and elder groups
- Skilled nursing facilities: administrators, social workers
- Specialty clinic/program managers, e.g., cancer center, etc.
- Subacutes/transitional care units: administrators, social workers
- Volunteers

MARKET TRENDS AND FORCES

The health care marketplace is dynamic with constant changes. New roads and relationships are built. New developments occur. Construction and maintenance along familiar routes might force some rerouting. Customers may move or close their businesses, and new customers may take their places.

To complete a market analysis, home care providers have to understand that the home care industry has became increasingly complex. Multiple customers with diverse needs and goals must be satisfied simultaneously. A side issue for many home care providers during the last decade has been managing enormous growth. Although that growth may level off for many agencies during the next decade, they must still grapple with a rapidly changing environment being reshaped by nine major trends and forces:

1. *Competition.* With the number of home care companies across the country increasing, competition is a central force in all but the most rural markets. Competition will be a factor in reducing the overall number of home care providers by causing weaker, less resourceful agencies to close or merge.

2. *Managed care.* Managed care brings a cost consciousness about the utilization of resources and a demand for accountability. For home care providers, the increasing presence of managed care not only realigns relationships and decision makers, but also requires data and measurements that demonstrate the performance of one provider over another. More important, the guiding principles of managed care have begun to spill over into other payer sources, including Medicare, Medicaid, and indemnity insurers that will increasingly demand similar cost consciousness and outcomes measurement.

3. *Consolidation.* A side effect of competition and managed care, consolidation has become a major trend in home care as agencies pursue mergers, acquisitions, and affiliations to strengthen market positions, streamline operations, and achieve economies of scale.

4. *New decision makers.* With the onset of managed care, payers have begun wielding more power as decision makers.

Exhibit 55-2 Elements of a Home Care Market Analysis

Identify and gather the following information to develop a home care market analysis.

Internal

- Current referral patterns, e.g., volume from specific referral sources, patient diagnoses, revenue per referral source, revenue per patient diagnosis, costs per patient, etc.
- Current referral sources
- Existing patient demographics
- Customer relationships and satisfaction rates
- Payer mix
- Agency strengths and weaknesses
- Profile of agency capabilities and services

External

- Decision makers for home care referrals
- Potential referral sources
- Relationships among referral sources as well as among competitors, e.g., networks, affiliations, integrated delivery systems, etc.
- Profile of patient demographics for each referral source
- Level of consumer choice
- Service area demographics
- Disease incidences within service area
- Health care market trends, e.g., shorter lengths of stay for inpatients, decreasing inpatient volume for hospitals, etc.
- Regulatory issues and developments
- Competitor analysis
- Customers' unmet needs and/or problems
- Managed care penetration
- Top hospital DRGs
- Number of patient discharges to home care
- Home care utilization for service area
- Community and industry leaders

Although hospital continuing care staff may have had significant influence in directing referrals to specific home care providers, now those decisions are determined before the patients are even admitted to the hospital. Managed care organizations establish contracts with providers, creating panels of accepted home care providers from which patients and their caregivers must choose. The redistribution of decision making is even creeping into Medicare and Medicaid programs as some states allow managed care organizations to participate in those programs. The shift in decision makers means home care providers must shift their marketing efforts to focus on these new powerbrokers.

5. *Technology.* Advances in technology have been a significant boon to home care, enabling ever more sophisticated capabilities to be delivered in the home setting. Technology has also changed the way information is captured, stored, and communicated. A decade ago facsimile machines dramatically altered communication between referral sources and home care providers. Now the Internet, e-mail, cellular phones, telemedicine, laptop computers, and hand-held electronic devices promise to do the same. Technology can be a competitive advantage, reducing costs, eliminating redundant procedures, and streamlining administration.

6. *Aging population.* The fastest growing segment of the U.S. population is the age 85 and over group. The irony of this public health success story is that, as elders live longer, they are often living longer with chronic health conditions that may limit their ability to care for themselves independently in the community. For home care providers, the aging population ensures that demand for home care services will continue. However, the flip side of that equation is that often these individ-

uals have complex conditions that may not fit within narrow boundaries for insurance coverage or may be more costly to treat.

7. *Integrated delivery systems.* As managed care has introduced risk-sharing and capitated payment methodologies, health care providers are looking for ways to streamline operations and more completely manage patients' care as they move from one care setting to the next. The result has been the rise in integrated delivery systems (IDS)—vertical arrangements of different types of providers through contract or formal affiliation. The creation of an IDS can either suddenly constrict the referral stream or expand it for home care providers, depending on whether the agencies are on the outside or the inside of the new system.

8. *Acceleration.* The pace of health care delivery today is faster, faster, faster. Patients who are admitted to inpatient facilities find they are discharged much sooner in their recuperation. The turnaround time from admission to discharge is dramatically shorter, leaving less time for inpatient staff to provide patient education, establish a discharge plan, or even identify that a patient may need home care services. For home care providers, the result has been that patients sometimes fall through the cracks and others go home "sicker and quicker." At the same time, patients are discharged whenever they receive their physicians' approvals—evenings, weekends, and holidays as well as normal business hours. Gone are the days of keeping a patient an extra day to avoid a weekend discharge. To respond, home care providers have extended their office hours and added regular evening and weekend staff to handle the off-hour referrals and admissions.

9. *Educated consumers.* Changes in the health care system have created an impetus for consumers to become better advocates for themselves. They ask more questions, demand more information, may challenge a health care professional's guidance, command greater knowledge of health care issues and options, and are asserting their rights more adamantly.

MARKET PREPARATION AND PLANNING

Once the marketplace has been analyzed, the next step is to create a marketing plan. The marketing plan takes the market analysis and weaves it with the organization's self-assessment to create a snapshot of the agency's current market position. The plan also outlines the agency's strengths and weaknesses as well as its opportunities and threats and should detail the primary and secondary customers, ranking them by priority and identifying the agency's marketing goals for each.

The market analysis also gives the home care provider the opportunity to assess whether its marketing goals are on track or need some adjustment. For example, if one of the agency's goals is to increase referrals from a specific hospital by 20 percent, it may find the goal is no longer realistic given that the hospital has merged with another hospital that has its own home care department—or it may find that the hospital's inpatient census has dramatically decreased so an increase of 20 percent may be unrealistic. More important, the home care agency will want to rededicate its resources to goals that will have a better return on investment.

The process of developing the marketing plan can be as important as the finished plan. By involving various frontline staff members along with the marketing coordinator and other appropriate managers, the agency can gain different perspectives while establishing consensus on where the agency is headed and the steps required to get there. The process can foster staff participation and buy-in with the marketing effort. Based on the snapshot created by the market and organizational analysis, the home care staff select the marketing tactics that will move the agency toward its goals. Those tactics are chosen based on the resources available, the potential return on investment, the customers involved, and the marketing goals. For example, a home care agency may decide that while a newsletter published four times a year is a great public awareness tool, it has become a costly endeavor in a market where there is little consumer choice. Instead, the agency may want to invest the resources usually spent on developing and distributing a quarterly newsletter toward building stronger relationships with specific physicians and case managers.

The marketing plan becomes a road map, outlining the obstacles and opportunities as well as the steps to circumvent the pitfalls and grab the opportunities (see Exhibit 55-3).

This is the stage where an agency must determine where to focus its effort. With limited time and resources, it will have to make some difficult decisions about where to channel its resources. Ideally, it wants to build on its strengths. It can be very expensive and time consuming to challenge a market leader or established home care provider without having a major competitive advantage or added-value capability.

THE MARKETING MIX

Marketing involves developing the right *product*, offering it in the right *place* at the right *price* with the right mix of *promotional* activities. Examining each of these four Ps of marketing more closely helps reveal their interrelationship.

Product

What products and capabilities will the agency offer and what competitive advantage do those capabilities hold? How will services be packaged and presented? How will the agency position itself in the market? What identity will it project? The demand for various products and capabilities varies over time. Different home care providers may serve different segments of the market. The environment changes and mar-

ket forces fluctuate, creating shifts in what customers seek. A home care provider needs to continually assess its market to determine how those changes affect its products and packaging.

The product is much more than just the services a home care provider supplies. It is the sum of all the parts within the home care agency—how the phone is answered, how accurate the billing is, and how easy it is to get questions answered. The product also involves the segment of the market that the home care agency strives to serve—children, elders, people with specific diagnoses, and so on. The product is a critical decision point in marketing. It determines what the organization is "selling" and who will potentially buy it. Ideally, the agency will build on its strengths and minimize its weaknesses to maximize customer satisfaction. However, the decision about the product needs to take into account the organization's mission, culture, organizational leadership, resources, and capabilities.

Packaging is how the product is presented to the customer. Is it simply skilled nursing or specialized certification in diabetic nursing? Is it the array of standard home care services (i.e., skilled nursing, home health aide, etc.) or is it a clinical pathway that more clearly defines what set of services a patient with a particular diagnosis will receive? Packaging is also an aspect of assigning specific home care nurses as liaisons to specific doctors. The doctor's liaison nurse builds a stronger relationship with the doctor and serves as the doctor's home care resource. That package of personal attention to the physicians adds value to the home care provider's product and makes it more attractive to the customer.

One of the most common marketing pitfalls for home care providers is the failure to establish a competitive advantage. To many customers—patients, families, physicians, payers, and so on—most home care providers look alike. In their eyes, home care has become a commodity product. Quality is not a competitive advantage in the current health care market; it is a baseline expectation. How an agency de-

Exhibit 55-3 Elements of a Marketing Plan

- **Marketing plan overview/summary**
- **External market analysis**
  - major referral sources
  - decision makers
  - market relationships
  - payer sources
  - service area demographics
  - disease incidence statistics
  - market trends
  - threats
  - opportunities
  - competitor analysis

- **Internal market analysis**
  - mission and business goals
  - existing referral sources and referral patterns
  - revenue per patient by diagnosis
  - patient profiles and demographics
  - strengths
  - weaknesses
  - customer feedback
- **Priority customers**
- **Key marketing messages**
- **Marketing goals and marketing activities for each goal**
- **Action plan**

fines and demonstrates quality, though, can be a competitive advantage. The competitive advantage is what sets a home care agency apart from its competitors. What added value does it bring to its customers? How does it help its customers achieve their goals? What special strengths does the agency have and how do those strengths benefit the customers?

Competitive advantages come in many shapes and sizes. Special clinical skills or programs, rapid response time, streamlined paperwork, electronic medical records, laptop computers in the field, superior clinical outcomes, cross-training of staff, service guarantees, discount prices, vast service areas, disease management programs or clinical pathways for high-cost complex diagnoses, one-stop shopping, and follow-up phone calls are all examples of different competitive advantages. The competitive advantage depends on the customers involved and how they perceive the advantage.

Place (Distribution)

Place represents where and how the home care services are offered, which can be another differentiating factor. Many home care providers are forming networks and alliances to give managed care organizations and IDSs a larger ser-

vice area for contracts. The alliances may also provide one-stop shopping, offering an array of services through a single access point. The location of an agency's main office can give it increased community visibility, as can the location of its satellite or branch offices. Place can also relate to the relationships a home care provider has. For example, a hospital-based provider has a distinct advantage in its market because of its relationship with the hospital, a relationship that places the agency in the path for referrals from the hospital. A home care provider that assigns a liaison nurse to specific physicians' offices has multiplied its distribution network by creating an extension of its office within the physician practices.

Price

Pricing is a new arena for most home care agencies. Until managed care burst on the scene, the major issue related to fees was fine tuning the cost report for the best reimbursement rate. There were no negotiations and no real pricing strategies involved. Pricing, though, has moved to center stage in many health care markets as home care providers struggle to offset price concessions with added-value capabilities that may allow them to secure higher prices. Price is the combination of costs and value. Traditionally, home care providers have not had a good understanding of either, which has left them vulnerable to the new pricing methodologies such as risk sharing and capitation.

Pricing methodologies in home care currently range from discounted fee-for-service arrangements, per diem payments, and episodic case rates to risk sharing, performance-based compensation, and capitation. As home care providers try to negotiate higher prices from managed care organizations, they learn that price is often the only factor that differentiates home care providers from one another. Until recently, there has been little available data about home care and few benchmarks that enabled managed care organizations to compare apples to apples among home care providers. To move beyond price as a differentiating factor, home care agencies need to offer other capabilities that are perceived as having value by the customers.

Promotion

The mix of marketing activities an agency selects to engage its various customers and move toward its marketing goals is called the *promotional mix*. The following is a sampling of promotional activities that a home care provider may select.

Media relations. News releases, television and radio public service announcements (PSAs), and feature stories have been standard elements in home care marketing outreach. A relatively low-cost promotional method, media relations have been effective in creating and maintaining the company's identity but are perhaps less effective in influencing which agencies end up on a managed care organization's provider panel. Some of the newest media avenues—the Internet and online forums—are low cost and offer ample opportunity for one-to-one contact with customers. Use of the media can be effective in reaching out to consumers, influencing patient choice, providing consumer education, and fostering the agency's identity.

Advertising. Advertising has become more prevalent in home care as some providers try to differentiate themselves from an increasing field of competitors and establish a market advantage. Interestingly, several managed care organizations have used home care success stories in their own advertising to consumers. A capital-intensive medium, advertising relies on the frequency of the ad placement and the ad size (or duration in broadcast media).

Community relations. The general public remains a pivotal audience for every home care provider even though the public's ability to choose a specific provider may be eroded through managed care contracts. Community education programs, screenings, and immunization clinics help position an agency as a community resource. Speakers' bureaus enable the agency to present a variety of topics related to home care and general health. For those providers affiliated with an integrated delivery system, the home care agency can provide the infrastructure for the system's community outreach efforts. For free-standing agencies, the community represents a major marketing audience.

Professional relations. As decision makers have become more diverse, home care providers have placed more emphasis on professional education and networking. Health care professionals often misunderstand home care. Hospital staff and physicians who must refer patients to home care may hold outdated notions of home care and its capabilities. Education efforts must bridge this gap while engaging professionals who may feel they already know all there is to know about home care. The relationship-building process fosters an exchange of information that will help the home care provider more fully understand the health care professional's needs and concerns, thereby enabling the agency to translate its home care services into appropriate benefits based on those needs and concerns.

Special events.   Although often labor intensive, special events can generate substantial
public and professional awareness of home care.
They can help publicize a specific service or capability and help with fund-raising.

Marketing communications.   Print communication has long been the mainstay of health care
marketing—brochures, annual reports, newsletters, and marketing collaterals. Print communication remains a strong component in home care
marketing but is taking more of a supportive role
to interpersonal marketing strategies such as
sales and one-to-one education efforts. At the
same time, the forums for marketing communications have expanded with the advent of videos,
e-mail, Web sites, and interactive software.

Contract negotiations and management.   One
of the newest dimensions of home care marketing, contract negotiations enable a home care
provider to more fully represent itself and its
capabilities with payers and other providers during the contract development. In addition, once
a contract is in place, the complexities of a contract extend beyond the legal nuances and into
the areas of service definition and compliance.
The ability to understand, interpret, and comply
with a contract can give a home care provider an
advantage over competitors.

Sales.   Structured sales efforts have become a
familiar factor in home care marketing as many
agencies have discovered that relationship
building demands one-to-one interactions. The
downfall of many home care sales efforts,
though, is that interactions are not focused on
achieving a particular goal or eliciting specific
information. By asking questions and proposing
case examples, sales representatives can lead
health care professionals and other referral
sources to a greater understanding of how home
care can solve problems they face. The questions help the sales representatives to better understand the customers' roles and perspectives,
enabling the sales representatives to then tailor

their home care messages and examples to the
customers' specific situations.

Fund-raising.   For not-for-profit home care
providers, fund-raising efforts form the cornerstone of much of their marketing outreach. Fund
development can be exercised at various levels
of sophistication from special events to finely
timed annual appeals. For fund-raising to be
successful, the target public must know and
have some type of vested interest in making a
donation. As a result, fund-raising efforts should
be closely coordinated with the rest of the organization's marketing outreach, to provide consistent messages and leverage the potential of
other marketing efforts.

Investor relations.   Investors are a critical
source of support for privately held and publicly
traded home care providers. The ongoing communication with these key audiences often takes
the form of marketing communications and relationship building.

IMPLEMENTATION

Focus

Once the marketing plan is complete, one of the
toughest marketing challenges for home care
providers is to maintain their marketing focus.
Too often they try to be all things to all customers. The result: Resources are spread too thin
and the impact of their marketing investment is
diluted. More important, by narrowing their targets, home care providers reduce the likelihood
that they'll be overwhelmed by their marketing
responsibilities, which often causes marketing
tasks to be placed on the back burner. Instead of
targeting 50 doctors, it may be more realistic for
a home care agency to target 5. They can launch
a more comprehensive campaign with the five
doctors, focus a greater proportion of resources
on building solid relations with those physicians,
and working with five physicians can seem much
more "doable" for home care providers already
saddled with other responsibilities.

Local Markets Demand Local Strategies

What works in one geographic area may not work in the neighboring service area. Each health care community has its own distinct needs and issues. Home care providers that operate several offices or regional networks know that each market demands its own version of the agency's overall marketing plan. The goals may remain the same, but the strategies and tactics may vary. In some markets, though, the goals may vary as well. Certain markets may have no need for a pediatric asthma program while other markets may find those programs flourishing.

A Living Document

The marketing plan should change over time, just as the market does. It is meant to be a living, breathing document. While the overall strategies should remain sound as long as the market doesn't undergo dramatic upheaval, the tactics should be adjusted to match the changing environment. Consider a situation where one marketing goal is to develop specialty programs, and the marketing plan originally recommended developing a pediatric asthma program. Then soon after the marketing plan is complete, the major referral source develops its own pediatric asthma program. The agency must adapt its marketing plan. It can either discontinue the pediatric asthma effort, investigate how it may be able to align with or augment the referral source's program, or develop new sources of referrals by expanding its service area.

One way to keep the marketing plan from sitting on a shelf is to transform the finished plan into an action plan that lists activities that need to be accomplished month by month with the names of the individuals responsible for accomplishing those tasks (see Exhibit 55-4).

Marketing Structure

The structure of a home care provider's marketing effort will affect its ability to implement its marketing tactics and achieve its goals. The structure should match the marketplace and the

Exhibit 55-4 Marketing Action Plan

January		February		March	
Action	**Responsible**	**Action**	**Responsible**	**Action**	**Responsible**
Meet with the three doctors in the new multigroup practice	Liaison nurse and clinical supervisor	Begin developing new agency capabilities sheet for physicians	Community relations director	Meet with three doctors in the new multigroup practice to explain new physician liaison program	Liaison nurse and clinical supervisor
Hold first meeting to develop physician liaison program	Liaison nurse, clinica supervisor, community relations director, and executive director	Compile list of physicians to be sent new capabilities sheet	Community relations director and administrative assistant	Mail new capabilities sheet to physicians	Administrative assistant

goals. For example, if there is a growing presence of managed care, the home care provider needs to send staff on marketing visits to build relationships with the increasing array of decision makers such as physicians, case managers, managed care contract managers, and subacute care managers.

Some agencies have decentralized their marketing effort by assigning marketing responsibilities to several staff members who also shoulder other agency responsibilities. Other agencies have designated a single individual as the marketing coordinator. Even in agencies with more extensive marketing departments, it can still make sense to decentralize some of the marketing responsibilities because this encourages staff participation in and understanding of the agency's marketing efforts.

MEASUREMENT AND ADAPTATION

Once a structured marketing effort is implemented, the evaluation begins. Evaluation and feedback enable the agency to determine not only whether its marketing efforts are working, but also whether its marketing goals are on track with any changes in the marketplace. Evaluation can occur through customer satisfaction surveys, data collection of key performance indicators, informal feedback from customers, market intelligence gathered through the media and other reports, and structured market research. Exhibit 55-5 offers a list of key indicators that can help measure marketing efforts.

Marketing in some respects is experimental, making it more an art than a science. Different

Exhibit 55-5 Key Performance Indicators

- Referral volume per referral source
- Revenue per patient
- Revenue per patient per diagnosis
- Revenue by payer/referral source
- Costs per patient
- Costs per patient by diagnosis
- Costs per patient by payer/referral source
- Agency revenue
- Patient volume
- Patient volume by diagnosis
- Customer satisfaction rates
- Visit utilization per patient
- Visit utilization per patient by diagnosis

products and promotional activities work in different situations. That's one reason why measurement is so important. Home care providers need to check whether their marketing efforts are working.

CONCLUSION

Marketing is a natural aspect of business, whether or not a home care provider consciously structures a marketing effort. However, by structuring a marketing effort that begins with analysis and continues through measurement and adaptation, the home care organization will move along the steps toward its marketing goals. The marketing plan becomes the road map, helping the agency navigate its changing health care landscape, understand and satisfy its customers' needs, and achieve its marketing goals.

BIBLIOGRAPHY

Bowen, D., and B. Schneider. 1995. *Winning the service game.* Boston: Harvard Business School Press.

Clampitt Douglas, L., P. Edwards, and S. Edwards. 1991. *Getting business to come to you.* Los Angeles: Jeremy P. Tarcher.

Collins, J. 2001. *Good to great: Why some companies make the leap . . . and others don't.* New York: Harper-Collins.

Collins, J., and J. Porras. 1994, 1997. *Built to last: Successful habits of visionary companies.* New York: Harper-Business.

Conrad Levinson, J. 1993. *Guerrilla marketing excellence: Fifty golden rules for small-business success.* Boston: Houghton Mifflin.

Drucker, P. 1964, 1986. *Managing for results.* New York: Harper & Row.

Drucker, P. 1990. *Managing the non-profit organization: Principles and practices.* New York: HarperCollins.

Fuld, L. 1995. *The new competitor intelligence.* New York: John Wiley & Sons.

Gumpert, D. 1992. *How to really create a successful marketing plan.* Boston: Inc. Publishing.

Hawken, P. 1987. *Growing a business.* New York: Simon & Schuster.

Kawasaki, G. 1991. *Selling the dream.* New York: HarperBusiness.

Kotler, P. 1996. *Marketing management: Analysis, planning, implementation, and control.* 9th ed. Englewood Cliffs, NJ: Prentice Hall.

McKenna, R. 1991. *Relationship marketing: Successful strategies for the age of the customer.* Reading, MA: Addison-Wesley.

Newsom, D., and A. Scott. 1976. *This is PR: The realities of public relations.* Belmont, CA: Wadsworth Publishing.

Peppers, D., and M. Rogers. 1993. *The one to one future: building relationships one customer at a time.* New York: Currency Doubleday.

Reilly, R. 1987. *Public relations in action,* 2nd ed. Englewood Cliffs, NJ: Prentice Hall.

Ries, A., and J. Trout. 1993. *The 22 immutable laws of marketing.* New York: HarperBusiness.

Sewell, C., and P. Brown. 1990. *Customers for life.* New York: Pocket Books.

Tracy, B. 1995. *Advanced selling strategies.* New York: Simon & Schuster.

Whitely, R. 1991. *The customer driven company: Moving from talk to action.* Reading, MA: Addison-Wesley.

CHAPTER 56

The Internet in Home Health and Hospice Care

Linda Q. Thede and Virginia K. Saba

INTRODUCTION

Ten years ago the Internet was something that was used mostly by academics and scientists for communication. Today, the Internet is changing how we live. We shop online, we communicate online, and we look for information online. It is slowly transforming health care and has given birth to a new term, *e-health*. Most health care agencies now have a World Wide Web presence and patients and health care professionals both look to the Internet for health care information.

The Internet grew from a 1969 Department of Defense network known as the Advanced Research Projects Agency Network (ARPANET) that was designed to transmit digital data from one computer to another. In the 1970s and 1980s as computer use grew, several other large regional networks were developed to provide researchers access to supercomputer and networking ability. The term *Internet* was first used in 1983 to describe the National Science Foundation network that in the late 1980s replaced ARPANET. In the early 1990s, the various networks coalesced into one network that we today know as the Internet.

There are many ways that the Internet and the Web can be useful in home health and hospice care. The following are some examples:

- Rapid and large-scale dissemination of information about nearly any aspect of home health or hospice care for health care professionals such as prevention of tuberculosis and other common secondary infections. Sites such as http://www.ahcpr.gov/clinic/epcix.htm provide easy access to evidence-based practice reports and to guidelines for care.
- Provision of information for the health care consumer about disease conditions, and services offered by home health and hospice agencies.
- Virtual visits, or visits in which the client and caregiver communicate via the Internet. Interactive monitoring devices that transmit vital signs and other clinical data allow home health care personnel to conduct post-surgical check-ups. By lowering the cost per visit, virtual visits can provide more visits per patient and increase the quality of life for those with chronic conditions (Thede, 2003).
- Support groups for patients and lay caregivers such as the one for caregivers of Alzheimer's patients. The Internet can also be used to provide grief counseling or support groups for those with the same condition or disease, such as one for people who have spinal cord injuries.
- Educating patients via the Internet. For example, patients and their families can be taught appropriate range of motion exercises, enterostomal care, or urinary catheterization with follow-up provided

by e-mail. Or a Web page with more information about a topic can be used. Web sites can also provide the ability for users to ask questions.

- Manage chronic illness and prevent frequent hospitalizations.
- Health care professionals can use the Internet for collaboration on care plans or manuscripts for publication.

WHAT IS THE INTERNET?

The Internet is a worldwide connection of computer networks that is similar to the telephone system. It links millions of local networks together and is the electronic information highway used to communicate, transmit, and retrieve digital data. It is similar, but different, from telephone networks. Telephone networks use online *analog* (sound wave signals) communication while electronic data is *digital*. The Internet is in essence a "free" worldwide electronic communication network that is not controlled by any single organization or country.

Internet connectivity is obtained via an Internet service provider (ISP), roughly analogous to a long-distance telephone service provider. Many educational and health care institutions act as an ISP for faculty, staff, and students. Other providers are nationally accessible value-added ISPs such as America Online and Microsoft Network. They primarily serve up a wide range of options for information, opinion, and products. They also provide some access to the Internet. ISPs can be national, regional, or local. Their primary purpose is to provide access to the Internet. Detailed information about thousands of ISPs and the information for accessing each is available at http://www.thelist.com.

Computers connected to the Internet are of various sizes and makes, and may be connected with each other by relatively expensive high-capacity fiber optics, telephone lines, or satellites. Over 100 countries are presently connected to the Internet and more join each year. Many third-world nations, however, do not yet have access. Still, when access becomes necessary in a situation, such as it was in the Ebola outbreak in Kikwit, Zaire, in the mid-1990s, portable satellite phones and cellular technologies can be added to enable connectivity.

Beyond selecting an ISP, there are several choices for connecting to the Internet. Many people still use POTS (plain old telephone service) through a dial-up modem. This provides a relatively slow connection, the standard today being 56 kilobits per second. In some locations faster connections using a telephone line can be achieved by using a digital subscriber line (DSL). Although this technology allows much higher transmission speeds over ordinary telephone lines, it requires users to live within 20,000 feet of a central telephone office. An even faster connection can be obtained with a modem that uses cable TV lines. Many TV cable companies now offer this option.

The Internet supports several different applications. The two most well known are e-mail and the World Wide Web (WWW). The WWW, which is often referred to simply as the Web, was preceded by Gopher, a program developed at the University of Minnesota (home of the Golden Gophers). Although Gopher supported hypertext, or the ability to point and click with a mouse, it was strictly text based and was supplanted by the Web. Another older format still used occasionally is Telnet. In this type of communication, the user connects with a computer and uses the files and programs provided on the distant computer as though they were on the user's own computer. Another older format, but one that is still used on the Internet, is the File Transfer Protocol (FTP). It is used for transferring files from one computer to another.

E-mail

Everyone who has Internet access has access to electronic mail (e-mail). The software that provides this function is part of all the popular Web browsers. Separate e-mail packages such as Qualcomms' Eudora, which is available both as a free download and for purchase, are also used. Although originally just text based, most e-mail packages now support text formatting and the inclusion of pictures that are in a format that is supported by the Web such as JPEG or GIF files

Attachments

Files created with other software, such as word processed documents or spreadsheets, can be sent via e-mail as an attachment. In most cases, recipients must have the program that created the file or they will be unable to use the attachment. For example, a file created in one brand of word processor may not be readable with a word processor from a different vendor. Some universal file types exist, such as rich text format (RTF). This format can be created by most word processors and allows files to be read by most word processors regardless of what program was used to create them. For example, if a user saves a file created with Corel's Word Perfect as an RTF, a person who uses Microsoft Word will be able to read and edit the file and vice versa.

E-mail Addresses

When sending e-mail, the e-mail address must always be accurate to the last character. To facilitate this, e-mail packages allow users to create address books of e-mail addresses that are used frequently. Some provide the user with the ability to right click on an address in a received mail and add it to the address book. Address books also provide the ability to create groups, or a list of e-mail addresses to use when certain messages need to be sent. For example, a supervisor who often sends messages to all staff nurses may create in the address book a group that contains all the e-mail addresses of the staff nurses. When he or she needs to communicate with this group, the supervisor only needs to enter the group name in the address bar instead of each nurse's e-mail address. See Figure 56-1.

Communicating Via E-mail

E-mail communication is different from other means of communication. In face-to-face meetings, one receives not only verbal input, but also

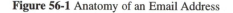

> Cbarton@redcross.org
>
> Cbarton = user ID
> @ = separates the user ID from the domain name of the computer
> .org = the top level domain

Figure 56-1 Anatomy of an Email Address

body language. In telephone conversations, verbal inflections are present. Although e-mail may seem analogous to letter writing, it is different in that it is generally done quickly; there is a tendency to use abbreviations and sentences may be terse. All of these differences can lead to difficulties. Add to this the ability of any e-mail message to be instantly forwarded to one or thousands of people and it becomes obvious that thought should be given to what an e-mail message contains. A good rule of thumb is that if you do not wish to read something in the morning newspaper, do not put it in an e-mail message. If you are bothered by something and a little short tempered, wait before firing off that message. Once sent, an e-mail message is irretrievable.

To help make e-mail a viable format for communication, guidelines have been created. Known as *e-mail etiquette*, they are available from many sites on the Web including http://www.kassj.com. Two important rules are to use a subject line and a signature. A brief title of a message in the subject line allows the recipient to handle the e-mail more effectively. Also, messages without subjects are often deleted without reading. E-mail messages without a signature are confusing and may also be deleted without reading. Because it is so easy to forget a signature, e-mail packages provide the ability to create a signature that is automatically added to all e-mail messages. E-mail software also provides a spell check and the ability to have it automatically check each message before it is sent. It is strongly suggested that the user sets the e-mail package to spell check automatically.

E-mail Viruses and Other Internet Hazards

In the "olden" days (until the late 1990s), computer viruses were usually spread from one computer to another by an infected disk. Today, most viruses arrive in the form of an e-mail attachment.

Although these nuisances are generally referred to as viruses, not all behave in the same manner. Worms and viruses are pretty similar in that both replicate themselves and perform malicious actions, such as using up the computer's resources or even shutting down the computer. Another type of destructive program is known as a Trojan horse. Trojan horses masquerade as benign applications but in reality are programs that create problems like deleting files. Unlike viruses and worms they cannot replicate themselves. Trojan horses can be avoided by not downloading or accepting programs from any source that does not have a sterling reputation, preferably a well known and respected company.

The first line of defense for viruses and worms is a good antivirus program such as Symantec's Norton Anti-Virus or McAffee's Antivirus program. Antivirus programs, however, are only effective against the viruses that they "know." Given that 3 to 10 new viruses are discovered each day, it follows that these programs are not effective if not updated. Both of these programs provide easy mechanisms for updating; some programs will automatically update themselves provided the computer is on and connected to the Internet at the time set for updating. Backing up an antivirus program with a healthy paranoia regarding e-mail attachments will help to keep your computer virus and worm free.

Under no circumstances should you open an e-mail attachment if you do not know what it contains and you are not expecting it. Knowing the sender is no guarantee of safety; most viruses not only do their damage, but also are programmed to open a user's e-mail address book and send themselves to all the addresses it contains.

Further protection is available through a device known as a *firewall*. Although it protects any Internet connection, it is a vital ingredient when one connects via either DSL or cable. A firewall can be either a piece of hardware or software. They operate either by examining all messages entering or leaving the system and blocking those that do not meet specific criteria or by denying entrance to messages if the destination port is not acceptable at the time an attempt is being made to contact it (Thede, 2003). One of the most popular firewalls is Zone Alarm (http://www.zonelabs.com), which is available both as a free download and in a professional version for which there is a charge.

It is not unusual for e-mail users to receive a message from a friend warning of an e-mail virus that will destroy one's computer. This message looks official and contains information that Microsoft, IBM, or some other well-respected source has provided these facts. They are almost always hoaxes. Never pass one on unless you check its authenticity with a Web site such as the U.S. Department of Energy's Computer Incident Advisory Capability (CIAC) Hoaxbusters page at http://hoaxbusters.ciac.org.

A new scam that has appeared on the Internet involves identity theft. An individual receives an e-mail message with a subject line about an account somewhere, for example a credit card or bank account. When the message is read, the user is directed to a specific site that appears almost identical to the legitimate site, but is not the real site. The user is then asked to enter personal information such as social security number, account numbers, and so on that can be used to steal the person's identity. This is easily avoided if one will remember not to provide this type of information without first calling the actual agency that has the account in question.

Personal and Group Networking

The Internet provides more formal ways of networking beyond e-mail. These include newsgroups, forums, and electronic mailing lists. They differ in how they are used, but all share the goal of fostering networking between those with similar interests. One has to actively access newsgroups and forums, but electronic mailing lists send messages directly to the subscriber.

Newsgroups

Newsgroups began in 1970 at the University of North Carolina as a forum for discussing politics, religion, and other subjects (Thede, 2003). Although the term "news" is in the title, in reality the news is messages sent by anyone who selects the group and decides to *post*. Reading newsgroups requires special software, but most e-mail software contain these readers. The main nursing newsgroup is sci.med.nursing. Messages in a newsgroup are *threaded* or organized by the topic in the subject line. These groups are generally completely unmoderated and information may or may not be accurate.

Forums

Many professional groups offer forums for discussion of topics pertaining to the group. Participation generally involves registering and selecting a password (Peters and Saba, 2001). Often these forums are moderated to a certain degree and may be an excellent source of information.

Electronic Mailing Lists

Although the term *mailing list* conjures up images of unwanted mail, electronic mailing lists are Internet interest groups. In these groups, members use e-mail to engage in asking and answering questions, as well as discussing subjects related to the topic of the group. There are many lists that pertain to all aspects of health care. Rod Ward at http://nmap.ac.uk maintains a list of health-related electronic mailing lists.

The term used for joining a mailing list is to *subscribe*; however, the subscription is free. Once one subscribes, all messages posted to the group are sent to each member of the group. E-mail lists have two addresses: one for members to use for sending messages to the list and one for the software that manages the list. The first address, or *posting address*, is the one that is used to send messages to the group and from which all received messages originate. The second address, or the one to which one sends a request for subscription, is for the software that manages the list. The software at this address handles not only subscriptions, but also setting e-mail preferences and "unsubscribing." When a list is joined, this software also sends out an automatic note providing information about how to use these features. Save this message; it saves you from showing your ignorance by posting to the group a request to be unsubscribed or asking how to use another feature of the list. The original software for managing these lists was called "Listserv," which is why these lists are often called *listservs*. Today there are many other software packages that manage lists, such as Majordomo and Mailserv. Often the type of software used is evident by the address that one uses to subscribe.

WORLD WIDE WEB

There is a tendency to think of the Internet and the Web as the same entity, but in fact, they are two separate entities. The Internet is simply a connection, or *network*, between millions of computers located all over the globe. Information that passes over this network adheres to prescribed *protocols*, or prescriptions for how to send and receive messages. The World Wide Web, or Web as it is often called, is a tool used on the Internet to access information. The Web is best described as an information-sharing tool built on top of the Internet (Webopedia, 2003).

Browsers

The Web is accessed using software called a *browser*. The two most popular browsers today are Microsoft's Internet Explorer, which is a feature in the Microsoft Windows Operating System, and Netscape's Communicator, which can be downloaded free from the Netscape Web site. Documents available on the Web are formatted with *tags*, which are invisible when a Web document is read, but tell the browser how the document should look and provide links to other Web pages. These tags comprise the *Hyptertext Mark-up Language* (HTML).

URLs

A *uniform resource locator* (URL) is the address used by Web software to find a given resource. Each URL has several basic components that are structured in a standardized manner. The combination of characters http:// www.nursingworld.org/ojin/index.htm is the address or URL for the *Online Journal of Issues in Nursing*. Each slash and period in a Web address is a demarcation between parts of the address. A breakdown of this URL is seen in Figure 56-2.

Web addresses are generally case sensitive; that is, the pattern of upper- and lower-case letters must be followed when entering the URL. Although one may be able to locate the page at the URL represented by the letters after the double forward slash and before the first single forward slash without paying attention to case, file directories and names, or those letters after the leftmost forward slash, are often case sensitive. Given the sensitivity of URLs to any variations in entering them, Web browsers provide ways to remember URLs of sites that are visited frequently. Called Favorites (Internet Explorer) or Bookmarks (Netscape), these tools record the exact URL of a site. They also provide a way of organizing these sites so that they are easily located when one wishes to access a site that has been recorded. Most e-mail packages transmit messages in a format such that if the message includes the full URL (that is, it starts with http) of a Web page, the recipient only needs to click on it for the browser to open the page. Whenever one has to copy an URL, the best way to do it is to use the copy and paste feature of the operating system.

Finding Information on the Web

The Web can be described as a gigantic encyclopedia that offers a wealth of information, but unfortunately given the different forms of infor-

▸http:// = indicates that the hypertext transfer protocol should be used to send this document. The colon and two forward slashes are used in Web addresses to separate the way the document should be transferred and the name of the computer. Sometimes you will see "ftp" or "https" instead of "http."

▸www = says that this is a document on the World Wide Web. Not all URLs use this designation.

▸nursingworld.org = is the domain name of the site. The last 3 letters of this URL, "org," referred to as the top level domain may designate the type of site, e.g. org may mean a non-profit organization, gov a government site, com a commercial site and edu an educational institution. These are not as strictly adhered to as in the past. Sometimes this location instead has a two letter code that indicates the country of origin.

▸ojin = the name of the directory or location in the computer containing the document where the document is stored.

▸index.htm = the name of the file that belongs to that URL. "Index" is a file name often used to denote the top page in a Web site, or the home page.

▸#Name (not in the above URL) = the pound sign followed by letters indicates that the location is a specific place within that document in the URL.

Figure 56-2 Anatomy of a URL

mation that can be found there, it lacks the neat organization of an encyclopedia or of bibliographic references. To find information on the Web, a search tool is used. Search strategies on the Web are a little different than those one would use for searching in an electronic bibliographic database. One not only has to select the appropriate term, but also select the appropriate type of tool as well as the best search engine for the task. A tutorial at http:// www.lib.berkeley.edu/TeachingLib/Guides/ Internet/Strategies.html (U.C. Berkeley Library

[2001]) provides a step by step guide to both of these tasks.

In the mid- to late 1990s, search tools could be neatly categorized as either directories, search engines, or meta-search tools. A *directory* only searched pages that it had personally examined and categorized, a *search engine* used a given algorithm (series of rules) to find pages that then were often ranked by another algorithm, and a *meta-search tool* searched many different search engines. Today, the borders between these tools has eased. Yahoo! (http://www.yahoo.com), which used to be a directory search tool, now defaults to the search engine Google when needed, and Google now offers a directory. Users generally develop a favorite search tool and depend on it. One of the most popular today is Google (http://www.google.com). If one is searching for health Web sites for both client and professional use, the sites at http://www.healthatoz.com and http://www.lib.uiowa.edu/hardin/ are very helpful. Additionally, using the Health section in a directory such as Yahoo! is very helpful.

Search tools will find all types of Web files that meet the search criteria, such as sites with products for sale and documents written by anyone who can post a Web page. Although much of it is valuable, it should not be equated with peer-reviewed journals. There are online search tools that search only journal articles or bibliographic databases. Many of the well-known ones such as CINAHL (http://www.cinahl.com) are fee based. Most academic institutions and some health care agencies maintain subscriptions to one or more of these bibliographic databases for use by students or employees. Individuals also can purchase time for many of these tools. For the most part, these tools do not provide access to the full text of an article, but instead the bibliographic information and abstracts if they are available.

The U.S. government provides a free biomedical journal bibliographical database called PubMed. The primary one, named Entrez (http://www3.ncbi.nlm.nih.gov/entrez/query.fcgi?db=PubMed), searches the entire biomedical literature, while a new search tool, Entrez Home (http://www3.ncbi.nlm.nih.gov/entrez/query.fcgi?db=pmc), searches for articles that journals have made available for free online. The Directory of Open Access Journals (http://www.doaj.org) is a free bibliographic search tool that provides searching and access to full text for articles in scientific and scholarly journals that are freely available online. A British site, Medic8, (http://www.medic8.com/Search.htm) provides many helpful tools for health care professionals and also publishes articles by professionals on various health-related topics. Searching effectively requires preplanning (Figure 56-3). Most search tools, both for Web documents and for bibliographic articles, provide help for using the tool. It is often advantageous to spend time reading this information before embarking on a search.

Journal Information on the Web

Many journals only publish online. Some are subscription based, but most are freely available. The Global Nursing Knowledge Network (http://www.gnkn.org) was created in 2002 to encourage authors who receive no remuneration for their articles from most print journals to publish online, where their articles will be freely available. A list of links to many online nursing journals can be found at http://junior.apk.net/~lqthede/Informatics/Chap06/OnlineJournals.htm.

> ▸Analyze the topic for possible terms to use in searching
> ▸ Select the correct search tool.
> ▸Learn and revise as the search proceeds (UC Berkeley Library, 2001).

Figure 56-3 Searching Steps

Evaluation of Web Information

Web pages range from peer-reviewed journal articles to advertising to an individual's ranting opinions. The purpose of the page can be advocacy of a cause, business, or marketing scheme; news; personal information; or general information on just about any topic. Designers of these pages include individuals, commercial establishments, governments, educational agencies, health care institutions, and organizations. Given the wide range of information plus the many applications for Web information, there is no one method for evaluating Web pages, although there are some general standards that are helpful.

Some items to consider when evaluating a Web page are credibility, content, disclosure, links, and navigation (Ambre et al., 1997). When considering credibility, one should take into account not only the context, currency, and relevance of the information, but also the source of the document. Accuracy of the content, especially health-related documents, can be evaluated based on whether there are sources included with the information plus one's own knowledge. Accuracy is sometimes affected by timing, thus looking for a date on which the information was last updated may be helpful. Knowing who sponsors the site is another lead in evaluating. Information on a site that is primarily for marketing, although it may present helpful information, needs to be evaluated with the goals of the publisher in mind. One can also evaluate the links that are on the site, not only for their pertinence and appropriateness, but also by whether most of them still work. Web sites are extremely fluid and sites are often reorganized, resulting in new locations for original documents that render links invalid. A site with many links that do not work is probably several years old. Navigability is also often used as a criterion in evaluating a Web site. The weight that one puts on links and navigability depends on the purpose for which the information on the page will be used. If the Web site of concern is a document, then the information is of primary concern, not the links and navigability. If, however, a site is more of a jumping off point for a topic, then the availability of the links and navigation are important.

Various proposals to promote reliability of health information on the Web have been offered. Most provide an examination of the page by an independent group, then if the page meets the group's criteria, the site is permitted to display the logo of the evaluating group. The logo links the site to a page of criteria and provides information for users who believe that the criteria have been violated to report the violations. The Health on the Net Foundation (http://www.hon.ch) applies this method. Their goal is to ensure that readers know the purpose and source of the information. They do not rate the medical accuracy, appropriateness, or validity of the information (Health on the Net Foundation, 2002), but rather set basic ethical standards that must be followed, such as making sure that readers know the purpose and source of information that they find.

Developing a Web Presence

Most health care agencies have a Web presence in the form of a home page. They are extremely useful for providing information about the services the organization offers as well as directions for driving to the agency. Some agencies also provide health information or links to Web pages that they feel would be valuable to their clientele.

Web sites are organized in a hierarchical fashion. The home page is the "top" of the hierarchy (see Figure 56-4). It is generally the domain name of the organization, such as "nursingworld.org" in the URL http://www.nursingworld.org/ojin/index.htm. The site then has directories, or named entities that hold either other directories, files, or both. Agencies usually "buy" a domain name that reflects the name of the organization to use as the home page. For example, the Visiting Nurses Ass-

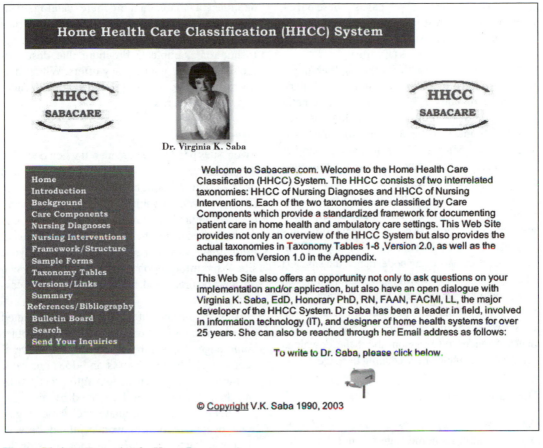

Figure 56–4 An Example of a Home Page

ociation of Cleveland, Ohio's home page is http://www.vnacleveland.org.

Many agencies hire outside firms to create their pages, or they may have someone on their staff who has this as part of their job responsibilities. Creating a Web page is only part of the tasks associated with a Web presence. Updating the information on the page is necessary as well as periodically checking the links attached to the page. If the page provides a way for users to contact the agency, it is necessary to have a method for responding. Not receiving an answer when one takes the time to send an e-mail or fill out a form creates a bad impression of the agency.

Until the late 1990s, most Web pages were created from scratch; that is, by an individual manually marking up documents with the necessary tags. Sometimes a software HTML editor was used that automated some of the coding process. What you see is what you get (WYSIWYG) Web page creators that behave similarly to word processors have since become the most popular method for creating a Web page. All modern software applications such as word processors, spreadsheets, and presentation programs provide a quick way of creating Web pages. These pages, however, often have substandard mark-up language plus generally suffer from overcoding that creates a larger than necessary file.

The price of software for creating Web pages varies from free to several thousand dollars. Netscape includes a WYSIWYG page creator free as part of its browser. One author has used this and found it to be adequate for small personal pages. Microsoft's Front Page is another Web page creator. It integrates extremely well with any page created with a Microsoft Office page. However, pages created using Front Page require special software on the server, thus they are not universally acceptable. Macromedia's Dreamweaver is more expensive than Front Page, but it creates clean code, hence the smallest files. File size affects download time, and although more and more people are using connections faster than POTS, the majority of users still have dial-up connections. Some software for creating Web pages provides information about the download time for a file while one is creating the page.

Design of a Web Page

At least seven major rules should be considered when designing a home page for an Internet resource or service: (1) purpose, (2) scope, (3) structure, (4) enhancements, (5) links, (6) forms, and (7) maintenance.

Purpose

Why do you want to share your information? Who is your audience? What does your audience want to know? Generally you create a home page to share and inform the world of your resources or services. Your home page should be designed to assist users in accessing information about what you have to offer. Remember, you should focus on the product being marketed.

Scope

What information do you want to share? Generally, it is the information that you disseminate and make available in a brochure, catalog, manual, or other printed documents. Such materials can serve as the primary focus of the home page menu; for example, a brochure that describes the services that your agency offers. When sharing printed documents, you need to consider copyright concerns.

Structure

Two issues need to be considered when deciding the structure of a Web site: organization and page design. Although organizing a Web page similar to your organizational chart may seem the most logical to you and your colleagues, this method often is not the best for the user. Instead, think about why someone would come to your site. What information will they want? How can this best be organized so the user will find it easiest to use?

How should the information to be presented appear? You can learn a lot by looking at other home pages for similar agencies. Have several people evaluate what works and does not work on these pages. Much insight into what works and does not work can be gained by having a few potential users evaluate the same pages. What designers think is wonderful can be very disconcerting to a user. Having those outside the agency test preliminary designs for your Web site as well as the finished product will make the site much more helpful (Krug, 2000).

After this step, make some preliminary designs on paper. It is important for all the pages on the same site to have a similar look and feel. For this reason, many of the WYSIWYG page creators include the ability to create a template that can be used for all the pages. Some items to consider are how to organize the menus, whether to use graphical or textual buttons, where to place the links, the colors of the page, what graphics to use, and whether to use frames. It is important to follow Web conventions; for example, changing the format for links from the conventional blue underlined text confuses users who have many other enticing sites to visit.

Enhancements

What enhancements, if any, should be used? Will graphics (pictures) enhance the information? How will the page look with and without the graphics? Turn off the graphics in your browser and look at the page because some users will view the home page using a text browser such as Lynx. Also consider download time; the transforming of graphics to a digital format requires a great deal of storage and takes a considerable time to appear on the user's screen.

Although it is possible to include audio and video files on your pages, only include these if they add good value to the message because they add to download time. If a page takes too long to download, users will not stick around to see the final result. The rule of "Because you can, does not mean you should," needs to be carefully weighed in all these decisions.

Links

Two types of links exist: (1) those that link to other files on the same site (that is, they all are hosted under the same domain name) and (2) links to sites outside the organization. Inside links are the easiest to manage. External links present several decisions. What purpose will be served by adding external links? If links will be used, what guidelines will be used to decide which ones to include? Will there be detailed notes so that users can more easily decide whether to follow them? All links, internal and external, need to be checked for accuracy. Many of the Web design software packages provide a feature that allows users to perform this task. It needs to be done initially and periodically. Free software for checking outside links is available at http://home.snafu.de/tilman/xenulink.html.

Forms

If the agency believes that users may want to request additional information, then a form can be included on the site. The form can be designed to be downloaded by a user to mail or fax or it can be designed to be filled out online. For online forms, information received can be programmed to be automatically entered into a database, or the information on the form can be sent as an e-mail to the agency. If forms are included, then have a staff member assigned the task of processing the requests. Forms can serve as an excellent source of feedback on use by others.

Maintenance

Maintenance of the site requires that procedures be established to support and update the content and links as well as handle requests from users. Pages should be dated so that a user will know how current they are. Additionally, an agency may wish to place a counter on each page to record how many times each page is used. There are many free counters, some of which create pop-up ads on your site. The counters can provide not just a count of how many visitors the site had, but extensive data about visitors such as where they are from, by what page they were referred, and what time they visited. An extensive list of these can be found at http://www.thefreesite.com/Webmaster_Freebies/Free_counters_and_trackers/.

It is also necessary to publicize a Web site. The URL can be placed on all printed material distributed by the agency, stationery, and business cards. Getting the page into a search tool's database is another matter. Some agencies advertise that they can make sure that your page is rated in the top 10 for your area, but these are expensive and are not effective for the long term. All search engines work in different ways, thus what works for one site does not necessarily work for another. One trick is to place words that people use to search in the title that appears on the top of the screen when a page is visited (Sullivan, 2002). Some search tools also look at the first few paragraphs of a page to determine if the page is a match. Other tools rank by how many pages have links to your site. In health care, there are pages that provide links to Web pages for various types of agencies. For example, the Web page at http://directory.google.com/Top/Health/Home_Health/Home_Care/Service_Providers/ provides links to as many home health and hospice agency's Web pages as they know about. You may wish to notify them of your agency's Web page. The Visiting Nurse Association of America site (http://www.vnaa.org) can only be accessed with Internet Explorer or Netscape 6.0 or higher, but provides users the ability to search for visiting nurse associations by city or ZIP code. It does not, however, provide links to Web pages.

Accessibility Issues

Given that many users of Web pages for health-related information may have some physical handicaps, the design of the page should take that into consideration. Web sites can be designed to facilitate their use by those with visual or physical handicaps. The World Wide Web Consortium (http://www.w3.org/TR/WCAG20/), also known as W3C, has guidelines for developers in designing accessible pages. The W3C consortium provides some tips such as using the *alt* attribute for all images, and using hypertext links that make sense (W3C, 2003). Under Section 508 of the Rehabilitation Act Amendments of 1998, federal agencies are required to have their electronic sites accessible to people with disabilities.

Many things need to be considered when designing for those with disabilities. Color can be confusing to those who are color blind, flickering items can cause epileptic seizures, and neurological disabilities can make it difficult for a user to use the keyboard or a mouse (Thede, 2003). Devices are available that make it easier for those with disabilities to use the Internet. Health care professionals may find the need to provide information about these devices to clients. Links to some of these devices

can be found at http://junior.apk.net/~lqthede/Informatics/Chap07/Chap07.htm#handicapped.

Internal Web Pages

Most agencies today have a computer network. This network can also function as an *intranet*, or a network within an agency that is available only to users within the agency. Documents on intranets can be formatted using HTML tags, allowing users to access them using a Web browser. This format can be extremely useful for documents that need frequent updating, such as policies and procedures. Placing documents on the intranet avoids the hassle of distributing printed sheets, placing them in a notebook, and being sure that the notebook is always complete.

An intranet can also be expanded to an *extranet*, or an intranet that permits use of the network from outside the agency. In this mode, personnel in the field could quickly access up-to-date information such as social agencies that a client might need as well as policies. Time reports can also be filed using an extranet.

Extranets, as well as intranets, require appropriate security such as logins, passwords, and firewalls. When Web technology is used for an intranet, agencies can save money on paper as well as make the job of finding information easier for their staff.

CONCLUSION

The worldwide connection of computers known as the Internet can be a valuable resource in home health and hospice care. The e-mail services it provides can facilitate communication among staff and between personnel and clients. The World Wide Web, a service on the Internet, provides access to a wealth of information. The Web also can provide health care agencies with a means to promote their services. How much benefit an agency derives from the Internet and its associated tools depends not only on the tools available, but also on the inventiveness that is used in applying them.

REFERENCES

Ambre, J., R. Guard, F. M. Perveiler, J. Renner, and R. Rippen. 1997. *Criteria for assessing the quality of health information on the Internet*. White paper. Retrieved March 4, 2003, from *http://hitiweb.mitretek.org/docs/criteria.html*.

Health on the Net Foundation. 2002. *Responsible self regulation*. Retrieved March 2, 2003, from *http://www.hon.ch/HONcode/method.html*.

Krug, S. 2000. *Don't make me think: A common sense approach to Web usability*. Indianapolis, IN: New Riders Publishing.

Peters, D. A., and V. K. Saba. 2001. Community health applications. In V. K. Saba and K. A. McCormick (eds.) *Essentials of computers for nurses: Informatics for the new millennium*. New York: McGraw Hill, pp. 265–295.

Sullivan, D. 2002. *How search engines rank Web pages*. Retrieved March 2, 2003, from *http://www.searchenginewatch.com/webmasters/rank.html*.

Thede, L. Q. 2003. *Informatics and nursing: Opportunities and challenges*. Philadelphia: Lippincott, Williams & Wilkins.

University of California, Berkeley Library. 2001. *Recommended search strategy*. Retrieved March 2, 2003, from *http://www.lib.berkeley.edu/TeachingLib/Guides/Internet/Strategies.html*.

W3C. 2003. *Quick tips to make accessible Web sites*. Retrieved March 2, 2003, from *http://www.w3.org/WAI/References/QuickTips/*.

Webopedia. *The difference between the Internet and the World Wide Web*. Retrieved February 26, 2003, from *http://www.webopedia.com/DidYouKnow/Internet/2002/Web_vs_Internet.asp*.

RESOURCES

Finding an ISP

Detailed information about thousands of ISPs and their direct access is available at *http://www.thelist.com*.

Guidelines for Designing Accessible Web Pages

From the World Wide Web Consortium *http://www.w3.org/TR/WCAG20/*

Home Health Care Agency Pages

Provides links to all Web pages for VNAs and home health agencies about which they know. *http://directory.google.com/Top/Health/Home_Health/Home_Care/Service_Providers/*

Link Checking

Free software for checking links—*http://home.snafu.de/tilman/xenulink.html*

Online Journals

Global Nursing Knowledge Network *(http://www.gnkn.org/)*—information about online publishing—*http://junior.apk.net/~lqthede/Informatics/Chap06/Online Journals.htm*—A list of links to many online nursing journals

Search tools for Online Medical Articles (Note these search only journal articles)

http://www.medic8.com/Search.htm

http://www.advantage-healthcare.net/search.html

Searching Strategies

Links to sites that provide information about successful searching. *http://junior.apk.net/~lqthede/Informatics/Chap06/Chap06.htm#Search*

Some Search Tools

Google *(http://www.google.com/)*

Yahoo *(http://www.yahoo.com/)*

Visiting Nurse Association of America

http://www.vnaa.org/ (Not accessible with versions of Netscape lower than 6.0)

*Note, some of these entries are news groups and forums. If you click on the link for a list you will be able to subscribe on the spot.

CHAPTER 57

Disease Management Programs

Miriam Cannon Wagner

INTRODUCTION AND HISTORY

Disease management has emerged as one of the most important approaches to the delivery of health care. Disease management is an integrated approach to health care because it is based on the normal course of disease and treats the person as a whole.[1] Successful disease management programs address the disease along the continuum of care in a manner that includes both clinical and nonclinical interventions essential to obtain effective outcomes. In disease management, the emphasis is on prevention and proactive case management. The successful implementation of the disease management program depends on the commitment and capability of the organization utilizing effective data collection and reporting mechanisms.

One of the primary reasons for the emergence of disease management is the growth and burden of chronic disease in the United States. Over 125 million persons are afflicted with a chronic disease.[2,3] Chronic, disabling conditions cause major limitations in activity for 1 out of every 10 Americans or 30 millon people.[2] Chronic illness accounts for more than 75 percent of all medical care costs each year. In 2003, cardiovascular diseases and stroke accounted for an estimated $351.8 billion in health care costs and lost productivity.[2] In 2002, the Centers for Disease Control's report, *The Burden of Chronic Disease and Their Risk Factors,* re-

ported that chronic diseases such as heart disease, cancer, and diabetes are the leading cause of disability and are responsible for 7 of every 10 deaths in the United States.[4] In 2001, the total healthcare cost was $104 trillion or an average of $5,035 for each American.[2] In addition, hospital readmission rates are as high as 50 percent for patients with a chronic disease such as heart failure.[5,6] Due to the increased life expectancy of the aging baby boomer generation and improved survival rates, there will be significant increases in the prevalence and incidence of chronic diseases over the next 25 years.[7,8]

The second primary reason why disease management programs began to emerge was due to the growing health care costs in the 1980s. Disease management's response was utilization reduction through managed care.[9,10,11] As health care costs continued to rise in the 1990s, health plans, employer groups, and others turned to disease management as a way to rein in costs, as well as to improve outcomes.[10,11] Initially, disease management programs were developed as an extension of pharmaceutical companies but evolved into disease-specific programs and more recently into comprehensive condition management programs. In 1997, revenues in the disease management industry were $77 million and they are projected to grow to over $500 million in 2001.[13,14] This revenue growth will be spread to more than 160 disease management companies.[14] Disease management providers are targeting persons with diabetes, congestive heart failure, asthma, depression, and other chronic conditions to secure part of the current $750 billion chronic disease market. The expected increased expenditures for disease management programs demand a greater need to prove the value (e.g., cost effectiveness) of these diverse programs in the marketplace (see Table 57–1).[15,16]

Table 57–1 Benefits of Disease Management

- Manages high cost or chronic illness in a systematic approach
- Prevents exacerbation or complications of diseases
- Improves health outcomes and reduces costs
- Targets interventions that affect health care costs
- Coordinates care with multidisciplinary groups
- Continuous care from prevention, diagnosis, treatment, follow-up
- Utilizes patient education to enhance program effectiveness
- Provides tools to enhance compliance and lifestyle adjustments
- Uses tools such as clinical practice guidelines
- Utilizes outcomes, disease modeling, and risk stratification
- Utilizes case management, telephonic, and home care interventions
- Provides data to forecast how to manage future high costs
- Organizes systems for the less urgent problems of the chronically ill
- Uses behavior intervention to improve adherence/self-management

Source: Adapted by Miriam Cannon Wagner, RN, from the Centers for Disease Control's National Center for Chronic Disease Prevention and the Disease Management Association of America.

PUBLISHED DISEASE MANAGEMENT PROGRAM RESULTS

A number of large government-sponsored evaluations of disease management programs are underway. These include studies funded by the Agency for Healthcare Research and Quality, the National Institutes of Health, the Centers for Medicare and Medicaid, and the Department of Health and Human Services as well as nongovernment sources such as the Robert Wood Johnson Foundation. The Centers for Medicare and Medicaid Services (formerly HCFA) awarded grants for coordinated care demonstration projects in its fee-for-service population to evaluate costs and patient outcomes in the elderly.[17] The Institute of Medicine (IOM) released the *Crossing the Quality Chasm: A New Health System for the 21st Century* report that supports the expansion of disease management programs.[18] The report requests that nurses, physicians, other clinicians, health organizations, and purchasers improve care for common chronic conditions such as heart disease, diabetes, and asthma that result in loss of quality of life, decreased work productivity, and elevated health care costs. The Task Force on Community Preventive Services strongly recommends disease and case management to improve outcomes, both in the home and in community gathering places.[19]

Numerous studies have been done to evaluate the impact of disease management programs but the quality of the studies have varied considerably.[15,20–24] Two review articles for the diagnosis of heart failure and coronary artery disease examined the methods used to evaluate the impact of multidisciplinary disease management programs.[25,27] In an article by Rich[20], a systematic review of the literature from 1983 to 1998 uncovered 10 nonrandomized observational studies and only 6 randomized clinical trials for multidisciplinary heart failure disease management programs. Dr. Rich stated that the randomized trials strongly supported the positive results of the observational studies. He also concluded that they provided convincing evidence of the positive impact of multidisciplinary heart failure disease programs in selected patient populations. The limitations of the randomized trials include their relatively small, highly select patient populations; their inability to generalize to more diverse populations; and use of various methods or interventions to provide care. Finlay[25] reviewed 12 randomized clinical trials of disease management programs in patients with coronary heart disease that were identified in the literature (1966 through 2000). The authors reported that these studies were generally positive, but again sample sizes were small and the interventions varied substantially across programs.

Numerous studies document the impact of nursing care provided in the home for various disease state management programs. One study reported improved outcomes in an intensive home care program focused on elderly heart failure patients. The program continued for 12 months and demonstrated a 62 percent reduction in total number of hospitalizations and a 77 percent reduction in total hospital days as well as a significant improvement in functional status. The 12-month before- and after-program effects were reported.[26] Another randomized controlled study design for heart failure patients utilized a nurse–pharmacist team approach for home-based intervention and education. This study realized 42 percent fewer hospitalizations and hospital days compared to the control group.[27]

Rich and associates reported 56 percent fewer rehospitalizations for heart failure, 61 percent fewer multiple hospital admissions, and a 36 percent reduction in hospital days; improved quality of life; and lower costs compared with the usual group in a randomized controlled trial.[6] The program consisted of inpatient analysis of medication prescriptions, inpatient education by a cardiovascular nurse, diet instruction by a dietitian, social services, discharge planning, intensive follow-up by home health services, and follow-up through home health visits and telephonic contact. West and colleagues also reported improved outcomes compared to

12 months before program enrollment. Patients exhibited an 87 percent reduction in heart failure rehospitalization and a 74 percent reduction in total admissions. After an initial visit, patients were educated via weekly telephone calls for 6 weeks to enhance compliance using behavior techniques.[29] In another study in heart failure, Shah and associates provided home-based telephonic interventions, weekly educational mailings, and a pager reminder system for medication compliance. The average follow-up was 8.5 months and realized a 67 percent reduction in cardiovascular hospitalizations and 92 percent fewer hospital days.[30] In an advanced practice nurse intervention study, patients were randomly assigned to the program or usual care. Discharge planning and 4 weeks of home care emphasized patient and caregiver self-management. The intervention group was less likely to have a hospital readmission and had fewer hospital days.[31]

Diabetes disease management programs have had similar results. Sidorov and colleagues reported results of cost savings of program participants versus usual care in a managed care organization. The program patients' claims per member per month were $394.62 versus $502.48 for nonprogram patients due to decreased inpatient care and fewer emergency room visits.[33] The disease management program patients also had higher Health Plan Employer Data and Information Set (HEDIS) scores for HbA1c testing (glycemic control) as well as for lipid, eye exam, and kidney screenings.[34] The Task Force on Community Preventive Services, supported by the U.S. Department of Health and Human Services and the Centers for Disease Control and Prevention (CDC), strongly recommends disease and case management to improve outcomes in diabetes.[24]

Asthma disease management programs for children and their parents and adult asthmatics have been effective in reducing the financial burden and improving the clinical outcome. In one study, low-income asthma patients experienced improved health status and health care costs were lowered in a disease management program that taught physicians new skills. Rossiter and associates reported a 41 percent reduction in emergency room visits that resulted in direct savings of $3 to $4 for every incremental dollar spent. The 2002 paper described improved health status for participants and new skills in disease management for physicians.[35] Another paper by Taitel reported significant savings for an adult asthma self-management program that taught symptom management, medication adherence, and life-style modification. The cost-benefit analysis after 1 year revealed a reduction in treatment costs of $472 per patient; hospital admission costs decreased from $18,488 to $1,538 per patient; lost income from asthma reduced from $11,593 to $4,589 per patient; and the cost ($208) to benefit ratio was 1 to 2.28.[36]

Patient compliance is a major determinant for the development of disease management programs. For example, Tsuyuki and colleagues concluded that 22 percent of heart failure exacerbations requiring hospitalizations were caused by noncompliance with salt restriction. Noncompliance with sodium restriction, the primary precipitating cause of hospitalization in this study, could be reduced by providing education, regular telephone contact for coaching and support, and a 24-hour support line for early interventions when symptoms present.[32]

DEFINITION OF DISEASE MANAGEMENT

The Disease Management Association of America defines disease management as a "system of coordinated healthcare interventions and communications for populations with conditions in which patient self-care efforts are significant."[37]

SETTING UP A DISEASE MANAGEMENT PROGRAM

The major force behind developing disease management programs has been the concern about health care expenditures. Disease management is focused toward systems of care in a less-fragmented approach, therefore, there is a greater potential for financial savings and quality improvement. It is coordinated interventions and communications that promote empowering patients and preventing exacerbations for chronic conditions. Successful implementation of a disease management program requires implementation within 1 year, high levels of patient enrollment, improvement in process and outcome measures of quality, reduced total patient cost, improved functional status, and increased patient and provider satisfaction.[38]

Select a Disease or Condition to Manage

Several chronic diseases are commonly chosen for disease management programs but the list continues to grow. The most common diagnoses include congestive heart failure, asthma, diabetes, cancer, coronary artery disease, and chronic obstructive pulmonary disease. Specific criteria need to be evaluated when selecting a disease or condition to manage (see Table 57–2). The condition should meet at least most, if not all, of the selected criteria to assure successful program results. Heart failure is one of the most common conditions addressed in disease management programs. Heart failure meets all of the criteria in Table 57–2, and the savings translate to decreased inpatient utilization that can be clearly measured. Physicians and health plans can easily identify the patients with frequent exacerbations or hospitalizations. Therefore, readmission rates can be reported as early as 30 days from the index or baseline hospitalization in most instances.

Successful disease management programs have researched the clinical and financial aspects of the disease such as the incidence, prevalence, and severity of illness and have determined the levels or chronic and acute parameters of the clinical condition. Does it have stages or levels that impact clinical management?

Many conditions have functional status limitations that affect the care delivered and greatly influence outcome reporting. For example, a

Table 57–2 Disease or Condition Selection Criteria for Disease Management

- Chronic disease state with documented high prevalence
- Identification easy through claims or diagnosis/procedure codes
- Substantial economic burden
- Potential for treatment variations
- Potential for lifestyle modifications to improve outcomes
- Documented compliance issues that can be improved
- High risk of negative outcome
- Cost savings can be generated within 1 year of implementation

Source: Adapted by Miriam Cannon Wagner, RN, from the Centers for Disease Control's National Center for Chronic Disease Prevention and Health Promotion and the Disease Management Association of America.

reduction in hospitalizations for a New York Heart Association (NYHA) class I heart failure patient (symptoms only with strenuous activity) would not be impressive as compared to a NYHA class IV patient (symptoms at rest).[39] The rehospitalization rate for NYHA class IV is 50 percent in 6 months, and several studies report 30 percent to 50 percent readmission rate at 30 days following the index hospitalization.[5,6,29,40] The hospitalization rate for NYHA class I, if admitted, may not be reported as heart failure because it may not be the primary diagnosis (another diagnosis may be primary). Therefore, the baseline data will be "unbalanced" and the cost-benefit ratio will be reported incorrectly. Determine if the customer wants the total population included or just the more severe cases of NYHA class III or IV heart failure. A patient with NYHA class III or IV heart failure is the most common type of patient enrolled in a disease management program.

Scope of the Program

The scope of a disease management program can be broad or confined to one aspect of care such as home care. Once the specific disease or population to manage is chosen, additional disease-specific identification measures, patient education tools, process measures, and outcome measures can be added to the program. If the scope is narrow, such as home care for heart failure patients, the operational issues are minimized. The operational issues can be great if the program is a large population of various conditions and multiple levels of care. An efficient disease management program should significantly reduce medical and administrative costs, while enriching the physician–patient communication and improving health conditions. It aims to improve the patient's health by continuously assessing clinical and economic outcomes.

The scope of management must be compared to the expected outcomes so that each program component can be evaluated. Inpatient and outpatient case management, discharge planning, telephonic interventions and education, telemonitoring, Web-based Internet intervention and education, home visits, and/or physician or clinic visits are all aspects of disease management. Inclusion or exclusion of these components will impact program outcomes and pricing. Other considerations for inclusion are claims review and stratification, predictive modeling for population-based programs, quality of life, screening or other risk survey questionnaires to identify patients (for example, SF-12 survey[41]), and distribution of patient tools or products (weight scales, pill boxes, education booklets, other durable medical equipment). The decision to include or exclude some of these components will directly affect the cost effectiveness of the program. Process measures such as the number of outbound and inbound calls between physicians, patients, and health plans should be evaluated. The number of mailed materials and outcome-reporting capabilities (computer systems, software, statisticians) need to be anticipated and included in overall program costs (see Table 57–3).

The Patient Identification Process

The identification process to determine enrollment criteria can be prospective, concurrent, retrospective, or a combination of all three for specific disease states or populations. The identification process can also be patient self-report, physician referral, case manager report, or claims review and screening. In a program designed to treat one disease process, prospective methods include patient self-report questionnaires for a total population base such as in a health plan.

Health status questionnaires can identify patients through telephonic methods and then screen for exclusions. For example, a questionnaire process may ask if the person has ever been told that they have heart disease, heart failure, diabetes, chronic lung disease, or other functional limitations. Follow-up questions can include more details about the specified response such as when the person was hospitalized or if medications are prescribed for the condition. Additional questions can assist with the evaluation of program exclusion criteria.

Other methods of prospective identification are to evaluate claims from physician office visits and past hospitalizations. A person may have had a hospital admission diagnosis for the selected disease or condition in the past year. This person may be prospectively selected for the disease management program, even if the disease process is stable at the current time.

Concurrent identification includes direct enrollment from a health plan, hospital, or physician office for an acute exacerbation of the condition or patient education needs. These referrals can be telephoned, e-mailed, or faxed. The enrollment process may be simplified due to the confirmation of the diagnosis and the severity of the illness.

Retrospective enrollment includes claims review for all patients admitted to the hospital with a specific diagnosis. The claims retrieval process needs to be automated with specific Diagnosis-Related Groups (DRGs) or International Classification of Diseases (ICD-9) diagnoses defined for a specific time period. The time period for review can be up to 2 years with the ICD-9 diagnosis as either the primary or secondary diagnosis.

Claims review should be followed by a qualification telephone call to the prospective patient. The patient may have disenrolled from the plan, died, or moved to another area of the country. The patient may also have been diagnosed with another disease that affects enrollment such as cancer, renal dialysis, severe chronic obstructive pulmonary disease, and new or severe cardiac disease (if not the primary disease state selected).

Inclusion criteria define the parameters for enrollment into the disease management program such as age, discharge diagnosis code, medications, and utilization parameters such as when the patient was admitted. Exclusion criteria define the reasons why certain patients cannot be included into the program. Examples of exclusion criteria include another dominant diagnosis such as cancer, the patient on a heart transplant list, inactive member of the health plan (or disenrollment), or no evidence of the condition as per the participant or physician, the transfer to a skilled nursing facility, or no telephone or the inability to communicate by telephone. After initial identification and prior to program enrollment, all potential patients should be contacted to screen for inclusion and exclusion criteria.

The Enrollment Process

The enrollment process includes documented screening for inclusion and exclusion criteria and collection of demographic data. All enrollment data should be computerized for access and retrieval. All patients that have been screened need to be data entered so that if a case manager refers the same patient 3 months later, the

Table 57–3 Components of a Disease Management Program

- Identification Measures
  - Claims Review—Inpatient or Outpatient
  - Pharmacy Claims
  - Case Manager Referral Process
  - Physician Referral Process
  - Questionnaires to Identify Disease or Functional Impairment
  - Stratification by Severity of Illness
- Patient Education, Equipment, and/or Tools
  - Telephonic, Web, or Home-Based Education
  - Weight Scales, Pillboxes, and Calendars to Record Findings
  - Booklets, Pamphlets, Newsletters, or Other Visual Aids
- Process Measures for Delivery of the Program
  - Hours of Operations, including 24-Hour On-Call
  - Symptom Monitoring and Management
  - Triage and Post-Hospital Visits
  - Telephonic Contacts and Follow-up Parameters
  - Medication Management—Guideline Recommendations
  - Laboratory Assessment and Reporting
  - Physician Communication—Initial, Monthly, and/or Quarterly
  - Process Reports—Number of Visits or Telephone Contacts
  - Reports—Referrals, Enrollments, Discharges, and Deaths
  - Home Health Aides and Physical or Occupational Therapy
- Outcome Reporting
  - Inpatient Admissions and Length of Stay
  - Emergency Room Utilization
  - Medication Utilization
  - Quality of Life Survey Analysis
  - Clinical Outcome Measures (Blood Pressure and Weight)
  - Immunization Status (Flu and Pneumococcal)
  - Functional Status
  - Satisfaction Results
  - Cost Savings

Source: Adapted by Miriam Cannon Wagner, RN, from the Joint Commission on Accreditation of Healthcare Organizations and the American Accreditation Healthcare Commission's Disease Management Accreditation Standards.

screening process will be eliminated and then the patient does not need to be contacted again.

Patient status can be categorized as one of the following: Pending, Active, Discharged, or Disqualified. Each of those categories can be further described with dates and reason codes. For example, three patients were disqualified due to another dominant diagnosis such as cancer or renal dialysis. Enrollment status lists can be sent to the health plan, for instance on a weekly or monthly basis, to be billed accordingly (see Table 57–4).

Table 57–4 Enrollment Data to Collect

- Name, Address, Telephone Number (Home, Cell, and Work)
- Social Security Number and Date of Birth
- Martial Status and Spouse's Name
- Emergency Contact—Not Living at the Same Address
- Employer—Name, Address, and Telephone Number
- Referring Physician Name, Address, and Telephone
- Primary Physician Name, Address, and Telephone
- Specialist Physician Name, Address, and Telephone
- Insurance Information—Case Manager Contact If Applicable
- Insurance Type (HMO, PPO, or Medicare)
- Insurance Benefits—Pharmacy and Medical Equipment Coverage
- Program Coverage (Home Visits, DME, Education Tools)
- Primary Diagnosis—List as ICD-9 Code: Program Specific
- Secondary Diagnosis—List as ICD-9 Code: Unlimited

Source: Miriam Cannon Wagner, RN

Program Implementation

The nurse is an integral element in the disease management program. These nurses can be called disease managers, case managers, clinical educators, home care clinicians, telephonic managers, outcome facilitators, or any name that is deemed appropriate for their role in the program. They will be called nurses in this chapter. Once the patient is enrolled in the program, the nurse begins a long-term process of building a relationship with the patient and the patient's physician. All nurses need training and experience in the selected clinical aspect as well as detailed training in the disease management program. Disease management training should include data collection process procedures with special emphasis on how outcomes are "pulled" and what information is essential to reporting.

The nurse plays a variety of roles in the management process. They initially collect and synthesize information on the patient's clinical condition, current treatment regimen, lifestyle, and psychosocial issues. On an ongoing basis, they are integrally involved in treatment planning with the physician, educating as well as "coaching" and motivating patients. Nurses also evaluate patient needs and make recommendations for other patient support services (such as physical therapy, counseling, and home health aids). When necessary, they also coordinate the provision of these services. In short, nurses provide comprehensive care management for their patients.

Nurses should be encouraged to build strong relationships with patients and may develop their own individualized motivational tools such as personalized postcards celebrating patient achievements or special patient-specific compliance ideas. Additionally, as the contact with nurses may become increasingly telephonic, the nurse may use other ways to personalize their interactions, such as sending pictures of themselves with brief biographies or remembering something special about the patient.

The initial disease management program intervention may provide a home visit of 1.5 to 2 hours conducted by a home-care nurse within 1 week of enrollment. The initial evaluation can include a history and physical examination, a psychosocial evaluation, a review of medications, and an assessment of dietary habits, including the types of food available in the home.

At the first visit, the patient is given any tools necessary to manage their disease such as a scale, pillbox, glucose monitor, education booklets, or other teaching tools included in the program. Distribution of program-specific materials is determined by contract for enrolled patients at a specific health plan. Questionnaires may be given to the patient at the first visit to gather baseline data and at regular intervals thereafter. Questionnaires can be administered initially, monthly, quarterly, every 6 months, or yearly. Many questionnaires are disease specific while others are general in scope to address many chronic conditions.

A phone follow-up contact is suggested within the next 2 to 3 days. This phone contact can focus on continued training and education initiated during the first visit and an assessment of patient's progress with adherence to medical therapy such as daily weight, blood glucose monitoring, or dietary intake.

A second home visit could be conducted within 1 week of the initial visit. This visit may include a follow-up history and physical examination, a reevaluation of patient's medications, a review of diet and weight patterns, and additional counseling. For example, with a heart failure patient, special emphasis can be placed on monitoring of body weight and symptom management. Patients can be instructed to contact the nurse for increased shortness of breath or if their weight increases 2 pounds overnight or 5 pounds during a week. Other home visits and follow-up telephone contacts can be scheduled according to the program guidelines.

The nurse is responsible for gathering clinical and other data about patients' status and the current treatment they are receiving. Nurses play an integral role in managing the patient by comparing and contrasting the current treatment to disease-specific clinical practice guidelines and

bringing discrepancies with their recommendations to the patient's physician. Particularly complex cases can be referred to a clinical team, supervisor, pharmacist, or a medical director who may contact the patient's physician for a consultation.

The nurse should be in regular contact with the patient's physician (or his or her office). It is recommended that the nurse provide written and phone reports to the physician regarding the patient's status on an ongoing basis. Any changes in the patient's treatment regimen are implemented with signed orders from the physician.

Advanced age, multiple comorbidities, or a lack of family care and support may increase follow-up home visits instead of telephonic intervention. As part of the ongoing management, nurses continue the patient educational process, provide reinforcement teaching, evaluate patients' treatment plan compliance and response to therapies (or lack thereof), and ensure that necessary follow-up testing takes place. Follow-up testing may include laboratory tests, diagnostic testing, or monitoring of any clinical parameter such as HbA1c testing for diabetic patients.

Ongoing communication with patients is essential to increase compliance. Newsletters are valuable because of their easy-to-read format, and they can provide ongoing education about diet, exercise, physician communication, medication management, and early treatment of signs and symptoms. The monthly or quarterly newsletter can also have fun-filled facts about health, disease-specific facts, low-fat recipes, smoking cessation programs, or exercise tips. Patients learn best with a variety of different teaching methods and small segments of information at a time. Research with social learning theories and stages of change models have shown that the greatest impact on behavior occurs in patients who already display a readiness to change and confidence that the change is important.[42,43,44]

Patients with chronic disease are at greatest risk of decreased compliance due to many factors. One of the most common reasons is due to lack of understanding and lack of education about their disease process and the medications or treatments recommended. Patients become confused about their treatments due to frequent hospitalizations and the many changes that occur with each hospitalization. If the patient is not provided home care or other teaching programs to educate about these changes, incorrect medications or treatments can occur. Patients with chronic disease enter the vicious cycle of hospitalization, lack of understanding, and then back to the hospital again. Current health care financial systems only provide for short-term education and follow-up following hospitalization and many require ongoing support to prevent exacerbation and hospitalization. Disease management programs address long-term management and have achieved good results.

Follow-up contacts are scheduled according to the disease management program schedule (contract specific) and are usually of decreasing frequency unless warning signs appear or the patient's condition significantly worsens. For patients who are rehospitalized, home visits or telephonic contacts are usually increased. Additionally, patients can be advised to contact the on-call nurse, if applicable, 24 hours a day, 7 days a week in cases of exacerbation or if questions arise. If program guidelines permit, the home care nurse may make an emergency visit to evaluate, triage, and treat the patient.

The length of program enrollment depends on the contract utilized, if applicable. Disease management is concerned with the long-term management of patients, and program length should be determined prior to implementation. Some programs advocate that patients remain in the program until death for specific conditions such as heart failure and severe chronic obstructive pulmonary disease. Conditions such as childhood asthma and diabetes usually have a defined education period and long-term follow-up period (up to 2 years) with decreasing points of communication to assess ongoing compliance. Other conditions such as post-myocardial infarction, adult onset diabetes, and hypertension may require education and compliance monitoring for 3 months to 1 year. Longer is better, but many

health plans cannot calculate cost savings in the long term because the interventions for these conditions may not be evident for years to come (another heart attack, heart disease due to long-term hypertension, end-organ disease from diabetes). The return on investment may not be evident because financial return is related to the prevention of high-cost care, not a reduction in conditions that may arise in the far future. Many health plans will not enroll patients with conditions unless the inpatient costs are high. Some independent disease management companies have been able to secure 5-year contracts and have negotiated a risk arrangement. The visit and telephone schedule is set by the disease management provider and all patients are included for the length of the program. The program is responsible for all inpatient and outpatient costs so that the health plan can pay a "per-member per-month" fee, hence their risk is minimal. The home care industry has been contending with the issue of limited visits and time constraints for many years in Medicare-insured patients. Many of those patients are admitted back to the hospital after the home care visits end and the vicious cycle continues. In the mid-1990s, Medicare-risk contracts through managed care provided some flexibility for home visits and management for the elderly Medicare patients.

Utilizing Clinical Practice Guidelines

Evidence-based practice guidelines are utilized in most disease management programs and are recognized as the "gold standard" for clinical management. These guidelines are published in clinical journals or by the appropriate medical society. Large, internationally recognized groups such as the Centers for Disease Control (CDC);[45] American Heart Association (AHA);[46] National Institute of Health (NIH); National Heart, Lung, and Blood Institute (NHLBI);[47] and the National Guideline Clearinghouse (NGC) (Agency for Healthcare Policy and Research [AHCPR])[48] include inpatient, outpatient, and long-term care as well as prevention strategies for disease processes. Their guidelines are found at their Internet sites.

Not all guidelines can be implemented in disease management programs, specifically the inpatient or procedure type guidelines. If a drug or procedure is advised within 24 hours of hospital admission, it is not advantageous to incorporate these guidelines into the program. Outpatient or long-term care guidelines are appropriate.

In the program design, review the disease-specific guidelines and retrieve all recomended medications, lab testing, immunizations, exercise, and dietary goals to constitute the patient education and outcome tools. A medical director or medical advisory board should review and approve the education, data collection, and process tools as compared to the clinical guidelines available.

Physician Communication and Marketing

A key factor in the successful implementation of a disease management program is physician awareness and a thorough understanding of the program. Providing information prior to implementation is a critical step in accomplishing this goal.

Follow-up communication with physicians could include a summary of clinical findings, suggested medications or lab parameters based on clinical practice guidelines, and the follow-up visit or contact schedule for that patient. A one-page copy of the applicable clinical practice guidelines, sent to physicians, will assist with ongoing management. The physician needs to know what you will be doing for his or her patient, what information you will be teaching, and the long-term goals. Yes, this information may be sent in an order sheet for signature, but it is also advisable to send a clear, eye-pleasing summary sheet of the program that lets the physician know that you will be calling again at regular intervals, if the program requires it.

Marketing to physicians can greatly increase enrollment into the program. If the disease management program is in conjunction with a health plan, this task may be easier and the health plan may assist with the communication via letters or meetings. If the program is affiliated with a hospital, the medical staff or advisory board may provide physicians' names and addresses for the program to send written announcements. If the program is via an independent home health agency, letters could be sent to all physicians that have previously sent patients or the medical director may select key physicians to contact. Physician "buy-in" is essential to develop and implement the program. A program announcement letter, a welcome packet, a newsletter announcement, or program awareness meetings are just a few ways to communicate the new program.

Retention of patients and referring physicians is essential to the success of the program. A balance must be achieved between too much and too little communication via telephone or mailings. Physicians can be contacted to ascertain how often they would like to be updated on specific patients or for the program as a whole. Communication within the program or agency to disseminate these findings is imperative.

Many disease management programs keep detailed contact logs via a database not only to monitor process outcomes, but also to understand potential problems that arise with physicians and patients. A large physician practice may have 30 patients in the program, followed by different nurses, and have the potential to receive 30 copies of mailed material, such as clinical practice guidelines. Systems to "link" physicians within groups must be initiated to prevent the numerous calls and mailings that have been cited to cause retention problems.

Types of Disease Management Contracts

Contracts within the disease management community vary depending on the level of risk each party is willing to take and the case mix of the group or the selected population to be managed. Contracts can cover the whole population of a health plan for a disease management company that has multiple programs for most significant health conditions, called condition or population management, or cover only one condition or diagnosis.

In population management, the disease management company or program is responsible for evaluating the case mix of the group, which can be millions of members, and provide education and clinical support for each respective diagnosis. These companies, usually at full risk, must use predictive modeling to determine how many members have a specific disease or condition in the group and calculate how many hospital admissions for the diagnosis are expected to occur within the year. Predictive modeling for population management requires a robust clinical data system to identify those health plan members who will use expensive resources and stratify all members by risk level. Members can be identified as high, moderate, or low risk for utilization of health care services. If members of a health plan are identified as low risk, expensive contacts, mailings, and education tools are not effective and are costly.

Another type of contract is a global, high-risk contract for a specific disease or condition. This contract includes a per-member per-month fee or a fee for service for each provision of care for members. A patient is identified by diagnosis via retrospective claim review, patient self-referral, or case manager or physician referral. Patients would not be included in outcomes analysis or payment until they are enrolled and receive services.

The term of the contract can be for 1 year or longer with an automatic renewal each year. The terms of the contract can include a savings guarantee or risk arrangement. A savings guarantee is determined by both parties and compares the cost of care to the baseline for all enrolled members. For example, if the average cost of a heart failure patient in the baseline year is $8,000 and cost of care for the second year is $6,000, the savings for cost of care is $2,000. The savings, minus program costs, can be split between the health plan and the disease management company. These savings are called operational savings and can be reconciled on an annual basis.

Another common risk arrangement is to provide penalties if certain outcome parameters are not met. These are called performance contracts. For example, a diabetic patient in a high-risk program may be priced at $100 per month but the contract states that the program guarantees an annual A1c level performance. The penalty could be a 3 percent reduction in fees if less than 75 percent of the patients have annual lab results. The program may have enrolled 500 patients and if the outcomes are not met, they will lose $18,000 ($600,000 per year for 500 patients minus 3 percent). Many risk contracts have multiple clinical and operational penalties as well as volume discounts for the number of members enrolled.

Exclusivity is a contract clause that many health plans will not guarantee. Health plans will contract with several providers to compare and evaluate the outcome results at the end of the contract year. Health plans will also contract with different providers for different disease states due to the program's specialty or proven success.

OUTCOME COLLECTION AND REPORTING

Outcome reporting is the most important aspect of disease management and the primary measure of success. It is critical to document improvement in care as evidenced by indicators of clinical and economic outcomes, quality of life, and patient satisfaction. Successful disease management programs will use continuous improvement programs to determine the ongoing changes necessary to provide the most cost-effective health care management.

Quantitative data provides the what, who, when, and where of health-related events or outcomes. They are measurable and tangible. Health outcome data includes many aspects of care such as the regular use of a prescription drug, restricted activity days, absence from work or school, lung function, blood pressure, cholesterol levels, mental status, and quality of life.

Risk-factor data includes those aspects of care that encompass direct causes, personal characteristics, or environmental factors that make patients more prone to a disease or exacerbation of an existing condition. Examples of direct causes would be high blood pressure and high cholesterol; behavioral causes such as noncompliance with diet or medications; smoking; lack of exercise and personal characteristics; or social-demographic factors such as elderly age, gender, race, poor financial status, and living alone.

Resource data describes the services available to patients and includes process measures such as the number of visits, telephone calls, clinic visits, and educational material mailed as well as personnel to develop and maintain the program. Information about the cost of providing the program is dependent on resource data and will determine the cost effectiveness of one intervention compared to another or the cost of the same intervention provided in alternate ways (telephone versus home visit).

Development of outcome measures for the program should begin with a list of measures or data to report. Analyze how and what is already collected and plan to add additional measures as necessary. All data must be computerized in a database. The database should be one of the first tools developed so data collection can begin immediately. An initial draft of a data list can be developed following a review of what is already available from nationally recognized measures such as the Health Plan Employer Data and Information Set (HEDIS), developed by the National Committee of Quality Assurance (NCQA).[34]

NCQA produces a yearly report called *The State of Managed Care Quality* using HEDIS guidelines that measure different activities that have a high financial cost to health care systems, purchasers, or consumers of health care. Commercial, Medicare- and Medicaid-managed health care plans may apply for HEDIS performance-based accreditation. The federal Centers for Medicare & Medicaid Services (CMS) have required annual HEDIS and the Consumer

Assessment of Health Plan Study (CAHPS) reporting for all plans since 1998, but accreditation is not yet required.[50,51] Most HEDIS measures are determined by accepted standards of health care practice and require that eligible plan members receive appropriate health care services. NCQA reports HEDIS Effectiveness of Care Measures such as childhood immunizations, cervical cancer screening, controlling high blood pressure, comprehensive diabetes care, beta-blocker treatment care after heart attack, asthma medications use, lipid screening and management, and many other measures to monitor clinical care, access, and physician ratings. CAHPS is a consumer survey that evaluates consumers' experience and level of satisfaction with the plan, its health care providers, customer service, and claims processing.

Disease management programs that have contracts with any managed care organization may be responsible to report HEDIS measures to the health plan on a regular basis. The health plan relies on the disease management program to report findings with the same specifications that HEDIS requires, so it is essential that the program adhere to these standards. Specifications can be found at the NCQA Web site (http://www.ncqa.org).[34]

Many of the HEDIS measures are specific to prevention and screening. For example, the cholesterol management measure is collected for health plan members who are 18 to 75 years of age who had evidence of an acute cardiovascular event (hospitalization for acute myocardial infarction, coronary artery bypass graft, or percutaneous transluminal coronary angioplasty). The percentage of those members who had a lipid panel drawn and whose LDL-C was screened and controlled to less than 130 mg/dL in the year following the event is reported. To collect this measure, for instance, the following data would be necessary for reporting: age, procedure or diagnosis and date, lab data, date of lab data, and a method for calculating the 1-year follow-up date for the cardiovascular event. If quarterly outcomes are reported, only some members will fit the criteria at each time interval. Methods to collect and report these parameters are necessary for all disease management programs depending on the population and the contract specifications (see Table 57–5).

Outcome Measures

Reported outcome measures should display a detailed description of the analytics, data sources, evaluation timeframes, and process flows associated with producing baselines, targets, and the actual statistics. Different measures may have different evaluation timeframes to allow the programs to have impact. Denominators can be determined by either member months or membership numbers to calculate outcome results.

Member months is based on the number of months each patient is enrolled into the specific program, while membership reflects all patients in the program regardless of time enrolled. For example, if 50 patients were admitted, the hospitalization rates are reported differently depending on the denominator used. If 500 patients are enrolled into the program and 100 have been enrolled for over 90 days, the hospitalization rates can be reported two ways. For member-months calculation, 20 patients admitted to the hospital who were enrolled for 90 days can be reported as follows: 100 patients for 3 months = 300 member-months, and 20 different patients would translate to 0.0067 admissions per member per month (20 ÷ 300). In comparison, the hospitalization rate for the total membership would be: 500 patients enrolled with a total of 50 admissions = 0.1 admissions per member (50 ÷ 500), and is usually reported as the hospital admissions per thousand or 100/1000 (0.1 × 1000).

The reporting method can greatly impact the final reported value of the program due to significant differences in the outcome methodology. Many programs use a member-month calculation for all reporting but have specific guidelines for what constitutes a month. Each patient may have to reach each 30-day timeline in order to qualify. For example, if a patient has been enrolled for 45 days, they would be included in 30-day reporting only. The data collection program should be set up to automatically calculate member-months for reporting.

Financial Impact of the Outcomes in Disease Management

One survey of chief medical officers found that they generally agreed that a positive return on investment is essential for disease management programs. They want a balance between costs and outcome improvement.[52]

Most studies assessing the financial impact (e.g., cost savings, return on investment) of disease management programs generally use one of three methods. The method generally acknowledged as the "gold standard" is the randomized-control study. For disease management programs, performing randomized control studies is not feasible due to ethical or moral reasons such as having some individuals receive usual care while others receive enhanced care. Retrospective randomized studies can also be expensive and time consuming.

A second and common method used by the disease management industry and others to estimate the savings associated with a disease management program is by comparing preprogram intervention costs to post-program intervention costs.[53–58] This method cannot determine the effect of a program intervention because other factors may have caused the improved outcomes, rather than the intervention itself. "Regression-to-the-mean," which is the tendency of extreme values to become less extreme on follow-up measurements, is a major problem with a simple prepost comparison.[60,61] For example, if 10 percent of the heart failure patients in the program had a significant number of admissions (greater than 3 in 90 days) prior to program enrollment, enrolled, and were not admitted in the next 90 days, a reduction of 100 percent in hospitalization could be reported for those patients. If those same patients were not admitted to a disease management program,

Table 57–5 Sample Outcome Measures

a. Global Clinical Measures Reported for All Patients in All Programs

Hospitalization and Emergency Room Usage Rate
Hospital Readmission Rates (Within 30, 60, or 90 Days of Discharge)
Productivity Measures—Missed Work or School Days
Influenza Vaccination
Number of Smokers Referred to Smoking Cessation
Quality of Life
Patient, Physician, and Health Plan Satisfaction

b. Process Measures: All Patients—Sort by Program or Intensity Level

Number of Outbound and Inbound Calls, Home Visits, and/or Ancillary Visits
Inappropriate Emergency Room Visits
Number of Products or Tools Dispensed (Scales, Pillboxes, Videos, Booklets)
Number of Alternate Products or Tools Dispensed for Nonprimary Condition
Number of People (Physicians, Case Managers) Receiving Mailings About the Program
Number of Referrals to Case Management
Number of Patients Called within 48 Hours of Hospital Discharge or Program Enrollment
Number of Patients Enrolled, Discharged, or Disqualified

c. Program-Specific Measures
Heart Failure

Left Ventricular Ejection Fraction Percent and Percent Systolic Dysfunction
Percent of a Vasodilator and Beta-Blocker Medication
New York Heart Association Functional Classification (NYHA)
Percent with Significant Co-Morbid Diagnosis (COPD, Diabetes, Asthma, HTN, or CAD)

Coronary Artery Disease

Percent on Antiplatelet, Beta-Blocker, and/or ACE Inhibitor Medication
Percent on Anti-Lipid Medication
Percent with Annual Lipid Lab Result
Percent with LDL <100 or 130mg/dL or Report HDL, Total Cholesterol, or Triglycerides

Diabetes—Adult Onset-Type 2

Percent with Annual Dilated Eye and Foot Exam, Annual Microalbumin Test
Percent with Annual A1c Lab Test and Result
Percent with Glucose Monitoring at Home
Percent with Annual Lipid Lab Result and LDL <100mg/dL
Percent with Controlled Blood Pressure (<130/80mm/Hg)

continues

Table 57–5 continued

Chronic Obstructive Pulmonary Disease

Percent Who Report Oxygen Use
Percent on Bronchodilator and Inhaled Steroid Medication
Percent on Oral Corticosteroid

Asthma

Percent with Sleep Disruption
Percent and Frequency of Asthma Attacks
Percent on Regular Bronchodilator Medication
Percent with Regular Inhaled Steroid Medication

Source: Adapted by Miriam Cannon Wagner, RN, from the American Heart Association's Clinical Practice Guidelines (Heart Failure, Coronary Artery Disease, Diabetes, Asthma, and Chronic Obstructive Pulmonary Disease).

would they be hospitalized or not? Regression to the mean analysis shows that most patients move toward the mean or average value over time regardless of interventions.

Another factor in financial outcome reporting is that the varied "mix" of patients is constantly changing because patients are discharged and admitted at different times. Most programs report total hospital admissions for each period; as patients are enrolled longer, subsequent data may change dramatically. Reporting patient outcomes by admission dates and functional or clinical status can reduce some of the data problems; however, many health plans report that patients move to the "mean" with or without program intervention.

A "retrospective prepost control group comparison study" is another alternative to report outcome changes, and may be more valuable and feasible than a randomized control trial or a prepost comparison.[12,16,57] Many studies, using this type of methodology, have been done.[13,18,58,61,62] Two important aspects need to be considered for a retrospective prepost study to

be successful. The first important factor is to identify, retrospectively, a control group that is similar to the intervention group in demographics, comorbidities, utilization data, and other clinical variables. The second factor is self-selection bias, which is found by comparing the intervention group to a group that chooses not to participate in the program.[13,58,63] It is also important to have a large enough sample (about 100 patients) in the intervention and control groups to be able to draw statistically sound conclusions regarding the impact of the intervention on the outcomes (see Exhibit 57–1).[64]

SUMMARY

Disease management is one of many options for the delivery of health care. It has emerged as a vital force to decrease the high cost of acute and chronic illness. The providers of disease management must ensure that outcomes are collected in a methodical way in order to report effective change in clinical care. The financial aspects of disease management programs

Exhibit 57–1 Sample Outcome Charts

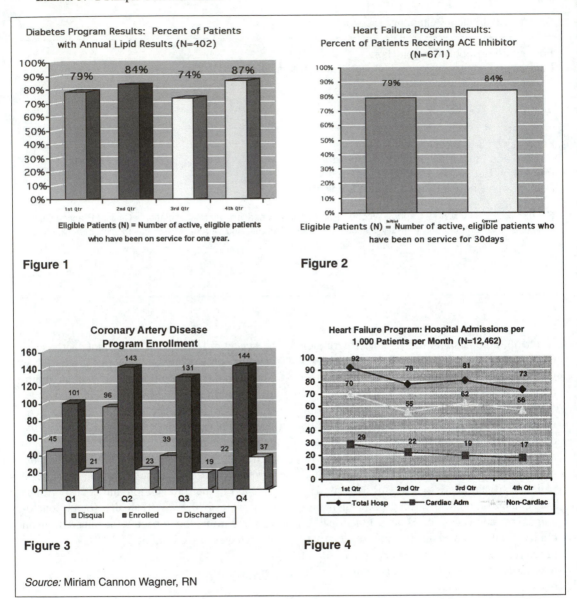

Source: Miriam Cannon Wagner, RN

continue to struggle to report savings and long-term improvements for all patients that utilize these services. The patients and their families will benefit from the broad aspects of disease management because it provides care in a proac-tive way. The focus of care expands not only to immediate post-hospital acute care, but also ad-dresses prevention and long-term strategies to prevent exacerbation of disease and promote health maintenance.

ENDNOTES

1. Gurnee, M. C., and R. V. DaSilva. 1997, June. Constructing disease management programs. *Managed Care.* Available online at *http://www .managedcaremag.com/archiveMC/9706/9706 .disease_man.shtml* (Accessed March 23, 1999).

2. Centers for Disease Control and Prevention. 2003, February. *The power of prevention. reducing the health and economic burden of chronic disease.* Atlanta: Department of Health and Human Services, Centers for Disease Control and Prevention.

3. Hoffman, C., D. Rice, H. Y. Sung. 1996. Persons with chronic conditions: Their prevalence and costs. *Journal of the American Medical Association* 276: 1473–1479.

4. Centers for Disease Control and Prevention. February 2002. *The burden of chronic disease and their risk factors: National and state perspectives.* Department of Health and Human Services, Centers for Disease Control and Prevention.

5. Krumholz, H. M., E. M. Parent, N. Tu, V. Vaccarine, Y. Wang, M. J. Radford, J. Hennen. 1997. Readmission after hospitalization for congestive heart failure among Medicare beneficiaries. *Archives of Internal Medicine* 157: 99–104.

6. Rich, M. W., V. Beckham, C. Witteberg, C. L. Leven, K. E. Freedland, R. M. Carney. 1995. A multidisciplinary intervention to prevent the readmission of elderly patients with congestive heart failure. *New England Journal of Medicine* 333: 1190–1195.

7. O'Connell, J. B. 2000. The economic burden of heart failure. *Clinical Cardiology* 23 (Suppl. III): III-6–10.

8. Grady, K. L., K. Dracup, G. Kennedy, D. K. Moser, M. Piano, L. W. Stevenson, J. B. Young. 2000. Team management of patients with heart failure: A statement for health care professionals from the cardiovascular nursing council of the American Heart Association. *Circulation* 102: 2443–2456.

9. Bodenheimer, T. 2000. Disease management in the American market. *British Medical Journal* 320: 563–566.

10. Bodenheimer, T. 1999. Disease management—Promises and pitfalls. *New England Journal of Medicine* 340(15): 1202–1205.

11. Rhinehart, E. 1998. DM payoffs include lower costs and better utilization: Disease management programs benefit payers, providers, patients and their families. Managed Healthcare 5(6): 20–22.

12. McAlearney, A. S. 2000. Designing and developing effective disease management programmes. *Disease Management and Health Outcomes* 7: 139–148.

13. Berger, J., J. Slezak, N. Stine, P. McStay, B. O'Leary, J. Addiego. 2001. Economic impact of a diabetes disease management program in a self-insured health plan: Early results. *Disease Management* 4: 65–73.

14. Downey, C. 2001. Disease management uses Web to net savings. *Managed Care* 10. Available online at *http://www.managedcaremag.com/archives/0107/01 07.online_dm.html* (accessed September 3, 2003).

15. Krumholz, H. M., D. W. Baker, C. M. Ashton, S. B. Dunbar, G. C. Friesinger, E. P. Havranek, M. A. Hlatky, M. Konstam, D. L. Ordin, I. L. Pina, B. Pitt, J. A. Spertus. 2000. Evaluating quality of care for patients with heart failure. *American Heart Association/American College of Cardiology Conference Proceedings.* Circulation 101: 1–19.

16. DM outcomes: Industry's "seamy underside," Critics say. 2001. *Disease Management News* 20: 1, 4.

17. Centers for Medicare and Medicaid Services. 2002, February 22. Demonstration project for disease management for severely chronically ill Medicare beneficiaries with congestive heart failure, diabetes and coronary heart disease [CMS-4030N]. Centers for Medicare and Medicaid Services, Department of Health and Human Services; *Federal Register*: 67 (36): 8267–8270.

18. Institute of Medicine. 2001. *Crossing the quality chasm: A new health system for the 21st century.* Washington, DC: National Academies Press.

19. CDC. 2001. *Strategies for reducing morbidity and mortality from diabetes through health-care system intervention: diabetes self-management education in communities: A report on recommendations of the Task Force on Community Preventive Services* 50(RR16): 1–15.

20. Rich, M. W. 1999. Heart failure disease management: A critical review. *Journal of Cardiac Failure* 5: 64–75.

21. Riegel, B., B. Carlson, D. Glaser, and P. Hoadland. 2000. Which patients with heart failure respond best to multidisciplinary disease management. *Journal of Cardiac Failure* 6: 290–299.

22. McAlister, F. A., F. M. E. Lawson, K. K. Teo, and P. W. Armstrong. 2001. Randomized trials of secondary prevention programmes in coronary heart disease: Systematic review. *British Medical Journal* 323: 957–962.

23. DeBusk, R. F., N. H. Miller, R. Superko, C. A. Dennis, R. J. Thomas, H. T. Lew, W. E. Berger, R. S. Heller, J. Rompf, D. Gee, H. Kreamer, A. Bandura, G. Ghandour, M. Clark, R. V. Shah, L. Fisher, C. B. Taylor. 1994. A case management system for coronary risk factor modification following acute

myocardial infarction. *Annals of Internal Medicine* 120: 721–729.

24. Miller, N. H., K. M. Parker, D. Senneca, G. Ghandour, M. Clark, G. Greenwald, R. S. Heller, M. B. Fowler, R. F. DeBusk. 1997. A comprehensive management system for heart failure improves clinical outcomes and reduces medical resource utilization. *American Journal of Cardiology* 79: 58–63.

25. Finay, F. A., F. M. E. Lawson, K. K. Teo, and P. W. Armstrong. 2001. Randomized trials of secondary prevention programmes in coronary heart disease: systematic review. *British Medical Journal* 323: 957–962.

26. Kornowski, R., D. Zeeli, M. Averbuch, A. Finkelstein, D. Schwartz, M. Moshkovitz, B. Weinreb, R. Hershkovitz, D. Eyal, M. Miller, Y. Levo, A. Pines. 1996. Intensive homecare surveillance prevents hospitalization and improves morbidity rates among elderly patients with severe congestive heart failure. *American Heart Journal* 129: 762–766.

27. Stewart, S., S. Pearson, and J. D. Horowitz. 1998. Effects of home-based intervention among patients with congestive heart failure discharged from acute care hospital. *Archives of Internal Medicine*; 158: 1067–1072.

28. Rich, M. W. 1999. Heart failure disease management: A critical review. *Journal of Cardiac Failure* 5: 64–75.

29. West, J. A., N. H. Miller, K. M. Parker, D. Senneca, G. Ghandour, M. Clark, G. Greenwald, R. S. Heller, M. B. Fowler, and R. F. DeBusk. 1997. A comprehensive management system for heart failure improves clinical outcomes and reduces medical resource utilization. *American Journal of Cardiology* 79: 58–63.

30. Shah, N. B., E. Der, C. Ruggerio, P. A. Heidenreich, and B. M. Massie. 1998. Prevention of hospitalization for heart failure with an interactive home monitoring program. *American Heart Journal* 135: 373–378.

31. Naylor, M. D., D. Brooten, R. Cambell, B. S. Jacobson, M. D. Mezey, M. V. Pauly, and J. S. Schwartz. 1999. Comprehensive discharge planning and home follow-up of hospitalized elders. *Journal of the American Medical Association* 281: 613–620.

32. Tsuyuki, R. T., R. S. McKelvie, M. O. Arnold, A. Avezum, A. C. Barretto, A. C. Carvalho, D. L. Isaac, A. D. Kitching, L. Sl. Piegas, K. K. Teo, and S. Yusuf. 2001. Acute precipitants of congestive heart failure exacerbations. *Archives of Internal Medicine* 161: 2337–2342.

33. Sidorov, J., R. Shull, J. Tomcavage, S. Girolami, R. Harris, and N. Lawton. 2002. Does diabetes disease management save money and improve outcomes? *Diabetes Care* 25(4): 684–689.

34. National Committee for Quality Assurance. 2003. The health plan employer data and information set (HEDIS). Available at *http://www.ncqa.org/Programs/HEDIS/index.htm* (accessed June 28, 2003).

35. Rossiter, L. F., M. Y. Whitehurst-Cook, R. E. Small, C. Shasky, V. E. Bovbjerg, L. Penberthy, A. Okasha, J. Green, I. A. Ibrahim, S. Yang, and K. Lee. 2000. The impact of disease management on outcomes and cost of care: A study of low-income asthma patients. *Inquiry* 37(2): 188–202.

36. Taitel, M., H. Kotses, I. L. Bernstein, D. J. Berstein, and T. Creer. 1995. A self-management program for adult asthma. Part 1: Development and evaluation. *Journal of Allergy and Clinical Immunology* 95: 529–540.

37. Definition of Disease Management. Disease Management Association of America. Available at *http://www.dmaa.org/definition.html* (accessed June 14, 2003).

38. Leider, H. L., and K. Krizan. (2001). Disease management: A great concept, but can you implement it. *Disease Management* 4(3): 111–119.

39. The Criteria Committee of the New York Heart Association. 1964. *Diseases of the heart and blood vessels: Nomenclature and criteria for diagnosis* (6th ed.). Boston, MA: Little Brown.

40. Vinson, J. M., M. W. Rich, J. C. Sperry, A. S. Shah, and T. McNamara. 1990. Early readmission of elderly patients with congestive heart failure. *Journal of the American Geriatric Society* 38: 1290–1295.

41. Ware, J. E., M. S. Kosinski, and S. D. Keller. 1998. *How to score the SF-12 physical and mental health summary scales* (3rd ed.). Boston, MA: The Health Institute, New England Medical Center.

42. Bandura, A. 1977. *Social learning theory*. Englewood Cliffs, NJ: Prentice Hall.

43. Bandura, A. 1986. *Social foundations of thought and action: A social cognitive theory*. Englewood Cliffs, NJ: Prentice Hall.

44. Prochaska, J. O., and C. C. DiClemente. 1983. Stages and process of self-change of smoking: Toward an integrative model of change. *Journal of Consulting and Clinical Psychology* 51: 390–395.

45. Centers for Disease Control, Disease Prevention and Health Promotion, Atlanta, GA. Available at *http://www.cdc.gov/nccdphp/* (accessed June 14, 2003).

46. American Heart Association Web site. Available at *http://www.americanheart.org* (accessed June 14, 2003).

47. National Institutes of Health, National Heart, Lung, and Blood Institute Web site. Available at *http://www.nhlbi.nih.gov* (accessed June 14, 2003).

48. Agency for Healthcare Research and Quality National Guidelines Clearinghouse Web site. Available at *http://www.ngc.org* (accessed June 16, 2003).

49. National Committee for Quality Assurance. 2002. The State of Managed Care Quality. Available at *http://www.ncqa.org/sohc2002* (accessed June 28, 2003).

50. Centers for Medicaid and Medicare Web site. Available at http://www.cms.gov; Medicare Managed Care Manual; Chapter 5, Quality Assessment. Rev 29 (accessed August 1, 2003). Available at *http://cms.hhs.gov/manuals/116_mmc/mc86c05.asp* (accessed June 14, 2003).

51. National Committee for Quality Assurance. 2003. The State of Managed Care Quality. Available at *http://www.ncqa.org/sohc2002/SOHC_2002_CAHPS_METHOD.html* (accessed June 28, 2003).

52. Xu, G., L. E. Paddock, J. P. O'Connor, D.B. Nash, M. Zitter. 2001. Chief medical officer's perceptions of disease management programs. *Disease Management* 4: 19–24.

53. Selecky, C. 2001. Integrating technology and interventions in the management of diabetes. *Disease Management and Health Outcomes* 9 (Supp. 1): 39–52.

54. Gomaa, W. H., T. Morrow, and P. Muntendam. 2001. Technology-based disease management. *Disease Management and Health Outcomes* 9: 577–588.

55. Eliaszadeh, P., H. Yarmohammadi, H. Nawaz, J. Boukhalil, and D. L. Katz. 2001. Congestive heart failure case management: A fiscal analysis. *Disease Management* 4: 25–32.

56. Hannumanthu, S., J. Butler, D. Chomsky, S. Davis, and J. R. Wilson. 1997. Effect of a heart failure program on hospitalization frequency and exercise tolerance. *Circulation* 96: 2842–2848.

57. Hershberger, R. E., H. Ni, D.J. Nauman, D. Burgess, W. Toy, K. Wise, D. Dutton, K. Crispell, M. Vossler, J. Everett. 2001. Prospective evaluation of an outpatient heart failure management program. *Journal of Cardiac Failure* 7: 64–74.

58. Whellan, D. J., L. Gaulden, W. A. Gattis, B. Granger, S. D. Russell, M. A. Blazing, M. S. Cuffe, C. M. O'Connor. 2001. The benefit of implementing a heart failure disease management program. *Archives of Internal Medicine* 161: 2223–2228.

59. Kane, R. L. 1997. *Understanding health care outcomes research*. Gaithersburg, MD: Aspen Publishers, Inc.

60. Lang, T. A., and M. Secic. 1997. *How to report statistics in medicine: Annotated guidelines for authors, editors, and reviewers*. Philadelphia: American College of Physicians.

61. Schulman, K. A., D. B. Mark, and R. M. Califf. 1998. Outcomes and costs within a disease management program for advanced congestive heart failure. *American Heart Journal* 135: S285–S292.

62. Vaccaro, J., J. Cherry, A. Harper, and M. O'Connell. 2001. Utilization reduction, cost savings, and return on investment for the PacifiCare chronic heart failure program, "Taking Charge of Your Heart Health." *Disease Management* 4: 131–142.

63. Heidenrich, P. A., C. M. Ruggerio, and B. M. Massic. 1999. Effect of a home monitoring system on hospitalization and resource use for patients with heart failure. *American Heart Journal* 138: 633–640.

64. Rubin, R. J., K. A. Dietrich, and A. D. Hawk. 1998. Clinical and economic impact of implementing a comprehensive diabetes management program in managed care. *Journal of Clinical Endocrinology and Metabolism* 83: 2635–2642.

CHAPTER 58

The Process of Visiting Nurse Association Affiliation with a Major Teaching Hospital

Marilyn D. Harris

PREFACE

It has been 16 years since the Visiting Nurse Association (VNA) of Eastern Montgomery County affiliated its programs and services with Abington Memorial Hospital (AMH) to become Abington Memorial Hospital Home Care (AMHHC). In retrospect, this was, and continues to be, a win-win decision. The AMHHC and hospice programs, with the support of the hospital's administration, physicians, staff, and referral sources, continue to expand their programs and staff to meet the needs of patients and their families. Examples of additional programs and services are: Home Infusion Company, expanded maternal-child health program, Congestive Heart Failure program, Palliative Care Team, Safe Harbor (see Chapter 67), and the addition of butterfly gardens throughout the hospital as one aspect of the Animal-Assisted Therapy program.

Balotsky and Smith (see Chapter 54) report that home health merger and acquisition (M&A) activity remains a consistent but maturing strategic response; after peaking at 137 transactions in 1997, activity decreased to 28 mergers in 2002. Another consultant reported that there is resurgence in new home health agencies, and many agencies are diversifying into private duty

services. I have included my positive experience with this M&A process because M&As continue to be one aspect of the strategic planning process for home health agencies in the 21st century.

HISTORICAL PERSPECTIVE

Affiliation among agencies with differing staff, resources, organizational structures, policies, and programs is never easy. This chapter discusses major components of an affiliation between a VNA and its former competitor, a major teaching hospital.

The VNA of Eastern Montgomery County was no stranger to corporate restructures. It had successfully completed five restructures since it was founded in 1919. Although I focus on the hospital affiliation in 1988, some comments apply to the three restructures that occurred since I became the director of the agency.

In 1988, the VNA was a voluntary, certified accredited home health agency and hospice that provided in-home and community health services. The VNA received referrals from physicians, hospitals, community agencies, and individuals.

Abington Memorial Hospital, a 500-bed teaching hospital, opened its doors in 1913 and

Source: This chapter was originally published as an article in 1992 in the Journal of Nursing Administration and has been updated to reflect the current status of AMHHC 16 years after the affiliation. Reprinted with permission from M. D. Harris, "The Process of Visiting Nurse Association Affiliation with a Major Teaching Hospital," *Journal of Nursing Administration* 22(7–8): 51–60 © 1992, J.B. Lippincott Company.

established a home care department in 1979. Home care services were made available through contracts with certified agencies for all disciplines. Occupational and physical therapy services were also offered through the hospital's rehabilitation department. In 1988, the hospital had a home care director, five home care coordinators, and support staff. Although informal discussions had taken place for several years and the VNA was the hospital's contractor for home care service, formal discussions regarding affiliation did not begin until 1985.

During June 1985, when affiliation discussions began, the VNA provided services to patients referred by multiple hospitals and physicians. Staff made 4,685 visits to 646 individuals. Referrals from AMH resulted in 1,765 visits (37 percent of total) to 236 individuals (36 percent of total). The VNA had 76.6 full-time equivalent employees and made 59,294 home visits during the fiscal year.

Although the VNA was a financially sound organization when discussions began in 1985, 1988 was a deficit year. This was due in part to the large percentage of fixed-rate, rather than cost-based, reimbursement from the VNA's contract with the hospital while the negotiations were taking place.

THE NEGOTIATION PROCESS

The VNA board received a formal letter from AMH's administrators in July 1985 outlining a proposal for merger. The board met to discuss the letter, and several VNA board members and the administrative staff scheduled a meeting with the hospital's executive vice president (EVP) and vice president for nursing to discuss the proposal. The hospital's president, EVP, and comptroller were invited to meet with the VNA board. After this meeting, an ad hoc committee including legal counsel was formed with representatives from the VNA and AMH. Regularly scheduled meetings were held with established agendas.

One of the first tasks was discussing the options available to the hospital and the VNA. There were at least four options for the VNA: (1)

to remain as is (i.e., the hospital would expand its own program and compete with the VNA); (2) a merger (dissolution of its present entity and a merger into one agency with the hospital); (3) a joint venture with the hospital, where each organization would keep its own identity; or (4) an affiliation with a division of services. The options for AMH were to expand its existing home care department separate from the VNA or to consider an affiliation with the VNA. The advantages and disadvantages of each option had to be identified.

From the start, both organizations felt that the VNA should continue to provide service to those patients who were referred by others in the community, including hospitals and physicians. There was concern that other facilities and referral sources might be reluctant to refer to the VNA if skilled service were offered through AMH (i.e., fear of loss of control of patients). Therefore, this issue was one of the topics for discussion. As of 2003, the AMHHC continues to receive referrals from other agencies/facilities.

The VNA also addressed the financial impact that any decision would have on its funding sources. The executive director (ED) contacted the United Way, Office on Aging, and municipal managers to determine what effect, if any, the various corporate structures would have on current and future funding. Certifying and accrediting agencies were also contacted to discuss the impact of restructuring. The VNA management staff determined that the least adverse effects were associated with the affiliation option.

Meanwhile, in 1986, while discussions were taking place with AMH, the VNA completed a planned internal corporate restructure. A parent company, VNA-Health Management Services (VNA-HMS), was formed with two subsidiaries, the VNA (the Medicare-certified home health agency) and VNA-Community Services, Inc. (VNA-CS), to provide the support and health promotion services. The three VNAs had separate boards of directors but shared the same administrative staff through a management agreement. A lease was established for rental space between the corporations that were housed in the same office buildings. This fact is mentioned because this internal corporate restructure with the resulting division of health care services was important in light of the decision made to affiliate the VNA with the hospital in 1988.

THE DECISION-MAKING PROCESS

The VNA and AMH mutually agreed to use a health care consulting firm to assist with data collection and analysis. The anticipated benefits of a cooperative effort were as follows:

- combined effort of two well-respected organizations
- continuation of needed patient services in a coordinated manner
- ability of the VNA again to realize costs for services by discipline rather than a fixed rate
- ability of AMH to maximize reimbursement
- opportunities for expansion of in-home and community services

The ad hoc committee met again after receipt of the consultant's report. Although the consultant recommended a community-based agency, the hospital administration determined that it would retain a hospital-based agency. Hospital administrators believed that a hospital-based agency would be financially beneficial because home care was reimbursed on a cost basis. A time frame was established for the VNA board to share its decision with hospital administration. The VNA board, in cooperation with the administrative staff, made the decision to affiliate the VNA services and personnel with the hospital. VNA-CS would remain a free-standing community-based agency with its own board of directors.

The VNA administrative staff developed a list of operational issues that were to be included in the affiliation agreement. These included use of the VNA's organizational chart, computer system, fiscal intermediary (FI), professional advisory committee, policy and procedure manual, and name. After legal counsel for both organizations finalized the agreement, the boards of the three VNAs approved the agreement on February 16, 1988. The hospital's board of

trustees approved the agreement the following week.

THE TRANSITION PROCESS

The transition period between February 25 and May 31, 1988, was extremely busy. In addition to the day-to-day operations of the three VNAs, the administrative staff had 30 meetings with hospital staff to facilitate the smooth transfer as of June 1, 1988. The reasons for meeting with the various departments are summarized here.

Nursing Administration

In 1988, the hospital's home care department director reported to the nursing department's business manager. As of June 1, 1988, the director would report to the hospital's EVP and chief operating officer. Many meetings were held to make sure that all the necessary details were completed. There was a good working relationship with the nursing department as personnel, clinical records, physical space, and the need for a smooth transition of patient care from one to another were addressed. Much time was devoted to the placement of existing home care personnel within the new home care department.

One major project was combining two policy and procedure manuals and obtaining approval of the professional advisory committee. The professional advisory committees of both organizations had overlapping membership. The existing VNA professional advisory committee membership was expanded to include the hospital's members.

Social Service Department

Before the affiliation, two discharge-planning nurses reported to the director of the social service department. One of the terms of the affiliation was that these two nurses plus three additional nurses responsible for the nursing aspect of discharge planning would report to the VNA. Numerous meetings were held with the director of social services and the director of professional service (DPS) at the VNA to develop mutually acceptable policies and procedures that identified areas of responsibilities. It was imperative that administrative-level personnel be aware of the sensitive nature of positions that overlapped or had similar areas of responsibilities.

Therapy Department

The VNA provided all therapy services through contracts. The hospital's home care department had, in addition to purchasing services from the VNA, purchased service from the hospital's occupational and physical therapy departments. The therapists were assigned to the home care department on a rotating basis. The VNA agreed to continue with this arrangement, although most services would still be provided through contract service because of the shortage of staff therapists.

Medical Record Committee

All clinical record forms had to be approved by the hospital's medical record committee. This meant that all the VNA forms had to be reviewed by this committee. Forms were sent to the committee chair, who circulated them to members. The ED, DPS, and supervisor for quality assessment (QA) attended the meeting to explain the forms and answer questions.

The administrative staff also met with the director of the hospital's medical record department to review the current record system and format, the storage of closed records, and the requirements to meet Joint Commission on Accreditation of Healthcare Organizations (JCAHO) standards. The VNA record format remained the same. The closed records are stored off site, in keeping with policy.

The VNA addressed the issue of custodian of the records as of May 31, 1988. The affiliation agreement included reference to clinical records. The hospital's medical record department agreed to accept, and the VNA board agreed to transfer, all active records with the effective date of the affiliation. All closed records were made available to the hospital.

The VNA also transferred active hospital home care patients to the VNA fiscal intermediary as of June 1, 1988. The hospital agreed to request an early transfer to the identified regional FI. This provided for continuity of clinical and billing aspects of care because the VNA was currently served by this FI. All these transactions were accomplished without major problems.

Pastoral Care

A meeting was scheduled with the ED, the DPS, and the assistant chaplain of the hospital to discuss how the VNA's certified hospice program would interface with the hospital's in-house program for terminally ill patients. We determined that the hospital's chaplains would not make home visits on a regular basis, nor would the VNA's hospice chaplain follow patients when they were hospitalized. Continuity of care is provided through the hospice coordinator, who attends both the in-house palliative care team meetings and the VNA's hospice interdisciplinary team meetings. In specific situations, the chaplain's visits may be interchangeable. The hospital's chaplain would continue to assist with the hospice's bereavement group meetings.

QA and Utilization Review

The VNA's QA program was extensive but had to be revised to meet Joint Commission and hospital standards. The ED, DPS, and QA supervisor attended several formal presentations on the JCAHO standards and QA and met with the hospital's director of QA and the staff. The administrative and supervisory staff rewrote the QA policy and procedures, identified specific aspects of care to be monitored, identified indicators and thresholds, and revised the yearly calendar for reporting outcomes. The VNA's QA report is presented to the hospital's board of trustees quarterly through established committees. The VNA's DPS and discharge planner (DP) nurse supervisor participate in regularly scheduled, hospital-wide, multidisciplinary meetings to address the DP process and current utilization of hospital days.

The VNA had been accredited by the National League for Nursing (NLN), now the Community Health Accreditation Program (CHAP) since 1967. Following the affiliation, the administration staff prepared for a site visit from the JCAHO surveyors to coincide with the hospital's survey cycle.

Volunteers

The hospital had an active volunteer program. The VNA's hospice volunteer program is directed by its own volunteer director. Meetings were held prior to the affiliation to formalize policy and procedures to enable VNA volunteers to visit hospice patients who are admitted to the hospital. Arrangements were also in place to allow a hospice volunteer to begin visits while the patient was still in the hospital, if this was indicated (Harris and Groshens, 1985).

Additional meetings were held to update these procedures. Mutually agreeable procedures were implemented. Hospice volunteers visited with patients at home and in the hospital. The VNA also had a friendly visitor program that was expanded to serve more patients. In 1996, a six-bed designated hospice unit was identified in the hospital. Hospice-trained volunteers are available to be on the unit during the morning, afternoon, and evening hours.

Communications

Numerous meetings were held with the director of communications to discuss multiple issues. The VNA would continue to occupy two offices off the hospital campus. One office was located two blocks from the hospital while the second office was 7 miles from campus. The physical location of the DP nurses' office within the hospital was moved. Arrangements had to be made to increase the number of telephones and to change the location. The hospital's telephone directory

was being updated, and the timing enabled the new numbers for all the DP nurses to be included. Arrangements were discussed for a future hookup between the VNA's computers and the hospital computer system. Discussions were held to arrange for dedicated telephone lines when the hospital expanded its system.

Additional pocket pagers were ordered and air time was coordinated because the hospital and the VNA used different systems. It was cost-effective to purchase new beepers and to purchase air time from the hospital's system.

The hospital initiated a voice mailbox system. The VNA was able to obtain voice mailboxes for most of its administrative staff, clinical supervisors, and all DP nurses. Staff nurses were added in November 1991. In 1997, this communication device made it easy to accept and leave messages while decreasing telephone tag for staff and contractors. As of 2002, all nursing staff have pagers and cell phones to provide for improved communications.

Internal communications were an important part of the VNA operation. For several years, weekly announcements had been held at a specific time. The two VNA offices were equipped with speaker telephones so that the entire staff could hear. These weekly staff announcements were taped and transcribed and made available on the bulletin boards for everyone to read. This method of communication continued even though all personnel were located in the same building, but in two separate offices.

Public Relations

The ED met with the director of public relations to discuss the current public relations activities and the procedures to be followed in the future. Discussions included public relations budget, news releases, articles, pictures, brochures, and handouts. Parameters were established for those activities that could be accomplished in-house and those that had to be done through freelance writers. Time frames were established for preparing new brochures and other promotional materials.

Fund-Raising

The VNA's ED and finance director met with the hospital's director of fund development to discuss the establishment of designated restricted funds specifically for the hospice program. The VNA's current fund-raising activities were also shared with the fund development director.

Personnel

The establishment of a good working relationship with the personnel department at the hospital was important before, during, and after the affiliation. Before a decision was made on the affiliation, it was important to meet with the vice president of human resources to share information about benefits available from both organizations and to make comparisons. It was important to bring the VNA benefits in line with the hospital's benefits while seeking to preserve existing benefits at current levels. The hospital and the VNA made a comparative chart for review by the hospital's administration and the VNA's board. There was a genuine interest and concern from both organizations to preserve the best of both policies. This was accomplished to the satisfaction of both parties and the staff.

Once the decision had been made to affiliate and the VNA board had agreed to the benefits package, administrators communicated this decision to staff. The hospital's vice president of human resources and his staff met with VNA staff to review the details and answer questions. Before the meeting, information packets were distributed to all staff including information about the available hospitalization, dental plans, and other benefits. This meeting was beneficial because it enabled the VNA staff to meet with the personnel department staff and get direct answers to their questions.

Payroll

The hospital was changing from a weekly to an every-other-week payroll schedule to coincide with the planned affiliation. The VNA was al-ready on a 2-week pay schedule with a different service bureau. Therefore, the VNA continued to prepare its own payroll for approximately 3 months. The delay in the transfer to the hospital's system allowed time for the hospital to transfer its 2,500 employees to a new system without disrupting the VNA payroll. The VNA payroll transfer occurred as planned. There were some problems encountered, most of which were related to accrual of time benefits and deductions. These problems were resolved after several pay periods.

The VNA staff lost the benefit of direct deposit for several months because the hospital did not have this program in place. It was instituted by the hospital about 6 months later.

Hiring

As the director of a community-based agency, I had the authority to hire staff to fill budgeted positions. This process changed with the affiliation. The employment process was now the responsibility of the personnel department. Vacant positions must be posted in the hospital for 5 days. Internal applicants are given the opportunity to interview for a position. A classified ad is placed if no internal transfers are received.

At times, applicants apply at the VNA office. When this occurs, the applicant is given general information and asked to contact the hospital's personnel department to complete forms and discuss salary and benefits. Interviewing is done at the VNA by the DPS and supervisors. The VNA staff has the final decision on which of the applicants will be offered employment. Also, all new positions must be approved through the budgeting process.

Staff Orientation

All VNA employees must attend selected sections of the hospital's orientation program in addition to job-specific orientation. Joint Commission standards state that specific items must be included in orientation, such as safety and infection control. To orient all VNA staff in

1988, a special orientation in-service was planned at the VNA office in cooperation with the personnel department. Representatives from AMH administration were also available. New employees attend the monthly orientation scheduled at AMH, which consists of 2 days of general orientation. Additional orientation is then done at the VNA. Other personnel issues included the development of criteria-based job descriptions for all positions and understanding of the performance-appraisal system for hourly and salaried personnel. We also had to determine how to assimilate the VNA staff into the hospital's wage and bonus system the first year. We decided that the VNA board would provide an increase as of May 31, 1988. The VNA staff would not be eligible for an increase in September 1988 that first year, although hourly rates would be adjusted at such time that overall increases were granted or the base was increased.

Finance Department Billing Activities

Continuity of business activities had to be maintained with the effective date of the affiliation. On June 1, 1988, there were two sets of bills that one VNA staff was responsible for processing. The VNA had to bill its May 1988 visits with one FI. It also had to bill the hospital's visits with a second FI. The non-Medicare billing also had to be done.

For many months, the administrative, business, and clinical supervisory staff had to deal with two FIs to answer questions on previous bills, denials, and requests for information on 485 forms. We also had two post-payment compliance audits within a short period of time from two different FIs. We also received requests from Keystone Peer Review Organization for charts for quality of care reviews for both hospital and VNA patients.

Check Requisition

Checks are issued once per week (except in an emergency). Based on internal operations, the requests must go to the VNA finance director on

Tuesday. Then they are processed and sent to the hospital finance department on Wednesday, which enables processing of the checks on Thursdays. Checks can be issued and available Friday morning. This requires advanced planning, such as for last-minute registration fees, which was a change for the staff. This timing also changed the way contractor checks were processed.

Budget/Reports

The VNA prepared its own budget, which was submitted as part of the total hospital budget. Departments are expected to live within these approved budgets unless additional personnel will generate additional revenues. Reports based on budget versus actual expenses and staffing hours on a monthly and year-to-date basis are available to administrative staff. The VNA handles its own billing and posting of accounts receivable and submits monthly reports to the hospital. Cost reports are prepared by the hospital's finance department.

Contract/Policy Approval

As the director of a community-based agency, I was accustomed to receiving or gathering information, seeking staff opinions, obtaining legal advice, and presenting findings to the board for approval. I had the authority to carry out the board's action.

In a larger bureaucratic system, more departments are involved in the process, and thus it moves more slowly. Also, specific contracts may have impact on the larger organization. Therefore, all aspects must be explored, not just those of the home care agency. Administrative approval is obtained at stated meetings that the director has with the EVP every 2 weeks or more frequently if needed.

Other Departments

Meetings were held with the nutrition department to discuss arrangements for the hospice program. An interdepartmental agreement was arranged for a registered dietitian to be available for the hospice program. Meetings were held with pharmacy personnel to discuss services available to the hospital's home care and hospice patients and to make billing arrangements. We made arrangements to obtain the daily census sheets of admissions and current patients for the DP nurses.

I, as well as the administrative team, met regularly with the hospital administration, including the EVP and the directors of finance, personnel, and nursing, to make sure that everyone was aware of all the transition activities.

The hospital's educational department offers many excellent in-service programs each month at no cost to the departments. Programs are available for the nurses as well as clerical and business office staff. I met with the director to determine how the VNA staff would access these programs. I also met with the director of media services to become familiar with the services available to the VNA, such as videotaping, in-house television programs, and preparation of slides.

The VNA would be ordering patient and office supplies through the hospital's purchasing department. We had to prepare policy and procedures and become familiar with time frames (e.g., length of time between placing an order and receiving it).

External Contacts

In addition to the meetings with AMH staff, it was essential to determine that the hospital and the VNA continued to meet all federal and state requirements during the transition process. This required early notification of the state licensing/certifying agency and the FIs.

State Certifying Agency

The hospital and VNA home care directors contacted the Pennsylvania Department of Health/ Division of Home Health. The hospital had to continue to provide those services for which it was certified during the transition phase. The VNA had to advise the state agency that it planned voluntarily to terminate its participation in the Medicare program as of May 31, 1988. Because the hospital did not have a Medicare-certified hospice, the VNA's Medicare hospice was transferred to the hospital by completing change in ownership forms. These changes were forwarded by the Pennsylvania Department of Health to the federal agency. The action required a completion of the civil rights compliance forms.

State Medical Assistance Office

The VNA's existing medical assistance (MA) number had to be relinquished when it went out of existence on May 31, 1988. Although the hospital had an MA number for the home care department, it could not be used as of June 1, 1988, because MA numbers are issued in Pennsylvania by address codes. The VNA/AMH home care department was no longer going to be located in the hospital. Therefore, the VNA had to apply for a new number for services provided as of June 1, 1988. MA billing had to be held for several weeks until the new number was issued.

FI

The hospital had its own FI. The VNA had Blue Cross of Greater Philadelphia, now Independence Blue Cross (IBC), as its FI. The affiliation agreement provided that the hospital would request an early transfer to IBC, one of the 10 regional FIs. The VNA had been with IBC since 1967. The hospital and VNA administrators wrote the necessary letters to both FIs. The hospital received permission to transfer to IBC. The transfer was easy to accomplish. All active hospital patients were transferred to IBC with a new form 485 as of June 1, 1988. All the VNA's patients continued on service. The transfer to the hospital's home care identification number was facilitated through a cooperative effort among the VNA, IBC, and Delta Computer System (Altoona, Pa.). The VNA's agency identification number was changed on the electronic billing that was completed as of June 1, 1988. Needless to say, there was some confusion until everyone became aware of the affiliation.

Accrediting Organizations

The VNA had been accredited by the National League for Nursing (NLN) since 1967. The hospital's home care department is accredited by the Joint Commission. The VNA submitted its annual report to the NLN spring board of review. Because the VNA would no longer exist as of May 1988, it would have to apply for NLN CHAP status as a new agency in the future.

Meanwhile, the hospital was scheduled for a Joint Commission survey in July 1988. The home care site visit was delayed until December 1988. At that time, the VNA had a successful three-day site visit.

State/National Associations

Letters were sent to the Pennsylvania Association of Home Health Agencies and the National Association for Home Care informing them that the VNA would become a hospital-based agency effective June 1, 1988.

United Way

The VNA had frequent, informative meetings with the staff at the local United Way organization. As noted earlier, the VNA completed a corporate restructure in 1986. Before 1986, the VNA was the United Way Member Agency. Funding was received for its health promotion and support services. These services were assumed by VNA-CS in 1986, when the three VNAs were formed. In 1986, VNA-CS became the United Way Member Agency because this agency provided the supported services. Therefore, in 1988 there was no change in the United Way relationship because VNA-CS remained a free-standing community-based agency.

Contracting Agencies

The VNA director wrote letters informing all individual and group contractors of the change

process. Letters of renewal sent to all contractors indicated that the hospital would be the new contracting entity. There was a slight change in the payment schedule to coincide with the hospital's weekly check processing system but there was no change in the clinical aspect of service.

Identification Numbers

It must be noted that many of the third-party payers and regulatory agencies required new agency/department identification numbers. It was important to notify all staff of the impending changes and new numbers. This was especially important in the instance of patient identification numbers. All care providers, nurses, aides, therapists, and medical record department personnel had to be aware of the change in VNA patient numbers so that clinical records and billing were correct. This took a few weeks, and some corrections or combinations of bills had to be made until all the patients were on the VNA's system.

"FEELINGS": THE IMPACT ON BOARD AND STAFF

At the board level, there was at least one resignation during the negotiating process. The plan of the VNA-CS board members was to enable interested members from the VNA and VNA-HMS boards to join the VNA-CS board as of June 1988. Although a few members chose not to continue, the board's size was increased from 15 to 22 members.

The VNA administrative staff was cognizant that the greatest impact of the affiliation would be felt at this level. The ED, director of finance (DF), and DPS felt that they had lost control in several areas. In the financial area, administrative personnel were accustomed to an internally generated monthly financial report showing income and expenses, profits and loss. Now, although we have control of the budget versus actual expenses, we do not have control of the bottom line.

In relationship to operating within a larger, more bureaucratic system, the administrative staff had to learn the process. For a while, I felt totally inadequate; I had to learn what forms to use to requisition the forms I needed to requisition the clerical and clinical supplies and checks! Timing and planning ahead were critical. I went to in-services for new managers to become familiar with all the details of hospital expectations in addition to the one-to-one meetings discussed earlier.

The VNA staff involved with clinical services and related issues (computer input, billing, and medical record) felt the impact with a change in volume of Medicare business from 30 percent in May 1988 to 70 percent in June 1988. This change resulted from the loss of the hospital's home care contract services, which represented about 50 percent of the VNA's business before June 1988.

There was a significant increase in the paperwork that had to be done by the VNA staff. As noted earlier, we also had to deal with two FIs for clinical and reimbursement purposes for many months. There were also some changes that were initiated to meet JCAHO requirements. The DPS and ED met with the hospital's chief of staff to review the existing procedure to make referrals for home care services and to verify physician credentials to meet Joint Commission requirements.

Once the decision to affiliate was announced, there were some resignations within the home care department. This occurred even though all employees of the VNA and the hospital's home care department were offered positions in the new home care department. Some employees chose to interview for the new position of DP nurse within the home care department. All these nurses were hired. Some took other positions in the hospital.

ADJUSTMENTS FOR STAFF

I asked the VNA staff to share written comments with me concerning the impact of the change from a community to a hospital-based agency. Exhibit 58–1 shows these selected observations and comments from staff at all levels in the organization. Personally and professionally, this was one of my most challenging experiences. Although I knew I was not personally responsible for the current health care climate, in which affiliations were common, I felt responsible for the agency's future direction because the board depended on the administrative staff and me for direction. The process could not have been accomplished without the support and expertise of the VNA's DPS and DF.

CHANGE IN PROFESSIONAL RELATIONSHIP WITH PEERS

Ongoing professional relationships are often organized under an agency's auspices. This occurs at the local, state, and national levels. A business decision is based on facts and is made after the pros and cons have been identified and discussed. Because the staff, more than the board, are usually involved with their peers on an ongoing basis, administrative staff must be prepared for changes in professional relationships. This change occurred at the VNA when I informed organizations of the agency's planned change and requested a decision concerning future membership based on interpretation of the bylaws. Based on these interpretations, some organizational relationships were terminated as a result of our restructure.

By the time the affiliation decision was made, I felt comfortable with the terms of the affiliation and the impact it would have on our daily operations. We were prepared for our new responsibilities and the change this might require in current relationships. The reactions of administrative colleagues ranged from "You sold out" to "I envy you. You know in what direction you're headed."

One relationship that did not change in 1998 was the one with the VNA-CS board. Before the affiliation, the administrative staff was accustomed to managing both in-home and community services through a management agreement. As of June 1, 1988, a management agreement was continued. VNA-CS had a management agreement with AMH for the administrative staff's time to manage its programs and services. The workload greatly increased, however,

Exhibit 58–1 Selected Observations and Comments from Staff

Emotional Aspects

- Coming to grips with feelings, specifically anger. It took the 3 years from 1985 to 1988 to move through the stages to acceptance.
- Looking at the environment and dealing with reality.

Organizational Considerations

- Excellent educational opportunities.
- Increase in income commensurate with hospital salaries is a plus!
- Less autonomy.
- Connected to the hospital and included in the activities.
- Involved in hospital politics.
- Trust in VNA administration to have the best interest of employees at heart.
- Confidence that concerns about the history and philosophy of the agency and the focus on quality of care have been addressed.

Operational Issues

- Identify the costs/benefits to the organization and individuals.
- Attend in-services and conferences to become familiar with new external organizations, such as the JCAHO and new reporting requirements.
- Stockpile supplies to allow time to fit into new time frame.

- Create position for Quality Assessment supervisor or new personnel before change.
- Get to know new players (e.g., department directors).
- Prepare for increased number of meetings.
- More departments to deal with.
- Increased need to justify requests for additional positions.
- Decreased overall control.
- Biggest frustration is waiting for answers.
- The autonomy of day-to-day decision making in the provision of patient care has remained intact, dispelling fears that the hospital system would alter this autonomy.
- Difficulty adapting to new payroll regulations, benefits, and especially leaving the flexibility of a small office to join a large, more inflexible organization. Yet, the hospital administration has seemed to strive to make the changes as easy as possible and has been accessible to staff when questions arise.
- Suddenly you are working for a whole new organization and management team. It's like starting a new job when you really haven't. The adjustments required can be formidable.

---

because there were now both hospital and community agency budgets, personnel policies, meetings, QA programs, accreditation standards, and public relations. The VNA administrative staff continued to interact with the United Way, Office on Aging, county/municipal offices, and the hospital administrator. The role of the ED was, and continued to be, a busy but enjoyable one to fill. The management agreement was not renewed by the hospital in 1993. My communications with, and access to, the hospital's

EVP were excellent. This positive working relationship continues in 2004 with the current AMHHC executive director and the hospital's EVP. The EVP is readily available by telephone or by voice mail. Pertinent written materials and articles related to home care and hospice are shared. Administrative staff is included on selected committees and asked to share ideas on issues within the hospital at the hospital-wide department director's meetings that are held every 2 weeks.

CONCLUSION

I believe that the VNA's decision to affiliate its skilled home care services with AMH was the result of a sound strategic planning process. The mission and purpose of the new entity are consistent with those of the two organizations involved. The affiliation met the needs of the staff, responded to market realities, and was accomplished in projected time frames. The budget projections and visit volumes have exceeded initial projections. The AMHHC has grown both in volume of patients served and visits and in full-time equivalents (FTEs) since the 1986 restructure and after the affiliation with AMH in 1988. The management team is committed to meeting the challenges that continue to present themselves each day. The honest discussion and compromises from both the VNA and AMH made it possible to achieve a workable and balanced approach to some difficult economic and sensitive organizational issues. I share this experience with you to assure you that there is life after affiliation with a major hospital.

REFERENCE

Harris, M., and M. Groshens. 1985. A cooperative volunteer training program. *Home Healthcare Nurse* 3: 37–40.

PART IX

Other Types of Relationships

CHAPTER 59

Grantsmanship in Home Health Care: Seeking Foundation Support

Jennifer W. Campbell

Wendy Yallowitz

Jane Isaacs Lowe

In today's environment, nonprofit organizations need to be innovative and effective in raising funds to fulfill the mission of the agency and its programs. There are two main categories of fundraising. The first is soliciting funds from individuals and community groups. Agencies need to demonstrate strong support from the individuals they serve. In addition, the agency must show that members of the community support the work done by the agency and are willing to demonstrate this support financially. These individuals and groups are important sources of agency funds, which are solicited through a variety of donor campaigns and solicitations.

The second approach, and the focus of this chapter, is grantsmanship, a term that represents a set of techniques and events that takes place in philanthropic giving. Grantsmanship includes the process of securing resources and generating revenues to support various aspects of a program. Grantsmanship is a complex process of interrelated activities. None of these activities happen in a linear fashion, but rather occur over time and are interrelated with many aspects of agency structure and function. Home care agencies, like all other organizations seeking funds, must approach fund-raising strategically. They must demonstrate a finely nuanced understanding of the agency's strengths and of the industry's trends in order to engage funders in a dynamic process of working together to address social-health issues inherent in home care.

This chapter will address the following aspects of seeking and securing grant funds from foundations:

- Assessing the agency infrastructure, including the mission, capacity, and community support
- Identifying ideas that are fundable
- Researching funding agencies
- Approaching funders versus responding to requests for proposals
- Preparing and writing the proposal
- Tracking grants and building a relationship with funders

This chapter does not address governmental grants, although these aspects of grantsmanship might apply.

ASSESSING THE AGENCY INFRASTRUCTURE: MISSION, CAPACITY, AND COMMUNITY SUPPORT

The infrastructure of the agency is a key and often overlooked aspect of successful funding. When starting an effort to secure grant funding, it is important to have a realistic internal assessment of the strengths and weaknesses of the home care organization, as well as an understanding of the industry's trends. The result of this assessment will provide the basis for creating a funding agenda. It also will determine whether the grant funds sought will strengthen the internal workings of the organization (e.g., a capacity-building grant), build new initiatives, or develop new alliances.

The core of the agency, also referred to as the *infrastructure,* is articulated in its mission statement. It is important that the agency mission be clearly stated and consistently implemented. If the agency has strayed from its original mission, it may need to rethink its direction and focus before applying for grant funding. Many agencies revisit their mission at regular intervals to ensure the dynamic strategic direction of the organization. Changing the agency mission can be a sign of a healthy and dynamic organization. Likewise, an outdated mission, which is no longer relevant to the organization, is a sign of an organization that is unfocused and may have trouble implementing new programs.

The demonstrated capacity of the organization to successfully undertake new programs is also important. What is the track record of the agency with new initiatives? If the agency has launched only small initiatives and is now considering a large undertaking, what proof exists to demonstrate that the agency is capable of this bigger step? If the new initiative under consideration is in building a partnership with another community agency, what successes has this organization had in this arena?

Finally, agencies must demonstrate strong community support for the current programs, as well as potential support for any new initiatives under way. People who are served by the agency, their family members, and the agency's referral sources are potential supporters of the agency's work. In order to be successful at grantsmanship, this support must be clear and evident. Are there actions that the agency can take to demonstrate this support? Are individual and community donations reflective of the level of support the agency receives? For some agencies, the volume of volunteer effort in the agency is a good indicator of strong community support.

Thus, an accurate analysis of the strengths and weaknesses of an organization can provide an opportunity to strengthen the profile of the agency so that when the organization is ready to engage in seeking grants, it can provide a stronger case to a potential funder. Understanding the home care industry's trends, demonstrating a clearly realized agency mission, ensuring that the organization has the capacity to effectively engage in new initiatives, and documenting community support to pursue new goals are all vital to entering into a successful grantsmanship effort.

IDENTIFYING IDEAS THAT ARE FUNDABLE

Philanthropy has a strong preference for developmental funding. For the most part, foundations conceptualize their role as making key investments in society to build new capacity, competence, and innovation in human service delivery. For home health agencies, this means being seen as a resource for testing, researching, and instituting new concepts and ideas to help individuals receive the care they need to restore their health and/or maintain independence. Foundations are most interested in funding demonstration programs to determine how to best develop models or programs that could benefit the agency's mission as well as the funder's goals.

Reviewing a foundation's request for proposals (RFP), sometimes called a call for proposals (CFP), often stimulates agency discussion about ways in which that particular initiative would fit into the overall funding goals of the agency. However, in order to have a successful funding strategy, the agency should have a wide range of potential programs that would move the agency forward in meeting its mission by utilizing outside funding. The mistake many agencies make in grant writing is trying to fit themselves into existing RFPs that are not a good match for their particular organization, thus wasting valuable staff time in preparing unsuccessful grants. A good grant seeking initiative builds on the strengths of the agency, including programs in which the agency already has a demonstrated interest and experience, and is closely aligned with furthering the realization of the mission of the organization. An example of a well-matched program and funding opportunity is as follows:

A home care agency had been meeting with local leaders of the Korean community to discuss the service barriers to providing home health care for Korean elderly. During the course of their discussions, they discovered that the home care agency's catchment area includes the largest population of Koreans in the city. As a result of their initial meetings, a task force emerged consisting of Korean community leaders, clergy, and leaders as well as staff of the home care agency. The task force compiled a list of barriers to home health care for the Korean community including language, cultural understanding of the Korean concept of aging and caregiving, and access to services. When an RFP to improve access to care for non-English–speaking populations was issued by a local funder, this home care agency opted to partner with a Korean service organization that proposed establishing a Korean caregiver training program for the Korean homebound population. The home care agency was able to document a prior commitment to the population, provide a clearly articulated understanding of the problems and issues to be addressed, and present a plan for launching a new program. Enthusiastic letters of support from leaders in the Korean community strengthened the grant application.

Although agencies often need support for general operating costs, it is unlikely that this need will be met through grants. Foundations, corporate giving, and organized philanthropy rarely provide general operating support. Likewise, only a few philanthropic organizations exist that will support capital projects. Therefore it is critical to research carefully the history of the foundation to better understand the types of support that can be considered fundable from a particular funder.

RESEARCHING FUNDERS

It is important to research each funder and know as much as possible about the history and intent of the funding agency, including past grants, the size of the grants, and the purpose for which the grants were given. In this way the agency seeking funds can be sure that the proposed program, agency, and approach are compatible with the funder's past record and future plans. Submitting grants to a funding organization that are a poor match for the agency or program initiative not only wastes the time of the agency seeking funding in preparing the grant, but it also reflects poorly on the agency seeking the funds.

Many sources of information about funders exist. The most obvious is searching the Web for specific names of funders and carefully reading the materials about the organization, the funder's mission, current grantees, and the structure of the grant process. Annual reports and publications listed online can provide additional information about the funder's interests.

When researching funders for specific programs, there are databases that can be helpful in winnowing down the options. The Foundation Center operates a Web site for conducting national searches for American funders. It can be accessed through the Web at http://fdncenter.org. They have a wealth of information, although some of it can be accessed only via subscription. The Foundation Center has offices in New York City, Atlanta, Cleveland, San Francisco, and Washington D.C., where materials can be reviewed. In addition, many libraries maintain a subscription to the services so that the enhanced information may be available locally. The Foundation Center maintains information on foundations categorized according to the amount of funds they have for giving: under $1 million, $1 to $2 million, and above $2 million. Utilizing the materials produced by the Foundation Center can be daunting at first, but those who work frequently with them develop expertise. To help grant seekers make the most of these resources, the center conducts periodic workshops (Geever and McNeill, 1997, p. 197).

Other avenues for help with seeking grants and getting assistance with searching also exist. The Grantsmanship Center at http://www.tgci .com is a register for federal RFP updates. Its Web site also provides links to information on potential grants and resources for nonprofits. Basic searches can be completed using keywords such as grants, foundations, funding resources, and philanthropy. Foundations are required to submit to the Internal Revenue Service (IRS) their annual information returns on the 990-Pf forms. You can review these forms at http://www .guidestar.org to help you identify possible funding prospects and whether the foundation is interested in the agency's specific field.

APPROACHING FUNDERS VERSUS RESPONDING TO REQUESTS FOR PROPOSALS

Foundations usually conduct their grantmaking in two ways, solicited and unsolicited grants. A solicited grant is when the philanthropy has an idea and disseminates an RFP that responds to specific criteria. They will send out an RFP, which will outline the goals and requirements for the grant, issuing a deadline for proposals as well as a timeline for the foundation to respond to the request.

An unsolicited grant is the term utilized when a proposal is sent to the foundation without a specific request from the foundation. The agency seeking a grant has researched the interests of the foundation, and has developed a proposal they anticipate will be in keeping with the foundation's goals and philanthropic mission.

Some foundations develop a portfolio of ideas in a specific area they are interested in funding, while other foundations depend almost entirely on applicants who bring innovative ideas to the foundation. An important grantmanship strategy is to get to know the foundations that are interested in a particular service sector, monitor the RFPs issued, and match program needs with potential unsolicited opportunities for funding. Many organizations exist that give grants that are interested in health care initiatives and they may be extremely interested in the home care segment. In addition, foundations are present that are committed to serving a particular population that home care agencies provide care for, such as developmentally delayed children, patients with spinal cord injuries, or homebound elderly. Still other organizations are interested in different staffing models for health care delivery, and thus may be interested in initiatives that use advanced practice nurses or provide innovative training for home health aides. Researching and understanding who these funders are and their timelines and requirements for their funding cycles will provide multiple opportunities for a home care agency to secure grant funding.

PREPARING AND WRITING THE PROPOSAL

Preparing and writing the proposal is an important aspect of grantsmanship. For solicited grants, most foundations develop RFPs with specific requested information, organized in a specific format. For an unsolicited proposal, the following list outlines the sections that should be included in a grant request:

- Nature of the problem
- History of efforts to address the problem
- Proposed project or program
- Goals and objectives of the project
- Agency mission, capacity, and community support for the program
- Potential sustainability of the project once funding is over

- Plan for evaluating the results of implementing the program
- Timeline for the proposed project
- Detailed budget for the proposed project
- Staffing for the proposed project

Whether writing for a solicited or an unsolicited grant, the following questions should be addressed in the proposal:

- *Respond to the theme in the CFP or in the foundation's statement of giving.* In the opening sentence, make it clear that this proposal speaks directly to themes outlined by the foundation. If not responding to an RFP, the opening sentence should show the connection between the funds requested and the foundation's stated philanthropic mission.
- *Quantify the problem when possible.* When describing the problem include statistics that support the statement of the problem, and, if possible, quantify the degree of success anticipated if the project is funded.
- *What is innovative about this program?* Has this type of approach been tried before? What was the result of previous attempts? Why is this agency the right agency to try this particular approach?
- *What are the goals, objectives, and expected outcomes of this project?* What results are expected? Who will be affected? What will change? How will achievement of these goals be measured?
- *Be realistic.* Reviewers will be looking carefully at how well the timeline is anticipated, the resources required, and the outcomes that are expected. Overly ambitious proposals raise the question of whether the agency knows what it is doing.
- *Demonstrate that you have* already *invested considerable time and resources in working on the problem.* Demonstrate that the problem has been well thought through, the right people convened to address the problem, and staff time already

invested in devising a thoughtful solution. Document successful efforts at partnering with other agencies to addressing the problem.

- *A conclusion must answer the question "So what?"* Make sure that the conclusion is a logical outgrowth of the problem statement and that the project will make a significant difference. A good summary should appeal to the values that the agency or program is striving to accomplish.
- *Budget.* Include a line-item budget by year including in-kind support and other funding sources. Pay careful attention to the foundation's guidelines about funding. Some foundations will not cover overhead cost, while others will not pay for equipment. How much staff time is needed and what will that cost? What are the administrative costs for this project? What materials, items, tools, or office supplies are needed at what cost? What about travel costs and consulting fees? Can this project be sustained at the end of the funding period, and if so, how?
- *Qualifications of the agency.* The qualifications of the agency applying for a grant is key. Does this project idea fit within the agency's mission and goals? Why is this agency appropriate to conduct this project? Is there evidence that this agency has successfully implemented programs before? What aspects of the agency are advantages to fulfilling the goals of this program? Who will staff this project and what is the staff's experience? Include resumes to illustrate areas of expertise as an attachment.

When compiling the proposal, follow these steps:

- *Schedule enough time to construct a good grant.* Grantsmanship is an expensive endeavor in terms of staff time and energy. Make sure the agency gets the most return from the investment by allowing more than enough time to produce a quality product. It takes times to revise drafts. Unanticipated events will occur (people get sick, the copier breaks, hard drives fail). Give the grant writing process the time and energy it needs so the agency doesn't risk submitting a poor representation of the agency and its vision.

- *Follow the directions.* Follow the organization suggested by the RFP *exactly.* Don't make the reviewers hunt for the required information. When using agency boilerplates (routine statements about the agency, community, etc.), make sure it really responds to the information requested by the foundation.
- *Each grant is unique.* When lifting information from one grant to insert in another, make sure that the names and titles of programs have been changed and the grant being submitted is truly unique and doesn't appear as a "cookie-cutter" approach to grantsmanship.
- *Make the grant easy to read.* Make the grant easy to read so reviewers can find key information quickly: Use bold face, underlining, bullets, and a table of contents. Bolding the first, carefully crafted sentence of each paragraph enables reviewers to skim the grant and get the gist quickly.
- *Paint a compelling picture.* A good grant application is a page turner and reads like a novel. Make sure the grant reflects the passion of the agency's mission and vision of service. Describe the people affected by the problem concisely, and then present a logical and well-organized way to successfully respond to the problem.
- *Attachments.* Attached to the proposal should be a copy of your Section 501(c)(3) of the IRS code, proof of tax-exempt status. Enthusiastic letters of support from key affected community and government stakeholders should be included. Also include resumes of key staff members and proposed consultants.

TRACKING GRANTS AND BUILDING A RELATIONSHIP WITH FUNDERS

Once a grant is submitted, the funder may contact the agency for additional information or clarification. These requests should be responded to promptly. From the moment that an agency is notified about receiving a grant, specifics about the dispersion of funds and the funder's expectations should be clarified. Sometimes grants will be funded but will be reduced from the amount initially requested. It is important to work closely with the foundation in reducing the expected results on the grant accordingly, putting all changes in writing to ensure no misunderstandings occur.

During the course of receiving funding, it is important to develop a relationship with the funder. Take this opportunity for the foundation liaison to gain a better understanding of your agency, the problems it faces, the successes it has had, and the foundation funding's impact on the agency's ability to provide services. Sharing good news (newspaper clippings, a particularly poignant letter of thanks from a consumer, etc.) is an important aspect of building the relationship.

To ensure timely compliance with agency expectations for funding, it is important to develop a tracking system for grant deadlines, expected calls for proposals, progress report due dates, and so forth. Developing a relationship with a funder means paying attention to the funder's requirements and demonstrating competency in meeting deadlines and delivering on expectations. When there are changes that occur in the agency that will impact on the grant, it is important to contact the grant's officer immediately, explain the issue, and reach a satisfactory understanding. Putting these resolutions in writing diminishes the chance that misunderstandings will occur.

If a grant is rejected, it is often appropriate to ask for feedback from the funding agency as to why it was rejected. Sometimes reviewers' comments will be shared, and other times a grant's officer will provide an overview of the review process and why this grant was rejected. If the foundation is willing to share this information, it is an invaluable opportunity to gain insight into the grantmanship process and to further refine grant-writing skills. Even if the foundation will not share reviewers' comments, a detailed analysis of the successfully funded projects will provide an important learning opportunity.

CONCLUSION

In summary, grantsmanship is a dynamic and challenging set of interrelated activities that require a high level of creativity, political acumen, and technical expertise. Home care agencies have many options in terms of seeking funding opportunities. Successful grantsmanship includes having a critical understanding of the strengths and weaknesses of the organization, an ability to identify problems and innovative solutions that are fundable, researching and refining a list of potential funders, and preparing a compelling proposal. The grant cycle then continues while funding is being received and flows into the building of the relationship between the agency and the funder toward future projects.

REFERENCES

Firstenberg, P. 1996. *The 21st century nonprofit: Remaking the organization in the post government era*. New York: The Foundation Center.

Geever, J., and McNeill, P. 1997. *Guide to proposal writing*. New York: The Foundation Center.

CHAPTER 60

Home Care Volunteer Program

Carol-Rae Green Sodano

THE NOTION OF VOLUNTEERISM

Old sailors know never to volunteer for anything. The implication is that volunteering places one at risk. Volunteering makes one vulnerable to the experience of injustice, a risk that is prevalent enough in all human interaction but is intensified by the intrinsic nature of volunteering. To volunteer means to offer one's services out of one's own volition with no guarantee of reciprocity.

To volunteer means to generate a proactive statement of commitment based on faith, belief, and individually felt principle. It is a projection of personal quality, which normally can remain hidden and safe from public perusal, into a concrete act that becomes visible and subject to public judgment. To volunteer is to make an open statement of principle. It makes the individual visible and accountable and consequently binds him or her by honor to the fulfillment of a promise. Here again is the potential for felt injustice. The volunteer risks visibility and public judgment by his or her own volition; he or she stands alone. The volunteer risks exposure and judgment from those who can shout their condemnation from the anonymous safety of the crowd. The volunteer is always vulnerable to the statement, "You offered."

Most individuals volunteer with the hope, perhaps even the belief, that they will feel the balance of their risk in received appreciation. Sometimes this payback comes through, but often it falls short. The self-perception of one as a volunteer can easily slip to a self-perception of one as a victim.

It is precisely this issue, keeping the volunteer a volunteer and not a felt victim, that is the key to a successful volunteer program. The object is to attract qualified, committed individuals who will risk the public statement of volunteering, to stimulate and support these individuals into working at maximum levels of investment and productivity, and finally to maintain their involvement over an extended period of time. Recruiting quality volunteers, stimulating them into maintained production, and retaining them demand a recognition of the risks incurred by the volunteer and responding to those risks by working toward a reciprocity of justice. A fundamental goal for any successful volunteer program must be mutuality: a mutuality of acted-out commitment by both volunteer and agency, a shared justice and fairness that precludes victimization.

Volunteerism is an American cultural trait and a well-established American tradition. The cultural demand to volunteer one's time, energy, and talent seems to be rooted in the American interpretation of the Protestant work ethic. In America, not only are you expected to work hard with every anticipation of financial and spiritual reward but, once your rewards have been recognized, you are expected to share the wealth, both material and moral. In America, once the individual is in a position of relative financial stability, he or she is expected to give time and talent for the general social good and for the good of individuals who are less fortunate. Considerable social pressure to share the wealth exists; individuals who, because of the time restrictions created by their success, cannot give directly of their skills are expected to surrogate this donation

778

with money. Government supports this practice by making contributions of this sort tax deductible, and in so doing concretely acts out the social sanction of this unique value.

Money is fine, but time is better. Direct action volunteerism has always held cultural esteem in our society. Interestingly, although it has usually been a predominantly female prerogative, volunteerism has consistently been encouraged of men as well. Often men volunteer for positions that hold significant social status (e.g., volunteer heads of foundations, social and cultural committees, or political and economic organizations), whereas women often volunteer for direct service functions (e.g., the Gray Ladies, institutional fund-raising committees, and volunteer services in schools and welfare agencies). All individuals are expected to participate, and if there are inequities in the volunteer system in America, they are inequities reflective of the general social system rather than those specific to volunteerism. The culture is consistent.

In summary, volunteerism in America is a well-established cultural trait rooted in moral sanction and perpetuated through significant social pressure. Volunteerism is a collective charge, a cultural norm propounded to all members of the society with every expectation that the individual will meet every challenge to the best of his or her ability.

HEALTH CARE VOLUNTEERISM

During the 20th century, the health care institution in America gained tremendous esteem. The post-World War II period saw a dramatic rise in social and political power for the health care community, a rise that seemed to reach its peak in the mid-1970s. This rise in power and esteem appears to be rooted in the notion, perpetuated in the latter half of the 20th century, that medical personnel can do more than mitigate pain, that they can, in fact, defeat death. With the "magic" powder of antibiotics tightly in hand, medicine in the post-World War II era came close to gaining religious prestige. Before this period, the power of life and death was pretty much in God's hands; now God seemed to have the assistance of a physician.

The public has done a great deal to increase the prestige of the health care community. It makes sense that, if you stand just under God's right hand or if the public believes that this is your designated position, you acquire a considerable amount of respect and a considerable amount of power. Add to this set of perceptions the popular American image of the life saver as a romantic hero, and you are well on your way toward sanctification.

The whole notion of a collective cultural fantasy spinning around a hero who exercises power over death is an intriguing cultural phenomenon. This fantasy allows the individual to bask in the warm light of public acclaim, of public recognition and esteem, and of direct ego gratification at the highest level through the performance of an act that by its nature is the ultimate in moral behavior. Give back to an individual that which is most morally valued, most ethically weighed—his or her life—and you earn the right to direct ego gratification. It is a point of curiosity that, for many of us in America, to free ourselves, even in our fantasy, to claim recognition on our own behalf we must pay the cost of performing an act that comes conceptually close to divine.

It should therefore not be surprising that volunteerism in health care settings has been consistently popular in America. Volunteering for service in a hospital or geriatric facility, for example, fulfills the requirement to give back to society and at the same time allows the individual to gain permitted self-gratification by engaging in good work. Whether one agrees with the ethical system or not, a system operative exists, and its reality must be recognized and worked within. Furthermore, an ethical system that manifests through altruism certainly is far better than a system that is nonaltruistic or anti-altruistic in its expression. Perhaps our motives are a bit bent, but better bent than crooked.

HOME CARE VOLUNTEERISM

Outpatient care is a growing movement in the current health care spectrum. In-home care has always been present, to a greater or lesser degree, in the general health care scene in America. Today, however, because of DRGs (Diagnosis Related Groups) and the payment policies they impose, more and more individuals find themselves at home at stages of more and more acute caretaking need. In addition, the growth of the hospice movement, which in America is predominantly of the in-home care variety, has vastly contributed to the need for trained volunteers for in-home care service.

Home care volunteerism makes good sense. If properly administrated, it is cost-efficient and delivers a quality of care that can be acquired in no other way. The patient who is clinically appropriate for in-home care has the advantage of being in the security of familiar surroundings, in an environment in which he or she can usually exercise a fair degree of individual control and can remain among those who are most significant, most trusted, and most nurturing in every sense. Well-trained and well-supervised volunteers, through their facilitation, can maximize the quality of the in-home care experience, and in many cases they do more than facilitate the process: They are essential to its very existence.

In-home care volunteers come in several varieties: individuals who volunteer their time to provide companionship for the at-home patient, and individuals who volunteer their professional services and skills. Without these donations of personal resources by volunteers, many patients and their families would not be able to function effectively in the in-home setting; responsibilities would be too demanding, and costs would be too consuming.

In-house care that incorporates the efficient use of volunteers has every potential to increase the possibility and quality of good patient care and at the same time to stabilize or lower cost. There are some risks, however, that cannot be ignored.

The first issue is the possibility of legal liability. When the volunteer is sent into the patient's home, institutional environmental control is given up, and this creates a degree of risk. In addition, in-home volunteers, unlike most volunteers working in institutional settings, usually hold an extraordinary degree of personal responsibility for the patient's well-being. Often the in-home volunteer is the only individual present and responsible for the patient. This singularity of responsibility demands that the degree of trust and confidence placed in in-home volunteers be extraordinary and in the extraordinary is risk. The second issue is the problem of burnout. In-home volunteers are giving a great deal of themselves in relatively intense doses; there is a risk of losing them or their quality if they are not treated with some degree of reciprocity and nurturing.

When the effect is balanced against the risk, most in-home care agencies choose in favor of volunteer involvement in patient care plans. Volunteers do not need to be present in every case handled by an agency to be perceived as earning their salt. They need to be present when their presence is critical and/or appropriate. In addition, they can provide peripheral services such as bookkeeping, secretarial, or library tasks, which usually translate into all-around increased quality of service. The bottom line is that volunteers enhance service at every level with a minimal cost in terms of both money and overhead.

THE PHILOSOPHICAL BASIS FOR A SUCCESSFUL VOLUNTEER PROGRAM

Program Goals

A well-organized volunteer program is designed to meet four basic program goals. These goals are internal and aimed at the creation and preservation of a productive, stable volunteer corps that in turn will provide quality service both to the service agency and, more important, to the public. Well-managed volunteer programs focus on meeting the demands of quality in (1) recruitment, (2) service, (3) retention, and (4) cost-effectiveness.

Quality in recruitment demands that the agency knows what it wants and expects from its volunteer corps and then aims its recruitment campaigns at populations best able to meet these expectations. Targeted recruitment, although demanding a greater effort and time investment up front, pays back with volunteers who bring in skills and who are more likely to remain in the program because they are wanted. They come to understand that they are wanted, and they value this recognition.

Another advantage of targeted recruitment is that only individuals appropriate to the function of the agency are approached, thus eliminating the problems that surface when large numbers of individuals who have nonspecific skills are recruited and the agency must find a use for all of them. Often it is discovered that there are too many individuals who are able to fulfill one task and not enough to fill another; consequently, more volunteers need to be recruited while volunteers already trained must remain idle. This policy is both monetarily inefficient and corrosive to morale.

Quality in service demands that volunteers be well trained and well supervised. Individuals recruited into a volunteer corps must be taught, and taught clearly, what is expected of them and how they are to meet these expectations. Little if anything should be left to chance. It is unfair to assume that the volunteer knows precisely what you want and how you want it done, even if he or she has a professional handle on a given skill. The volunteer must be helped to integrate this skill into the personality and function of the agency. Training is as much a function of integration as it is the communication of information. Similarly, the function of supervision is more guidance and development than discipline and judgment. Supervision policy and process must encourage the volunteers in the performance of their tasks and assist their growth in both skills and self-assurance.

Quality in retention suggests that skilled and well-functioning volunteers remain in a program not by accident but by design and effort. Because the economic investment in volunteers is primarily in their training and only secondarily in their supervision, it makes good fiscal sense to work consciously to maintain the fruits of the initial investment. The longer a volunteer remains productively a part of the corps, the lower the cost to train that volunteer and the lower the cost of the services provided by the volunteer. More important, the longer the volunteer remains in the

corps, the greater his or her skill and adaptability to work within the process of the agency become as he or she develops into an incorporated member of the team. It takes time and effort to train new people continually; it takes time, effort, and loss of service to integrate new individuals into a team continually.

The quality of a volunteer program is often measured by its cost-effectiveness. Although cost considerations need not be the only rationale for a volunteer program, they are certainly important. Any quality program will be designed to achieve the best service for the least amount of money. Volunteer programs have their cost in the staff necessary to train and supervise them. Effective programs that result in a volunteer corps characterized by skill, adaptability, variability, and creativity will be quite cost-efficient. The measure of the cost-effectiveness of a volunteer program is not so much what it costs to create and maintain the corps but how much the corps can provide in both quality and variability of service, or what the corps allows you to offer to the public that could not be offered without it.

Basic Premises Necessary to Attain Goals

Successful attainment of these goals through a system that does not rely on monetary incentive falls just short of being an art form. Volunteerism depends virtually exclusively on an affirmative relational process to attain its specified goals. This process is a skill under any circumstance, but in the context of volunteerism, unobserved by economic support, it becomes critical.

The relational process necessary to create and maintain a successful volunteer program must flow from a clear, committed philosophical basis. This basis consists of two concomitant sets of premises: the ethical and the relational. The ethical premises, those of integrity, justice, and humanism, are the philosophical foundation for the process. The relational premises, those of trust, fairness, mutuality, reciprocity, and dialogue, are the actuating behavior of the process. The ethical premises form the essence of the process, and the relational premises form its actuality.

The Ethical Premises

The ethical premises form the value system that directs the process of interpersonal relationship. It is the commitment to these values that determines the criteria against which behavior is judged and decisions of policy and procedure are made. Successful volunteer programs are based on policies and procedures that remain committed and faithful to integrity, justice, and humanism.

Ethical integrity is a commitment to reality, consistency, and truthfulness. Integrity demands that individuals and the systems they create recognize the nature of reality and, having recognized that nature, work compatibly and affirmatively with that reality. Integrity demands that reality not be denied, mutilated, or distorted but rather it be honored and credited for its existence and its essence. Integrity demands consistency, that actions match spoken words and understood agreements, and that policy mirrors principles. Integrity demands that truth be honored and continuously respected in thought and deed.

Specific to a volunteer program, integrity demands that administration have a realistic understanding about what is needed and what will be required to meet the need; that these requirements be clearly stated to both the client and the volunteer so that communication is kept open, clear, and appropriate; that what is asked of the volunteer is what is wanted and possible with no hidden messages, motives, or circumstances; and that feedback given to the volunteer is inclusive, direct, and always truthful.

Justice is a commitment to fairness, to making a return on what is received, to giving credit when credit is due, and to critiquing when critiquing is deserved. Justice flows from integrity, and although the two are separate in essence, they are experienced simultaneously. Justice in a volunteer program demands that all sides are heard and credited, that treatment of the volunteer is fair and equitable in every circumstance, and that there is recognition of earned trust and reliability as well as open, clear statements of complaints.

Humanism is the capacity to see and respect others for the honor and dignity they hold by virtue of their status as human. Humanism demands respect, honor, empathy, and judgment that is recognized as individual and subjective, not authoritarian and absolute. Humanism in a volunteer program demands that each individual in the corps be continuously seen, perceived, and responded to with consideration and conscious recognition of his or her human dignity and needs. Humanism demands that administration relate through constructive processes with the volunteer; by doing so, administration earns the right to similar consideration from the volunteer.

Relational Premises

The relational premises are the modes of behavior that concretize and make experiential the abstract principles of ethics. They are the particulars of the processes that form and maintain relationship; they are the actions and exchanges that engender union and encourage its continuity.

To maintain itself and to create a constructive history, a relationship must be founded on trust. Trust building consequently becomes a critical dynamic in the relational process. Trust is earned over time and with experience. Trust generates out of mutual, constructive interaction that binds individuals in a common history. Trust cannot be rushed; neither can it be given away and remain in character. Trust demands mutual disclosure of individual truths; it demands that the individual speak and act with integrity, justice, and humanism. Trust demands appropriate self-disclosure and a corresponding willingness to be held accountable. Trust demands the courage to know one's truth, to say and act one's truth, to hear the other's response to one's truth, and to credit the legitimacy of the other's side.

The creation and maintenance of trust are essential to a successful volunteer program. The trust building must be mutually engaged in by volunteer and agency as well as mutually earned and mutually felt. The building of trust demands a mutually created history of integrity, of honest statements openly given and carefully adhered to over time.

Fairness encourages trust. Crediting others' positions recognizes their presence and honors their intrinsic value. Fairness encourages reciprocal behavior and works to ensure a future in the relationship.

The volunteer must be treated with fairness based on a commitment to justice. Fairness to volunteers includes working with them to help make their experience personally enriching, openly recognizing their accomplishments and their contributions, clearly communicating direction, delivering honest critiques with sensitivity and encouragement, and recognizing that they are entitled to something back for what they give.

Reciprocity is the give and take necessary to maintain the momentum of the relationship. Reciprocity is the interchange within which fairness is experienced and trust evolves. The balance that creates reciprocity actuates in the willingness to give and to receive information and assistance and to encompass attitudes and events. Reciprocity must have the perceived experience of equality, but it does not need to be tit for tat. It is the recognition of entitlement both in the other and in oneself and the capacity to act on that entitlement.

Reciprocity in the volunteer corps requires that the volunteers be encouraged to share their side and that, when they share, they be legitimately heard and considered. In turn, the agency also has its right to have its side stated, heard, and worked through to mutual understanding. Reciprocity demands again those volunteers receive from their experience as well as give and that the agency appreciates and credits what it receives from the volunteers.

Reciprocity requires mutuality. Mutuality is recognition of relational reality and a willingness to work cooperatively with that reality. Mutuality demands that all parties affected by a given process or decision be consciously and actively included in the evolution of that process or decision. Mutuality precludes authoritarianism and the dictatorial imposition of one's wants on another. Mutuality demands that all parties involved be given an opportunity to contribute to the processes that will directly affect them, thereby encouraging their sense of inclusion, cooperation, and adaptation. Mutuality forestalls resentment, resistance, and no cooperative reaction; it assists in creating a smooth administrative process.

Mutuality with the volunteer corps requires stated recognition of the volunteers' existence and contribution to the process of the organization. It requires that volunteers be included in the development of policy that will directly affect them as individuals or the nature and manner of their work. Throughout the evolution of this process, they must be given legitimate attention and consideration; spoken to with honest, direct statements; and heard with openness and sincerity. This willingness to engage in an authentic, mutual process does not preclude the legitimate power of the agency to make final policy decisions; in fact, mutuality demands that the volunteer recognize and respect the rights of the agency to exercise its administrative function. The volunteer must credit the administration's side as honorably as the administration credits the volunteer's position.

Trust, fairness, reciprocity, and mutuality are clearly interdependent, each being interlocked and supportive of the others in a productive process of human relationship. Key to the actuality of this process is the additional premise of commitment to dialogue. Dialogue—the concrete, mutual, reciprocal, and fair exchange of each individual's "I" truths—may not guarantee universal positive resolution, but it will generate trust and consequently lay the foundations for a process that is most often constructive, most often progressive, and most often highly productive.

Dialogue not only encourages cooperation and integration, but also generates creativity. It is out of dialogue that new perceptions, new insights, and new approaches find their way into consideration and, often, productive implementation. Dialogue engenders the productiveness of a team model. Dialogue is the essential dynamic of team process, and an attempt to create and maintain a team approach without dialogue is doomed to failure.

Dialogue must be encouraged with and from the volunteer corps. Volunteers must be given, in understandable vocabulary, the position of the agency, particularly on issues that directly affect them. In turn, their "I" statements must be given a time and place in which to be voiced and the credit they warrant. Volunteers must be known, they must be spoken with, and they must be credited. In turn, the agency must also be known, heard, and credited. This requires a system of practices that consciously and deliberately encourages dialogue, including support groups, in-service programs, retreats, one-on-one interviews, and reasonable access to volunteer supervisors and agency personnel. The time commitment this requires is balanced with a relatively smooth and productive process. It is much easier, and much less costly in terms of time and money, to forestall personnel problems proactively than to attempt to counter and correct problems reactively.

PROGRAM DESIGN

What has been discussed so far is a consideration of desires and premises, wants and beliefs that form the abstract foundations for a successful volunteer program. How to make these principles concrete in both design and execution needs to be addressed next. With concreteness and effectiveness in mind, we now turn our attention to the specifics of program design.

Director of Volunteers

Any program, no matter how well designed, is only as effective as the individuals involved in its execution. With this postulate in mind, it seems appropriate to begin a discussion of program design with a description of expectations and responsibilities associated with the creation of the position of director of volunteers and a description and recommendations about the nature and capability of the individual hired to serve in this function. Both these points warrant careful consideration because, realistically, the function given to the position of volunteer director and how that function is executed greatly determine the success of a volunteer program.

Job Description

The director of volunteers is usually responsible for recruitment, selection, placement, supervision, and evaluation. In addition, many programs are designed so that training is included as the director's responsibility, although this can be contracted out. The advantage of facilitating new members' entry and bonding into an established corps is obviously hampered to some degree, however, when training is done by an outside individual.

The director of volunteers should hold equal status to other divisional directors in an agency and should be directly responsible to the administrative director. It must be remembered that the volunteer director will be responsible for the administration of a division that houses a significant number of people; in fact, in many home care agencies the volunteer corps represents, in gross number of personnel, the largest division in the agency. The degree of responsibility held by the director is measured by the number of functions he or she is accountable to perform, the number of personnel under his or her supervision, and the fact that personnel in this division usually have the greatest amount of contact hours with the public and consequently represent significant risk if mismanaged.

The director of volunteers is usually responsible to the executive or managing director of the agency. Occasionally the position of director of volunteers is combined with or responsible to the social services division or, in a few instances, to the pastoral unit. In still other instances, the position of director of volunteers is filled by a volunteer, an arrangement that works well provided that nothing major occurs for which the director needs to be held accountable. When this position is held on a volunteer basis, it limits the power of the executive administration to hold the division accountable; this is a subtle point but warrants careful consideration before one institutes a totally volunteer division.

In addition to administrative and educational responsibilities, the director of volunteers ideally should perform a counseling function. The capacity to defuse psychodynamic problems as they begin to evolve is invaluable in the administration of a problem-limited agency. The director of volunteers, like any director of any division, needs to be able to keep problems from developing, and must be aggressively proactive in philosophy and policy so that there is need for only a limited amount of reactive administrative decisions. This helps keep the general balance of administrative power in place and helps the executive director maintain an effective and assertive leadership role.

In most home care agencies, teamwork is essential. First, it is the volunteer director's responsibility to inculcate and nurture a cooperative team interaction within the corps itself. Second, the director must function as the chief catalyst to assist in the integration of the corps into the general agency team. The director's responsibility is to help the corps remain cognitively, emotionally, and functionally integrated with the agency as a whole. Finally, it is the obligation of the volunteer director to ensure that the corps's function meets and matches the service needs of the agency in general and of other divisions in specifics; the director is responsible for seeing that the corps delivers, and delivers with some skill, the services requested by the various divisions of the agency.

Special Skills Required

Ideally, the individual who functions as volunteer director should have administrative (particularly in health care or social areas), educational, and psychotherapeutic (counseling) skills. It is difficult to find one individual who has talent, experience, and training in all three of these areas, so compromises must often be made. It must be remembered, however, that the more compromises agreed to, the weaker the structure and the greater the potential for problems. With this in mind, a good rule of thumb is that any individual hired to act as director of volunteers should be skilled in performing at least two of the three ideal functions of the job. In addition, no compromise should be made on administrative capability. Individuals who are skilled in administration and education would be suitable; the psychothera-peutic function could be addressed by the social service division. Alternatively, individuals who are skilled in administration and psychotherapy could forfeit the educational function to an outside contract. It is risky, however, to have as director an individual who has only administrative skills; this cre-

ates too weak a structure by dividing responsibility and thereby accountability. It is difficult, if not impossible, to administer an integrated division if the majority of responsibilities are farmed out, along with their accountability and control.

The individual should be empathetic, perceptive, and capable of being supportive to others; should have well-developed listening and communication skills; and should be relatively charismatic or at least capable of stimulating bonding, cohesion, and commitment in a group. In addition, the individual should be skilled in evaluation and decision making, should be capable of exercising his or her responsibility with decisiveness, and should have the strength and the courage to accept responsibility and be held accountable.

Ideally, the individual should hold at least a master's degree in psychology, sociology, human services, administration, or related fields and should have a minimum of 3 years of experience in working with groups and/or the public. The credentials are important, but the bottom line is the effectiveness of the individual in the job; consequently, exceptions to specific credentials are always possible.

Structure of the Corps

The structure of the corps must be logically and thoughtfully developed. This structuring begins with a careful evaluation of what is expected in performance from the corps, or what the volunteers will be doing. Their various functions should be conceptualized in terms that are concrete and specific (e.g., cataloging books for a library, cooking, or filling in for personnel shortages in other divisions, such as social service or nursing). Once it is determined what the corps is expected to do, then an educated guess about how many individuals will be needed to fulfill the functions listed must be made. What should be avoided is having too many volunteers who can serve a function for which there is limited use and not enough volunteers to fill functions where there is demand.

Home care volunteer corps should contain individuals who are proficient in general social skills, homemaking, child care, fine arts, and fund-raising. In addition, a percentage of the corps should have professional skills in nursing, social work, geriatric care, business, law, library science, or virtually any area in which the agency sees itself potentially involved. The greater the versatility of the corps, the greater the agency's potential for service and for lowering the costs of service. A volunteer corps should be envisioned as a pool of resources in terms of both the skills of the individuals themselves and the potential that these individuals offer through the networking of their contacts. These individuals bring not only themselves and their skills into the corps, but also their world.

All volunteers enlisted into the corps should be required to attend a training program designed by the agency to orient the individuals to the expectations and procedures of the organization. The training program should be structured so that the focus includes orientation and group integration in addition to factual data. The skills and talents brought into the corps by the volunteers must be recognized and credited, and training programs must be flexible enough to enhance and facilitate a variety of volunteer offerings; they must never suffocate, mutilate, denigrate, or disregard what the volunteer offers as his or her own. Training programs must come from a position of respect, reinforcement, and facilitation rather than from a position of haughty authoritarianism and unilateral righteousness.

PROGRAM STRUCTURE

Recruitment

Appropriate time and consideration given to a recruitment campaign can save a great deal of time, effort, and money later on in the management of the volunteer corps. As described before, targeted recruitment is well worth the time and effort it involves because it guarantees an appropriately populated resource pool and aids morale by ensuring that those recruited will be appreciated and used.

In-home care agencies should begin their recruitment programs with a careful examination of the services they offer and those that can legitimately be expected from a volunteer corps: what the corps can be expected to do for the agency, and what it can be trained to do for the public served by the agency. The outline in Table 60–1 is generally adaptable and serves as a base for virtually any in-home care volunteer corps. An attempt should be made to recruit individuals who have specialties within areas that are concurrent with the specialties of the agency. For example, if a particular agency specializes in the care of terminally ill children, then individuals who are familiar with nursing, psychotherapy, and physical therapy specific to children should be sought.

Obviously, familiarity with the structure and service function of the agency is important when one is choosing a recruitment target, but equally important is a familiarity with the demographic nature of the population served by the agency. A concerted effort must be made to recruit a complementary, representative sample of the service population. Here the issues relevant to the client population that must be considered include the following:

- Number of males and females in the client population
- Age factors
- Racial and ethnic factors
- Educational factors
- Socioeconomic factors
- Religious factors
- Neighborhood ethnocentric factors

Every attempt should be made to recruit volunteers from each demographic group perceived as essential and representative of the client population. Good recruitment policy should result in a corps that has flexibility, adaptability, and enough variety in resources to meet creatively virtually any challenge of service offered by the population. In short, the corps should match in demographic make-up the make-up of the population served and should match in resources the wants and needs of the agency's clients.

Recruits can be gathered from a variety of sources. Individuals with professional and semi-

Table 60–1 Volunteers Who Have Skills Most Appropriate for the Agency and the Public

For the Agency	*For the Public*
Librarians	Nurses
Accountants	Physician assistants
Lawyers	Physical therapists
Bookkeepers	Educators
Grant writers	Social workers
Fund-raisers	Clergy
Secretaries	Psychotherapists
Computer operators	Homemakers
Publicity personnel	

professional skills can be acquired by tapping into business and industry volunteer programs, professional service organizations and clubs, and professional schools, particularly for combined volunteer/internship programs. Contact with these sources should be personal and ongoing, and the director of volunteers must be responsible for the cultivation of a wide-ranging, solidly woven network of personal contacts in each of these recruitment areas. In addition, volunteers from the existing corps can be trained to speak to religious groups, women's organizations, general social service clubs, and special interest groups that might have an interest in the function and services offered by the agency. The development of a speaker's bureau within the corps is an excellent technique. This involves the development of a brochure listing a variety of topics on which members of the corps are willing and capable to talk, circulating these pamphlets in appropriate places (many groups are looking for speakers), and following up with phone calls and personal arrangements for bookings.

Publicity is an important factor in the recruitment plan. It is a good idea to begin by seeking out for recruitment an individual who has some degree of skill in creating, developing, and executing publicity campaigns. This individual might be someone who is actually in public relations but may also be someone familiar with newspaper writing, advertising, and the like. Once this individual is in place, then he or she can carry the ball in designing public relation programs aimed at general recruitment. In addition, remember that every constructively used and credited volunteer in the corps will recruit for the corps through his or her spoken enthusiasm.

Good recruitment demands that you know what you are doing as an agency and that you have a good idea where you are going and how you are going to get there. How you are going to get there should include the creation of a corps that has as its goal not only service, but also the capacity to be self-generating. When you begin by recruiting individuals who are skilled in recruitment, you are well on your way; simply credit their skill, maintain basic guidance and cohesiveness, and allow your original recruits to do what they do best: recruit.

Evaluation

Evaluation is one of the more difficult functions of the volunteer director. Bad decisions can be costly in many ways; consequently, it is essential that the volunteer director have some basic familiarity with standard evaluation instruments and techniques and also have well-developed and well-tested visceral reactions.

Every candidate should be required to have a private initial interview with the director. At this point, the candidate should be evaluated for basic social skills, generally appropriate behavior and expression, and the identification of any gross problems that would make the candidate inappropriate for recruitment. A conversational interview of about 30 to 45 minutes is usually enough to give you a general sense of the individual's personality. If there is a desire to be more clinical, any one of the standard personality tests could be administered at the end of the interview, and the individual could then be told that he or she will hear from the agency about the decision as to his or her status.

The guideline for this evaluation must be appropriateness for the program, not whether the director likes the individual. Evaluations must be kept as fair as possible, and that requires looking at what is needed to do the job and how much the individual being interviewed fits the need.

Once past the initial interview, the candidates should be informed that they will be under ongoing evaluation during the training period. This is one of the reasons why it is a good idea to have training periods that extend over time (4 to 6 weeks); it gives the extended opportunity necessary for a fair and accurate evaluation.

During the training period, candidates should be evaluated in terms of their creativity, insightfulness, perception, cooperativeness, empathic capacity, adaptability, and capability to integrate relatively easily into the group. In addition, attention should be given to identification of leadership potential in general and of particular talent areas. It is an excellent idea to include a practicum period at the conclusion of the training course. This practicum should include at least 6 hours of on-site observation and supervised participation by the candidate in activities appropriate for the volunteer corps. Candidates should be evaluated by their practicum supervisor, and this evaluation should be handed in and reviewed by the volunteer director before the closing interview.

The closing interview must be perceived and conducted as a mutual dialogue between the candidate and the volunteer director. Both parties must present their side with reasonably open disclosure. If a candidate has proved less than appropriate for a particular volunteer program, the individual should be credited for skills that he or she does hold, an explanation given for why this particular program is not a particularly good context for his or her offerings, and constructive suggestions given for situations that might prove more fulfilling. Candidates who appear to be appropriate need to be credited, and clear statements must be made about how their skills will be incorporated into the program and what their rights and responsibilities are as members of the corps. Time must be given in all cases to hear and process candidates' concerns, questions, and opinions. In ad-

dition, candidates should be reminded of the fact that they are subject to continuous evaluation and that there is a mutual right to terminate the relationship at any point if either volunteer or agency finds that necessary. Finally, a contract stipulating the rights, responsibilities, and terms of the relationship should be jointly signed, and each participating party should receive a copy.

Training Program

The goals of a well-developed and welldelivered training program must be the integration of the recruit into the system and structure of the agency, the inculcation of necessary skills and pertinent information, and the encouragement and direction of preexisting skills and information brought into the program by the recruit. Training programs should be aimed at enhancement and integration rather than reformation and visionary indoctrination, at development and adaptability rather than reconstruction and remodeling. A syllabus that has proved successful with a variety of training classes is presented in Exhibit 60–1.

The case review is a method of engendering thematic cohesiveness throughout the lectures. In addition, it is an excellent method of integrating new members into the ongoing work experience of the agency. A current case seen as didactically appropriate should be chosen and introduced with initial relevant data at the second session, and then in each session thereafter the material being presented that day should be applied to the ongoing case study. The result should be clarity, concreteness, and a growing familiarity with agency process; in addition, there should be a distinct evolution of identification, inclusiveness, and integration and a feeling of developing familiarity and confidence within the volunteer candidates.

The practicum, as just discussed, gives the agency a unique opportunity for on-site evaluation. In addition, it offers the volunteer candidates a chance to experience concretely what they might have only imagined. Experiencing

Exhibit 60–1 Syllabus for Volunteer Training Program

Structure: Twenty-four hours of class time divided into 2-hour sessions for 6 weeks and 6 hours of practicum experience for a total of 30 instructional hours.

Delivery: Appropriate team members with one core instructor to provide continuity and integration as well as group cohesion. Methods should include lecture and discussion, demonstration and guided hands-on experience, and group process.

Content Breakdown:

- *Session 1*—general introduction (focus primarily on structure, function, and general process of agency, including introduction of personnel and demonstration of procedures)
- *Session 2*—context presentations (what they will do, where they will do it and with whom, and how the current program integrates with work they have already done in other areas), group process session, case review and process session, case review and process demonstration
- *Session 3*—history of the movement in which they are involved (e.g., if hospice groups, a full explanation and differentiation of types, forms, and methods of hospice care), discussion of philosophical roots of program, notion and practice of confidentiality and professional responsibility, group process, case review
- *Session 4*—presentation of materials by the social service division, including policy, practice, and issues of integration and cohesiveness; group process; case review
- *Session 5*—presentation by the medical division, including material on pain control, psy-

chiatry, and other relevant medical issues; group process; case review

- *Session 6*—presentation and demonstration of material from the nursing division, including basic information about lifting the patient, making a bed, etc.; group process; case review
- *Session 7*—consideration of basic sociological issues surrounding in-home care, general information and significant demographics in the catchment area served by the agency, discussion of social and legal issues, group process, case review
- *Session 8*—communication skills, including nonverbal communication; listening skills and basic evaluation methods (fact, cognitive, and affect levels of evaluation); group process and practice; case review
- *Session 9*—communication skills, including demonstration and practice in content and affect responses; application of methods to various psychological situations (e.g., responding to an agency patient); group process and practice; case review
- *Session 10*—presentation and consideration of issues on family dynamics; variability in family structure and function; what might they find, how must they adjust, and when they need to refer; group process; case review
- *Session 11*—consideration of religious dynamics and their function and influence on patient and family, presentation by chaplain, group process, case review
- *Session 12*—ethical issues (suicide, euthanasia, confidentiality, integrity, responsibility), general review, closure

the reality allows the candidates to discover whether they really want to do this work; it is one thing to imagine a role, another to live it.

There are two formats that the practicum can follow: accompanying as an observer an in-home care nurse as he or she makes rounds, or assisting a working volunteer. Ideally, both formats can be included with the nursing observation as the

formal practicum experience and the volunteer assistance a primary step in actual volunteer function. It is important for the volunteer director to do a debriefing with each candidate as he or she completes the nursing observation; this gives the candidate a chance to work through any surfaced concerns or anxieties and at the same time allows the volunteer director to acquire necessary firsthand feedback from the experience.

It is important that clear recognition and crediting be given to the volunteers who successfully complete the training program. This is a factor of both incorporation and morale. Successful candidates should be formally issued certificates of completion at a graduation ceremony. It is not at all inappropriate to schedule an evening event, off site at a town hall or a church auditorium, with a guest keynote speaker, the distribution of certificates to each graduate, and a reception. Graduation should be seen as a rite of passage or initiation marking a distinct shift of status based on the recognition of skill. It is a formal recognition of the incorporation of the candidates as fully functioning members of the corps; it is a statement of welcome, trust, and inclusion.

Retention

The capacity to retain individuals who do their jobs with skill and dedication is always a goal for volunteer programs. Retention is usually important in any personnel program because it should guarantee a maintenance of quality in service or product. Consistency, commitment, personal identification, and consequent responsibility, loyalty, and increased skill that come from experience are all excellent reasons for encouraging retention. In a volunteer program, the economic factor makes retention programs essential. The cost of volunteer labor is primarily in recruiting and training. Once the initial investment has been made, the cost of supervision should be significantly lower. Because the largest cost invested in an individual volunteer comes up front, and because maintenance costs are significantly lower, it stands to reason that the longer the individual remains in active and productive service, the greater the return on the initial cost. The expense of training an individual is clearly and significantly diminished by the length of his or her service.

The key to a strong retention program is a commitment by the agency to a policy of equability, mutuality, and fairness. It is essential to remember that, although volunteers are not paid, they do need paybacks. It is essential that individuals get something back for what they give. If this balance of giving and receiving is not maintained, it will not be long before corps members will begin to feel victimized. Volunteers want to feel useful, not used.

Payback is given in recognition, reward, and authenticity of respect. Recognition demands that volunteers, both collectively and individually, be credited for the nature and quality of what they do. Individuals need to have communicated to them that their immediate supervisor and the agency see and understand what they are actually producing. The volunteer needs to know—by being told—that the director is aware and appreciative of the difficulties involved in the volunteer's performance of responsibilities. Recognition demands that the director be familiar with the person and performance of the volunteer and that this understanding be communicated to the volunteer as acknowledged praise and/or direction at regular intervals.

Rituals of reward are part of the paycheck in volunteerism. Open, formal, public rewards for quality of service are necessary for morale and to help maintain retention. Rewards, whatever specific form they take, should always involve some degree of public recognition for the individual and the corps and for the quality of their work.

Authenticity of respect can only be communicated if the director truly knows the volunteer and his or her work and takes the time and effort to communicate that familiarity. Authenticity of respect demands that the director perform his or her job responsibilities with a high degree of commitment and involvement. It is the director's responsibility to develop appropriate relationships with each volunteer and, within the context of this relationship, to understand perceptively the capacity and character of each corps member. Authenticity communicates when it exists; if the goal is to communicate authentic respect, then the director must be committed to behavior that engenders an honest and appropriate knowledge of and appreciation for each individual member of the corps. Basically, the issue here is integrity of behavior, an integrity that is quickly recognized by the volunteer and is responded to with appreciation, trust, and mutuality.

The question still remains as to how specifically the director can apply recognition, reward, and authenticity of respect toward a goal of retention. Basically, this goal can be accomplished through structures of interchange, which fall into two broad categories: those activities that are the specific personal efforts of the director, and those activities that involve the participation of the agency and the corps.

Under the first category, it is essential that the director know the members of the corps. A file should be kept on each member containing as much relevant data as can be acquired. Information that is standard to a resume obviously should be present in this file, but the profile should be broadened to include details of life events, personal traits, unique characteristics and relationships, and anything and everything that will help the director know and understand the individual with whom he or she is working; obviously, all information should be kept confidential. A complete medical and psychological history should be acquired if possible, enhanced by an appropriate social history. Updates as to addresses, phone numbers, changes in name, marital status, and jobs are essential. The record should include basic information about the volunteer's mate and family so that a sense of the volunteer's social context and needs is continuously and accurately maintained.

The director must make every effort to keep the dialogue open with members of the corps. The maintenance of dialogue involves time, relational skill, and commitment to the process.

Approximately 25 percent of the director's time should be dedicated to the "cultivation of the garden." This cultivation involves time spent in direct interchange with the volunteers as individuals and as a group. Individual time can be created in a variety of ways. It is a good idea periodically to schedule lunch with individual

members of the corps at the initiative of the director. The lunches should be informal and conducive to open dialogue. They should occur at least once a year and more frequently if the calendar permits. Individual lunches offer time and opportunity for personal disclosure, for needed recognition, for mutual evaluation, and for defusing and affirmation. In addition, they serve to enhance and maintain the bonding and integration of the volunteer with the program and as such are a major tool in retention.

It is important that the director advocate on behalf of volunteers, as individuals and as a group, to the agency. The corps needs someone to speak on its behalf, to exhibit concern for its interests, and to act as a peer representative within the management level of the agency. This can be a delicate balance for the director who is obligated to meet the needs of the agency as well as those of the corps. Every attempt must be made to keep the corps bonded and integrated with the agency so that goals become reciprocal and mutual. The director must be open and truthful in all communications, both to the corps and to the agency; this includes making statements of the inability to disclose when permission to discuss an issue has not been received from involved parties. Basically, it must be recognized that it is the responsibility of the director to safeguard the fair treatment of corps members and to work to maintain trust, equability, and mutuality.

In the same vein, it is the responsibility of the director to maintain clear communication between the agency's administration and the corps. Weekly meetings with the executives are quite appropriate when possible. These discussions should center on a mutual exchange of information, interest, and concern in which management is kept informed as to the function and character of the corps and the director can in turn be informed as to management's attitude and insights concerning the corps.

In addition, it is the responsibility of the director to meet with the corps, ideally on a weekly basis. These meetings should function as an open exchange of information and attitudes. They should be conducted as open dialogues directed toward goals of understanding and cohesion. These discussions are clearly an essential tool in maintaining good communication, but in addition they serve to identify and defuse problems of anxiety, insecurity, rumor, and discontent before they fester into major administrative difficulties.

Just mentioned was the director's responsibility for the organization and facilitation of collective methods to assist retention. These collective tools include operating a weekly support group, conducting recognition events, offering periodic in-service programs, and awarding certification and credentials when possible.

Support groups are essential in maintaining an effective volunteer program. Ideally, the support group should meet once a week and be open to all volunteers. The group should not exceed 20 participants; if it does, a second group should be formed. The group must have a professional facilitator; if the director is not qualified to act in this capacity, someone who is credentialed should be brought in. The presence of a professional is required because the basic function and nature of the group are therapeutic rather than self-help. The issues that surface from in-home care volunteerism are often heavily psychologically laden and warrant therapeutic response. A well-conducted support group can forestall numerous problems, some of a serious nature, before they have a chance to begin. The group should function therapeutically (defusing emotional or conceptual issues before they evolve into a crisis), educationally (with continued instruction included that is relevant to the volunteers' current experiences), and cohesively (as members begin to identify with and support each other as a group).

Group meetings should be 1.5 hours in length. This gives enough time for all members to participate if they so choose. It is helpful to have a therapeutic theme for each session. For example, the issue of the volunteers' self-confidence might be chosen. The facilitator then introduces the theme, and as the group progresses with discussion around the individual volunteer's experiences and concerns, the facilitator clarifies, interprets, and interconnects individual contributions along thematic lines. This process serves to educate, affect therapeutically, and encourage the group in terms of identification and cohesion.

Alternatively, the thematic line can be extracted by the facilitator from the group process. In this case, the group begins its process immediately, and the facilitator, having paid close and perceptive attention, extracts whatever thematic thread begins to surface, mirrors it back to the group, clarifies, elaborates, and again reinforces the theme as the group process continues. Here again, the same positive effect of education, therapy, and cohesion can be achieved with a final result of minimal crisis and burnout within the corps.

We all need to feel a sense of accomplishment and competency, regardless of what it is we have chosen to do; this is especially true for volunteers. For this reason, recognition events are essential to maintain individual involvement in the volunteer corps. Recognition events should include graduation, an awards lunch, a Christmas or other holiday event, a mates dinner, and a summer picnic hosted by the agency.

Graduation, as discussed previously, should be a specific event, held off site in the evening, with a guest speaker and the distribution of certificates of completion. A reception after the ceremony always is well received and serves to enhance group identity and belonging.

An awards lunch, given by the director usually in the early spring or fall, serves to affirm publicly the director's recognition and appreciation for the corps and its members. The lunch is for the corps, and outside individuals should be invited only at the initiative of the volunteers; this includes invitations extended to other members of the agency. The lunch provides an excellent opportunity for a review of in-house corps business and the highlights of the preceding year of service. In addition, specific awards for contributions and performance can be given, with care being taken that presentations are always given in fairness and justice. The main theme, however, should be the affirmation of the corps as a unit, and an open statement of appreciation for the quality of the corps' performance and commitment should be the central focus of the luncheon.

A mates dinner is essential for any assertive retention program. In-home care volunteers have a degree of involvement in their work that is rivaled by few paid employees. The work tends to hold the volunteers emotionally and intellectually. It is as though a piece of them were put aside especially for this work, and those who are close to them are acutely aware of this surrender. Mates may become uneasy, competitive, and in some case jealous of the volunteers' time and vested concern. Often the mate may experience the volunteer's new commitment as a personal loss and may subtly or aggressively agitate for the volunteer to resign from the corps. This agitation can be eased by giving recognition and credit to the mate's position. A dinner, sponsored by the agency and hosted by the corps, given in February or March, again off campus, usually works exceptionally well. The months of February and March tend to be depressed periods, times when issues that are grains of sand during the rest of the year become pebbles or perhaps rocks to stumble over. It is quite appropriate for all agency administrators to be invited, and the executive administrator as well as the director of volunteers should be asked to address the group. Regardless of the general theme chosen for the evening, it is essential that direct recognition of the mates' position and difficulties be expressed. Statements must be open and discussion direct, not subtle or alluding.

The mates' side must be clearly credited, and it is essential that the agency thank these individuals for their support and recognize them as non-rostered members of the team. Again, the goal is cohesion and dissipation of dissatisfaction before it blossoms into crisis; in addition, the dinner serves an advocacy function for the volunteers and consequently directly bolsters their adhesion to the program by increasing their trust in the agency as a concerned personal resource.

Holiday parties and summer picnics are events best sponsored by the agency. The holiday party may include only agency personnel; the summer picnic may include family members, mates, and children. Again, the purpose is cohesion, affirmation, recognition, and nurturing of group identification. In these two events the emphasis is cohesion and identification with the agency as well as with the corps.

In-service programs provide continuing education for the corps in addition to a psychodynamic function. A full-day in-service program in the fall, planned and prepared by the volunteers, works well. A central theme, a guest speaker, and appropriate representation from the agency are the basic ingredients. The day can be broken into a morning and afternoon session with a luncheon in between; it is a good idea to leave plenty of time for group process and participation. What is important here is that the volunteers get something, learn something, from whatever is offered and that the corps be involved in every aspect of the planning and presentation, that they own the day as their own. The goal, here again, is to reinforce involvement and commitment and to stimulate the enthusiasm and spirit of the corps with new learning, new insights, and new possibilities.

A feeling of belonging, of being an integral, appreciated part of the team, is an essential dynamic in retention. Consequently, it is important that a conscious and consistent effort be made by the agency as a whole continuously to integrate the volunteers into the spirit and function of the agency. This is as much an attitude as it is a mode of behavior, an attitude that must pervade policy and be actively present in the day-to-day operation of the agency. The bottom line is that volunteers remain present and active if they feel useful, appreciated, and rewarded and perceive themselves as active, necessary parts of the team.

Volunteers who remain with the corps need to feel competent and successful. With this need in mind, the director of volunteers should make every effort, when placing the individual volunteer on an assignment, to place the volunteer for success. Placing a volunteer for success demands that the director know each volunteer, know the particulars of each case, and carefully match the volunteer and his or her skills and personality to the needs of the placement case. It is helpful to envision each case as a context in which the volunteer must function. The object is to choose an individual who, when placed in the case context, will connect and engage in a positive, productive process that will culminate in positive resolutions for everyone, or at least almost everyone.

Placement must begin with an evaluation visit to the family by the director of volunteers. Evaluation data to be considered should include a consideration of the following:

- The patient's physical and psychosocial needs
- The family's physical and psychosocial needs
- The family structure and basic dynamics
- Relevant demographic data, such as socioeconomic level of the family, education, ethnicity, religion, race, and the like

Once this material has been gathered, a general profile of family needs and functions can be created and a volunteer chosen who is perceived as compatible with the case dynamics. A great deal of this process is procedural, but there must be, present and active on the part of the director, an intuitive capacity for matchmaking. No matter how many data are collected, and no matter how documented and procedural the evaluation is, success often rests on the intuitive, perceptual capacity of the director to match precisely the right volunteer with the right case context. If the match is fundamentally compatible, the success of the case, in terms of resultant positive resolutions, is close to guaranteed barring introduced or unforeseen circumstances.

Once placement has been made, a schedule for supervision contact must be followed. Ideally, it is good for the director to accompany the volunteer on an introductory visit to the family. This gives the director an on-site opportunity to make sure that there is, in fact, basic compatibility between the volunteer and the context. On the day when the volunteer actually begins his or her assignment, a brief visit or phone call to the volunteer while he or she is working on the case is both affirming and supportive. Thereafter, periodic on-site visits for evaluation and morale are appropriate. The frequency of these visits depends on the complexity of the case and its length. Cases that are complicated demand more attention, and cases that extend over lengthy durations demand periodic visits to sustain volunteer morale. In addition, periodic brief meetings in the office for review and suggestions are appropriate.

The volunteer should be present at team meetings and encouraged to participate in the case report. Here again, it is the director's responsibility to facilitate this participation and to evaluate its content and process for accuracy, compatibility, and effectiveness. The director then needs to feed back appropriate critiques or affirmation privately to the volunteer about his or her contribution, remembering always that the main objects of supervision include education and development of the volunteer as well as quality service to the client.

Times exist when cases do not work out as anticipated, no matter how carefully the preparatory work has been done. It is the director's responsibility to initiate and facilitate the exit of a volunteer in these cases. Circumstances that warrant this intervention include situations where the health and safety of the volunteer are at risk, situations where gross incompatibilities of personalities develop, and situations where the family dynamic is fundamentally dysfunctional and threatens the general procedure of the case.

It is the responsibility of the director to advocate on behalf of the volunteer to the family and to the agency in these circumstances and in any situation where it is critical that the volunteer's side be heard. In this regard, the director is answerable for the creation and maintenance of an open, constructive dialogue. This demands a degree of diplomatic skill and courage. In the end, however, it takes less courage to deal directly with each crisis as it arrives than to let discontent and antagonism grow to proportions of a major incident and then attempt to deal with it. Again, the object is to keep problems from ever developing rather than to figure out how to cope with them after the fact. The object is to be consistently proactive and consistently in control and thereby to minimize the necessity to respond reactively, subjugated to control by the situation.

CONCLUSION

A successful volunteer program demands that the agency in general, and the director in particular, have a clear, mutual understanding of a relational ethic that is conscientiously and consistently concretized in program design and process. There must be an active commitment to

the ethical values of integrity, justice, and humanism. These values must influence policy and decision making at every level, acting as an integrating thread of uniformity and consistency. In addition, there must be an active commitment by all involved parties to the relational premises of trust, fairness, mutuality, reciprocity, and dialogue, premises that must be experienced in and through the daily process of the program. The bottom line is that quality recruits who are appropriately and skillfully trained and supervised are retained and remain productive, thereby increasing the quality of service and the cost-efficiency of a good volunteer program.

Fair treatment and experienced justice for all parties involved pay dividends on every level in every way, regardless of the currency used, whether monetary or relational, to ensure the magnitude of the result.

BIBLIOGRAPHY

Benton, R. 1978. *Death and dying: Principles and practices in patient care.* New York: Van Nostrand Reinhold.

Boszoimenyi-Nagy, I., and B. Krasner. 1986. *Between give and take.* New York: Brunner/Mazel.

Chapman, J., and H. Chapman. 1975. *Behavior and health care: A Humanistic Helping Process.* St. Louis, MO: Mosby.

Danish, S. J., and A. C. Haner. 1976. *Helping skills: A basic training program.* New York: Human Services Press.

Doka, K. J. 1998. *Living with life-threatening illness: A guide for patients, their families and caregivers.* San Francisco: Jossey-Bass.

Fisher, J. C., and K. M. Cole. 1998. *Leadership and management of volunteer programs: A guide for volunteer administrators.* San Francisco: Jossey-Bass.

Levin, M. 1992. *The gift of leadership: How to relight the volunteer spirit in the 21st century.* Columbia, MD: BAI Publishing.

Logan, M., and E. Hunt. 1978. *Death and the human condition.* North Scituate, MA: Duxbury.

Mann, R. 1967. *Interpersonal styles and group development: An analysis of the member-leader relationship.* New York: John Wiley & Sons.

Mezey, M.D. (ed.). 2002. *Ethical patient care: A casebook for geriatric health care teams.* Baltimore, MD: Johns Hopkins University Press.

National Hospice and Palliative Care Organization. 2002. *Hospice volunteer program resource manual.* Alexandria, VA: National Hospice and Palliative Care Organization.

Schein, E., and W. Bennis. 1965. *Personal and organizational change through group methods.* New York: John Wiley & Sons.

Schmolling, P., M. Youkeles, and W. Burger. 1989. *Human services in contemporary America,* 2nd ed. Pacific Grove, CA: Brooks/Cole.

CHAPTER 61

The Manager as Published Author: Tips on Writing for Publication

Suzanne P. Smith

Writing for publication is a process: It can be learned and it can be mastered. Although understanding the writing and publishing process can increase your chances of being a published author, it cannot replace experience.

Think of the processes, skills, and techniques mastered during your nursing education; for example, giving injections. Knowledge of physiology, pharmacology, anatomy, biology, and psychology gave you needed conceptual skills. Knowing how and actually doing, however, were two different things. To develop proficiency, you actually had to administer drugs and observe client reactions.

Likewise, writing for publication has a conceptual and an experiential component. Although resources related to writing, such as this chapter, will give you information you need to write for publication, it is practice that leads to success.

BLOCKS TO WRITING

When I ask nurse administrators and managers why they do not write for publication, I get answers such as I can't seem to get started; I'm not motivated; I can't write at work; I'm not creative; I can't write at home; Other things seem more important each day; I have nothing unique to share; I don't write well; My first paper was rejected; and I'm too busy.

These reasons for not writing fall into three main categories. The first is lack of motivation

stemming from inexperience, past rejection of a manuscript, and negative feedback on your writing. The second hindrance is your workload and how you choose to prioritize. The third reason is procrastination. Here are some suggestions to overcome these personal blocks to getting started.

Inexperience

If lack of motivation is due to inexperience or poor writing, take a writing or journalism course at a local college or attend seminars on writing for publication. A source of motivation and support is colleagues who have already published. Many neophyte authors attribute their success in publishing to being mentored by a nationally known and well-published nurse. This relationship is most often initiated by the neophyte author asking the expert for advice. Do not hesitate to establish contact with published experts in your content area. They most often appreciate the opportunity to share their knowledge with and help develop others.

Another source of motivation can be a writers' support group. Find colleagues who are interested in writing but, like you, can't seem to get started. Form a group and meet on a regular basis. Share resources, critique small writing projects (such as an abstract or an interoffice memo), develop interesting and innovative topics, write query letters to editors about your ideas, and co-author manuscripts. For assistance in structuring a writers' support group, read Valente's article (2003) on journal clubs.

Workload

Overcoming the second block, setting workload priorities, involves deciding what activities you want in your life. You have to be honest about the value of writing for publication to you, your life, and your career. Do you really want to make writing a priority over reading a good novel, a trip to the gym, or a long bath? Time is always found to do what we want and value. Once you take writing into your life, when and where is it going to be done? How will you set your priorities and manage your time?

Procrastination

Overcoming the third block, procrastination, is the same as overcoming procrastination in your daily life. You have to know what motivates you, and what works to get you started on projects.

Strategies

Here are some techniques to overcome blocks to getting started; all can work if you use them consistently, in a disciplined way:

- Set aside a specific period of time to write, preferably a time when you are at your peak. Write in a place that is conducive to work and where you will not be interrupted by family, colleagues, or telephone calls.
- Break your writing into reasonable time blocks. Trying to find 8 hours of uninterrupted time in a busy schedule is impossible and demotivating. Instead, for example, set aside 30 minutes every other day. Work exactly 30 minutes and stop, even if you are in the middle of a thought. This will motivate you to return to the work the next time.
- Use a tape recorder to dictate your first draft. Transcribe, cut, paste, and edit that material. This approach avoids the blank piece of paper and the "where should I start?" syndrome.

- For those who cannot work until the first sentence is perfect, start in the middle of your paper. The introduction and conclusion of a paper are often the hardest to do. Leave them until the end.
- Start in a small way by writing a query letter about your topic to the editors of several journals. A positive response from an editor can be the motivation to write the whole paper.

Another less intimidating way to overcome writing inertia is to write short, concise letters to the editor. To be timely, the letter should be written soon after the journal publishes the article you wish to critique. An effective letter will contain information that sheds additional light on the topic rather than just praises the article.

Most journals have specific departments—such as executive development, education for administration, professional innovations, and news, notes, and tips—that accept brief manuscripts in the one- to five-page range. Peruse journals to assess the fit of an idea you have with the department's purpose.

Use behavior modification to establish a reward system for every so many pages you write. Rosenberg and Lah (1985), using this approach, lead the reader through an analysis of tasks and overt and covert reinforcements and distractions. With this analysis, the would-be author develops a self-modification timetable and a reinforcement and evaluation schedule.

Finally, if lack of spontaneity and creativity seem to be the problem, Rico's (2001) book is a must. A well-known nurse editor referred this book to me after I asked her how she managed to write consistently interesting editorials. Rico presents a creative, developmental, step-by-step process for making writing easier. The book is interactive: As you read, you are asked to do brief writing exercises. The book's approach can be used for any type of writing.

REJECTION

Manuscript rejection can be a major block to continued writing. Too many first-time authors who have their first manuscript rejected by an editor never try again. Rather than seeing rejection as a chance to learn from mistakes, improve ideas through the use of feedback, and master a process, authors are personally crushed by their perceived failure.

Rejection of any kind sets up a grieving process. Symbolically, rejected manuscripts are seen as an attack on one's ideas and perhaps even on one's life's work. Even though it was the paper, not you, that was rejected, you still have to deal with an emotional reaction.

If your manuscript is rejected, avoid the urge to destroy it immediately. Instead, give yourself time to deal with the shock, hurt, and anger. After your disappointment has subsided to a manageable level, analyze why the paper was rejected. Ask a trusted colleague to critique the manuscript in light of the reasons given for rejection. The perspective of a person more distant from your work can be helpful as well as supportive.

If you want more feedback from the editor as to why your paper was not acceptable, call or write the editor. A large part of an editor's role is as a teacher. Ask for guidance. If you have enough feedback and your idea is still timely, revise the paper, improving your ideas and their presentation. If the editor expressed interest in your idea, resubmit the revised and improved version of your manuscript to the same journal. If the journal's editor did not indicate an interest in seeing the revised paper, submit your paper to another journal. Revise the paper based on the first journal's feedback or submit the original paper. Using either approach, you will continue to receive feedback so that you can perfect your idea and its presentation.

If your paper is rejected by several journals, you must seriously reconsider the approach, validity, and importance of your topic. At some point, cut your losses, move on to another topic of interest, and start the process again. You will be wiser and the process will become easier. Do not quit, no matter how you are feeling.

Reasons for Rejection

Although it is important to be mentally prepared to deal with rejection, it is equally important to know and avoid the major reasons why manuscripts are rejected. Manuscripts are sometimes rejected because a journal has recently published or is soon to publish an article on a similar topic. A query letter to the editor helps avoid this reason for rejection.

Manuscripts are also rejected because the content is outdated, not important, not appropriate (e.g., a clinical topic for a management journal), too technical or too basic for the journal's readers, inaccurate, undocumented or poorly documented, or fabricated. A research paper is most often rejected because of poor research design. Finally, a poorly organized and poorly written paper is almost always rejected.

Minimizing Rejection

These reasons for rejection imply some obvious solutions. Know what the journal has published in the last several years related to your topic, know who the primary audience of the journal is, know the types of positions held by and the average educational preparation of the readers, and do not write a research paper for a national journal if your sample is small and geographically isolated or your methodology is flawed. If grammar, spelling, and composition are not your strengths, get editorial assistance.

MANUSCRIPT CRITIQUE

Before you complete the final version of a manuscript, have it critiqued for content, style, and relevance to the reader. Although one person might be able to evaluate all these areas of your manuscript, I recommend three different people; the task is more manageable for each, and you will receive more and better criticism than if one person does all.

First, have a content expert read your paper for the information's accuracy and completeness. The content expert should be concerned only with the paper's technical content. For example, if your topic is using financial spreadsheets, your agency's financial officer might be the reviewer.

Second, have a style reviewer read the paper for clarity, flow, organization, and grammar. This person might be a teacher or student of journalism or English, or perhaps just a friend who has good writing and organizational skills.

Third, a colleague who represents the journal's primary reader should review the paper for appropriateness and relevance of focus. If you are not the journal's primary reader, your content might be too dogmatic, might be above or below the readers' knowledge level, or might attack "sacred cows." For example, imagine that as a graduate student, a faculty member, or clinical nurse specialist, you write a manuscript on budgeting for *The Journal of Nursing Administration* (JONA). Because JONA is edited for top-level administrators and you are not in that position, find an agency administrator to check the content's level of sophistication and appropriateness for the reader.

GETTING STARTED

Many excellent resources exist that discuss critical elements in the writing and publishing process (Barnum, 1995; Daly, 2000; Fondiller, 1999; Grant, 1998; Huth, 1999; Oermann, 2001; Sheridan and Dowdney, 1997; Zilm, 1998). The following highlights a few areas.

Generating Ideas

How many times have you read an article and said, "I've been doing that for years," or "I could have written that article"? The difference between you and published authors is that they actually did it. Too often, we feel that our ideas are commonplace. A better thought to have is, "If I have a problem, other people around the country probably have it too. If I have a solution that's working in my institution, other people would probably be interested in hearing about it." A few telephone calls to colleagues will confirm the validity and timeliness of your idea.

If you do not have an idea, become a critical reader and observer. As you read professional and nonprofessional literature, ask what the implications of the information are to you, your institution, other nurses, and the profession. What

problems are common at work and how are they being addressed? What trends are emerging that will affect how nursing is practiced and how can we be proactive now? What have you learned through your work with community and professional groups? How could that knowledge be applied to the profession or your work situation? Answering these questions can be the basis of a publishable idea.

The often maligned technique of brainstorming is always a good way to generate ideas alone or in groups. Brainstorming works when care is taken to avoid premature criticism of ideas. Productivity is increased by brainstorming answers to a specific question. For example, what is the most difficult job-related problem you expect to face in the next 3 years? Answers to questions such as this can lead to interesting, innovative, and visionary manuscripts.

Selecting an Idea

Before committing to an idea, assess it for timeliness, focus, interest to readers, and interest to you. You need to know why your idea is important (perhaps because of recent advances in technology or new legislation or because it is a new way to do an old thing). To pinpoint hot topics, go to the literature. You probably have a hot topic if there is little to nothing in the professional literature.

The best articles also have a specific slant. Article titles and abstracts often reveal an article's focus. Know the particular point your article will make before you start writing. For example, a manuscript on developing a capital budget will be easier to write and more likely to be accepted for publication than a broad-based manuscript on financial management. Your topic's focus will emerge as you review the literature and identify missing information.

When you know who the primary reader of a journal is (staff nurses, first-line managers, academic educators, or clinical nurse specialists), tailor your ideas to their needs for certain information. Find out who the primary reader of a journal is by reading the journal and its instructions for authors. If still in doubt, call or write the editor.

Finally, pick an idea that is personally interesting. The publishing process is lengthy, often 12 to 18 months from manuscript submission to publication. Your interest and motivation have to be sustained over a long period of time. Avoid writing about past experiences if they are not relevant to your personal or professional life. For example, if you were a practitioner involved in a complex clinical problem and are now in a new management position, removed from day-to-day clinical contact, it will become harder and harder for you to write the clinical paper. Your attention and commitment will be directed toward acquisition of new management skills.

Developing Your Idea

The best idea in the world can lack substance, interest, and clarity if it is poorly developed. Your comprehensive review of the literature occurs when you are committed to one topic. It is during this period that your ideas are refined. You should emerge from the literature review phase by being able to answer these questions:

- What purpose do you hope to achieve by writing on a particular topic with a particular slant? (e.g., you want to change the way administrators evaluate the performance of staff)
- What is the point you want to make? (e.g., this paper will show administrators how to establish a nonthreatening environment for evaluation of staff)
- How does your idea relate to trends that affect health care and nursing?
- How does your idea differ from present practice?
- What examples illustrate the idea and its usefulness?
- What aspects of your idea are original and unique?
- Who would be interested in reading about the idea? Administrators? Faculty? Staff educators? Staff nurses? Students?

- What information about your topic is not in the literature?

Answering these questions as you review the literature will give you an idea of the depth of your knowledge of the topic as well as gaps in your understanding. Answers to these questions also give you the information you need to query the editor, write a working abstract, and begin the paper.

SELECTING THE APPROPRIATE JOURNAL

Most people are aware of only the few journals that they read. By knowing all the journals that might be appropriate for your idea, you will increase your chances of getting your paper published. The most useful sources of information about nursing journals are Daly's book (2000), Northam and associates' article (2000), and Allen's (2000) and Johnson's (2003) Web sites. In addition to listing numerous journals by specialty area (e.g., administration, gerontology, and maternal-child health, to name a few), these sources provide a variety of demographics about each journal in categories, such as number of subscribers, issues per year, desired manuscript length, need for query letter, length of time for the review process, and length of time from acceptance until publication. McConnell (1995) provides similar information for 42 nursing publications outside the United States.

Use these sources to identify potential journals that, by title, seem appropriate for your topic and target readers. When potential journals have been identified, it is critical that you obtain and examine copies of the journals; many are now available online at the journal's Web site. Photocopy or download the instructions for authors' guidelines and note the editor's name and address from the most recent issue. Rank the best to the least likely fit of your topic with the journal. Consider the following items.

Readership

Know for whom you are writing and how your paper will meet the information needs of the journal's primary readership. Determine the audience's educational level, degree of expertise, and special interests by scanning journal article titles, abstracts, and contents. Note this information because later your query letter, your abstract, and your article will all have to be tailored to this particular group.

Circulation

How much of your target audience is reached by the journal? Only a small percentage of home health care administrators subscribe to generic nursing journals such as the *American Journal of Nursing* (AJN) or *Nursing*. A manuscript with an administrative focus has a better chance of being accepted if it is submitted to a journal that is read only by administrators (e.g., *The Journal of Nursing Administration*) or has an exclusive home health care focus (e.g., *Home Healthcare Nurse*).

Yearly Journal Page Count

The more pages a journal publishes in a year, the more manuscripts it can accept. Multiply the number of article pages in an issue by the number of issues published in a year to derive total editorial pages. All other factors being equal, choose the journal that publishes the most number of pages per year over one that has significantly less pages.

Refereed or Peer Review Status

A refereed journal, also referred to as a peer reviewed journal, publishes manuscripts that have been reviewed by members of a journal's advisory board or manuscript review panel. These reviewers represent a broad range of expertise in the journal's subject matter. In academic settings, publication and promotion committees give more weight to articles published in refereed journals. If you now or ever intend to work in a school of nursing, this factor is an important journal selection criterion.

Format

Examine at least two issues of all your potential journals. Make a note of the style and the average length of an article, language complexity and style, length and format of the abstract, title, biographical statement, introduction, conclusion, structure of tables and figures, and use of photographs and illustrations. Will your topic, as you envision it being developed, fit into the journal's overall style and format? For example, if your article uses photographs to show how a procedure is done, does the journal publish photographs? If no, would the journal publish photographs if asked, or could you make your point through line drawings instead?

Type of Article

Is your article going to be conceptual, practical, how-to-do, or research oriented? Does it have a clinical, management, staff, or academic focus? Make sure your plan for developing an idea for a specific journal fits into the journal's approach to contents.

Author Payment

Although some journals pay authors a certain amount of money per printed journal page, most simply provide reprints of the article or copies of the issue in which the article appears.

Time Frames

The length of time it takes to review and publish a manuscript is a critical journal selection criterion depending on the timeliness of your idea. For example, a manuscript on time management can tolerate a longer time frame than a paper dealing with a strategy to comply with a new federal regulation. If possible, write for journals with the shortest time frames.

Acceptance Rates

Specialty journals and new journals tend to have higher acceptance rates than generic journals (such as the *American Journal of Nursing* or *Nursing*) and well-established journals (such as *The Journal of Nursing Administration* and *Nursing Research*). Two reasons contribute to this phenomenon: Compared with a generic journal, specialty journals have a smaller group of people with expertise in the subject matter, whereas mature, well-established journals are the first journals that come to all authors' minds.

Interest in Your Idea

To assess a journal's interest in your idea, query the editor via e-mail, telephone, or letter. In the query, briefly explain the problem or issue that the readership faces and how the reader will be better off after reading your solution or approach. You can gauge interest in your idea by how quickly and in what manner the editor responds—from an impersonal form letter to a personalized, encouraging e-mail to a telephone call.

Decision Making

Assess these journal selection factors and their relative importance to you. Rank your potential journals from first to last choice. Write query letters to the editors of all your potential journals. As soon as your number one–ranked journal responds positively to your manuscript query, finalize the draft of your paper with that journal's specific formatting requirements.

WRITING THE PAPER

Several methods exist that you can use to organize your content before actually writing. The most well known is the standard outline. The outline is useful, however, only if you outline with ideas rather than words. It is useless to have Roman numeral I of your outline be "Introduction." That doesn't assist you in writing the introduction or anyone else in knowing what you want to do. Instead, have each step of the outline highlight a major point. Now, Roman numeral I might

be "Avoiding prospective payment system denials due to incorrect ICD-9-CM coding."

Another outline approach is the use of index cards. Each key idea of your content is written in a sentence at the top of the card. These key ideas are each paragraph's topic sequence. Below each sentence, jot down the key points you wish to make in the paragraph. Shuffle the cards to organize and reorganize the content, and start the writing process. This modular approach to organizing content allows you to write any part of the paper first. If one card's key concept eludes you, pick another card.

A good approach to organizing content for a visual person is the hurricane method. Using a brainstorming approach, quickly write all your ideas about your topic on a large piece of paper. Then, using different colored crayons or markers, circle similar concepts in the same color. To define each idea further, a second round might include taking each word in a color set, for example all the words marked in green, and repeating the exercise. You would quickly brainstorm all ideas related to the green words, and color code the subset. Do this until you feel you are ready to write using your color-coded pages.

For those who actually have to write the paper before they can do an outline, try the following methods for organizing content. Write your paper without much attention to fine details. Just get your ideas down on paper. Then copy the paper and cut it into pieces, grouping the paragraphs with similar ideas together and throwing away redundant information. As with the index card approach, rewrite the paper, and repeat the process.

For help with style, format, and grammar, refer to the style book recommended in your target journal's instructions for authors. Two popular manuals are those of the American Psychological Association (2001) and the American Medical Association (1998). After writing the last draft of your paper, have it critiqued by the three types of reviewers previously discussed. When you are done writing, refer to the journal's instructions for authors and the most recent copy of the journal to prepare the manuscript for submission.

SUBMISSION CHECKLIST

If the instructions for authors' guidelines and an issue of the journal do not give you the following information, telephone the editorial assistant and ask for the journal's procedure.

Electronic and Paper Copies

For journals that still require submission of paper copies, at a minimum, most journals require three copies; some require five or more. For Web-based manuscript submission, follow the instructions, noting special requirements for electronic file formatting.

Abstracts

Three basic types of abstracts exist: descriptive, structured, and benefit oriented. The descriptive abstract is most often seen in a research journal. It outlines the major elements of the manuscript and can be up to 250 words in length. The structured abstract, again used most often by research journals, describes the content using these headings: objective, methods (sample, procedures, analysis), results, and conclusions. The benefit-oriented abstract stresses the article's outcomes for the reader (how the reader will be better off after reading the content). It is usually 100 words or less and states the importance of a problem or issue to the reader and how the reader will be more effective after reading the author's solution to the problem. It does not give many details about the approach or solution.

Illustrations

Tables and figures should each be placed on separate pages that follow the reference list. Give a title as well as a page number to each illustration. Make sure every illustration has a reference in the text. Most journals require camera-ready illustrations, which are black type or ink on white paper or black-and-white glossy photographs. Diagrams, graphs, and line drawings should be professionally drawn or laser generated.

Reference Style

Make sure your references are formatted correctly according to the style manual used by your target journal. Although many journals use the style manual of the American Psychological Association, many journals use other styles, such as the *Chicago Manual of Style* or the *American Medical Association's Manual of Style*. Style manuals specify how referencing should be done in the text as well as in the reference list at the end of the manuscript. Instructions will address the correct order of the elements that comprise a reference citation (e.g., the authors' names, article title, journal name, volume numbers, and the year of publication) and the punctuation that should be placed between the elements.

Headings

Divide manuscript content by using headings and subheadings. This makes it easier for the reader to follow your main points. The subdivision of the content by headings is similar to a standard outline except that the Roman numerals, numbers, and letters are eliminated. All headings and subheadings should be grammatically similar.

Biographical Statement

Some journals use three- or four-sentence narrative biographical statements; others simply use name, credentials, title, and place, city, and state of employment. Some publish a photograph of the author. The ideal photograph is a black-and-white glossy photograph of the head and shoulders. For as little as $100, professional photographers will provide you with 10 wallet-size publicity photos. Ask the photographer also to provide you with a computer diskette containing your digitalized photograph files, in a common file format such as JPEG.

Computer Disks

Most publishers will ask you to submit a computer disk containing your manuscript file. Although each journal has specific formatting details for electronic copy, in general, you need to label the disk indicating which word processing software version you used and what you named your file. Unless the instructions for authors state otherwise, the computer disk is submitted only after review and acceptance of your manuscript.

Copyright Transfer

Just by producing a work, you hold its copyright. At some point, the editor will require transfer of your copyright to the journal's publisher. Some journals wish the transfer to be made when you submit the manuscript; others will require this only if the paper is accepted for publication. If transfer is to be made with your paper, the instructions for authors will provide the correct wording or tell you how to obtain the form online.

Use of Copyrighted Material

To use material already published by someone else, you must have permission from the copyright holder. It is your responsibility to write the copyright holder, requesting permission and indicating exactly how you will use the material. In addition to sending a copy of your manuscript highlighting the borrowed materials, send a copy of the original material indicating its source (because most copyright holders are publishers of many journals and books).

Copyright law does not specify how much material you can borrow without requesting permission. A general rule is that you need permis-

sion to borrow any element that is self-standing (such as a poem, a cartoon, a photograph, a figure, or a table) or that represents a significant percentage of the whole (three words of a four-word poem). When you directly quote narrative, a general rule of thumb is to request permission when quoting more than 250 words.

Finally, if you are a published author, you still have to get permission to quote yourself. Even though your ideas are always yours to be used at will, the exact words in published material belong to the copyright holder. Do not be guilty of self-plagiarism.

Cover Letter

When submitting your manuscript, include basic information in a cover letter or e-mail. The cover letter should highlight the importance of the manuscript's content to the reader in two or three brief sentences. It should include the title of the article and with whom the editor should correspond if there is more than one author. If you previously queried the editor, refer to that communication.

Appearance

I often receive manuscripts with no cover letter, too few copies, incorrect formatting, hard-to-read photocopies, and no author address (except that the institution and city might be mentioned in the biographical statement or somewhere in the manuscript). Papers received through our Web-based submission system frequently do not conform to our electronic file requirements. Failure to adhere to guidelines and to present yourself and your manuscript in a professional way at best reflects poorly on you and at worst is a cause of rejection. When two papers with equally good but similar content are being assessed, the editor will always choose the one that followed the instructions for authors' guidelines.

Web-Based Manuscript Submission

Journals allow authors to submit manuscripts via the postal service, e-mail attachment, or a

Wed-based system; however, a growing number of journals are allowing Web-based submissions only. Web-based manuscript tracking systems always require some formatting variation that differs from the traditional paper-copy method. As an example, each of the following manuscript elements may have to be placed in separate files: title/author biography, abstract, text, references, acknowledgments, figures/exhibits, and tables. Graphic files may have to be saved in special file formats, such as TIFF. Each line of the text file may have to be sequentially numbered. To see one journal's Web-based systems requirements go to http://jona.edmgr.com and download the instructions for authors.

RESEARCH

Research reports, theses, and dissertations have a different style and format from what is required by journals. For example, most research reports have lengthy background narrative and literature reviews. These two items are dramatically reduced in papers written for journal publication.

Nursing journals vary in how they report research projects and in the emphasis each wants placed on major elements. Before writing a manuscript about your research, study articles in your target journals, and note how the article is formatted, how long various sections are, and what sections are stressed the most.

In *The Journal of Nursing Administration*, which is not a research journal, we want the research reported in as brief a way as possible, with the author stressing the implications of the study, answering the "so what" question. We are not as concerned with a literature review section as we are with the literature being integrated into the narrative to support the author's ideas. Many other journals want a comprehensive but synthesized literature review section that highlights major literature in the topic area.

Student Research Projects

Publishing reports of research done as a student can be difficult. Because of limited resources,

the student's sample is usually small, which hampers the ability to generalize the findings and limits the scope of the research problem. In this case, local publications (newsletters and journals published by area schools of nursing institutions or professional associations) can be an appropriate outlet.

Also, the style and format for writing school papers, particularly theses and dissertations, differ from what is required by journals. The academic paper tends to be written in a passive, third-person voice ("It was believed that . . .") rather than the active first-person voice ("The investigator believes . . .") wanted by journals. The school paper's literature review is lengthy to show the professor that you have a full grasp of your topic. Editors of nursing journals assume that you know the published material and seek to have you add to the literature rather than repeat it.

School papers generally are lengthy and redundant because key ideas are said many times in different ways. Editors want concisely written papers; every extra word and redundant idea in a manuscript takes editorial space away from others waiting to be published. Use the smallest number of words to convey your message.

Last, many student authors are not members of the journal's readership group. This often leads to manuscript content that is not sufficiently sophisticated and relevant for the readers. This problem can be overcome through co-authorship with, or review of the manuscript by, a member of the journal's prime readership.

Although it can be difficult, it is possible to get work accomplished as a student published in nursing journals. Those who wish to turn theses, dissertations, and research reports into publishable manuscripts will find the work of Dunkin (1999) and Mateo and colleagues (1999) helpful. Tornquist (1999) discusses each element of a research report and then highlights approaches to rewriting the material for nursing journals.

Agency Data

Every agency has research data (e.g., number of staff, number of visits, code numbers, or type of client). Often, data are manipulated to see what will happen. Will the number of client visits increase if the staff only come into the agency once a week? Will the staff be any happier? Will patients be better off? Will office efficiency increase? Many times, the methods used to assess the intervention are informal. When this is the case, do not try to write a research article. The flawed methodology and inability to generalize the findings will lead to rejection.

The outcomes of your intervention probably are of interest to others, however. Many journals welcome manuscripts that discuss one agency's experience with an emerging problem or issue. It is acceptable to support discussion of the problem and the solution with agency data, even if data collection tools only had face validity. Readers can decide whether they want to test your ideas in their agency. Never feel hesitant about sharing what works for you with others; just do not try to disguise informal problem solving and data collection as a formal research project.

THE PUBLISHING PROCESS

When you submit your manuscript, it is critiqued by the editor and selected members of the manuscript review panel. If your manuscript is rejected, you will be told why. If you are not clear why your manuscript was unacceptable, write or call the editor.

Most accepted manuscripts require at least one revision based on the editor's and reviewers' feedback. If suggestions are extensive, you may actually have to rewrite the paper. All revision suggestions should be carefully considered while keeping two thoughts in mind: It is better to address a criticism or question before publication than after, and the point of review, feedback, and revision is to make your manuscript as good as it can be, thus making you and the journal look good.

Once your paper is acceptable to the editor, you will wait from 6 months to 2 years to see it published. The production process (copy editing, composition, proofing, and preparation of art work) takes approximately 3 to 4 months. The remaining time is accounted for by all the other manuscripts accepted before yours that are not yet published. If you did your preliminary work in selecting a journal, you should not be one of the people waiting 2 years.

Manuscripts are edited to improve clarity, conciseness, grammar, and expression of ideas. You will be asked to approve the copyedited manuscript before publication. The copyeditor will probably have questions for you, asking you to supply missing information or to clarify your intent. Because the published paper reflects your views, always feel free to contest copyediting that changes your meaning.

Up to 4 months before the scheduled publication date, information in the manuscript can be changed. Editors want manuscripts to be as up to date as possible. If there is a new development on your topic, ask whether you can add a paragraph to the paper. If new information has just been published on your topic, ask whether you can add the resource to your reference list. Finally, if you change jobs or addresses, notify the editorial office so that your biographical statement can be updated.

ETHICS

Authors make many decisions during the process of writing for publication. Some decision making is straightforward: Should a query be made to the editor? What graphs best illustrate the material? These decisions do not involve a moral right or wrong. Other decision-making points involve legal and ethical considerations. For example, all authors should know from reading the instructions for authors' guidelines and publishing agreements that editors assume that they are considering and publishing original material unless told otherwise (Blancett et al., 1995). This means you will submit your manuscript to only one journal; if it is rejected, you may submit then to another journal.

If you do write highly similar papers for two journals serving different readership, let each editor know of the existence and similarity of the other paper. Make sure that each paper cites the other paper as being under review to avoid any perception of duplicate publication. Doing so will help you avoid what editors perceive as unethical and often illegal behavior. For example, it is illegal to use copyrighted material, even if it is your own, without permission from the copyright holder. Most often the copyright holder is the publisher. Second, authors, even if pleading ignorance of copyright stipulations, should cite other similar manuscripts. And, finally, when submitting your paper, inform editors of all prior public dissemination of similar information. This allows the editor (and later reviewers) to assess your new paper in light of the prior dissemination of some of its content.

To add another dimension to this issue, what should you do if you see almost identical articles in two journals by a colleague and note that neither article refers to the other? Notify the editor? Confront your colleague? Write an anonymous letter to your colleague or to your colleague's boss? Do nothing? Living with the possible implications of any choice is not easy. Not doing anything, however, whether as author, editor, or reader, clutters the literature with already published ideas and impedes the publication of someone else's original contribution.

Another ethical problem area involves entitlement to authorship. A common assumption exists that people listed as authors have made a substantial contribution to the work. However, many times this is not the case. A research director lists as an author a staff nurse who did some peripheral work to reward and motivate the nurse to continue scholarly pursuits. To thank an agency director for support, an author lists the director as an author.

Although it is noble and generous of the real authors to be so thoughtful, honorary authorship can also be viewed as diluting the work of the real author, giving credit where credit is not due, and deceiving the editor and readers. The ethical problem is whether to tell the editor that there are honorary authors.

Another area in which authors and editors make an ethical decision relates to informed consent. Should an author inform the editor, and the editor, in turn, inform readers, that the author of an article about a new and innovative staffing software package consults for the company that produced the software? If the content of the article is peer reviewed, accurate, and seemingly unbiased, does it matter that the author can gain financially?

Legal and ethical decision making is often difficult because there are always two or more interested parties, ethical principles can compete with each other in any given situation, and laws are open to interpretation. A key in making the right decision legally and the best decision ethically when writing and publishing is being informed and having a decision-making framework. I recommend that you read Silva (1990) for a clear decision-making framework and Blancett (1991), Erlen et al. (1997), King et al. (1997), Rennie et al. (1997), White et al. (1998), and Yarbro (1995) for information about ethical issues in writing and publishing.

THE BENEFITS OF PUBLISHING

How often do you use ideas in your management practice that come from nursing books and journals? As you read and think about ideas in the literature, you probably adapt and further develop them so that they work better. However, did you take the final step in developing and refining nursing knowledge—that of disseminating knowledge? Our obligation to contribute to the ongoing development of the profession's body of knowledge implies that we should not only develop, but also share our expertise. Writing for publication is the ideal medium through which nursing knowledge can directly advance professional practice and the health of the nation.

When we publish our ideas, we increase the effectiveness and efficiency with which professional, program, and agency development occur. Publishing your work decreases the amount of time all professionals spend addressing the same problem. As an additional benefit, published authors receive feedback from colleagues on their work and thus further develop their own ideas and approaches.

Writing for publication also brings recognition for your institution. As competition and concern with image increase, having details of an institutional program or event in the national press is a boost for public relations. Institutional visibility through the publications of staff implies a visionary, supportive environment and can be used as a recruiting tool for new staff.

Publications often lead to reader requests for more information. Authors are asked to speak and consult. Agencies are asked to share programs and tools.

Personal satisfaction with seeing one's name in print and claiming an idea as one's own is both a benefit of writing and a motivator to write. In addition, publication is a mark of professional skill and is often a performance evaluation criterion for nurse administrators and expert practitioners. A list of publications on a curriculum vita may assist in job security, promotion, and research funding.

CONCLUSION

Writing for publication can be an exciting process. Knowledge combined with experience and perseverance is a powerful tool for effecting change. Just as it works in your personal and professional life, it can work to make you a published author.

REFERENCES

Allen, P. 2000. Key nursing journals: Characteristics and database coverage. Available at *http://nahrs.library.kent.edu/resource/reports/keyjnls200012.pdf* (accessed May 16, 2003).

American Medical Association. 1998. *Manual of style,* 9th ed. Baltimore, MD: Author.

American Psychological Association. 2001. *Publication manual of the American Psychological Association,* 5th ed. Washington, DC: Author.

Barnum, B. S. 1995. *Writing and getting published: A primer for nurses.* New York: Springer Publishing Co.

Blancett, S. S. 1991. The ethics of writing and publishing. *The Journal of Nursing Administration* 21(5): 31–36.

Blancett, S. S., A. F. Flanagin, and R. K. Young. 1995. Duplicate publication in the nursing literature. *Image: The Journal of Nursing Scholarship* 27(1): 51–56.

Daly, J. M. 2000. *Writer's guide to nursing periodicals.* Thousand Oaks, CA: Sage.

Dunkin, A. M. 1999. Authorship, dissemination of research findings, and related matters. *Applied Nursing Research* 12(2): 101–106.

Erlen, J. A., L. A. Siminoff, S. M. Sereika, and L. B. Sutton. 1997. Multiple authorship: Issues and recommendations. *Journal of Professional Nursing* 13(4): 262–270.

Fondiller, S. H. 1999. *The writer's workbook: Health professionals guide to getting published,* 2nd ed. Sudbury, MA: Jones and Bartlett.

Grant, J. S. 1998. Writing manuscripts for clinical journals. *Home Healthcare Nurse* 16(12): 813–822.

Huth, E. J. 1999. *Writing and publishing in medicine,* 3rd ed. Baltimore, MD: Williams & Wilkins.

Johnson, S. H. Nursing Editors On-Line index. Available at *http//members.aol.com/suzannehj/naed.htm* (accessed January 5, 2003).

King, C. R., D. B. McGuire, A. J. Longman, and R. M. Carroll-Johnson. 1997. Peer review, authorship, ethics, and conflict of interest. *Image: Journal of Nursing Scholarship* 29(2): 159–162.

Mateo, M. A., S. P. Smith, and D. L. Flarey, D. L. 1999. Disseminating research: The medium and the message. In M. A. Mateo and K. Kirchhoff, eds. *Conducting and using nursing research in the clinical setting,* 2nd ed. Baltimore, MD: Williams & Wilkins, pp. 339–352.

McConnell, E. A. 1995. Journal and publishing characteristics for 42 nursing publications outside the United States. *Image: The Journal of Nursing Scholarship* 27(3): 225–229.

Northam, S., M. Trubenbach, and L. Bentov, L. 2000. Nursing journal survey: Information to help you publish. *Nurse Educator* 25(4): 227–236.

Oermann, M. H. (2001). *Writing for publication in nursing.* Philadelphia, PA: Lippincott.

Rennie, D., V. Yank, and L. Emanuel. 1997. When authorship fails: A proposal to make contributors accountable. *Journal of the American Medical Association,* 278(7): 579–585.

Rico, G. L. 2001. *Writing the natural way,* 2nd ed. Available at *http://www.gabrielerico.com/Main/AboutGabriele Rico.htm* (accessed May 15, 2003).

Rosenberg, H., and M. Lah. 1985. Tackling writer's block: Suggestions for self-modification. *The Journal of Nursing Administration* 15(3): 40–42.

Sheridan, D. R., and D. L. Dowdney. 1997. *How to write and publish articles in nursing,* 2nd ed. New York: Springer.

Silva, M. C. 1990. *Ethical decision making in nursing administration.* Norwalk, CT: Appleton & Lange.

Tornquist, E. M. 1999. *From proposal to publication: An informal guide to writing about nursing research.* Boston: Pearson Addison Wesley.

Valente, S. M. 2003. Creative ways to improve practice: The research journal club. *Home Healthcare Nurse* 21(4): 271–274.

White, A. H., N. A. Coudret, and C. S. Goodwin. 1998. From authorship to contributorship: Promoting integrity in research publication. *Nurse Educator* 23(6): 26–32.

Yarbro, C. H. 1995. Duplicate publication: Guidelines for nurse authors and editors. *Image: Journal of Nursing Scholarship* 27(1): 57.

Zilm, G. 1998. *The SMART way: An introduction to writing for nurses.* Toronto, Ontario, Canada: Saunders.

CHAPTER 62

Student Placements in Home Health Care Agencies: Boost or Barrier to Quality Patient Care?

Ida M. Androwich and Pamela A. Andresen

The placement of students in a home health care agency has the potential to both help and hinder the work of the agency. In this chapter, these boosts and barriers to quality patient care are addressed by two nursing faculty members who have taught community health administration courses using home health care agencies as clinical sites (Androwich and Andresen, 1986). One faculty member was formerly the director of a Medicare-certified home health care agency involved with student placements and currently teaches graduate students in home health care administration. The other faculty member is the current director of Loyola University's faculty nurse-managed center and has extensive experience as a staff member in a large visiting nurse association.

BOOSTS

A major benefit of student placements is the collaboration or marriage between education and service. Motivators for this union include the need for home care for the sick and the desire for faculty-student shared clinical practice. Opportunities for sharing of information and expertise between these disciplines are great. Nurse educators offer clinical expertise, research skills, a desire to test new models of nursing practice, and students who can make reimbursable home visits and assist with specific projects. The home care agency brings to the marriage an available clinical site, a population of patients and qualified nursing personnel and support services.

A second benefit to the agency is increased staff support. A typical group of 8 to 10 students is able to visit at least that number of patients during a clinical day. Not only can this produce revenue for the agency, but it also conserves staff resources, allowing staff to pursue other endeavors. For example, having students make visits can permit staff to complete outstanding paperwork or to attend continuing education programs without an accompanying drop in the agency's productivity.

Depending on the type or level of student (e.g., associate degree [AD], bachelors of science in nursing [BSN], or graduate student) and the length of the clinical experience, creative use of students can provide assistance to the agency in many other ways besides making visits. Home health agencies frequently receive requests to participate in community programs (e.g., health fairs, blood pressure screenings, and health education for community groups) that do not generate revenue for the agency but enhance good community relations. Students can be used to help meet these requests. This type of contact with community groups provides students with a well-rounded view of different roles in community health nursing.

Medicare provides coverage for medically ordered services; however, students may be used

810

to fill the Medigap by providing additional visits for nonreimbursable services. For example, the health promotion needs of other family members may be addressed. Chronically ill adults could be visited by students after discharge by the primary nurse for reimbursable visits. The agency might also accept referrals for nonreimbursable visits that would otherwise be refused. These are just a few examples of how students can be used to expand the agency's services without placing further demands on the staff.

Harris (1984) describes two outcomes of student experiences that have the advantage of being mutually beneficial to both learner and service agency. Graduate students can provide assistance with several types of administrative projects, such as completing needs assessments and quality review audits, developing management information systems, and conducting program planning and evaluation of existing programs. Graduate students in clinical specialty programs can also assist with staff inservices and serve as consultants to the staff.

Staff usually benefit from student placements. They are given an opportunity to serve as role models for students and are typically rewarded with gratitude and admiration from those students. Students are impressed by the independent judgment and high degree of professionalism demonstrated by the community health nurse. Staff may feel renewed by exposure to student enthusiasm.

The nursing care plan for a patient cared for by a student is developed by the student in conjunction with the primary nurse and the instructor, either a masters or doctorally prepared expert in community health nursing. Thus the patient then receives the benefit of staff, faculty, and student input with a fully comprehensive plan of care as a result.

Productivity, in terms of the number of patients whom students visit per day, is typically not a priority of nursing education. Therefore, a student who visits only one or two patients per day has much more time to spend preparing for the visit as well as more actual visit time compared to a staff nurse visiting five or more patients on the same day. This is another benefit to the client and can be particularly helpful with cases requiring lengthy teaching such as new diabetics.

After students have completed their clinical experiences, home health administrators may find that the best and most enthusiastic of the students return as employees after graduation. This can facilitate not only recruitment, but also retention, because the student and staff already know each other. Expectations of the staff nurse role should be clearer to these new graduates because they are familiar with the agency and orientation time is typically decreased.

Before graduation, students may be able to work temporarily as home health aides, offering flexible staffing in this area. The Loyola University Community Nursing Center uses students quite successfully for staffing periods of the year when clinical courses are not in session. Registered nurse (RN-BSN) completion students or graduate students looking for part-time or flexible hours may be hired on a fee-for-visit basis. Many of these students work in or have had experience in critical care settings and are qualified to deliver high-technology care in the home. Again, because they are familiar with the agency, the quality of their work will probably be superior to that of a nurse hired on a contract basis who has never been oriented to the agency.

Beyond the contact with students and faculty during clinical experiences, the home health administrator and agency staff can benefit from their relationship with a university and its school of nursing. Some degree of prestige is associated with having a university affiliation. Administrators are frequently offered clinical faculty appointments and are often invited to participate in university programs and continuing education. Formal or informal consultations may be provided to the agency by faculty. An administrator can also develop working relations with faculty from other departments within the university (e.g., social work, psychology, medicine, and business). Unique experiences can be offered to students from these departments that fulfill their objectives as well as meet the needs of the agency. Graduate students from Loyola's School of Business provided the university's nurse-managed center with extensive consultation in the area of marketing. Students from the psychology department have visited caregivers of elderly family members in need of support. These are just two examples of the many possibilities available to an agency affiliated with a university.

BARRIERS

Despite the many benefits, there are drawbacks to student placements. Perhaps the greatest barrier is presented by the increasing complexity of technology delivered in the home. Staff nurses with or without critical care backgrounds often require extensive training in technical areas (e.g., intravenous therapy, Total Parenteral Nutrition) in order to adapt these procedures to the home environment. Students and faculty without recent acute care experience may be unprepared to provide high-tech care in the home. Therefore, great consideration needs to be given to the individual nurse's skills when assigning a technically complex patient. RN students enrolled in BSN completion programs are not consistently prepared in these technical skills, and faculty may rely on one or two students to visit patients requiring, for example, venipuncture. Developing a caseload for a group of traditional undergraduate students can become an overwhelming task for both the instructor and nursing supervisor. Yet, the pairing of students with staff nurses for all home visits may be an unacceptable solution from the viewpoint of both the instructor and the home care supervisor. From the instructor's perspective, the student placed in the role of follower is unlikely to develop the case management skills necessary to meet the objectives of his or her community health nursing practicum. From the agency perspective, the decrease in productivity may be unacceptable because the time demands this arrangement places on the staff nurse may be extraordinary.

Although an adequate caseload must be available for student experiences, a second issue deals with orienting students to written documentation. If visits are not documented correctly, denials for Medicare reimbursement may follow. With new regulations in the recent Health Insurance Portability and Accountability Act (HIPAA) of 1996, both the agency staff and the faculty need to provide adequate oversight and education to students to ensure compliance with agency policies. For example, a faculty member may request that students chart in-depth information on a family's psychosocial status. This could lead Medicare reviewers to believe that the patient is being followed primarily for nonreimbursable mental health needs rather than for an unstable physical condition. As previously mentioned, student visits have the potential to generate revenue for the agency. Although the instructor should review student documentation, the home health administrator must determine who within the agency, such as the primary nurse, will also review student charting.

In addition to communicating through written documentation, many agencies have automated documentation systems. The type and amount of documentation in the computer-based patient record that students complete needs to be negotiated. In any event, students need to have a clear mechanism for communicating pertinent information to the primary nurse and physician. The danger of misinterpretation of patient data arises if information is relayed through a circuitous route. For example, communication may flow from the student (who actually made the visit and assessed the client) to his or her instructor to the nursing supervisor to the primary nurse to the physician, with each step increasing the opportunity for miscommunication. This is not an unlikely scenario, because a student's clinical hours often do not coincide with a primary nurse's time in the office. Further communication gaps may occur when students are not present in the agency on days when support staff, such as the rehabilitation team, are available.

Although the strengths and goals of nursing education and service complement one another, they may also create conflict. For example, a faculty member may wish to use the agency as a site for testing a new model for nursing practice. The time required to orient staff to assist with the research may conflict with the administrator's need for the nurses to maintain a certain level of productivity. Communications may be another pitfall. Community health nurses have long valued team conferences as a means for receiving input when managing caseloads. Students are continuously in a team environment that includes their instructor and other students. A student seeking advice from diverse sources may find it difficult to develop one comprehensive nursing care plan with clear long-term goals for the patient.

A quality of care concern is discontinuity. A student bringing much time and energy to a case may also create discontinuity because the patient wonders what has happened to his or her "regular" nurse whom he or she knows and trusts. Patient visits must also fit into the student's schedule because students are rarely in an agency 5 days per week. Students are also present in an agency for a limited number of weeks. A student may have just established a good working relationship with a client or family when it is time for the student to move on to his or her next clinical experience. Discontinuity may also occur when students are not present in the agency on days when support staff, such as the rehabilitation team, are available.

Environmental or space problems may be a minor but constant irritant. It is obviously not cost-effective for an agency to maintain more space than needed, so that, when a team of 10 or 11 students and their instructor is added to a space meant to house 11 fewer people, crowding occurs.

GRADUATE STUDENTS

The previous boosts and barriers apply to both undergraduate and graduate students from a va-

riety of disciplines. Certain differences are considered when one is planning for a graduate student experience.

The graduate student experience is different from the undergraduate experience in two main ways. First, it is usually organized on a one to-one basis with a specified preceptor. The preceptor, student, and faculty work jointly to outline the practicum parameters. Graduate students are usually at the agency for longer periods of time and can assume leadership roles in specified projects. The relationship that develops between the preceptor and the student will have a major impact on the satisfactory outcome of the experience.

Preceptor Considerations

The preceptor serves as role model, facilitator, supervisor, educator, resource, and sounding board for the student. It is critical that the preceptor be committed to the experience and be aware at the outset that having a student will require additional time and reorganization of daily schedules. Different preceptors have successfully used a number of strategies to integrate the student's experience into the agency routine. Depending on the time parameters of the practicum, a preceptor might lay out his or her calendar for the student to select the most interesting and useful meetings to attend. One preceptor had the student begin each day as she did, by sorting the in basket and discussing plans to address each item on the calendar. Wide variation exists in the techniques that can be used to promote the student's learning.

Lettow (1991), a graduate student in home health care, cited three aspects of the student–preceptor relationship: (1) as a contract, with formal structure, guidelines, concrete objectives, mutually developed outcomes, and the preceptor as the senior member of the relationship; (2) as a partnership, with mutual benefits and respect for the experiences and position of the other; and (3) as a commitment, with respect for the other's time and efforts, self-direction on the student's part, and support on the preceptor's part.

The student–preceptor relationship develops as trust is established. A major ingredient in this trust building is the assurance of confidentiality. Strict confidentiality is stressed with the students as an essential component of the practicum and one that may not be violated. It is helpful to discuss this issue during the first joint meeting with the preceptor, student, and faculty present. On occasion, a potential conflict may develop when the student is employed at a competing agency. If this type of potential conflict is present, these competing interests should be addressed and managed with either an alternative placement for the student or clear guidelines as to what information is to be treated with confidentiality. In our experience, students at this level have uniformly responded with noteworthy sensitivity and discretion.

Another issue concerning preceptors is related to the evaluation of the experience. It is important for the preceptor to be clear as to the type and weight of any expected student evaluation. Thoughtful analysis of the student's strengths as well as areas and skill sets to enhance can be extremely useful to the student. A strategy that has proved successful is for the student and preceptor to discuss their perceptions of the experience before the final faculty conference. Most preceptors elicit student feedback about components of the practicum and the types of support that were most beneficial to the student. This allows for an open sharing without concern for the valuative nature of grading considerations to interfere.

Setting Objectives

The second major characteristic distinguishing graduate from undergraduate students involves the type of objectives and projects to be accomplished. Whereas the undergraduate students are concerned with visiting patients, the graduate student will be more apt to work on broader projects or programs. Preceptors and faculty must work together to assist the student in developing achievable goals.

The worst projects are those that are vague, amorphous, and linked to others' schedules and approvals with little opportunity for the student to exercise independent decision making. Frequently the student may arrive with the idea that he or she would like to do something in the area of quality improvement and monitoring (QI). If the agency has struggled for the last 10 years with developing continuous quality improvement (CQI) and has no more than a minimum QI program, help the student accept that such a program will not be achieved in the next 3 months. It may be possible to accommodate the student's interests by carving out a discrete piece of QI, or it may be best to have alternative suggestions.

The best projects are small, limited in scope, self-contained, allow the student to work independently within broad parameters, and yield a tangible result. In addition to the projects mentioned earlier, some that have been successful for both the student and the agency are as follows:

- assessing needs for health care among retirement home dwellers
- developing an orientation/preceptor's book for new agency staff
- outlining a marketing plan for a new program
- assessing the reliability and validity of a newly developed QA (quality assessment) audit tool
- analyzing the cost-benefit of a proposed hospice program
- assessing mature nurses' employment needs
- developing specific policy (e.g., do not resuscitate orders, home health aide program)
- developing a pro forma business plan for opening a branch office

Numerous others exist, and one that blends agency needs with student goals usually can be found.

It is important that the student be involved in a project that is perceived to be worthwhile; that is, not artificially created as busywork for the student. One way to achieve this is to discuss how the project output will be used by the agency. This will also ensure that the information the student produces is in a practical form.

RECOMMENDATIONS

From these just-listed advantages and disadvantages, a set of recommendations has been developed. First, faculty need to be oriented to the agency before the student begins the experience. It is recommended that faculty not only be oriented to the organizational structure, policies, and documentation, but also be given the opportunity to make joint home visits with a staff nurse. The administrator and educator should jointly develop a plan for orienting students in these areas, with each party's role in the orientation being clearly spelled out. Some agencies may use faculty in practice roles or to serve on various agency committees, such as the audit committee or the professional advisory committee. Faculty who are knowledgeable concerning the mechanics of operations and reimbursement benefit the agency by providing improved student guidance and decreasing the amount of time staff need to spend with students and faculty.

Orientation is only one area for which accountability must be determined. Accountability for documentation (other than progress notes), Medicare form completion, communication with support services and the physician, and case finding are just a few of the many points to be addressed. From the start, a plan should be developed for evaluation of the experience, including feedback from students, faculty, nursing staff, and administration.

Planning for the student experience must begin far in advance of its start. It is standard practice in universities to solidify contractual arrangements during the spring semester preceding a fall semester experience. During the summer months, faculty should meet with administrators to discuss the needs of each party in terms of case finding, space, the orientation process, and so forth.

Contractual Arrangements

It is to each party's advantage to have respective responsibilities clearly delineated in the form of a contract or letter of agreement. In many cases, this will be initiated (and required) by the school or university. Typically this contract is negotiated to outline each party's areas of accountability—the agency assuming primary responsibility for the quality of patient care and education assuming primary accountability for student supervision. In *Bottorf v. Waltz*, the Pennsylvania superior court ruled that teachers have three main areas of responsibility to their students (Van Biervliet and Sheldon-Wildgen, 1981):

1. to provide adequate supervision
2. to exercise good judgment
3. to provide proper instruction, especially when potentially hazardous conditions exist

Implications of this ruling include the need for agency staff to assist faculty in meeting their responsibilities in this area. Often agency staff are in a better position to evaluate client needs and characteristics and can guide faculty in the selection of appropriate clients for the student's level of skill.

Other components of a contract or letter of agreement are the following:

- a statement as to the scope and duration of the agreement
- a nondiscriminatory statement
- liability and insurance documentation
- the agency's responsibilities (e.g., ultimate responsibility for patient care; provision of general orientation to aspects of the agency, policies, and procedures; emergency care, if needed; and space for faculty and students)

- the educational institution's responsibilities (e.g., providing an educational program meeting accrediting body standards; providing appropriate, qualified registered nurse faculty as a specified faculty–student ratio and designated availability, such as on-call, etc.; informing the agency of the student and program educational objectives; assuring that the students meet identified health and other requirements; and participating in joint evaluation)
- the appropriate privacy requirements to meet the HIPAA legislation

Even with extensive planning, unanticipated problems are certain to occur. Not only must communication be open, but also the channels of communication must be determined ahead of time. Considerations include whether students should communicate patient problems, issues, or questions directly to the staff nurse or to their instructor first. The second route may prevent the constant bombardment of staff with diverse student questions. A plan for reporting off at the end of the day should be developed for both students and faculty. Faculty should be advised of agency policy and preferences for reporting problems and communicating concerns.

Finally, assume that students will create a space problem to some degree. Even with unlimited space, students are often perceived as invading the staff's territory. During planning sessions, the administrator and educator should designate which space and telephones are available for student use.

COST-BENEFIT CONSIDERATIONS

It is extremely difficult to generalize a cost-benefit analysis from agency to agency because there are so many factors that are unique to each agency yet must be considered in an assessment of costs and benefits of student experiences. In a health care environment that is rapidly moving to managed care, individual agency incentives and ability to provide student placements will vary.

The first of these variables is the organizational structure and environment of the agency. At what stage of development is the agency? The stress of accommodating student placements in a new agency may prove to be overwhelming in an agency where systems have yet to become smooth. How adequate is staffing? Is there an individual with primary responsibility for coordinating student–faculty communications? An individual designated in this role can assist in the integration of students into the agency routine. Can provisions for alternative staff activities be made while students are in the agency? Unless the agency is seriously understaffed (not a desirable situation with students), staff will receive the same salary irrespective of student visits, and the total agency visits will not increase. If staff can be scheduled for continuing education/staff development, to use time as a "breather" and to catch up on documentation, or to assist with program/policy and procedure development or to audit records in the agency, the time can be maximized. The amount of documentation that is expected of students will also influence the time that staff spend with student cases. Does the agency desire or need the public relations exposure of a university affiliation? Is the potential for staff recruitment from student populations present?

A second major consideration is the type of faculty and students. Generic, RN-BSN completion, or graduate students may make a difference in the reimbursement. Medicare will reimburse for all nursing student visits, but other third-party payers may require registered nurse licensure for reimbursement; thus only RN or graduate students would be reimbursed for visits. The faculty supervisor's familiarity with the agency and its clients and his or her general proficiency and experience in home care will influence the time required by the agency in orientation and assistance with documentation and care planning. Faculty who can assume the bulk of the student's orientation and can oversee charting and client care services will reduce the amount of time spent by agency personnel in these activities.

Consequently no single answer exists for every agency, or even for the same agency at different time periods. Overall, the consensus among the agencies with whom we have had the good fortune to be affiliated is that the boosts and benefits of having students in the environment far outweigh the barriers.

REFERENCES

Androwich, I. M., and P. A. Andresen. 1986, May. *Student placements in home health care agencies: Boost or barrier to quality patient care?* Poster presented at the Second National Symposium of Home Health Nursing, Ann Arbor, MI.

Harris, M. 1984. Student programs benefit nursing service agencies. *Home Health Care Nurse* 2: 34–35.

Lettow, J. 1991, February. *The preceptor role in home health care administration: The student perspective.* Paper presented at the University of Illinois, College of Nursing, Chicago, IL.

Van Biervliet, A., and J. Sheldon-Wildgen. 1981. *Liability issues in community-based programs.* Baltimore, MD: Brooks.

BIBLIOGRAPHY

Androwich, I. M. 1989. Creative utilization of staff. In L. Benefield (ed.), *Home health care management* (pp. 180–199). Englewood Cliffs, NJ: Prentice Hall.

Hackbarth, D., and I. M. Androwich. 1989. Graduate nursing education for leadership in home care. *Caring* 2: 6–11.

CHAPTER 63

A Student Program in One Home Health Agency

Marilyn D. Harris

The Abington Memorial Hospital Home Care (AMHHC) has an active student program. Each year educational facilities place students with the AMHHC for observational or practical experience variable periods of time each year.

The AMHHC offers educational opportunities for diploma, baccalaureate, graduate, and doctoral student nurses; medical students and residents; and health care administration students. The AMHHC has developed manuals that include a statement of the philosophy and objectives for the overall program (Exhibit 63–1). Goals and objectives for each level of the student programs also exist. The educational facilities are asked to submit program objectives and curriculum outlines to the agency. Affiliation agreements are approved and signed by both the AMHHC and the school. These are reviewed annually and renewed on a periodic basis. A new affiliation agreement was written to comply with the Health Insurance Portability and Accountability Act (HIPAA) of 1996 that became effective April 14, 2003 (Exhibit 63–2). The contract lists the responsibilities of both organizations, the number of students to be assigned to the agency at any one time, and other pertinent terms of the affiliation. The AMHHC has an interdepartmental arrangement with the Abington Memorial Hospital (AMH) Dixon School of Nursing (Exhibit 63–3).

In some instances, guidelines for cooperative relationships between the clinical setting and the graduate program (Exhibit 63–4) are shared and agreed upon. These guidelines include information related to agency selection, qualifications of the preceptor, functions of the agency preceptor, expectations of the graduate students, responsibilities of the faculty preceptor, and the placement process.

The contractual relationships are the responsibility of the administrator at the AMHHC. The determination of the number of educational institutions and students that will affiliate at the AMHHC each year is the responsibility of the Education and Research Coordinator (ERC). The ERC makes this decision in consultation with the director of professional services and the clinical supervisors. The ERC is responsible for orientation of the faculty and students to the AMHHC each semester.

Each student who affiliates with the AMHHC is required to sign a Student Pledge and Confidentiality Statement (Exhibit 63–5). Patients must give written permission for home visits by the students. A Client Authorization for Home Visit form (Exhibit 63–6) is obtained by the nurse or therapist prior to the joint or independent visit.

Evaluation of the student placements is an integral part of the total annual evaluation process at the AMHHC. As part of the evaluation process, students complete, and the schools forward to the AMHHC, evaluations of the experience.

These evaluations are shared with the staff. In general, the students, patients, and staff indicate

Exhibit 63–1 Student Program

PHILOSOPHY

We, the AMHHC, believe that our student program is a vital component of our home health and hospice program and is mutually beneficial to both the student and our agency. Furthermore, we believe that it is a valuable experience because it provides the student with a broader perspective of the health care system by incorporating a uniquely different health component. It also provides an opportunity for practical application of the theory gained through an academic program. Finally, we value highly the information exchange that occurs as a result of our experiences with the students.

PURPOSE

The primary purpose of the program is to provide the student with an opportunity to augment his or her perspective of the health needs of the aggregate population as well as of the client and family in the community setting. The program also allows the student an opportunity to gain a better understanding of the role of a community nursing organization in meeting these health needs.

OBJECTIVE

The individual student experiences are based upon and consistent with the course objectives of the various academic institutions that participate in our program.

Origin: 2/83
Revised: 6/93
Revised: 6/03

Source: Reported with permission of Abington Memorial Hospital Home Care, Willow Grove, Pennsylvania.

---

that student affiliations are a valuable aspect of the total AMHHC service.

CONSIDERATIONS FOR THE ADMINISTRATOR

The changing health care climate presents several areas of consideration for the home health agency administrator in relationship to student programs. Staff productivity is one of these areas. Students do affect the productivity of staff. Even though a representative from the educational institution is on site, staff are involved in student orientation to both agency and patients. Having someone accompany the nurse on home visits on a regular basis slows down the nurse. The Medicare regulations allow for student nurses to provide billable services under a general supervision provision (U.S. Department of Health and Human Services, 1989). Physical therapy students must work under the direct supervision of the licensed therapist. Once again, this requires the time of the licensed therapist in the home and office.

Documentation is another area for consideration. Documentation must be reviewed to determine that it meets agency standards, professional standards, and reimbursement standards. Agencies cannot afford to have visits denied on a medical or technical basis. Therefore, additional supervisory time and expenses are incurred to review and verify that all student documentation meets established criteria.

Another consideration regarding documentation at the AMHHC is related to the computerized clinical documentation system. Students do not have access to laptop computers for documentation; therefore, all manual documentation completed by the students has to be input into the computerized system by the AMHHC staff.

Exhibit 63–2 Affiliation Agreement

Abington Memorial Hospital Home Care

Affiliation Agreement

THIS AGREEMENT, made this tenth day of April 2003, by and between Abington Memorial Hospital Home Care (AMHC), a corporation organized and existing under the laws of the State of Pennsylvania ("the Agency") and XYZ University, an educational institution organized and operated under the Commonwealth of Pennsylvania, (University).

WITNESSETH

WHEREAS, it is of mutual interest and advantage to the parties that students enrolled in the University's College of Nursing be given the opportunity and the benefit of the Agency's clinical facilities for experience in the practice of nursing.

NOW, THEREFORE, in consideration of the good and valuable consideration each to the other provided for hereunder and intending to be legally bound hereby, the parties agree as follows:

1. Provision of Clinical Facilities and Instruction. The Agency agrees to provide clinical facilities and nursing experience for University students and the University agrees to provide instruction, guidance and evaluation of its nursing students by University instructors all in accordance with the terms and conditions of this Agreement. Additional particulars with respect to this agreement, if any, are set forth on Exhibit A attached hereto and made a part hereof.

2. Responsibility of Agency. The Agency shall be responsible for:

   a) supplying, to the best of its ability, to University students and faculty, emergency medical care or, if advisable, a prompt referral to the nearest appropriate medical facility in any emergency requiring medical attention.
   b) providing conference room space for University nursing students and faculty when required.
   c) serving as a clinical laboratory in which University nursing students may be assigned for educational experience.

---

continues

Exhibit 63–2 continued

d) providing sufficient staff time for planning with the University faculty for student learning experiences.

e) providing sufficient staff time for the orientation of the University faculty to the Agency's facilities and policies.

3. <u>Responsibilities of University</u>. The University shall be responsible for:

a) Maintaining a record of complete physical examination of each student inclusive of PPD and immunization records. Records to be keep on file at University and available to Agency upon request.

b) Providing a copy of professional license (when applicable) in advance of the clinical placement.

c) Have available upon request to agency a criminal background check (for students visiting patients without direct supervision).

d) Providing evidence that the student is certified in Basic Cardiac Life Support.

e) Informing its students of their obligations to abide by the general policies of the Agency regarding patient care.

f) Carrying malpractice liability coverage at state mandated levels, which covers students during course related clinical experience in an agency in amounts to be determined by the University. University shall provide proof of such insurance at request of Agency and must notify Agency in the event of lapse or change in policy.

g) Notifying the Agency of the approximate number of students who will be having clinical experience in nursing and the times the students will report.

h) Assume any and all obligations imposed by Workmen's Compensation Law of Pennsylvania, and carry necessary Workman's Compensation Insurance, insofar as a member of its faculty may sustain injury or disability arising out of or in the course of, instruction by a member of its faculty.

4. <u>Patient Care</u>. The University will assume the responsibility for the education of the students in the specified clinical areas as described in paragraph 1 herein, provided, however, that ultimate responsibility for patient care remains with the Agency staff.

5. <u>Withdrawal of</u>

a) The University will withdraw upon recommendation of the Agency any student who fails to abide by the regulations respecting student personnel or

continues

Exhibit 63–2 continued

who otherwise fails to fulfill the personnel and/or professional requirements of the Agency.

b) In the event that, in the University's judgment, a change in the learning environment of the Agency should occur that would be disruptive, or that might interfere with the achievement of the objectives of the clinical experience, the University, after consultation with the Agency, may withdraw students from the Agency.

6. Coordinating Committee. The parties shall form a coordinating committee of University and Agency representatives to meet when necessary to discuss problems and plans and to insure the effective functioning of both institutions with regard to the matters covered by this Agreement.

7. Non-Discrimination. The University and Agency agree that discrimination against any student or faculty member on the basis of race, religion, national origin, age, handicap or sex will not be tolerated. Each of the parties affirms that its policies prohibit discrimination.

8. Termination. Either party may terminate this Agreement upon six months notice in writing to the other, or immediately upon written notice of the other party's material default of an obligation under this Agreement.

9. Notices. All notices of default or other communications regarding contract renewals or terminations required or permitted under this Agreement shall be deemed duly given if in writing and delivered personally or sent by registered or certified mail, return receipt requested, first-class postage prepaid,

(A) If to the Agency, to the Executive Director, 2510 Maryland Road, Suite 250, Willow Grove, PA 19090. and
(B) If to the University, to Dean, Department of Nursing, _____
_____ .

Notices will be deemed given on the date of delivery (in the case of personal delivery) or at the time of mailing (in the case of mail delivery). Either party may change its notice address by giving the other party notice of such change.

10. Renewal. This Agreement may be renewed for additional academic year or years upon the mutual agreement of authorized representatives of the Agency and the University. The Agency and the University shall use their best efforts to monitor their needs over the term of this Agreement in order to facilitate timely coordination of renewals or extensions of this Agreement.

11. Indemnification.

continues

Exhibit 63–2 continued

a) The Agency agrees to indemnify and hold the University harmless from any claims, demands, causes of action or damages (including reasonable attorney fees) arising out of, or resulting from, the activities of its employees, staff and agents at the Agency which are related to this agreement.

b) The University agrees to indemnify and hold the Agency harmless from any claims, demands, causes of action or damages (including reasonable attorney fees) arising out of, or resulting from, the activities of its faculty members and students at the Agency which are related to this Agreement.

11. <u>Governing Law</u>. This Agreement shall be construed and enforced in accordance with the laws of the Commonwealth of Pennsylvania. Any action brought under this Agreement shall be brought in the courts of the Commonwealth of Pennsylvania.

BUSINESS ASSOCIATE PROVISION

This section sets forth the terms and conditions pursuant to which Protected Health Information ("PHI") that is provided by, or created or received by, UNIVERSITY (BUSINESS ASSOCIATE) from or on behalf of HOSPITAL, will be handled between both parties and with third parties. The parties mutually agree to incorporate the following into the Master Agreement and that all other provisions of the Master Agreement will remain unchanged unless specifically addressed below:

1. DEFINITION:

PHI – Protected Health Information. Information that relates to a person's physical or mental health, the provision of health care, or the payment of health care that identifies, or could be used to identify, the person who is the subject of the information and that is created or received by HOSPITAL or by another person or entity on behalf of HOSPITAL. Information that is de-identified does not constitute PHI and is not subject to the terms of this Agreement.

2. PERMITTED USES AND DISCLOSURES OF PROTECTED HEALTH INFORMATION

a) <u>Services</u>. Pursuant to the Master Agreement, BUSINESS ASSOCIATE provides Services for Hospital that involves the use or disclosure of PHI. Except as otherwise specified herein, BUSINESS ASSOCIATE may make any and all uses of PHI necessary to perform its obligations under the Master Agreement. All other uses not authorized by this Agreement are prohibited.

a) <u>Business Activities of BUSINESS ASSOCIATE</u>. The BUSINESS ASSOCIATE may use PHI in its possession for its proper management and administration and to fulfill any present or future legal responsibilities of the BUSINESS ASSOCIATE provided that such uses are permitted under state and federal confidentiality laws.

continues

Exhibit 63–2 continued

3. OBLIGATIONS OF BUSINESS ASSOCIATE

BUSINESS ASSOCIATE hereby agrees to:

a) Use and disclose PHI only as necessary for the provision of Services under the Master Agreement, unless otherwise required by law. BUSINESS ASSOCIATE may not use or disclose PHI in such a manner that a similar use by HOSPITAL would violate the HHS regulation entitled "Standards for Privacy of Individually Identifiable Health Information" at 45 CFR Parts 160 and 164.

b) Obtain written Agreements with any person or entity to whom it delegates a function, activity, or service for which it is responsible for under this contract that provides for the same terms and conditions on the use and disclosure of PHI that apply to the BUSINESS ASSOCIATE in this Agreement. Evidence of such Agreements shall be provided to HOSPITAL.

c) Timely provide PHI to HOSPITAL to accommodate an individual requestor, if the PHI requested relates to that individual unless access to such information is restricted by law.

d) Make PHI available to HOSPITAL for amendment of such information upon request of HOSPITAL and to incorporate any such amendment into the PHI controlled by BUSINESS ASSOCIATE.

e) Upon prior written request, make available during normal business hours at BUSINESS ASSOCIATE's offices all records, books, agreements, policies and procedures relating to the use and/or disclosure of PHI to the HOSPITAL within 30 days for purposes of enabling the HOSPITAL to determine the BUSINESS ASSOCIATE's compliance with the terms of this Agreement.

f) Provide any information requested by HOSPITAL within 45 days that is required to make a proper accounting of the disclosures of an individual's PHI.

g) Make its books and records available to the Secretary of HHS for purposes of determining HOSPITAL compliance with the HHS regulation entitled "Standards for Privacy of Individually Identifiable Health Information" at 45 CFR Parts 160 and 164 or for any other purpose required by law.

h) Employ commercially reasonable safeguards designed to protect PHI from disclosures that are not authorized by this section. BUSINESS ASSOCIATE agrees to report to HOSPITAL, in writing, any use and/or disclosure of PHI that it reasonably believes is not permitted or required by this Agreement of which BUSINESS ASSOCIATE becomes aware within 10 days of the

continues

Exhibit 63–2 continued

BUSINESS ASSOCIATE's discovery of such unauthorized use and/or disclosure.

i) Return or destroy all PHI in its possession at the termination of the contract, but if such return or destruction is not feasible, the privacy protections contained in this section continues for as long as the BUSINESS ASSOCIATE retains the information.

j) Develop policies and procedures to provide for appropriate discipline for employees of BUSINESS ASSOCIATE that violates the provisions of this Agreement.

4. OBLIGATIONS OF HOSPITAL

HOSPITAL hereby agrees to:

a) Inform BUSINESS ASSOCIATE of any relevant changes in the form of notice of privacy practices that HOSPITAL provides to individuals and provide the BUSINESS ASSOCIATE with a copy of said notice.

b) Inform BUSINESS ASSOCIATE of any relevant changes in, or withdrawal of, the consent or authorization provided to HOSPITAL by individuals pursuant to 45 CFR §§ 164.506 or 164.508.

5. TERM AND TERMINATION

a) Term. This Agreement shall become effective on the Effective Date and shall continue in effect until all obligations of the Parties have been met, unless terminated as provided in this Section 5. In addition, certain provisions and requirements of this Agreement shall survive its expiration or other termination in accordance with Section 7 herein.

b) Termination by Hospital. If the BUSINESS ASSOCIATE has breached any material term of this section, HOSPITAL will terminate this Agreement and the Master Agreement, if feasible, thirty days after the breach becomes known, if the breach is not cured during this thirty day period. If such a termination would be unreasonably burdensome to HOSPITAL, HOSPITAL must notify the Secretary of Health and Human Services about such breach.

c) Termination by Either Party. If the HOSPITAL, at its sole discretion, determines that a modification to this Agreement is required due to a change in any law, regulation or guidance or a reasonable change in interpretation of any law, regulation or guidance and the parties cannot agree to the execution of an amendment representing such modification within sixty (60) days of such notification by Hospital, either party may terminate this Agreement and the Master Agreement with thirty (30) days notice.

continues

Exhibit 63–2 continued

d) <u>Automatic Termination</u>. This Agreement will automatically terminate without any further action of the Parties upon the termination or expiration of the Master Agreement.

6. INDEMNIFICATION

BUSINESS ASSOCIATE hereby agrees to indemnify, hold harmless (including reasonable attorney's fees) HOSPITAL, and any officer, employee or agent thereof, (each of the foregoing being hereinafter referred to individually as "Indemnified Party") against all claims of, and liability to, third parties, including but not limited to those of Federal, State and Local governments, (other than liability solely and entirely the fault of the Indemnified Party) arising from or in connection with BUSINESS ASSOCIATE or its officers, employees or agents, using or disclosing PHI in any way that violates the terms of this section. BUSINESS ASSOCIATE obligation to indemnify, hold harmless and defend any Indemnified Party shall survive the expiration or termination of this Agreement by either party for any reason.

7. MISCELLANEOUS

a) <u>Survival</u>. The respective rights and obligations of BUSINESS ASSOCIATE and HOSPITAL solely with respect to PHI that BUSINESS ASSOCIATE retains in accordance with Section 3(i) because it is not feasible to return or destroy such PHI shall survive the termination of this Agreement indefinitely.

b) <u>Amendments; Waiver</u>. This Agreement may not be modified, nor shall any provision hereof be waived or amended, except in writing duly signed by authorized representatives of the Parties. A waiver with respect to one event shall not be construed as continuing, or as a bar to or waiver of any right or remedy as to subsequent events.

c) <u>No Third Party Beneficiaries</u>. Nothing express or implied in this Agreement is intended, nor shall anything herein confer, upon any person other than the Parties and the respective successors or assigns of the Parties, any rights, remedies, obligations, or liabilities whatsoever.

continues

Exhibit 63–2 continued

IN WITNESS WHEREOF, the parties have executed this Agreement on the date given under their names.

AGENCY   UNIVERSITY

_____   _____
Executive Vice President   Name/Title

_____   _____
Date   Date

Source: Reprinted with permission of Abington Memorial Hospital Home Care, Willow Grove, PA.

Exhibit 63–3 Operational Agreement with the Abington Memorial Hospital Dixon School of Nursing

---

OPERATIONAL AGREEMENT WITH THE ABINGTON MEMORIAL HOSPITAL DIXON

SCHOOL OF NURSING

PURPOSE: To provide a clinical facility for observation of the skills necessary for the nursing of clients in the home.

**RESPONSIBLE
PERSONNEL:**   Home Care Executive Director; Director, School of Nursing; Director of Education and Quality Assessment/Improvement and Staff Development; Education and Research Coordinator.

POLICY: Observational experience limited to two days per student and subject to procedures listed below, will be made available to students.

PROCEDURE	RATIONALE
1. The number of students sent to the Home Care Dept. by the School of Nursing shall not exceed three (3) or four (4) on any one day.	1. This is the maximum number of students that can be accommodated by the nursing staff.
2. The Home Care Dept. will provide each student with orientation and observation under the direction of a registered nurse.	2. The nurse serves as a role model for students.
3. The School of Nursing will provide the Home Care Dept. with a master schedule listing names of student nurses and dates of the planned experience prior to beginning of observation. In the event of any change in schedules, either party may notify the other of the change verbally or in writing.	3. The advance notice allows time for the nurses to schedule student visits.
4. The School of Nursing agrees to have its students:	
a. abide by general policies of the Home Care Dept. when visiting patients by direction of registered nurse with whom students are observing.	a. The care of the patient is foremost.
b. keep confidential all knowledge and records of patients.	b. This meets certification, accreditation and professional standards.

continues

Exhibit 63–3 continued

PROCEDURE	RATIONALE
5. The Home Care Dept. will make available to students and faculty all pertinent educational material during period of observation.	5. The Home Care Dept. is a partner in the educational process.
6. In the event of accident, injury or illness of student on observation experience, the Home Care Dept. will notify School of Nursing and plans for student's return to School of Nursing will be made on an individual basis dependent on situation. The School of Nursing shall assume responsibility for care and emergency transportation of student.	6. This meets hospital's policies/procedures.
7. The faculty of the School of Nursing agrees to present the terminal evaluation of the observation experience to the Executive Director of the Home Care Dept. within thirty days of its completion.	7. The evaluations by students are included as one aspect of the total annual agency evaluation process.
8. School of Nursing students will provide individual malpractice insurance coverage.	8. Meets hospital requirements.

Origin Date: 9/80
Revision Date: 5/91, 5/94, 1/97, 6/03

Source: Reprinted with permission of Abington Memorial Hospital Home Care, Willow Grove, PA.

Exhibit 63–4 Guidelines for Cooperative Relationship between Villanova University College of Nursing and Practicum Agencies

---

SELECTION OF AGENCY—The agency must be:
1. Willing to cooperate with the university in providing learning experiences for a graduate nursing student.
2. Willing to offer opportunities for a student to implement specified skills in an administrative, teaching, or clinical role.
3. Approved/accredited by the appropriate state/national agencies.
4. Willing to sign a contract or letter of agreement with Villanova University as per the criteria for selection of agencies.

QUALIFICATION OF THE AGENCY PRECEPTOR—The agency preceptor:
1. Must hold a minimum of a Master's degree in nursing.
2. Must have demonstrated expertise in the specific practicum area.
3. Must be willing to serve as a preceptor and be a role model for the student.
4. Is designated by the agency's nursing department head.

FUNCTIONS OF THE AGENCY PRECEPTOR—The agency preceptor is expected to:
1. Participate with the designated faculty member and student to plan the practicum experience.
2. Assist the student in achieving practicum objectives through facilitating his or her involvement in various relevant activities within the agency.
3. Assume a liaison role in clarifying the expectations of students as learners compared with expectations of employees.
4. Participate in the evaluation of the practicum process and the preceptorship program.

EXPECTATIONS OF THE GRADUATE STUDENT—The student is expected to:
1. Submit a resume and evidence of a current registered nurse license in the state where the practicum experience occurs, current malpractice insurance, a current health examination, and current certification in CPR (basic life support).
2. Write specific practicum plan, including personal learning objectives, process and outcome activities, a time frame, and how he or she will comply with the agency's expectations.
3. Serve as the liaison between the agency preceptor and the faculty member.

RESPONSIBILITIES OF THE FACULTY MEMBER—The Villanova University faculty member is responsible for:
1. Planning the practicum experience with the student and agency preceptor.
2. Monitoring the implementation of the practicum.
3. Evaluating the student's achievement of practicum objectives.
4. Conducting periodic supervision/teaching/consultation visits with the student at the agency and being available for interim consultation.
5. Assisting the student to reorder and reorganize current knowledge and to apply new knowledge throughout the practicum.
6. Evaluating the practicum experience.

PLACEMENT PROCESS—The following process is to be followed to arrange practicum placements:
1. The director of the graduate program will initiate contacts with the agency and determine the feasibility of placement of students in any given academic year.
2. The faculty member will initiate contacts with the agency preceptor for specific practicum planning.
3. The assistant to the dean will initiate interagency contracts or letters of agreement.

Source: Courtesy of the Villanova University College of Nursing, Villanova, Pennsylvania.

Exhibit 63–5 Student Pledge and Confidentiality Statement

STUDENT PLEDGE AND CONFIDENTIALITY STATEMENT

PLEDGE: I agree to abide by all Abington Memorial Hospital rules and regulations. I understand that if I fail to abide by these rules and regulations, I may be terminated by the hospital at any time.

I agree to return all hospital property loaned to me such as identification badges, uniforms, parking cards, etc. to the Volunteer Resources Department.

I affirm that all the information on this statement is true and correct.

COMMITMENT TO CONFIDENTIALITY: I understand my obligation to maintain complete confidentiality of information in order to protect patients and their families, as well as all members of the Abington Memorial Hospital family from improper disclosure of information given in confidence, particularly when the information is related to the health, business or personal matters of the patient, patient's family, associates, volunteers or members of the board or medical staff.

Signature:_____Date:_____

Source: Reprinted with permission of Abington Memorial Hospital Home Care. Willow Grove, PA.

Exhibit 63–6 Client Authorization for Home Visit

CLIENT AUTHORIZATION FOR HOME VISIT

I understand the purpose of the observation and educational experience for prospective

employees and students at Abington Memorial Hospital Home Care (AMHHC) and

consent to

_____joint home visit(s) on _____with an AMHHC nurse/therapist.

_____independent student home visit(s).

The pledge of confidentiality has been explained to me and I understand the

applicant's/student's obligation to abide by the rules and regulations of AMHHC

including a commitment to maintain confidentiality of patient information.

Patient Signature:_____Date:_____

In the event the patient is unable to sign, a responsible person is to sign below:

_____   _____   _____

Signature   Relationship   Date

Reason patient us unable to sign:_____

Source: Reprinted with permission of Abington Memorial Hospital Home Care. Willow
Grove, PA.

Students do have access to their patient's computerized documentation from previous visits to obtain pertinent clinical information prior to the home visit.

The financial impact of student programs must also be considered. To date, there is minimal or no financial compensation available to agencies that cooperate in student programs. Financial consideration for clinical experience should be discussed with each institution and included in the agreement whenever this can be negotiated. This compensation could be in the form of actual dollars or free attendance at continuing education programs for a specific number of staff from the cooperating agency.

Another form of payment could be the free use of audiovisual equipment, services, or faculty participation in agency projects. This matter should be discussed each time the contract is renewed.

CONCLUSION

Student programs in home health agencies are beneficial for staff, patients, students, and the educational facilities. Although administrators must be cognizant of the various challenges that exist, they should take the opportunity to participate in the education of future home care staff.

REFERENCES

U.S. Department of Health and Human Services. Health Care Financing Administration. 1989. *Medicare home health agency manual* (Transmittal 222, Section 205.1 (14)). Baltimore, MD: Department of Health and Human Services.

CHAPTER 64

The Role of the Physician in Home Care

Todd R. Cote and Leona Wilneff

While the duration of hospital stays decreases and the size of our aging population increases, where will we find the necessary resources to care for our aging ill and medically needy?

Harrison's Principles of Internal Medicine (Massey and Johnson-Hurzeler, 1997) does not mention care of the patient at home in its over 2,000 pages, but does address the physician's role. We can't conclude that home care as a delivery system to health care is inferior to the current models that are familiar to us. This chapter will help us realize that home care has a way to go before it's fully integrated into society's concept of medical care. And to get there, physicians must take an active role in the process so they can develop and implement certifiable and accredited home care programs.

INTRODUCTION

Home care administrators continue to be faced with many challenges—nursing shortages, decreasing reimbursement, and constant regulatory changes to mention a few. Unlike hospital billing in the form of diagnosis-related groups (DRGs) that are based on diagnosis, home care reimbursement with the onset of the Prospective Payment System (PPS) is based on an assessment of patients' needs and physical limitations. The outcome, however, is often more indicative of the nurse's skill of assessment than it is the true need of the patient.

A common sentiment exists among home care administrators today, and that is "we are learning to do more with less." In no other area of health care is an administrator required to have such a diverse and expansive set of skills including a high level in understanding assessment, care planning, technology, regulatory compliance, and fiscal management. All of this is coupled with a growing population of people requiring the need of home care services (Smith-Stoner, 2002).

As we proceed through the concepts of where home care is and where it is headed, we will consider how the physician can play a more active role in caring for patients out of the structured acute care setting and the confines of the physician's office.

In order to help identify the benefits and challenges of having a physician as an active participant on the home care team, we must look at what will contribute to success and failure, how this role will be defined, and what organizational investments will be required to ensure the benefits of the cost.

IS ANYONE HOME?

The geriatric population in the United States will continue to grow. Individuals aged 65 and older represented 5.4 percent of the nation's total population in 1930, 11 percent in 1980, and an estimated 21 percent in 2038 (Page et al., 1988).

Along with exacerbation of acute illness requiring hospitalization, this population also makes up the homebound chronically ill and those who have a progressive disease to which there is no cure or irreversibility to the disease process. With DRG-prospective reimbursement decreasing, and the concomitant shorter lengths of hospital stays and long waiting lists for access to skilled nursing facilities, patients are requiring more care at home.

"There is no place like home" is a cliché often heard from the lips of those patients required to consider living options other than home. A "typical" home care patient is the elderly woman who has a low income, high physical limitations, and may or may not have a caregiver. It's also probably that, even in her weakened state, she cares for her elderly husband with health issues. This type of home care patient poses a challenge for physicians and home care agencies. It is often difficult for these patients to get to the doctor's office, and while at home, the need for support and resources are great.

Two types of programs exist that could support the need of a home care patient just described. One program would be straightforward home health care, and the other would be a more specialized hospice program. The differences between the two are not relevant as each provides in-home care for the patient. The downfall and potential limitation to these programs? Physicians don't understand the criteria for referring their patients to home care, not to mention the inability of the patient to get to the physician and the physician to get to the patient.

Patients feel reassurance under the care of a physician, but one of the greatest dissatisfactions among those who are seriously ill is the care they receive during the last days of their lives (Ogle and Plumb, 1996). In a recent study of terminally ill patients, only 3 percent of those patients preferred institutional care over home care (Massey and Johnson-Hurzeler, 1998). Since home care is preferred over institutional care for the comfort it provides, physicians look for ways to honor this choice and remain a symbol of hope in the patient's eyes.

BENEFITS OF HOUSE CALLS

The office of inspector general of the Department of Health and Human Services states that 40 percent of Medicare patients did not see a physician for an average of 3 months after admission into home care. Many reasons exist for continued lack of physician involvement in home care. Whether real or perceived, home care administrators continue to be faced with the challenge of getting the physician involved at the "home" bedside.

Patients are not ill in a vacuum—they are surrounded by friends and relatives; in other words, caregivers. According to a long-term care study, caregivers provide unpaid help that amounts to an average of 30 to 60 hours of caregiving per week (Thobaben, 2001). This places caregivers in a scary and unfamiliar role. In turn, this places the additional burden on health care professionals to share their expertise to caregivers to help them understand and cope with ever-changing uncertainties of illness and caregiver demands.

In an attitude assessment of fourth-year medical students, they noted the myriad advantages of including house calls in their future practice: enable the physician to integrate psychosocial and medical issues in a treatment plan; provide support to caregivers; gather pertinent knowledge of family relationships; provide continuing comprehensive healthcare; and develop a comprehensive view of the patient (Page et al., 1998).

No dispute exists. Most healthcare providers agree that performing a patient assessment in the home care environment contributes greatly to one's insight into the factors that contribute to that individual's health and/or illness. Home visits enable the physician to evaluate the patient's social and family network of support and the patient's ability to perform activities of daily living.

PHYSICIAN EDUCATION

Among health care providers, physicians are usually prepared with more advanced education and training. This education, however, lacks formal exposure to home care. Home care experiences are often an elective part of the physician's education. Unless the soon-to-be physician realizes the benefits of this experience to his or her future practice, he or she may not elect this as part of their study. The next opportunity to be involved with home care might be when they are required to be involved with their patient's care from the distant and uniquely different environment of their own practice. The physician's lack of understanding of home care regulations, reimbursement, and clinical operations require home care providers to take the additional time necessary to teach physicians how to expedite something as basic as medication orders.

Educational approaches to promoting physician involvement in home care needs to have a two-fold approach. First, medical students should be exposed to home care within their educational curriculum. This will help eliminate ambivalence to the validity of its importance and facilitate a comfort level with the home environment. In a study of 18 fourth-year medical students, home visits were considered the most valuable method for educating about home care (Humphrey, 2002). The responsibility of the second approach lies with the home care administrator. It is here that physicians learn about the variety of ways that home care can be delivered. The "rules of the road" are defined by the many entities that reimburse for home care services. Regulatory and accreditation agencies have their sets of rules. And, when the rules are clearly understood from a regulatory standpoint, it is then the challenge of the administrator to teach the home care physician how to network and become familiar with surrounding hospitals, vendors, community programs, and so forth.

Home health care takes advantage of all available resources that can contribute to a patient's health at home. This approach to care takes into consideration the physical, psychosocial, and spiritual well-being of both the patient and the caregiver. Not unlike the hospice model of care that incorporates the many disciplines required to achieve this, home care requires the physician not only to assess the patient in a more comprehensive manner, but also to further understand the role of the other disciplines in the health care process.

CHANGING TRENDS IN HOME CARE

Models of broader approaches to care are evident in today's health care settings. With heightened awareness and expectations, patients and families have become more versed in their rights and needs in home health delivery. It is not uncommon for patients and families to greet the nurse with statements of how many home health aide hours to which they are entitled. Patients and families are strong advocates for their health care needs, and physicians often act on the suggestion of families to make referrals to home health programs.

As data continue to be collected and compiled to evaluate quality and as benchmarking activities increase to identify quality home health providers, home care administrators will continue to look for ways to provide quality and cost effective care. As evidence-based practice leads to improved clinical care, the physician's role promises a clinical expertise that can contribute to stronger clinical programs. This is more easily possible with advances in technology and telehealth communications. It is not uncommon or difficult to equip ourselves with portable diagnostic gadgets that can enable a physician to diagnose in the home care setting. Many procedures can now be done at home: X-rays, intravenous therapies, mechanical ventilation, and advanced pain management by way of infusion pumps to mention a few.

Home care reimbursement is inadequate in any attempt to attract physicians to home care. Although reimbursement rates are on the rise, it is still not sufficient to compete with hospital and private practice funding. Therefore, home care agencies looking to incorporate physicians to the home care team need to look at all avenues of reimbursement.

Home care agencies have not been successful at defining productivity from the perspective of nursing visits. As the "holy grail" of best home care practices, the National Association for Home and Hospice Care lays out productivity, staff expectations, salaries, and overall issues that impact good management and cost effectiveness of programs and agencies, aggregating data and experiences from coast to coast. Even here we are just beginning to imagine what a physician on staff may do to boost best practices and support community physicians, as well as the home care programs and the patients they serve.

HOME HEALTH PARALLEL

It's reasonable to understand that people are fearful of the unknown, yet we have grown frustrated and unsympathetic of the community physicians who have difficulty treating the home care patient who may have been missing from the physician's radar for quite some time. It may be possible with the assistance of home care resources that the patient can get to the physician, but often that isn't the case. It is not uncommon for patients to enter the last stages of a progressive disease and not have the ability to be physically attended to by their physician. The hope of any successful outcome in this situation will depend on the physician's trust of the skills of the home care providers along with their own willingness to participate in a plan of care that they might not fully understand.

It is important for the home care administrator to recognize the need to educate the primary care physician of a suitable program that can address the complete needs of the patient and family. It will be your challenge to convey the confidence you have in the ability to provide excellent quality care despite the lack of an acute care setting. You will also be faced with the challenge of breaking down some barriers and myths about what end of life care is and isn't.

Example of Two Common Myths

Myth 1: Hospice care means abandoning the patient.

Reality: Hospice care does not mean that the physician has given up on the patient or that the patient is foregoing treatment. Rather, it sees the patient within their family unit and strives to maximize the quality of their final days. The earlier hospice care is initiated, the more effective pain management can be, resulting in the highest quality of life during the final days.

Myth 2: Hospice puts patients in a drug-induced coma.

Reality: Hospice care does not rely solely on the use of narcotics to alleviate patient pain. Palliative care becomes like bad drug therapy only when it is initiated so late in the disease process that there is too little time remaining for other treatments to have any pain alleviating effect. The beauty of hospice care is that it uses so many modalities to enhance patient comfort including art therapy, pastoral care, social work, and trained volunteers.

Chronic illness, be it cancer, dementia, end-stage congestive heart failure, chronic obstructive pulmonary disease, or acquired immune deficiency syndrome at some point reach a degree of severity that requires specialized home care. Many home care agencies have realized this and have developed palliative care programs. For example, the Connecticut Hospice has developed a palliative care program called "Can Support Care" that community physicians can refer their patients to when chronic disease has progressed to the point that close titration of the treatment regime is required.

The time and manner in which this approach takes place varies depending on a range of factors that include the physician's, patient's, and family's understanding of the disease; prior and proposed treatment approaches; spiritual and religious orientation; the degree of symptomatology; and the physician's relationship with the patient (Ogle and Plumb, 1996).

CONCLUSIONS

At all levels of health care, change needs to occur to be more open to direct physician care in the home care setting. Legislatively we need to recognize that quality care can extend beyond the walls of hospitals and doctors' offices and further develop structured reimbursement models that promote physician involvement.

Education is lacking, not only in teaching medical students how to conduct home care, but also in teaching home care administrators how to incorporate the physician into the home care model. Physicians can function in two different capacities regarding the home care patient's plan of care. This is done either by direct management of all orders for disciplines involved in the plan of care or a community physician may decide to work collaboratively with the home care physician to maintain the plan of care.

The industry is very clear about the outcome it wants: to provide patients with the option of having excellent quality home care. What it is not clear about is how this can be obtained with the inclusion of a home care physician as part of the unit of caregiving.

The industry needs to further recognize the need to increase the acceptance and availability of home care services, and physicians as an active and coordinating member on the home care team. Physicians are the directors of the orchestra, and the orchestra consists of the many other support services that make a home care model. Home care success will depend greatly on society's acceptance and understanding of the important role of home care, thus supporting its growth through public support at all levels.

As a home care administrator, you may want to evaluate your current program and how you could enhance your program with direct physician involvement. Take the self-assessment survey (Exhibit 64-1) found at www.hospice.com, and evaluate if bringing a physician into your organization will prove beneficial.

Exhibit 64–1 Survey Questions

1. How do you obtain medical orders after hours and would your community physician like an after-hour partnership?
2. When your patient's symptoms need close titration, do you receive quick physician response?
3. Do your nurses face emergencies that need the clinical expertise of a physician? Could you and your agency benefit from physician administrative leadership?
4. Could you and your agency benefit from physician administrative leadership?
5. Could you benefit from physician-to-physician relationships to promote new and existing programs?
6. Have you ever been asked to provide home care services to people entering into your area with no physician?
7. How do your homebound and/or frail patients receive physician assessments?
8. Would a physician on your team be helpful with your marketing efforts to other physicians?
9. Do you need medical certification for a hospice-benefit population of patients?
10. Could your education department benefit from more advanced in-service training?

REFERENCES

Humphrey, C. J. 2002. The current status of home care nursing practice. *Home Healthcare Nurse* 20(11): 741–747.

Massey, R., M.D., and R. Johnson-Hurzeler. 1998, May/June. Hospice and Palliative Care. *Cancer Therapeutics* 61(2): 773–826.

Ogle, K. S., and J. D. Plumb. 1996. The role of the primary care physician in the care of the terminally ill. *Clinics in Geriatric Medicine* 12(2): 267–279.

Page, A. K., et al. 1988. A program to teach house calls for the elderly to fourth-year medical students. *Journal of Medical Education* 63(1): 51–58.

Smith-Stoner, M. 2002. There's still no place like home. *Home Healthcare Nurse* 20(10): 657–662.

Thobaben, M. 2001. Family home care providers. *Home Care Provider* 9: 180–181.

CHAPTER 65

Research in Home Health Agencies

Karen Beckman Pace

INTRODUCTION

The purpose of this chapter is to introduce basic research concepts that can be applied to practice in the home health care setting. Home health agency involvement in research can range from research utilization to participating in or conducting research studies. Most home health agency (HHA) administrators are not developing proposals and conducting research, but increasingly they are receiving requests to participate in research studies. Further, all HHAs can benefit when research methods are applied to investigating and evaluating operations and practice. With an emphasis on evidence-based practice, staff also need to be educated consumers of research literature.

DEFINITION OF RESEARCH

Research is a systematic investigation designed to contribute to generalizable knowledge (Powers and Knapp, 1995; Protection of Human Subjects, 2001a, 2001b). Two conditions must be met to be considered research: (1) a systematic investigation and (2) a design that contributes to generalizable knowledge. Systematic investigation refers to using an orderly approach to study a question of interest. Although research methods can be applied to investigating agency-specific problems and issues, the process would not be considered research if the intent were not to produce knowledge that was generaliz-

able beyond that specific agency. Examples of situations where an agency administrator might use research methods for internal agency purposes rather than for creating generalizable knowledge include program evaluation and quality improvement.

That does not mean that studies undertaken in a single agency cannot contribute to generalizable knowledge; they do. They can be viewed as contributing to a body of knowledge on a particular subject, likened to adding one brick to a wall at a time. Sound research methods are imperative to make a contribution to knowledge, but they can be useful in addressing an agency-specific issue as well.

POTENTIAL ROLES IN RESEARCH

In this day and age, it is impossible to escape some involvement in research. Even if agency staff are not actively involved in research studies, they should, at a minimum, be educated consumers of research findings. Clinical practice should be based on the best available evidence. Other aspects of the organization such as management, leadership, information technology, supervision, and staff education also can benefit from findings from research studies. The ways that home health agencies can be involved in research range from research utilization to participating in, collaborating in, or conducting research studies.

RESEARCH UTILIZATION AND EVIDENCE-BASED PRACTICE

Research utilization refers to using research findings as a basis for practice. Today there is an emphasis on "evidence-based" practice, which incorporates research utilization and allows for other types of evidence such as clinical expertise, scientific principles, and pathophysiology (Jennings and Loan, 2001). Although there is considerable variation in the interpretation of evidence-based practice, a key component is rating the strength of the evidence for a particular clinical practice. Randomized controlled clinical trials often are considered the gold standard of evidence. However, as will be discussed later, randomized controlled trials are not always possible, or the best way, to investigate a particular research question. Regardless of the terminology, providing current quality care requires use of the increasing volume of research literature. Of particular interest to practicing nurses are systematic reviews in which results from original studies are synthesized to derive an overall finding (McKibbon and Marks, 1998) and meta-analyses where statistical techniques are used to quantify the effect size across several studies.

Key Questions

1. Is there research literature on the topic?
   a. Were the research methods sound?
   b. Are the results generalizable?
2. Is there clinical literature on the topic of interest?
   a. Is there a sound rationale for the care practice?
   b. Is the context comparable to my practice?

PARTICIPATING/COLLABORATING IN RESEARCH

Some agencies may choose to participate or collaborate in research studies. This is an excellent way for home health agencies to be involved in advancing knowledge without taking on all the responsibilities for conducting a research study.

Activities can range from supporting masters or doctoral students in conducting research studies in the home care setting to being a more active partner with a principal investigator of a larger multisite study.

Key Questions

1. Is the research design sound?
2. Are human subjects protected?
3. What agency resources are required?

CONDUCTING RESEARCH

Some agencies may have the expertise and resources to be more actively involved in designing research proposals and conducting studies. The size and complexity of the project can range from single-agency research projects to large multisite studies. Agencies seeking to conduct research studies will be interested in exploring potential funding sources. Small agency studies are more likely to be supported by local foundations. Funding from the federal government or national foundations is extremely competitive based on a rigorous review process. However, small single-agency studies can lay the groundwork for larger studies that are eligible for funding.

TYPES OF RESEARCH

To many people, the term *research* evokes visions of a scientist in a laboratory or randomly assigning patients to treatment and control groups, but there are many other types of research designs. Nursing administrators are likely to encounter secondary data analysis, evaluation, survey, and health services research. One of the primary research design distinctions is made between quantitative and qualitative research. Quantitative research is what many associate with the term *research* or the scientific method. Quantitative research is concerned with objective measurement and quantification, replicability, prediction, and control and encompasses a variety of designs (Powers and Knapp, 1995). Qualitative research is a broad term that encompasses many methodologies such as ethnography, phenomenology, and grounded theory. Qualitative research is characterized by personal involvement of the investigator and methods such as in-depth interviewing and observation with analysis of large volumes of narrative data (Powers and Knapp, 1995). However, these distinctions alone are not sufficient because quantitative methods could be employed in a primarily qualitative study and vice versa. A philosophical distinction between quantitative and qualitative research is in the investigator's worldview, ranging from the viewpoint that there is one knowable truth that can be discovered to there is only truth as perceived by the participants in a particular phenomenon (Lincoln and Guba, 1998). A substantial body of literature on the qualitative research traditions exists, which is beyond the scope of this chapter. However, from a practical standpoint, it is the research question that should drive the research approach. For example, if the question is "how do patients with a terminal prognosis continue to find meaning in their lives," then a qualitative approach with in-depth interviews is likely to be a better match than constructing some quantitative questionnaire.

Another way to categorize research is based on the amount of control an investigator can exert over the environment. Control is greatest in experimental studies, exemplified by laboratory studies. With studies involving human subjects, the randomized controlled trial provides the most control. In these trials, the investigator carefully controls the experimental treatment, and random assignment of subjects to a treatment or control group theoretically balances all the human subject factors that can't be directly controlled or manipulated. On the other end of the control continuum are observational or nonexperimental studies where the investigator uses real-life situations, sometimes referred to as natural experiments. Comparing outcomes from two home health agencies that are known to have different models of organizing their nursing care would be an example of an observational study. Quasiexperimental research falls

somewhere in the middle of the control continuum. Research designs categorized as quasiexperimental use treatment and control conditions just as in experimental research, but subjects are not randomly assigned to those groups (Polit and Hungler, 1999). An example of a quasiexperimental design would be where patients from designated HHAs served as the control group and received usual care and patients from other designated agencies received an experimental treatment, such as a new teaching protocol for congestive heart failure. An experimental treatment is carried out, but the patients were not randomly assigned to groups.

There are many descriptions of research designs and classifications (Burns and Grove, 1997; LoBiondo-Wood and Haber, 1998; Polit and Hungler, 1999). Each discipline tends to have its own research traditions and ways of gaining knowledge. In 1978 Carper identified the ways of knowing in nursing as empirics (science), aesthetics (art), personal knowledge of self, and ethics (moral knowledge). These ways of gaining knowledge are still accepted today and underscore the need for a variety of study approaches and methods.

RESEARCH PROCESS

The research process provides a systematic way to investigate questions. Although presented in a linear stepwise fashion, one step may lead to rethinking a previous step. These steps are essential for developing a sound study and also can be used as a guide for critiquing research articles or reviewing a research proposal when considering agency participation. The study proposal or description needs to show logical consistency from problem identification through the study design and interpretation of the findings.

Identify and Define the Problem

Identifying a problem in practice is often the spark for a good research study. The problem needs to be clearly delineated in order to move forward with a manageable research study.

Key Questions

1. Is the problem delineated?
2. Is the problem stated clearly?

Review the Literature

The literature is reviewed to determine the current state of knowledge on a topic of interest. Gaps in knowledge and a foundation for the proposed study are identified, as well as the significance or importance of addressing the problem.

Key Questions

1. Is the research topic important?
2. Is what is known, as well as gaps in knowledge, identified?

Identify the Conceptual/Theoretical Framework

A conceptual framework need not be a formal model or theory; however, it is important to place the research problem in a context that helps identify the key variables and their hypothesized relationships. A conceptual framework also helps with interpreting findings. Findings from studies that are undertaken without some conceptual framework remain isolated and do not contribute to knowledge about a subject. In health services research, Donabedian's (1966; 1992) classic Structure-Process-Outcome Model for Quality Assessment often is used. The basic tenet of this model is that organizational and delivery system structures influence the process of care between providers and patients, which in turn influences patient outcomes. Theories and conceptual models do not explicitly drive qualitative studies, but a conceptual framework might be used to help form initial questions and later in analysis and interpretation (Marshall and Rossman, 1995).

Key Question

1. In quantitative research, are the variables and hypothesized relationships logically derived from a conceptual model?

Formulate the Research Question or Hypothesis

If possible, a research hypothesis should be generated. A hypothesis is a statement of the expected relationship between variables (incluing a treatment intervention) based on previous knowledge, observations, or theoretical and conceptual frameworks (Powers and Knapp, 1995). Some exploratory studies use a research question because the investigator does not have an expectation about the relationships among the variables. The population of interest also should be identified in the hypothesis. An example of a research hypothesis is:

> Home health patients with pressure ulcers who receive more elements of care outlined in the Agency for Healthcare Policy and Research (AHCPR) guidelines are more likely to improve as measured by Outcome and Assessment Information Set (OASIS) item on the status of healing.

Qualitative studies will have a broad question or problem statement that focuses on understanding interactions and processes in social systems, but not specific variables or hypothesized relationships (Marshall and Rossman, 1995). An example of a qualitative research question is:

> What are the relevant behaviors, events, beliefs, attitudes, structures, and processes occurring with implementation of a congestive heart failure (CHF) critical pathway in a home health agency?

Key Questions

1. Does the hypothesis include dependent and independent variables, their relationships, and the population of interest?
2. In a qualitative study, is the question broad enough so as not to prematurely delimit the study yet manageable in scope?

Develop the Research Design

The research design should flow from the previous steps. Research design elements include the overarching approach such as qualitative or quantitative and experimental, quasiexperimental, or observational. Practical considerations also play a role in the ultimate selection of the research design. For example, it may be unethical, impossible, or too costly to randomly assign subjects to various treatment conditions.

Operationalize the Variables and Establish Protocols

In a quantitative study, the variables of interest need to be operationalized; that is, measured. If pressure ulcers are the focus of study, how are they measured and classified? In an experimental or quasiexperimental design, the treatment protocol is defined and standardized. Data collection procedures also are specified. In a qualitative study, the approaches for data collection include in-depth interviews, observation, and document review.

Key Questions

1. Is the measure reliable (consistent) and valid (measure the construct of interest)?
2. Is the treatment condition described in detail?
3. Are data collection protocols specified?

Determine the Sample

Usually it is not possible to study the entire population of interest, so a sample is identified. The goal is to be able to make inferences about the population from studying a sample; therefore, a probability sample is ideal whenever possible. Probability sampling means that each subject has a known probability of selection; in the case of simple random sampling, each has an equal probability of selection (Powers and Knapp, 1995). However, practical considerations often necessitate nonprobablity or convenience sampling, such as when using volunteers or one particular site. In qualitative research, purposive sampling is used where the respondents are selected purposely to gain the most information about the phenomenon of interest (Patton, 1990). Any time a study involves humans either through intervention or interaction, identifiable private information procedures to protect human subjects need to be addressed (Protection of Human Subjects, 2001b).

Key Questions

1. Is the sampling method appropriate?
2. Is the sample adequately described?
3. Are human subjects protected?

Specify the Analysis Plan

The analysis plan should logically flow from the hypothesis, measures, and research design. In quantitative studies, descriptive, parametric, and nonparametric statistics may be used. The specific analytic procedure is based on the type of measures, proposed relationships among the variables, and the sample size and distribution (Polit, 1996). In qualitative studies, various approaches to analyzing large quantities of narrative data are available, but all entail various methods for coding and categorizing the content, often referred to as data reduction, then reorganizing it into various displays to identify patterns and themes that advance understanding of the phenomenon (Glesne and Peshkin, 1992).

Key Questions

1. Are the appropriate statistical analyses performed?
2. In qualitative studies, is it evident that analysis moved beyond simple coding and categorization?

Conduct the Study, Collect Data, and Analyze the Data

This phase involves carrying out the research design. Procedures for maintaining the integrity of the research protocols and managing the data are essential. Invariably a research study requires modification as it progresses. It is critical to maintain an audit trail of these modifications and decisions about protocols and analysis. Qualitative studies are considered to have an emergent design that unfolds as the investigator gains more understanding of the phenomenon being studied (Marshall and Rossman, 1995).

Interpret the Results and Disseminate the Findings

Analysis generates volumes of additional information and output. These statistical tables and data displays need to be interpreted to explain the findings. The study conclusions need to be supported in the data and should be placed in the context of the conceptual framework and literature. The investigator also critically evaluates the methods used and decisions made during the course of the study that result in limitations and identifies potential alternatives for future research on the topic. Research that is not published cannot contribute to our collective knowledge or ultimately influence our practice so it is imperative to communicate research findings.

Key Questions

1. Are the data fully presented?
2. Are conclusions supported in the data?

VALIDITY OF RESEARCH DESIGN

Research design validity is concerned with the questions of (1) whether the effect on a dependent variable can be attributed to the independent variables (including intervention) or whether there are plausible alternative explanations, and (2) to what extent the findings can be generalized beyond the research setting to the population of interest. Cook and Campbell (1979) wrote a classic treatise on quasi-experimental design validity examining these questions. The first question has to do with controlling confounding factors in the environment and in the subjects that could influence the dependent variable, and the second has to do with

using a representative sample. Lincoln and Guba (1985) referred to the question of establishing the soundness of a qualitative study as determining its trustworthiness. This is accomplished by addressing credibility, transferability, dependability, and confirmability.

STATISTICAL CONCEPTS

Quantitative studies will employ a variety of statistical procedures and analyses. A few important concepts are identified here.

Variable

Variables are constructs on which the population under study varies or takes on different values. The dependent variable is the variable of primary interest and is hypothesized to depend upon other variables, referred to as independent variables. Independent variables influence the dependent variable and are manipulated or controlled in the study. In an experimental study, assignment to the treatment or control group is the variable of interest.

Types of Measures

Variables are measured on various scales that can be characterized as continuous (1.2, 5.6, etc.), ordinal (1, 2, 3, 4, 5), dichotomous (0, 1), or categorical (race) (Polit, 1996; Waltz et al., 1991). The type of measure will influence the type of statistical analysis that is appropriate. The two primary concerns with measures are reliability and validity. Reliability is concerned with consistency in assigning scores (i.e., items within a scale, scores over time or across raters). Validity is concerned with whether the measure is truly capturing the concept of interest (e.g., does a particular instrument identify patients with depression).

Statistical Significance Testing

Statistical significance testing is performed to determine the likelihood that the observed results for a sample are due to chance. Statistical testing cannot definitively prove a finding, but can demonstrate that a null hypothesis of no relationship has a high probability of being incorrect. The probability for determining significance, referred to as alpha, is set by the researcher, and .05 often is used. If a result is significant at the .05 level it means that there is a 5 percent chance of obtaining the study result if, in fact, the null hypothesis of no relationship were true. In other words, if the experiment were repeated 100 times, in 5 of the experiments we would erroneously reject the null hypothesis when the null hypothesis was true.

Sometimes an overemphasis can be placed on statistical significance (Rothstein and Tonges, 2000). The power to detect statistically significant differences is influenced by sample size and effect size. Thus, the larger the sample, the more likely it is to have a statistically significant result even for very small differences. Therefore, it is important to think about the clinical or substantive significance of research findings in addition to statistical significance. For example, is a change of 1 point on a depression scale clinically important even if it is statistically significant?

USING RESEARCH METHODS IN AGENCY PRACTICE

The research concepts and principles discussed thus far can be applied to agency practice and operations. Applying research methods to addressing agency problems or issues in practice or organizational operations can enhance the results. The following are some examples where research methods might be applied.

Annual Program Evaluation

Medicare regulations require an annual program evaluation, but the methods for doing so are left to each agency to determine. Using some of the research methods can enhance this process.

1. Formulate the research question or hypothesis. For program evaluation, clearly identify what you are evaluating—quality, patient satisfaction, financial status, or some combination of these.

2. Develop the research (evaluation) design. Although not a research study, the same types of elements need to be identified. Do any of your questions require a qualitative approach, such as open-ended interviews with patients or staff?

3. Operationalize the variables and establish protocols. If you are evaluating quality, how will it be measured? How will you collect the data and at what time intervals?

4. Determine the sample. If you are not using entire agency data, how is the sample being drawn?

5. Specify the analysis plan. How will the data be analyzed? If you are using your outcomes data, you could consider identifying the percentage of outcomes for which the agency is statistically significantly superior to the reference and inferior to the reference.

6. Conduct the study, collect the data, and analyze the data. Make sure that the specified design is carried out and the data are collected and available for analysis.

7. Interpret the results and disseminate the findings. It is not sufficient to just present tables of data. The results need to be placed in the context of the home health care environment and local market. With an agency program evaluation, the findings are disseminated primarily to an internal audience.

PRODUCT EVALUATION

Many agencies are in the position of choosing which supplies or products they will stock for use by their staff. In some instances, staff are asked to use different brands of a particular device and provide feedback in an effort to help with the purchasing decision. These evaluations could be more effective if research methods were applied. Identifying the question and variables and specifying the measures, sample, data collection protocols, and analysis plan will enhance the possibility of obtaining results that can guide the decision.

QUALITY IMPROVEMENT/ PERFORMANCE IMPROVEMENT

Quality improvement and performance improvement activities will be more likely to succeed if research methods are used. The chapter on outcome-based quality improvement (OBQI) provides an example of using research methods in quality improvement activities. Some of the research elements already have been specified in the Medicare national outcome-based quality improvement system, such as data collection, outcome measures, and statistical testing. In most cases, quality improvement activities are not considered research studies. Reinhardt and Ray (2003) identified four criteria for differentiating quality improvement and research. Quality improvement activities:

1. do not test new interventions; they focus on evaluating existing or accepted practices.

2. do not pose *any* risk to the subjects.

3. are intended to inform the organization, not the scientific community.

4. are designed for a single organization.

CLINICAL INTERVENTION EVALUATION

Agencies may want to evaluate clinical interventions such as specific treatment or teaching interventions, or broader interventions such as case management or telephone follow-up. These studies could have broader implications beyond the agencies where they are conducted. These types of evaluations would be considered research studies and should employ the research methods discussed in this chapter. It is important

that they be conducted with appropriate human subject protections. Sound research methods increase the likelihood the study will contribute to the body of knowledge related to home health care and can be disseminated through the peer reviewed literature.

ETHICAL/REGULATORY CONCERNS

As with providing health care services, research involving an agency's patients is subject to regulation. The most important are those related to research involving human subjects including informed consent and the privacy of health information.

Human Subjects

The National Commission for the Protection of Human Subjects of Biomedical and Behavioral Research issued the Belmont Report in 1979 that identified the three major ethical principles involved in research with human subjects as (1) respect for persons (i.e., autonomy), (2) beneficence, and (3) justice (Penslar, 2001). The principle of autonomy is the basis for voluntary informed consent and requires the protection of persons with diminished autonomy, such as children, the mentally handicapped, and prisoners. The principle of beneficence and its counterpart nonmaleficence require that subjects be protected from harm and efforts be made to secure their well-being. The principle of justice directs that the benefits and burdens of research should be distributed equally without bias. Home health agencies that undertake research studies should have procedures in place to protect human subjects. If they partner with universities or federally funded studies, they will encounter specific regulations related to institutional review boards and required training on human subjects protection.

Privacy of Health Information

Regulations under the Health Insurance Portability and Accountability Act (HIPAA) protect the privacy of individually identifiable health information (AcademyHealth, 2003). The Office of Civil Rights in the Department of Health and Human Services has authority for oversight and enforcement. Health care providers such as home health agencies are "covered entities" and must follow the rules for how and when protected health information (PHI) may be disclosed. Researchers will have to either gain consent from each person whose information is sought or obtain a waiver of consent from an institutional review board or privacy board. However, de-identified information is not protected and can be made available.

CONCLUSION

Research provides the scientific basis for the practice of nursing and the means to solve our most challenging problems. All nurses have the responsibility to utilize research in their practice and identify problems that warrant investigation. Home care administrators are in a unique position to promote the value of and use research findings in all aspects of the organization operations, but most importantly in the area of clinical practice. With the complexity of health care and the health care delivery system it is imperative that our practice be scientifically based to the extent that current knowledge allows.

RESOURCES

Following are some web sites and journals for more information on research issues and nursing research studies.

Web sites

Office for Human Research Protections, U.S. Department of Health and Human Services, http://ohrp.osophs.dhhs.gov.

Self-instructional slide show on human subject requirements, http://ohrp.osophs.dhhs.gov/humansubjects/assurance/sbirsttr/sbir2003_files/frame.htm.

National Institute of Nursing Research, http://www.nih.gov/ninr/.

Office of Civil Rights in the Department of Health and Human Services information on HIPAA, http://www.hhs.gov/ocr/hipaa/.

AcademyHealth, http://www.academyhealth.org.

Sigma Theta Tau International, http://www.stti.org.

Agency for Health Care Research and Quality, http://www.ahrq.gov.

Journals

Advances in Nursing Science

Annual Review of Nursing Research

Applied Nursing Research

Evidence-Based Nursing

Journal of Nursing Scholarship

Nursing Research

Research in Nursing and Health

Western Journal of Nursing Research

REFERENCES

AcademyHealth. 2003, April. Playing by new rules: Privacy and health services research. Background paper. Available at *http://www.academyhealth.org/privacy/backgroundpaper.pdf* (accessed July 2003).

Burns, N., and S. K. Grove. 1997. *The practice of nursing research: Conduct, critique, and utilization.* Philadelphia: Saunders.

Carper, B. A. 1978. Fundamental patterns of knowing in nursing. *Advances in Nursing Science* 1(1): 13–23.

Cook, T. D., and D. T. Campbell. 1979. *Quasi-Experimentation: Design and analysis issues for field settings.* Boston: Houghton Mifflin Co.

Donabedian, A. 1966. Evaluating the quality of medical care. *Milbank Memorial Fund Quarterly* 44(Part 2): 166–206.

Donabedian, A. 1992. The role of outcomes in quality assessment and assurance. *Quality Review Bulletin* (November): 356–360.

Glesne, C., and A. Peshkin. 1992. *Becoming qualitative researchers: An introduction.* White Plains, NY: Longman.

Jennings, B. M., and L. A. Loan. 2001. Misconceptions among nurses about evidence-based practice. *Journal of Nursing Scholarship* 33(2): 121–127.

Lincoln, Y. S., and E. G. Guba. 1985. Establishing trustworthiness. In Y. S. Lincoln and E. G. Guba (eds.), *Naturalistic inquiry.* Beverly Hills, CA: Sage, pp. 289–331.

Lincoln, Y. S., and E. G. Guba. 1998. Competing paradigms in qualitative research. In Y. S. Lincoln and N. K. Denzin (eds.), *The landscape of qualitative research.* Thousand Oaks, CA: Sage Publications, pp. 195–220.

LoBiondo-Wood, G., and J. Haber. 1998. *Nursing research: Methods, critical appraisal, and utilization,* 4th ed. St. Louis, MO: Mosby.

Marshall, C., and G. B. Rossman. 1995. *Designing qualitative research,* 2nd ed. Thousand Oaks, CA: Sage Publications.

McKibbon, K. A., and S. Marks. 1998. Searching for the best evidence. Part 2: Searching CINAHL and Medline. *Evidence-Based Nursing* 1(4): 105–107.

Patton, M. Q. 1990. *Qualitative evaluation and research methods,* 2nd ed. Newbury Park, CA: Sage.

Penslar, R. L. 2001. *Institutional review board guidebook.* Office for Human Research Protections. Available at *http://ohrp.osophs.dhhs.gov/irb/irb_guidebook.htm* (accessed July 2003).

Polit, D. F. 1996. *Data analyses and statistics for nursing research.* Stamford, CT: Appleton & Lange.

Polit, D. F., and B. P. Hungler. 1999. *Nursing research: Principles and method,* 6th ed. Philadelphia: Lippincott.

Powers, B. A., and T. R. Knapp. 1995. *A dictionary of nursing theory and research,* 2nd ed. Thousand Oaks, CA: Sage.

Protection of Human Subjects, 45 Part 46 *Code of Federal Regulations,* Sec. 46.102(d). 2001a (accessed July 2003).

Protection of Human Subjects, 45 Part 46 *Code of Federal Regulations,* Sec. 46.102(f). 2001b (accessed July 2003).

Reinhardt, A. C., and L. N. Ray. 2003. Differentiating quality improvement from research. *Applied Nursing Research* 16(1): 2–8.

Rothstein, H., and M. C. Tonges. 2000. Beyond the significance test in administrative research and policy decisions. *Journal of Nursing Scholarship* 32(1): 65–70.

Waltz, C. F., O. L. Strickland, and E. R. Lenz. 1991. *Measurement in nursing research,* 2nd ed. Philadelphia: F. A. Davis.

CHAPTER 66

Hospice Care
Pioneering the Ultimate Love Connection About Living, Not Dying

*Rosemary Johnson-Hurzeler, Judith A. Conley,
Rosemary Franco, David R. Goldfarb, and Ronny J. Knight*

*Death occurs in a moment and all that time that
stretches from birth until that moment is, in fact, life
in which choices need to be made.*

Thomas Hoyer (1997)

Pioneering for the last 30 years, hospice in America has taught us that the satisfaction of patients with a progressive, irreversible illness and their families is the ultimate goal. Wellness comes with more rather than less hospice care (Bradley et al., 2002a). The strength of an institution's connectedness and relationships to the community and its physicians assures a seamless continuum of good care, a good death, and life without, because hospice care is the last frontier and the ultimate referral service.

INTRODUCTION

In the dawn of the 21st century with the global trends of population aging, longer life expectancy, fewer traditional community and family support systems, and the technological advances in medicine, it is hoped that every patient and family would be aware of physician assisted living (PAL) (Exhibit 66–1) (Thomson et al., 1997).

The initiative is a joint effort between the office of the State of Connecticut Attorney General, the Hospice Institute for Education Training and Research (the Institute), and the Connecticut Bar Association, and is supported by clergy and other leaders, demonstrating the kind

of broad power elicited by this concept. The *Journal of the Connecticut State Medical Society* published and thereby helped launch this initiative in the winter of 1997.

A BETTER WAY

Clinically, PAL is an initiative committed to allowing patients and families to meet life until death in the most dignified, supportive, and pain-free way possible, surrounded by loved ones under a rigorous medical direction; anticipate bereavement; and grieve.

Educationally, the initiative is committed to principles of hospice and palliative care through a legally nonbinding advance directive. In May 2003, at the conference of the National Association of Attorneys General (NAAG), Connecticut's Attorney General Richard Blumenthal stated:

> Through the PAL initiative individuals may express a preference for hospice care, before the onslaught of pain and depression, through a document similar to the living will and power of attorney for health care instruments. PAL includes a document entitled notice for desire of hospice care [Appendix 66-A] as well as a consumer brochure that explains the need for end-of-life planning. PAL is

Exhibit 66–1 Physician Assisted Living

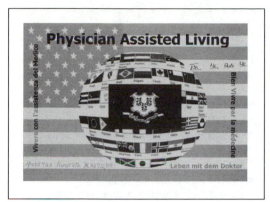

Exhibit 66–2 J-Jibe: A Relationship Modeling Diagram

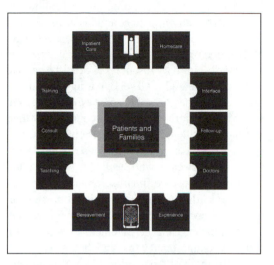

an instrument designed to help the medical professional communicate with their patients about their needs. PAL provides a message of hope that is durable and doesn't respect time. The PAL concept creates a means for each patient through collaboration with their physician to view the broadest array of care options.

Thus, the challenge to the hospice movement in the United States is to get involved with PAL so that there is knowledge of hospice for those 3 million people in the country who will die each year and their families, and so that they will have a better life because of this philosophy. The challenge is to make hospice care an integral, seamless part of the health care delivery system.

In this chapter, we will define a framework for the anticipatory adoption of hospice care (PAL), present a definition of hospice care, discuss the relationships needed for access to hospice care (Exhibit 66–2), provide examples of two environments within the model, and conclude with an overview of an education, training, and research platform.

A FRAMEWORK TO PARTNER PAL

Professionals representing medicine, law, nursing, social sciences, theology, and the arts designed the PAL Partners Initiative to achieve the following objectives:

1. Assure that potential patients and their families are aware of their full range of health care options when a disease is diagnosed as irreversible.
2. Create greater access to hospice care by advising all potential patients of the availability of the hospice option, preferably well before they need hospice care or are experiencing serious illness.
3. Afford the mechanism and opportunity for all patients to designate their preference for hospice care in writing as an advance directive.
4. Educate patients and health care providers regarding the benefits of hospice care as an early intervention for patients with advanced irreversible illness, and the appropriate clinical decision-making processes to facilitate transition to PAL partners' caregiving through a hospice program.
5. Encourage dialogue, both at the patient and provider level, around the principles of hospice care and how care might be optimized during an advanced, progressive, irreversible illness.
6. Inspire all physicians to continue to collaborate with patients regardless of length of life.

HOSPICE DEFINED

Hospice is a specialized program of health care for the terminally ill patient and his or her family (Exhibit 66–3). For these patients, management of their end of life care requires clinical expertise and interdisciplinary resources to offer the patient and family the highest level of caring in a limited time period. The goals of hospice care are directed toward palliation of pain and control of other symptoms, rather than toward curative measures. Hospice care is appropriate for those patients with progressive disease who need the full complement of the hospice interdisciplinary approach, which extends beyond the traditional home care model to encompass medicine, pastoral care, the arts, volunteers, and bereavement in addition to skilled nursing, social work, and therapies.

The strength of the relationship between community physicians and the hospice team under the leadership of a hospice medical director is a critical aspect of the interdisciplinary team function. Close communication and interaction with community physicians and the caregiving community facilitates patient, family, and staff education as well as the refinement of the patient care plan (Exhibit 66–4).

The role of pastoral care in the interdisciplinary team is to offer support to meet the sensitive spiritual needs of the patient and family. The arts program also provides a venue that heightens the spiritual awareness of many hospice patients. The creative blend of music, literature, and the creative arts enhances the ability of patients and families to express themselves and the deep feelings they are experiencing.

Volunteers are an essential component of the hospice team. The commitment and the dedication of specially trained lay and professional volunteers augment the care of staff.

An integral part of any hospice program is comprehensive bereavement follow-up to assist families with grief and loss. This is the dimension of hospice care that can be regarded as preventive care. An effective bereavement program enables individuals who have experienced loss

Exhibit 66–3 Commonly Used Terms

Palliative care is comfort-oriented tending directed to the alleviation of pain and control of other symptoms experienced by a patient in advanced stages of disease.

Hospice care incorporates both palliative and end-of-life care (the other end of life from birth, whether young or old, is close, usually measured in months, weeks, or days) with a focus on the family as well as the patient. Includes an interdisciplinary approach in a comprehensive, structured program. Although nurse-driven and medically directed, most hospice care occurs at home.

Source: Courtesy of the Connecticut Hospice.

to assimilate that loss and promotes wellness in the future.

Hospice care is primarily a home care program but necessarily includes an inpatient component to meet the more complex needs of some patients and families. The hospice program of care enables the patient to remain at home for as long as possible. Hospice caregivers encourage and support the patient and family to participate in decisions about the patient's care and assist in caring for the patient.

Hospice home care can also be available to residents of skilled nursing and extended care facilities, providing that the resident's room and board as well as care not related to their terminal illness are not reimbursed by Medicare. With the appropriate agreements in place to coordinate the work of the hospice home care team and the work of facility personnel, full-scope hospice home care can be effectively rendered to residents of skilled nursing facilities.

Regulations

The three components to any health care delivery system today are licensure, certification, and accreditation.

Exhibit 66–4 Ten Principles of Hospice Care

1. Patient and family are regarded as the unit of care.
2. Services are physician directed and nurse coordinated
3. Emphasis is on control of symptoms (physical, sociological, spiritual, psychological)
4. Care is provided by an interdisciplinary team.
5. Trained volunteers are an integral part of the team.
6. Services are available on a 24/7, on-call basis with emphasis on availability of medical and nursing skills.
7. Family members receive bereavement follow-up.
8. Home care and inpatient care are coordinated.
9. Patients are accepted on the basis of health needs, not on ability to pay.
10. There are structured systems for staff support and communication.

Source: © 1974 The Connecticut Hospice

Licensure

State licensure plays an important role in monitoring quality of care and performance improvement. The licensure requirements for hospice were first adopted in Connecticut and serve as a model for home care and inpatient. Most states have now adopted their own licensure requirements.

Certification

Certification, which happened under the federal Tax Equity and Fiscal Responsibility Act of 1974, makes a unique distinction between that certification and one of certified home care. Under certification for hospice care, not only was a new payment mechanism created, to be known as perspective pay per day, but also the requirement known as "essentially home bound," still in effect today for home care certification, was removed. This requires a patient to stay at home, presumably because of their great sickness, and enables a patient to leave the home only to visit with the physician. If the patient violates this and it is discovered, the patient is no longer considered eligible for home care. It also introduced for the first time the concept of the interdisciplinary team and the requirement that families be followed for 1 year during their bereavement. Another unique feature of this certification program for those 65 years and over (imitated by many private insurance companies) was the requirement to assure that patients had access to an institutional environment of care if they were on hospice home care and required institutionalized care. Volunteers were also introduced as members of this interdisciplinary team.

Accreditation

By 1995, the Joint Commission on Accreditation of Health Care Organizations (JCAHO) reinstated accreditation for hospice home care by incorporating it as a dimension of care within the 1995 JCAHO Accreditation Manual for Home Care.

Under this design, documented performance improvement, which is measurable, leads to outcomes that create best practice; coupled with the unique requirements under state licensure, this assure patients and families that every effort is made to make things better today and tomorrow.

Privacy and Confidentiality

The requirement for privacy and confidentiality at a most intimate and vulnerable time in people's lives has now come under federal legislation that requires all providers of care, especially in the technological age, to have systems in place that will protect confidentiality. The Health Insurance Portability and Accountability Act (HIPAA) of 1996 established standards of privacy of health care information regarding electronic health care transactions.

POPULATION DEFINED

"Dress for the game" (be prepared) and, in this case, life as it certainly is a journey that requires great fortitude. As noted, "dressed" with regulations, hospice care involves the realization that the fulfillment of human life is only in relation to others. In fact, every human being is who he or she is because of their relationships to others.

The following four characteristics identify the stages and the acuity of the disease and the range of ages for those with disease.

1. Adult and Pediatric—Patient and Family

The impact on the patient as well as the impact on family members that care for them is the focus of hospice care.

In 1980, when the first palliative care hospital/hospice first opened, a licensed preschool for children 3 to 4 years of age was integral to the intergenerational activity that allowed the children to say "they had many patients in their school." Ten years later, the hospice home care staff demanded a special place for young patients when inpatient care was a necessity. The staff would have control over the plan of care when the situation required utilization. The original school, known as Charlie Mills, was closed to make way for "The Children's Place." In 1995, the American Hospital Association Hospital Awards program recognized The Connecticut Hospice for its Rocker Program, in which a volunteer corps of senior citizens spends time rocking extremely ill infants.

2. Malignant and nonmalignant
3. Staged: Progressive, Irreversible

When hospice care is required, the severity of illness places these patients in the 92nd percentile in the classification of case-mix index—severity of illness. Over the year, the Federal Register publishes the ranking of all hospitals in the United States for the purpose of Medicare reimbursement. In particular, the ICD-MC (International Classification of Disease Clinical Modification) is the basis for the diagnosis-related groups, which is the basis for Medicare reimbursement for hospitals. When hospitals are ranked in the Federal Register, this classification ranks them based on the ICD-CM on what the mortality and the morbidity is within the institution. That relative number helps establish one or two components for reimbursement.

4. Diagnosis made years to weeks before death

Institutional relationships, between provider (community physicians and acute care hospitals) enable hospice, whether a palliative care unit within the palliative hospital, a unit connected with the hospital, or home care, to know one another so that 24/7 during a critical time in a patient's disease process, a referral can be made with confidence, so that (a) the institution will receive and give the higher care during a critical care time, and (b) the institution can be assured that every active medical practice towards cure has been initiated on behalf of the patient and it has been determined that cure is no longer possible.

A COLLABORATIVE ENERGIZED BY PATIENT/FAMILY DECISIONS

The therapeutic care envisaged in *Advanced Care 2001 Summary Guidelines* (Appendix B) involves a one-on-one response to the patient. With the assessment tool, the palliative care consultative service (PCCS) may recommend post-hospital transfer to CanSupport, a home care program for advanced care, where patients undergoing aggressive curative therapy in or out of clinical trials receive clinical management in their homes so they can return to clinic, office, and rehospitalization when necessary. The PCCS will also recommend treatment for symptoms of all advanced diseases, whether malignant or nonmalignant, cancer or noncancer. The "trigger points" clearly define the appropriate timing of an intervention based on specific clinical criteria. The dynamic of PCCS is therapeutic options (Exhibit 66–5). During this period, a change in the focus of treatment may occur. At a time just before entering a discussion with the patient and family, the physician prepares for the discussion with the family by posing the questions:

1. What does this patient and family understand?
2. What do the patient and family want?
3. What degree of futility is there in further therapeutic events?
4. What and how severe are the patient's symptoms?
5. What is the progression over the last few weeks or months?
6. Can I anticipate how or when the patient will die?
7. What are reasonable goals?
8. Could I make this patient worse by whatever I do?

9. What do I do if the patient and family disagree with my recommendation?
10. What are the specific ways to involve the patient and family in decision making?

EXAMPLES OF POTENTIAL ENVIRONMENTS OF CARE

CanSUPPORT CARE

CanSupport Care is a disease management program where home care is available to support patients early in the course of their disease. Patients enter the program while they are participating in clinical trials. With the addition of telemedicine, psychological counseling, transportation to doctors' offices, and 24/7 availability for a home visit from a trained palliative care physician (without taking an ambulance to the nearest emergency room), a patient is supported and their quality of life and choices they have made are honored.

How Do People Access CanSupport?

Referring to the J-Jibe (a Relationship Model), a palliative care consult is requested by the regular medical management team. This service can be provided by the hospice or others and indeed, a palliative care clinic can be established at various cancer centers, neighborhood health centers, and hospital sites, so that on a routine basis physicians would have a referral mechanism. As one can infer from the J-Jibe, a consultation could then be called, with the derivative being the patient leaving the hospital sooner and still receiving excellent home care for pain and symptoms, and being able to continue with therapeutic modalities appropriate for their disease management. In this way, the patient and their family is assured, on a timely basis, access to the most appropriate level of palliative and hospice home care, while not being separated or distanced from treatments that may make a difference in the course of their life. This mechanism to assure continuity of

Exhibit 66–5 The Refocus Zone: Therapeutic Options

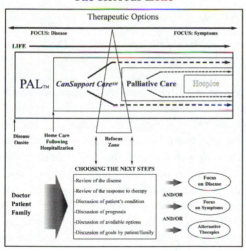

Source: Courtesy of The Connecticut Hospice

care depends on relationships, and is particularly important if one's hospice is close to a community or comprehensive cancer center.

HOSPAL™

The use of physical space and beauty to facilitate patient and family care helps enact the values that are reflected in hospice care: the underlying belief in the sanctity of life from beginning to end and the importance of caring. Exhibit 66–6 displays design concepts of a palliative and hospice care setting to be considered when reconstructing, renovating, remodeling, or building from scratch.

EDUCATION, TRAINING AND RESEARCH

Education and Training

Many derivatives exist from the research that families have participating in over the last decade. The most exciting finding has been that the more hospice care a patient receives during the appropriate time, the better the family survives in regard to major depression, days lost from work or school, and time spent on emergency room visits.

The scoring guidelines in this will help all families to recognize that hospice is a program of wellness, not only for the physical and spiritual components of the program, but for the benefits that the family will receive in the long term. Academic (medical school appointments) and/or community (family and/or internal medicine) physicians who are not directly linked to hospice and palliative care work are currently participating in programs of academic excellence with associated credit units as well as selected residency clerkships and internships for those still in school. Through the John D. Thompson Hospice Institute for Education, Training and Research, Inc., which is associated with The Connecticut Hospice and its Ac-

creditation Council for Continuing Medical Education (ACCME), the courses listed in Exhibit 66–7 have been found helpful and are going to be repeated, with upgrades, in upcoming years.

The accreditation program provides continuing medical education credits to physicians in varying sums of credit, depending on the amount of educational material presented and the amount of activity. In 2001, over 580 continuing medical education units in Category I for physicians were granted as well as 137 credit hours in Category I for advanced practice registered nurses and 470 contact hours for registered nurses.

Residencies, clerkships, and internships occur with a variety of academic institutions in clinical settings (Exhibit 66–8). The Connecticut Hospice, together with other hospices throughout the country, offer these programs and they are usually described in the academic institution's catalog; for example, Yale Medical School has a fourth year elective in which the student can take one month at The Connecticut Hospice. The University of Connecticut Health Sciences PharmD Program describes in their catalog that every PharmD student must take one month clinical rotation to graduate.

Research

Institutional review boards assess the practical, legal, and ethical issues surrounding each potential research project. Once initiated, projects often need to be incorporated into day-to-day activities, including anticipatory bereavement. Research that is conducted in this way appears to benefit from the understanding that the patients and families are the best teachers, and whether coincident or longitudinal, research with patients and families pose many challenges. If the study is successfully concluded and the data are found statistically significant, various new profiles, instruments, and initiatives all geared toward improving not only pain, symptom management, and the environment of

Exhibit 66–6 A Palliative Hospital Hospice

Enhancing quality of life via connection with nature
- interior skylight
- patients brought outside
- patient rooms with "greenhouses"
- ocean views
- beach and deck access with ramps

Giving choice for patients and family via space variety
- family lounges
- commons
- chapel
- outdoors

Respecting family desire for involvement
- pantries, fireplaces

Source: Courtesy of The Connecticut Hospice

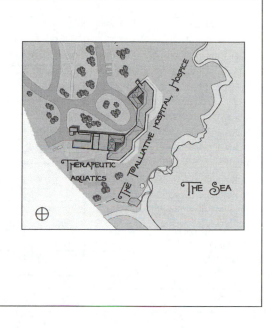

care, but also the wellness of the caregiver can be put forth for the benefit of the community. Evidence exists that families (caregivers) involved in such research continue to seek guidance and "counseling" time from the research affiliate because they believe that their feelings matter and they are able to express themselves more clearly as time goes by.

Exhibit 66–7 Educational Courses

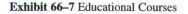

The Doctor–Patient Encounter
Hospice Care and End-Stage Dementia
Living, Not Dying with ALS: The Role of Hospice
A Hospice Care Journey
Exploring Grief and Loss Through the Hospice Philosophy
A Tale and Approach to Pain Management
Redefining the Focus of Hope

These data, once analyzed, lead to publications that may be found useful by the provider community. The following is a selection of research objectives, findings, and implications published between 1997 and 2002:

Objectives: To assess the influences of self-rated knowledge and attitudes on physicians' discussions and referrals for hospice care (Bradley et al., 2002b).

Findings:
- In a study of 233 physicians working in Connecticut hospitals, about half of the physicians agreed or strongly agreed that they were well-trained to take care of symptoms of terminally ill patients. Almost 75 percent agreed or strongly agreed that they were knowledgeable enough to discuss hospice with patients.

Exhibit 66–8 Selected Academic Affiliations for Residencies, Clerkships, and Internships

Affiliation	Public Health	Medicine	Nursing	Social Work	Pharmacy	Arts	Spiritual
Yale School of Public Health	X						
Yale School of Medicine		X					
Yale School of Nursing			X				
UConn School of Social Work				X			
UConn School of Pharmacy					X		
UConn School of Medicine		X					
Fordham University				X			
Southern Connecticut State University	X		X	X		X	
Albertus Magnus College				X		X	X
Quinnipiac University	X		X			X	
Wesleyan University				X			X

- Overall, physicians had very positive attitudes concerning hospice. Most agreed or strongly agreed that hospice care meets the needs of the patient and their families better than conventional care.
- However, almost half of the physicians agreed or strongly agreed that telling patients and family members that a patient is dying was difficult.
- Both self-rated knowledge and attitudes may influence physician practices for patients with terminal illnesses.

Implications:
- Study demonstrates that physicians' knowledge and attitudes can influence hospice referrals and identifies gaps in some physicians' knowledge and understanding of hospice.
- Findings support current efforts to change medical school curric-

ula and develop continuing education programs that focus on many aspects of caring for terminally ill patients, including the use of hospice.

Objectives: To estimate the proportion of terminally ill inpatients whose physician discusses prognosis and hospice with patient or family members, to describe the nature and correlates of such discussions, and to assess the association between documented discussions about prognosis and subsequent advance care planning (Bradley et al., 2001a).

Findings:
- Random sample of terminally ill, hospitalized patients.
- Documentation of discussions about prognosis by physicians in the hospital setting with patients with terminal cancer is infrequent

and vague in nature, rarely giving time frames.

- When discussions do occur, a physician is rarely involved. In these cases, either a social worker or a nurse was the clinician involved in the discussion of prognosis with the patient or family.
- Patients are often omitted from such discussions in the hospital setting; most discussions were between clinicians and family members.
- Having a documented discussion about prognosis was more likely to occur if there were discussion about life-sustaining treatments or having do-not-resuscitate orders.

Implications:
- Encouraging more explicit discussions about prognosis with patients and families may improve patients' abilities to express their preferences for care, and the clinicians' likelihood of meeting those preferences for care at the end of life.[1]

Objectives: To examine the frequency, nature, and correlates of palliative care practices used by nurses in the acute care setting. The study also explored training and knowledge about hospice and their influences on palliative care practices among acute care nurses (Bradley et al., 2001b).

Findings:
- In a study of 180 acute care nurses working in Connecticut hospitals, a little more than half of the nurses reported they never discussed hospice and over 25 percent did not discuss prognosis with their patients.

- Most nurses (88.5 percent) reported using palliative care practices when caring for terminally ill patients. Some of these practices included active/passive listening (86.45 percent), requesting increased doses of pain medication to ensure patients were pain free (81.8 percent), and supportive counseling (53.8 percent).
- Nurses with more knowledge of hospice, who had hospice training in the last 5 years, and who were younger were more likely to include palliative care practices in their care of hospitalized patients.

Implications:
- Palliative care practices are commonly used by nurses in the acute care setting,
- However, limited communication among nurses and patients or families continues to be a problem in preparing families for hospice care.
- Evaluation of palliative care practices in the acute care setting should be a focus in future studies assessing the integration of palliative and acute care.[2]

Objectives: To estimate the proportion of terminally ill patients who are referred to hospice and to identify physician factors associated with increased referrals for hospice care (Bradley et al., 2000a).

Findings:
- In a random sample of Connecticut physicians, physicians report that on average they refer just over half of their terminally ill patients for hospice care.

1. *Source:* Paper presented at the 2000 Gerontological Society of America Conference.
2. *Source:* Paper presented at the 1999 Gerontological Society Association conference.

- Over 26 percent of the physicians referred fewer than one quarter of their terminally ill patients for hospice.
- Cardiologists, pulmonologists, and other subspecialists were particularly less likely to use hospice for terminally ill patients, as compared to internists and oncologists.
- Some of the common reasons physicians report for nonreferral included the patient refused or was not interested in hospice, the family refused or was not interested in hospice, and the physician believed hospice was not appropriate or applicable for the patient.

Implications:
- Many terminally ill patients who are eligible for hospice do not receive it.
- The study identifies physician-groups to target with interventions to enhance the appropriate use of hospice.[3]

Objectives: To develop and test a concise and easily administered instrument to measure physicians' and nurses' attitudes toward care at the end of life (Bradley et al., 2000b).

Findings:
- Three attitudinal constructs were identified in the development of the instrument:
  1. The extent of professional responsibility in the care of dying patients (what roles and responsibilities medical professionals have in providing care at the end of life)

2. The efficacy of hospice (the degree to which one believes that hospice meets the needs of patients and their families, as opposed to continuing more traditional medical care)
3. The importance of clinician–patient communication about dying (the role and importance of communication about discussions of prognosis, hospice, or advance care planning)

Implications:
- The instrument was found to have both test-retest reliability and construct validity, suggesting it might be useful in evaluating the impact of initiatives to affect clinicians' attitudes toward terminal care and in improving the quality of care at the end of life.[4]

Objectives: To examine patient preferences for life-sustaining treatment and how treatment burden and expected outcomes influence those preferences. (Freid et al., 2002a).

Findings:
- The burden of treatment (length of hospital stay, extent of testing, invasiveness of the treatment), the expected outcome, and the uncertainty concerning outcomes all influence patients' preferences.
- The majority of patients (98 percent) said they would choose to receive the treatment if the burden was low and their current health would be restored.
- If the outcome was survival but with severe functional disability, most patients (90 percent) would choose not to receive the treatment. Likewise, if the outcome

3. *Source:* Paper presented at the 1999 Gerontological Society Association conference.

4. *Source:* Paper presented at the 1999 Gerontological Society Association conference.

was survival with cognitive impairment, about 75 percent of the patients would not choose the treatment.

Implications:
- The provision of care at the end of life should take into account the patient's preferences. The findings suggest that understanding patients' preferences depends on assessing how they view the burden of treatment in relation to all possible outcomes. The possibility of functional or cognitive impairment is an important determinant of patients' preferences and needs to be taken into consideration in end-of-life care planning.

Objectives: To develop an instrument designed to measure patients' treatment preferences across a range of diseases, based on evaluating patients' attitudes toward treatment burden compared to a variety of treatment outcomes (Freid et al., 2002a).

Findings:
- The WALT (Willingness to Access Life-Sustaining Treatment) instrument was developed.
- The instrument evaluates patients' attitudes toward (1) the burden of treatment; (2) health states (severity of functional or cognitive impairment) and length of life following treatment; and (3) likelihood of treatment outcomes.

Implications:
- The WALT was found to have good test-retest reliability and construct validity.
- The instrument can be used by clinicians to enhance physician–

patient communication about treatment decision making.

Objectives: To examine the relationship between dying at home and a set of demographic, disease-related, and health resource factors among individuals who died of cancer (Gallo et al., 2001).

Findings:
- The sample included 4,766 individuals who died of cancer-related causes in 1994, had been diagnosed with cancer in Connecticut, and were 18 years or older at the time of death. Of these, 42 percent died in a hospital, 17 percent died in a nursing home, and 11 percent died in an inpatient hospice facility.
- Individuals who were married, female, white, or living in a higher income area were more likely to choose to die at home.
- Patients surviving 1 to 5 years after being diagnosed with cancer were more likely to die at home than those surviving less than 1 year. Individuals whose cause of death was colorectal cancer were more likely to die at home than those with other cancers.
- In addition, individuals who resided in an area with greater availability of hospice providers *and* less availability of hospital beds were more likely to die at home, rather than in a hospital or inpatient hospice.

Implications:
- The findings of this study identify groups (men, unmarried individuals, and those living in lower income areas) at higher risk of dying in an institution.

- Knowing which groups might be at risk of institutional death allows clinicians to provide possible interventions to promote home death if that is the preference of the patients and their families.
- The site of death is related to the available health resources.[5]

Objectives:
- To highlight the current efforts that measure quality of life in the end of life and suggest ways to enhance the measurement.
- To discuss gaps in current research about quality of life in the end of life and what this area of research can contribute to future policy and practice (Bradley et al., 2000c).

Findings:
- Efforts measuring quality of life have generated several points: (1) the idea that there is a pattern of decline in health status prior to death for many patients and that this decline is not always predictable; (2) quality of life in the end of life is multidimensional; and (3) measurement of quality of life in the end of life fails to recognize the changing needs of individuals and families over the course of terminal illness.

Implications:
- There are many dimensions to quality of life in the end of life and that there may be ways to enhance the quality in that portion of life. This recognition has been a major contribution to the hospice movement and philosophy.
- Many of the components of quality of life in the end of life come from the community and family efforts. Social support is an important component to quality of life in the end of life.
- Quality of life in the end of life will continue to be a major area for future research. Recognizing that quality of life in the end of life is multidimensional is central to designing ways to enhance quality of life in that portion of life.

---

5. *Source:* Paper presented at the 2000 Gerontological Society of America Conference

State of Connecticut Physician Assisted Living (PAL) Directive

State of Connecticut

RICHARD BLUMENTHAL
ATTORNEY GENERAL

Hartford

TO MY PHYSICIAN:

There may be a time in my life when I am incapacitated to the point when I can no longer actively take part in decisions for my own life and am unable to direct my physician as to may own medical care, I wish that this document stand as a testament to my wishes.

Subject to the provisions of a living will or other legal health care directive, if I have a terminal medical condition, I desire that hospice care, as guided by the ten principles below, be provided.

The ten principles of hospice care are: (1) patient and family are regarded as the unit of care; (2) services are physician-directed and nurse coordinated; (3) symptom control is emphasized through physical (including the provision of medication), sociological, spiritual and psychological care; (4) care is provided by an interdisciplinary team; (5) trained volunteers are an integral part of the team; (6) services are available on a continuous basis; (7) family members receive bereavement followup; (8) home care and inpatient care are coordinated; (9) patients are accepted on the basis of health needs, not on ability to pay and (10) there are structured systems for staff support and communication.

I understand that this document is not legally binding and that there may be extenuating family, financial, or medical circumstances that would make other forms of treatment more appropriate. However, I urge you, my physician, family members and any person authorized to be involved in health care decisions on my behalf to work together to comply with my desires as expressed in this document.

_____

_____

PATIENT SIGNATURE/DATE

Summary Guidelines for Initiation of Advanced Care

Disease Category	Refer to Advanced Care Upon			
Cancer	Initial Diagnosis	Recurrence	Progression	Critical Clinical Decision
Brain/CNS Tumor	●			
Breast			2	
Colorectal			2	
Esophagus		1		
Gallbladder	●			
Head and Neck		1		
Lukemia				
Liver			2	
Lung		1		
Lung-inoperable	●			
Melanoma			2	
Ovarian-inoperable	●			
Ovarian/GYN			2	
Pancreatic	●			
Prostate/GU			2	
Renal		1		
Sarcoma			2	
Stomach		1		
End-Stage Diseases				
Neurological: Alzheimers Disease			3	
ALS			4	
CVA				5
MS				4
Congenital, Infectious, or Traumatic Disability				6
Heart Failure			7	
Lung-COPD			8	
Liver Failure			9	
Kidney Failure				10
AIDS			11	

Initial Diagnosis: The first diagnosis of disease by a physician.

Recurrence: Subsequent diagnosis of same disease resulting from limited response to additional therapy expected and not durable.

Progression: Continuation of disease process.

Critical Clinical Decision: Consensus decision made by physician, patient, and family that want to forego any continuing curative or rehabilitative treatment.

Footnotes

1. Limited response to additional therapy expected and not durable.

2. First-line salvage therapies have failed. Less than 20% response to second-line or other therapy expected and not durable.

3. Dementia beyond State 7 of the Functional Assessment Staging Scale for Alzheimer's Disease or Multi-symptoms present and declining functional status (Karnofsky <50% and when there is partial or total dependence in ADLs).

4. Progressive nerve degeneration with resultant partial/total paresis or paralysis of extremities and muscles of respiration. Optimal therapy reached (i.e. no further response to therapies expected), with major symptoms present and declining functional status (Karnofsky <50% and when there is partial or total dependence in ADLs).

5. Massive CVA with no rehabilitation potential; patient unable to eat. Optimal therapy reached (i.e. no further response to therapies expected), with major symptoms present and declining functional status (Karnofsky <50% and when there is partial or total dependence in ADLs).

6. Congenital defects, complication of infections, or trauma based upon individual case review.

7. Long-standing history of congestive heart failure or multiple MI. Class IV NY Heart Association Symptoms and ejection fraction <20%. No further responses expected to medical therapy and no options for CABG, grafting, angioplasty, pacemaker, or transplant. Any one of the following dyspnea, angina, othopnea, edema. Any two of the following: Karnofsky<50%, minimal activity tolerance, dependence on 2 or more ADLs.

8. Degradation of PFTs: FEV1 after bronchodilator <30% of predicted, decrease in FEV1 on yearly serial testing of >40ml/year, Cor Pulmonale, Hypoxemia, Significant CO2 retention as measured by ABGs. Optimal therapy reached with multiple bronchodilators and steriod dependence with dyspnea (of any kind) and O2 dependence. Declining functional status including Karnofsky <50%, chairbound, minimal activity tolerance, and dependence on 2 or more ADLs.

9. Worsening LFTs and documented evidence of disease (utilizing abdominal ultrasound, CT, HIDA Scan, Cholangiography, ERCP or any appropriate diagnostic imaging demonstrating biliary obstruction, hepatic vein occlusion, hepatic artery thrombosis, hepatocellular dysfunction. No expectation of success from medical management and/or surgical intervention. Presence of any one major symptom and declining functional status (Karnofsky <50% and dependence on 2 or more ADLs).

10. Decision made to stop dialysis with one of the following conditions: chronic dialysis necessary to sustain life, disease progression despite interventions, intolerable associated medical complications of non-renal disease. In addition, at least one of the following: peripheral vascular disease degradation, hypotension, dementia, depression, resistance to dialysis Rx; and, declining functional status.

11. CD4<50 with concurrent ongoing major infections, and the presence of at least one of the following: lymphoma, Kaposi's Sarcoma, PML, HIV encephalopathy, HIV wasting syndrome. Progression of disease on antiretroviral therapy and the presence of major symptoms with declining functional status.

Important Note on These Guidelines: The footnotes above are an integral part of these guidelines. They must be used in conjunction with the matrix on the left

REFERENCES

Bradley, E. H., E. Cherlin, R. McCorkle, T. R. Fried, S. V. Kasl, D. V. Cicchetti, R. Johnson-Hurzeler, and S. M. Horwitz. 2001b. Nurses' use of palliative care practices in the acute care setting. *Journal of Professional Nursing* 17: 14–22.

Bradley, E. H., D. Cicchetti, T. Fried, D. M. Rousseau, R. Johnson-Hurzeler, S. Kasl, and S. Horwitz. 2000a. Referral of terminally ill patients for hospice: Frequency and correlates, *Journal of Palliative Care* 16: 20–26.

Bradley, E. H., D. Cicchetti, T. Fried, D. M. Rousseau, R. Johnson-Hurzeler, S. Kasl, and S. Horwitz. 2000b. Attitudes about care at the end of life among clinicians (ACE-C): A quick, reliable, and valid assessment instrument. *Journal of Palliative Care* 16: 6–14.

Bradley, E. H., Cramer, L. D., Bogardus, S. V., Kasl, S. V., Johnson-Hurzeler, R. and Horwitz, S. M. 2002b. Physicians self-rated knowledge and attitudes and end-of-life care practices. *Academic Medicine* 77:305–311.

Bradley, E. H., T. R. Fried, S. V. Kasl, and E. L. Idler. 2000c. Quality-of-life trajectories in the end of life. In M. P. Lawton (ed.), *Annual Review of Gerontology and Geriatrics.* 20: 64–96 New York: Springer.

Bradley, E. H., A. G. Hallemeier, T. R. Fried, E. J. Cherlin, S. V. Kasl, R. J. Hurzeler, and S. M. Horwitz. 2001a. Discussing prognosis: Communication with elderly patients at the end of life. *American Journal of Medicine* 111: 218–223.

Bradley, E. H., H. Prigerson, E. Cherlin, R. Johnson-Hurzeler, and S. V. Kasl. 2002a. Delayed hospice enrollment and caregiver well being. *Gerontologist* 254: 254.

The Connecticut Hospice. 1993. Ten principles of hospice care. *Critical Care Nurse* 26: 1.

Freid, R. R., Bradley, E. H., Towle, V. R. 2002a. Assessment of patient preferences: integrating treatments and outcomes. *Journals of Gerontology: Psychological Sciences & Social Sciences* 57B: S348–S354.

Freid, T. R., Bradley, E. H., Towle, V. R., Allore, H. 2002b. Understanding the treatment preferences of seriously ill patients. *New England Journal of Medicine* 336, 1061–1066.

Gallo, W. T., Baker, M. J., Bradley, E. H. 2001. Factors associated with home versus institutional death among cancer patients in Connecticut. *Journal of the American Geriatrics Society* 49: 771–777.

Hospice Association of America. 2002. *Hospice facts and statistics (November 2002).* Washington, DC: Hospice Association of America/National Association for Home Care.

Hoyer, Thomas. 1997. Physician assisted living: The PAL initiative. *Connecticut Medicine:* 61(12).

Thomson, G. E., R. Johnson-Hurzeler, G. Fraunhar, and K. Howe. 1997. Physician assisted living: The PAL Initiative. *Connecticut Medicine* 61(12): 789–791.

CHAPTER 67

Safe Harbor

A Bereavement Program for Children, Teens, and Families

Elissa Della Monica

To companion bereaved children means to be an active participant in their healing. When you as a caregiver companion grieving children, you allow yourself to learn from their unique experiences. You let them teach you instead of the other way around. You make the commitment to walk with them as they journey through grief.

Alan D. Wolfelt, Ph.D (1996, p. ix)

THE BEREAVED CHILD

Our culture struggles with embracing the pain of grief, thus, leaving children in a difficult position to address their thoughts and feelings. Modern medicine has created an environment in which children rarely experience death during their formative years. Technology has resulted in decreased infant and children mortality and increased life expectancy. Today's children have become the first "grief-free generation" (Wolfelt, 1996, p. 8), frequently being excluded from the death of a loved one. Our society has difficulty dealing with grief in a child; hence, mourning a death is not encouraged. Alan Wolfelt (1996) defines *grief* as the thoughts and feelings that are experienced within children when someone they love dies and *mourning* as the expression of the internal experience of grief (p. 15). To ensure healing, a healthy environment must be created for the bereaved child to effectively mourn.

Bereaved children have the ability to grow during the grieving process. Surrounding a death event, messages are frequently given to children to deny or avoid the pain of grief as adults are struggling with their own grief. When bereaved children internalize messages that encourage the repression, avoidance, and denial of grief, they lose the ability to heal themselves. This may result in children expressing their grief in destructive ways. Children must be helped to slowly embrace the pain and depth of their loss and grow in the process (Wolfelt, 1996).

Bereaved children may experience emotional, physical, and behavioral changes. Emotional changes can be manifested in shock, denial, and an apparent lack of feeling, depression, and anxiety; physical manifestations may be physical symptoms, lack of energy, and inability to sleep. Behavioral changes may be reflected in regressive behavior, explosive emotions, depression, acting out, and hyperactivity. Articulation of emotions is difficult for children, especially in the presence of a grieving adult. The manifestations of these behaviors are a call for help and is a way for children to express their feelings (Wolfelt, 1996).

The Dougy Center, The National Center for Grieving Children and Families, believes that children's feelings are their allies and that feelings help the child to pay attention and understand their loss (The Dougy Center, 2003). The Dougy *Skills Development Training Manual* (2003) identifies fear, guilt, anger, and sorrow as the feelings most expressed through behavior. The most basic expression of loss for a child is that of fear: Who will die next? Who will take care of me? and Will I die? Guilt is usually felt as an unrealistic sense of responsibility for the death. Anger is a means by which the child may protest the death and the lack of dependability of life, and finally sorrow and acceptance occur when the child is ready to accept the truth of the loss without protest and learn to live with or accept the death (The Dougy Center, 2003).

SAFE HARBOR PROGRAM DEVELOPMENT

Recognizing the work of Dr. Alan Wolfelt in *Healing the Bereaved Child* (1996) and having a commitment to creating an environment for the bereaved child to mourn, Safe Harbor, a bereavement program for children, teens, and families, was developed as an extension of the Abington Memorial Hospital Home Care (AMHHC) and Hospice bereavement program. It was the dream of the hospice's director of volunteers who studied under Dr. Wolfelt, a renowned thalantologist, to create this program to serve the children of the community.

Development of the AMHHC program was based on Dr. Wolfelt's personal tenets on grief and the bereaved child. Dr. Wolfelt (1996) believes that we have a responsibility to create a safe environment for the bereaved child to do the work of mourning; that a child's understanding of death depends upon his or her developmental level; that play is the child's natural method of self-expression and communication; that some children do the work of mourning well in the safety of a group experience; that the ultimate responsibility for healing lies within the child; and that we must create a social context that allow bereaved children to mourn openly and honestly (Wolfelt, 1996, p. 12).

Abington Memorial Hospital (AMH) is an accredited, not-for-profit, teaching hospital located in Abington, Pennsylvania, that provides comprehensive health care services for residents in Montgomery, Bucks, and Philadelphia counties. The mission of AMH is to meet the health care needs of the community by providing high-quality health care services to patients in a compassionate, caring, and cost-effective manner. The AMH opened in 1914 in response to the need for medical service in the growing area of suburban Philadelphia. Safe Harbor was established in January 2001 as an outgrowth of Abington Memorial Hospital Home Care and Hospice, which was begun in 1979 to offer home health, hospice, and bereavement services. In recent years, the home care and hospice programs witnessed an increase in the incidence of young hospice patients dying, leaving behind a spouse and family. In addition, the hospice bereavement program began receiving community requests for pediatric bereavement services from schools, funeral homes, pediatricians, and parents or caregivers. A community-needs assessment identified only one pediatric bereavement program in the Philadelphia area serving children and families. It was quickly determined that there was no program in the communities directly serviced by AMH. Letters were sent to local schools, funeral directors, and pediatricians introducing the concept and informing them of the plans. The hospice director of volunteers prepared a program description, identifying the preliminary mission statement, goals, projected resource needs, and preliminary cost. In addition to the hospice director of volunteers, staffing consisted of two part-time coordinators, both prepared at the masters' level. One coordinator possessed a masters degree in social work and the other a masters degree in counseling psychology. Both were active participants in the AMH hospice volunteer program and had proved themselves as effective leaders, well-versed in the counseling of the bereaved and grief recovery. Recognizing the need in the community and the quality of program leadership, hospital administration quickly gave their approval and offered full support of the program.

PROGRAM STARTUP

The AMH hospice program is highly successful and provides care for over 700 patients per year. (AMHHC 2003 Annual Report). Families express their appreciation for the excellent care provided to their loved ones through donations to the hospice memorial fund. Because Safe Harbor is an extension of the AMH hospice bereavement program, a decision was made to use monies from the hospice memorial fund for program startup. The AMH properties corporation found unused office space in a building on the hospital satellite campus and offered the space at no cost to the program. Money from the hospice memorial fund was used for room renovations, furniture, supplies, and salary expenses for the part-time program coordinators. The AMH fund development department received a grant from a local foundation to purchase toys, dolls and dollhouses, a puppet show, art supplies, television and audio equipment, and air hockey and foosball tables. Safe Harbor staff approached the community for donations of used toys and stuffed animals. The response was overwhelming, allowing Safe Harbor to open with limited expenditures for required toys. The AMH women's board contributed dollars for the volcano room (described later in the chapter) and the butterfly garden.

The Safe Harbor coordinators notified area schools of the upcoming program. The local high school contacted Safe Harbor to identify service-learning opportunities for their students. Six of their students contributed their artistic talent by assisting with the painting of murals in the children and teen rooms. A local artist volunteered her time to coordinate the activities of the students in addition to completing the more difficult portions of the artwork. A group of troubled teens from an art school contributed their artistic talent in painting murals in the teen room. Other schools and churches donated money, art sup-

plies, and hand-made stuffed animals. Hospice and bereavement program volunteers contributed materials and "handyman" time to building shelves, hanging pictures and wallpaper, and many other small jobs. The tremendous response from the churches, schools, and local communities demonstrated acceptance and support of our project and validated the need for this program in the community.

PROGRAM DESIGN

Safe Harbor is modeled after the internationally recognized Dougy Center, The National Center for Grieving Children and Families. A consultant from the Dougy Center in Portland, Oregon, was contracted to train the staff and volunteers using the *Dougy Center for Grieving Children Program Development Manual* (1995). The AMH program teaches children how to grieve, preventing destructive or depressed behavior, and teaches parents and caregivers how to manage the bereaved child while confronting their own grief. Safe Harbor provides ongoing support to children ages 3 to 18 who are grieving the death of a parent, caregiver, sibling, grandparent, or friend. In addition, the program provides parents with the necessary tools to understand and assist their grieving children. Safe Harbor provides these services to any family requiring assistance at no cost. The program does not provide therapy, but rather it offers a safe environment for the peer group to express their feelings and thoughts about the death. Following a family-needs assessment, the completion of a family intake questionnaire, and a grief assessment questionnaire, children are assigned to age-appropriate support groups. Each group meets biweekly for 1.5 hours in the evenings on alternating Tuesday, Wednesday, and Thursday evenings. The support groups are arranged for ages 3 to 5, 6 to 9, 10 to 13, and 14 to 18, plus a group for parents. A parent or caregiver must always accompany the child and agree to be an active participant in the program.

The children's groups, ages 13 and under, include talking circles and time for unstructured play activities. Play is a very important part of grief work, allowing children to express their grieving through the powerful language of creative play. Play opportunities include an art room, puppet theater, sand tray, music, and pretend play. Animal-assisted therapy is also available, using trained therapy dogs. Trained bereavement volunteer facilitators and volunteers assist in talking circles. Children always have the option of choosing whether they want to talk.

The teen groups are structured to provide time to discuss issues with peers and trained facilitators. Teens can choose to talk or engage in other unstructured activities such as art, music, foosball, air hockey, and other activities. Volunteers supervise all children groups.

The adult groups meet at the same time as the children and teen groups. These support groups provide an opportunity for the adult to meet with other adults in a similar situation, to discuss concerns about parenting grieving children and teens. Parents are given an opportunity to share their own experiences of grief and provide mutual support. A trained bereavement facilitator aids the adult group.

With funding from the AMH women's board, Safe Harbor recently opened the volcano room. The volcano room measures approximately 14 by 16 feet with padded walls and floors. It is equipped with a hanging punching bag, boxing gloves, a tumbling mat, huge stuffed animals, a stuffed mannequin, and soft foam balls. Grief counseling may trigger the emotions of anger and fear. The volcano room offers the structure and place for the safe expression of these painful feelings and serves to channel a release from the turmoil and conflict grieving children experience. When the children tire of the physical activity, the facilitators talk about the experience and help the child or teen discuss their feelings. By having a place for these thoughts and feelings to be expressed, children learn that their feelings are not bad and they can be directed to safely channel these emotions.

Confidentiality is of paramount importance in the Safe Harbor program. The staff will discuss their impressions of the child or teen with the parents in a general manner, but will not disclose specifics of what is said or done in the groups. In addition, the child or teen can share what he or she said, but may not share what others said. No written records are kept on what the child, teen, or adult discusses in the group. The only time information will be disclosed to the parent is when safety issues become a concern. Safe Harbor does not provide therapy or private counseling. In the event that counseling or private therapy is needed, the parent or caregiver is provided with a list of several therapists. Each family is responsible for selecting the therapist of their own choice.

EVALUATION

Safe Harbor is an open-ended support group, with children and teens progressing in their grief recovery at their own pace. A review of the child's, teen's, and adult's progress is made in cooperation with the families and the Safe Harbor staff when the child or teen is ready to leave the program, or at specific intervals throughout the program. These intervals may be after several months or a year. The staff and facilitators use questionnaires that measure growth in family and personal relationships, school or work performance, sleeping and eating habits, need for counseling or antidepressant medications, and destructive behavior such as drug or alcohol use. Each questionnaire is treated confidentially to ensure honesty; however, information is shared with the facilitators. Parents do not have access to the information on the questionnaire. The questionnaire is then compared with the intake questionnaire that was completed when the child or teen entered the program. The Safe Harbor team, including an AMH psychiatrist who is the designated medical director, reviews and compares the questionnaires to help determine the client's bereavement status. If the results do not yield a measurable improvement, recommendations are made for referral to a therapist. Because of the extended waiting list and the need to open the program to other children in need, the staff is considering evaluating all children on an annual basis, and encouraging separation when indicated. Staff also utilizes an in-session satisfaction survey in which parents have the opportunity to evaluate their child's support group. In addition, an overall family satisfaction survey is used at the completion of the program. The parent and family satisfaction surveys provide valuable insight into participant perception of the quality and effectiveness of the program.

The co-coordinators along with the program director are responsible for analyzing data from the questionnaires and satisfaction surveys and making appropriate changes to the Safe Harbor program. Review and analysis of the overall program is ongoing as the program continues to grow and mature.

PROGRAM STAFFING AND VOLUNTEERS

Safe Harbor is staffed by approximately three full-time equivalents. The hospice director of volunteers functions as the program director and is responsible for overall program management and supervision of the co-coordinators. The two part-time co-coordinators are responsible for the daily management of the program. Responsibilities include developing, planning, and managing the support group program; handling the initial contact with families and their placement in the support groups; supervising facilitators and volunteers, including initial and ongoing training; and designing and implementing community outreach to schools, community organizations, and other interested organizations. Three staff facilitators support the program in various activities and function as lead facilitators for the weekly groups. The staff facilitators work 8 hours per week in preparing the newsletter, creating and managing school in-service programs, and facilitating ongoing training for new and current volunteers.

Trained bereavement volunteers are the heart of the Safe Harbor program. Recruitment, training, and retention of volunteer staff facilitators are essential in supporting the existing program and accommodating growth. Volunteers are recruited from schools, hospitals, churches, and the community. Two types of volunteers exist: facilitators and lay volunteers. Facilitators have a background in counseling or therapy or have worked with children in a mental health facility. The lay volunteers have a personal bereavement experience through the loss of either a parent, spouse, or child. Lay volunteers assist the facilitators and provide supervision during activities.

Facilitators work to establish a climate of trust and safety, initiate and promote interaction among participants, set limits and rules, conduct various activities, and share personal impressions of what is happening in the group with the co-coordinators. Volunteer facilitators work 4 hours a night every other week and are extensively trained in a 21-hour comprehensive training program. Training also includes observation and active participation with existing volunteers and groups.

Ongoing trainings are offered, providing volunteers with updated knowledge and skills on such topics as coping with traumatic loss and suicide, play therapy, sand tray therapy, and the use of humor in therapy. Social workers and guidance counselors receive continuing education credits for participation in training programs. The AMH chairperson of the department of psychiatry, a specialist in adolescent and child development, supports the Safe Harbor staff and volunteers through biannual meetings. He is readily available to address problems, issues, or concerns and provide guidance and advice to Safe Harbor staff or volunteers. Safe Harbor collaborates with school counselors, principals, funeral homes, and pediatrician offices, which all serve as valuable referral sources. Safe Harbor maintains a relationship with other pediatric bereavement programs as well as parenting programs and other community youth resource centers.

FUNDING

Although AMH is willing to financially support the program, Safe Harbor is strongly encouraged by AMH administration to secure funding to offset the cost of the program. A variety of methods are being used to secure funding including contributions from individual donors; earned income from bereavement seminars to schools, colleges, and social support agencies; grants from private and community foundations and corporations; contributions from individual donors to the hospice memorial fund; and annual fund raising activities.

SUMMARY

Since its inception in January 2001, Safe Harbor has successfully grown and was awarded the Hospital Association of Pennsylvania Achievement Award for Community Stewardship in May 2002. The program has grown from 48 children and teens in 2001 to 117 children and teens and over 80 parents and caregivers in 2003 (AMHHC, Annual Report, 2003). After only 2 years, the demand for Safe Harbor services exceeded the program's capacity. Staff facilitators have developed age-specific educational programs on pediatric grief and recovery for local schools and colleges. These educational programs are offered for a small fee as training programs for student teachers and continuing education for teachers and school counselors.

Recognizing the success of the program and the need for controlled program growth, a donor recently funded a strategic planning consultant to identify priorities, assess and evaluate the current structure of the program, analyze the external environment, and develop plans for future growth and funding. The updated strategic plan will include specific action steps: time frames, intended outcomes, and resource development strategies to secure funding needed to fulfill the plan's goals.

The success of this program is a tribute to the staff of Safe Harbor and the volunteers who have contributed many hours to nurture and support the bereaved child and their families as they grow through the grief process.

REFERENCES

Abington Memorial Hospital Home Care Annual Report. 2003. Willow Grove, PA: Author.

The Dougy Center for Grieving Children. 1995. *Program development manual*. Portland, OR: Author.

The Dougy Center, The National Center for Grieving Children and Families. 2003. *Skills development training manual*. Portland, OR: Author.

Tantum-Hollish, Barbara. 2001. *Abington Memorial Hospital Home Care and Hospice request for proposal for Safe Harbor funding*. Abington, PA: Author.

Wolfelt, Alan D. 1996. *Healing the bereaved child*. Fort Collins, CO: Companion Press.

CHAPTER 68

Planning, Implementing, and Managing a Community-Based Nursing Center: Current Challenges and Future Opportunities

Katherine K. Kinsey and Patricia Gerrity

INTRODUCTION

The concept of a successful community-based nursing center is not new. In fact, the concept began with Lillian Wald and like-minded nurses in the 1890s. Wald founded the Henry Street Settlement House in response to the evident public health needs of New York City poor and émigré families. Through street outreach, culturally sensitive initiatives, and community activism, Wald and colleagues engaged community members in nursing and social services. Such services improved the well being of individuals as well as the health of the community. The spread of infectious diseases and school absenteeism declined, obstetrical care became more of a norm, housing improved, and family life stabilized (Buhler Wilkerson, 1993).

Wald's vision of nursing practice moved beyond individualized care for the sick and infirm. Her prevention and advocacy perspective encompassed a reform agenda in the areas of health, education, industry, recreation, and housing. She actively campaigned for the social betterment of all (Reverby, 1993).

This nursing model of direct access to health care services in home and community settings when combined with social activism is as essential today as it was more than a century ago. In fact, given the changing health care delivery systems and funding sources, such a nursing service model may be the linchpin in planning and providing optimal health care to diverse populations in community settings (Anderko, 2000).

Nurses and others who expand Wald's vision will create models of care that offer culturally appropriate preventive and primary health services. These proactive models will then engage the larger infrastructure of medical care and social institutions in the provision of cost-effective services.

Home health agencies are in ideal positions to develop such centers of care. In fact, many home health agencies have the needed resources to initiate such models. These resources include staff, internal agency structures, and recognized histories of successful clinical services in varied home and community settings.

Despite the current reimbursement limitations on holistic nursing practice in home and community settings, this is the opportune time for agencies to make prevention and social activism essential core activities. Agencies committed to change rather than the status quo may be better positioned to survive in this time of health care reform (Christensen et al., 2000).

The commitment to change and transformation is risky, but it is also challenging. One challenge will be to create a nurse-managed public health and primary care service model in tandem with a sick care model. Another challenge will be to marshal the human resources and capital necessary for such risky transformation.

One of the most valuable capital investments that a home health agency has is in its staff. Wald contended that public health nurses were doers, educators, advocates, and creators. She saw their creative work as the start of broader community work. This broad work linked agencies and groups committed to the social betterment of all (Berkman and Lochner, 2002). Home health agencies that view their staff as positive change agents will maneuver through and survive these uncertain times.

Maneuvering through any system is risky, particularly when there are few guidelines. In fact, there was substantial risk taking and no guidelines for faculty, students, and staff to fall back on when La Salle University Neighborhood Nursing Center (LSNNC) was established in June 1991.

OVERVIEW

This chapter briefly describes the evolution of LSNNC as a nurse-managed health center in a challenging urban setting. Strategies and issues influencing the ongoing development of this and other centers are highlighted. These include (1) conducting a practical assessment of community and agency assets, (2) prioritizing needs and interests of specific groups, (3) initiating a strategic plan, and (4) developing realistic service programs and evaluation criteria. The challenges to cost-effective administrative and fiscal management processes and sustainability are highlighted. Advocacy approaches and future opportunities are discussed.

EVOLUTION OF ONE URBAN ACADEMIC NURSING CENTER MODEL

La Salle University Neighborhood Nursing Center is unique in the city of Philadelphia. This primary health care model emerged from the private faith-based university's school of nursing and its commitment to the community and conversely, the community's interest in LSNNC's outreach, health promotion, disease/injury prevention initiatives, and primary health care services. The nursing center model extends Wald's model of culturally sensitive services and social activism in an at-risk community.

The evolution of LSNNC built on the creative work of public health nursing faculty, students, and volunteers. Previously, there were limited opportunities to expose students to citywide public health nursing experiences; therefore, the faculty designed prevention and health promotion programs to actively involve students in community initiatives. Through these community initiatives, the health risks of individuals and families were further documented. It was evident that faculty and students should develop the resources to improve the health of community members over time.

A feasibility study to implement a nursing center was undertaken. This study was supported by a grant from the William Penn Foundation. This support enabled school of nursing faculty to further examine community needs and resources, propose internal administrative restructuring, develop an initial mission statement and goals, initiate program planning for particular populations, establish a marketing plan, project financial support, and identify key community members to participate in the development of LSNNC.

Based on this feasibility study, the nursing center was formally established in June 1991 and is one of the four divisions of the school of nursing. The other divisions are the undergraduate, graduate, and certificate programs. Each program director reports to the dean of the school of nursing. The school of nursing faculty directs the LSNNC programs. LSNNC staff consists of full- and part-time faculty, advanced practice nurses including public health nurses and nurse practitioners, substance abuse and mental health counselors, social workers, operations/business managers, community health outreach workers, and affiliated graduate and undergraduate students in nursing, pharmacy, social work, busness, and medicine. The diverse staff composition fosters collaborative work. Emphasis is placed on holistic services that focus on relevant and appropriate community health care initiatives. This model is adaptive and can be designed to meet the needs of other diverse urban populations as well as rural and suburban communities. It is not the traditional model of one-site primary care services or home health care administrative offices; therefore, it was critical to develop mission, vision, and purpose statements that captured the essence of the model. The mission statement reflects the school and university's mission and represents the collective work of faculty, staff, students, and volunteers (see Exhibit 68–1).

Diverse populations and settings are targeted for services. Settings include the home; school; day care; Head Start programs; Women, Infants, and Children (WIC) nutrition sites; recreation centers; prenatal centers; faith-based organizations; and so forth (Gerrity and Kinsey, 1999). Outreach, case finding, case management, quality public health nursing services, and collaborative community work are hallmarks of LSNNC programs and are framed by LSNNC goals. The LSNNC goals are dynamic in nature and are constructed on agency and community assets. Based on the dynamic processes of goal development, staff continually monitors community needs, interests, and the influences of external forces (i.e., natural and man-made disasters). These assessments reveal the need for amendments or changes to goals. Exhibit 68–2 displays current LSNNC goals.

Since the center's inception, emphasis has been placed on collaborative, multidisciplinary efforts to improve the health of underserved residents in this culturally diverse community. This work is demonstrated by the types of federal, state, regional, and city grants and contracts awarded to the center for its collaborative, community-focused initiatives. Funding support includes Department of Health and Human Services (DHHS), Bureau of Health Professions, Division of Nursing, Special Projects grants to establish and extend primary health care ser-

Exhibit 68–1 Mission, Vision, and Purpose Statements

MISSION

The La Salle Neighborhood Nursing Center supports and enhances the teaching, learning and service mission of the School of Nursing and the University through the development and implementation of exemplary health care and educational programs.

VISION

The School of Nursing and its Neighborhood Nursing Center will be positioned as a nationally recognized provider of quality health care services in urban settings.

PURPOSE

The organization's general purpose is to provide access to public health, educational, counseling and primary care services to under-served populations residing in a multicultural, diverse urban community. Emphasis is placed on health promotion, disease and injury prevention, screening, detection, early intervention and rehabilitation.

Source: Courtesy of La Salle University, Neighborhood Nursing Center, 2003, Philadelphia, PA.

---

vices in noninstitutional settings; DDHS; Office of Minority Health: North Philadelphia Cancer Awareness Prevention Program; Commonwealth of Pennsylvania Departments of Health, Insurance and Public Welfare; City of Philadelphia Departments of Health and Human Services; Independence Foundation; the Patricia Kind Family Foundation; William Penn Foundation; the Robert Wood Johnson Foundation; and others.

These collaboratives, as well as the mission and goals, have evolved from much inter- and intraorganizational work and time. Such work demands the input of others outside the university and the school of nursing. The development of realistic goals relates to the contributions of

Exhibit 68–2 2003 Goals

- To exemplify Lasallian values in everyday life.
- To provide optimal community-based educational experiences for students and clients
- To improve the health of individuals, families, and communities
- To provide direct access to primary health care services to underserved individuals, families, and groups
- To emphasize disease prevention and health promotion initiatives
- To incorporate Healthy People 2010 goals and objectives in individual, group, and community programs

- To involve those at highest risk and least likely to be served by existing health care programs through outreach and case finding
- To promote 100 percent access, 0 percent disparity for all
- To provide community consultation
- To evaluate program services and population outcomes
- To promote organizational, environmental, and public policy change
- To share evidence-based practice and program outcomes in regional and national forums

Source: Courtesy of La Salle University Neighborhood Nursing Center, 2003, Philadelphia, PA.

community members. Community involvement continues to represent one of the most significant contributions to LSNNC sustainability. No nursing center can sustain itself in a particular locale if community representatives are excluded from the processes of assessment and program development. In fact, it might be prudent to involve community representatives at every point of center work.

However, such involvement can influence staff contributions and perspectives. These influences may be positive or negative. Skillful home health agency administrators must be sensitive to adverse or positive influences on staff productivity and relationships with community members. For example, staff that do not live in the immediate community (point of service) might be viewed by community members as less informed or insensitive to their concerns about daily life. In addition, staff and community members who do not share similar cultural or racial backgrounds, religious orientations, or work experiences may find it challenging to develop productive relationships. Common interests and bonds can be established. Still, the

labor to nurture productive relationships is time consuming. Constructive outcomes may ultimately evolve only if all parties want things to happen—and often those at the table may not yet know what those "things" might be.

For example, one of the "things" that happened to create LSNNC was the expressed community interest in ongoing primary health care services. Initially, a neighborhood faith-based organization committed space for renovation as a nursing center site. This site became the hub of faculty and student activity. Through such activity, it became evident that community members, in particular young women and their children, had unmet needs.

Interestingly, the opportunities for possible funding sources surfaced as the need for more services was documented. In part, these possibilities occurred in the form of request for proposals (RFP) calls from public and private organizations; however, much emerged through networking with community agencies and multidisciplinary collaboratives. The current LSNNC programs have evolved from a variety of these possibilities. What the staff has realized is never to underestimate the value of relationship building and the potential to work together to create relevant health services for targeted populations.

Many LSNNC services have taken much time and effort to build; others have seemingly evolved serendipitously. However, in retrospect, even those services have emerged from much community and staff work. For example, the 2000 to 2003 Healthy Me + Healthy You = Healthy Schools & Healthy Neighborhoods Initiative funded by the Robert Wood Johnson Foundation through the Association of Supervision and Curriculum Development (ASCD) started from community and school work to engage minority low income youth in a health career program. Funding enabled LSNNC advanced practice nurses and undergraduate students to work with more than 400 children in one public school on health-related activities and academic goal setting beyond high school. This initiative was 1 of only 10 to be funded across the nation with more than 180 organizations invited to submit proposals to ASCD (Smith, 2003). Many academic and professional lessons have been learned from this work and many challenges to implementation and evaluation of this initiative had to be overcome. Two of the more notable challenges included (1) the below-grade-level preparation of 7th and 8th graders in English, math, and science; and (2) the foster and kinship family compositions in this area of the city that limited parental involvement in career and goal setting activities.

Although LSNNC evolved from an academic model of teaching, learning, and service, the model could have just as well emerged from a home health agency. Different missions, goals, reimbursement structures, and program designs may appear obvious, yet the commitment across organizations to improving personal and family life is evident. What can influence the evolution of a similar model in a home health agency might be the agency's principal source of funds being linked solely to restorative and curative care. If sick care is the principal focus of an agency, a thorough community and agency assessment must be conducted before undertaking such a contrasting enterprise.

ASSESSMENT

Frequently, assessments are targeted outward toward the community of interest and do not include internal agency audits of resources, skills, interests, or needs. It is important to conduct concurrent internal agency review and external community assessments. Such information will be invaluable in constructing a realistic portrait of the feasibility of establishing a nursing model focusing on preventive health measures, not a disease and illness orientation of a community (Campbell, 2000).

At the community level, assessments focus on current health data, population demographics, specific needs by locale or neighborhood, resources, environmental characteristics, explicit and implicit needs, and interests of residents, workers, and so forth. In addition, barriers to services need to be identified. Such barriers may range from lack of public transportation to low literacy levels of adults to state changes in Medicaid coverage for low-income families.

The internal agency assessment will examine resources, staff skills, and limitations. This assessment should include (1) services currently in place, (2) services severely restricted by third-party payers, (3) services expanded to meet third-party requirements (i.e., more paperwork), and (4) services that have the potential to be more responsive and comprehensive to families.

Community assessments and resource analyses have always been strengths within nursing. Public health nurses in particular are prepared to take a holistic approach regarding health and ascertain the community's perspective on needs and problems. Holistic nursing assessments encompass more than health. Other factors that contribute to a community's health status include social, environmental, educational, employment, and demographic characteristics. Without such information, a community assessment is lacking and powerless to support agency change.

The purposes of the community and agency assessment must be forthright. Community members involved in such assessments may be skeptical about the motive and, if suspicious, less inclined to contribute. Their skepticism may be due to past experiences with ineffectual community assessments. Open dialogue about agency interests and commitment can mobilize residents to work with staff throughout this phase.

The assessment phase should include careful consideration of locales for services. For example, should there be maternal-child health nurses who follow families until their youngest child has completed the primary immunization series? Should there be a source and site for low-cost pregnancy tests and counseling, particularly for adolescents? Should there be open immunization hours for school-age children so they can be "caught up" and enrolled in school immediately? Should there be primary care providers closer to clients in need of such services?

This internal assessment may lead to some clarity about agency interest in establishing a site for one or multiple services—or the audit may suggest that there should be an array of additional services but not necessarily more service sites. If there is an interest in establishing a site for services, the external assessment phase should not concentrate solely on "vulnerable" populations or socioeconomically depressed areas. All communities—be they urban, rural, or suburban—have interests and needs for accessible primary health care services. Community members, if asked, often provide invaluable insights as to where such a service site could be established and perceived as "user friendly."

In addition, the assessment phase should not exclusively focus on what nurses offer to the community. The assessment forums must be open to community needs. It may be that in the eyes of the consumer, the concept of a "nursing center" is archaic. For example, LSNNC has an array of staff. The staff includes nursing, medical, and allied health personnel and others. Such a multidisciplinary, collaborative model of preventive health care may be a difficult concept for the consumer to understand—and the name "nursing center" might limit consumers' ideas about what is available. Careful thought should be given to naming the center. What the service or site is called may influence consumer use and acceptance. It can also raise community awareness about what nurses and other health professionals can do in this era of change.

Further phases emerge if internal agency and external community data document need and interest. One phase can be viewed as a secondary process of assessment. It is now the time to gauge the amount of time, effort, and expertise necessary to develop a strategic plan. One essential step is to select a person or persons to spearhead this strategic plan. In addition, restructuring roles and responsibilities to lead this initiative must occur concurrently. Selected individuals must have sufficient time and resources to develop the strategic plan. If this work is simply added to a person's current responsibilities, there may be too little effort allocated to this initiative. This work must be viewed as essential and integral to moving the agency forward.

The secondary assessment phase allows for further examination of resources and possible influences on the development of this nursing service model. Is a site critical for the model? Are staff skills and interests sufficient in developing this model? Will other disciplines be critical to programmatic design? Is more staff needed? Can staff be retrained? How can the collaborative nature of this model be nurtured?

Professional barriers to model development might include lack of state prescriptive power for nurses, definition of "primary care provider" in managed care legislation, lack of or inadequate reimbursement for health promotion and health education, lack of physical space to provide on-site services, and the like. Community barriers could be escalating violence in the immediate target areas, commuting distances to service sites, inadequate networking with other community and institutional services, the increasing acquisition of hospitals, and medical practices by for-profit companies.

The transition from secondary assessment into strategic planning may be effortless if the commitment to develop this model is clear, resources are available, and barriers seem surmountable. On the other hand, there will be agencies who will struggle with the question, should we or shouldn't we? The transition will then be more labor intensive. In fact, the process may be abruptly arrested.

STRATEGIC PLANNING

In the strategic planning phase, the agency's mission and vision need reexamination. The mission, vision, and values of the home health agency will strategically position the organization to develop a public health or a primary care model or blend features of each.

Current nursing centers, freestanding or housed within an academic center, are not alike. Some are based on the public health model in which services are designed for all those who need care whether or not the consumers present themselves for such services, such as an ambulatory care center. This public health model requires that outreach, case finding, and public health nursing case management be integrated components in any population- or health-focused service.

Primary care services that involve on-site nurse practitioners—pediatric, adult, or family—may develop accessible, affordable, user-friendly on-site programs. Such programs may not include outreach and community-based case finding. Other centers blend the models of public health and primary care and provide primary health care services. These services include population-focused outreach, case finding, and case management as well as on-site and in-home primary care services.

Service sites also vary from center to center. Rural agencies may consider a mobile van an essential source of care. Thus, the van can be scheduled for services in strategic geographic points to reach the most people (Hurst and Osban, 2000). An urban agency might consider multiple sites as point of contact. Some

urban sites include schools, senior housing complexes, recreation centers, churches, and day care centers.

Throughout the strategic planning phases, the identification of agency collaborators will be critical. Home health agencies do not need to do this in isolation of other organizational resources. In fact, other organizations may have similar interests in extending relevant community services to those in need. Your agency may have to assume the risk in reaching out to other organizations and sharing ideas, but the yield might be great. For example, social service agencies and home health agencies have resources that complement each other. The nursing center model has the possibility of sharing resources. The sharing of such resources is economically sound and expands the nature of community-focused services.

The reimbursement struggle for newly proposed services now begins. The strategic plan and specific program development must constantly wrestle with this dilemma. Some state agencies provide direct reimbursement for primary care services to advanced practice nurses; thus, the idea of establishing a primary care site staffed by nurse practitioners may be immediately feasible. However, health promotion, education, and disease prevention, hallmarks of public health and holistic nursing practice, are seldom directly reimbursable from state agencies. The possibility of contracting with local or regional agencies, public and private, for such public health services must be explored. These services could include immunization, outreach, and perinatal home-visiting services (Swan and Catroneo, 1999).

When direct reimbursement for proposed services is not evident, the agency must commit to moving forward with grant and contract proposals. Funding services through grants and time-limited service contracts allow for program implementation, but the lack of predictability of these funding streams is stressful. Agency staff must be continually vigilant about possible funding changes and other opportunities to seek alternative fiscal support.

PROGRAM DEVELOPMENT AND INFORMATION SYSTEMS

The transition to program development will be based on critical factors identified throughout the assessment and strategic planning phases. Agency resources and locus of services, be it one site, multisite, all community based, or in-home, will need to be built into each program developed. Therefore, staffing expertise, work patterns, familiarity with program development, strategic planning, the services the agency and its collaborators can provide, the community receptivity, and reliable reimbursement sources are all concerns.

Again, it may be prudent for the agency to determine what services could be shared with other providers. For example, social workers and public health nurses together can develop holistic care models that address individual and family issues. Rather than agencies working in isolation, communication and care patterns improve, and ultimately the client benefits from the dual nature of the work.

If there are one or more services in place, the agency must begin to measure client- or population-based outcomes. The methods of documenting the nature of services, client outcomes, and the costs of such services should be built into each program. Unfortunately, many outcomes have been based on medical models that do not capture the nature of public health work. Data will be needed not only to evaluate outcomes and improve quality, but also to cost out services, to provide data for policy development, and to conduct research.

The struggle to simultaneously determine what data points to collect and at what intervals and what system to use will be ongoing. Centers that blend public health and primary care services, in addition to home health services, will be additionally challenged. Data from health promotion, disease prevention, education, outreach, and case-finding activities should be maintained as well as the curative, restorative primary care data. What should be entered, how much should be entered, who enters the data, who analyzes the data, what are the data expectations of the funders, and what equipment is necessary to enter these data are major questions.

Some concerns may be dismissed early on but reemerge later as fundamental barriers to data analysis. For example, the assumption that the person who enters the data may be a low-level staff person may spell disaster. If there is lack of understanding of the nature of data and missing data, the retrievable information may be limited in scope—and many hours of professional labor may be invested later to retrieve data. In other words, cheap investments do not always pay off.

In addition, the scope of services may defy easy data computation. The complexity of nursing and allied roles continues to evolve. The escalating advances in the areas of telecommunication, including the Internet, raise serious questions about how to "capture" client encounters, the services provided, and client, family, and community outcomes. Despite the technological advances made, many staff and their clients may not be computer literate and may not have an interest in learning these skills despite agency advocacy. In addition, some communities do not have the resources to support or secure expensive technology.

However, home health administrators appreciate the programmatic demands placed on them by particular funders. Careful thought must be given to the modalities the agency can use for data collection and what would be wise investments. Two current possibilities are (1) to purchase a commercial computer product and customize data collection for particular programs with this product or (2) to have a consultant work with the staff to develop an agency-specific system.

Commercial products are now quite good in capturing primary care data, particularly as it relates to sick care and current International Classification of Diseases billing codes. Such products rarely include nursing and health promotion activities. On the other hand, the customized product may be quite costly. In addition, this product may require the ongoing services of that particular company or consultant. Does the agency want to have a continuing expense? Furthermore, developing the customized computer program may be a tedious process requiring much staff work.

Another consideration will be the multiple sites that may be targeted for services. The more sites involved, the less manageable the data entry, collection, and analysis. Should data be entered into a portable system and moved from site to site? Should there be paper records and data entered later at a central site? What are the expenses involved in setting up computer support at each site? What happens if sites change? Multiple sites complicate an already complex issue. These issues and questions do not have easy answers.

It may be that resolution is directly related to agency resources and experiences with computerization and data collection. Another alternative is an agency directive to move forward. Then, there is no dispute about computerization. It is then a question of how much and when.

HUMAN RESOURCE AND FISCAL MANAGEMENT

Sound program development will be directly related to the agency's human resource and fiscal management services. This model is not inexpensive to initiate and sustain. For many home health agencies, such a model is beyond the scope of their services and mission. Other agencies may commit to this model because their resources are greater or the client and/or community need is so great.

For a nursing center model to be successful, the staff must envision themselves responsible and responsive to human need and interest without self-imposed boundaries. The attitude that "that is not my job" does not create the necessary esprit de corps. Flexibility, adaptability, the notion of transcending boundaries and bureaucracies, creativity, and commitment to the untried will be critical staff characteristics. Matching staff with new programs and the new ways of doing business at one or multiple sites is critical. The staff can make or break this new

initiative. In fact, the agency and the staff must be risk takers together.

Part of the risk with introducing this model will be whether services are separated from or integrated into currently funded services. It may be a blend of each. On-site services for lead screening may be part of an overall lead toxicity prevention program. In-home services for mothers and their infants may also include education regarding lead and its effects on young children. This intervention may cross several programs. The nurse who understands that the intervention can be conducted several different ways, in several different places, and with multiple clients is the person for the job. The staff that want discrete roles and responsibilities, who become anxious with newness, and who are uncomfortable making independent decisions will undermine this initiative.

Agencies may be severely tested in recruiting staff for this model. Staff assignments without an interviewing and selection process may yield disappointing results. The staff must be the front-line marketers and representatives of this initiative and the agency. Putting the best foot forward is a necessary step in this process.

Also critical are sound fiscal management and solid grant-writing skills. Home health agencies interested in developing this nursing model must reach out to nontraditional sources of funding. Grantsmanship will be critical as will staff investment of time, energy to write proposals, and the ability to accept the rejects with the acceptances. In addition, agency administrators must know the costs and charges associated with such an endeavor. Nothing is for free, even if it appears so to the public (Hansen-Turton and Kinsey, 2001).

Current knowledge about managed care contracts in your state, county, and city will be the responsibility of the fiscal manager and senior staff. In addition, how to project budgets based on certain health mandates or contract languages will increasingly be an expectation. Maximizing staff skills in these turbulent times will be challenging but is possible. Reallocation of resources, be they personnel, space, or equipment, is also the purview of the fiscal manager and senior staff.

Careful consideration of budgets, financial opportunities, and constraints must be ongoing. Conferences with the fiscal manager should be routinely scheduled. Senior staff should actively participate and be aware of productivity, client outcomes, program costs, personnel costs (including benefits), the status of accounts receivable, the prospects of future funding, and so forth. No one person should assume total responsibility for this model's fiscal viability. This, too, is a shared enterprise.

Nurses and other allied health professionals have seldom been involved in the planning and managing of budgets. This may be a first for some of the agency's staff. As such, staff may be reluctant to learn and may withdraw from the process. This would be detrimental to all. Through learning and sharing, expenses can be managed, programs can be provided, and positive outcomes can be documented.

Any plan for this nursing model must be realistic. Some voluntary programs may emerge from internal agency reserves but such reserves may not be sustainable. Long-term sustainability may emerge from productive provider and community relationships and their interests in working together to achieve common goals through shared resources.

THE FUTURE OF ADVOCACY AND NURSING CENTERS

Throughout the assessment, strategic planning, program development, information systems, human resource, and fiscal management phases, client advocacy prevails. If the agency loses sight of what the clients' needs and interests are, the viability and long-term sustainability of this nursing model is jeopardized.

Lillian Wald's advocacy prototype should be one of the agency's core activities, regardless of program, site of service, or targeted outcome. This activity should involve clients, staff, community members, and agency affiliates. Changes in staff roles and responsibilities can

emerge through advocacy work. Even venues of services as well as the name for this nursing model may change over time. Being in tune with the community will help the agency move in concert with others interested in preserving and sustaining health.

It may be that the home health agency starting this nursing model is now better positioned to work with local health care institutions than to plan major moves into the community. The institutions may be seeking practice opportunities, and the agency may need skilled staff. These are ideal opportunities to share rather than create more resources in isolation.

In recent years, it has been increasingly difficult for free-standing nurse-managed health centers to remain financially viable. Many centers have opened with specific grant or contract-funding streams only to learn over time that the reimbursement for primary care services is insufficient for low-income persons and that the number of insured presenting for care constantly strains the budget. The constant demands of seeking new and ongoing sources of funds places pressure on finite staff resources and, inevitably, some programs end.

Successful centers have taken advantage of opportunities to collaborate with other service providers and organizations either through sub-contracts or joint-funding sources. Several centers have been awarded federally qualified health center (FQHC) status, which provides cost-based reimbursement for Medicaid patients and, depending on the type of FQHC status, grant monies to offset the cost of care to the uninsured. Centers have applied for this status independently or have linked with an existing FQHC. This opportunity should be examined by home health agencies. Thoughtful scrutiny of the proposed board composition and bylaws structure must be conducted. FQHC status requires that community board members be active and equal participants in the governance of the FQHC. The board is responsible for fiduciary oversight and hiring and/or dismissing the executive director. These two requirements may be counter to the current governance of the nonprofit agency.

The evolution and future of nursing centers rest mainly on the targeted community, the agency, staff, and consumers. In the future, nursing centers may be hubs of health care with more work to accomplish than the large tertiary care institutions around the corner. Nursing cen-

ters will then be the stepping stones for other social and health enterprises.

The possibilities are limitless. Is your home health agency up for the challenge? Lillian Wald would say so.

REFERENCES

Anderko, L. 2000. The effectiveness of a rural nursing center in improving the health care access in a three-county area. *Journal of Rural Health* 16(2): 177–184.

Berkman, L., and K. Lochner. 2002. Social determinants of health: Meeting at the crossroads. *Health Affairs* 21(2): 291–293.

Buhler Wilkerson, K. 1993. Bring care to the people: Lillian Wald's legacy to public health nursing. *American Journal of Public Health* 83(12): 1778–1786.

Campbell, B. 2000. Preventive health service outcomes in three government funded health centers. *Family & Community Health* 23(1): 18–28.

Christensen, C., R. Bohmer, and J. Kenagy. 2000. Will disruptive innovations cure health care? *Harvard Business Review* 78(5): 102–112.

Gerrity, P., and K. Kinsey. 1999. An urban nurse-managed primary health care center: Health promotion in action. *Family & Community Health* 21(4): 29–40.

Hansen-Turton, T., and K. Kinsey. 2001. The quest for self-sustainability: Nurse-managed health centers meeting the policy challenge. *Policy, Politics & Nursing Practice* 2(4): 304–309.

Hurst, C., and L. Osban. 2000. Service learning on wheels: The Nightingale mobile clinic. *Nursing and Health Care Perspectives* 21(4): 184–187.

Reverby, S. 1993. From Lillian Wald to Hillary Rodham Clinton: What will happen to public health nursing? *American Journal of Public Health* 83(12): 1662–1663.

Smith, J. 2003. *Education and public health: Natural partners in learning for life.* Alexandra, VA. Association for Supervision and Curriculum Development.

Swan, B., and M. Catroneo. 1999. Financing strategies for a community nursing center. *Nursing Economics* 17(1): 44–48.

CHAPTER 69

Adult Day Services—The Next Frontier

Nancy Brundy, Judith A. Bellome, and Paulette Bryan

Adult day services have become masters at managing their clients' chronic health conditions over time. Adult day services are community-based group programs designed to meet the needs of adults with physical and cognitive impairments through individual plans of care. Adult day centers' teams of professionals assess the needs of participants and provide services to meet those needs. These structured, comprehensive, nonresidential programs offer a variety of health, social, rehabilitative, and related support services in a protective setting. By supporting families and other caregivers who choose home and community-based services, adult day services enable participants to live in their communities (National Adult Day Services, 1997).

The current surge of interest in adult day services can be attributed to the versatility and the cost-effectiveness of these programs. In fact, at an average cost of $56 per day (Cox, 2002), adult day services are the health care bargain of the decade. With health care costs soaring, the need for health care services growing, and the older population booming, adult day services are becoming the new choice of the health care industry. Adding to the popularity of the program is the fact that these programs, like home care, help to keep elderly and disabled adults in their homes and communities—where they choose to be.

HISTORY OF ADULT DAY SERVICES

In the United States, adult day services began as psychiatric day hospitals, such as the Yale Psychiatric Clinic in the 1940s, primarily to assist patients following release from mental institutions. In the 1950s, Dr. Lionel Cosin's geriatric day hospital programs at sites in England inspired interest in creating adult day services in this country. He established his model of day programs in the Cherry State Hospital in North Carolina in the 1960s. During this decade, the day care concept shifted from its single psychiatric focus to other health maintenance issues. The growth in the number of centers was significant over the next three decades. In 1975, there were only 15 adult day centers (Cox et al, 1995). The number had grown to 1,200 in 1985, 2,100 in 1989, and 3,000 in 1994. Today there are over 3,400 centers nationwide. Continued growth of centers has been hindered by the lack of adequate third-party payment.

In the late 1960s, adult day service centers responded to the need for supportive care outside of institutions. By the 1970s, it was recognized that institutions such as nursing homes were being overused. The cost of institutional care was so high that, as an alternative, adult day service centers began offering skilled health services. Into the 1980s, Medicaid still remained the primary source of funding in addition to private pay. Today, additional sources of revenue that continue to foster growth in the adult day services industry include the Medicaid Home and Community-Based Waiver; state and local programs; USDA/CACFP (food program); Title III of the Older Americans Act and the National Family Caregivers Support Program (NFCSP); Veteran's Administration—VA Millennium Act; Medicaid Personal Care; Title XX—Social Services Block Grant; Comprehensive Outpatient Rehabilitation Facility

(CORF), under Medicare, for outpatient therapies; county and state levies; long-term care insurance; and managed care reimbursement for skilled services including restorative and functional maintenance rehabilitation. The last frontier for adult day care covered services is Medicare and other health insurances.

THE ADULT DAY CARE SERVICE MARKET

Dr. Burton V. Reifler, director of Partners in Caregiving: The Dementia Services Program, predicted a need for 10,000 adult day care centers by the year 2000 (Cox et al., 1995). With approximately 3,400 adult day centers existing in 2003, an abundance of business opportunity exists.

A profile of current providers reveals that 70 percent of the centers are affiliated with a larger parent organization including community-based service organizations, hospitals, and nursing homes. Seventy-seven percent are located in urban areas and 23 percent in rural areas. Centers provide a wide array of services, including substantial health care and rehabilitation (Figure 69–1) (Cox, 2002).

A profile of day center participants, done by the same study, shows the average age of the adult day care client is 72, with 93 percent of those participants served having some type of dementia or frailty, resulting in the client requiring assistance. Over the past 20 years, the industry has responded to the decrease in functional level and independence of their target population. The National Adult Day Services Association (NADSA) revised its *Standards and Guidelines for Adult Day Services* (1997) in response to the increasing number of centers and clients' increasing acuity levels, by creating the following structure of health care levels. There are three levels of care that describe the needs and interventions required for individuals:

1. The client at *Level of Need 1* or *Core Services Level* is in need of socialization, some protective supervision, supportive services, and minimal assistance with activities of daily living (ADLs). This client is medically stable and does not need nursing observation or intervention on a regular basis.

2. The client at *Level of Need 2* or *Enhanced Services Level* is in need of moderate assistance and may need—in addition to health assessment—nursing oversight, therapy services at a maintenance level, and moderate assistance with one to three ADLs. The participant may have difficulty communicating and making appropriate judgments, and may periodically demonstrate disruptive behavior that can be managed.

3. The client at *Level of Need 3* or *Intensive Services Level* is in need of maximum assistance. The participant's medical condition is not stable and requires regular monitoring or intervention by a nurse. Therapy services are needed at a rehabilitative or restorative level. There may be a need for total care in one or more ADLs. The individual may display frequent disruptive behavior requiring staff intervention and may be unable to communicate needs.

These standards are not meant to define levels of need or serve as an inflexible guideline by which to provide care. Instead, they emphasize the importance of individual assessments and individualized plans of care.

STATE REGULATIONS AND ADULT DAY SERVICES

State regulation of adult day services varies, with only 26 states requiring licensure and 24 states having some type of certification regulations. Regulations regarding staff support ratios and square footage requirements are established by each state, *but at a minimum*, the staff to participant ratio should be one to six (National Adult Day Services Association, 1997). As the number and severity of participants with functional impairments increase, the staff to participant ratio should be adjusted accordingly. For example, more specifically, the National Study of Adult Day Services, conducted by the Robert Wood

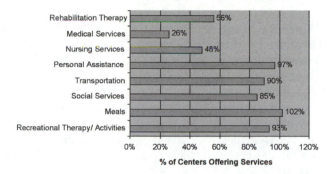

Services Offered by Adult Day Services Programs

Service	%
Rehabilitation Therapy	56%
Medical Services	26%
Nursing Services	48%
Personal Assistance	97%
Transportation	90%
Social Services	85%
Meals	102%
Recreational Therapy/ Activities	93%

% of Centers Offering Services

Figure 69–1 Services Offered by Adult Day Service Programming

Source: Partners in Caregiving: The Adult Day Services Program. (2003). *A National Study of Adult Day Services, 2001–2002.* Winston-Salem, NC: Wake Forest University School of Medicine.

Note: Data include all levels of adult day services, including specialty centers (e.g., HIV and dementia care).

Johnson Partners in Caregiving Program, revealed that the direct care staffing ratio for dementia-specific centers is 1:6.5, for social model programs the ratio is 1:7.3, for combination model programs the ratio is 1:7.4, and for medical model programs the ratio is 1:7.8 (Cox, 2002). The important aspect to keep in mind is that as these figures are reviewed, it is the acuity levels of the center population that must be evaluated individually.

The average required space for participant usage is 60 square feet per participant (National Adult Day Services Association, 1997). In centers that serve a significant number of people with cognitive impairment or who use adaptive equipment for ambulation or medical equipment for support, a higher level of square footage is recommended. Other regulatory requirements may mandate minimum services and staff credentials. Some regulations may prevent adult day service centers from being part of an existing nursing home structure while others may require it. Standardization in the area of regulatory requirements is a goal of NADSA.

FINANCING ADULT DAY CARE

Financing an adult day services business is a challenge. The challenge includes an average start-up time of 2 to 3 years before full census (35 participants per day) is achieved, an operating cost of at least $200,000 to $250,000 per year, and poor third-party reimbursement. Traditionally, adult day service centers have been started and managed by not-for-profit organizations that served the low-income, Medicaid-eligible client. Because state Medicaid programs, the largest source of third-party payment, usually pay less than the cost of care, these providers covered their start-up, maintenance, service, and transportation costs with grants and fund-raising activities. As these philanthropic dollars have become more challenging to obtain, centers have sought more private-pay opportunities. As of this printing, Medicare does not cover the cost of adult day services, and affordable long-term care insurance policies that cover this kind of care are still fairly rare.

MARKETING AND PROMOTIONS

As in all successful business practices, having a sound business plan is critical to planning and operations. Key elements in the business plan are the completion of a comprehensive market assessment and marketing/promotion plan, both of which will help in the identification and development of the center's market share, which will determine the sustainability of the adult day services business. Community awareness and name recognition for the adult day services industry still presents a challenge. One of the key elements in a comprehensive marketing plan is a strong emphasis on building media relationships. Human-interest stories about clients and their families often attract media attention. Compelling stories can develop into press opportunities that are newsworthy, translating into coverage and visibility for the adult day center. Some additional, low-cost marketing options include phone book advertisements and distribution of attractive, professional brochures.

More informal and personal mechanisms of marketing adult day services involve the utilization of existing networks of social service and health care providers. Attendance at meetings and membership in service organizations helps to increase contacts that can lead to referral sources. Targeting family practice physicians and other physicians with practices that include older adults and disabled adults, gerontologists, local area Agency on Aging offices, and discharge planners in hospitals, home health, and long-term facilities is essential to a successful marketing plan. Building collaborative relationships with home health agencies, assisted living facilities, and retirement communities may also lead to an integrated system of referral and support, establishing more formal alliances or networks that can lead to increased managed care and insurance contracts for services. These efforts should have a positive effect upon your census development and ultimately the center's bottom line.

FINANCIAL MANAGEMENT

Beyond the selling of the services lies the issue of financial management. Maintaining the delicate balance of multiple revenue streams and expenses is the administrator's task. Basic business principles support knowing your unit cost and making sure fees are set *at* or *above* unit cost. Adherence to these principles should enable the business to achieve good financial standing. His-

torically, many adult day services organizations have charged less than the cost of care, due to the mistaken belief that most clients and families are unable to afford the cost of care. Fund-raising and grant writing have been the primary mechanisms by which costs were subsidized. However, in today's market, many philanthropic sources have cut back on their giving.

The National Adult Day Services Association supports the premise that the business of adult day services should follow the example of children's day care. Child day care clients pay the service fee in advance and receive no refunds, even if the client does not attend as scheduled. By following this example, cash flow remains positive and human resource management becomes manageable. Predictable staffing patterns enhance quality of care and consequently support the stabilization of an otherwise volatile long-term care workforce. Continuing in the footsteps of child day care, the adult day center's hours of operation should reflect those of the local child-care centers in order to accommodate working caregivers.

Transportation is necessary to ensure the success of any center, but can be one of the greatest expenses and challenges to the program. Many centers recommend contracting for the transportation services with existing community businesses, due to the high cost of wheelchair accessible multi-passenger vans, high insurance rates, vehicle maintenance, driver availability and reliability, and issues surrounding scheduling. Facilities that are centrally located and close to major roads and highways make accessibility easy and convenient for the contracted transportation or family-arranged rides.

ATMOSPHERE AND DESIGN

A great many adult day experts regard the environment, or milieu, of a day center as an essential part of the therapeutic process. Additionally, these same experts also recognize the tremendous impact that atmosphere and design can have on the center's earning power. Both of these points of view will be discussed here.

The Americans with Disabilities Act (ADA) of 1990 and Section 504 of the Rehabilitation Act of 1973 contain provisions requiring that facilities design their surroundings to be accessible for people with disabilities. However, a distinction is made between older buildings and new construction. Federal barrier-free standard requirements and specifications are more stringent for new construction. The regulations state that removal of barriers in a structure already built is necessary only if "already achievable" and carried out without difficulty or extraordinary expense. Additionally, physical facilities need to be in compliance with applicable state and local building regulations and zoning, and fire and health codes or ordinances. When possible, the center should also be located on street level and have its own separate, identifiable entrance and space, enabling ease of accessibility and visibility.

Keeping federal and state regulations in mind, the facility, to be therapeutically effective, needs to have sufficient space to accommodate the full range of planned activities, services, and staff. When all of these allowances are made to work in concert with each other, a center can then begin to realize the power of economies of scale. True economies of scale can be achieved by increased square footage, and proper utilization of paraprofessional staff to client ratios are maximized for enhanced quality of care. Such economies make it possible to serve a higher census, thus improving operating margins.

HIPAA AND ADULT DAY SERVICES

The National Adult Day Services Association's *Standards and Guidelines* (1997) state: "Each adult day center shall maintain a participant record system." In this standard is the guideline that "a written policy on confidentiality and the protection of records . . . be maintained" (National Adult Day Services Association, 1984). Recently, the Health Insurance Portability and Accountability Act of 1996 (HIPAA) has been amended with new protections. This law has always held that identifiable health information about participants be kept confidential. HIPAA law has been expanded to include electronic transmittals and businesses that have not previously been considered health care entities. Adult day services have prepared for these changes.

NATIONAL ACCREDITATION

The National Adult Day Services Association selected the Commission of Accreditation for Rehabilitation Facilities, the Rehabilitation Accreditation Commission, to provide national accreditation for the field of adult day services. The number of centers seeking accreditation is growing, as there is increasing recognition that third-party payers, as well as many consumers, look for accreditation as a measure of quality in services provided and in their business operations. States and the federal government are also looking at accreditation as a way to ensure quality and/or provide oversight without having to expand or create licensing and certification programs.

CONSUMER DEMAND

Few experts in the field of aging deny that the population is aging. The need for more long-term care services and care options will grow with this population of health care consumers. However, such professional organizations as the National Adult Day Services Association and the National Association for Home Care and Hospice have also found that consumer awareness is also a primary determinant of consumer demand for adult day and home health services. A recent study, completed by Georgetown University's Long-Term Care Financing project, found that "well-informed applicants are likely to fare better . . . in the long-term care continuum. Officials noted that the outcome of inquiries made by the families . . . regarding the availability of long-term care services might depend on how savvy, connected, or aware they are regarding the availability of services. If they were able to ask about specific programs and request pertinent information on those programs they may have a more favorable outcome [in obtaining services]" (Georgetown University, 2003).

Consumer demand appears to be stronger among caregivers seeking respite from the responsibilities associated with dementia care. Supported by the Robert Wood Johnson Foundation, the National Partners in Caregivers Project identified three target markets within the caregiver group: (1) care seekers, who want full-day, center-based services and are potential heavy users; (2) respite seekers, who seek occasional breaks rather than daily care and are potential moderate users; and (3) information seekers, interested in information but unsure if their loved one needs care. Despite consumer demand for day care services being somewhat higher among dementia caregivers, direct consumer referrals from family, friends, and co-workers accounted for only 19 percent of total referrals. Seventy-five percent of referrals typically come from formal sources: health care professionals, social service agencies, and the Alzheimer's Association (Reifler,1995).

In addition to the lack of consumer awareness, there are two other formidable barriers to use of adult day services. To many older people, the notion of regular attendance at a center, even when transportation is provided, is an unfamiliar one. Participation in most day care programs requires a commitment of a certain number of days per week; services are rarely provided on a drop-in basis. If a client has never visited a center, he or she may not be responsive initially to the service, expressing a preference to have services brought into the home. However, after attending the center for just a few days, a client quickly realizes the advantages of the group activities, social interchange, and the services available at the center. For this reason, most centers have prospective clients spend a few days on a trial basis so that both the client and the provider can determine the appropriateness of this type of service.

The out-of-pocket cost to the consumer is another formidable barrier. As just noted, Medicaid is the only significant third-party payer of

adult day services at the present time, leaving most of the cost to be paid directly by clients and their families. Although a daily cost of $56 per day covers several services and reflects an hourly rate of less than $10, families with fixed incomes or limited resources may find the total monthly cost to be substantial. Many not-for-profit centers have traditionally been reluctant to set their standard fee equal to or greater than cost for this reason, denying them the opportunity to have willing clients pay what the service actually costs.

THE HOME CARE–DAY SERVICE CONNECTION

Home care companies traditionally view day services as either a competitor or a service to which they can refer once skilled care is completed. The competitive view is reinforced by some fiscal intermediaries' interpretation of Medicare's homebound requirement in such a way as to render an adult day service client ineligible for home health agency services. New provisions in interpretation of P.L. 106-554: Homebound Clarification Act, allow "any absence from home attributable to need to receive healthcare treatment shall not negate the beneficiary's homebound status—including regular absences to participate in therapeutic, psychosocial or medical treatment in adult day services program" (Medicare, 2000). The home care and day service industries worked together to remove this barrier. As home care assumes an increasingly important role within integrated delivery systems, incentives are created for home care companies to develop cooperative partnerships with day service providers. For example, a home care company operating under a health maintenance organization (HMO), traditional insurance plan, or Medicare under prospective payment can expand services to the patient by coordinating the care plan site of service between home and the adult day center. A patient requiring three nursing visits and three therapy visits in the home can receive additional care on the 2 days of attendance to the adult day center without jeopardizing the homebound status or impacting the payment to the home care agency.

The National Adult Day Services Association is sponsoring federal legislation that would enable a patient to receive home health level of care in the adult day service center. This will provide opportunities for home health providers to develop partnerships with adult day service centers or to establish their own adult day service centers. The benefit to the patient and family is increased choice as to the setting of care. In addition, the individual and family will receive a broader range of service than home care alone can provide. For example, twice-a-day dressing changes could be accomplished in the home and in the day service center under the same plan of care.

As home care assumes an increasing role within integrated delivery systems, health plan capitation would be interested in a home care day service care package if it effectively met clients' needs at a lower cost than home care alone. For a client receiving several skilled services per week, the cost of providing such treatment in a congregate group setting could provide significant savings. While a home care nurse might see 5 to 7 clients a day, a nurse in the adult day health center can provide skilled services to 15 a day. In this instance, the home care company would pay for the day services out of its capitation.

Most of the creative managed care opportunities for day service providers are in the skilled services arena, stimulating interest on their part in developing the health services component of these programs. Home care companies can enter into contractual arrangements to provide nursing and therapy staff to day centers or provide additional training to existing center staff to strengthen their hands-on skills.

ADULT DAY SERVICES IN A NEW HEALTH CARE MARKET

Will the significant growth that the adult day services field has seen over the last few years be helped or hindered by health care reform and market changes? Can a traditionally public-funded and subsidized service attract both the private pay and insurance dollars required for expansion? These authors predict that adult day services will experience significant growth and development over the next five years as providers become part of integrated delivery systems and increasingly seek to manage chronic illness and disability through utilization of alternate levels of care.

Management of a stroke within an integrated delivery system provides an illustrative example. The traditional plan of care following the acute episode usually involves rehabilitation in a skilled nursing facility (SNF), followed by several weeks of home health care involving multiple disciplines. An alternative plan is to bypass or significantly shorten the SNF stay, replacing it with a combined home care/day services plan that utilizes the time spent in the center for aggressive rehabilitation, skilled nursing, and personal care, supplemented by supportive home care services. The costs of a day care service/home care package are significantly less than the costs of the SNF alone or home health care alone.

Although adult day service is not yet a covered Medicare or traditional insurance benefit, HMOs, including Medicare HMOs, have the flexibility to "go outside of benefit." Some third party insurers will pay the cost of the rehabilitation component of adult day health services, under their policies' outpatient benefits. Likewise, provider delivery systems that operate under full capitation have incentives to pay for day services if they effectively substitute for higher-cost services. To build the case, adult day service providers are busy trying to identify the types of clients and conditions that will benefit most from an alternative treatment plan. Outcome measurement is in its infancy in the adult day services field, and the definitive data that HMOs want is generally not yet available.

Coverage under long-term care policies is much more common but less visible because of the small number of policyholders that currently use such benefits. California, for example, requires that adult day service be part of the benefit package under all its "certified" long-term care policies. The newer long-term care policies include adult day services and home care in addition to nursing home placement. The projected growth of long-term care insurance will undoubtedly expand the day service market.

The national trend toward Medicaid-managed care may well be the most significant factor fueling the growth of the day service field. Medicaid currently spends 74 percent of its budget on long-term care costs, primarily nursing homes. While the potential of adult day service to reduce acute care costs is yet untapped, its ability to prevent or postpone nursing home use for certain populations is well recognized. Because those states that have a Medicaid adult day service benefit usually require that the client be "nursing home certifiable" to become eligible, day service providers have substantial experience with this frail population. When the states include long-term care under their Medicaid-managed care initiatives, insurers and Medicaid nursing home providers will suddenly have huge incentives to utilize adult day services.

This country's leading example of a fully capitated system of primary, acute, and long-term care for frail elders is the Program of All Inclusive Care for the Elderly (PACE). PACE is the national replication of the On-Lok model, developed in San Francisco, and is now provided by a number of organizations across the country. A PACE provider receives a monthly capitation from Medicare and Medicaid for each client and is responsible for providing the full spectrum of medical, health, and social services, including acute and nursing home care if necessary, all aimed at making it possible for clients who would otherwise be in a nursing home to stay in the community. PACE services focus on clients' regular attendance at an adult day health center, combined with home care. All primary medical care and most skilled nursing care are provided on site at the center.

Based on all these factors, several companies, coming out of the home health and rehabilitation arenas, have developed large numbers of adult day services. These currently include Active Services Corporation, Almost Family, and Senior Care Centers of America. Many nonprofit providers of adult day services have also expanded with multiple centers and, in some cases, PACE programs. Easter Seals has a network of over 45 adult day centers as well.

CONCLUSION

Adult day services will continue to develop and expand as long-term care needs, managed care pressures, and integrated health care system trends exert their collective influence to shape new forms of care. For home care providers, adult day services are a logical addition and a significant business opportunity. The combination of day services and home care services may well become the core of America's future long-term care system.

REFERENCES

Adult Day Services and Home Care: Setting A New Standards in Community Based Care. (1996, December). *CARING Magazine* 12.

Cox, Nancy. 2002. *National study of adult day services 2001–2002 (CD)*. Partners In Caregiving: Robert Wood Johnson Foundation. North Carolina.

Cox, Nancy, Rona Smyth Henry, and Burton Reifler. (1995). *Adult day services in America*. Robert Wood Johnson partners in Caregiving: The Dementia Services Program. North Carolina.

Laura Sumner. May 2003. Georgetown University Long-Term Care Financing Project. *http://ltc.georgetown.edu/pdfs/choicesexec.pdf*.

Medicare, Medicaid and SCHIP Benefits Improvement and Protection Act, P.L. 106-554. 21 December 2000. Section 507 114 Stat. 2763A-532, 2763A-533 Department of Health Care Human Services Health Care Financing Administration. (2001, February 6). Clarification of the Homebound Definition under the Medicare Home Health Benefit. Program Memorandum: Intermediaries Transmittal A-01-21.

National Adult Day Services Association. 1984, 1997. *Standards and guidelines*. Washington, DC: The National Council on the Aging.

New Frontier for Home Care: Adult Day Care Comes of Age. 1996. *Home Health Business Report III* 5: 12–14.

Reifler, B.V. May, 1995. What I want if I get Alzheimer's disease. *Archives of Family Medicine* 4(5): 395–6.

CHAPTER 70

Partners in Healing: Home Care, Hospice, and Parish Nurses

Karen Cassidy

A creative way to support patients in self-care strategies is to work with the parish nurse as a practice partner. This chapter shares approaches and innovative ideas on how home care and hospice nurses can work effectively with parish nurses.

Prospective payment systems (PPS) have greatly impacted the provision of all services, especially the need for every visit to be cost effective and to enable the patient to become self-sufficient as soon as possible. More now than before, nurses must find creative ways to provide continued services while using their professional expertise to offer skilled services in the most effective and efficient manner. Nurses must work closely with families and other support systems from the first visit to assist in an effective discharge that facilitates patient goals. The parish nurse can be an effective support system with whom the nurse can coordinate services and who the patient and family can use as a resource for self-care.

A BRIEF HISTORY OF PARISH NURSING

Sending church women into parishioners' homes to provide health care dates back to the third century. By the 19th century, religious denominations in the United States were implementing health ministry programs within congregations (Zersen, 1994). The trend toward health care for the whole person has led to the development of an independent nursing practice role called parish nursing (Matteson, 1999).

The latest parish nursing movement in the United States is credited to the work of the Reverend Dr. Granger Westberg, a Lutheran minister, hospital chaplain, and medical school professor who established the first institutionally based parish nurse program with six churches in 1984 in Chicago, Illinois. Dr. Westberg believed that these nurses combine two critical languages—the language of science and the language of spiritual care (McGee, 1998). In the 1990s, public health programs began using churches for health programs, targeting minority groups especially for cancer and hypertension control and detection (Davis et al., 1994; Edwards, 1995).

ROLES AND RELATIONSHIPS

Parish nursing is a unique, specialized practice of professional nursing that holds the spiritual dimension as central to practice (Matteson, 1999). Based in a faith community, the parish nurse specialty is a needed safety net in an increasingly complex health care delivery system (Abbott, 1998). The parish nurse promotes wellness in the physical, social, emotional, and spiritual realms.

Parish nurses do not perform hands-on care or reimbursable skilled-nursing services, nor do they take the place of home care nurses (see Figure 70-1). Instead, parish nurses focus on health

	Parish Nurse	Home Care Nurse
Types of Nursing Services	No hands-on services; praying with patients	Skilled-nursing services; billable services only
Focus of Care	Focus on health promotion, disease prevention, with emphasis on spiritual care	Focus on nursing problem list, specific problems
Accountable to	Patients, faith-based community, ministerial team, or hospital-based team	Patients, home care agency
Doctors Order and Plan of Care	Not needed	Mandatory
Functions	Counselor, referral source, educator, advocate	Case manager, direct caregiver
Client's Payment Method	No payment from client health agency or insurance	Client billed through home
Nurse's Payment Method	Volunteer, or paid by faith community	Salary from home health agency
Nurse-Client Relationship	Member of client's faith community, may know family and friends	Professional relationship, based on personally therapeutic relationship
Location of Visit	Home, nursing home, hospital, screenings, and health fairs	Home visit
Visit Limit	Variable, one visit to ongoing	Restricted, 60-day maximum

Figure 70–1 Role Comparison of the Parish Nurse and Home Care Nurse

promotion and disease prevention—an aspect of care that home care nurses wish they had time to do. A parish nurse focuses on the promotion of health within the context of the values, beliefs, and practices of a faith community, such as a church, synagogue, or mosque. The nursing practice provided includes the faith community's mission and ministry to its members, the families, individuals, and community it serves (HMA/ANA, 1998). A parish nurse brings together knowledge from the humanities and sciences, works collegially with both health professionals and clergy, and perceives nursing as a service in the spirit of personal faith (Westberg, 1990).

A parish nurse's job description is continually developing to respond to the needs of the congregation served. Typically, a parish nurse assesses the needs of a particular congregation in a holistic manner with the goal of meeting the needs of members of all ages. The most common interventions that arise from this assessment require the nurse to function as educator, counselor, referral agent, advocate, and facilitator.

One parish nurse described a day of practice:

I have just completed a weekly phone conversation with a woman whose husband, suffering from severe memory loss, is awaiting placement in a nursing home. Alerted by our senior pastor, we identified her need for someone to talk to regularly and freely through this crisis period. . . . I also assist two other elderly couples to connect with services they need in order to continue living in their own homes. . . . These couples become part of my "hello rounds" before each Sunday. (Scott, 1995)

Coenen and associates (1999) describe the parish nurse practice using the framework of the Nursing Minimum Data Set. Nineteen parish nurses practicing in 22 faith communities collected data using standardized nursing classification systems and developed a database for quantitative analysis. Parish nurses recorded 1,557 encounters for services provided to 77 individuals. The most frequent nursing diagnoses and nursing interventions emphasized health promotion and illness prevention. The roles of educator, counselor, referral agent, and advocate/facilitator found in this study were consistent with the parish nurse role.

Parish nurses are willing partners in caring for the home and hospice patient. If a client is a member of a faith community, he or she may know if the congregation has a parish nurse; however, many elderly or inactive parishioners may not realize that this resource is available. Because parish nurses are independent care providers, a doctor's order is not needed. However, confidentiality must be honored. Be sure to obtain prior approval from the patient before contacting the parish nurse.

IS THERE A NEED FOR PARISH NURSING?

Many events in health care illustrate the need for parish nurses (Schank, 1996):

- The public has an increased interest in health promotion and disease prevention.
- There has been an increased awareness of the problematic fragmentation of the current health care system.

- The concept of "wholeness" has reemerged, with particular emphasis on self-care and individual responsibility.
- The elderly population has grown significantly, resulting in increases in the prevalence of many chronic illnesses.
- Health care trends, such as managed care and reduced length of hospital stay, in addition to limited resources and reimbursement, increase the need for nurses in community roles.

Parish nurses frequently coordinate volunteers for patient assistance such as grocery shopping, meal preparation, and house cleaning. Services such as daily contacts and transportation to the physician's office may be provided when eligibility for home care expires, and before and after home care nurses are involved in providing care.

THE ROLE AND FUNCTION OF THE PARISH NURSE AS CARE PARTNER

Parish nurses are eager to work in professional relationships with home and hospice nurses to enhance care delivery to members of their faith communities, and more than 40 percent attend a worship service at least weekly (Schank et al., 1996). A parish nurse is a friendly face seen by parishioners as they worship. The nurses usually know the client's family and friends and are invaluable in assessing needs and linking the client with care providers, such as church members, community resources, or health care institutions (Abbott, 1998).

The parish nurse is a registered nurse who must fulfill (1) state-mandated expectations as required by the Nurse Practice Act, (2) the *Scope and Standards of the Parish Nursing Practice* (HMA/ANA, 1998), and (3) the interdisciplinary role as member of the ministry team of the faith community.

Most parish nurses work on a part-time, voluntary basis. To be effective, the parish nurse must possess many competencies. Nursing expertise must be combined with ministry skills and theological adequacy. The parish nurse must have a clear sense of pastoral identity and ministry presence (Mustoe, 1998).

With the client's informed consent, the parish nurse can assist the home and hospice nurse as a qualified, additional set of "eyes and ears" (Penner and Galloway-Lee, 1997). Observing the client's and family's functional levels and coping mechanisms can be as much a part of the parish nurse's home visit as that of the home care nurse, with referral to other providers as indicated. Contacting discharge planners, case managers, and home and hospice providers when clients are hospitalized and likely to require services after discharge is a function that parish nurses can perform well because of their clinical backgrounds (Penner and Galloway-Lee, 1997). Parish nurses can provide care before and during home care services, not merely when Medicare or insurance coverage has expired.

The majority of nurses believe in holistic health—the integration of the physical, psychological, social, and spiritual aspects of patients and their families within the community. Such integration allows harmony with self, others, the environment, and God and creates a sense of "wholeness, salvation, or shalom" (HMA/ANA, 1998). This bond between practitioners provides a platform of communication that enables both types of professional to work more effectively together.

HOW TO WORK WITH PARISH NURSES

Here are some tips that might be helpful for nurses seeking to collaborate with parish nurses:

- Consult with parish nurses between home visits and especially at the time of discharge.
- Remember, these nurses have the valuable skills of observation and assessment. They can be your teammate to observe wounds, eating habits, mobility, and support systems as well as to refer patients to other agencies and support groups.
- For the patient experiencing exacerbations and remissions of chronic illness, networking with parish nurses can result in a

continuing emphasis on living within limitations within the community (Thomas and King, 2000).

- When the curing of disease holds little hope or when spiritual care is especially important, consider contacting the parish nurse. Her emphasis is on overall care and praying with the patient.
- Contact the parish nurse when the patient continues to require assistance after home care discharge.
- When the patient seems to be healing physically but coping poorly with the emotional aspects of their condition, consider asking if they belong to a faith community that has a parish nurse.

BARRIERS AND ASSUMPTIONS

Often parishioners believe the hospital will automatically notify their church, synagogue, or parish. Due to HIPAA policies, hospitals cannot provide access to patient records. Patients must give permission to share information with any individual or organization. Many clergy have insufficient time to make home visits, but also fail to understand the role or potential benefit of a parish nurse. In addition, hospital and home care chaplains and discharge planners are often unaware of the emerging role of parish nursing.

SUMMARY

Parish nurses have the potential to reduce the cost of health care and to improve the quality of life by focusing on the prevention of disease before the need for expensive treatment. They can assist clients to learn new lifestyle behaviors (and to modify current ones) and help the elderly remain in their homes, thus reducing the cost of institutionalization. Foremost, the parish nurse is a resource for promoting optimal self-care and efficient use of resources to prevent complications and reoccurrence, especially in cases of chronic and functional disability (Schank et al., 1996).

PARISH NURSING ONLINE RESOURCES

www.marguette.edu/dept/nursing/
parish.html
www.carroll.edu/parishnurse/
GettingStarted.htm
www.stfx.ca/academic/extension/
continuing/parish/html
www.mabc.bc.ca.biblio/parish.htm
ocprint.otterbein.edu/grad/
nursing/parishnursing.htm
parish.nurse.resource.center
@worldnet.att.net

TIPS FOR WORKING WITH PARISH NURSES

Talk with your agency chaplains and discharge planners to determine if they are aware of the concept of parish nursing. Show them this chapter.

Together with the chaplains and discharge planners, conduct a community assessment of the faith communities in your area; contact them to determine if they have parish nurses. Develop a list all can use.

Consider having the parish nurse visit clients during your home visit (after consulting with and obtaining permission from the client). Your clients can benefit from the parish nurse's skills of assessment and observation between your visits.

If you belong to a faith community or have the opportunity to support a parish nurse, do so for the health of your clients, as well as for the health of the overall community. Support parish nurses as part of the ministry team and as a part of your team.

A CONVERSATION BETWEEN A HOME HEALTH NURSE (HHN) AND A PARISH NURSE (PN)

HHN: What can you really do to help me?

PN: From what I understand about home care nursing today, you have a heavy caseload and *you can't spend more that 60 minutes with a patient. I can spend a longer period of time, without having a caseload for the day that I must visit. I can listen to what is bothering our patient. I can help you by visiting with you. I can arrive at the beginning, middle, or end of your visit and you can use me to observe what is important to you in between visits. Remember that I am a nurse! I have had health assessment and have observational skills like you. Tell me what you want me to observe. I can reinforce whatever you are teaching the patient.*

HHN: How does your visiting my patient help the patient?

PN: You may be aware of the research that connects the mind and body and the powerful effect of mental attitude on effective healing. The lower the anxiety and fear, the better the healing. I will pray with our client and ask their Higher Power to assist them in the healing. If our patient is a member of a faith community, praying with another member— particularly a parish nurse—can be very helpful.

My visit will support the healing of the mind, body, and spirit. By praying with our patient, I assist the patient to turn their fears over to God. Together we can help our patient heal holistically.

Acknowledgment

The author extends her appreciation to Mary Oppelt, RN, Parish Nurse, St. Francis of Assisi Catholic Church, Louisville, Kentucky, for her assistance with this chapter.

REFERENCES

Abbott, B. 1998. Parish nursing. *Home Healthcare Nurse* 16(4): 265–267.

American Nurses Association/Health Ministries Association. 1998. *Scope and standards of parish nursing practice*. Washington, DC: ANA.

Coenen, A., D. M. Weis, M. J. Schank, and R. Matheus. 1999. Describing parish nurse practice using the Nursing Minimum Data Set. *Public Health Nursing* 16(6): 412–416.

Davis, D. T., A. Bustamenta, C. P. Brown, G. Walde-Tsadik, and E. W. Savage. 1994. The urban church and cancer control: A source of social influence in minority communities. *Public Health Reporter* 109: 500–506.

Edwards, C. H. 1995. Emerging issues in lifestyle, social and environmental interventions to promote behavioral change related to prevention and control of hypertension in the African-American population. *Journal of National Medical Association* 87(8S): 642–646.

Matteson, P. S. 1999, March. Parish nursing—A new, yet old model of care. *Massachusetts Nurse* 69(3): 5.

McGee, A. K. 1998. Parish nursing brings health care closer to home. *Texas Nursing* 72(6): 12.

Mustoe, K. J. 1998. Parish nursing is becoming an important stage in the healthcare continuum. *Health Progress* 79(3): 47.

Penner, S. J., and B. Galloway-Lee. 1997. Parish nursing opportunities in community health. *Home Care Provider* 2(5): 244–249.

Schank, M. J., D. Weis, and R. Matheus. 1996. Parish nursing: Ministry of healing. *Geriatric Nursing* 17(1): 11–13.

Scott, R. S. 1995. A day in the life of a parish nurse. *Minnesota Nursing Accent* 67(2): 1.

Thomas, D. J., and M. A. King. 2000. Parish nursing assessment: What should you know? *Home Healthcare Manager* 4(5): 11–13.

Westberg, G. A. 1990. A historical perspective: Wholistic health and the parish nurse. In A. Solari-Twadell, A. M. Djupe, and M. A. McDermott (eds.). *Parish nursing: The developing practice*. Park Ridge, IL: Lutheran General Health Care System, pp. 27–40.

Zersen, D. 1994. Parish nursing: 20th century fad? *Journal of Christian Nursing* 11(2): 19–21.

PART X

Strategies for Success

Meeting the Present Challenges and Continuing to Thrive in the Future: Tips on How to Be Successful as an Administrator in Home Health and Hospice Care

Marilyn D. Harris

TODAY'S HEALTH CARE CLIMATE

Changes in health care financing methods continue to have an impact on in-home services. One of the most obvious ones is that patients continue to be discharged more quickly and need more intensive levels of care. From the patient's and family's viewpoints, patients require skilled and support services, many of which they expect will be paid by Medicare or other third-party payers. This is not the case. For the administrator, more intensive levels of care may equal longer visits and decreased productivity for staff.

Another consideration is fixed payment as determined by the third-party payer and increased costs. Although the homebound elderly represent a majority of home care patients, there are other age groups that benefit from home care services.

The administrator faces several challenges:

- to provide high-quality home health and hospice care in a continuously changing and uncertain economic and regulatory climate
- to continue to meet certification, accreditation, and licensure standards
- to keep the home health agency fiscally sound and solvent
- to retain and attract qualified professional and support staff
- to maintain staff productivity
- to keep the staff and supervisors content and happy
- to maintain a sense of humor and perspective
- to consider the ethical issues that affect patients, families, staff, and the home health agency

These issues include the increased responsibilities that are placed on families as a result of high-technology procedures in the home as well as administrative issues, such as who will receive care in light of shrinking financial resources and how this care will be distributed in order to meet the health care needs of patients.

The staff members face still other dilemmas:

- how to provide quality care to patients under increased pressures from internal and external sources
- how to keep up with all the regulations regarding the provision of care and the ever-changing coverage issues

- how to document care for reimbursement purposes, not only for clinical, legal, and professional purposes
- how to master computerized clinical documentation systems
- how to maintain productivity standards established by and communicated to them by their administrators and supervisors
- how to maintain their sense of humor and proper perspective amid all the internal and external demands placed on them

Patients and families face still other issues:

- increased responsibilities to care for acutely ill individuals in the home
- scattered nuclear family members, who make it more difficult to coordinate care
- lack of financial resources to pay for needed services that are not covered by third-party payers
- lack of public or private funds to pay for long-term care

Although the prospective payment system (PPS) for home health care was implemented in 2000, some terms continue to surface in Medicare-funding proposals, including copayments. In addition to the financial challenges and uncertainties that administrators face each day, there are the clinical issues. For those administrators who are nurses, the American Nurses Association's *Scope and Standards for Nurse Administrators* delineates five primary domains of activity (ANA, 1996, p. 6): (1) leading, (2) collaborating, (3) integrating, (4) facilitating, and (5) evaluating. The nurse executive provides leadership and vision for nursing's philosophy, development, and advancement within the organization in particular and for the society at large. As an administrator, the nurse executive promotes a practice environment that empowers nurses to provide effective, compassionate, and efficient nursing care.

STRATEGIES FOR SURVIVAL

In spite of the many uncertainties in the 21st century, home health care and hospice adminis-

trators continue to survive the present and thrive in the future. To accomplish these goals, both long- and short-term strategies must be in place and utilized. All the issues addressed in this book are important for administrators to use as survival strategies. In review, these include the following issues, which are not listed in priority order, except for number 1:

1. Provide cost-effective, high-quality care (which is an expectation), ever mindful that the main reason why a home health agency and/or hospice exists is that there are patients who need the services that the agency's staff can provide. This multidisciplinary care must be flexible to meet the needs of individual patients and their families. Patient safety and satisfaction are priorities.

2. Evaluate the care rendered in terms of patient-focused outcomes. Administrators must collect and analyze manual or computerized data that will assist with the documentation of these patient outcomes.

3. Be totally familiar with the certification and accreditation standards that affect home health and hospice services.

4. Establish or improve methods to maintain fiscal stability. This includes the use of a management information system to monitor the myriad patient-related activities, payer sources, and demographic data to provide vital information that must be reported and on which to base sound management decisions.

5. Retain and attract qualified staff and contractors.

6. Manage fluctuating caseloads that can be financially and psychologically devastating to administration and staff. This may include alternative staffing patterns as discussed in this book.

7. Consider diversification or corporate reorganizations, if indicated.

8. Use a patient classification system (PCS), standardized flow sheets (SFS), nursing diagnoses (ND), and/or a computerized system to document patient care and pa-

tient outcomes. The use of these tools makes it possible for staff to address all the parameters that contribute to quality patient care. Staff know what parameters have to be addressed to meet the agency's quality assessment/performance improvement program's patient outcome criteria, which are based on certification and accreditation standards.

9. Provide disease management programs.

10. Be alert to legislative and regulatory issues that affect home care and hospice. It is most important to keep in contact with local, state, and national elected officials through letters and personal visits. It is also important to be a member of the state and national trade organizations that have established hotline communication networks to address pertinent issues on a timely basis.

11. Participate in research in the administrative and clinical aspects of home health and hospice care.

12. Develop and use patient education materials to maintain or increase the quality of care provided to patients to become even more efficient in the delivery of services.

13. Select carefully the other providers with whom you do business. Home care staff need good equipment and services to meet patient and staff needs. The nurse or patient needs only one bad experience, such as not having the proper equipment in the home or all the supplies for a specific procedure, as reason not to use a specific company or contractor. Waiting for service or equipment affects patients, families, public relations, productivity, and everyone's satisfaction with the home care services.

14. Develop a sound business and marketing plan for your particular home care agency's services in this era of competition. This is especially important when the issue of cost or price is eliminated.

15. Network with other home care providers. This is accomplished through attendance at local, regional, state, and national conferences. This is also accomplished through sharing information about successes and failures, developing useful tools, sharing research findings, and making suggestions for improvements in the delivery of services through publication of these results in professional journals.

16. Understand the importance of the educational and professional preparation of the administrative and supervisory staff of the home health agency. Clinical staff must be competent in their areas of expertise. Clerical and billing staff are also of the utmost importance to the overall quality of the agency.

17. Know individual state professional licensing regulations and professional practice acts.

18. Establish positive working relationships with the fiscal intermediary and referral sources.

19. Embrace the new technologies that are available for patient care.

20. Benchmark with similar agencies.

21. Be innovative and creative. Help to shape the future of home health care.

22. Be involved. Make positive things happen professionally, legislatively, and personally.

SUCCESSFUL ADMINISTRATORS SHARE THEIR STRATEGIES

I invited several colleagues who are successful administrators and with whom I have worked and served over the years to share their strategies for success in the 21st century. All of them referred to similar challenges. I included excerpts from their responses and their strategies that address the innumerable responsibilities and issues that administrators face every day.

Reverence for Our Workforce

In reflecting on my 25 years in the profession of home care, I realize that what successes I've been a party to have all been driven by a reverence for our workforce. What impact our agency has on the world around us is achieved by the hands-on efforts of our nurses and home care aides. The average tenure for our 350 home care aides is over 8 years with many here longer than my quarter century. Their collective experiences and ever-growing sense of caring have been nurtured at our organization. That's why they stay. I believe our staff understands in a very visceral way that they are appreciated. I know they know that their work is important and that this organization cares about them as people. This sense of belonging and being cared about fosters caring in them and that comes out in how they treat their patients.

I believe, therefore, that when you look at a successful home care organization, you are looking at a place where concern for the workforce is primary. It is easy to take staff for granted when constantly dealing with in-your-face problems of technology, politics, and regulation. But somewhere along the way I got the message: "It's the workforce. . . ."

Ken Wessel, MSW, ACSW, LSW
Executive Director
HomeCare Options
Paterson, New Jersey

Know Your Values and Manage by Them

Don't lose sight of them in the shifting landscape of home care under the prospective payment system—instead, use them as your anchor and decision-making tool. Roy Disney, chief financial officer of Disney Enterprises for many years, observes: ". . . when you know what your values are, decision making is easier" (Vance and Deacon, 1995). And it works; when confronted with a dilemma, ask how your decision would serve your values. Stand up for your values in turbulent times as well as good ones. If your values are worth believing in, they are worth fighting for.

Deliver quality care; respect your employees; know resource utilization and management; strive to deliver what your client needs—not less and not more; stay on top of technology; collaborate with your competitors to better serve your communities; plan to be in home care for the long haul, not for the quick payoff; get involved personally; and serve your community in some way outside of your office.

Margaret J. (Peg) Cushman, MSN, RN, CHCE, FHHC, FAAN
Former Executive Director, Home Health Care Agency

Ability to Constantly Defend Patient Care Plan Decisions and Practice Criteria

In the current era, we have seen a tremendous increase in the regulatory mandates and paperwork burden, the need for constant preparedness for bioterrorism and ever-growing inadequacy in reimbursement from all payers. These restraints, added to a severe shortage of nurses (with half of the existing working registered nurses to retire within the next 10 years in many states), create major challenges for administrators and their leadership staff. Administrators need to constantly defend patient care plan decisions and practice criteria.

Virginia S. Humphrey, MPH, BSN, RN, F.H.H.C.
Retired Executive Director
Connecticut Association for Home Care

Health and Well-Being of the Patients, Especially the Aging Population, Financing Health Care, Management of a Culturally Diverse Workforce and Movement, Nursing Shortage, and More Community-Based Care

The 21st century promises to be as challenging and thought provoking as the 20th century. Nursing leaders: (1) are confronted with innumerable responsibilities and issues as noted in the title; (2) must prepare their operations, the human and physical resources, to manage and care for the ever-increasing chronically ill and the expanding frail elderly populations; (3) are plagued with escalating labor costs, unfunded mandates from all manner of regulatory entities, soaring vacancies and increasing legal costs; (4) must be skilled negotiators for scarce fiscal resources; and (5) must set the standard and put into operation a tolerant workplace environment or the scarce fiscal resources, already mentioned, will simply be wasted.

I have never regretted my decision to become a registered nurse. I am infinitely proud of the difference I know I made to patients and families and what I have accomplished in my career. I wish all who read this the same pride and fulfillment.

Susan Craig Schulmerich, RN, MSN, MBA, CNA
Vice President, Community Health Services
ELANE, Inc. Goshen, New York

MEETING THE CHALLENGES

As noted in the introduction to this book, there are primary and secondary cluster areas of knowledge and skills recommended for home care administrators. In addition to these cluster areas, textbooks indicate that a nurse administrator should be a leader of a clinical discipline, a problem solver, a facilitator, a teacher, a scholar, and a manager and should be able to do budgeting, staffing, and labor relations and meet regulatory demands. The basic attributes that are desirable in an administrator were listed 27 years ago in a 1977 National League for Nursing publication titled *Characteristics of the Home Health Agency Administrator.* Some of the personal characteristics listed are the following: exhibits a strong commitment to and abundant energy for the task (that "extra something" required to achieve goals), shows emotional stability, possesses the ability to operate under pressure, and shows initiative, enthusiasm, pragmatism, and creativity. These attributes are as important in the 21st century as they were in 1977. In reality, the administration of home health and hospice care services, plus the expanded areas of responsibilities, includes variable percentages of all these.

Ben Leichtling (2003) notes that there is no best leadership style or model. Leaders of successful agencies have opposite personalities, leadership styles, and business strategies. He states: "However, across the board, inside and outside home care, successful leaders have the same qualities, characteristics, and operational goals. They are highly driven, self-disciplined, focused, relentless, enduring, demanding, hardnosed, straight shooting, and thrive on challenges" (pp. 44–45).

The stress level is often high for administrators, supervisors, staff, physicians, patients, and families. The important thing to remember is that the provision of high-quality health care services is a team effort. Staff must hear about those issues that could and probably will affect their work and stress level. Staff from all levels and departments within the agency must also be involved in the identification of the challenges that may adversely affect patient care and the solutions to meet these challenges. Working together as a team, successful administrators, staff, and governing bodies will be able to survive and thrive in the current health care climate.

In 1600 B.C., King Solomon said, "Have two goals: wisdom—that is, knowing and doing right—and common sense. Don't let them slip away, for they will fill you with living energy, and bring you honor and respect" (Proverbs 3:21–23. *The One Year Bible*. 1985). These two goals—wisdom (including all the information that has been shared in this book) and common sense—were important to me as an administrator of home health and hospice care and health care in the community.

Pulliam (1989) shared *Survival Skills for a Fast-Forward Society*. Three of her suggestions are as essential today as they were in 1989:

1. Let go of what's no longer working. Make room for what will work.
2. Take risks. In an era of diminishing guarantees, it's necessary to do so in order to not only survive, but also thrive.
3. Make friends with this changing world.

Carney (2004) noted that the home care marketplace is dynamic; it doesn't stand still. There are constant changes with new roads and relationships to build. New developments occur. Construction and maintenance along familiar routes might force some rerouting.

In her *Notes on Nursing,* Florence Nightingale (1859;1992) shared her thoughts on management (p. 20):

All the results of good nursing, as detailed in these notes, may be spoiled or utterly negated by one defect, viz: in petty management, or, in other words, by not knowing how to manage that what you do when you are there, shall be done when you are not there. The most devoted friend and nurse cannot be always there. Nor is it desirable that she should. But, in both let whoever is in charge keep this simple question in her head, not, how can I always do this right thing myself, but, how can I provide for this right thing to be always done?

CONCLUSION

Administrators must manage the agency in an effective and efficient manner in spite of multiple internal and external changes, current economic conditions, regulations, and budget constraints. The information presented in this book should help students understand the many details involved with the administration of home health care and hospice services. The assimilation of the contents of this book into daily practice should enable administrators to be confident that the multifaceted responsibilities involved with home health care and hospice administration, as well as the expanded community-centered care, are carried out when they are present and when they have delegated these responsibilities to competent staff members in their absence.

REFERENCES

American Nurses Association. 1996. *Scope and standards for nurse administrators*. Washington, DC: Author.

Carney, K. 2004. Marketing: An overview. In M. Harris (ed.). *Handbook of home health care administration,* 4th ed. Sudbury, MA: Jones and Bartlett.

Leichtling, B. 2003. Best leadership style and "caretaker mentality." *CARING* XXII(6): 44–45.

National League for Nursing. 1977. *Characteristics of the home health agency administrator* (Publication No. 21-1681). New York: Author.

Nightingale, F. 1859;1992. *Notes on nursing. What it is and what it isn't.* Philadelphia: Lippincott-Raven.

Pulliam, L. 1989. *Survival skills for a fast-forward society.* Chapel Hill, NC: Pulliam Associates.

Vance, M., and D. Deacon. 1995. *Think out of the box.* Franklin Lakes, NJ: Career Press, p. 181.

The One Year Bible (The Living Bible. A Thought-for-Thought Translation). 1985. Wheaton, IL: Tyndale House Publishers.

Abbreviations

AAA—Area Agencies on Aging

AAAHC—Accreditation Association for Ambulatory Health Care

AAPI—American Accreditation Program Inc.

ABC—Activity-Based Costing

ABM—Activity-Based Management

ABMS—American Board of Medical Specialties

ABNS—American Board of Nursing Specialties

ACCME—Accreditation Council for Continuing Medical Education

ACHC—Accreditation Commission for Health Care, Inc.

ACHE—American College of Healthcare Executives

ACOG—American College of Obstetricians and Gynecologists

AD—Associate Degree

ADA—American Diabetes Association

ADA—Americans with Disabilities Act

ADLs—Activities of Daily Living

ADRs—Additional Development Requests

AHA—American Hospital Association

AHA—American Heart Association

AHCPR—Agency for Health Care Policy and Research

AHRQ—Agency for Healthcare Research and Quality

AIDS—Acquired Immune Deficiency Syndrome

ALJ—Administrative Law Judge

ALOS—Average Length of Stay

ALS—Amyotrophic Lateral Sclerosis

AMA—American Medical Association

AMCRA—American Managed Care and Review Association

AMH—Abington Memorial Hospital

AMHHC—Abington Memorial Hospital Home Care

ANA—American Nurses Association

ANCC—American Nurses Credentialing Center

ANSI—American National Standards Institute

ANSI HISB—American National Standards Institute Healthcare Informatics Standards Board

APN—Advanced Practice Nurse

ARPANET—Advanced Research Projects Agency Network

ASCA—Administrative Simplification Compliance Act

ASCD—Association of Supervision and Curriculum Development

ASCII—American Standard Code for Information Interchange

AVPD—Average Visits per Day

AWP—Any Willing Provider

BA—Business Associate

BBA of 1997—Balanced Budget Amendment of 1997

BBRA—Balanced Budget Refinement Act of 1999

BOR—Board of Review

BP—Blood Pressure

BSN—Bachelor of Science in Nursing

C—Competent
CAC—Consumer Advocacy Center
CAD—Coronary Artery Disease
CAHPS—Consumer Assessment of Health Plans Study
CAMHC—Comprehensive Accreditation Manual for Home Care
CAPD—Continuous Abdominal Peritoneal Dialysis
CARF—The Rehabilitation Accreditation Commission
CCMC—Commission for Case Management Certification
CCO—Community Care Option
CDC—Centers for Disease Control
CEO—Chief Executive Officer
CEU—Continuing Education Unit
CFO—Chief Financial Officer
CFP—Call for Proposal
CHAP—Community Health Accreditation Program
CHCE—Certified Home Care Executive
CHCL—Center for Health Care Law
CHE®—Certified Health Executive Diplomat
CHF—Congestive Heart Failure
CHHA—Certified Home Health Aide
CHINs—Community Health Information Networks
CHIRS—Community Health Intensity Rating Scale
CIAC—Computer Incident Advisory Capability
CINAHL—Cumulative Index to Nursing and Allied Health Literature
CL/WLA—Caseload/Workload Analysis
CLAS—Culturally and Linguistically Appropriate Services
CLIA—Clinical Laboratories Improvement Act
CMP—Civil Money Penalties
CMS—Center for Medicare and Medicaid Services
CMV—Cytomegalovirus
CNA—Certified Nursing Administration
CNA, BC—Certification in Nursing Administration, Board Certified
CNAA—Certified Nursing Administration, Advanced

CNAA, BC—Certification in Nursing Administration, Advanced, Board Certified
CNPII—Committee for Nursing Practice Information Infrastructure
COBRA—Consolidated Omnibus Budget Reconciliation Act
COPs—Conditions of Participation
COPD—Chronic Obstructive Pulmonary Disease
CORF—Comprehensive Outpatient Rehabilitation Facility
CPAP—Continuous Positive Airway Pressure
CPEC—Contractor Performance Evaluation Criteria
CPI—Consumer Price Index
CPI—Continuous Process Improvement
CPM—Continuous Passive Motion
CPR—Cardiopulmonary Resuscitation
CPR—Computer-Based Patient Record
CPU—Central Processing Unit
CQI—Continuous Quality Improvement
CRT—Computer Readout Terminal
CVA—Cerebrovascular Accident
DC—Discharge
DEA—Drug Enforcement Administration
DHEW—Department of Health, Education, and Welfare
DHHS—Department of Health and Human Services
DME—Durable Medical Equipment
DP—Discharge Planner
DPS—Director of Professional Services
DPW—Department of Public Welfare
DRGs—Diagnosis-Related Groups
DSL—Digital Subscriber Line
E—Exceeds Requirements
EAP—Employee Assistance Program
EBP—Evidence-Based Practice
ED—Executive Director
EDI—Electronic Data Interchange
EEOC—Equal Employment Opportunity Commission
EIN—Employer Identification Number
EKG/ECG—Electrocardiogram
EMR—Electronic Medical Record
EMS—Emergency Medical Services
EOB—Explanation of Benefits
EPA—Environmental Protection Agency

EPO—Exclusive Provider Organization

ERISA—Employee Retirement Income Security Act

ESC—Evidence of Standards Compliance

EVP—Executive Vice President

FACHE—Fellow—American College of Healthcare Executives

FAI—Functional Assessment Instrument

FBI—Federal Bureau of Investigation

FCA—False Claims Act

FDA—Food and Drug Administration

FI—Fiscal Intermediary

FIM—Functional Independence Measure

FISS—Fiscal Intermediary Shared System

FMR—Focused Medical Review

FOCUS—Find, Organize, Clarify, Understand, Select

FQHC—Federally Qualified Health Center

FT—Full Time

FTE—Full-Time Equivalent

FTP—File Transfer Protocol

FY—Fiscal Year

GAO—General Accounting Office

GE—Graduate Equivalency Degree

GHAA—Group Health Association of America

GI—Gastrointestinal

GIGO—Garbage In/Garbage Out

GNP—Gross National Product

GQS—Generic Quality Screens

GUI—Graphical User Interface

HAVEN—Home Assessment Validation and Entry

HCA—Home Care Aide

HCBS—Home and Community-Based Services

HCCM—Home Care Case Manager

HCFA—Health Care Financing Administration

HCU—Home Care University

HDL—High Density Lipoproteins

HEDIS—Health Plan Employer Data and Information Set

HELLP—Hemolysis-Elevated Liver Enzyme-Low Platelets

HHA—Home Health Agency

HHA—Home Health Aide

HHC—Home Care Coordinator

HHCC—Home Health Care Classification

HHCC—Home Health Care Component

H-HHA—Homemaker-Home Health Aide

HHN—Home Health Nurse

HHNA—Home Healthcare Nurses Association

HHPPS—Home Health Prospective Payment System

HHQI—Home Health Quality Initiative

HHRG—Home Health Resource Group

HHS—Health and Human Services

HIC—Health Insurance Claim

HIM—Health Insurance Manual

HIPAA—Health Insurance Portability and Accountability Act of 1996

HIV—Human Immunodeficiency Virus

HL7—Health Level 7

HMA—Health Ministries Association

HME—Home Medical Equipment

HMEAA—Home Medical Equipment Association of America

HMO—Health Maintenance Organization

HR—Heart Rate

HR—Human Resources

HTML—Hypertext Markup Language

HTN—Hypertension

HV—Home Visit

I-9—Immigration and Naturalization Form

IBC—Independence Blue Cross

ICD-9—*International Classification of Diseases, 9th Edition*

ICD-10-CM—*International Classification of Disease and Health-Related Problems*

ICN—International Council of Nursing

ICNP—International Classification of Nursing Practice

ICNP—International Classification in Nursing Project

IDDM—Insulin-Dependent Diabetes Mellitus

IDS—Integrated Delivery System

IDT—Interdisciplinary Team

INS—Intravenous Nurses Society

IOM—Institute of Medicine

IPA—Independent Practice Association

IPO—Independent Physician Organization

IPS—Interim Payment System

IRB—Institutional Review Board

IRS—Internal Revenue Service

IS—Information Services

ISO—International Standards Organization

ISP—Internet Service Provider
IV—Intravenous
JCAHO—Joint Commission on Accreditation of Healthcare Organizations
J-Jibe—Hospice Care
JRN—Joints R Us
LAN—Local Area Network
LBW—Low Birth Weight
LDL—Low Density Lipoproteins
LE—Lower Extremity
LEP—Limited English Proficient
LOINC—Logical Observations, Identifiers, Names, and Codes
LOS—Length of Stay
LPN—Licensed Practical Nurse
LSNNC—LaSalle University Neighborhood Nursing Center
LUPA—Low-Utilization Payment Adjustment
M&A—Merger and Acquisition
MA—Medical Assistance
MAE—Management and Evaluation
MBA—Master of Business Administration
MCH—Maternal-Child Health
MCO—Managed Care Organization
MD—Medical Doctor
ME—Mistaken Entry
MFCUs—Medicaid Fraud Control Units
MIS—Management Information System
MSN—Master of Science in Nursing
MSO—Management Service Organization
MSW—Medical Social Worker
NA—Not Applicable/Not Assessed
NAAG—National Association of Attorneys General
NAHC—National Association for Home Care and Hospice
NADSA—National Adult Day Services Association
NANDA—North American Nursing Diagnosis Association
NAPHN—National Association for Public Health Nursing
NAQA—National Association for Quality Assurance
NASA—National Aeronautical and Space Administration

NCCA—National Commission for Certifying Agencies
NCQA—National Committee for Quality Assurance
ND—Nursing Diagnosis
NFCSP—National Family Caregivers Support Program
NGC—National Guideline Clearinghouse
NHCC—National Home Caring Council
NI—Needs Improvement
NIC—National International Classification
NICU—Neonatal Intensive Care Unit
NIDSEC—Nursing Information and Data Set Evaluation Center
NLM—National Library of Medicine
NLN—National League for Nursing
NLRB—National Labor Relations Board
NMDS—Nursing Minimum Data Set
NOC—Nursing Outcome Classification
NP—Nurse Practitioner
NPPN—National Preferred Provider Network
NPR—Notice of Program Reimbursement
NVRA—National Voter Registration Act of 1993
NYHA—New York Association Functional Classification
OASIS—Outcome and Assessment Information Set
OBQI—Outcome-Based Quality Improvement
OBQM—Outcome-Based Quality Monitoring
OBRA—Omnibus Budget Reconciliation Act
OCESSA—Omnibus Consolidated and Emergency Supplemental Appropriations Act of 1999
OCR—Office for Civil Rights
OEC—OASIS Education Coordinator
OIG—Office of Inspector General
OJCI—Online Journal of Clinical Innovations
OJKSN—Online Journal of Knowledge Synthesis for Nursing
OMH—Office of Minority Health
OSHA—Occupational Safety and Health Administration
OT—Occupational Therapist
OTR—Occupational Therapist Registered

PAC—Political Action Committee
PAC—Professional Advisory Committee
PACE—Program for All-Inclusive Care for the
 Elderly
PAL—Physician Assisted Living
PB—Privacy Board
PC—Personal Computer
PCA—Philadelphia Corporation on Aging
PCA—Professional Care Aide
PCCS—Palliative Care Consultative Service
PCDS—Patient Care Data Set
PCM—Payer Case Manager
PCO—Patient Classification Outcome
PCP—Primary Care Provider/Physician
PCS—Patient Classification System
PDA—Pennsylvania Department of Aging
PDCA—Plan, Do, Check, Act
PEP—Partial Episode Payment
PHI—Protected Health Information
PHO—Physician Hospital Organization
PI—Performance Improvement
PI—Program Integrity
PICC—Peripheral Insertion Central Catheter
PIH—Pregnancy Induced Hypertension
PIP—Periodic Interim Payment
PN—Parish Nurse
P.O.—Per Os (by mouth)
POA—Plan of Action
POC—Plan of Care
POR—Problem-Oriented Record
POS—Point of Service
POT—Plan of Treatment
POTS—Plain Old Telephone Service
PPD—Purified Protein Derivative
PPO—Preferred Provider Organization
PPS—Prospective Payment System
PRO—Peer Review Organization
ProPAC—Prospective Payment Assessment
 Commission
PRRB—Provider Reimbursement Review
 Board
PSDA—Patient Self-Determination Act
PT—Part Time
PT—Physical Therapist
PTA—Physical Therapy Assistant
PTO—Paid Time Off

QA—Quality Assurance
QA/PI—Quality Assessment/Performance
 Improvement
QI—Quality Improvement
QIO—Quality Improvement Organization
QRR—Quarterly Record Review
QUIGs—Quality Indicator Groups
RAM—Random-Access Memory
RAP—Requests for Anticipated Payments
RD/ED—Regional Director/Executive Director
RFP—Request for Proposal
RHHI—Regional Home Health Intermediary
RN—Registered Nurse
ROC—Resumption of Care
ROM—Range of Motion
ROM—Read-Only Memory
RR—Respiratory Rate
RTF—Rich Text Format
SCHIP—State Children's Health Insurance
 Program
SCIC—Significant Change in Condition
SEIU—Service Employees International Union
SF-12—Short Form—12
SHMO—Social Health Maintenance
 Organization
SN—Skilled Nursing
SNF—Skilled Nursing Facility
SNOMED RT—Systematized Nomenclature
 of Medicine Reference Terminology,
 Systematized Nomenclature of Veterinary
 Medicine Reference Terminology
SOAP—Subjective, Objective, Assessment,
 and Planning
SOC—Start of Care
SP—Speech Pathology
S/P—Status Post
s/s—Signs and Symptoms
SSI—Supplemental Security Income
ST—Speech Therapist
SW—Social Worker
SWOT—Strengths, Weakness, Opportunities,
 Threats
TB—Tuberculosis
TEFRA—Tax Equity and Fiscal
 Responsibility Act of 1982
TPA—Third-Party Administrator

TPN—Total Parenteral Nutrition
TPO—Treatment, Payment, Operations
TQM—Total Quality Management
UB-92—Uniform Bill–92
UE—Upper Extremity
UMLS—Unified Medical Language System
UNLS—Unified Nursing Language System
UPS—Uninterruptible Power Supply
UR—Utilization Review
URAC—Utilization Review Accreditation
  Commission
URLs—Uniform Resource Locator
USDA/CACFP—United States Department of
  Agriculture/Child and Adult Care Food
  Program

VNA—Visiting Nurse Association
VNA-CS—Visiting Nurse Association—
  Community Services
VNA-HMS—Visiting Nurse Association—
  Health Management Services
W3C—World Wide Web Consortium
WALT—Willingness to Access Life-
  Sustaining Treatment
WANs—Wide Area Networks
WIC—Women, Infant, and Children
WOCN—Wound and Ostomy Continence
  Nurses Society
WWW—World Wide Web
WYSWIG—What You See Is What You Get

Index